Renal Cell Cancer

Jean J.M.C.H. de la Rosette, Cora N. Sternberg,
and Hein P.A. van Poppel (Eds.)

Renal Cell Cancer

Diagnosis and Therapy

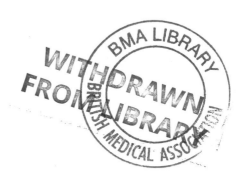

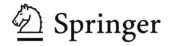

Springer

Editors

Jean J.M.C.H. de la Rosette, MD, PhD
Chairman
Department of Urology
Academic Medical Center University Hospital
Amsterdam
The Netherlands

Hein P.A. van Poppel MD, PhD
Chairman
Department of Urology
University Hospital of Katholieke
 Universiteit Leuven
Leuven
Belgium

Cora N. Sternberg MD, FACP
Chairman
Department of Medical Oncology
San Camillo and Forlanini Hospitals
Rome
Italy

ISBN: 978-1-84628-385-7   e-ISBN: 978-1-84628-763-3
DOI: 10.1007/978-1-84628-763-3

British Library Cataloguing in Publication Data
Renal cell cancer : diagnosis and therapy
   1. Renal cell carcinoma - Treatment 2. Renal cell carcinoma
   - Diagnosis
   I. Rosette, Jean J. M. C. H. de la II. Sternberg, Cora N.
   III. Poppel, Hein P. A. van
   616.9'9461
ISBN-13: 9781846283857

Library of Congress Control Number: 2007937488

Springer Science+Business Media
springer.com

Preface

Although the first nephrectomy was performed as early as 1867 by Spillgeberg, it was not until 1903 that Gregoire performed the first formal nephrectomy. It was, however, six decades later that Robson published his radical nephrectomy series. Since then radical nephrectomy has become the cornerstone of the surgical treatment of renal cell carcinoma.

During the past decade, urology has been facing rapid changes in the understanding of oncological urology. Changes in surgical treatment strategies accompanied by the availability of newer effective medical therapies have led to improved results. In addition, laparoscopic radical nephrectomy has become the standard of care for the treatment of localized renal cell cancer.

The expanded use of imaging techniques has resulted in detection of an increasing number of small renal cell cancers. For the majority of these tumors, radical nephrectomy is considered overtreatment, and nephron sparing surgeries such as partial laparoscopic nephrectomy or tumor ablative surgery, using various different energy sources, has become routine.

The medical management of renal cell carcinoma has recently experienced an exciting revolution with approvals of new pharmaceuticals in a disease that was previously considered refractory to most therapies. Increasing understanding of the molecular biology of kidney cancer has led to this remarkable progress. Several biologic agents aiming at angiogenesis, growth factors and their pathways have produced extremely dramatic results. In addition, newer sophisticated radiological methods are increasingly being used to evaluate tumor blood flow and response to therapy.

In addition to better treatments this textbook also explores upon improving, making a proper precocious diagnosis and optimizing follow-up. To accomplish this, specific markers need to be developed and imaging modalities should be improved.

This textbook aims at covering the entire field of the current knowledge of renal cell cancer, presented by some of the finest experts in the field. In addition to reflecting upon past and present achievements, this work also aims at addressing possible future developments in this field.

Jean J.M.C.H. de la Rosette
Cora N. Sternberg
Hein P.A. van Poppel

Contents

Contributors

Ferran Algaba, MD
Section of Pathology, Fundació Puigvert, Barcelona, Spain

Gerasimos J. Alivizatos, MD, PhD, FEBU
Department of Urology, Athens Medical School, Sismanoglio Hospital, Athens, Greece

Ernst P. Allhoff, MD
Department of Urology, Otto-von-Güricke-University, Magdeburg, Germany

Yolanda Arce, MD
Section of Pathology, Fundació Puigvert, Barcelona, Spain

Richad K. Babayan, MD
Department of Urology, Boston Medical Center, Boston University School of Medicine, Boston, MA, USA

Doddametikurke R. Basavaraj, MS, FRCS
Pyrah Department of Urology, St James University Hospital, Leeds, UK

Arie S. Belldegrun, MD
Department of Urology, David Geffen School of Medicine, University of California, Los Angeles, CA, USA

Axel Bex, MD, PhD
Department of Urology, The Netherlands Cancer Institute, Amsterdam, The Netherlands

Michael L. Blute, MD
Mayo Medical School, Mayo Clinic, Rochester, MI, USA

Morton A. Bosniak MD
Department of Radiology, New York University Medical Center, New York, NY, USA

Patrick M.M. Bossuyt, MD, PhD
Clinical Epidemiology and Biostatistics, Academic Medical Centre, University of Amsterdam, Amsterdam, The Netherlands

Sarah K. Ceyssens, MD
Department of Nuclear Medicine, Antwerp University Hospital, Edegem, Belgium

Gayun Chan-Smutko, MS, CGC
Massachusetts General Hospital Centre for Cancer Risk Analysis, Boston, MA, USA

Richard W. Childs, MD
Hematology Branch, National Heart, Lung, and Blood Institute, National Institutes of Health, Bethesda, MD, USA

Allen W. Chiu, MD, PhD
Department of Urology, Taipei City Hospital, Taipei, Taiwan, Republic of China

Benjamin I. Chung, MD
Department of Urology, Lahey Clinic, Burlington, MA, USA

Jose R. Colombo Jr., MD
Section of Laparoscopic and Robotic Surgery, Glickman Urological Institute,
The Cleveland Clinic Foundation, Cleveland, OH, USA

Gijsbert C. de Gast, MD, PhD
Department of Medical Oncology, The Netherlands Cancer Institute, Amsterdam,
The Netherlands

Jean B. deKernion, MD
Department of Urology, David Geffen School of Medicine, University of California,
Los Angeles, CA, USA

Jean J.M.C.H. de la Rosette, MD, PhD
Department of Urology, Academic Medical Centre, University of Amsterdam,
Amsterdam, The Netherlands

Theo M. de Reijke, PhD
Department of Urology, Academic Medical Centre, University of Amsterdam,
Amsterdam, The Netherlands

Meaghan L. Douglas, BSc Hons, PhD
School of Medicine, Southern Clinical Division, University of Queensland, Princess
Alexandra Hospital, Brisbane, Queensland, Australia

Tibet Erdogru, MD
Department of Urology, SLK-Klinikum Heilbronn, University of Heidelberg, Germany

Bernard Escudier, MD
Department of Oncology, Institut Gustave Roussy, Villejuif, France

Robert A. Figlin, MD
Department of Medicine, David Geffen School of Medicine, University of California,
Los Angeles, CA, USA

Robert C. Flanigan, MD, FACS
Department of Urology, Loyola University Medical Center, Maywood, IL, USA

Bernhard Frankenberger, PhD
Institute of Molecular Immunology, GSF National Research Center for Environment and
Health, Munich, Germany

Elmar W. Gerharz, MD, PhD
Department of Urology, Bavarian Julius-Maximilians-University Medical School,
Würzburg, Germany

Inderbir S. Gill, MD, MCh
Section of Laparoscopic and Robotic Surgery, Glickman Urological Institute, The
Cleveland Clinic Foundation, Cleveland, OH, USA

Mary K. Gospodarowicz, MD, FRCPC
Department of Radiation Oncology, Princess Margaret Hospital, University of Toronto,
Toronto, Ontario, Canada

Alexander V. Govorov, MD
Department of Urology, Moscow State Medical University, Moscow, Russia

Ali S Gözen, MD
Department of Urology, SLK-Klinikum Heilbronn, University of Heidelberg, Germany

Georges-Pascal Haber, MD
Section of Laparoscopic and Robotic Surgery, Glickman Urological Institute,
The Cleveland Clinic Foundation, Cleveland, OH, USA

Hans Heinzer, MD
Department of Urology, University Medical Centre Hamburg, Hamburg, Germany

Simon Horenblas, MD, PhD
Department of Urology, The Netherlands Cancer Institute, Amsterdam, The Netherlands

Yi-Hsiu Huang, MD
Department of Urology, Taipei City Hospital, Taipei, Taiwan, Republic of China

Edith Huland, MD, PhD
Department of Urology, University Hospital Hamburg, Hamburg, Germany

Hartwig Huland, MD, PhD
Department of Urology, University Medical Centre Hamburg, Hamburg, Germany

Peter Hulick, MD
Center for Genetics and Genomics, Harvard Medical School, Boston, MA, USA

Othon Iliopoulos, MD
Hematology-Oncology Unit, Harvard Medical School, Boston, MA, USA

Brant A. Inman, MD
Department of Urology, Mayo Clinic College of Medicine, Rochester, MN, USA

Gary M. Israel, MD
Department of Radiology, Yale University School of Medicine, New Haven, CT, USA

Didier Jacqmin, MD, PhD
Department of Urology, Hopitaux Universitaires de Strasbourg, Strasbourg, France

Adrian Joyce, MS, FRCS(Urol)
Pyrah Department of Urology, St James University Hospital, Leeds, UK

Fiebo J.W. Ten Kate, MD, PhD
Department of Pathology, Academic Medical Centre, University of Amsterdam,
Amsterdam, The Netherlands

Emil Kheterpal, BS
Boston Medical Center, Boston University School of Medicine, Boston, MA, USA

Ziya Kirkali, MD
Department of Urology, Dokuz Eylul University School of Medicine, Inciralti, Izmir,
Turkey

Intan P.E.D. Kümmerlin, MD
Department of Urology, Academic Medical Centre, University of Amsterdam,
Amsterdam, The Netherlands

Brunolf W. Lagerveld, MD
Department of Urology, Academic Medical Center, University of Amsterdam,
Amsterdam, The Netherlands

M. Pilar Laguna, MD
Department of Urology, Academic Medical Center, University of Amsterdam,
Amsterdam, The Netherlands

John S. Lam, MD
Department of Urology, David Geffen School of Medicine, University of California,
Los Angeles, CA, USA

Johan S. Laméris, PhD
Department of Radiology, Academic Medical Centre, University of Amsterdam,
Amsterdam, The Netherlands

Benjamin R. Lee, MD
Department of Urology, North Shore-Long Island Jewish Medical Center, New Hyde
Park, NY, USA

Bradley C. Leibovich, MD
Mayo Medical School, Mayo Clinic, Rochester, MI, USA

John T. Leppert, MD
Department of Urology, David Geffen School of Medicine, University of California,
Los Angeles, CA, USA

John A. Libertino, MD
Department of Urology, Lahey Clinic, Burlington, MA, USA

Louis S. Liou, MD, PhD
Department of Urology, Boston Medical Center, Boston University School
of Medicine, Boston, MA, USA

Allan Lipton, MD
Milton S. Hershey Medical Center, Division of Oncology, Hershey, PA, USA

Martijn P. Lolkema, MD
Department of Medical Oncology, University Medical Centre, Utrecht, The Netherlands

Andreas E. Lundqvist, PhD
Hematology Branch, National Heart, Lung, and Blood Institute, National Institutes
of Health, Bethesda, MD, USA

Andrea Mancuso, MD
Department of Medical Oncology, San Camillo and Forlanini Hospitals, Rome, Italy

Michael Marberger, MD, FRCS (Ed)
Department of Urology, University of Vienna, Vienna, Austria

Surena F. Matin, MD, FACS
Department of Urology, University of Texas M. D. Anderson Cancer Center, Houston,
TX, USA

Gerald H.J. Mickisch, MD, PhD, FRCS
Center of Operative Urology, Academic Hospital Bremen "Links der Weser," Bremen, Germany

Luc Mortelmans, MD, PhD
Department of Nuclear Medicine, University Hospital Leuven, Leuven, Belgium

Masaru Murai
Department of Urology, Keio University School of Medicine, Shinjuku-ku, Japan

Stephen Y. Nakada, MD
Division of Urology, Department of Surgery, University of Wisconsin-Madison Medical School, Madison, WI, USA

David L. Nicol, MBBS, FRACS
School of Medicine, Southern Clinical Division, University of Queensland, Princess Alexandra Hospital, Brisbane, Queensland, Australia

Els L.F. Nijs, MD
Department of Radiology, University Hospitals Gasthuisberg, Katholieke Universiteit, Leuven, Belgium

Can Öbek, MD, FEBU
Department of Urology, University of Istanbul, Atasehir, Istanbul, Turkey

Michael C. Ost, MD
Department of Urology, North Shore-Long Island Jewish Medical Center, New Hyde Park, NY, USA

Mototsugu Oya, MD
Department of Urology, Keio University School of Medicine, Shinjuku-ku, Japan

Raymond H. Oyen, MD, PhD
Department of Radiology, University Hospitals Gasthuisberg, Katholieke Universiteit, Leuven, Belgium

Sascha Pahernik, MD
Department of Urology, Johannes Gutenberg University Medical School, Mainz, Germany

Gyan Pareek, MD
Division of Urology, Department of Surgery, Brown Medical School, Providence, RI, USA

Saffire S.K.S. Phoa, MD, PhD
Department of Radiology, Academic Medical Centre, University of Amsterdam, Amsterdam, The Netherlands

Dmitry Y. Pushkar, MD
Department of Urology, Moscow State Medical University, Moscow, Russia

Jens Rassweiler, MD
Department of Urology, SLK-Klinikum Heilbronn, University of Heidelberg, Germany

Karen L. Reckamp, MD, MS
Department of Medicine, David Geffen School of Medicine, University of California, Los Angeles, CA, USA

Dick Richel, MD
Department of Internal Medicine, Academic Medical Centre, University of Amsterdam, Amsterdam, The Netherlands

Hubertus Riedmiller, MD, PhD
Department of Urology, Bavarian Julius-Maximilians-University Medical School, Würzburg, Germany

Alexander Roosen, MD
Department of Urology, Bavarian Julius-Maximilians-University Medical School, Würzburg, Germany

Catherine Roy, MD
Department of Radiology, University Hospital of Strasbourg, Strasbourg, France

Fred Saad, MD FRCS
Centre Hospitalier de l'Université de Montréal, Hôpital Notre-Dame, Montréal, Quebec, Canada

Ignace R. Samson, MD
Department of Orthopaedic Surgery, University Hospital Leuven, Pellenberg, Belgium

Dolores J. Schendel, MD, PhD
Institute of Molecular Immunology, GSF National Research Center for Environment and Health, Munich, Germany

Avigdor Scherz, PhD
Department of Plant Sciences, Weizmann Institute of Science, Rehovot, Israel

Michael Schulze, MD
Department of Urology, SLK-Klinikum Heilbronn, University of Heidelberg, Germany

Fred Schuster MD
Depatment of Urology, Städtisches Klinikum Dresden-Friedrichstadt, Dresden, Germany

Friedl C. Sinnaeve, MD
Department of Orthopaedic Surgery, University Hospital Leuven, Pellenberg, Belgium

Andreas Skolarikos MD, PhD, FEBU
Department of Urology, Athens Medical School, Sismanoglio Hospital, Athens, Greece

Walter M. Stadler, MD, FACP
Departments of Medicine and Surgery, University of Chicago, Chicago, IL, USA

Frank Steinbach, MD
Depatment of Urology, Städtisches Klinikum Dresden-Friedrichstadt, Dresden, Germany

Cora N. Sternberg, MD, FACP
Department of Medical Oncology, San Camillo and Forlanini Hospitals, Rome, Italy

Robert M. Strieter, MD
Department of Medicine, David Geffen School of Medicine, University of California, Los Angeles, CA, USA

Marto Sugiono, MBChB, FRCS (Eng)
Department of Urology, SLK-Klinikum Heilbronn, University of Heidelberg, Germany

Dogu Teber, MD
Department of Urology, SLK-Klinikum Heilbronn, University of Heidelberg, Germany

Joachim W. Thüroff, MD
Department of Urology, Johannes Gutenberg University Medical School, Mainz, Germany

Isabel Trias, MD
Department of Pathology, Clínica Plató, Fundació Privada, Spain

Otto M. van Delden, PhD
Department of Radiology, Academic Medical Centre, University of Amsterdam, Amsterdam, The Netherlands

Hein P.A. van Poppel, MD, PhD
Chairman Department of Urology, University Hospital, Katholieke Universiteit Leuven, Belgium

Raf van Reusel, MD
Department of Urology, University Hospital, Katholieke Universiteit, Leuven, Belgium

Sreenivas N. Vemulapalli, MD
Department of Urology, University of Oklahoma Health Sciences Center, Oklahoma City, OK, USA

Bryan B. Voelzke, MD
Department of Urology, Loyola University Medical Center, Maywood, IL, USA

Emile E. Voest, MD, PhD
Department of Medical Oncology, University Medical Centre, Utrecht, The Netherlands

Padraig R. Warde, MB, MRCPI, FRCPC
Department of Radiation Oncology, Princess Margaret Hospital, University of Toronto, Toronto, Ontario, Canada

Margot H. Wink, MD
Department of Urology, Academic Medical Centre, University of Amsterdam, Amsterdam, The Netherlands

Michael Zimmer, PhD
Hematology-Oncology Unit, Harvard Medical School, Boston, MA, USA

1
Epidemiology of Renal Cell Carcinoma

Intan P.E.D. Kümmerlin, M. Pilar Laguna, Jean J.M.C.H. de la Rosette, and Patrick M.M. Bossuyt

Incidence, Mortality, and Survival

The incidence of renal cell cancer (RCC) is increasing worldwide. RCC accounts for 2% of the world total of all adult malignancies (Parkin, 2005). In 2005, RCC will be diagnosed in approximately 36,000 patients in the United States of which 22,000 are males and 14,000 females (Jemal, 2005). It is estimated that 8000 men and 5000 women will die from the disease. Since 1973, the incidence has increased by 43% (Fig. 1-1) and the death rate by 16% (Fig. 1-2) (Ries, 1997) . The rise in incidence is greatest for African-American women and men (Jemal, 2005).

Incidence and mortality data from Europe for 1997 point to 30,000 male cases, 17,000 female cases, and 14,000 deaths in men and 9000 in women, respectively (Bray, 2003). Mortality rates from kidney cancer increased throughout Europe until the 1990s (Levi, 2004). After the mid-1990s mortality rates have leveled of. Kidney cancer mortality declined by over 10% over the past 5 years for both sexes. The largest decreases were seen in Germany, Denmark, and the Netherlands. The highest cancer incidence in Europe in 1995 was observed in the Czech Republic. The lowest incidence was seen in the Southern European countries: Portugal for males and Greece for females (Bray, 2002). This may be partly explained by differences in autopsy rates in these countries.

The estimated global incidence and mortality numbers are 208,000 and 102,000:129,000 and 63,000 for men and 79,000 and 39,000 for women, respectively (Parkin, 2005). The highest incidence rates are observed mainly in developed countries like North America, Australia, New Zealand, and western, eastern, and northern Europe. The lowest incidence rates are seen in Africa, Asia (except for Japanese males), and the Pacific (Parkin, 2005) countries.

The increasing discovery of RCC is due to the widespread use of abdominal imaging. In 1970 approximately 10% of the RCC were found incidentally compared to 61% in 1998 (Jayson, 1998). Yet Hock et al. (2002) found no significant difference in cancer stage at presentation. To determine if the increase in RCC cases truly reflects a rising incidence or has to be attributed to increased abdominal imaging, Mindrup et al. (2005) compared the proportion of RCC detected at autopsy from only two periods. A true increase in clinical incidence of RCC should not influence the number of previously undiscovered RCC cases found only at autopsy. Mindrup and colleagues found that the number of tumors, benign and malignant, discovered at autopsy only was declining. This could be due to better detection before death. As the proportion of occult renal cancer per 100 autopsies did not change significantly between the two periods, a true increase in the incidence of clinical detected renal cancer could be present. This suggests that the biology of this tumor is changing deleteriously, perhaps due to environmental factors such as tobacco use, diet, or exposure to other carcinogens.

The incidence of RCC has risen 3-fold in comparison to the mortality rate, which in itself suggests an improvement in survival over the last 25 years (Ries, 1997). The 5-year relative survival rate has increased from 34% in 1954 to 62% in 1996 (Pantuck, 2001). The improved survival is mostly attributed to earlier diagnosis (Chow, 1999). This theory is supported by several studies, where an increase in the percentage of organ-confined tumors has been shown (Chow, 1999; Lee, 2000).

Gender and Age

Age-specific RCC rates for men are about 2-fold higher than in women, but recent data show that the gap is narrowing (Parkin, 2005). RCC occurs predominantly between the sixth to eighth decades of life with a median age of 65 years. Children are very rarely diagnosed with RCC with the exception of Wilms tumor. Familial tumors are more common in young adults (Eggener, 2004).

Risk Factors

A comprehensive and systematic review of the literature through literature searches in the National Library of

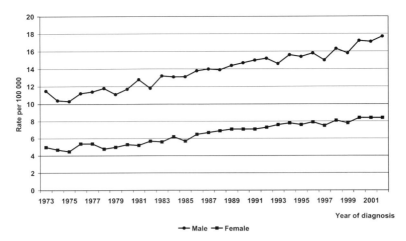

FIGURE 1-1. Age adjusted incidence rates for kidney cancer per 100,000 person-years. Data extracted from the National Cancer Institute's Surveillance, Epidemiology, and End Results (SEER) program (Ries, 1997).

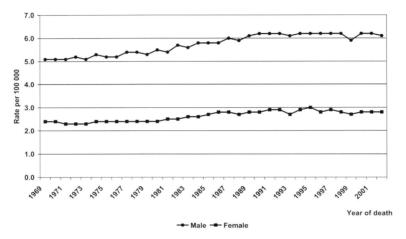

FIGURE 1-2. Age adjusted mortality rates for kidney cancer per 100,000 person-years. Data extracted from the National Cancer Institute's Surveillance, Epidemiology, and End Results (SEER) program (Ries, 1997).

Medicine was carried out to identify studies of putative risk factors for RCC. Potentially eligible articles were screened for inclusion.

Although epidemiological studies identified several risk factors that may relate to the development of RCC, the full etiology of RCC is still unknown and a causative factor has not yet been identified. Identifying risk factors is hampered by potential confounders, like age, race, education, marital status, smoking status, physical activity, alcohol use, aspirin use, and/or fat consumption and several risk factors act synergistically such as smoking, obesity, and hypertension. The evidence for most reported associations has been inconsistent or equivocal.

Smoking

Consumption of tobacco products increased dramatically in the second half of the nineteenth century. Over the past few decades tobacco consumption has decreased in the United States and some European countries by 50% (Sasco, 2004).

Smoking tobacco is associated with an increased risk for several malignancies (IARC, 2004; Sasco, 2004), in particular, malignancies of the lung, upper respiratory system, and the digestive system.

The causative role of tobacco use in the etiology of RCC is not clear. It may be relatively moderate compared to some of the neoplasms mentioned above (Tavani, 1997). Hunt et al. (2005) published a meta-analysis of 24 studies in which they analyzed the risk of RCC associated with tobacco smoking. They evaluated hospital-based case–control studies, a registry based case–control study, population based case–control studies, and prospective cohort studies. Several case–control studies showed that tobacco smoking was associated with a statistically increased risk for RCC. The relative risk (RR) for RCC calculated by Hunt et al. was 1.38 for ever smokers as compared to never smokers. The RR for male smokers was 1.54 and for female smokers was 1.22.

It seems evident that smoking tobacco significantly increases the risk for RCC, although moderately so. Risk increased with intensity and duration. There is a higher RR for men compared to women, even when equal doses were considered. This difference may be related to a true increased risk for men, but it can also be explained by the maturity of the smoking trends in the studied populations. An analysis that considers dose and duration of exposure (e.g., pack-years) would be more accurate than a simple comparison by cigarettes consumed a day. Such an analysis could result in an RR that is equal for both sexes. Both active and passive smoking might play a role in the etiology of RCC (Hu, 2005).

Although the association between smoking and RCC is not confirmed by all studies, the causal relationship between tobacco and kidney cancer has recently been established by the International Agency for Research on Cancer (IARC, 2004). Tobacco smoking seems to be the strongest risk factor for RCC, as this met their criteria: consistency of the studies, dose-dependent effect, and strength of the association.

Tobacco contains carcinogens that may induce cancer in several organs. Its toxicological mechanism in renal cancer has not been elucidated yet. It is known that the urine of smokers contains mutagenic activity (Yamasaki, 1977).

The increase in incidence of RCC in mainly industrialized countries led to the hypothesis that certain environmental carcinogens may affect the occurrence of RCC. The enzymes responsible for the breakdown of these environmental carcinogens are usually polymorphic and may therefore play a role in the variable susceptibility to RCC. *N*-Acetyltransferase is an enzyme that plays a role in the detoxication and/or metabolic activation of certain drugs, chemicals, and carcinogens. There are two isoforms (NAT1 and NAT2) that are products of different genes (Roden, 2002). *N*-Acetyltransferase 2 (NAT2) was selected as a genetic susceptibility marker because this enzyme is polymorphic in a large proportion of the population (Longuemaux, 1999). There are slow and rapid NAT2 genotypes. Slow acetylator genotypes affect NAT2 enzyme activity, which reduces the detoxification capacity of NAT2 substrates, like tobacco smoke. Semenza et al. (2001) have proposed that subjects with slow genotypes, could be at increased risk for developing RCC when they smoke. Approximately 50% of whites and African-Americans are "slow" acetylators, a phenotype that is rare among Asians. There could be a relationship between the low incidence of slow acetylators and RCC in Asians and the high incidence of slow acetylators in whites and African-Americans.

Smoking cessation results in a decline of RCC risk. Parker et al. (2003) concluded that cessation of smoking is associated with a linear decrease in risk for RCC after adjustment for potential confounders such as obesity, hypertension, and age. Cessation of smoking longer than 20 years reduces the risk for RCC to the level of nonsmokers, even after adjustment for life-time smoking intensity and duration. A shorter cessation of smoking results in a moderate decrease in risk for RCC.

The prevalence of smoking has declined in the past decades (Sasco, 2004). This seems in contrast with the increasing incidence of RCC. The long latency of tumor development and the differences in smoking behavior for those who have not quit may have contributed to the increase in RCC.

We now know that smoking tobacco is the greatest risk factor for developing RCC. Smoking prevention or cessation would not only decrease the risk for RCC, but would also lower the global burden of cancer and other chronic diseases associated with smoking tobacco.

Obesity

Elevated BMI (body mass index = the weight in kilograms divided by the square of the height in meters) is known to be associated with overall mortality (Calle, 1999). Obesity is defined as a BMI of greater than 30 kg/m². Just as RCC, obesity is increasing worldwide (Calle, 2004). The prevalence of obesity among adults is high in high-income countries while it is relatively uncommon in China and most parts of Africa. It is estimated that globally 2 million deaths each year are caused by inactivity (Ezzati, 2002).

In a quantitative review by Bergstrom et al. (2001), increased BMI was found to be associated with an increased risk for RCC in both sexes, which is supported by work from Bianchini et al. (2002). These authors examined the published evidence for obesity and the risk of cancer. Almost all studies with more than 100 cases have shown an increase in risk with increasing BMI for RCC (summary RR 1.7 for men and RR 2.0 for women). The severely obese have a much higher risk, suggesting that extreme obesity may play the greatest role in the development of RCC (Dhote, 2000).

Although many epidemiological studies have shown that obesity increases the risk of RCC (Bergstrom, 2001; Chow, 2000), particularly among women (Calle, 2003; Chow, 1996), the evidence for men is weaker. In general, the risk for obese women for developing RCC seems greater than for obese men. An explanation could be the differences in distribution of BMI among women and men and the hormonal levels. Women tend to be more obese and this could result in a higher relative risk for women.

With regard to kidney cancer, there is no direct evidence on how the mechanism of obesity could promote the development of RCC. Several hormonal abnormalities have been associated with obese people. They tend to have an elevated insulin, free insulin growth factor-I (IGF-I), and estrogen level and lower insulin growth factor binding protein (IGFBP) level (Calle, 2004).

IGF-1 is an important mutagen that affects the cell cycle. It stimulates cell proliferation and inhibits apoptosis. Insulin and free IGF-I interact with and regulate the synthesis and bioavailability of sex steroids that affect the development and progression of certain cancers such as breast cancer, prostate cancer, and colorectal cancer (Giovannucci, 1999). More recently, Cheung et al. (2004) suggested that IGF-I and several of its binding proteins are upregulated in clear cell RCC.

Free estrogens might also increase the risk for RCC. Animal studies have shown an association between increased levels of free estrogen and the risk of developing RCC (Hodgson, 1998). In human epidemiologic studies, no such association has been found between women using exogenous estrogens and their risk for developing RCC (Gago-Dominguez, 1999a; Lindblad, 1995).

Obesity is a risk factor for non-insulin-dependent diabetes (Overweight, obesity, and health risk. National Task Force on the Prevention and Treatment of Obesity, 2000), which is associated with insulin resistance and hyperinsulinemia. Chronically increased insulin concentrations will reduce the synthesis of IGFBP, which in turn will lead to increased IGF-I activity. Diabetes and thus chronic hyperinsulinemia could be a risk factor for RCC. A population-based retrospective cohort study (Lindblad, 1999) and an international case–control study (Schlehofer, 1996) both showed that an increased risk was observed for RCC, although the latter failed to show significance.

Obesity also contributes to the development of hypertension (Overweight, obesity, and health risk. National Task Force on the Prevention and Treatment of Obesity, 2000). Hypertension has been identified as a risk factor for the development for RCC (see "Hypertension"). The prevalence of hypertension is higher among blacks, which could explain the higher incidence of RCC among blacks. The same survey has also shown that black women tend to be more obese than white women (Hedley, 2004). As obesity is a risk factor for RCC and is more prevalent among blacks, we could expect the upward trend in incidence to be reflected in an upward trend in obesity. So far, the trend in obesity has been shown to vary little with race and sex (Flegal, 1998). Chow et al. (2000), found the obesity-associated risk of RCC to be independent of blood pressure, so hypertension and obesity could influence RCC though different mechanisms.

It is reported that obese people have an increased glomerular filtration rate and renal plasma flow independent of hypertension, which may be a risk for kidney damage (Ribstein, 1995) and therefore make the kidneys more vulnerable for carcinogens.

The role of active vitamin D_3 (VD) has also been suggested. VD can inhibit the growth of murine RCC (Fujioka, 1998). Although the mechanism is unknown, obese people have in general lower vitamin D levels than normal and serum vitamin D levels are also significantly lower than in patients with RCC (Fujioka, 2000).

In summary, increased body weight is associated with an increased risk for developing RCC among women and men. This finding is of great public health relevance because it suggests that developing RCC can be prevented by lifelong maintenance of a normal body weight or, when people have become overweight, by avoiding further weight gain and weight reduction, if possible.

Hypertension

Hypertension, which has a higher prevalence in men than in women (Burt, 1995), has been associated with a low-grade risk factor for malignancies, particular RCC (Grossman, 2002). Grossman et al. (2002) identified 13 case–control studies of the association between hypertension and RCC. In all 13 studies hypertension was associated with RCC with an unadjusted pooled odds ratio of 1.62 and an adjusted odds ratio of 1.75.

Chow et al. (2000) showed a clear dose–response relationship over a wide range of blood pressure levels. A decrease in blood pressure over time decreased the risk for RCC, although more investigations are needed to confirm this finding. Even though this finding was seen in men, it may not apply to the same extent in women. In a systematic review by Dhôte et al. (2000), hypertension could only be classified as a risk marker, not as a risk factor, because no dose-dependent effects were observed.

It should be noted that the association between hypertension and RCC can partly be explained by two facts: patients with hypertension are under stronger medical surveillance than persons who are not being treated for hypertension, and RCC is more likely to be diagnosed in the first group.

There are several other risk factors that are common in hypertensive people, such as obesity, smoking, and diabetes. The association between hypertension and malignancy could be due to confounding. The use of antihypertensive therapy may also confound the relationship between hypertension and malignancy. A comprehensive review of Grossman et al. (1999) analyzed the relation between diuretic therapy and malignancy. Diuretic therapy could be associated with the risk for RCC, particularly in women, although this study did not definitively prove or rule out a causal relationship between diuretics and RCC. The major limitations of most of these studies are incomplete adjustment for potentially confounding factors, in particular hypertension.

Despite the lack of an unambiguous association between diuretics and RCC, there is evidence of a possibly increased risk for the development of RCC that cannot completely be neglected.

There are various explanations for a putative carcinogenic mechanism of diuretics. A plausible anatomical link is that RCC arises from the renal tubular cell, the main target for the pharmacological effect of diuretics (Lip, 1999). Chronic use of diuretics for years and decades and the associated chemical attacks of this cell could lead to a low-grade carcinogenic effect. Another hypothesis points to the toxic metabolites of thiazides and loop diuretics, in particular the mutagenic N-nitroso derivatives, which are assumed to be tumor promoters (Gold, 1977). Hydrochlorothiazide as a cyclic imide can be converted in the stomach to a nitroso derivative.

In most studies women on diuretics were found to be at higher risk than men (Grossman, 1999). There are several potential explanations for this difference. Women use twice as many diuretics as men (Burt, 1995). Women also use more analgesics that are RCC risk factors (see "Analgesic Abuse Nephropathy"). In animal studies, estrogens have been found to potentiate the action of thiazide in the distal tubule in ovariectomized rats (Verlander, 1998), which could contribute to a higher risk for women to develop RCC.

In summary, most epidemiological studies showed that hypertension is a risk factor for RCC, although the association is weaker than for smoking and obesity. Diuretics can be considered as a risk marker rather than a risk factor for RCC, particularly in women, although it must be emphasized that diuretics may increase the risk of RCC but also prevent strokes, heart attacks, and cardiovascular deaths in a much larger proportion, which affects the risk/benefit ratio. Although there are several plausible hypotheses for the etiology of hypertension and antihypertensive medications, the etiology remains largely unknown.

Renal Replacement Therapy

The prevalence of RCC in patients with renal replacement therapy (RRT) is ~40–100 times greater than in the general population (Denton, 2002; Doublet, 1997; Hoshida, 1999). The term RRT is used to describe hemodialysis, peritoneal dialysis, and kidney transplantation. Denton et al. (2002) performed a nephrectomy of the ipsilateral native kidney before transplantation to study the prevalence of RCC in patients with end-stage renal disease (ESRD). They found a prevalence of 4.2% of RCC.

The risk of developing RCC seems greater for patients after renal transplantation than for patients treated with dialysis (Hoshida, 1999), probably because the majority of patients with ESRD receive dialysis before receiving a renal transplant. Patients with ESRD are frequently found to have acquired cystic kidney disease (ACKD) (Bennett, 2003), which is considered to predispose to RCC (Truong, 1995), especially papillary RCC (Peces, 2004). The development of ACKD in patients with ESRD can begin before and after the introduction of RRT (Peces, 2004), but its incidence rises with time on dialysis (Stewart, 2003). Patients treated with dialysis for ESRD are at increased risk for several forms of cancers, especially in the kidneys (Maisonneuve, 1999). The risk of cancer does not depend on the type of dialysis (Stewart, 2003), so it is assumed that the uremic state, rather than any treatment-related phenomenon, is the cause of the increased risk (Maisonneuve, 1999). The pathogenesis of ACKD and the carcinogenic process of dialysis on the kidneys are not completely understood.

Patients undergoing renal transplantation show a higher risk of developing cancer (London, 1995), which is attributed to the associated immunosuppressive treatment and concurrent infections (Andres, 2005). The prior period of uremia and dialysis could also be a cofactor. One of the increased risks includes malignancies of the native kidney (London, 1995; Neuzillet, 2005), with high grade and papillary tumors being particularly common (Neuzillet, 2005). The tumors are often early stage lesions with high grade malignancies, reflecting the potential aggressiveness of the native renal malignancies. RCC of transplanted kidneys is rare.

Occupational Exposure

Unlike urothelial malignancies, RCC is not considered an occupationally related tumor. Yet a number of studies have provided evidence that substantial exposure to metals and solvents can be nephrocarcinogenic, with the highest RR for cadmium (Mandel, 1995; Pesch, 2000), which is known to affect the DNA. An international multicenter population-based case–control study by Mandel et al. (1995) suggested that occupation was more important in the etiology of RCC than previously considered, although no specific agent has been definitively established as causative in RCC.

Analgesic Abuse Nephropathy

There are four major classes of analgesics: aspirin, nonsteroidal antiinflammatory drugs (NSAID), acetaminophen, and phenacetin. Phenacetin has been linked to the development of renal failure and renal pelvis cancer and has been designated as a human carcinogen in 1987 by the International Agency for Research on Cancer. This led to its removal as an analgesic compound in many European countries and the United States. The role of chronic use of the three other analgesics for the risk for RCC remains controversial (Gago-Dominguez, 1999b; McCredie, 1995; Tavani, 1997). They can be nephrotoxic in humans and in animals and nephrotoxic agents are known to be potential nephrocarcinogens.

Genetic Factors

Endogenous risk factors include hereditary familial forms of kidney cancer as the von Hippel–Lindau disease (VHL), familial papillary renal cell carcinoma (HPRCC), hereditary leiomyoma RCC (HLRCC), the Birt–Hogg–Dubé syndrome (BHD), and tuberous sclerosis (TS). These hereditary factors will be extensively discussed in Chapter 7a, but will be briefly introduced here.

VHL disease is an autosomal dominant disorder characterized by several neoplasms, including RCC. There is an abnormality on chromosome 3, especially on chromosome 3p, on which the VHL tumor suppressor gene is located. The gene is involved in both spontaneous and hereditary RCC. Patients with VHL have an inactivation of both copies of the VHL tumor suppressor genes in the tissue of all VHL-associated kidney cancers and in 45–90% of sporadic RCC by deletion, and/ or by hypermethylation (Clifford, 1998). Mutations on this gene are associated almost exclusively with the clear cell type of RCC.

A second form of familial RCC is the HPRCC, characterized by multiple, bilateral papillary renal tumors. Instead of inactivation of a tumor suppressor gene, this tumor is associated with activation of a protooncogene. Mutations in the tyrosine kinase domain of the c-MET protooncogene at chromosome 7 lead to constitutive activations. The product of this gene is the hepatocyte growth factor receptor, which plays a significant role in the regulation of the proliferation and differentiation of epithelial and endothelial cells in a wide variety of organs, including the kidney (Olivero, 1999; Schmidt, 1997, 2004).

HLRCC, also known as the Reed syndrome, is an autosomal dominant disorder characterized by smooth-muscle tumors of the skin and uterus and RCC (Launonen, 2001). Mutations in the fumarate hydratase (FH) gene are considered to predispose to HLRCC (Toro, 2003). The mechanisms by which these mutations lead to carcino-genesis are unknown.

The BHD syndrome is an autosomal dominant disorder predisposing to cutaneous fibrofolliculomas, pulmonary cysts, spontaneous pneumothorax, and renal tumors (Pavlovich, 2005). It is thought that the BHD gene might be a tumor suppressor gene (Nickerson, 2002) mapped to chromosome 17p11.2 (Schmidt, 2001).

Tuberous sclerosis is an autosomal disorder with gene abnormalities localized on two different loci, one on chromosome 9 and one on chromosome 16p. The latter is located adjacent to the gene that is responsible for the most common form of polycystic kidney disease (Identifi-cation and characterization of the tuberous sclerosis gene on chromosome 16. The European Chromosome 16 Tuberous Sclerosis Consortium, 1993; Brook-Carter, 1994). These genes might function as tumor suppressor genes. Tuberous sclerosis is characterized by the formation of angiomy-olipomas or tubers in the skin (called adenoma sebaceum), brain, kidneys, and other organs.

Others

Several case–control studies have investigated the role of medical conditions (Schlehofer, 1996), diet (Wolk, 1996), female hormones (Chow, 1995), and education and socioeco-nomic factors (Mandel, 1995). Moore et al., (2005) described in their review article among other things life-style factors and exposures. In these studies a number of relatively moderate positive associations between these factors and RCC have been found, with issues of mechanism and causality remaining open to discussion. The evidence for most reported associations has been inconsistent or equivocal.

Conclusions

The incidence of RCC is increasing worldwide, with an improvement in survival. Smoking seems to be the main independent risk factors for RCC. Several other risk factors, such as obesity, hypertension, RRT, occupational exposures, and use of analgesics, may be involved, although their contri-bution is minor compared to smoking. An enhanced risk of RCC is observed in certain hereditary disorders such as VHL, HPRCC, HLRCC, BHD syndrome, and TS.

References

Andres A. Cancer incidence after immunosuppressive treatment following kidney transplantation. Crit Rev Oncol Hematol 2005;56:71–85.

Bennett WM, Rose BD. Acquired cystic disease of the kidney in adults. UpToDate online 13.1. 7-10-2003.

Bergstrom A, Hsieh CC, Lindblad P et al. Obesity and renal cell cancer—a quantitative review. Br J Cancer 2001;85:984–990.

Bianchini F, Kaaks R, Vainio H. Overweight, obesity, and cancer risk. Lancet Oncol 2002;3:565–574.

Bray F, Sankila R, Ferlay J et al. Estimates of cancer incidence and mortality in Europe in 1995. Eur J Cancer 2002;38:99–166.

Bray F, Guerra YM, Parkin DM. The comprehensive cancer monitoring programme in Europe. Eur J Public Health 2003;13:61–66.

Brook-Carter PT, Peral B, Ward CJ et al. Deletion of the TSC2 and PKD1 genes associated with severe infantile polycystic kidney disease—-a contiguous gene syndrome. Nat Genet 1994;8: 328–332.

Burt VL, Whelton P, Roccella EJ et al. Prevalence of hypertension in the US adult population. Results from the Third National Health and Nutrition Examination Survey, 1988–1991. Hyper-tension 1995;25:305–313.

Calle EE, Thun MJ, Petrelli JM et al. Body-mass index and mortality in a prospective cohort of U.S. adults. N Engl J Med 1999;341:1097–1105.

Calle EE, Rodriguez C, Walker-Thurmond K et al. Overweight, obesity, and mortality from cancer in a prospectively studied cohort of U.S. adults. N Engl J Med 2003;348:1625–1638.

Calle EE, Thun MJ. Obesity and cancer. Oncogene 2004;23: 6365–6378.

Cheung CW, Vesey DA, Nicol DL et al. The roles of IGF-I and IGFBP-3 in the regulation of proximal tubule, and renal cell carcinoma cell proliferation. Kidney Int 2004;65:1272–1279.

Chow WH, McLaughlin JK, Mandel JS et al. Reproductive factors and the risk of renal cell cancer among women. Int J Cancer 1995;60:321–324.

Chow WH, McLaughlin JK, Mandel JS et al. Obesity and risk of renal cell cancer. Cancer Epidemiol Biomarkers Prev 1996;5: 17–21.

Chow WH, Devesa SS, Warren JL et al. Rising incidence of renal cell cancer in the United States. JAMA 1999;281:1628–1631.

Chow WH, Gridley G, Fraumeni JF, Jr. et al. Obesity, hyper-tension, and the risk of kidney cancer in men. N Engl J Med 2000;343:1305–1311.

Clifford SC, Prowse AH, Affara NA et al. Inactivation of the von Hippel-Lindau (VHL) tumour suppressor gene and allelic losses at chromosome arm 3p in primary renal cell carcinoma: Evidence for a VHL-independent pathway in clear cell renal tumourigenesis. Genes Chromosomes Cancer 1998;22:200–209.

Denton MD, Magee CC, Ovuworie C et al. Prevalence of renal cell carcinoma in patients with ESRD pre-transplantation: A patho-logic analysis. Kidney Int 2002;61:2201–2209.

Denton MD, Magee CC, Ovuworie C et al. Prevalence of renal cell carcinoma in patients with ESRD pre-transplantation: A patho-logic analysis. Kidney Int 2002;61:2201–2209.

Dhote R, Pellicer-Coeuret M, Thiounn N et al. Risk factors for adult renal cell carcinoma: A systematic review and implications for prevention. BJU Int 2000;86:20–27.

Dhôte R, Pellicer-Coeuret M, Thiounn N et al. Risk factors for adult renal cell carcinoma: A systematic review and implications for prevention. BJU Int 2000;86:20–27.

Doublet JD, Peraldi MN, Gattegno B et al. Renal cell carcinoma of native kidneys: Prospective study of 129 renal transplant patients. J Urol 1997;158:42–44.

Eggener SE, Rubenstein JN, Smith ND et al. Renal tumors in young adults. J Urol 2004;171:106–110.

Ezzati M, Lopez AD, Rodgers A et al. Selected major risk factors and global and regional burden of disease. Lancet 2002;360: 1347–1360.

Flegal KM, Carroll MD, Kuczmarski RJ et al. Overweight and obesity in the United States: prevalence and trends, 1960–1994. Int J Obes Relat Metab Disord 1998;22:39–47.

Fujioka T, Hasegawa M, Ishikura K et al. Inhibition of tumor growth and angiogenesis by vitamin D3 agents in murine renal cell carcinoma. J Urol 1998;160:247–251.

Fujioka T, Suzuki Y, Okamoto T et al. Prevention of renal cell carcinoma by active vitamin D3. World J Surg 2000;24: 1205–1210.

Gago-Dominguez M, Castelao JE, Yuan JM et al. Increased risk of renal cell carcinoma subsequent to hysterectomy. Cancer Epidemiol Biomarkers Prev 1999a;8:999–1003.

Gago-Dominguez M, Yuan JM, Castelao JE et al. Regular use of analgesics is a risk factor for renal cell carcinoma. Br J Cancer 1999b;81:542–548.

Giovannucci E. Insulin-like growth factor-I and binding protein-3 and risk of cancer. Horm Res 1999;51(Suppl 3):34–41.

Gold B, Mirvish SS. N-Nitroso derivatives of hydrochlorothiazide, niridazole, and tolbutamide. Toxicol Appl Pharmacol 1977;40:131–136.

Grossman E, Messerli FH, Goldbourt U. Does diuretic therapy increase the risk of renal cell carcinoma? Am J Cardiol 1999;83:1090–1093.

Grossman E, Messerli FH, Goldbourt U. Does diuretic therapy increase the risk of renal cell carcinoma? Am J Cardiol 1999;83:1090–1093.

Grossman E, Messerli FH, Boyko V et al. Is there an association between hypertension and cancer mortality? Am J Med 2002;112:479–486.

Hedley AA, Ogden CL, Johnson CL et al. Prevalence of overweight and obesity among US children, adolescents, and adults, 1999–2002. JAMA 2004;291:2847–2850.

Hock LM, Lynch J, Balaji KC. Increasing incidence of all stages of kidney cancer in the last 2 decades in the United States: An analysis of surveillance, epidemiology and end results program data. J Urol 2002;167:57–60.

Hodgson AV, yala-Torres S, Thompson EB et al. Estrogen-induced microsatellite DNA alterations are associated with Syrian hamster kidney tumorigenesis. Carcinogenesis 1998;19:2169–2172.

Hoshida Y, Nakanishi H, Shin M et al. Renal neoplasias in patients receiving dialysis and renal transplantation: Clinico-pathological features and p53 gene mutations. Transplantation 1999;68: 385–390.

Hu J, Ugnat AM. Active and passive smoking and risk of renal cell carcinoma in Canada. Eur J Cancer 2005;41:770–778.

Hunt JD, van der Hel OL, McMillan GP et al. Renal cell carcinoma in relation to cigarette smoking: Meta-analysis of 24 studies. Int J Cancer 2005;114:101–108.

IARC. Tobacco Smoke and Involuntary Smoking, in IARC Monographs on the Evaluation of Carcinogenic Risk to Humans. IARC, Lyon, France, 2004, 339–355.

Identification and characterization of the tuberous sclerosis gene on chromosome 16. The European Chromosome 16 Tuberous Sclerosis Consortium. Cell 1993;75:1305–1315.

Jayson M, Sanders H. Increased incidence of serendipitously discovered renal cell carcinoma. Urology 1998;51:203–205.

Jemal A, Murray T, Ward E et al. Cancer statistics, 2005. CA Cancer J Clin 2005;55:10–30.

Launonen V, Vierimaa O, Kiuru M et al. Inherited susceptibility to uterine leiomyomas and renal cell cancer. Proc Natl Acad Sci USA 2001;98:3387–3392.

Lee CT, Katz J, Shi W et al. Surgical management of renal tumors 4 cm. or less in a contemporary cohort. J Urol 2000;163:730–736.

Levi F, Lucchini F, Negri E et al. Declining mortality from kidney cancer in Europe. Ann Oncol 2004;15:1130–1135.

Lindblad P, Mellemgaard A, Schlehofer B et al. International renal-cell cancer study. V. Reproductive factors, gynecologic operations and exogenous hormones. Int J Cancer 1995;61:192–198.

Lindblad P, Chow WH, Chan J et al. The role of diabetes mellitus in the aetiology of renal cell cancer. Diabetologia 1999;42:107–112.

Lip GY, Ferner RE. Diuretic therapy for hypertension: A cancer risk? J Hum Hypertens 1999;13:421–423.

London NJ, Farmery SM, Will EJ et al. Risk of neoplasia in renal transplant patients. Lancet 1995;346:403–406.

Longuemaux S, Delomenie C, Gallou C et al. Candidate genetic modifiers of individual susceptibility to renal cell carcinoma: A study of polymorphic human xenobiotic-metabolizing enzymes. Cancer Res 1999;59:2903–2908.

Maisonneuve P, Agodoa L, Gellert R et al. Cancer in patients on dialysis for end-stage renal disease: An international collaborative study. Lancet 1999;354:93–99.

Mandel JS, McLaughlin JK, Schlehofer B et al. International renal-cell cancer study. IV. Occupation. Int J Cancer 1995;61: 601–605.

Mandel JS, McLaughlin JK, Schlehofer B et al. International renal-cell cancer study. IV. Occupation. Int J Cancer 1995;61: 601–605.

McCredie M, Pommer W, McLaughlin JK et al. International renal-cell cancer study. II. Analgesics. Int J Cancer 1995;60: 345–349.

Mindrup SR, Pierre JS, Dahmoush L et al. The prevalence of renal cell carcinoma diagnosed at autopsy. BJU Int 2005;95:31–33.

Moore LE, Wilson RT, Campleman SL. Lifestyle factors, exposures, genetic susceptibility, and renal cell cancer risk: A review. Cancer Invest 2005;23:240–255.

Neuzillet Y, Lay F, Luccioni A et al. De novo renal cell carcinoma of native kidney in renal transplant recipients. Cancer 2005;103: 251–257.

Nickerson ML, Warren MB, Toro JR et al. Mutations in a novel gene lead to kidney tumors, lung wall defects, and benign tumors of the hair follicle in patients with the Birt-Hogg-Dube syndrome. Cancer Cell 2002;2:157–164.

Olivero M, Valente G, Bardelli A et al. Novel mutation in the ATP-binding site of the MET oncogene tyrosine kinase in a HPRCC family. Int J Cancer 1999;82:640–643.

Overweight, obesity, and health risk. National Task Force on the Prevention and Treatment of Obesity. Arch Intern Med 2000;160:898–904.

Pantuck AJ, Zisman A, Belldegrun AS. The changing natural history of renal cell carcinoma. J Urol 2001;166: 1611–1623.

Parker AS, Cerhan JR, Janney CA et al. Smoking cessation and renal cell carcinoma. Ann Epidemiol 2003;13:245–251.

Parkin DM, Bray F, Ferlay J et al. Global cancer statistics, 2002. CA Cancer J Clin 2005;55:74–108.

Pavlovich CP, Grubb RL, III, Hurley K et al. Evaluation and management of renal tumors in the Birt-Hogg-Dube syndrome. J Urol 2005;173:1482–1486.

Peces R, Martinez-Ara J, Miguel JL et al. Renal cell carcinoma co-existent with other renal disease: Clinico-pathological features in pre-dialysis patients and those receiving dialysis or renal transplantation. Nephrol Dial Transplant 2004;19:2789–2796.

Pesch B, Haerting J, Ranft U et al. Occupational risk factors for renal cell carcinoma: Agent-specific results from a case-control study in Germany. MURC Study Group. Multicenter urothelial and renal cancer study. Int J Epidemiol 2000;29: 1014–1024.

Ribstein J, du Cailar G, Mimran A. Combined renal effects of overweight and hypertension. Hypertension 1995;26: 610–615.

Ries LAG, Eisner MP, Kosary CL et al. SEER Cancer Statistics Review, 1975–2002. National Cancer Institute, Bethesda Maryland, 1997.

Roden DM. Genetic determinants of drug metabolism. UpToDate online 13.1. 4–12–2002.

Sasco AJ, Secretan MB, Straif K. Tobacco smoking and cancer: A brief review of recent epidemiological evidence. Lung Cancer 2004;45(Suppl 2):S3–S9.

Schlehofer B, Pommer W, Mellemgaard A et al. International renal-cell-cancer study. VI. The role of medical and family history. Int J Cancer 1996;66:723–726.

Schmidt L, Duh FM, Chen F et al. Germline and somatic mutations in the tyrosine kinase domain of the MET proto-oncogene in papillary renal carcinomas. Nat Genet 1997;16:68–73.

Schmidt LS, Warren MB, Nickerson ML et al. Birt-Hogg-Dube syndrome, a genodermatosis associated with spontaneous pneumothorax and kidney neoplasia, maps to chromosome 17p11.2. Am J Hum Genet 2001;69: 876–882.

Schmidt LS, Nickerson ML, Angeloni D et al. Early onset hereditary papillary renal carcinoma: Germline missense mutations in the tyrosine kinase domain of the met proto-oncogene. J Urol 2004;172:1256–1261.

Semenza JC, Ziogas A, Largent J et al. Gene-environment interactions in renal cell carcinoma. Am J Epidemiol 2001;153: 851–859.

Stewart JH, Buccianti G, Agodoa L et al. Cancers of the kidney and urinary tract in patients on dialysis for end-stage renal disease: Analysis of data from the United States, Europe, and Australia and New Zealand. J Am Soc Nephrol 2003;14: 197–207.

Tavani A, La VC. Epidemiology of renal-cell carcinoma. J Nephrol 1997;10:93–106.

Toro JR, Nickerson ML, Wei MH et al. Mutations in the fumarate hydratase gene cause hereditary leiomyomatosis and renal cell cancer in families in North America. Am J Hum Genet 2003;73:95–106.

Truong LD, Krishnan B, Cao JT et al. Renal neoplasm in acquired cystic kidney disease. Am J Kidney Dis 1995;26: 1–12.

Verlander JW, Tran TM, Zhang L et al. Estradiol enhances thiazide-sensitive NaCl cotransporter density in the apical plasma membrane of the distal convoluted tubule in ovariectomized rats. J Clin Invest 1998;101:1661–1669.

Wolk A, Gridley G, Niwa S et al. International renal cell cancer study. VII. Role of diet. Int J Cancer 1996;65:67–73.

Yamasaki E, Ames BN. Concentration of mutagens from urine by absorption with the nonpolar resin XAD-2: Cigarette smokers have mutagenic urine. Proc Natl Acad Sci USA 1977;74: 3555–3559.

2
Natural History of Renal Cell Carcinoma

Mototsugu Oya and Masaru Murai

Introduction

With the increasing use of imaging modalities such as ultrasonography and computed tomography as screening modalities, renal cell carcinoma (RCC) can now frequently be detected asymptomatically in the early stages. As a consequence, the rate of incidental detection has increased from 10% to greater than 60% over the past 30 years (11, 16), thus resulting in a significant downward stage migration (18). In the era when such modalities were not available, RCC tended to be diagnosed based on the local symptoms of the patients including hematuria, flank pain, and a palpable mass. Occasionally, surgical procedures were not performed in these patients because they had metastatic lesions or because they were too ill to withstand such procedures. Generally, these patients did not live long enough to observe the natural history of the untreated RCC. Since the standard management of most renal masses is an immediate surgical extirpation, the natural history of these lesions has thus remained unknown. Furthermore, although the pathological findings including the tumor grade and stage provide prognostic information, the outcome for patients with RCC is occasionally unpredictable (21). Now, with the increasing number of incidental discoveries of small low-grade and stage renal tumors, the opportunities to observe the growth rate of these tumors has become possible. The data on growth rates mainly come from elderly patients or patients with complications that are too serious for them to undergo surgical procedures. A key consideration of these RCCs detected by serendipity is the nature of these lesions (10). Do these tumors progress until they threaten the life of the patients? What percentage of such RCC has an aggressive phenotype that will result in metastasis? Do patients need to have surgical operations to cure RCC that might remain dormant for decades and never become clinically evident during their lifetime? To date, there are no precise answers to these questions. However, recent publications have shed some light on these issues.

Small Incidentally Detected Renal Tumors

RCCs comprise up to 85% of all solid renal tumors (4). The widespread use of imaging modalities has now enabled us to detect small RCCs. Duchene et al. (4) indicated that in surgically treated tumors measuring 4 cm or less in size, 18 (20%) of 90 were benign tumors including oncocytoma and angiomyolipoma. It is therefore challenging for radiologists and urologists to distinguish small oncocytomas from RCC preoperatively. Small angiomyolipomas, if the components are dominantly smooth muscles, are also difficult to distinguish from RCC (12). These small benign tumors are usually treated as if they are RCC. We should keep in mind that about 20% of all small renal tumors include benign tumors. We should also keep in mind that regarding the histological classification, RCC includes several subtypes. A clear cell histology accounts for 70–80%, followed by papillary (10–15%) and chromophobe (5%) types (27).

Excellent Prognosis of Small Renal Cell Carcinoma

Hafez et al. (8) retrospectively analyzed the outcome of 485 patients with RCC treated with nephron sparing surgery. The cancer-free survival was significantly better in patients with tumors measuring 4 cm or less in size. The five-and 10-year survival rate was 99% and 94%, respectively, in 142 patients with tumors measuring 2.5 cm or less in size. Yamada et al. (31) also reported an excellent prognosis of small RCC less than 25 mm in size. Of 17 tumors, 13 were incidentally detected. All tumors demonstrated a low grade and stage, and the 10-year survival rate was 100%.

Aggressive Nature of Small Renal Cell Carcinoma

Small renal tumors smaller than 3 cm in size have long been regarded as adenomas because they seldom metastasize. In 1987, Aizawa et al. (1) reported that 7 out of 40 RCCs had metastasis including the lymph nodes, bone, and chest wall. Surprisingly, one patient with clear cell RCC measuring 8 mm in size had bone metastases and died 7 months after presentation (1). Eschwege et al. (5) showed the long-term follow-up results of patients treated with a radical nephrectomy for RCC measuring 3 cm in size or smaller. At their institute out of 850 patients who underwent a radical nephrectomy, 74 RCCs were 3 cm or smaller in size (8.7%). Ninety-three percent of the tumors were clear cell type. The average follow-up was 101 months (range 10–236). Out of the 74 patients, 11 patients died of disease progression. Five patients had metastatic disease at diagnosis. The overall cancer-specific survival rates were 81% at 5 years, and 72% at 10 and 20 years. This study suggests that clear cell type tumors measuring 3.0 cm or less in size have a potential to metastasize (5). They concluded that small RCC is not a benign disease and that there was a risk of metastatic disease. Notably, their series included only 22 incidentally detected cases (29.7%). This is in contrast with Yamada's series, mentioned above, which demonstrated a 100% 10-year survival rate. Their series included 13 incidental cases out of 16 RCCs (81.2%). The contrast between the two series may be due to the rate of incidentally detected RCC. In fact, the lower malignant potential of incidental RCC was pointed out in another study (29). Biological differences might also exist between incidental and symptomatic RCC. Hsu et al. (10) described the pathological characteristics of 50 small RCCs measuring 3 cm in size or less. Nineteen (38%) had extension outside the renal capsule and 14 (28%) showed a high nuclear grade. Lesions measuring 3 cm in size or less and those ranging from 3 cm to 5 cm in size did not differ statistically regarding the T stage and nuclear grade. These reports all note that some small RCCs have a potentially aggressive nature when left in place.

Latent Renal Cell Carcinoma Diagnosed at Autopsy

The question remains whether small RCC may eventually cause the death of a patient if left in place. This question is analogous to occult prostate cancer discovered at autopsy. Regarding the prostate, most latent cancers are well differentiated and do not threaten the patient's life. A report from an autopsy series by Hellsten et al. (9) before the widespread use of imaging modalities showed that about 67% of RCC remained undetected until death and that 24% of undiagnosed RCC were related to the patient's death. This rate seems high in the era when incidentally RCCs are routinely found. Mindrup et al. (19) compared the rate of RCC from two periods, 1955–1960 and 1991–2001. The rate of RCC detected only at autopsy was 0.91 vs. 0.72 per 100 autopsies. The mean size of the latent RCC detected at autopsy was smaller in the more recent group, thus suggesting a better detection of latent RCC before death (19). Kihira et al. (15) reported a series of 7970 autopsies examining the histological types of RCC found incidentally and those found clinically. Of the 51 cases 25 were found at autopsy. The mean tumor size of the latent RCC was 2.6 ± 2.5 cm. This was significantly smaller than that of the clinically identified RCC (7.3 ± 2.8 cm). Grade 1 and clear cell type was more predominant in occult RCC. One case in the latent RCC had a solitary metastasis to a pulmonary hilar lymph node. This tumor was the largest latent RCC measuring 8 cm in diameter and a grade 2 clear cell type. Of note, no difference was shown between the clinical group and the latent group regarding age. This fact suggests that latent cancer might have a different character from clinical RCC. If the latent RCC is merely early small RCC, then the mean age of patients with latent RCC should be younger than the patients with clinical RCC because such tumors need time to grow. They concluded that the incidental tumors tended to have a less malignant potential (15). This finding supports the clinical observation that the age at diagnosis is lower in symptomatic patients than in patients with incidentally detected masses (18). These observations found both clinically and at autopsy do not support the concept that incidental RCCs eventually grow into symptomatic RCCs. Latent RCCs do not exhibit an aggressive nature any more at present when screening is widespread. The natural history of clinical RCCs might therefore be different from latent or incidental RCCs.

Impact of the Size on the Natural History of Renal Cell Carcinoma

Tumor size has been used to stratify the different pathological stages: pT1 (7 cm or smaller) and pT2 (larger than 7 cm). Furthermore, pT1 is subdivided into pT1a (4 cm or smaller) and pT1b (larger than 4 cm). This staging system has recently been validated in terms of the prognosis (24). Frank et al. (6) suggested a further subclassification of pT2 into pT2a (less than 10 cm) and pT2b (10 cm or greater). The larger the tumor, the more likely it will metastasize and have a poorer prognosis. Conversely, the smaller the tumor, the more likely it will be a low-grade tumor that will not metastasize. It is known that the larger lesions tend to have a higher tumor grade; however, it is not clear whether the tumor changed the grade during tumor growth or whether the tumor had a higher grade from that initially observed and thereafter had grown more rapidly.

Symptoms in the Natural History of Renal Cell Carcinoma

Schips et al. (25) evaluated the impact of the cancer-associated symptoms present at diagnosis of RCC on the prognosis of 683 patients. At diagnosis 537 (79.2%) were asymptomatic and 141 patients (20.8%) presented with symptoms. The most frequent symptoms were gross hematuria in 65 (46%), flank pain in 29 (20.6%), and weight loss in 18 (2.6%). The receiver operating characteristics curve revealed an association between an increasing tumor size and symptoms. A cutoff value of 5 cm was most appropriate because the area under the curve was the largest based on this value (25). Patard et al. (22) separated symptoms into local and general. They stratified 388 RCCs into three groups: asymptomatic tumors, tumors with local symptoms, and tumors with systemic symptoms. In a multivariate analysis, the symptom classification was an independent prognostic factor as well as for stage and grade. This study implies that RCC causes local to systemic symptoms in the natural history of RCC (22). Sowery and Siemens (26) also showed that symptomatic lesions may be at higher risk for growth and metastasis despite the stage at presentation. Furthermore, Lee et al. (17) showed that a symptomatic detection of RCC was an independent prognosis factor. A symptomatic presentation had a larger percentage of a clear cell histology when compared to the incidental group. However, the biological differences between incidental and symptomatic RCCs remain to be elucidated. In other words, what factors accelerate the symptoms and worsen the prognosis remain unknown. Lee et al. (17) also showed that in comparison to incidental cases, a symptomatic presentation was predominantly detected in younger patients. This observation supports the idea that the natural history of symptomatic RCC in younger patients is different from the incidental RCC commonly detected in elderly patients.

Growth Rate of Small Renal Cell Carcinoma

Table 2-1 summarizes the reports describing the growth rate of RCC. It should also be noted that a pathological confirmation was not performed in every study. In other words, these tumors may include benign renal tumors such as oncocytoma and angiomyolipoma. The highest average tumor diameter was 4.08 cm in the series by Sowery and Siemens (26). The series included a relatively high rate of symptomatic cases. The average growth rate was 0.86 cm/year. This was highest in the reports shown in Table 2-1. The lowest growth rate was 0.1 cm/year by Volpe et al. (30). In this series all 29 cases were asymptomatic. The mean tumor diameter was 2.74 cm.

Bosniak et al. (2) reported a series of 40 renal tumors (37 patients) measuring 3.5 cm in size or smaller. A surgical removal was performed in 26 tumors. Notably, 4 tumors were oncocytomas while the remaining 22 tumors were all grade 1 or 2 RCC. The overall growth rate was 0–1.10 cm/year (mean 0.36 cm/year). They concluded that most small, incidentally found tumors grow slowly and are not an immediate threat to a patient's life. Watchful waiting might thus be appropriate in elderly patients or in those demonstrating a poor physical condition. However, lesions that measure more than 3.0 cm in diameter when initially seen or that are poorly marginated or contain necrosis cannot be viewed in the same way. They pointed out that lesions measuring larger than 3.5–4.0 cm in diameter are more likely to demonstrate a higher grade. Several lesions measuring more than 4.0 cm grew rapidly (>1.5 cm/year) and metastasized.

Oda et al. (20) reported a growth rate of 16 incidentally detected RCCs. The growth rate was 0.10–1.35 cm/year (mean 0.54 cm/year). In comparison to Bosniak's series, the growth rate was rapid. This may be due to differences in the pathological features between the two series. Oda's series included only pathologically proven RCCs, whereas Bosniak's series included pathologically unknown tumors and oncocytomas.

Kato et al. (14) reported the growth rate of 18 cases of incidentally detected RCC. All cases were pathologically diagnosed including 15 cases of clear cell type and 3 cases of papillary cell type. The average tumor growth rate was 0.42 cm/year. Of note, this series included three cases of grade 3 tumors. The mean growth rate of these grade 3 RCC was 0.93 cm/year. Bosniak's series and Oda's series did not include any grade 3 tumors. There was no difference between the grade 1 and grade 2 tumors in terms of growth rate. The tumor growth rate did not correlate with the Ki-67 positive ratio. In contrast, the TUNEL positive ratio correlated with the growth rate. Grade 3 tumors grew faster than grade 2 tumors. They concluded that most incidentally found RCCs were therefore slow growing; however, some RCCs were also found to grow rapidly and have a poor prognosis. They recommended that more attention be paid to the growth of small RCCs.

Kassouf et al. (13) reported a series of 24 renal tumors. Only five patients demonstrated tumor growth during the surveillance period. Only four patients underwent surgery because of tumor growth in two patients and two patients per request. Pathologically, three patients were clear cell and one was papillary. Sowery and Siemens (26) reported 22 cases with renal tumors managed conservatively. The overall tumor growth in 22 renal tumors was 0.86 cm/year. This series is unique because as many as nine cases had tumors measuring more than 4 cm in diameter at presentation. This report helps to evaluate the natural history of relatively large renal tumors. The mean tumor growth of this group was 1.43 cm/year. One patient underwent a nephrectomy due to rapid growth. One patient developed metastasis, although the growth rate was 0.2 cm/year. The size of the tumor at diagnosis was as large as 8.8 cm.

TABLE 2-1. Growth rate of renal cell carcinoma.

Authors	Publication year	Patient number male/female	Patient age average (range)	Follow-up period mean (range) months	Asumptomatic cases	Tumor diameter mean (range) cm	Tumor growth rate per year (cm)	Pathological confirmation	Subsequent metastasis
Kassouf et al. (13)	2004	24 (16/8)	68.3 (29–83)	31.6 (8–86)	22/24	3.3(0.9–10)	0.49	Partly	No
Kato et al. (14)	2004	18 (13/5)	56.5 (37–71)	22.5 (12–63)	18/18	2.0(1.0–3.4)	0.42	All	No
Volpe et al. (30)	2004	29 (25/4)	71 (27–84)	27.9 (5.3–143.0)	29/29	2.74(0.9–3.9)	0.1	Partly	No
Sowery and Siemens (26)	2004	22 (15/7)	77 (60–92)	26	16/22	4.08(2–8.8)	0.86	Partly	Yes, one patient
Oda et al. (20)	2001	16 (12/4)	54 (28–78)	25.2 (12–72)	16/16	2.0(1.0–4.5)	0.54	All	No
Rendon et al. (23)	2000	13(13/0)	69 (56–85)	42 (5–57)	7/13	2.7(0.9–4.0)	0.144	Partly	No
Bosniak et al. (2)	1995	37(26/11)	65.5 (42–84)	39 (21–102)	37/37	1.73(0.2–3.5)	0.36	Partly	No

In summary, most renal tumors, both benign and malignant, grow slowly. However, these retrospective analyses showed that some RCCs grow faster and metastasize. We do not have any way to predict the outcome. Symptomatic RCCs may tend to progress even if they are small. Grade 3 tumors therefore seem to have a different natural history even if they are incidentally detected.

Natural History of Renal Cell Carcinoma Arising in Patients with Acquired Cystic Kidney Disease

Acquired cystic kidney disease (ACKD) is a state of end-stage kidneys where numerous cysts are observed. It is commonly observed in patients undergoing hemodialysis. ACKD is frequently associated with RCC. Takebayashi et al. (28) reported a growth rate of 17 RCCs arising in ACKD followed for 2.1 years before they underwent a nephrectomy. Fifteen of the 17 RCCs measured less than 3 cm in size at the initial diagnosis. The overall volume growth rate was $0.07–17.34$ cm^3/year (mean, 4.14 ± 5.66) and the estimated volume-doubling time was $0.08–23.31$ years (mean, 5.09 ± 6.99 years). The mean growth rate of the three grade 3 RCCs was 6.01 cm^3/year, which was significantly greater than that of either grade 1 (0.40) or grade 2 (0.79). These observations suggest that RCCs from ACKD grew at variable rates compared to RCCs in the general population. The biological difference in the two groups remains unknown. It is commonly observed that incidentally detected RCCs include grade 3 tumors and such grade 3 tumors are known to grow more rapidly than grade 1 or 2 tumors.

Watchful Waiting: An Option

The increasing incidence of incidentally detected RCCs with a downward stage migration raises the possibility of overtreatment of more indolent RCCs. In elderly patients or in those with a poor physical condition, watchful waiting is often justified. However, there is little reason to choose watchful waiting in younger and otherwise healthy patients with RCCs measuring more than 1.5–2.0 cm in size. While the growth rate is slow, they do grow to reach a size that will metastasize. Furthermore, watchful waiting might change the surgical approach from a partial nephrectomy to a total nephrectomy when the tumor grows as large as about 4 cm in size. We cannot definitely determine which patients are good candidates for watchful waiting due to the lack of any clear association between the imaging features and the subsequent tumor growth. Presently, we do not have sufficient evidence to recommend watchful waiting as a safe management option for small RCCs.

Prospective Observation of Small Renal Masses

Rendon et al. (23) reported a prospective study including 13 patients with a 42-month median follow-up period. Five patients underwent surgery because of either an apparent tumor enlargement or a new onset of symptoms. All five cases were pathologically diagnosed to be RCC. No patients had metastases. Notably two cases were fast growing and those were the only cases in which symptoms developed. When these patients were excluded from the study, the average growth rate was not statistically different from a 0 slope or no growth. These findings suggest that the growth rate of RCC is variable: some tumors grow progressively and possibly metastasize early while most small RCCs grow at a low rate or not at all.

Volpe et al. (30) updated and expanded Rendon's study and prospectively followed 32 renal masses smaller than 4 cm in size. The average growth rate did not differ statistically from zero growth. Seven masses reached 4 cm after a 12–85 month follow-up. Nine tumors were surgically removed because of a rapid growth in five masses or due to the patients' request in four masses. Eight masses were clear cell RCC and one was oncocytoma. Four clear cell RCCs were high grade (grade 3 or 4 as Fuhrman's grade). No patient developed metastasis or died of RCC. A size of 4 cm might be the upper limit for surveillance. Further studies will be needed before we can clearly define the precise thresholds for treatment.

Growth Rate of Metastatic Lesions

Fujimoto et al. (7) investigated the growth rate of primary lesions (six cases) and pulmonary lesions (12 cases). The primary lesions grew slowly and the doubling time was 468 ± 84.6 days. Pulmonary lesions grew more rapidly with a doubling time 89.4 ± 43.0 days. Oda et al. (20) compared the growth rates of 16 primary RCCs and the same number of metastatic lesions. The growth rate of metastatic sites was 1.72 cm/year. This rate was about three times faster than for the primary lesions (0.54 cm/year). These two studies support our general impression that metastatic lesions tend to grow faster and threaten the patient's life.

Conclusions

The growth rate of RCC is variable. Most small incidentally detected RCCs grow very slowly and may not be a threat to the patient's life. Therefore, incidental RCC may not necessarily be a precursor to more aggressive, symptomatic RCC with metastatic potential. With the increasing detection of RCC in older patients or patients with comorbidities, watchful waiting should be considered. However, a few cases of RCC do have the potential to grow and develop into more aggressive disease, even if the tumors are detected at a small size in an early stage. At present we do not have any definite diagnostic modality to predict the natural history of RCC. Therefore, small RCC should be treated, especially in young patients. It is not known whether a tumor changes grade during growth or has a higher grade from the onset and then grows more rapidly than lower grade tumors. Aggressive RCC may therefore exist, including grade 3 tumors, even though they are small in size and incidentally detected.

References

1. Aizawa S, Suzuki M, Kikuchi Y et al. Clinicopathological study on small renal cell carcinomas with metastases. Acta Pathol Jpn 1987;37:947–954.
2. Bosniak MA, Birnbaum BA, Krinsky GA et al. Small renal parenchymal neoplasms: Further observations on growth. Radiology 1995;197:589–597.
3. Derweesh IH and Novick AC. Small renal tumors: Natural history, observation strategies and emerging modalities of energy based tumor ablation. Can J Urol 2003;10:1871–1879.
4. Duchene DA, Lotan Y, Cadeddu JF et al. Histopathology of surgically managed renal tumors: Analysis of a contemporary series. Urology 2003;62:827–830.
5. Eschwege P, Saussine C, Steichen G et al. Radical nephrectomy for renal cell carcinoma 30 mm. or less: Long-term followup results. J Urol 1996;155:1196–1199.
6. Frank I, Blute ML, Leibovich BC et al. pT2 classification for renal cell carcinoma. Can its accuracy be improved? J Urol 2005;173:380–384.
7. Fujimoto N, Sugita A, Terasawa Y et al. Observations on the growth of renal cell carcinoma. Int J Urol 1995;2:71–76.
8. Hafez KS, Fergany AF and Novick AC. Nephron sparing surgery for localized renal cell carcinoma: Impact of tumor size on patient survival, tumor recurrence and TNM staging. J Urol 1999;162:1930–1933.
9. Hellsten S, Berge T and Wehlin L. Unrecognized renal cell carcinoma. Clinical and pathological aspects. Scan J Urol Nephrol 1981;15:273–278.
10. Hsu MH, Chan DY and Siegelman SS. Small renal cell carcinomas: Correlation of size with tumor stage, nuclear grade, and histologic subtype. AJR 2004;182:551–557.
11. Jayson M and Sanders H. Increased incidence of serendipitously discovered renal cell carcinoma. Urology 1998;51:203–205.
12. Jinzaki M, Tanimoto A, Narimatsu Y et al. Angiomyolipoma: Imaging findings in lesions with minimal fat. Radiology 1997;205:497–502.
13. Kassouf W, Aprikian AG, Laplante M et al. Natural history of renal masses followed expectantly. J Urol 2004;171:111–113.
14. Kato M, Suzuki T, Suzuki Y et al. Natural history of small renal cell carcinoma: Evaluation of growth rate, histological grade, cell proliferation and apoptosis. J Urol 2004;172:863–866.
15. Kihira T, Shiraishi T, Yatani R et al. Pathological features of renal cell carcinoma incidentally discovered at autopsy. Acta Pathol Jpn 1991;41:680–684.
16. Konnak JW and Grossman HB. Renal cell carcinoma as an incidental finding. J Urol 1985;134:1094–1096.
17. Lee CT, Katz J, Fearn PA et al. Mode of presentation of renal cell carcinoma provides prognostic information. Urol Oncol 2002;7:135–140.
18. Luciani LG, Cestari R and Tallarigo C. Incidental renal cell carcinoma—Age and stage characterization and clinical implications: Study of 1092 patients (1982–1997). Urology 2000;56:58–62.
19. Mindrup SR, Pierre JS, Dahmoush L et al. The prevalence of renal cell carcinoma diagnosed at autopsy. BJU Int 2005;95:31–33.
20. Oda T, Miyao N, Takahashi A et al. Growth rate of primary and metastatic lesions of renal cell carcinoma. Int J Urol 2001;8:473–477.

21. Oya M and Murai M. Renal cell carcinoma: Relevance of pathology. Curr Opin Urol 2003;13:445–449.

22. Patard J-J, Leray E, Rodriguez A et al. Correlation between symptom graduation, tumor characteristics and survival in renal cell carcinoma. Eur Urol 2003;44:226–232.

23. Rendon RA, Stanietzky N, Panzarella T et al. The natural history of small masses. J Urol 2000;164:1143–1147.

24. Salama ME, Guru K, Stricker H et al. pT1 substaging in renal cell carcinoma: Validation of the 2002 TNM staging modification of malignant renal epithelial tumors. J Urol 2005;173:1492–1495.

25. Schips L, Lipsky K, Zigeuner R et al. Impact of tumor-associated symptoms on the prognosis of patients with renal cell carcinoma: A single-center experience of 683 patients. Urology 2003;62:1024–1028.

26. Sowery RD and Siemens R. Growth characteristics of renal cortical tumors in patients managed by watchful waiting. Can J Urol 2004;11:2407–2410.

27. Storkel S, Ebel JN, Adlakha K et al. Classification of renal cell carcinoma: Workgroup No. 1. Union Internationale Contre le Cancer (UICC) and the American Joint Committee on Cancer (AJCC). Cancer 1997;80:987–989.

28. Takebayashi S, Hidai H, Chiba T et al. Renal cell carcinoma in acquired cystic kidney disease: Volume growth rate determined by helical computed tomography. Am J Kidney Dis 2000;36:759–766.

29. Tsui KH, Shvarts O, Smith RB et al. Renal cell carcinoma: Prognostic significance of incidentally detected tumors. J Urol 2000;163:426–430.

30. Volpe A, Panzarella T, Rendon RA et al. The natural history of incidentally detected small renal masses. Cancer 2004;100: 738–745.

31. Yamada Y, Honda N, Mitsui K et al. Clinical features of renal cell carcinoma less than 25 millimeters in diameter. Int J Urol 2002;9:663–667.

3
Pathology of Renal Cell Carcinoma: Correlation of Morphology, Immunophenotype, and Genetic and Clinical Aspects

Ferran Algaba, Yolanda Arce, and Isabel Trias

Historical Perspective of the Pathology of Renal Cell Carcinoma

During the seventeenth and eighteenth centuries, both neoplastic renal masses and tumor-looking inflammatory processes were described. In 1826, Koenig published the first pathological classification of renal tumors and subdivided them into *scirrhous, steatomatous, fungoid,* and *medullary* forms[1] based on their macroscopic characteristics.

The microscopic characterization of renal tumors started in the mid-nineteenth century with the controversy aroused by Grawitz's hypothesis: in 1883 Grawitz stated that *"alveolar"* (clear cell) tumors, previously considered lipomas, originated in the neoplastic transformation of adrenal cortical residues into renal cortical residues. One year later he confirmed his theory when he found ectopic adrenal cortex in the renal cortex, and he differentiated these neoplasias from the *papillary* forms and pronounced them of renal origin.[2] This theory was readily opposed by Sudek, who considered that both tumors (alveolar and papillary) were mere variations of the same renal tubular origin.[3] The controversy between supporters and detractors of the Grawitz theory went on for decades. The term *hypernephroma* was introduced in 1909, and made reference to its adrenal origin.[4] Even though support for the supposedly adrenal origin started to grow weaker, publications still appeared during the first half of the twentieth century[5] that validated it; however, the end of the Grawitz theory was near, as shown by the classical book by Herbut[6] in which the generalized opinion appears that all renal tumors are of tubular origin; eventually the ultrastructural studies of Oberling et al.[7] put a stop to the argument when they demonstrated the tubular origin of renal carcinoma.

The international classifications unified all histological types under the common denomination of renal adenocarcinoma; this could be a clear cell or a granular cell carcinoma, its architecture could be tubular, papillary, or cystic, and its appearance was rarely sarcomatoid.[8] Even though the argument seemed ended by this homogenization, attempts to distinguish histological subtypes according to their supposed origins of different nephron stretches started to appear quite soon, correlating them to different clinical evolutions.

One of the major developments was Thoenes et al.'s description of the *chromophobe renal cell carcinoma*,[9] morphologically different from the clear cell carcinoma and probably originating in the intercalated cells of the distal nephron.[10] From this description (initially not accepted by the international classifications), the possibility of determining different origins of the histological subtypes started to be explored with monoclonal antibodies;[11] unfortunately, it was not possible to differentiate neat groups, so no modification of the established classification was finally determined.

Only when Kovacs' initial chromosome studies,[12] subsequently redefined by the Heidelberg classification,[13] were introduced were renal cancer microscopic subtypes taken into account again, as a correspondence was confirmed between genetic abnormalities and microscopic phenotype.

From the above considerations the latest World Health Organization (WHO)'s 2004 classification[14] emerges, which combines morphological and genetic characteristics and starts to recognize some variations with evidence of different immunophenotypes or molecular changes with clinical implications.

Nephrectomy Specimen Handling

The quality of any pathological evaluation depends on a careful macroscopic examination of the surgical specimens.[15] Basic for an efficacious pathological study are identification of the anatomical structures, preservation of the complete specimens (i.e., no cuts), and appropriate handling by urologists.

The specimens should be manipulated when fresh. Avoid stripping the capsule before sectioning the specimen, and identify the renal vein, the renal artery, and the ureter. Careful external inspection is basic for evaluating the radicality of the nephrectomy. The areas in which such radicality is dubious should be inked with India ink before sectioning.

The specimen should be sectioned every 10 mm including the perinephric fat tissue. Every tumoral nodule and anatomical structure should be identified and the specimen should be fixed and left overnight.

Samples for microscopy study should be selected and identified by means of identification labels, and they should include the following: (1) one tumor section per every centimeter of tumor diameter; (2) section of the tumor–fat tissue interface; (3) accurate study of the sinus fat tissue close to the tumor, with a sagittal section of this area;[16] (4) section of the renal vein, even if normal; and (5) two or three samples of normal kidney, close to the tumor and also distal to it. One of the objectives of this sampling is finding microvascular invasion: (6) adrenal gland section, even if the tumor is far from it; and (7) complete dissection including the lymph nodes. The number of lymph nodes to be dissected depends on the pathologist's motivation and the urologist´s skills. Generally the lymph nodes are rarely identifiable unless specifically dissected by the surgeon. In this case inclusion of the complete hiliar fat tissue is recommended.[16]

Margins are of the utmost importance. Positive margins are very rarely found in specimens from a radical procedure. If positive margins are found, their location and their extension should be reported.

The margins of a nephron-sparing nephrectomy are the renal parenchyma margin and the perinephric fat margin. It is advisable to ink the excision margins before dissection. The urinary tract wall should be considered a margin if the tumor extends into the calyceal system.[17]

Pathological Prognostic Markers of Renal Cell Carcinomas

The extension (staging) of the tumor continues to be the most important marker of pathological prognosis. Nuclear grading is useful even in localized tumors and histological subtypes also play a role in prognosis.

Staging

The global usefulness of TNM 2002 (Table 3-1)[18] is acceptable, but the prognostic validity of some individual variables is controversial in the literature.

By categories, the most debatable aspects include the following.

TABLE 3-1. TNM classification 2002 for renal tumors.

T category

TX Primary tumor cannot be assessed
T0 No evidence of primary tumor
T1a Tumor 4 cm or less
T1b Tumor more than 4 cm but not more than 7 cm.
T2 Tumor more than 7 cm in greatest dimension, limited to the kidney
T3a Tumor directly invades adrenal gland or perinephric tissues (*includes renal sinus*) but not beyond the Gerota fascia
T3b Tumor grossly extends into the renal vein (*includes segmental muscle-containing branches*) or vena cava or its wall below the diaphragm
T3c Tumor grossly extends into the vena cava or its wall above the diaphragm
T4 Tumor directly invades beyond the Gerota fascia
N category
NX Regional lymph nodes cannot be assessed
N0 No regional lymph node metastasis
N1 Metastasis in a single regional lymph node
N2 Metastasis in more than one regional lymph node
M category
MX Distant metastasis cannot be assessed
M0 No distant metastasis
M1 Distant metastasis

Category pT1

In 2002 classification, pT1 tumors are subclassified as pT1a (4 cm or less) and pT1b (larger than 4 cm but not larger than 7 cm). However, some authors have recently proposed that the cut-off should be higher,[19–21] and when the size is considered as a continuous variable, the 5.5 cm cut-off has a greater statistical significance (10-year cancer-specific survival in 87.9% with ≤ 5.5 cm tumors versus 73.9% with >5 cm tumors) than the 4 cm one.[22] This controversy regarding size is related to prognosis and should not influence the decision concerning nephron-sparing surgery.[23]

Category pT2

This category includes tumors larger than 7 cm at most, but limited to the kidney. Some authors are considering the possibility of stratifying this category in tumors larger than 7 cm but smaller than 10 cm, and 10 cm or larger (risk ratio 1.42 vs. 1.22).[21]

Category pT3a

The presence of renal capsular invasion is often difficult to be accurately determined; that is why definitive pathological criteria have been necessary. Some authors believe that absolute size has greater predictive value than renal capsular invasion.[24, 25]

However, *invasion of the sinus fat tissue* seems to entail greater aggressiveness (5-year specific survival 25.9%) than perinephric fat tissue invasion (5-year specific survival 50.9%),[26] probably because it contains a number of large thin-walled veins and lymphatics, and it is not separated from the renal cortex by a fibrous capsule.[27] All these data confirm the need for an accurate analysis of the surgical specimens according to international guidelines.[15]

The *ipsilateral adrenal gland invasion* is rare (2.5%). Its prognosis is worse than that of perinephric fat tissue invasion[28] and has no significant differences with pT4.[29]

Category pT3b

The *tumoral venous thrombus* apparently does not mean a poor prognosis in the absence of local invasion, as previously thought (5-year survival from 47 to 69%).[30]

Category pT3c

Tumor thrombus level in the inferior vena cava does not significantly affect long-term survival,[31] but these patients have a worse prognosis that those with pT3b.[29]

The *involvement of the pelvicalyceal system* is under discussion because authors believe it means a worse prognosis,[32] whereas others believe it does not represent an independent prognostic factor, except in organ-confined tumors.[33]

Category pN

Some authors find a statistically significant difference in the rate of lymph node metastasis between organ-confined patients with less than 13 nodes examined and those with 13 or more nodes studied (3.4% vs. 10.5%, $p <0.01$), and cases with locally advanced tumors (19.7% vs. 32.2% $p <0.05$).[34]

All of these considerations in the literature call for implementation of a future TNM classification.

Grading

Despite criticisms concerning the reproducibility of Fuhrman's nuclear grade (based on the size and shape of the nucleus and also on the presence or absence of nucleoli)[35] (Table 3-2 and Fig. 3-1) it is the most widely method used internationally.

It is a good prognostic marker with a 5-year cancer specific survival rate of 89%, 65%, and 46% for grades 1, 2, and 3–4, respectively.[36] The present trend is to subdivide the four Fuhrman's grades into low grade (grade 1 and 2) and

high grade (grade 3 and 4).[37] With this approach the interobserver and intraobserver variability is improved without loss of outcome discrimination.[38]

The wider use of ultrasound favors the detection of asymptomatic renal tumors[39] with a higher incidence of organ-confined carcinomas. In this situation the Fuhrman's grading can also be of help. A nuclear grade greater than 2 correlates with significantly shorter survival ($p = 0.018$) in Stage I tumors.[40]

At first the Fuhrman's grade was applied only to the clear cell renal cell carcinomas. Now the grading of all cell subtypes is recommended. But in some cell types (chromophobe renal cell carcinoma) irregular nuclei and prominent nucleoli are intrinsic. Hence the Fuhrman's grade is higher even with favorable outcomes. To overcome this obstacle some authors propose an adaptation of the classification for this subtype with redefinition of the grades in three levels and with the acceptance of a somewhat more nuclear pleomorphic aspect in low grades that correlates with the pT category and independently predicts the clinical outcome.[41] But this new approach should be validated by other series.

Microvascular Invasion

For quite some time now microvascular invasion of the peritumoral kidney parenchyma has been considered an important prognostic factor after radical nephrectomy for clinically nonmetastatic renal cell carcinoma, with a progression rate of 29–39.2% vs. 6.2–17% in cases with no microvascular invasion.[42, 43] But there are discrepancies among the authors as to whether this finding has any independent statistical significance[43–45]. So far there is no consensus about strict criteria for microvascular diagnosis and nontumoral kidney sampling. It is advisable to reach an agreement about this topic as soon as possible because an obvious clinical fact exists despite all the criticisms of the interobserver variability.

Tumoral Necrosis

Another prognostic marker with similar problems is tumor necrosis. Necrosis in the primary tumor is associated with survival in localized renal cell carcinomas (5-year cancer specific survival is 36% among patients with tumor necrosis vs. 75% among patients without it).[46] Necrosis correlates with a higher expression of the cell proliferation factor (Ki-67)[46] and the vascular endothelial growth factor.[47] These findings have encouraged us to reevaluate some morphological prognostic markers as their molecular basis may be directly involved in the molecular alterations of the cellular cycle.[48] Once again consensus methods for reproducible quantification criteria were established.

TABLE 3-2. Fuhrman system.

Grade 1	Round uniform nuclei approximately 10 μm in diameter; small or absent nucleoli
Grade 2	Slightly irregular nuclear contours and diameters of approximately 15 μm; nucleoli visible at ×400
Grade 3	Moderately to severely irregular nuclear contours and diameter of approximately 20 μm; Large nucleoli visible at ×100
Grade 4	Nuclei similar to grade 3 but also multilobular, multiple; bizarre nuclei and heavy clumps of chromatin

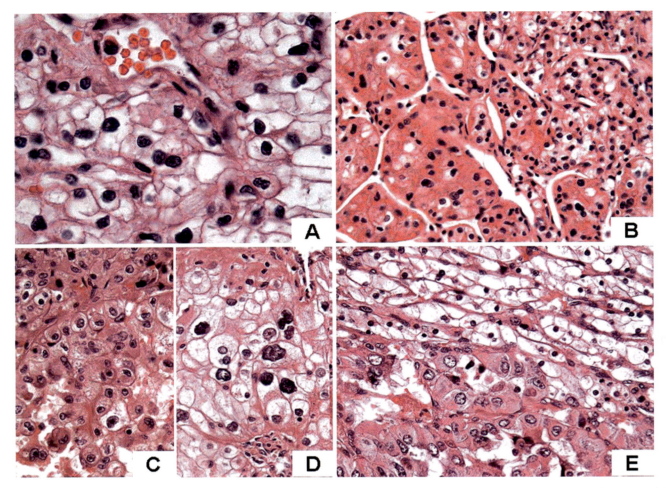

FIGURE 3-1. Nuclear grading in renal cell carcinoma (Fuhrman system). (**A**) Grade 1. (**B**) Grades 1 and 2. (**C**) Grade 3. (**D**) Grade 4. (**E**) Grades 1 and 3 in the same microscopic field.

Histological Subtypes

The WHO's 2004 classification makes a clear distinction between tumor subtypes having a better prognosis and others that do not. The differences regarding prognosis of the most usual forms are statistically significant at univariant studies,[49,50] but have no independent statistical significance in some other studies.[51] In spite of this, some cell subtypes do seem to be related to different carcinogenesis,[52] and their response to future therapies may be different too.[53] This is the reason why we must widely consider the morphology and the genetics of the different renal cell carcinoma subtypes.

WHO's Histological Classification of the Kidney Tumors

The WHO's primary classification criterion is the cell appearance, and the different variations of renal carcinoma are consecutively expounded (Table 3-3). However, there is presently enough genetic and immunohistochemical evidence to enable us to assign the different types to a nephron segment or to another one,[54] and for this reason the discussion below, even though it continues to be the WHO's, will be grouped according to these segments.

TABLE 3-3. WHO histological classification of renal cell tumors.

Clear cell renal cell carcinoma
Multilocular clear cell renal cell carcinoma
Papillary renal cell carcinoma
Chromophobe renal cell carcinoma
Carcinoma of the collecting ducts of Bellini
Renal medullary carcinoma
Xp11 translocation carcinomas
Carcinoma associated with neuroblastoma
Mucinous tubular and spindle cell carcinoma
Renal cell carcinoma, unclassified
Papillary adenoma
Oncocytoma

Pathology of Proximal Nephron Renal Cell Carcinomas

Clear Cell Renal Cell Carcinoma

Clinical Features

This is the most frequent subtype of renal carcinoma of the adult, representing around 66.8% of our cases (between 70% and 85% in the literature).[51,55] The sporadic forms appear during the sixth decade of life (global mean age 59.4 years for both sexes) and they are three times as frequent in men as in women.

Macroscopy

Tumors are usually single in the sporadic cases, with 4% multiplicity and 3% bilaterality. The tumor is well delimited by a pseudocapsule of fibrous tissue that is the consequence of compression of the surrounding tissues. Due to cytoplasm lipid accumulation the section surface is yellow. Hemorrhagic areas are frequent for the large vascular stroma

(Fig. 3-2A). Occasionally there are scar areas and some of them even include calcification. Necrosis is associated with more aggressive neoplasias.

The cystic appearance it sometimes adopts may be due to necrosis and liquefaction (pseudocysts) or because it is formed by genuine neoplastic cysts (Fig. 3-2B and C).

Among the cystic renal cell carcinomas there are cases of clear cell renal cell carcinomas with a wide cystic transformation, as well as cases with complete cystic appearance that lack a solid tumoral component.

The latter subtype has been called **multilocular cystic renal cell carcinoma**[56] (Fig. 3-2B). The cysts' wall exhibits isolated malignant cells (Fig. 3-2C). Macroscopically their appearance may be similar to that of a multilocular cyst (cystic nephroma). The excellent prognosis in a recent multi-institutional study suggests the possibility of considering it a low-malignant-potential carcinoma.[57]

Microscopy

As suggested by its name, this neoplasia consists of clear cytoplasm cells; they are clear due to their high content of

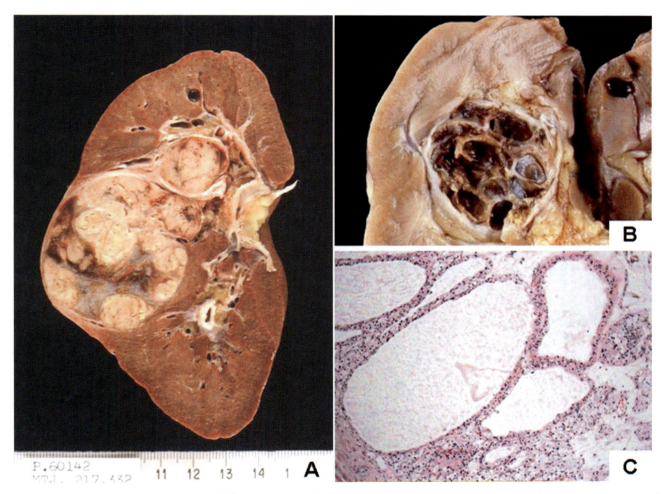

FIGURE 3-2. Clear cell renal cell carcinoma. (**A**) Solid tumor of yellow color with some hemorrhagic area. (**B**) Macroscopic aspect of a multilocular clear cell renal cell carcinoma. (**C**) Microscopic true neoplastic cysts without solid growth.

glycogen and lipids that dissolve in the course of histological processing (Fig. 3-3A). Cells with a higher mitochondrial content may be seen to acquire an eosinophilic or granular appearance (Fig. 3-3B). The predominance of this cell type is exceptional. Rounded or irregular eosinophilic cytoplasmic inclusions are rarely found. The nuclei are rounded and their characteristics depend upon their degree of differentiation. The most frequent arrangement forms a solid pattern. Tubular and occasionally microcystic patterns can also be present (Fig. 3-3C). Papillary areas are very rarely observed (Fig. 3-3D).[58] Five percent of cases are of the spindle cell (sarcomatoid) type.[59]

Immunophenotype

The cells more frequently express low-molecular-weight cytokeratins (CAM 5.2 around 60%) than high-molecular-weight cytokeratins (CK14 in 3.7%).[60] Vimentin is expressed in 82.6%,[61] CD10 in 94% (Fig. 3-4), RCC antibody in 85%,[62] epithelial membrane antigen (EMA) (MUC-1) in 85%,[63] and glutathione S-transferase-α (GST-α) in 82%.[64] From

adhesion molecules there is only 5% of E-cadherin[63] and kidney-specific cadherin (Ksp-cadherin) is negative.[65] Parvalbumin is expressed in 26% and β-defensin-1 in 13%.[61] Other markers such as c-kit, RON protooncogene, and p504S–α-methylacyl-CoA racemase (AMACR) are almost always negative.[66–68]

Genetic Changes

3p deletion (LOH 3p) is the most typical genetic abnormality of this carcinoma, present in 75.8% of cases,[69] but not exclusive to it.[70] Three genes have been located on the short arm of chromosome 3 that are probably involved in renal carcinoma. The suppressor gene in 3p25-26 (VHL) coincides with von Hippel–Lindau disease but is expressed in 34–56% of sporadic carcinomas,[71] and those located on 3p14.2 (potential gene FHIT) and on 3p.12, whose deletion is more frequent than that of the former. Other putative tumor suppressor genes at 3p such as RASSF1A and NRC-1 at 3p12 are reported.[72, 73]

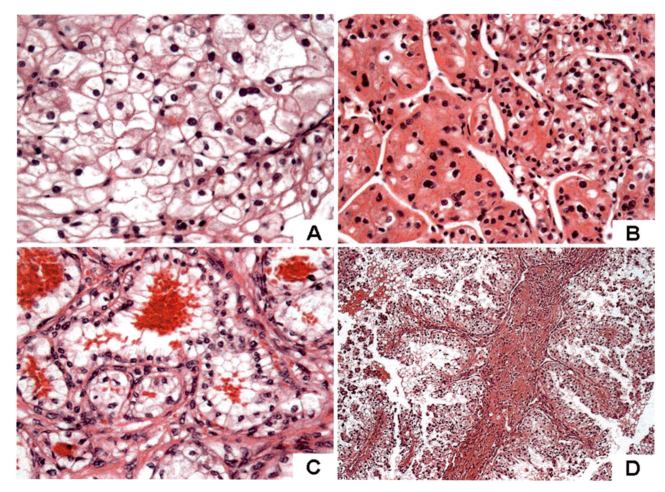

FIGURE 3-3. Clear cell renal cell carcinoma. (A) Clear cell (empty cytoplasm) in a solid pattern. (B) Eosinophilic cell variant in a solid pattern. (C) Tubular pattern. (D) Focal papillary pattern.

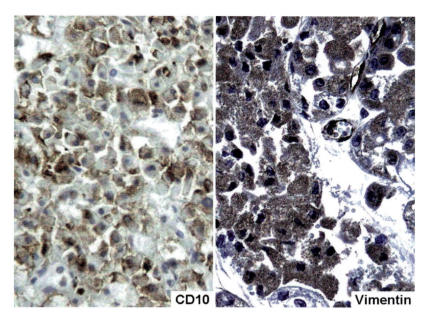

FIGURE 3-4. Clear cell renal cell carcinoma. Immunophenotype with cytoplasmatic expression of CD10 and vimentin.

LOH 3p interferes with the hypoxia-inducible pathway that activates vascular endothelial growth factor (VEGF) and platelet-derived growth factor (PDGF), both of which play an essential role in angiogenesis, glucose transport, glycolysis, pH control, epithelial proliferation, cell migration, and apoptosis, and can help the hypoxic adaptation of the clear cell carcinoma.[74] Therefore, a therapeutic multitargeted approach that selectively and simultaneously blocks these growth factors represents an attractive way of treatment.[75,76]

Papillary Renal Cell Carcinoma

Clinical Features

Twenty percent of our renal carcinoma cases are of the papillary type (oscillating in the literature between 7% and 15%).[55] The age of the appearance of sporadic forms is the same as for clear cell renal carcinoma (mean age 59.7 years for both sexes). In our experience, the male/female ratio is 7:1, but in the literature it is reported to be from 4:1[77] to 7:1.[78]

Macroscopy

They are usually well-delimited tumors and their section shows rather frequently necrotic and hemorrhagic areas. Their appearance is granular and pink colored (Fig. 3-5) and their consistency is softer than the other renal cell carcinomas. Multifocality is present in about 31.9% of the patients[78] and bilaterality in about 2%,[77] i.e., more frequently than in the clear cell renal cell carcinoma, even in sporadic cases. Small tumors of less than 5 mm, considered papillary adenomas, are frequent.

Microscopy

Some years ago this subtype was named *chromophilic carcinoma*.[79] Even though the general criterion for categorization of renal carcinomas continues to be the cell type, this tumor is now identified by cell distribution around the capillary cores (papillae) in at least 50–70% of the tumor,[55] thus distinguishing it from the occasional papillary areas that may be found in other types of renal carcinoma.[58]

In 73% of them the cells that cover such papillae are a single layer of basophilic cells (type 1) (Fig. 3-6A). In another 42% the papillae are covered by eosinophilic cells with nucleus pseudostratification (type 2) (Fig. 3-6B). Type 1 is more frequently multifocal than type 2.[80,81]

Cases of solid growth (Fig. 3-6D) with a vague tubular or micronodular pattern showing a compressed papillary architecture[82] can also be seen. Two percent to five percent of these tumors are spindle cell tumors.[59,80] These cytological and architectural variations, besides apparently having some prognostic significance,[80] should be known by the pathologist in order to avoid diagnostic error.

The stroma may be fibrous or edematous, and it is characteristic to find foamy macrophages (Fig. 3-6C), specifically in cellular type 1. Hemorrhage and necrosis with cholesterol clefts are frequent.[55]

Immunophenotype

Low-molecular-weight cytokeratins (Fig. 3-7): CAM 5.2 are usually expressed in most tumors, and CK7 in 75% of both subtypes,[65] and they are more frequent in type 1 tumors than in type 2 (87% vs. 20%).[83] High-molecular-weight cytokeratins are expressed in only 3% of cases.[83] Vimentin is

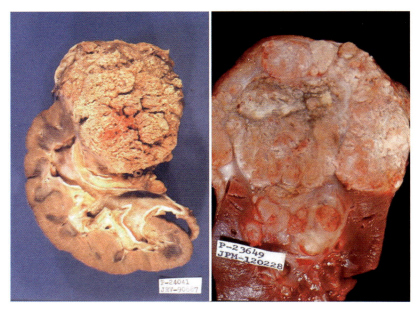

FIGURE 3-5. Papillary renal cell carcinoma. Macroscopic appearance with a solid, granular aspect.

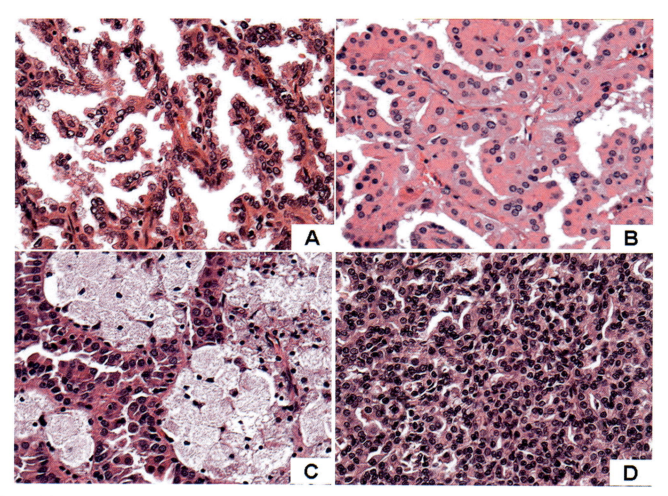

FIGURE 3-6. Papillary renal cell carcinoma. (**A**) Basophilic cells in a papillary growth (type 1). (**B**) Eosinophilic cells in a papillary growth (type 2). (**C**) Foamy cells in the stroma. (**D**) Solid variant of papillary renal cell carcinoma.

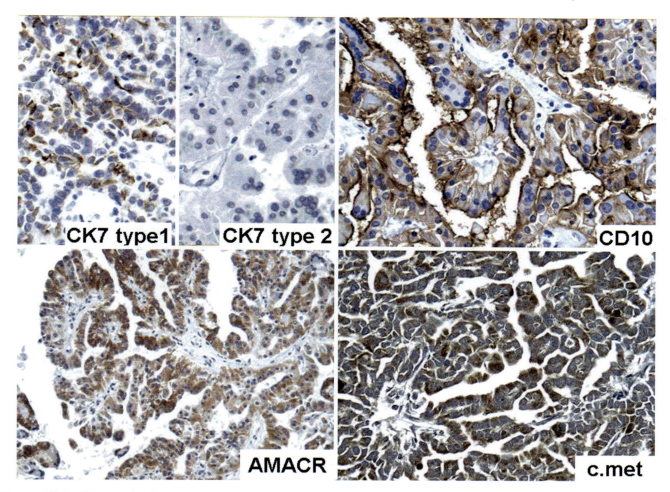

FIGURE 3-7. Papillary renal cell carcinoma. Immunophenotype with a cytokeratin 7 expression in type 1, no expression of cytokeratin 7 in type 2, and expression of CD10, AMACR, and c-met.

expressed in 85%,[61] CD10 between 63% and 93%,[62,84] renal cell carcinoma (RCC) antibody in 93%,[62] EMA (MUC-1) between 40% and 60% of all cases[63] but more frequently in type 1 than in type 2 (72% vs. 16.6%),[85] and GST-α in 20%.[64] Among adhesion molecules, E-cadherin is expressed in 67% of types 1 and not at all in types 2,[63] Ksp-cadherin only in 2.2%,[65] EpCAM in 90%,[86] parvalbumin in 71%, and β-defensin-1 in 100%.[61] P504S (AMACR) has recently been found to be expressed in all the cases.[68,87,88] Other markers such as c-kit, RON protooncogene and *Ulex europaeus* are mostly negative.[66,67]

Genetic Changes

Trisomy or tetrasomy 7, trisomy 17, and loss of chromosome Y are the most common genetic changes in papillary renal cell carcinoma.[89] These modifications have been related to the activation of the protooncogene *c-MET* (7q34) that codes HGFr,[90] which can be found both in the sporadic and in the familial forms. LOH 3p has also been detected in 59% of cases, more frequently LOH 3p25-26 (*VHL*), present in

53.8%. LOH 3p14.2 (*FHIT*) is observed in 40.7%.[70] Other trisomies, in 12, 16 and 20, were considered in connection with tumor progression.[89]

Recent studies have discovered that the allelic imbalances on 17q are almost exclusively confined to type 1 in contrast to the allelic imbalances on 9p, which are confined to type 2, suggesting that each of these cell types can originate from different molecular genetic pathways.[91]

Pathology of Cortical Distal Nephron Renal Cell Carcinomas

Chromophobe Renal Cell Carcinoma

Clinical Features

These tumors represent 7.3% of our cases (the literature reports 5–10%).[92] The age of presentation is similar to that of all renal carcinomas for both sexes. There is no sex predominance.

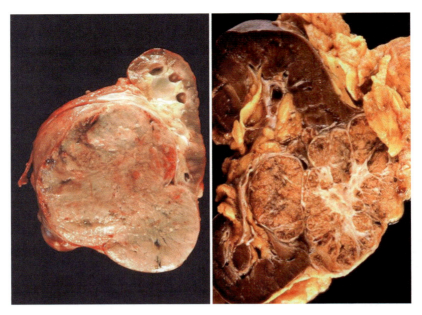

FIGURE 3-8. Chromophobe renal cell carcinoma. Brown solid tumor with a central scar in the left figure.

Macroscopy

The sporadic forms are commonly single,[77] well outlined, brown or tan colored, with an occasional central scar (Fig. 3-8).

Microscopy

The characteristic appearance of the cells includes large cell size, a polygonal shape with a good delimitation of the cytoplasmic membrane (that gives them the appearance of a plant cell), and plenty of pale reticulated cytoplasm due to the presence of abundant cytoplasmic invaginated 150- to 300-nm-diameter vesicles resembling those of type b interspersed cells of the cortical collecting duct.[93] These cells may have a clear cytoplasm (clear cell subtype) due to loose glycogen deposits[93] (Fig. 3-9A) (but not as clear as that of the clear cell renal cell carcinoma), or a more eosinophilic one (eosinophilic variant) (Fig. 3-9B and C), depending on the number of mitochondria.[94]

The eosinophilic variant has recently been subdivided into a further two forms, with cells smaller than the classic ones. The first form has a perinuclear halo (Fig. 3-9C) and the second one a more eosinophilic halo (Fig. 3-9B).[95] These differences correlate with ultrastructural changes,[96] and even though apparently they have no clinical or therapeutic significance, they are indeed worth knowing in order to issue a differential diagnosis versus oncocytoma (see below).

Sarcomatoid transformation (Fig. 3-9D) can occur in 8.7% of cases.[59] The stroma may have broad fibrotic septa with thick-walled hyalinized vessels.[97]

Histochemical Phenotype

The presence of cytoplasmic vesicles correlates with Hale's colloidal iron staining, and depending on their being more or less preserved, such staining will be either granular or diffuse (Fig. 3-10A and B).[98] However, as it is a mucosubstance staining sometimes there may also be colloidal iron deposits on other tumors (Fig. 3-10C and D), but with weak droplets,[99] and so the interpretation should be very careful.

Immunophenotype

Both the low-molecular-weight cytokeratins and the high-molecular-weight cytokeratins are almost always present: CAM 5.2 practically in 100% of cases, CK7 between 73% and 90%,[65,100] and CK14 in 100%[60] (Fig. 3-11). Other markers that generally are positive are EMA (MUC-1),[63,65,101] E-cadherin, Ksp-cadherin, Ep.Cam adhesion molecules (over 90%),[63,65,86] parvalbumin and β-defensin-1 (in 100%),[61] c-kit (88%),[66] and RON protooncogene (96%).[67] Vimentin is infrequently expressed (only in 9.7%).[61] RCC antibody is variably positive from 0%[62] to 45%.[102] GST-α[23] and p504S (AMACR)[68] are negative.

CD10 is usually negative,[62] but in some series it can be observed in up to 26% of cases, which generally correspond to the most aggressive forms.[84]

Genetic Changes

An extensive chromosomal loss in 1, 2, 6, 10, 13, 17, and 21 is present.[103] LOH 17 associates this tumor type with the Birt–Hogg–Dubé syndrome.[104]

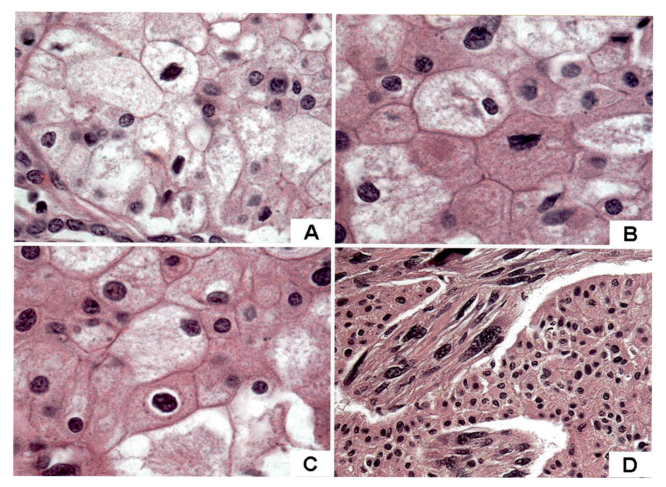

FIGURE 3-9. Chromophobe renal cell carcinoma. (A) "Clear cell" variant with a granular cytoplasmatic aspect. (B) "Clear cell" among eosinophilic cells. (C) Eosinophilic cells, some of them smaller and with a perinuclear halo. (D) Sarcomatoid component.

LOH 3p has also been found in 86.6%, and LHO 3p25-26 (71.4%) is more frequent than LOH 3p14.2 (66.6%).[69]

In 27% of the cases there is a *TP53* mutation,[105] and losses around *PTEN* were also appreciated.[106]

Pathology of Renal Cell Carcinomas of the Distal Medullary Nephron

Carcinoma of the Collecting Ducts of Bellini

Clinical Features

It is quite difficult to know the true incidence and clinical features of this neoplasia because it is mostly a diagnosis by exclusion. The diagnosis is difficult because the histology of this carcinoma can overlap urothelial cell carcinoma. This overlapping may be an expression of the same carcinogenetic process[107] (common wolffian origin of the collecting ducts and urothelium) or the result of confusing both neoplasias in a single group. This is why some authors require more strict criteria for the diagnosis of collecting duct carcinoma.[108]

Macroscopy

When the tumor is small it is located centrally in the medullary area. It has a poorly defined contour with an infiltrating appearance. A characteristic white color and a fibrillary surface are often present (Fig. 3-12).

Microscopy

The criteria for the diagnosis of this tumor are very poorly defined.[92] The WHO's definition includes major and minor criteria.[109] The six major criteria are (1) small tumors located in pyramid of medulla, (2) showing a typical histology with irregular tubular architecture and high nuclear grade, some of them with a hobnail appearance,[110] (3) with an inflammatory desmoplastic stroma with plenty of granulocytes, (4) immunohistochemically reactive to antibodies of high-molecular-weight cytokeratins, (5) and reactive to *Ulex europaeus* lectin, and (6) with no urothelial cell carcinoma (Fig. 3-13A–C). The four minor diagnostic criteria are (1) centrally located large tumors, (2) the papillary

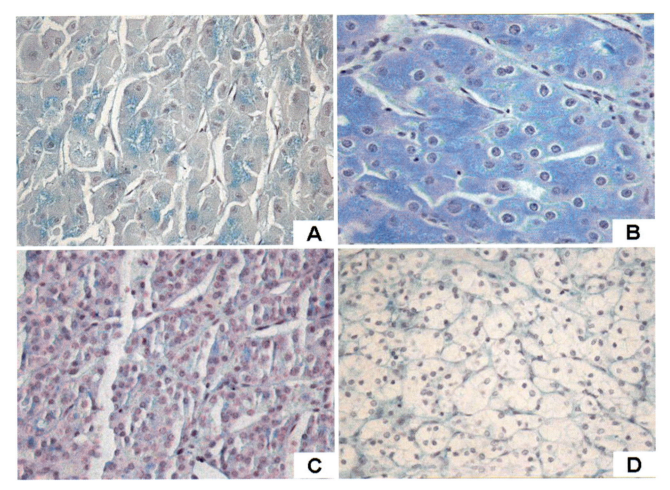

FIGURE 3-10. Colloidal Hale stain in renal tumors. (A) Chromophobe renal cell carcinoma with a cytoplasmatic granular stain. (B) Chromophobe renal cell carcinoma with diffuse cytoplasmatic staining. (C) Oncocytoma with a minimal cytoplasmatic stain. (D) Clear cell renal cell carcinoma without cytoplasmatic staining.

architecture shows thick fibrous stalks and a desmoplastic stroma,[111] (3) extensive and interglomerular infiltration into the glomeruli and tubules and extrarenal invasion with lymphatic and venous infiltration, and (4) intratubular epithelial atypia (hyperchromatic and/or enlarged nuclei with an irregular nuclear membrane and a prominent nucleolus) of the parenchyma adjacent to the tumor (Fig. 3-13D). PAS and mucicarmin positive material can be seen in the neoplastic tubular lumina.[111] A sarcomatoid appearance can be present in 29% of cases.[112]

Immunophenotype

The studies are scarce, and so the percentage of cases expressing different antibodies is relative. Considering this fact, the expression of high-molecular-weight cytokeratins (34βE12 and CK19) and of *Ulex europaeus* lectin in almost all cases has been observed,[113] which justifies including them as major criteria within the WHO classification[109] (Fig. 3-14).

CD10 and vimentin are variably positive,[65,114] CK7 and EMA in 33%.[65,114] p504S (AMACR) is negative.[68]

Genetic Changes

The cytogenetic studies are very scarce. Extensive chromosomal loss in 1q, 6p, 13q, 14, 15, 21q, and 22 is present.[116] HER2/neu amplification has been described.[117]

Renal Medullary Carcinoma

Clinical Features

This tumor was first described in 1995;[118] approximately 100 cases have since been described, all of them in young people (from 5 to 40 years of age), with men almost twice as frequent as women, most of them black people and with the sickle cell trait or disease.[119,120]

The symptomatology is the common one of renal neoplasias; however, there are cases that mimic an inflammatory process.[120] Mortality approaches 100% in a few months.[118–120]

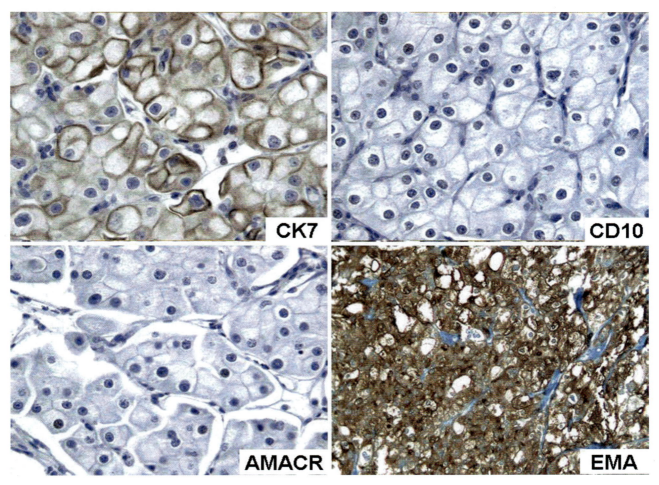

FIGURE 3-11. Chromophobe renal cell carcinoma. Immunophenotype with expression of cytokeratin 7 and epithelial membrane antigen and no expression of CD10 and AMACR.

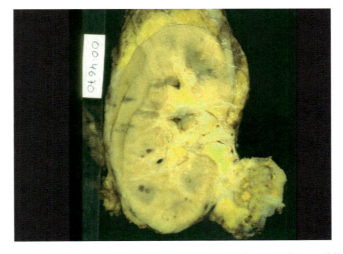

FIGURE 3-12. Carcinoma of the collecting ducts of Bellini. Irregular white tumor in the central area with extension to the renal parenchyma without mass effect.

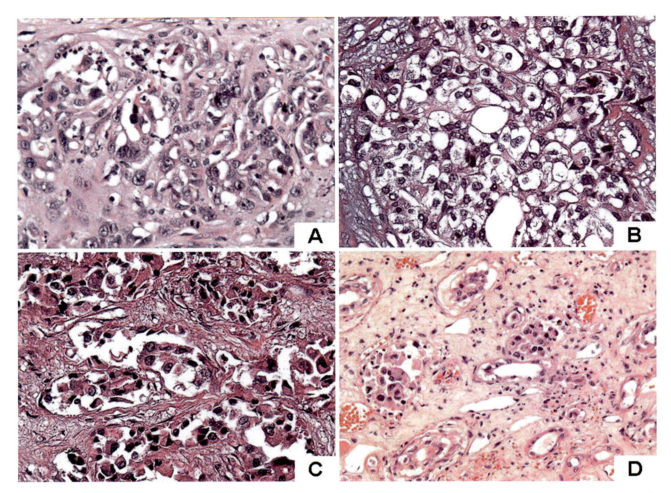

FIGURE 3-13. Carcinoma of the collecting ducts of Bellini. (**A**) Poorly differentiated eosinophilic cells. (**B**) Poorly differentiated vacuolated cells. (**C**) Angulated tubular pattern of the malignant growth. (**D**) Intratubular malignant cells in the collecting ducts of Bellini, near the tumor.

Macroscopy

A poorly circumscribed medullary mass (from 2 to 13 cm) of fibrillary white tissue is the typical appearance of the tumor.[118–120] The right kidney is involved three times more frequently than the left one.[119]

Microscopy

A reticular growth pattern and adenoid cystic tubular morphology are the common features. Clear and eosinophilic cells with a bizarre nucleus with nucleoli are present. Geographic necrosis and hemorrhage are frequent.[118,119] Sarcomatoid areas can be present.[120] The stroma is edematous and desmoplastic with acute and chronic inflammation.[118,120]

Immunophenotype

There are very few immunophenotype studies, but all of them coincide in the usual expression of the low-molecular-weight cytokeratins (CAM 5.2) and the negativity of the high-molecular-weight cytokeratins (34βE12)[120,121] as well as the EMA (MUC-1).[118,120,121] *Ulex europaeus* lectin is focally present in 50% of the cases.[120]

Genetic Changes

The data on genetic alterations of this tumor are very scarce, and the findings reported vary from normality to occasional translocation t(3;8)(p21;q24)[121] or monosomy for chromosome 11 (gene β-globin is found in 11p).[122] Some authors believe this tumor to be an aggressive variant of Bellini's collecting duct carcinoma,[123] a suspicion strengthened by a case of collecting duct carcinoma associated with the sickle cell trait,[124] and because its genetic expression is closer to the urothelial carcinoma than to the usual renal carcinomas.[125] These observations suggest a common carcinogenesis, as stated above.[107] No HER2/neu expression is present,[121] but immunohistochemical VEGF and HIF are.[121]

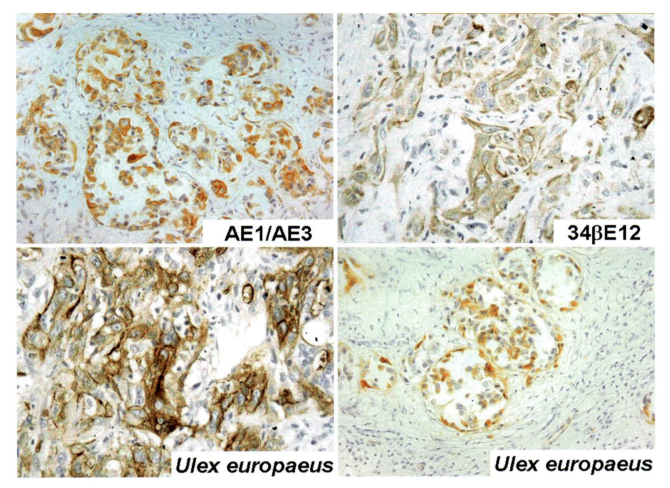

FIGURE 3-14. Carcinoma of the collecting ducts of Bellini. Immunophenotype with keratin expression (AE1/AE3 and 34βE12) and *Ulex europaeus*.

Mucinous Tubular and Spindle Cell Carcinoma

Clinical Features

The cases published are scarce but the female predominance is outstanding. The mean age is around 55 years and the symptomatology is the one common to renal neoplasias; however, its association with renal lithiasis is remarkable.[126] These tumors have an excellent prognosis,[127] even in isolated cases of local ganglion metastasis.[126]

Macroscopy

They are well-delimited tumors, 3–10 cm in size, with a homogeneous yellow-to-brown section surface.[128]

Microscopy

This subtype has recently been included in the WHO classification, after some studies had drawn attention to the fact that certain neoplasias with basophilic cells and an elongated tubular and/or spindle pattern showed a differential clinical behaviour.[129]

As suggested by its name, this neoplasia is characterized by cuboidal cells with scarce cytoplasm distributed in elongated tubules (Fig. 3-15A and B) intermingled with solid areas of spindle cells with a bland (nonsarcomatoid) nucleus (Fig. 3-15C and D). The stroma is edematous with extracellular mucin (Fig. 3-15B and C).[80] Foamy macrophages may be appraised.

Immunophenotype

It expresses CK7 (100%) far more frequently than high-molecular-weight cytokeratins (34βE12 in 33%) (Fig. 3-16).[130] Vimentin is expressed in all cases.[130] In 12 of our patients suffering from this tumor, CD10 and c-kit were always negative. But some authors find cases with CD10 expression.[131] EMA (MUC-1) was expressed in all of them but it was very extensive in only 50%; E-cadherin is focally expressed in 25%, but other authors find more positive cases.[131] It is worth remarking that p504S (AMACR) is present in 92% of the patients in an average 50% of the cells. *Ulex europaeus* lectin is negative.[132]

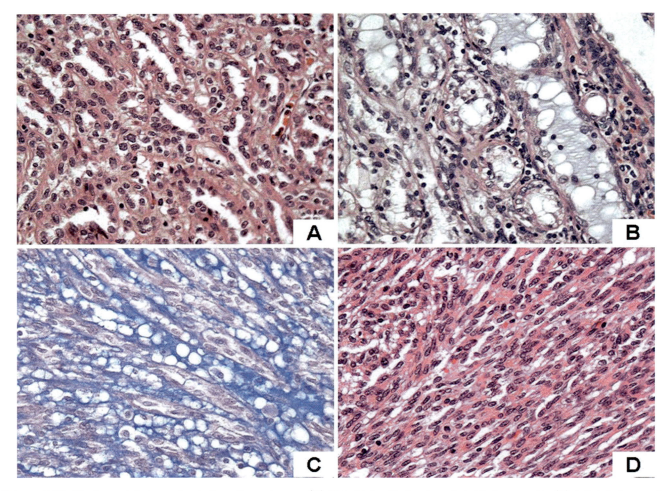

FIGURE 3-15. Mucinous tubular and spindle cell carcinoma. (A) Cuboidal cells in elongated tubular growth. (B) Intratubular mucin. (C) Intercellular mucin with Alcian blue staining. (D) Spindle proliferation with a bland nucleus.

Genetic Changes

The main chromosomal alterations are monosomies that can be found on 1, 4, 6, 8, 9, 13, 14, 15, and 22[128] that together with the above mentioned immunohistochemical characteristics support the tumor origin at the distal nephron. There was some speculation about the tumor generating at the Henle loop, but there is not enough evidence to confirm this.[127]

Other Histological Subtypes of Renal Cell Carcinomas

Renal Cell Carcinomas Associated with Chromosome Translocations (*TFE3* or *TFEB* Gene Fusions)

Clinical Features

These tumors occur in children and young adults. Some cases in older patients have also been described. They are more common among women, and we lack enough data to know their genuine biology,[133,134] but apparently they can be different according to the type of translocation.[135]

Macroscopy

The gross aspect looks like the clear cell renal cell carcinoma.

Microscopy

Some papillary and clear cell carcinomas with certain differential morphological characteristics[136] were described in 1968, but only in 1996[137] were the translocations of these carcinomas determined, thus giving raise to the entity included by the WHO in its classification in 2004.[133]

In these carcinomas the cells may be clear and eosinophilic with an ample voluminous, soap bubble-like cytoplasm and calcified psamoma bodies. A focal papillary pattern is almost always present among solid, tubular, acinar, and alveolar areas;[134] however, depending on the type of translocation, subtle microscopic differences are apparently present in the cell volume.[135,138]

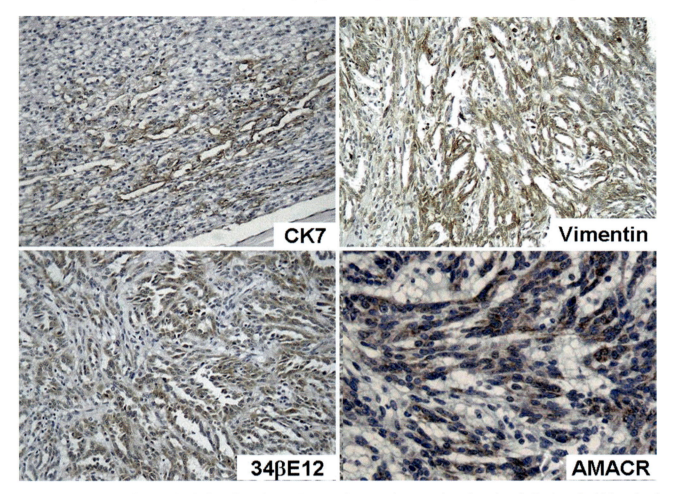

FIGURE 3-16. Mucinous tubular and spindle cell carcinoma. Immunophenotype in expression of cytokeratin 7, vimentin, high-molecular-weight cytokeratin (34βE12), and AMACR.

Immunophenotype

CAM 5.2 and CK7 are expressed in 45% of cases, in a local manner. Vimentin is expressed in 63%, CD10 and RCC antibody in 100%, and EMA (MUC-1) in 45%.[134] As a consequence of the translocations the gene fusion codes new chimeric proteins that preserve transcription factors *TFE3* or *TFEB*. We can detect these proteins in the tumor cell nuclei by immunohistochemical methods, whereas they very rarely are expressed in normal tissues.[135]

Genetics

Many different translocations involving chromosome Xp11.2 have been described, all resulting in gene fusions involving the TFE3 gene; these include t(X;1)(p11,2;q21) fusion *PRCC* and *TFE3* (the most frequent one); t(X;17) (p11.2; q25) fusion *ASPL* and *TFE3* (less aggressive);[135] t(X;1) (p11.2;p34) fusion *PSF* and *TFE3*; and Inv(X)(p11;q12)

fusion Non-O(p54nrb) and *TFE3*.[133] Another translocation is t(6;11)(p21;q12) fusion *TFEB*.[139]

Renal Cell Carcinoma, Unclassified

Every attempt of histological classification includes specific cases that are difficult to assign to any one of the groups; this fact has prompted the WHO's classification to accept unclassified renal cell carcinomas.

To be able to include a renal carcinoma in this group, numerous representative specimens of the whole tumor must have been taken.

The incidence of unclassified renal cell carcinomas oscillates between 3% and 5%.[140] If we analyze the cases included under this label, we will observe that they have various origins. This fact turns this group into a quite heterogeneous one, but its acceptance has enabled homogeneity within the other subtypes.

In addition, we may subdivide them in three groups with different clinical and prognostic implications.

Anaplastic and Purely Sarcomatoid Renal Cell Carcinomas

All histological subtypes may develop sarcomatoid forms.[59,112] Doubt appears regarding which methods should be applied to recognize the potential cellular origin of the undifferentiated form.[141] Anyway, the most undifferentiated cases are included under the "unclassified" denomination (Fig. 3-17A). They are locally invasive (42%) as well as metastatic in almost 50% of the cases, with a mean survival of 4.3 months.[140]

Renal carcinoma with rhabdoid features (cells with large, paranuclear intracytoplasmic hyaline globules, not related to pediatric rhabdoid tumors) (Fig. 3-17B) may be included within this group. It has been described as diverging clonal, particularly from clear cell and chromophobe renal cell carcinomas,[142,143] all of them showing great biological aggressiveness.[144]

Hybrid Tumors (Carcinomas)

Another unclassified carcinoma occurs when different cell types are mixed in a same tumor. The most common hybrid types are those produced by the overlapping distal nephron types, particularly *oncocytoma + chromophobe renal cell carcinoma* (Fig. 3-17C),[145] frequent in the Birt–Hogg–Dubé's syndrome.[146] Other hybrid types are composed by *oncocytoma + chromophobe renal cell carcinoma + collecting duct carcinoma*[147,148], and *collecting duct carcinoma + papillary renal cell carcinoma*.[149] Much rarer is the association of *clear cell renal cell carcinoma + mucinous tubular and spindle cell carcinoma*.[126]

These cases should be considered with caution because not all the papillary patterns belong to papillary renal cell carcinomas, and kidney-infiltrating urothelial carcinoma may show the appearance of a collecting duct carcinoma. Despite these considerations, transition forms do seem to exist,

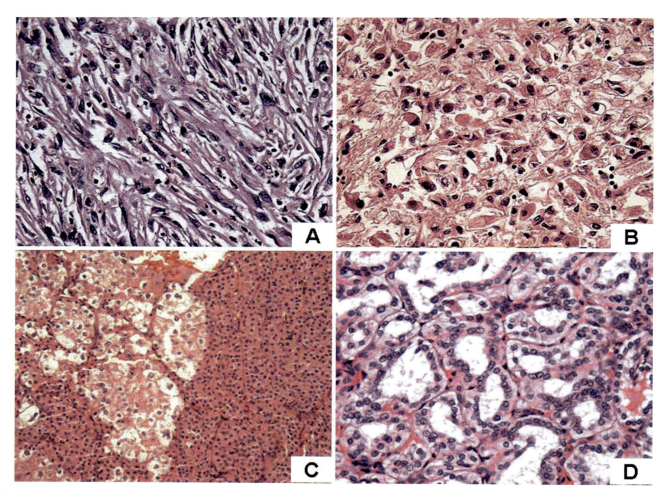

FIGURE 3-17. Renal cell carcinoma, unclassified. (**A**) Pure sarcomatoid carcinoma. (**B**) Poorly differentiated carcinoma with rhabdoid features. (**C**) Hybrid carcinoma with chromophobe renal cell carcinoma and oncocytoma. (**D**) Well-differentiated tubular carcinoma with distal nephron features.

justifiable by genetic alterations, as happens in the Birt–Hogg–Dubé's syndrome.

Another problem of hybrid tumors is prognosis. However, it would appear that the prognosis of the most frequent hybrid tumors (*oncocytoma + chromophobe renal cell carcinoma*) is the same as that of oncocytoma.[145]

Morphological Subtypes Not Recognized by the WHO Classification

In spite of the progressive inclusion of different tumor variants in the WHO's classification, the morphological changeability of renal carcinoma is such that different authors continue to publish their findings of morphologic forms not entirely attributable to any one of the groups already described.[150,151] These cases add to the controversy and are the origin of potential new entities. However, until consensus is reached they should be considered as unclassified.

Perhaps one of the most interesting among the latter morphological variants is *low-grade renal collecting duct carcinoma*[151] (Fig. 3-17D). This neoplasm had been described with the name *low-grade mucinous tubulocystic carcinoma*.[152] It is characterized by proliferation of low-grade neoplastic cells forming more or less dilated tubules that may exhibit a multicystic appearance,[151] without a spindle component[152] and with a distal nephron immunophenotype).[130,152]

The WHO's histological classification enables us to recognize a group of tumors with an excellent prognosis (papillary renal cell carcinomas type 1, mucinous tubular and spindle cell carcinomas), and also another very aggressive group (carcinoma of the collecting ducts of Bellini, renal medullary carcinoma). Sarcomatoid transformation, even in small areas, has a negative impact on prognosis.[112]

Renal Cell Carcinomas in Children and Adolescents

In children, less than 4% of sporadic renal tumors are carcinomas.

The literature data are contradictory. While some authors report a higher incidence of papillary renal cell carcinomas within this age group,[153] chromophobe renal cell carcinomas are found in a greater proportion by other authors.[154] Such discrepancies are a consequence of the scarcity of data and of the morphological heterogeneity in renal cell carcinomas associated with chromosomal translocations,[133] i.e., carcinomas arising from nephroblastoma or associated with neuroblastoma.[155]

A recent publication of 41 cases of renal cell carcinomas in children and adolescents disclosed that 14% were clear cell renal cell carcinomas, 22% were papillary renal cell carcinomas (with the same incidence for type 1 and type 2), 5% were chromophobe renal cell carcinomas, 5% were carcinoma of the collecting ducts of Bellini, 7% were renal carcinomas arising from nephroblastoma, 2% were postneuroblastoma renal carcinoma, 19.5% were translocation carcinomas, and 24% were unclassified.[138] Thus, we see that any kind of tumor may appear at these ages; however, translocation tumors are more typically found in children and adolescents.

Renal Adenomas and Their Relationship to Renal Cell Carcinomas

In the literature we may find extensive controversy regarding the existence or nonexistence of renal adenomas and their relationship to carcinomas. We should make it clear that at this moment the existence of clear cell adenomas is not contemplated since genetic changes of the clear cell renal cell carcinoma have been found in very small tumors (Fig. 3-18A).[156]

Papillary adenomas are papillary lesions with microscopic characteristics identical to those of type 1 papillary carcinomas (Fig. 3-18B) (but rarely of type 2), differentiated only by their size (maximum 5 mm). Chromosome 7 and 17 trisomies are genetically typical and for some authors the addition of chromosomal abnormalities may be a biological indicator of malignant evolution.[12]

Oncocytoma is characterized by a proliferation of eosinophilic cells with a bland nucleus with a solid, tubular pattern, fibrous stroma, and brown macroscopic appearance (Fig. 3-18C and D). The immunophenotype is similar to that of chromophobe renal cell carcinoma, so the differential diagnosis of such tumors is difficult. Apparently kidney-specific cadherin is able to recognize it.[65] Some authors believe that a subgroup of oncocytomas could exist that may be the adenoma form of chromophobe renal cell carcinomas.

Familial Renal Cell Tumors

Most of the variants described may be expressed in familial forms, amounting to 4% of all renal carcinomas.[54] Most frequently they are multiple, bilateral. They appear at earlier ages than their corresponding sporadic forms. Many of them are found among other neoplasias.

The following are the most significant forms recognised so far.[157]

Von Hippel–Lindau (VHL) disease is an autosomal dominant disorder. The VHL gene is located on chromosome 3p25. Retina hemangioma, *clear cell renal carcinoma*, cerebellar and spinal cord hemangioblastoma, pheochromocytoma, pancreas endocrine tumors, and epididymal cystadenoma are associated with this disease.[158] The mean age for expression of the renal carcinoma is 37, and the major cause of death is metastasis of the renal cell carcinoma.

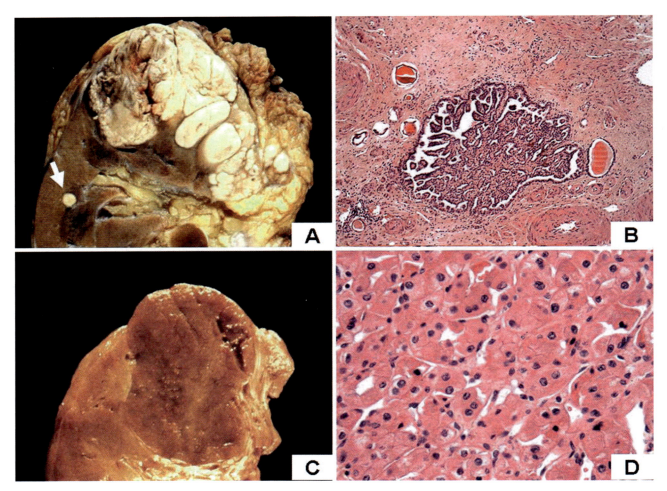

FIGURE 3-18. (A) Small clear cell renal cell carcinoma (arrow) in a patient with a large clear cell renal cell carcinoma. No clear cell adenomas are considered. (B) Papillary renal cell adenoma. (C) Oncocytoma. Macroscopic aspect with a uniform brown color. (D) Microscopic aspect of the oncocytoma with eosinophilic cells without nuclear atypia.

Hereditary papillary renal carcinoma is characterized by the presence of type 1 papillary renal cell carcinomas with genetic changes similar to the sporadic cases and occasional translocations.[159] The presence of numerous tumors of sundry sizes in both kidneys should raise the suspicion of this kind of syndrome. Even though isolated renal involvement is usually predominant, breast, pancreas, lung, skin, and gastric tumors have also been reported.

Tuberous sclerosis complex (TSC) is an autosomal dominant form with very wide affectation of different tissues by facial angiofibromas, subungual fibromas, flat cutaneous fibromas, hyperpigmented macules, kidney angiomyolipomas, and clear cell carcinomas (the latter only occasionally).[160] They are related to two genes: TSC1 (9q34) and TSC2 (16p13.3).

Birt–Hogg–Dubé's (BHD) syndrome is an autosomal dominant syndrome with a classical triad of multiple cutaneous lesions (fibrofolliculomas, trichodiscomas, and acrochordons) and multiple and bilateral renal tumors, primarily oncocytomas or chromophobe renal cell carci-

nomas, although clear cell and papillary renal tumors[104] have also been associated with colon cancer, multiple lipomas, and spontaneous neumothorax. The gene is located on 17q12-q11.2

The following are much more infrequent.

Leiomyomatosis and familial renal cancer are characterized by multiple uterine leiomyomas and type 2 papillary renal carcinoma. The gene has been found on 1q42-q44.[161]

The gene for thyroidal familial papillary carcinoma and renal papillary tumor has been found on 1q21, and this discovery raises the question of which role is this locus playing in the development of renal papillary carcinomas.[162]

Familial oncocytomas: some families with oncocytomas have been described, but certain cases have finally been described as Birt–Hogg–Dubé's syndrome; however, it is thought that this variant of the familial renal tumor may exist even though the gene location has not yet been found.[163]

Future Renal Cell Carcinoma Prognostic Markers and Classification

Various studies have shown that certain chromosomal alterations are associated with a better or a worse prognosis, and so in clear cell renal cell carcinoma the loss of 8p is frequently seen in the metastatic cases,[164] the loss of 9p is associated with poor prognosis in papillary renal cell carcinomas,[165] and the loss of 3 is a good prognostic marker of the chromophobe renal cell carcinomas.

Among the emerging molecular factors vimentin,[166] cell adhesion molecules, gelsolin, and VEGFR[28] are a few that can be interesting.

The inclusion of studies with tissue microarrays of various cell cycle markers, cell mobility, and the hypoxia pathway, not arranged according to previous morphological criteria, could determine clusters of renal cell carcinomas. One of the first findings is the differentiation of clear cell renal cell carcinomas from nonclear cell renal cell carcinomas, of low grade from high grade, with the grade 2 cluster having two clusters with different prognosis not explainable by morphological variations but by different markers (CA9-carbonic anhydrase and the gelsolin-acting-binding protein family).[167]

These findings suggest that the classical morphological markers will not be substituted with molecular and protein markers, but these will improve the former, so once again we confirm that the new discoveries improve but do not replace the already established knowledge.

References

1. Gilbert JB.: Diagnosis and treatment of malignant renal tumors. J. Urol. 1938; 39: 223–237.
2. Grawitz PA.: Die Entstehung von Nierentumoren aus Nebennierengewebe. Arch. Klin. Chir. 1884; 30: 824–834.
3. Sudeck P.: Ueber die Strucktur der Nieradenoma. Ihre Stellung zu den Strumae suprarenales aberrante (Grawitz). Arch. Pathol. Anat. Pysiol. Klin. Med. 1893; 133: 405–409.
4. Delahunt B, Thornton A.: Renal cell carcinoma. A historical perspective. J. Urol. Pathol. 1996; 4: 31– 49.
5. O´Crowley CR, Martland.: Adrenal heterotopia, rests, and the so-called Grawitz tumor. J. Urol. 1943; 50: 756–768.
6. Herbut PA.: Urological Pathology. Vol. I, p. 608. Lea & Febiger, Philadelphia, 1952.
7. Oberling C, Rivière M, Haguenan F.: Ultrastructure of the clear cells in renal carcinomas and its importance for the determination of their renal origin. Nature. 1960; 186: 402–403.
8. Bennington JL, Beckwith JB.: Tumors of the kidney, renal pelvis, and ureter. Atlas of tumor pathology. Second series. Fascicle 12 p. 130. AFIP Washington, 1975.
9. Thoenes W, Störtkel S, Rumpelt HJ.: Human chromophobe cell renal carcinoma. Wirchows Arch. (Cell Pathol.) 1985; 155: 277–287.
10. Störkel S, Pannen B, Thoenes W, Staert PV, Wagner S, Drenckhalm D.: Intercalated cells as a probable source for the development of renal oncocitoma.. Wirchows Arch. (B) 1988; 56: 185–189.
11. Liu GF, Song-Liang C, Bi-Juan C, Chieh-Ping W.: Cellular origin of renal cell carcinoma. An immunohistochemical study on monoclonal antibodies. Scand. J. Urol. Nephrol. 1991; 138 (S): 203–206.
12. Kovacs G.: Molecular differential pathology of renal cell tumours. Histopathology 1993; 22: 1–8.
13. Kovacs G, Akhtar M, Beckwith BJ.: The Heidelberg classification of renal cell tumours . J. Pathol. 1997; 183: 131–133.
14. Eble JN, Sauter G, Epstein JI, Sesterhenn IA.: World Health Organization Classification of Tumours. Pathology and Genetics Tumours of the Urinary System and Male Genital Organs. p. 10. IARC Press, Lyon, 2004.
15. Algaba F, Trias I, Scarpelli M, Boccon-Gibod L, Kirkali Z, Van Poppel H.: Handling and pathology reporting of renal tumor specimens. Eur. Urol. 2004; 45: 437–443.
16. Fleming S, Griffiths DFR.: Nephrectomy for renal tumour; dissection guide and dataset. J. Clin. Pathol. 2005; 58: 7–14.
17. Algaba F, Arce Y, Lopez-Beltran A, Montironi R, Mikuz G, Bono AV; European Society of Uropathology; Uropathology Working Group.: Intraoperative frozen section diagnosis in urological oncology. Eur. Urol. 2005; 47: 129–136.
18. Sobin LH, Wittekind CH.: Urological tumours. In: Sobin LH, Wittekind C. TNM Classification of Malignant Tumours. Geneva UICC, 2002: 179–206.
19. Ficarra V, Prayer-Galetti T, Novara G, Bratti E, Zanolla L, dak Bianco M, Artibani W, Pagano F.: Tumor-size breakpoint for prognostic stratification of localized renal cell carcinoma. Urology 2004; 63: 235–240.
20. Wunderlich H, Dreihaup M, Schlichter A, Kosmehl H, Reichelt O, Schubert J.: New cut-off point between T1 and T2 renal cell carcinoma—-Necessary for a better discriminatory power of the TNM classification. Urol. Int 2004; 72: 123–128.
21. Frank I, Blute ML, Leibovich BC, Cheville JC, Lohse CM, Kwon ED, Zincke H.: pT2 classification for renal cell carcinoma. Can its accuracy be improved?. J. Urol. 2005; 173: 380–384.
22. Ficarra V, Guille F, Schips L, de la Taille A, Prayer Galetti T, Tostain J, Cindolo L, Novara G, Zigeuner R, Bratti E, Li G, Altieri V, Abbou CC, Zanolla L, Artibani W, Patard JJ.: Proposal for revision of the TNM classification system for renal cell carcinoma. Cancer. 2005; 104: 2116–2123.
23. Patard JJ, Shvarts O, Lam JS, Pantuck AJ, K8im HL, Ficarra V, Cindolo L, Han KR, De la Taille A, Tostain J, Artibani W, Abbou CC, Lobel B, Chopin DK, Figlin RA, Mulders PF, Belldegrun AS.: Safety and efficacy of partial nephrectomy for all T1 tumors based on an international multicenter experience. J. Urol. 2004; 171: 2181–2185
24. Murphy AM, Gilbert SM, Katz AE, Goluboff ET, Sawczuk IS, Olsson CA, Benson MC, McKiernan JM.: Re-evaluation of the tumour-node-metastasis staging of locally advanced renal cortical tumours: absolute size (T2) is more significant than renal capsular invasion (T3a). BJU Int. 2005; 95: 27–30.
25. Siemer S, Lehmann J, Loch A, Becker F, Stein U, Schneider G, Ziegler M, StockleM.: Current TNM classification of renal cell carcinoma evaluated: revising stageT3a. J. Urol. 2005; 173: 33–37.
26. Bonsib SM.: The renal sinus is the principal invasive pathway: a prospective study of 100 renal cell carcinomas. Am. J. Surg. Pathol. 2004; 28: 1594–1600.

27. Bonsib SM, Gibson D, Mhoon M, Greene GF.: Renal sinus involvement in renal cell carcinoma. Am. J. Surg. Pathol. 2000; 24: 451–458.

28. Lam JS, Shvarts O, Leppert JT, Figlin RA, Belldegrun AS.: Renal cell carcinoma 2005: new frontiers in staging, prognostication and targeted molecular therapy. J. Urol. 2005; 173: 1853–1862.

29. Thompson RH, Cheville JC, Lohse CM, Webster WS, Zincke H, Kwon ED, Frank I, Blute ML, Leibovich BC.: Reclassification of patients with pT3 and pT4 renal cell carcinoma improves prognostic accuracy. Cancer 2005; 104: 53–60.

30. Zisman A, Wieder JA, Pantuck AJ, Chao DH, Dorey F, Said JW, Gitlitz BJ, deKernion JB, Figlin RA, Belldegrun AS.: Renal cell carcinoma with tumor thrombus extension: biological role of nephrectomy and response to immunotherapy. J. Urol. 2003; 169: 909 – 916.

31. Moinzadeh A, Libertino JA.: Prognostic significance of tumor thrombus level in patients with renal cell carcinoma and venous tumor thrombus extension. Is all T3b the same? J. Urol. 2004; 171: 598–601.

32. Palapattu GS, Pantuck AJ, Dorey F.: Collecting system invasion in renal cell carcinoma impact on prognosis and future staging strategies. J. Urol. 2003; 170: 768–772.

33. Terrone C, Cracco C, Guercio S, Bollito E, Poggio M, Scoffone C, Tarabuzzi R, Porpiglia F, Scarpa RM, Fontana D, Rocca Rossetti S.: Prognostic value of the involvement of the urinary collecting system in renal cell carcinoma. Eur. Urol. 2004; 46: 472–476.

34. Terrone C, Guercio S, De Luca S, Poggio M, Castelli E, Scoffone C, Tarabuzzi R, Scarpa RM, Fontana D, Roca Rossetti S.: The number of lymph nodes examined and staging accuracy in renal cell carcinoma. BJU Int. 2003; 91: 37–40.

35. Fuhrman SA, Lasky LC, Limas C.: Prognostic significance of morphologic parameters in renal cell carcinoma. Am. J. Surg. Pathol. 1982; 6: 655–663.

36. Tsui KH, Shvarts O, Smith RB, Figlin RA, deKernion JB, Belldegrun A.: Prognostic indicators for renal cell carcinoma: a multivariate analysis of 643 patients using the revised 1997 TNM staging criteria. J. Urol. 2000; 163: 1090–1095.

37. Algaba F.: Prognostic factors of epithelial tumours of the kidney. Pathologica 1999; 91: 51–53.

38. Al-Aynati M, Chen V, Salama S, Shuhaibar H, Treleaven D, Vincic L.: Interobserver and intraobserver variability using the Fuhrman grading system for renal cell carcinoma. Arch. Pathol. Lab. Med. 2003; 127: 593–596.

39. Bos SD, Mellema CT, Mensink HJ.: Increase in incidental renal cell carcinoma in the northern part of the Netherlands. Eur. Urol. 2000; 37: 267–270.

40. Gelb AB, Shibuya RB, Weiss LM, Medeiros LJ.: Stage I renal cell carcinoma. A clinicopathologic study of 82 cases. Am. J. Surg. Pathol. 1993; 17: 275–286.

41. Paner GP, Alvarado-Cabrero I, Moch H, Young A, Stricker H, Lyles R, Datta MW, Amin MB.: A novel nuclear grading scheme for chromophobe renal cell carcinoma. Prognostic utility and comparison with Fuhrman´s nuclear grading. Mod. Pathol. 2006; 19: 154 (711).

42. Van Poppel H, Vandendriessche H, Boel K, Mertens V, Goethuys H, Haustermans K, Van Damme B, Baert L.: Microscopic vascular invasion is the most relevant prognosticator

after radical nephrectomy for clinically non-metastatic renal cell carcinoma. J. Urol. 1997; 158: 45–49.

43. Sevinc M, Kirkali Z, Yorukoglu K, Mungan U, Sade M.: Prognostic significance of microvascular invasion in localized renal cell carcinoma. Eur. Urol. 2000; 38: 728–733.

44. Lang H, Lindner V, Saussine C, Havel D, Faure F, Jacqmin D.: Microscopic venous invasion: a prognostic factor in renal cell carcinoma. Eur. Urol. 2000; 38: 600–605.

45. Lang H, Lindner V, Letourneux H, Martin M, Saussine C, Jacqmin D.: Prognostic value of microscopic venous invasion in renal cell carcinoma: long-term follow-up. Eur. Urol. 2004; 46: 331–335.

46. Lam JS, Shvarts O, Said JW, Pantuck AJ, Seligson DB, Aldridge ME, Bui MH, Liu X, Horvath S, Figlin RA, Belldegrun AS.: Clinicopathologic and molecular correlations of necrosis in the primary tumor of patients with renal cell carcinoma. Cancer 2005; 103: 2517–2525.

47. Hemmerlein B, Kugler A, Ozisik R, Ringert RH, Radzun HJ, Thelen P.: Vascular endothelial growth factor expression, angiogenesis, and necrosis in renal cell carcinomas. Virchows Arch. 2001; 439: 645–652.

48. Algaba F.: Is tumor necrosis a predictor of survival in patients with renal cell carcinoma? Nat. Clin. Pract. Urol. 2006; 3: 196–197.

49. Amin MB, Amin MB, Tamboli P, Javidan J, Stricker H, De-Peralta Venturina M, Deshpande A, Menon M.: Prognostic impact of histologic subtyping of adult renal epithelial neoplasms. An experience of 405 cases. Am. J. Surg. Pathol. 2002; 26: 281–291.

50. Cheville JC, Lohse CM, Zincke H, Weaver AL, Blute ML.: Comparisons of outcome and prognostic features among histological subtypes of renal cell carcinoma. Am. J. Surg. Pathol. 2003; 27: 612–624.

51. Patard JJ, Leray E, Rioux-Leclercq N, Cindolo L, Ficarra V, Zisman A, de la Taille A, Tostain J, Artibani W, Abbou CC, Lobel B, Guille F, Chopin DK, Mulders PF, Wood CG, Swanson DA, Figlin RA, Belldegrun AS, Patuck AJ.: Prognostic value of histologic subtypes in renal cell carcinomas: a multicenter experience. J. Clin. Oncol. 2005; 23: 2763–2771.

52. Renshaw AA, Richie JP.: Subtypes of renal carcinoma. Different onset and sites of metastatic disease. Am. J. Clin. Pathol. 1999; 111: 539–549.

53. Motzer RJ, Bacik J, Mariani T , Russo P, Mazumdar M, Reuter V.: Treatment outcome and survival associated with metastatic renal cell carcinoma of non-clear-cell histology. J. Clin. Oncol. 2002; 20: 2376–2381.

54. Bodmer D, van den Hurk W, van Groningen JJ, Eleveld MJ, Martens GJ, Weterman MA, van Kessel AG.: Understanding familial and non-familial renal cell cancer. Hum. Mol. Genet. 2002; 11: 2489–2498.

55. Fleming S, O´Donell M.: Surgical pathology of renal epithelial neoplasms: recent advances and current status. Histopathology 2000; 36: 195–202.

56. Eble JN.: Multilocular cystic renal cell carcinoma. In Eble JN, Sauter G, Epstein JI, Sesterhenn IA. World Health Organization Classification of Tumours. Pathology and Genetics Tumours of the Urinary System and Male Genital Organs. p. 26. IARC Press, Lyon, 2004.

57. Suzigan S, Lopez-Beltran A, Montironi R, Drut R, Romero A, Hayashi T, Gentili AL, Fonseca PS, deTorres I, Billis A, Japp LC, Bollito E, Algaba F, Requena-Tapias MJ.: Multilocular cystic renal cell carcinoma: a report of 45 cases of a kidney tumor of low malignant potential. Am. J. Clin. Pathol. 2006; 125: 217–222.

58. Füzesi L, Gunawan B, Bergmann F, Tack S, Braun S, Jakse G.: Papillary renal cell carcinoma with clear cytomorphology and chromosomal loss of 3p. Histopathology 1999; 35: 157–161.

59. Cheville JC, Lohse CM, Zincke H, Weaver AL, Leibovich BC, Frank I, Blute ML.: Sarcomatoid renal cell carcinoma. An examination of underlying histologic subtype and analysis of associations with patient outcome. Am. J. Surg. Pathol. 2004; 28: 435–441.

60. Chu PG, Weiss LM.: Cytokeratin 14 immunoreactivity distinguishes oncocytic tumour from its renal mimics: an immunohistochemical study of 63 cases. Histopathology 2001; 39: 455–462.

61. Young AN, de Oliveira Sales PG, Lim SD, Cohen C, Petros JA, Marshall FF, Neish AS, Amin MB.: Beta-defensin-1, parvalbumin and vimentin. A panel of diagnostic immunohistochemical markers for renal tumors derived from gene expression profiling studies using cDNA microarrays. Am. J. Surg. Pathol. 2003; 27: 199–205.

62. Avery AK, Beckstead J, Renshaw AA, Corless CL.: Use of antibodies to RCC and CD10 in the differential diagnosis of renal neoplasms. Am. J. Surg. Pathol. 2000; 24: 203–210.

63. Langner C, Ratschek M, Rehak P, Schips L, Zigeuner R.: Expression of MUC1(EMA) and E-cadherin in renal cell carcinoma: a systematic immunohistochemical analysis of 188 cases. Modern Pathol. 2004; 17: 180–188.

64. Chuang ST, Chu P, Sugimura J, Tretiakova MS, Papavero V, Wang K, Tan MH, Lin F, The BT, Yang XJ.: Overexpression of glutathione S-transferase α in clear cell renal cell carcinoma. Am. J. Clin. Pathol. 2005; 123: 421–429.

65. Mazal PR, Exner M, Haitel A, Krieger S, Thomson RB, Aronson PS, Susani M.: Expression of kidney-specific cadherin distinguishes chromophobe renal cell carcinoma from renal oncocytoma. Hum. Pathol. 2005; 36: 22–28.

66. Petit A, Castillo M, Santos M, Mellado B, Alcover J, Mallofré C.: Kit expression in chromophobe cell carcinoma. Comparative immunohistochemical analysis of kit expression in different renal cell neoplasms. Am. J. Surg. Pathol. 2004; 28: 676–678.

67. Patton KT, Tretiakova MS, Yao JL, Papavero V, Huo L, Adley BP, Wu G, Huang J, Pins MR, Teh BT, Yang XJ.: Expression of RON-proto-oncogene in renal oncocytoma and chromophobe renal cell carcinoma. Am. J. Surg. Pathol. 2004; 28: 1045–1050.

68. Tretiakova MS, Sahoo S, Takahashin M, Turkyilmaz M, Vogelzang NJ, Lin F, Krausz T, Teh BT, Yang XJ.: Expression of alpha-methylacil-CoA racemase in papillary renal cell carcinoma. Am. J. Surg. Pathol. 2004; 28: 69–76.

69. Velickovic M, Delahunt B, Grebe SKG.: Loss of heterozygosity at 3p14.2 in clear cell carcinoma is an early event and is localized to the *FHIT* gene locus. Cancer Res. 1999; 59: 1323–1326.

70. Velickovic M, Delahunt B, Störkel S, Grebe SKG.: *VHL* and *FHIT* locus loss of heterozygosity is common in all renal cancer morphotypes but differs in pattern and prognostic significance. Cancer Res. 2001; 61: 4815–4819.

71. Schraml P, Struckmann K, Hatz F, Sonnet S, Kully C, Gasser T, Sauter G, Mihatsch MJ, Moch H.: *VHL* mutations and their correlation with tumour cell proliferation, microvessel density, and patient prognosis in clear cell renal cell carcinoma. J. Pathol. 2002; 196; 186–193.

72. Morrisey C, Martinez A, Zatyka M, Agathanggelou A, Honorio S, Astuti D, Morgan NV, Moch H, Richards FM, Kishida T, Yao M, Schraml P, Latif F, Maher ER.: Epigenetic inactivation of the RASSF1A 3p21.3 tumor suppressor gene in both clear and papillary renal cell carcinoma. Cancer Res. 2001; 61: 7277–7281.

73. Lott ST, Lovell M, Naylor SL, Killary AM.: Physical and functional mapping of a tumor suppressor locus for renal cell carcinoma within chromosome 3p12. Cancer Res. 1998; 58: 3533–3537.

74. Lam JS, Shvarts O, Leppert JT, Figlin RA, Belldegrun AS.: Renal cell carcinoma 2005: new frontiers in staging, prognostication and targeted molecular therapy. J. Urol. 2005; 173: 1853–1862.

75. Bergers G, Song S, Meyer-Morse N, Bergsland E, Hanahan D.: Benefits of targeting both pericytes and endothelial cells in the tumor vasculature with kinase inhibitors. J. Clin. Invest. 2003; 111:1287–1295.

76. Motzer RJ, Michaelson MD, Redman BG, Hudes GR, Wilding G, Figlin RA, Ginsberg MS, Kim ST, Baum CM, DePrimo SE, Li JZ, Bello CL, Theuer CP, George DJ, Rini BI.: Activity of SU11248, a multitargeted inhibitor of vascular endothelial growth factor receptor and platelet-derived growth factor receptor, in patients with metastatic renal cell carcinoma. J. Clin. Oncol. 2006; 24: 16–24.

77. Gudbjartsson T, Hardarson S, Petursdottir V, Thoroddsen A, Magnusson J, Einarsson GV.: Histological subtyping and nuclear grading of renal cell carcinoma and their implications for survival: a retrospective nation-wide study of 629 patients. Eur. Urol. 2005; 48: 593–600.

78. Chow GK, Myles J, Novick AC.: The Cleveland Clinic experience with papillary (chromophil) renal cell carcinoma: clinical outcome with histopathological correlation. Can. J. Urol. 2001; 8: 1223–1228.

79. Thoenes W, Storkel S, Rumpelt HJ.: Histopathology and classification of renal cell tumors (adenomas, oncocytomas and carcinomas). The basic cytological and histopathological elements and their use for diagnostics. Pathol. Res. Pract. 1986; 181: 125–143.

80. Delahunt B, Eble JN.: Papillary renal cell carcinoma: a clinicopathologic and immunohistochemical study of 105 tumors. Mod. Pathol. 1997; 10: 537–544.

81. Amin MB, Corless CL, Renshaw AA, Tickoo SK, Kubus J, Schultz DS.: Papillary (chromophil) renal cell carcinoma: histomorphologic characteristics and evaluation of conventional pathologic prognostic parameters in 62 cases. Am. J. Surg. Pathol. 1997; 21: 621–635.

82. Renshaw AA, Zhang H, Corless CL, Fletcher JA, Pins MR.: Solid variants of papillary (chromophil) renal cell carcinoma: clinicopathologic and genetic features. Am. J. Surg. Pathol. 1997; 21: 1203–1209.

83. Delahunt B, Eble JN.: Papillary renal cell carcinoma. In Eble JN, Sauter G, Epstein JI, Sesterhenn IA. World

Health Organization Classification of Tumours. Pathology and Genetics Tumours of the Urinary System and Male Genital Organs. p. 27. IARC Press, Lyon, 2004.

84. Martignoni G, Pea M, Brunelli M, Chilosi M, Zamó A, Bertaso M, Cossu-Rocca P, Eble JN, Mikuz G, Puppa G, Badonal C, Ficarra V, Novella G, Bonetti F.: CD10 is expressed in a subset of chromophobe renal cell carcinomas. Mod. Pathol. 2004; 17: 1455–1463.

85. Leroy X, Zini L, Leteurtre E, Zerimech F, Porchet N, Aubert JP, Gosselin B, Copin MC.: Morphologic subtyping of papillary renal cell carcinoma: correlation with prognosis and differential expression of MUC1 between the two subtypes. Mod. Pathol. 2002; 15: 1126–1130.

86. Went P, Dirnhofer S, Salvisberg T, Amin MB, Lim SD, Diener PA, Moch H.: Expression of epithelial cell adhesion molecule (EpCAM) in renal epithelial tumors. Am. J. Surg. Pathol. 2005; 29: 83–88.

87. Zhou M, Roma A, Magi-Galluzzi C.: The usefulness of immunohistochemical markers in the differential diagnosis of renal neoplasms. Clin. Lab. Med. 2005; 25: 247–257.

88. Paner GP, Srigley JR, Radhakrishnan A, Cohen C, Skinnider BF, Tickoo SK, Young AN, Amin MB.: Immunohistochemical analysis of mucinous tubular and spindle cell carcinoma and papillary renal cell carcinoma of the kidney: significant immunophenotypic overlap warrants diagnostic caution. Am. J. Surg. Pathol. 2006; 30: 13–19.

89. Kovacs G, Fucesi L, Emanual A, Kung HF.: Cytogenetics of papillary renal cell tumors. Genes Chromosomes Cancer 1991; 3: 249–255.

90. Schmidt L, Junker K, Weirich G, Glenn G, Choyke P, Lubensky I, Zhuang Z, Jeffers M, Vande Woude G, Neumann H, Walther M, Linehan WM, Zbar B.: Two North American families with hereditary papillary renal carcinoma and identical novel mutations in the MET proto-oncogene. Cancer Res. 1998; 58(8): 1719–1722.

91. Sanders ME, Mick R, Tomaszewski JE, Barr FG.: Unique patterns of allelic imbalance distinguish type 1 from type 2 sporadic papillary renal cell carcinoma. Am. J. Pathol. 2002; 161: 997–1005.

92. Renshaw AA.: Subclassification of renal neoplasms: an update for practicing pathologists. Histopathology 2002; 41: 283–300.

93. Störkel S, Steart PV, Drenckhahn D, Thoenes W.: The human chromophobe cell renal carcinoma: its probable relation to intercalated cells of the collecting duct. Virchows Arch. B Cell. Pathol. Incl. Mol. Pathol. 1989; 56: 237–245.

94. Thoenes W, Störkel S, Rumpelt H-J, Moll R, Baum HP, Werner S.: Chromophobe cell renal carcinoma and its variants—a report on 32 cases. J. Pathol. 1988; 155: 277–287.

95. Akhtar M, Kardar H, Linjawi T, McClintock J, Ali MA.: Chromophobe cell carcinoma of the kidney: a clinicopathologic study of 21 cases. Am. J. Surg. Pathol. 1995; 19: 1245–1256.

96. Latham B, Dickersin GR, Oliva E.: Subtypes of chromophobe cell renal carcinoma. An ultrastructural and histochemical study of 13 cases. Am. J. Surg. Pathol. 1999; 23: 530–535.

97. Störkel S, Martignoni G, van den Berg E.: Chromophobe renal cell carcinoma In Eble JN, Sauter G, Epstein JI, Sesterhenn IA. World Health Organization Classification of Tumours.

98. Bonsib SM.: Renal chromophobe cell carcinoma. The relationship between cytoplasmic vesicles and colloidal iron stain. J. Urol. Pathol. 1996; 4: 9–14.

99. DeLong WH, Sakr W, Grignon DJ.: Chromophobe renal cell carcinoma. A comparative histochemical and immunohistochemical study. J. Urol. Pathol. 1996; 4: 1–8.

100. Wu SL, Kothari P, Wheeler TM, Reese T, Connelly JH.: Cytokeratins 7 and 20 immunoreactivity in chromophobe renal cell carcinomas and renal oncocytomas. Mod. Pathol. 2002; 15: 712–717.

101. Abrahams NA, MacLennan GT, Khoury JD, Ormsby AH, Tamboli P, Doglioni C, Schumaker B, Tickoo SK.: Chromophobe renal cell carcinoma: a comparative study of histological, immunohistochemical and ultrastructural features using high throughput tissue microarray. Histopathology 2004; 45: 595–602.

102. McGregor DK, Khurana KK, Cao C, Tsao CC, Ayala G, Krishnan B, Ro JY, Lechago J, Truong LD.: Diagnosing primary and metastatic renal cell carcinoma: the use of the monoclonal antibody 'Renal Cell Carcinoma Marker.' Am. J. Surg. Pathol. 2001; 25: 1485–1492.

103. Speicher MR, Schoell B, du Manoir S, Schrock E, Ried T, Cremer T, Störkel S, Kovacs G.: Specific loss of chromosomes 1, 2, 6, 10, 13, 17 and 21 in chromophobe renal cell carcinomas revealed by comparative genomic hybridization. Am. J. Pathol. 1994; 145: 356–364.

104. Roth JS, Rabinowitz AD, Benson M, Grossman ME.: Bilateral renal cell carcinoma in the Birt-Hogg-Dubé syndrome Am. Acad. Dermatol. 1993; 6: 1055–1056.

105. Contractor H, Zariwala M, Bugert P, Zeisler J, Kovacs G.: Mutation of the p53 tumour suppressor gene occurs preferentially in the chromophobe type of renal cell tumour. J. Pathol. 1997; 181: 136–139.

106. Sukosd F, Digon B, Fischer J, Pietsch T, Kovacs G.: Allelic loss at 10q23.3, but lack of mutation of PTEN/MMAC1 in chromophobe renal cell carcinoma. Cancer Genet. Cytogenet. 2001; 128: 161–163.

107. Orsola A, Trias I, Raventós CX, Español I, Cecchini L, Orsola I.: Renal collecting (Bellini) duct carcinoma displays similar characteristics to upper tract urothelial cell carcinoma. Urology 2005; 65: 49–54.

108. Kafe H, Verbavatz JM, Cochand-Priollet B, Castagnet P, Viellefond J.: Collecting duct carcinoma: an entity to be redefined? Virchows Arch. 2004; 445: 637–640.

109. Srigley JR, Moch H.: Carcinoma of the collecting ducts of Bellini. In Eble JN, Sauter G, Epstein JI, Sesterhenn IA. World Health Organization Classification of Tumours. Pathology and Genetics Tumours of the Urinary System and Male Genital Organs. p. 33. IARC Press, Lyon, 2004.

110. Srigley JR, Eble JN.: Collecting duct carcinoma of kidney. Sem. Diagn. Pathol. 1998; 15: 54–57.

111. Kennedy SM, Merino M, Linehan WM, Roberts JR, Robertson CN, Neumann RD.: Collecting duct carcinoma of the kidney. Hum. Pathol. 1990; 21: 449–456.

112. De Peralta-Venturina M, Moch H, Amin M, Tamboli O, Hailemariam S, Mihatsch M, Javidan J, Stricker H, Ro JY, Amin MB.: Sarcomatoid differentiation in renal cell carcinoma. A study of 101 cases. Am. J. Surg. Pathol. 2001; 25: 275–284.

(Continued left column) Pathology and Genetics Tumours of the Urinary System and Male Genital Organs. p. 30. IARC Press, Lyon, 2004.

113. Fleming S, Symes CE.: The distribution of cytokeratin antigens in the kidney and in renal tumours. Histopathology 1987; 11: 157–170.
114. Mazal PR, Stichenwirth M, Koller A, Blach S, Haitel A, Susani M.: Expression of aquaporins and PAX-2 compared to CD10 and cytokeratin 7 in renal neoplasms: a tissue microarray study. Mod. Pathol. 2005; 18: 535–540.
115. Pan CC, Chen PC, Ho DM.: The diagnostic utility of MOC31, BerEP4, RCC marker and CD10 in the classification of renal cell carcinoma and renal oncocytoma: an immunohistochemical analysis of 328 cases. Histopathology 2004; 45: 452–459.
116. Füzesi L, Cober M, Mittermayer CH.: Collecting duct carcinoma: cytogenetic characterization. Histopathology 1992; 21: 155–160.
117. Selli C, Amorosi A, Vona G, Sestini R, Travaglini F, Bartoletti F, Orlando C.: Retrospective evaluation of c-erbB-2 oncogene amplification using competitive PCR in collecting duct carcinoma of the kidney. J. Urol. 1997; 158: 245–247.
118. Davis CJ, Mostofi FK, Sesterhenn IA.: Renal medullary carcinoma the seventh sickle cell nephropaty. Am. J. Surg. Pathol. 1995; 19: 1–11.
119. Dimashkieh H, Choe J, Mutema G.: Renal medullary carcinoma. A report of 2 cases and review of the literature. Arch. Pathol. Lab. Med. 2003; 127: 135–138.
120. Swartz MA, Karth J, Schneider DT, Rodríguez R, Beckwith JB, Perlman EJ.: Renal medullary carcinoma, pathologic, immunohistochemical, and genetic analysis with pathogenetic implications. Urology 2002; 60: 1083–1089
121. Rodriguez-Jurado R, González-Crussi F.: Renal medullary carcinoma. Immunohistochemical and ultrastructural observations. J. Urol. Pathol. 1996; 4: 191–203.
122. Avery RA, Harris JE, Davis CJ Jr, Borgaonkar DS, Byrd JC, Weiss RB.: Renal medullary carcinoma: clinical and therapeutic aspects of a newly described tumor. Cancer 1996; 78: 128–132.
123. Polascik TJ, Bostwick DG, Cairos P.: Molecular genetics and histopathologic features of adult distal nephron tumors. Urology 2002; 60: 941–946.
124. Yip D, Steer C, al-Nawab M, van der Walt J, Harper P.: Collecting duct carcinoma of the kidney associated with the sickle cell trait. Int. J. Clin. Pract. 2001; 55: 415–417.
125. Yang XJ, Sugimura J, Tretiakova MS, Furge K, Zagaja G, Sokoloff M, Pins M, Bergan R, Grignon DJ, Stadler WM, Vogelzang NJ, Teh BT.: Gene expression of profiling of renal medullary carcinoma: potential clinical relevance . Cancer 2004; 100: 976–985.
126. Hes O, Hora M, Perez-Montiel DM, Suster S, Curik R, Sokol L, Ondic O, Mikulastik J, Betlach J, Peychl K, Hrabal P, Kobec R, Struku L, Ferák I, Vrabec V, Michal M.: Spindle and cuboidal renal cell carcinoma, a tumor having frequent association with nephrolitiasis: report of 11 cases including a case with hybrid conventional renal cell carcinoma/spindle and cuboidal renal cell carcinoma components. Histopathology 2002; 41: 549–555.
127. Weber A, Srigley J, Moch H.: Mucinous spindle cell carcinoma of the kidney. A molecular analysis. Pathologe 2003; 24: 453–459.
128. Rakozy C, Schmahl GE, Bogner S, Störkel S.: Low-grade tubular mucinous renal neoplasms: morphologic, immuno-histochemical, and genetic features. Mod. Pathol. 2002; 15: 1162–1171.
129. Srigley JR.: Mucinous tubular and spindle cell carcinoma In Eble JN, Sauter G, Epstein JI, Sesterhenn IA. World Health Organization Classification of Tumours. Pathology and Genetics Tumours of the Urinary System and Male Genital Organs. p. 40. IARC Press, Lyon, 2004.
130. Skinnider BF, Folpe AL, Hennigar RA, Lim SD, Cohen C, Tamboli P, Young A, Peralta-Venturina M, Amin MB.: Distribution of cytokeratins and vimentin in adult renal neoplasms and normal renal tissue. Potential utility of a cytokeratin antibody panel in the differential diagnosis of renal tumors. Am. J. Surg. Pathol. 2005; 29: 747–754.
131. Ferlicot S, Allory Y, Comperat E, Mege-Lechevalier F, Dimet S, Sibony M, Couturier J, Vieillefond A.: Mucinous tubular and spindle cell carcinoma: a report of 15 cases and a review of the literature. Virchows Arch. 2005; 447: 978–983.
132. Parwani AV, Husain AN, Epstein JI, Beckwith JB, Argani P.: Low-grade myxoid renal epithelial neoplasms with distal nephron differentiation. Hum. Pathol. 2001; 32: 506–512.
133. Argani P, Ladanyil M.: Renal carcinomas associated with Xp11.2 translocations/TFE3 gene fusions. In Eble JN, Sauter G, Epstein JI, Sesterhenn IA World Health Organization Classification of Tumours. Pathology and Genetics Tumours of the Urinary System and Male Genital Organs. p. 37. IARC Press, Lyon, 2004.
134. Argani P, Antonescu CR, Couturier J, Fournet JC, Sciot R, Debiec-Rychter M, Hutchinson B, Reuter VE, Boccon-Gibod L, Timmons C, Hafez N, Ladanyi M.: PRCC-TFE3 renal carcinomas. Morphologic, immunohistochemical, ultrastructural, and molecular analysis of an entity associated with the t(X;1)(p11.2;q21). Am. J. Surg. Pathol. 2002; 26: 1553–1566.
135. Argani P, Lal P, Hutchinson B, Lui MY, Reuter VE, Ladanyi M.: Aberrant nuclear immunoreactivity for TFE3 in neoplasms with TFE3 gene fusions. A sensitive and specific immunohistochemical assay. Am. J. Surg. Pathol. 2003; 27: 750–761.
136. Imbert MC, Gerard-Marchant R, Schwesguth O.: Tubulopapillary carcinoma of the kidney in children: apropos of 9 observations. Ann. Pediatr. (Paris) 1968; 15: 1094–1104.
137. Sidhar SK, Clark J, Gill S, Hamoudi R, Crew AJ, Gwilliam R, Ross M, Linehan WM, Birdsall S, Shipley J, Cooper CS.: The t(X;1)(p11.2;q21.2) translocation in papillary renal cell carcinoma fuses a novel gene PRCC to the TFE3 transcription factor gene. Hum. Mol. Genet. 1996; 5: 1333–1338.
138. Bruder E, Passera O, Harms D, Leuschner I, Ladany M, Argani P, Eble JN, Struckmann K, Schraml P, Moch H.: Morphologic and molecular characterization of renal cell carcinoma in children and young adults. Am. J. Surg. Pathol. 2004; 28: 1117–1132.
139. Kuiper RP, Schepens M, Thijssen J, van Asseldonk M, van den Berg E, Bridge J, Schuuring E, Schoenmakers EFPM, van Kessel AG.: Upregulation of the transcription factor TFEB in t(6;11)(p21;q13)-positive renal cell carcinomas due to promoter substitution. Hum. Mol. Genet. 2003; 12: 1661–1669.
140. Zisman A, Chao DH, Pantuck AJ, Kim HJ, Wieder JA, Figlin RA, Said JW, Belldegrun AS.: Unclassified renal cell carcinoma: clinical features and prognostic impact of new histological subtypes. J. Urol. 2002; 168: 950–955.

141. Dijkhuizen T, Van Den Berg E, Van Den Berg A, Van De Veen A, Dam A, Faber H, Buys CH, Storkel S, De Jong B.: Genetics as a diagnostic tool in sarcomatoid renal cell cancer. Int. J. Cancer 1997; 72: 265–269.

142. Shannon B, Wisniewski ZS, Bentel J, Cohen RJ.: Adult rhabdoid renal cell carcinoma. Divergent differentiation of conventional (clear cell) carcinoma. Arch. Pathol. Lab. Med. 2002; 126: 1506–1510.

143. Shannon BA, Cohen RJ.: Rhabdoid differentiation of chromophobe renal cell carcinoma. Pathology 2003; 35: 228–230.

144. Gokden N, Nappi O, Swanson PE, Pfeifer JD, Vollmer RT, Wick MR, Humphrey PA.: Renal cell carcinoma with rabdoid features. Am. J. Surg. Pathol. 2000; 24: 1329–1338.

145. Tickoo SK, Reuter VE, Amin MB, Srigley JR, Epstein JI, Min KW, Rubin MA, Ro JY.: Renal oncocytosis. A morphologic study of fourteen cases. Am. J. Surg. Pathol. 1999; 23: 1094–1101.

146. Pavlovich CP, Walter MM, Eyler RA, Hewitt SM, Zbar B, Linehan WM, Merino MJ.: Renal tumors in the Birt-Hogg-Dube syndrome. Am. J. Surg. Pathol. 2002; 26: 1542–1552.

147. Lindgren V, Paner GP, Flanigan RC, Clark JI, Campbell SC, Picken MM.: Renal tumor with overlapping distal nephron morphology and karyotype. Arch. Pathol. Lab. Med. 2004; 128: 1274–1278.

148. Gong Y, Sun X, Haines GK, Pins MR.: Renal cell carcinoma, chromophobe type, with collecting duct carcinoma and sarcomatoid components. Arch. Pathol. Lab. Med. 2003; 127: 38–40.

149. Matei DV, Rocco B, Varela R, Verwei F, Scardino E, Renne G, De Cobelli O.: Synchronous collecting duct carcinoma and papillary renal cell carcinoma: A case report and review of the literature. Anticancer Res. 2005; 25: 579–586.

150. Amin MB, Michal M, Radhakrishnan A, Hes O, McKenney JK, Cheville JC.: Primary thyroid-like follicular carcinoma of the kidney: A histological distinctive primary renal epithelial tumor. Mod. Pathol. 2004; 17 (S1): 136A (A 567).

151. Farah R, Ben-Izhak O, Munichor M, Cohen H.: Low-grade renal collecting duct carcinoma. A case report with histochemical, immunohistochemical, and ultrastructural study. Ann. Diagn. Pathol. 2005; 9: 46–48.

152. MacLennan GT, Farrow GM, Bostwick DG.: Low-grade collecting duct carcinoma of the kidney: report of 13 cases of low-grade mucinous tubulocystic renal carcinoma of possible collecting duct origin. Urology 1997; 50: 679–684.

153. Renshaw AA, Granter SR, Fletcher JA, Kozakewick HP, Corless CL, Perez-Atayde AR.: Renal cell carcinomas in children and young adults. Increased incidence of papillary architecture and unique subtypes. Am. J. Surg. Pathol. 1999; 23: 795–802.

154. Gillett MD, Cheville JC, Karnes RJ, Lohse CM, Kwon ED, Leibovich BC, Zincke H, Blute ML.: Comparison of presentation and outcome for patients 18 to 40 and 60 to 70 years old with solid renal masses. J. Urol. 2005; 173: 1893–1896.

155. Medeiros LJ.: Renal cell carcinoma associated with neuroblastoma. In Eble JN, Sauter G, Epstein JI, Sesterhenn IA. World Health Organization Classification of Tumours. Pathology and Genetics Tumours of the Urinary System and Male Genital Organs. p. 39. IARC Press, Lyon, 2004.

156. Presti JC Jr, Moch H, Gelb AB, Huynth D, Wadman FM.: Initiating genetic events in small renal neoplasms detected by comparative genomic hybridization. J. Urol. 1998; 160: 1557–1561.

157. Merino MJ, Eccles DM, Linehan WM, Algaba F, Zbar B, Kovacs G, Kleihues P, Geurts van Kessel A, Kiuru M, Launonen V, Herva R, Aaltonen LA, Neumann HPH, Pavlovich CP.: Familial renal cell carcinoma. In Eble JN, Sauter G, Epstein JI, Sesterhenn IA. World Health Organization Classification of Tumours. Pathology and Genetics Tumours of the Urinary System and Male Genital Organs. p. 15. IARC Press, Lyon, 2004.

158. Maher ER, Kaelin WG.: von Hippel-Lindau disease. Medicine 1997; 76: 381–391.

159. Prat E, Bernues M, Del Rey J, Camps J, Ponsa I, Algaba F, Egozcue J, Caballin MR, Gelabert A, Miro R.: Common pattern of unusual chromosome abnormalities in hereditary papillary renal carcinoma. Cancer Genet. Cytogenet. 2006; 15; 142–147.

160. Sampson JR, Patel A, Mee AD.: Multifocal renal cell carcinoma in sibs from a chromosome 9 linked (TSC1) tuberous sclerosis family. J. Med. Genet. 1995; 32: 848–850.

161. Launonen V, Vierimaa O, Kiuru M, Isola J, Roth S, Pukkala E, Sistonen P, Herva R, Aaltonen LA.: Inherited susceptibility to uterine leiomyomas and renal cell cancer. Proc. Natl. Acad. Sci. USA. 2001; 13: 3387–3392.

162. Malchoff CD, Sarfarazi M, Tendler B, Forouhar F, Whalen G, Joshi V, Arnold A, Malchoff DM.: Papillary thyroid carcinoma associated with papillary renal neoplasia: genetic linkage analysis of a distinct heritable tumor syndrome. J. Clin. Endocrinol. Metab. 2000; 85: 1758–1764.

163. Weirich G, Glenn G, Junker K, Merino M, Storkel S, Lubensky I, Choyke P, Pack S, Amin M, Walther MM, Linehan WM, Zbar B.: Familial renal oncocytoma: clinicopathological study of 5 families. J. Urol. 1998; 160: 335–340.

164. Algaba F.: Modern molecular classification of renal cell carcinoma: relevance for urologists. In Progress and Controversies in Oncological Urology VII (PACIOU VII), edited by Bangma ChH, Newling DWW. pp. 286–290. The Parthenon Publishing Group, London, 2003.

165. Schraml P, Muller D, Bednar R, Gasser T, Sauter G, Mihatsch MJ, Moch H.: Allelic loss: the D9S171 locus on chromosome 9p13 is associated with progression of papillary renal cell carcinoma. J. Pathol. 2000; 190: 457–461.

166. Moch H, Schraml P, Bubendorf L, Mirlacher M, Kononen J, Gasser T, Mihatsch MJ, Kallioniemi OP, Sauter G.: High-throughput tissue microarray analysis to evaluate genes uncovered by cDNA microarray screening in renal cell carcinoma. Am. J. Pathol. 1999; 154: 981–986.

167. Shi T, Seligson D, Belldegrun AS, Palotie A, Horvath S.: Tumor classification by tissue microarray profiling: random forest clustering applied to renal cell carcinoma. Mod. Pathol. 2005; 18: 547–557.

4
Staging of Renal Cell Carcinoma

John T. Leppert, John S. Lam, and Arie S. Belldegrun

Introduction

Cancer of the kidney and renal pelvis is estimated to account for 36,160 new cases and 12,660 deaths in the United States in 2005.[43] Worldwide, 208,000 new cases and 102,000 deaths were attributed to kidney cancer in 2002, with the highest incidence in North America, Europe, and Australia.[82] Renal cell carcinoma (RCC) accounts for approximately 2–3% of all adult malignancies and is the most lethal of the urological cancers. More than 40% of patients with RCC will die from their cancer compared with the approximately 20% mortality rates associated with prostate and bladder cancers.[43] Approximately 20–30% of patients present with metastatic disease, and 20–40% of patients undergoing nephrectomy for clinically localized RCC will develop metastases.[41] The incidence of RCC is steadily increasing at a rate of about 2.5% per year across population groups.[10, 78] During the past 2 decades, significant advances in the diagnosis, staging, and treatment of patients with RCC have resulted in improved survival of a select group of patients and an overall change in the natural history of the disease.[78] However, despite advances in biological and immune-based therapies, response rates for patients with metastatic RCC remain modest. These data underscore the critical importance of staging systems for kidney cancer.

Staging systems for kidney cancer serve to provide (1) descriptive tumor characteristics, (2) aid in the selection of therapeutic options for the individual patient, (3) accurate prognostic information to stratify risk of disease recurrence or cancer-related death, (4) criteria to identify patient populations for specific adjuvant therapies, and (5) inclusion criteria for clinical trials.[62] With many new and promising adjuvant therapies on the horizon, staging systems will continue to play a pivotal role in the development of treatment strategies for RCC.[15]

RCC staging systems have evolved in parallel with the rapid increase in understanding of kidney cancer biology. As a result, staging systems, initially based on gross anatomic information, have been revised to include a myriad of pathological, histological, and clinical characteristics. High throughput tissue arrays have facilitated the rapid analysis of potential protein molecular markers. Similar recent advances in gene expression analysis have identified many candidate genetic markers in RCC. Combining tumor anatomy, pathology, histology, and molecular profiling has allowed for further improvement of staging constructs. We review the evolution of RCC staging systems and current controversies and highlight future directions and advances in the staging of kidney cancer.

Kidney Cancer Staging Systems

Anatomic Staging Systems

The first formal staging system was proposed by Flocks and Kadesky in 1958 and was based on the description of the tumor and location of cancer spread.[23] This system was later modified by Robson et al.[87] to consider the presence of vascular involvement) (Fig. 4-1). The Robson staging system stressed the importance of stratifying the anatomic spread of the tumor for the purpose of patient prognostication and improving surgical technique. While simple and easy to use, the Robson staging system groups tumor characteristics currently thought to have a dissimilar prognosis.[78]

Tumor, Nodes, Metastasis Staging System

Subsequent refinements of these anatomic based staging systems have led to the current tumor, nodes, metastasis (TNM) system proposed by the Union Internationale Contre le Cancer (UICC)[34, 94] Table 4-1. The TNM system is currently the most commonly used staging system for RCC and has been shown to accurately define patient prognosis. At UCLA, the 5-year cancer specific survival according to the 1997 TNM criteria for stage I to IV lesions was 91%, 74%, 67%, and 32%, respectively[104] (Fig. 4-2). Other investigators have reported similar survival results for the respective TNM stages.[27, 42] Despite its strengths, many elements of the TNM staging system are controversial and hotly debated. In 2002, the American Joint Committee on Cancer (AJCC) revised the TNM system and these most recent changes

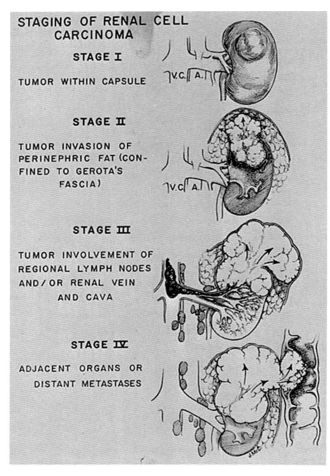

STAGING OF RENAL CELL
CARCINOMA

STAGE I

TUMOR WITHIN CAPSULE

STAGE II

TUMOR INVASION OF
PERINEPHRIC FAT (CON-
FINED TO GEROTA'S
FASCIA)

STAGE III

TUMOR INVOLVEMENT OF
REGIONAL LYMPH NODES
AND / OR RENAL VEIN
AND CAVA

STAGE IV

ADJACENT ORGANS OR
DISTANT METASTASES

FIGURE 4-1. Renal cell carcinoma staging.

are noted in Table 4-1. The 2002 TNM staging system has subsequently been externally validated[21] and found to offer improved prognostic ability when compared with the prior 1997 TNM criteria.[25]

Tumor Size

The size of the primary tumor has repeatedly been shown to be an important prognostic indicator[3,28,32,101] and has, therefore, become an integral part of the TNM system. The 1997 TNM staging system increased the cutoff size for T1 tumors from 2.5 cm to 7 cm as the lower size cutoff did not generate statistically significant survival differences.[33,40] Zisman et al.[111] evaluated the impact of the 1997 change in TNM staging criteria by retrospectively analyzing data from 661 patients who had undergone either partial or radical nephrectomy for RCC. They demonstrated that patients with T1 tumors larger than 4.5 cm experienced decreased survival times, higher recurrence rates, and higher rates of lymph node involvement and metastatic disease compared to patients with smaller T1 tumors. In addition, survival of patients with T1 tumors >4.5 cm was identical to the survival of patients

with T2 tumors. Several other recent studies have evaluated the optimal T1 size criteria for patients undergoing either partial or radical nephrectomy suggesting alternative cutoffs, which include 5,[60] 5.5,[22,51] 8[31] and 10[69] cm. While these studies disagree about the optimal cutoff, they all demonstrate that primary tumor size is an important determinant of prognosis. Based on its prognostic value, investigators have delineated a tumor size cutoff in determining eligibility for nephron-sparing surgery (NSS). Hafez et al.[35] attempted to better delineate the optimal cutoff size for tumors amenable to partial nephrectomy and, in so doing, demonstrated that patients with tumors less than 4 cm who underwent NSS had a significantly better survival rate than patients with larger tumors. In the past 10 years, evidence from major clinical series has shown the effectiveness and safety of NSS in the treatment of renal tumors 4 cm or less.[35,61,64] As a result, the American Joint Committee on Cancer (AJCC) amended the 1997 TNM staging system in 2002 to include T1a and T1b subcategories, based on a 4 cm size cutoff Table 4-1.[95]

Impact of Tumor Thrombus

RCC invades the venous system in 4–9% of newly diagnosed patients.[39,76] The presence and extent of tumor thrombus are recognized as a prognostic factor in the Robson and TNM staging systems. Moinzadeh and Libertino[73] recently reviewed 153 patients who underwent nephrectomy and tumor thrombectomy. They concluded that long-term survival in patients with right ventricle (RV) involvement was significantly greater than in those with inferior vena cava (IVC) involvement. Kim et al.[48] recently compared 226 patients who underwent nephrectomy and RV or IVC tumor thrombectomy with 654 patients undergoing nephrectomy without venous involvement. In those with localized RCC (N0M0) cancer-specific survival was similar in patients with RV (T3b) and IVC involvement below the diaphragm (T3b). However, patients with IVC involvement above the diaphragm (T3c) had significantly worse survival even after controlling for grade and Eastern Cooperative Oncology Group performance status (ECOG-PS) on multivariate analysis. The 3-year cancer-specific survival rates associated with RCC without thrombus, RV involvement (T3b), IVC involvement below the diaphragm (T3b), and IVC involvement above the diaphragm (T3c) were 89%, 76%, 63%, and 23%, respectively. Patients treated for metastatic RCC had a similar prognosis regardless of the level of venous involvement. The group concluded that local tumor stage and grade were better predictors of prognosis than the extent of venous involvement, supporting the current TNM classification of venous involvement. Based on these studies and others,[29,39,48,67,96] the revision that effectively downstaged supradiaphragmatic tumor thrombus in the TNM 1997 system seems appropriate. Recent studies have demonstrated 5-year survival rates of 47–69% in RCC cases with venous involvement and tumor limited to the kidney.[29,39,66,92,114]

TABLE 4-1. Comparison of the 1987 and 1997 UICC/AJCC and the 2002 AJCC staging systems.

Classification	1987 UICC/AJCC	1997 UICC/AJCC	2002 AJCC
T stage			
T1	Tumor >2.5 cm in greatest dimension, limited to kidney	Tumor >7 cm in greatest dimension, limited to kidney	Tumor >7 cm in greatest dimension, limited to kidney
T1a			Tumor >4 cm in greatest dimension, limited to kidney
T1b			Tumor >4 cm and >7 cm, limited to kidney
T2	Tumor >2.5 cm in greatest dimension, limited to kidney	Tumor >7 cm in greatest dimension, limited to kidney	Tumor >7 cm in greatest dimension, limited to kidney
T3	Tumor extends into major veins, adrenal gland, or perinephric tissues but not beyond Gerota's fascia	Tumor extends into major veins, adrenal gland, or perinephric tissue, but not beyond Gerota's fascia	Tumor extends into major veins, adrenal gland, or perinephric tissue, but not beyond Gerota's fascia
T3a	Tumor invades adrenal gland or perinephric tissues but not beyond Gerota's fascia	Tumor invades adrenal gland or perinephric tissues	Tumor invades adrenal gland or perinephric tissues
T3b	Tumor grossly extends into renal vein(s) or vena cava	Tumor grossly extends into renal vein(s) or vena cava below the diaphragm	Tumor grossly extends into renal vein(s) or vena cava below diaphragm
T3c		Tumor grossly extends into vena cava above the diaphragm	Tumor gross extends into vena cava above diaphragm
T4	Tumor invades beyond Gerota's fascia	Tumor invades beyond Gerota's fascia	Tumor invades beyond Gerota's fascia
N stage			
N0	No regional lymph node metastasis	No regional lymph node metastasis	No regional lymph node metastasis
N1	Metastasis in one lhymph node >2 cm in greatest dimensions	Metastasis in single regional node	Metastasis in single regional node
N2	Metastasis in one lymph node >2 cm but not >5 cm in greatest dimension, or multiple lymph nodes, none >5 cm in greatest dimension	Metastasis in more than one regional lymph node	Metastasis in more than one regional lymph node
N3	Metastasis in a lymph node >5 cm in greatest dimension		
M stage			
M0	No distant metastasis	No distant metastasis	No distant metastasis
M1	Distant metastasis	Distant metastasis	Distant metastasis

With modern advances in surgical technique, contemporary series demonstrate that surgical resection can be performed with acceptable morbidity.[81]

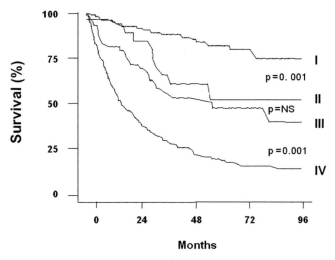

FIGURE 4-2. UCLA TNM stagings.

Adrenal Gland Involvement

Few patients present with ipsilateral adrenal gland involvement at the time of diagnosis.[52, 105] The current 2002 TNM staging system classifies these patients as T3a along with tumors demonstrating invasion into perirenal fat. Han et al.[37] reported significantly lower 5-year cancer-specific survival among patients with T3a tumors due to adrenal gland involvement when compared with perinephric fat invasion. This report demonstrated no difference in survival among patients with T3a tumors due to adrenal involvement when compared with those with T4 disease. Recently, Thompson et al.[103] found adrenal invasion of the tumor to be associated with a 20% 5-year disease-free survival, and recommended that these tumors be classified as T4 disease. The reclassification of adrenal involvement has also recently been suggested by Siemer et al. in a retrospective study of 241 patients with T3a disease.[89] In addition, the route of tumor spread to the adrenal gland may be important. Further investigation is needed to determine if the direct extension of tumor into the adrenal gland portends a prognosis similar to hematogenous metastasis to the adrenal gland.

Impact of Lymphadenopathy

The overall risk of lymph node (LN) metastasis is approximately 20% and the 5-year survival rate in patients with LN metastases is 11–35%.[79,80,108] However, the risk of LN involvement varies depending on primary tumor stage and size, RV involvement, metastases, and the extent of LN dissection (LND) performed.[79,102] Patients with clinically localized disease have a relatively low incidence (2–9%) of nodal involvement,[5,71,90,102] whereas the incidence in patients with metastatic disease or RV involvement is as high as 45%[6,79] Vasselli et al.[108] reported that patients with no preoperative evidence of LN involvement had significantly longer median survival than those with LN involvement (14.7 vs. 8.5 months). Pantuck et al.[79,80] retrospectively reviewed the impact of lymphadenopathy in relation to the response to immunotherapy and survival. In a review of 900 patients, positive LN status was associated with larger, higher grade, more locally advanced tumors that were more likely to demonstrate sarcomatoid features. Patients with lymphadenopathy were three to four times more likely to have distant metastatic disease. Patients with metastatic RCC and LN disease showed a significantly worse 5-year survival rate compared to patients with metastatic disease alone (15% vs. 23%). Importantly, patients with node-positive disease who underwent LND had better responses to immunotherapy and higher survival rates compared to patients in whom involved LNs were left in place.[79,80] The European Organization for Research and Treatment of Cancer (EORTC) is performing the only prospective, randomized, controlled study (EORTC 30881), comprising 772 patients with clinically localized disease randomized to nephrectomy with or without standardized LND.[5] Although the data are still immature, there were no differences in progression or survival between patients treated with or without LND at the 5-year median follow-up. The group has noted an excellent 5-year survival rate (82%) and longer follow-up may be needed to allow for a survival difference to become apparent.

Prognostic Factors Not Included in Anatomic Staging Systems

Tumor Grade

Nearly all histopathological tumor grading systems have shown independent prognostic value in studies that included grade as a variable.[54] Skinner et al.[91] noted the correlation between nuclear features and survival in 1971. Fuhrman et al.[26] then developed a 4 tier grading system based on nuclear and nucleolar size, shape and content that remains the most commonly used system in North America. Unfortunately, controversy exists concerning the inter-observer reproducibility of grading, and relevant cutoff points between the different grade classifications. Tsui et al.[104] noted a strong correlation between tumor grade and survival with 5-year

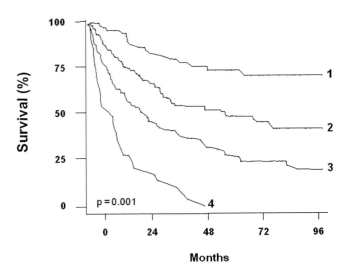

FIGURE 4-3. UCLA grade.

cancer specific survival rates of 89%, 65% and 46.1% for grades 1, 2 and 3 to 4, respectively (Fig. 4-3). Furthermore, 5-year cancer specific survival rates in patients with T1 tumors were 91%, 83%, 60% and 0% for grades 1 to 4, respectively, demonstrating the ability of histological grade to stratify survival even in patients with tumors of identical stage.

Histologic Subtype

Current histological criteria classify RCC into clear cell, papillary, chromophobe, and collecting duct subtypes.[56,97] Each subtype of renal tumor has distinguishing characteristics and patterns of disease that may be associated with prognosis.[2,75]

Clear cell (conventional) carcinomas account for 70–80% of RCCs. Multilocular RCC, a variant of clear cell carcinoma, may have a lower potential for recurrences and metastasis. In a recent review,[4] 96% of cases occurred in male patients, and nuclear grade and stage were lower than in patients with other types of RCC. Cystic RCC is another clear cell variant associated with a slower growth rate, improved prognosis, and longer survival than conventional RCC.[13,36]

Papillary RCC accounts for 10–20% of RCCs and is the second most common type of RCC. The clinical behavior of papillary RCC has been reported to be more aggressive than that of clear cell RCC;[85] however, there are more data in the literature indicating that the behavior of papillary RCC is less aggressive than that of clear cell RCC.[1,2,45] Papillary RCC is further divided into two types[1,16] Type 1 papillary RCC has been found to behave less aggressively than type[2,72] and a recent analysis of data from patients with these two morphotypes demonstrated that papillary tumor subtype 2 is a significant and independent predictor of survival.[17]

Chromophobe RCC accounts for approximately 5% of RCCs. The overall survival of patients with chromophobe RCC seems to be better than that of patients with other types of RCC.[2,72] However, chromophobe and papillary subtypes of RCC are associated with extremely poor responses to interleukin (IL)-2 therapy, with median survival times reported to be 11 months and 5.5 months, respectively.[75]

Collecting duct carcinoma is an aggressive and rare variant of RCC accounting for less than 1% of tumors. In patients with collecting duct carcinomas, systemic metastases tend to develop rapidly.[46]

The question of whether different histological variants of RCC portend different survival outcomes remains controversial. A retrospective review of 2385 RCC patients treated by radical nephrectomy at the Mayo Clinic demonstrated that cancer-specific survival was worse for clear cell RCC than for papillary or chromophobe RCC, with 5-year cancer-specific survival rates of 69%, 87%, and 87%, respectively.[9] This survival difference persisted after stratifying for TNM stage and nuclear grade. However, a recent international, multicenter study of 4063 RCC patients treated by surgical resection found all histological types had similar survival when adjusted for stage and grade.[83]

Presence of Sarcomatoid Features

The sarcomatoid variant is no longer considered a distinct histological subtype of RCC.[30] The spindle cell growth pattern typical of sarcomatoid features can be seen in any histological subtype of RCC, occurring in less than 5% of RCC cases.[7,88] The reported median survival of untreated patients diagnosed with the sarcomatoid variant is 3.8–6.8 months.[20] Ro et al.[86] noted that the amount of tumor necrosis and proportion of sarcomatoid tumor were independently predictive of a poorer prognosis in low stage disease. de Peralta-Venturina et al.[14] recently reviewed 101 cases of RCC with sarcomatoid features and reported 5- and 10-year survival rates of 22% and 13%, respectively.

Histological Tumor Necrosis

Recently, several publications have demonstrated the prognostic value of histological tumor necrosis.[2,8,14,24,72] Occurring in approximately one-third of RCC tumors,[8,72] histological necrosis is defined as any degree of microscopic tumor necrosis exclusive of degenerative changes such as hyalinization, hemorrhage, or fibrosis.[8] Amin et al.[2] analyzed the prognostic value of histological necrosis in 405 RCC specimens and multivariate analysis revealed that TNM stage, nuclear grade, and histological necrosis were associated with survival. Patients with necrosis in the pathology specimen had a 3-fold higher likelihood of cancer-specific death when compared with patients without histological necrosis. In 1801 patients at the Mayo Clinic with unilateral clear cell carcinoma, the presence of histological necrosis in tumor specimens was shown to be an independent predictor of survival associated with twice the risk of death from RCC compared to patients without necrosis.[24] A recent study at

UCLA in 310 patients with localized or metastatic RCC demonstrated that the presence and extent of histologic necrosis in tumor specimens were independent predictors of survival in localized (p <0.05), but not metastatic (p >0.05) patients.[59]

Collecting System Invasion

The invasion of the collecting system by RCC has been demonstrated to be a prognostic indicator.[77,107] Palapattu et al.[77] reviewed the records of 895 patients and demonstrated that patients with collecting system invasion had a significantly lower 3-year cancer-specific survival rate than their counterparts who did not have involvement of the collecting system (62% vs. 39%, respectively). This difference was particularly evident in patients with stage T1 tumors (81% vs. 67%, respectively). Multivariate analysis demonstrated that collecting system invasion was an independent predictor of survival associated with a 1.4-fold greater risk for death when compared with patients without collecting system invasion.

Performance Status

The Karnofsky or Eastern Cooperative Oncology Group performance status (ECOG-PS) scales are a convenient common denominator of the overall impact of multiple symptoms on patients. Several studies have demonstrated the ECOG-PS to be an independent prognostic factor of survival in patients with metastatic RCC at presentation with higher scores correlating with poorer survival[12,19,68] (Fig. 4-4). Recently, it has been suggested that the utility of the ECOG-PS as a prognostic factor can be extended to all stages of RCC.[113] Patients with RCC who had ECOG-PS values of 1 or greater were found to have a significantly lower 5-year survival rate of 51% when compared with the

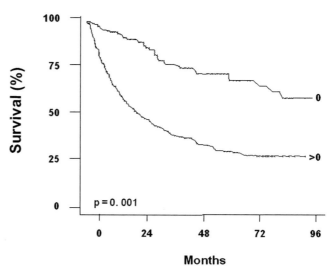

FIGURE 4-4. UCLA ECOG.

81% 5-year survival rate for patients with an ECOG-PS of 0, a difference that was found to be an independent prognostic factor of survival.

Other Patient Clinical Characteristics

Kim et al.[47,49] recently demonstrated in 1046 patients undergoing nephrectomy for RCC that cachexia, defined as hypoalbuminemia, weight loss, anorexia, or malaise, was an independent predictor of worse survival (hazard ratio = 2.8). The prognostic significance of cachexia in patients with stage T1 RCC was also evaluated. Multivariate analysis demonstrated that the presence of cachexia-related symptoms was associated with a poorer recurrence-free survival rate and disease-specific survival rate compared to patients without such symptoms.

Integrated Staging Systems and Nomograms

Comprehensive integrated staging systems were born from the addition of the numerous nonanatomic variables found to be significant prognostic indicators to traditional anatomic staging systems. Several of these prognostic tools were initially developed to determine eligibility of patients with metastatic disease for immunotherapy. Elson et al.[18] was the first to develop a scoring system to stratify patients with metastatic disease into five categories based on criteria such as ECOG-PS score, time from diagnosis to metastasis, weight loss, prior chemotherapy, and number of metastatic sites. Using this system, they demonstrated median survival times ranging from 2.1 to 12.8 months across the five categories. Using a similar approach Citterio et al.[12] identified prognostic subgroups based on ECOG-PS and serum hemoglobin.

More recently, Motzer et al.[74] created a model based on a study of 670 patients with advanced RCC treated at Memorial Sloan Kettering Cancer Center by defining the relationship of pretreatment clinical features and survival, which included risk factors such as low Karnofsky score or high ECOG-PS score, high serum lactate dehydrogenase levels, low hemoglobin levels, hypercalcemia, and prior nephrectomy (Fig. 4-5). Patients at poor risk with three or more risk factors had a median survival of only 4 months, whereas median survival improved to 20 months in those with no risk factors. Mekhail et al. recently examined this model in 353 patients with previously untreated metastatic RCC[70] In this patient population, the Motzer criteria, as well as the number of metastatic sites, were independent predictors of patient survival.

The Kattan postoperative prognostic nomogram[45] was created to predict the probability of tumor recurrence within 5 years in patients undergoing radical nephrectomy for RCC. The nomogram assigns numerical scores to various prognostic indicators, such as the presence of symptoms

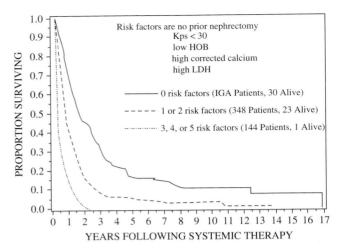

FIGURE 4-5. Relationship of pretreatment clinical features and survival based on risk factors.

(including local versus systemic), histology, tumor size, and the standard TNM staging criteria. In a study of 601 patients with RCC who were treated with nephrectomy, the nomogram appeared accurate and discriminating, with an area under the receiver operating curve, which compares the predicted probability with the actual outcome, of 0.74[45] (Fig. 4-6).

The Mayo Clinic also created a new, more extensive outcome prediction model for patients with clear cell RCC who were to be treated with radical nephrectomy.[24] According to an analysis of data from 1801 patients in the Mayo Clinic database, TNM stage, tumor size ≥5 cm, nuclear grade, and the presence of histological tumor necrosis were all found to be independent predictors of survival. These factors were combined into the stage, size, grade, and necrosis (SSIGN) scoring algorithm. Decreased survival was shown to correlate with increased SSIGN score, with scores of 0–1 and ≥10 correlating with 5-year cancer-specific survival rates of 99.4% and 7.4%, respectively (Fig 4-7).

At UCLA, an extensive prognostic system has been created for both localized and metastatic RCC designated the UCLA Integrated Staging System (UISS).[113] The UISS was developed to better stratify patients into prognostic categories using statistical tools that accurately define the probability of survival of an individual patient[113] (Fig. 4-8). Initially evaluated were a multitude of factors in 661 patients, including age, sex, Fuhrman grade, TNM stage, tumor size alone, ECOG-PS, laterality, bilaterality, smoking, number of presenting symptoms, weight loss alone, tumor histological type, administration of immunotherapy, IVC involvement, number of metastatic sites, sites of metastases, and time interval between nephrectomy and tumor recurrence to determine which factors had the greatest impact on the survival of patients with RCC. The initial UISS contained five groups based on TNM stage, Fuhrman grade, and ECOG-PS. Projected 2- and 5-year survival for patients in UISS groups I to V are 96% and 94%, 89% and 67%, 66%

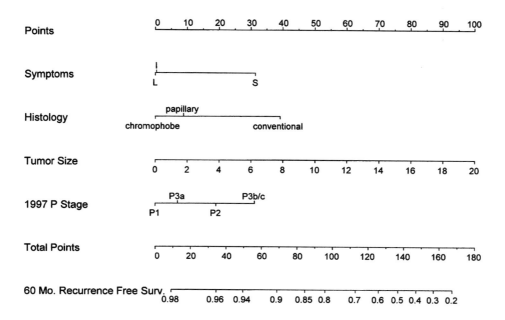

Instructions for Physician: Locate the patient's symptoms (I=incidental, L=local, S=systemic) on the Symptoms axis. Draw a line straight upwards to the **Points** axis to determine how many points towards recurrence the patient receives for his symptoms. Repeat this process for the other axes, each time drawing straight upward to the **Points** axis. Sum the points achieved for each predictor and locate this sum on the **Total Points** axis. Draw a line straight down to find the patient's probability of remaining recurrence free for 5 years assuming he or she does not die of another cause first.

Instruction to Patient: "Mr. X, if we had 100 men or women exactly like you, we would expect between <predicted percentage from nomogram − 10%> and <predicted percentage + 10%> to remain free of their disease at 5 years following surgery, though recurrence after 5 years is still possible."

FIGURE 4-6. Postoperative prognostic nomogram to predict tumor recurrence.

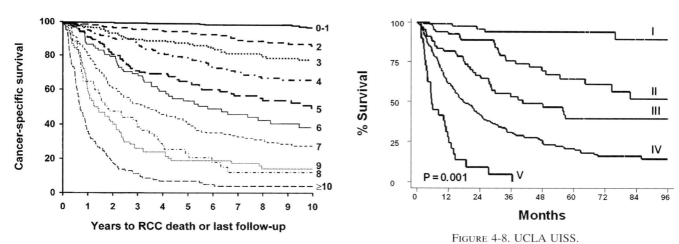

FIGURE 4-7. Clear cell SSIGN score.

FIGURE 4-8. UCLA UISS.

and 39%, 42% and 23%, and 9% and 0%, respectively. The UISS was internally validated using a bootstrapping technique and then using an expanded database of patients treated at UCLA between 1989 and 2000,[110] with external data from 576 RCC patients treated at MD Anderson Cancer Center and in Nijmegen, Netherlands,[38,93] and most recently with 4202 RCC patients from eight international centers.[84] The UISS has been subsequently modified into a simplified system, based on separate stratification of metastatic and nonmetastatic patients into low-, intermediate-, and high-risk groups.[112] A comprehensive algorithm was subsequently developed (Fig. 4-9), which consists of two decision boxes (one for patients with localized RCC and one for patients with metastatic RCC) that are used to assign patients to one of three risk groups (low, intermediate, and high) based on UISS criteria (Fig. 4-10). This provides a clinically useful system for predicting postoperative outcome, and provides a unique tool for risk assignment and outcome analysis to

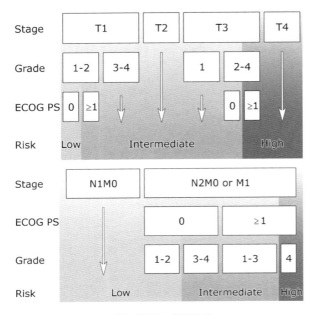

FIGURE 4-9. UCLA UISS diagram.

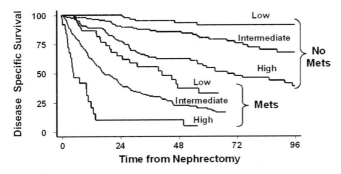

FIGURE 4-10. UCLA simplified UISS.

help determine follow-up regimens and eligibility for clinical trials.

A large European multicenter study compared the predictive performance of several integrated staging systems, including the Kattan nomogram and the UISS.[11] This affirmed the accuracy of these postoperative integrated systems with the Kattan nomogram and UISS performing best, with c-indexes of 0.706 and 0.683, respectively. In addition, the Kattan nomogram was found to work well to differentiate the patients classified as intermediate risk by the UISS.

Integrated Staging Systems and Selection for Adjuvant Therapy and Clinical Trials

In an effort to identify patients with RCC most likely to benefit from adjuvant therapy, investigators have defined predictive factors for recurrence. Several protocols based on reported prognostic factors and risk of recurrence have been proposed by a number of investigators.[57] Levy and

co-workers described aggressive patterns of RCC recurrence with advanced pathological staging.[65] Following radical nephrectomy, approximately 7% of patients with stage T1 disease experience a recurrence at a median of 38 months, whereas nearly 40% of patients with stage T3 disease experience a recurrence within a median of 17 months. Patients in the UISS nonmetastatic high-risk group had a high rate of systemic failure, suggesting the presence of occult metastasis at diagnosis.[112]

The Mayo Clinic has developed a simple scoring algorithm to predict progression to metastatic disease in patients that have undergone radical nephrectomy for clinically localized, clear cell RCC.[63] An evidence-based postoperative surveillance protocol based on the UISS risk group stratification system for patients with localized and locally advanced RCC has also been created by analyzing recurrence patterns between different risk groups following surgical resection.[58] Stratification of patients into risk groups allows for the prediction of disease recurrence, as well as the prediction of the time to tumor recurrence. This provides a clinically useful system for predicting postoperative outcome and a unique tool to help determine eligibility for adjuvant clinical trials.

Molecular Staging Systems

As research advances our understanding of the molecular and genetic biology of kidney cancer, inclusion of important genetic and protein molecular markers represents the next logical advance in RCC staging systems. Tissue array technology has facilitated the discovery of many molecular markers in RCC. Sections of the microarray provide targets for parallel in situ detection of DNA, RNA, and protein targets on an array containing hundreds of tumor specimens.[53] These data can then be correlated to clinical data with respect to disease progression, treatment response, and survival. Gene expression profiling offers the ability to analyze thousands of candidate genes and has led to a greater knowledge of the molecular genetics of RCC. The expression of these genetic/protein markers may provide prognostic information because they represent (1) surrogate markers of tumor aggressiveness, (2) antigens recognized by the host immune system, (3) a mechanism used by the tumor in growth or invasion, and (4) markers that predict response to treatment modalities. The incorporation of molecular tumor markers into future staging systems is expected to completely revolutionize the approach to diagnosis and prognosis.[18,24,45,74,78,113]

Carbonic Anhydrase IX as an Example Prognostic Molecular Marker

Significant attention has been paid to carbonic anhydrase IX (CA IX) (also known as G250 or MN), a member of the carbonic anhydrase family. CA IX is thought to assist in the regulation of intracellular and extracellular pH levels. In one study, CA IX was detected in 86% of RCC samples studied, but was found in only 9% of normal kidney tissue samples, suggesting that CA IX expression may be a useful diagnostic biomarker.[106] A study at UCLA found that 94% of clear cell RCC tumor samples stained positively for CA IX.[6] Low CA IX staining was found to be an independent prognostic indicator of poor survival in patients with metastatic RCC (hazard ratio = 3.10). For patients with localized, high-risk RCC lesions, low CA IX staining also implied a worse prognosis. CA IX, and many other individual markers, has shown the ability to stratify patient prognosis by marker data alone.

Protein Expression and Staging Nomograms

Recently, Kim et al.[50] combined multiple protein molecular markers and the UISS to create a Molecular Integrated Staging System. Immunohistochemical analysis of Ki-67, p53, gelsolin, CA IX, CA XII, PTEN, EpCAM, and vimentin was analyzed from 318 clear cell RCC tumors. Increased staining for Ki-67, p53, vimentin, and gelsolin correlated with worse survival, while the inverse was true for CA IX, PTEN, CA XII, and EpCAM. In multivariate analysis, the presence of metastasis, gelsolin, p53 expression, and CA IX remained significant predictors of survival and were used to create a prognostic model (marker model). This model, based entirely on molecular marker information, performed better than individual clinical variables, such as tumor grade and T stage, and was as powerful as the integrated UISS model. Combining clinical variables and marker data (clinical/marker model) resulted in a prognostic system for clear cell RCC that outperformed the UISS. This report demonstrates several important principles. First, molecular marker information can be a powerful tool in the staging of RCC. In addition, combining molecular marker information will further strengthen the prognostic ability of staging systems (Fig. 4-11).

Examining Gene Expression in Renal Cell Carcinoma

With the completion of the Human Genome Project, cancer research is being revolutionized by the ability to measure the expression of essentially all human genes at the level of messenger RNA simultaneously. Gene expression profiling offers the ability to analyze thousands of candidate genes in high-throughput arrays. This powerful technology can identify RCC subtypes, recapitulating and refining the current histological classifications. Gene expression analysis studies have also shown ability to define patient prognosis. Takahashi et al.[98] studied 29 patients with clear cell RCC. When compared with normal tissue samples, clear cell RCC tumors exhibited a high expression of markers such as vascular endothelial growth factor (VEGF) and ceruloplasmin and down-regulation of kininogen. Among

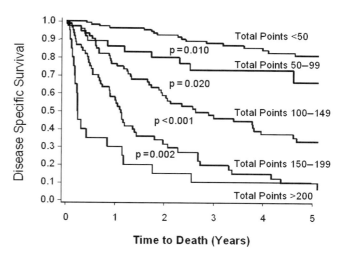

FIGURE 4-11. UCLA UISS.

these clear cell tumors, the 40 genes were identified that differentiated patients with the best prognosis. Increased expression of SPROUTY, an angiogenesis inhibitor, was associated with a good prognosis while loss of tumor growth factor (TGF)-β receptor II and metalloproteinase 3 were associated with poor outcomes. In a second study by Takahashi et al.,[99] a unique expression profile in clear cell tumors differentiated a poor-prognosis subcluster including the patients who died from their disease from patients with no evidence of metastasis. Jones et al.[44] also reported the ability of gene expression analysis within the primary tumor to identify a metastatic signature. Vasselli et al.[109] used gene expression to evaluate the prognosis for patients with metastatic RCC. They related 58 metastatic RCC specimens to global gene-expression patterns most correlated with patient survival. They divided 45 genes from separate patients into groups by prognosis. Increased expression of vascular cell adhesion molecule (VCAM)-1 was noted to be particularly powerful in selecting patients with improved prognosis. The International Kidney Cancer Study Group recently reported the ability of gene expression profiling to predict survival for patients with clear cell RCC.[100] Evaluating 110 primary tumors resulted in gene predictors of patient survival independent of traditional clinicopathological variables. Kosari et al.[55] were also able to identify 35 differentially expressed genes that allowed for clustering of nonaggressive clear cell RCC specimens separate from aggressive and metastatic tumors. The fact that aggressive but localized RCC samples demonstrated a gene expression profile similar to metastatic tumors presents an opportunity to identify patients at the highest risk of disease progression and recurrence, as well as those most likely to benefit from adjuvant therapies. These early reports suggest that within a short period of time, gene expression analysis will become an integral component of future kidney cancer staging systems.

Conclusions

Kidney cancer staging systems have developed from simple anatomical based constructs to include clinical and histopathologic data along with molecular prognostic factors. With new research insights, the staging of RCC will continue to be refined and improved. Staging systems remain an integral part of the application of current therapies and development of future treatment strategies for kidney cancer.

References

1. Amin MB, et al. Papillary (chromophil) renal cell carcinoma: histomorphologic characteristics and evaluation of conventional pathologic prognostic parameters in 62 cases. *Am J Surg Pathol* 1997; 21:621–635.
2. Amin MB, et al. Prognostic impact of histologic subtyping of adult renal epithelial neoplasms: an experience of 405 cases. *Am J Surg Pathol* 2002; 26:281–291.
3. Bell ET. A classification of renal tumors with observations on the frequency of the various types. *J Urol* 1938; 39:238–243.
4. Bielsa O, Lloreta J, and Gelabert-Mas. A Cystic renal cell carcinoma: pathological features, survival and implications for treatment. *Br J Urol* 1998; 82:16–20.
5. Blom JH, et al. Radical nephrectomy with and without lymph node dissection: preliminary results of the EORTC randomized phase III protocol 30881. EORTC Genitourinary Group. *Eur Urol* 1999; 36:570–575.
6. Bui MH, et al. Carbonic anhydrase IX is an independent predictor of survival in advanced renal clear cell carcinoma: implications for prognosis and therapy. *Clin Cancer Res* 2003; 9:802–811.
7. Cangiano T, et al. Sarcomatoid renal cell carcinoma: biologic behavior, prognosis, and response to combined surgical resection and immunotherapy. *J Clin Oncol* 1999; 17:523–528.
8. Cheville JC, et al. Stage pT1 conventional (clear cell) renal cell carcinoma: pathological features associated with cancer specific survival. *J Urol* 2001; 166:453–456.
9. Cheville JC, et al. Comparisons of outcome and prognostic features among histologic subtypes of renal cell carcinoma. *Am J Surg Pathol* 2003; 27:612–624.
10. Chow WH, et al. Rising incidence of renal cell cancer in the United States. *JAMA* 1999; 281:1628–1631.
11. Cindolo L, et al. Comparison of predictive accuracy of four prognostic models for nonmetastatic renal cell carcinoma after nephrectomy: a multicenter European study. *Cancer* 2005; 104:1362–1371.
12. Citterio G, et al. Reduction of brain metastasis following immunotherapy with interleukin-2 for stage IV renal cell cancer. *Acta Oncol* 1997; 36:228.
13. Corica FA, et al. Cystic renal cell carcinoma is cured by resection: a study of 24 cases with long-term followup. *J Urol* 1999; 161:408–411.
14. de Peralta-Venturina M, et al. Sarcomatoid differentiation in renal cell carcinoma: a study of 101 cases. *Am J Surg Pathol* 2001; 25:275–284.
15. deKernion JB. Reexamination of current staging for renal cell carcinoma. *J Urol* 2005; 173:680.

16. Delahunt B and Eble JN. Papillary renal cell carcinoma: a clinicopathologic and immunohistochemical study of 105 tumors. *Mod Pathol* 1997; 10:537–544.
17. Delahunt B, et al. Morphologic typing of papillary renal cell carcinoma: comparison of growth kinetics and patient survival in 66 cases. *Hum Pathol* 2001; 32:590–595.
18. Elson PJ, Witte RS, and Trump DL. Prognostic factors for survival in patients with recurrent or metastatic renal cell carcinoma. *Cancer Res* 1988; 48:7310–7313.
19. Fallick ML, et al. Nephrectomy before interleukin-2 therapy for patients with metastatic renal cell carcinoma. *J Urol* 1997; 158:1691–1695.
20. Farrow GM, Harrison EG, Jr., and Utz DC. Sarcomas and sarcomatoid and mixed malignant tumors of the kidney in adults. 3. *Cancer* 1968; 22:556–563.
21. Ficarra V, et al. Multiinstitutional European validation of the 2002 TNM staging system in conventional and papillary localized renal cell carcinoma. *Cancer* 2005; 104:968–974.
22. Ficarra V, et al. Proposal for revision of the TNM classification system for renal cell carcinoma. *Cancer* 2005; 104:2116–2123.
23. Flocks RH and Kadesky MC. Malignant neoplasms of the kidney; an analysis of 353 patients followed five years or more. *J Urol* 1958; 79:196–201.
24. Frank I, et al. An outcome prediction model for patients with clear cell renal cell carcinoma treated with radical nephrectomy based on tumor stage, size, grade and necrosis: the SSIGN score. *J Urol* 2002; 168:2395–2400.
25. Frank I, et al. Independent validation of the 2002 American Joint Committee on cancer primary tumor classification for renal cell carcinoma using a large, single institution cohort. *J Urol* 2005; 173:1889–1892.
26. Fuhrman SA, Lasky LC, and Limas C. Prognostic significance of morphologic parameters in renal cell carcinoma. *Am J Surg Pathol* 1982; 6:655–663.
27. Gettman MT, et al. Pathologic staging of renal cell carcinoma: significance of tumor classification with the 1997 TNM staging system. *Cancer* 2001; 91:354–361.
28. Giuliani L, et al. Radical extensive surgery for renal cell carcinoma: long-term results and prognostic factors. *J Urol* 1990; 143:468–473; discussion 473–464.
29. Glazer AA and Novick AC. Long-term followup after surgical treatment for renal cell carcinoma extending into the right atrium. *J Urol* 1996; 155:448–450.
30. Goldstein NS. The current state of renal cell carcinoma grading. Union Internationale Contre le Cancer (UICC) and the American Joint Committee on Cancer (AJCC). *Cancer* 1997; 80:977–980.
31. Green LK, et al. Role of nuclear grading in stage I renal cell carcinoma. *Urology* 1989; 34:310–315.
32. Grignon DJ, et al. Renal cell carcinoma. A clinicopathologic and DNA flow cytometric analysis of 103 cases. *Cancer* 1989; 64:2133–2140.
33. Guinan P, et al. Renal cell carcinoma: comparison of the TNM and Robson stage groupings. *J Surg Oncol* 1995; 59:186–189.
34. Guinan P, et al. TNM staging of renal cell carcinoma: Workgroup No. 3. Union International Contre le Cancer (UICC) and the American Joint Committee on Cancer (AJCC). *Cancer* 1997; 80:992–993.
35. Hafez KS, Fergany AF, and Novick AC. Nephron sparing surgery for localized renal cell carcinoma: impact of tumor

size on patient survival, tumor recurrence and TNM staging. *J Urol* 1999; 162:1930–1933.

36. Han KR, et al. Cystic renal cell carcinoma: biology and clinical behavior. *Urol Oncol* 2004; 22:410–414.

37. Han KR, et al. TNM T3a renal cell carcinoma: adrenal gland involvement is not the same as renal fat invasion. *J Urol* 2003; 169:899–903; discussion 903–904.

38. Han KR, et al. Validation of an integrated staging system toward improved prognostication of patients with localized renal cell carcinoma in an international population. *J Urol* 2003; 170:2221–2224.

39. Hatcher PA, et al. Surgical management and prognosis of renal cell carcinoma invading the vena cava. *J Urol* 1991;145:20–23; discussion 23–24.

40. Hermanek P and Schrott KM. Evaluation of the new tumor, nodes and metastases classification of renal cell carcinoma. *J Urol* 1990; 144:238–241; discussion 241–242.

41. Janzen NK, et al. Surveillance after radical or partial nephrectomy for localized renal cell carcinoma and management of recurrent disease. *Urol Clin North Am* 2003; 30:843–852.

42. Javidan J, et al. Prognostic significance of the 1997 TNM classification of renal cell carcinoma. *J Urol* 1999; 162: 1277–1281.

43. Jemal A, et al. Cancer statistics, 2005. *CA Cancer J Clin* 2005; 55:10–30.

44. Jones J, et al. Gene signatures of progression and metastasis in renal cell cancer. *Clin Cancer Res* 2005; 11:5730–5739.

45. Kattan MW, et al. A postoperative prognostic nomogram for renal cell carcinoma. *J Urol* 2001; 166:63–67.

46. Kennedy SM, et al. Collecting duct carcinoma of the kidney. *Hum Pathol* 1990; 21:449–456.

47. Kim HL, et al. Cachexia-like symptoms predict a worse prognosis in localized t1 renal cell carcinoma. *J Urol* 2004; 171:1810–1813.

48. Kim HL, et al. Prognostic significance of venous thrombus in renal cell carcinoma. Are renal vein and inferior vena cava involvement different? *J Urol* 2004;171:588–591.

49. Kim HL, et al. Paraneoplastic signs and symptoms of renal cell carcinoma: implications for prognosis. *J Urol* 2003; 170: 1742–1746.

50. Kim HL, et al. Using protein expressions to predict survival in clear cell renal carcinoma. *Clin Cancer Res* 2004; 10: 5464–5471.

51. Kinouchi T, et al. Impact of tumor size on the clinical outcomes of patients with Robson Stage I renal cell carcinoma. *Cancer* 1999; 85:689–695.

52. Kletscher BA, et al. Prospective analysis of the incidence of ipsilateral adrenal metastasis in localized renal cell carcinoma. *J Urol* 1996; 155:1844–1846.

53. Kononen J, et al. Tissue microarrays for high-throughput molecular profiling of tumor specimens. *Nat Med* 1998; 4: 844–847.

54. Kontak JA and Campbell SC. Prognostic factors in renal cell carcinoma. *Urol Clin North Am* 2003; 30:467–480.

55. Kosari F, et al. Clear cell renal cell carcinoma: gene expression analyses identify a potential signature for tumor aggressiveness. *Clin Cancer Res* 2005; 11:5128–5139.

56. Kovacs G, et al. The Heidelberg classification of renal cell tumours. *J Pathol* 1997; 183:131–133.

57. Lam JS, et al. Renal cell carcinoma 2005: new frontiers in staging, prognostication and targeted molecular therapy. *J Urol* 2005; 173:1853–1862.

58. Lam JS, et al. Postoperative surveillance protocol for patients with localized and locally advanced renal cell carcinoma based on a validated prognostic nomogram and risk group stratification system. *J Urol* 2005; 174:466–472; discussion 472; quiz 801.

59. Lam JS, et al. Clinicopathologic and molecular correlations of necrosis in the primary tumor of patients with renal cell carcinoma. *Cancer* 2005; 103:2517–2525.

60. Lau WK, et al. Prognostic features of pathologic stage T1 renal cell carcinoma after radical nephrectomy. *Urology* 2002; 59:532–537.

61. Lee CT, et al. Surgical management of renal tumors 4 cm. or less in a contemporary cohort. *J Urol* 2000; 163:730–736.

62. Leibovich BC, et al. Current staging of renal cell carcinoma. *Urol Clin North Am* 2003; 30:481–497, viii.

63. Leibovich BC, et al. Prediction of progression after radical nephrectomy for patients with clear cell renal cell carcinoma: a stratification tool for prospective clinical trials. *Cancer* 2003; 97:1663–1671.

64. Lerner SE, et al. Disease outcome in patients with low stage renal cell carcinoma treated with nephron sparing or radical surgery. *J Urol* 1996; 155:1868–1873.

65. Levy DA, et al. Stage specific guidelines for surveillance after radical nephrectomy for local renal cell carcinoma. *J Urol* 1998; 159:1163–1167.

66. Libertino JA, Zinman L, and Watkins E, Jr. Long-term results of resection of renal cell cancer with extension into inferior vena cava. *J Urol* 1987; 137:21–24.

67. Ljungberg B, et al. Vein invasion in renal cell carcinoma: impact on metastatic behavior and survival. *J Urol* 1995; 154:1681–1684.

68. Mani S, et al. Prognostic factors for survival in patients with metastatic renal cancer treated with biological response modifiers. *J Urol* 1995; 154:35–40.

69. Medeiros LJ, Gelb AB, and Weiss LM. Renal cell carcinoma. Prognostic significance of morphologic parameters in 121 cases. *Cancer* 1988; 61:1639–1651.

70. Mekhail TM, et al. Validation and extension of the Memorial Sloan-Kettering prognostic factors model for survival in patients with previously untreated metastatic renal cell carcinoma. *J Clin Oncol* 2005; 23:832–841.

71. Minervini A, et al. Regional lymph node dissection in the treatment of renal cell carcinoma: is it useful in patients with no suspected adenopathy before or during surgery? *BJU Int* 2001; 88:169–172.

72. Moch H, et al. Prognostic utility of the recently recommended histologic classification and revised TNM staging system of renal cell carcinoma: a Swiss experience with 588 tumors. *Cancer* 2000; 89:604–614.

73. Moinzadeh A and Libertino JA. Prognostic significance of tumor thrombus level in patients with renal cell carcinoma and venous tumor thrombus extension. Is all T3b the same? *J Urol* 2004; 171:598–601.

74. Motzer RJ, et al. Survival and prognostic stratification of 670 patients with advanced renal cell carcinoma. *J Clin Oncol* 1999; 17:2530–2540.

75. Motzer RJ, et al. Treatment outcome and survival associated with metastatic renal cell carcinoma of non-clear-cell histology. *J Clin Oncol* 2002; 20:2376–2381.

76. Pagano F, et al. Renal cell carcinoma with extension into the inferior vena cava: problems in diagnosis, staging and treatment. *Eur Urol* 1992; 22:200–203.

77. Palapattu GS, et al. Collecting system invasion in renal cell carcinoma: impact on prognosis and future staging strategies. *J Urol* 2003; 170:768–772; discussion 772.

78. Pantuck AJ, Zisman A, and Belldegrun AS. The changing natural history of renal cell carcinoma. *J Urol* 2001; 166: 1611–1623.

79. Pantuck AJ, et al. Renal cell carcinoma with retroperitoneal lymph nodes: role of lymph node dissection. *J Urol* 2003; 169:2076–2083.

80. Pantuck AJ, et al. Renal cell carcinoma with retroperitoneal lymph nodes. Impact on survival and benefits of immunotherapy. *Cancer* 2003; 97:2995–3002.

81. Parekh DJ, et al. Renal cell carcinoma with renal vein and inferior vena caval involvement: clinicopathological features, surgical techniques and outcomes. *J Urol* 2005; 173:1897–1902.

82. Parkin DM, et al. Global cancer statistics, 2002. *CA Cancer J Clin* 2005; 55:74–108.

83. Patard JJ, et al. Prognostic value of histologic subtypes in renal cell carcinoma: a multicenter experience. *J Clin Oncol* 2005; 23:2763–2771.

84. Patard JJ, et al. Use of the University of California Los Angeles integrated staging system to predict survival in renal cell carcinoma: an international multicenter study. *J Clin Oncol* 2004; 22:3316–3322.

85. Renshaw AA and Richie JP. Subtypes of renal cell carcinoma. Different onset and sites of metastatic disease. *Am J Clin Pathol* 1999; 111:539–543.

86. Ro JY, et al. Sarcomatoid renal cell carcinoma: clinicopathologic. A study of 42 cases. *Cancer* 1987; 59:516–526.

87. Robson CJ, Churchill BM, and Anderson W. The results of radical nephrectomy for renal cell carcinoma. *J Urol* 1969; 101:297–301.

88. Sella A, et al. Sarcomatoid renal cell carcinoma. A treatable entity. *Cancer* 1987; 60:1313–1318.

89. Siemer S, et al. Current TNM classification of renal cell carcinoma evaluated: revising stage T3a. *J Urol* 2005; 173: 33–37.

90. Siminovitch JP, Montie JE, and Straffon RA. Lymphadenectomy in renal adenocarcinoma. *J Urol* 1982; 127:1090–1091.

91. Skinner DG, et al. Diagnosis and management of renal cell carcinoma. A clinical and pathologic study of 309 cases. *Cancer* 1971; 28:1165–1177.

92. Skinner DG, et al. Vena caval involvement by renal cell carcinoma. Surgical resection provides meaningful long-term survival. *Ann Surg* 1989; 210:387–392; discussion 392–394.

93. Slaton JW, et al. Validation of UCLA integrated staging system (UISS) as a predictor for survival in patients undergoing nephrectomy for renal cell carcinoma. *J Urol* 2002; 167:192.

94. Sobin LH. TNM, sixth edition: new developments in general concepts and rules. *Semin Surg Oncol* 2003; 21:19–22.

95. Sobin LH and Wittekind C. *TNM Classification of Malignant Tumours*, 6 ed. Wiley-Liss: New York, 2002; p 193.

96. Staehler G and Brkovic D. The role of radical surgery for renal cell carcinoma with extension into the vena cava. *J Urol* 2000; 163:1671–1675.

97. Storkel S, et al. Classification of renal cell carcinoma: Workgroup No. 1. Union Internationale Contre le Cancer (UICC) and the American Joint Committee on Cancer (AJCC). *Cancer* 1997; 80:987–989.

98. Takahashi M, et al. Gene expression profiling of clear cell renal cell carcinoma: gene identification and prognostic classification. *Proc Natl Acad Sci USA* 2001; 98:9754–9759.

99. Takahashi M, et al. Molecular subclassification of kidney tumors and the discovery of new diagnostic markers. *Oncogene* 2003; 22:6810–6818.

100. Tan M. Gene expression profiling predicts survival in clear cell renal cell carcinoma. *J Clin Oncol* 2005; 23:4534.

101. Targonski PV, et al. Value of tumor size in predicting survival from renal cell carcinoma among tumors, nodes and metastases stage 1 and stage 2 patients. *J Urol* 1994; 152:1389–1392.

102. Terrone C, et al. The number of lymph nodes examined and staging accuracy in renal cell carcinoma. *BJU Int* 2003;91: 37–40.

103. Thompson RH, et al. Reclassification of patients with pT3 and pT4 renal cell carcinoma improves prognostic accuracy. *Cancer* 2005; 104:53–60.

104. Tsui KH, et al. Prognostic indicators for renal cell carcinoma: a multivariate analysis of 643 patients using the revised 1997 TNM staging criteria. *J Urol* 2000; 163:1090–1095; quiz 1295.

105. Tsui KH, et al. Is adrenalectomy a necessary component of radical nephrectomy? UCLA experience with 511 radical nephrectomies. *J Urol* 2000; 163:437–441.

106. Uemura H, et al. MN/CA IX/G250 as a potential target for immunotherapy of renal cell carcinomas. *Br J Cancer* 1999; 81:741–746.

107. Uzzo RG, et al. Renal cell carcinoma invading the urinary collecting system: implications for staging. *J Urol* 2002; 167:2392–2396.

108. Vasselli JR, et al. Lack of retroperitoneal lymphadenopathy predicts survival of patients with metastatic renal cell carcinoma. *J Urol* 2001; 166:68–72.

109. Vasselli JR, et al. Predicting survival in patients with metastatic kidney cancer by gene-expression profiling in the primary tumor. *Proc Natl Acad Sci USA* 2003; 100:6958–6963.

110. Zisman A, et al. Validation of the UCLA integrated staging system for patients with renal cell carcinoma. *J Clin Oncol* 2001; 19:3792–3793.

111. Zisman A, et al. Reevaluation of the 1997 TNM classification for renal cell carcinoma: T1 and T2 cutoff point at 4.5 rather than 7 cm. better correlates with clinical outcome. *J Urol* 2001; 166:54–58.

112. Zisman A, et al. Risk group assessment and clinical outcome algorithm to predict the natural history of patients with surgically resected renal cell carcinoma. *J Clin Oncol* 2002; 20:4559–4566.

113. Zisman A, et al. Improved prognostication of renal cell carcinoma using an integrated staging system. *J Clin Oncol* 2001; 19:1649–1657.

114. Zisman A, et al. Renal cell carcinoma with tumor thrombus extension: biology, role of nephrectomy and response to immunotherapy. *J Urol* 2003; 169:909–916.

5
Prognostic Factors: Markers

Benjamin I. Chung and John A. Libertino

Introduction

Renal cell carcinoma (RCC) is a neoplasm that still requires surgical extirpation as the mainstay in its cure. Currently, with the advancement of more sophisticated cross-sectional imaging modalities, it is a disease that has become more frequently diagnosed incidentally, prior to the development of symptomatic disease, with approximately 50% of cases diagnosed in this manner.[1] However, RCC is a potentially lethal entity, even in localized disease, with approximately 30% of patients developing tumor recurrence after radical nephrectomy for localized RCC.[2] The heterogeneity and unpredictability of RCC[3] make its natural history uncertain and determining accurate prognostic factors for survival is important and germane to contemporary practice, especially in counseling patients[1] and attempting to direct adjuvant therapy modalities to those who would benefit from them.[4]

Prognostic Factors

Prognostic factors can predict with accuracy the clinical course of a particular neoplastic process and the subsequent response by the host.[5] Such factors may include those that are involved with tumor growth, tumor aggressiveness, propensity for dissemination of metastases, or the patient's response to the neoplastic process.[5] Ideal prognostic factors should be clinically relevant, correlate with survival, and, on multivariate statistical analysis, have independent significance.[6] According to the College of American Pathologists, these factors fall under three categories. Category I is a marker that is well supported by the literature and generally used in patient management. Category II is a marker that has been extensively studied biologically and clinically, but is validated by few clinical outcome studies. Category III denotes a marker that does not meet criteria in Category I or II.[7] These are listed in Table 5-1.

Most factors that predict the patient's response to the neoplastic process fall into Category I. These include the Eastern Cooperative Oncology Group (ECOG) performance status, symptoms at presentation, weight loss, increased sedimentation rate, hypercalcemia, anemia, and increased alkaline phosphatase.[5] Some specific cancer-related factors also fall into Category I and these include pathological stage, grade, the presence of sarcomatoid histology, and the presence of metastases.[5] There are numerous other factors that are currently being studied and offer hope and promise, but have not been extensively validated and therefore fall into Category II or III. Category II prognostic factors include symptomatic presentation and performance status.[6] Tables 5-2 and 5-3 list patient-related and tumor-related prognostic factors.

Oncogenes

Abnormalities in chromosome structure or number are generally found to occur in many cancers[8] and current knowledge has led to the finding that the loss or inactivation of the short arm of chromosome 3 (3p) appears to be a necessary early step in the pathway to clear cell RCC.[5] Multiple authors have reported chromosome 3p aberrations and its consistent correlation with tumorigenesis.[8–10] Carroll and associates found an association with clear cell RCC and abnormalities in 3p. They also found that 3p abnormalities seemed to be limited to clear cell histology, with papillary RCC without 3p abnormalities.[8] Yoshida and associates discovered frequent 3p clonal abnormalities in their cytogenetic analysis of patients with nonfamilial RCC.[9] Also, in von Hippel–Lindau (VHL) syndrome, a gene has been identified, located on 3p, and deletions of this gene leads to RCC.[5]

Similarly, in other histological forms of RCC, other specific chromosomal abnormalities appear pathognomonic. In papillary or chromophillic RCC, several aberrations have been identified including loss of the Y chromosome and trisomy of chromosomes 3q, 7, 12, 16, and 20.[3,5] Speicher and associates examined the pattern of chromosomal abnormalities in chromophobe RCC and concluded that it is characterized by a pattern of multiple chromosomal losses in chromosomes 1, 2, 6, 10, 13, 17, 21, and Y and that this pattern may be helpful in distinguishing chromophobe from

TABLE 5-1. College of American Pathologists working classification for prognostic markers.

I	Well supported by the literature: generally used in patient management
II	Extensively studied biologically and/or clinically
	A. Tested in clinical trials
	B. Biological and correlative studies performed for clinical outcome studies
III	Currently do not meet criteria for Category I or Category II

TABLE 5-2. Patient-related prognostic factors.

Attribute	Unfavorable feature	Working classification
Demographic		
Age	–	III
Gender	–	III
Race	–	III
Geography	–	III
Socioeconomic	–	III
Patient-related		
Presentation	Symptomatic	I
Weight loss[a]	> 10% body weight	I
Performance status	ECOG 2–3	I
Acute phase reactants		
ESR	> 30	I
CRP	–	IIB
Anemia	< 10 g/dL female	I
	< 12 g/dL female	I
Serum calcium[a]	Hypercalcemia	I
Alkaline phosphatase[a]	↑	I

ECOG: Eastern Cooperative Oncology Group; ESR: erythrocyte sedimentation rate; CRP: C-reative protein.
[a]Applicable only in metastatic disease.

TABLE 5-3. Tumor-related prognostic factors.

Attribute	Unfavorable feature	Working classification
Macroscopic		
Surgical margins	Positive	I
Metastases		
No.	Multiple	I
Solitary	Unresectable	I
Location	Liver, lung	I
Microscopic		
pTNM	–	I
Grade	High grade	I
Histologic type	Conventional (clear);	I
	collecting duct	IIB
Architecture	Sarcomatoid	I
Nuclear morphometry	↑ area and shape variation	IIB
Biomolecular factors		
DNA content (ploidy)	Aneuploidy	IIB
Proliferation markers		
Ki-67 (MIB-1)	↑	IIB
AgNORs	↑	IIB
S-phase fraction	↑	IIB
PCNA	↑	IIB
Apoptosis markers		
p53	–	III
bcl-2	–	III
p21	–	III
Growth factors	–	III
Cell adhesion molecules	–	III
Angiogenesis	–	III
Host response factors	–	III
Tumors suppressor genes/ oncogenes	–	III
Resistance factors	–	III
Cytokines	–	III
Cytogenetic abnormalities/ loss of heterozygosity	–	III

AgNORs: argyrophilic nucleolar proteins; PCNA: proliferating cell nuclear antigen.

nonchromophobe RCC.[11] Also, at our institution, we have found an association with the tyrosine kinase gene Axl and upregulation with RCC.[12] However, the above information can help with the diagnosis of neoplasm, but cannot currently assist in the prediction of specific prognosis.

Ploidy

Ploidy of DNA has also been shown to predict the aggressiveness of RCC.[6] Aneuploidy refers to a situation in which the cell has deviated from an exact multiple of the normal haploid number of chromosomes. In such cases, the aneuploid cell may exhibit genomic instability, which predisposes it to enhanced survival and a propensity to metastasize.[13] Abou-Rebyeh and associates found that diploid tumors decreased as tumor size and pathological stage increased and also that aneuploidy increased as pathological stage increased. These authors also found that there were significant decreases in survival in patients with aneuploid tumors.[14] In papillary RCC, aneuploidy confers a poorer prognosis.[6] Grignon et al. reported that 10-year survival for diploid tumors was 79% versus 49% for nondiploid tumors. Also, mean time to death in diploid tumors was 62.3 months, compared with 34.1 in the nondiploid tumors. Not surprisingly, ploidy was an independent prognosticator of outcome.[15] However, in chromophobe RCC, a correlation between aneuploidy and prognosis has not been elucidated.[6] At this time, however, for RCC, there is not consistent agreement between all studies regarding the prognostic value of aneuploidy.[6] More studies are needed to confirm or deny the true value of aneuploidy.

Molecular Markers

The presence of accurate tumor markers could potentially make the identification of high-risk patients possible and allow for adjuvant therapeutic modalities. Also, tumor markers could provide novel sites for the targeting of new adjuvant therapies. Molecular markers that can be incorporated into future staging systems will hold great promise for the more accurate prognostic ability in RCC.[16] Advances in technology, such as gene arrays and high-throughput tissue arrays, make the detection of such markers more facile.[16] Microarray technology makes it possible to screen hundreds of different targets including DNA, RNA, and protein and rapidly analyze their clinical applicability.[16] Although no molecular markers currently fall into Category I status, many hold promise for achieving that status in the future. In other genitourinary cancers, specifically testicular cancer, biological markers do exist and can shape and guide management strategies. In RCC, we do not have the luxury of such markers, though promise does appear to be on the horizon of clinical applicability. As science and knowledge advances, the human genome project and microarray technology will exponentially expand what we know in a much more rapid fashion.[5]

Carbonic anhydrase IX (CA IX) is an enzyme that has recently been implicated in the pathogenesis of RCC. Its putative role is that of a regulator of intracellular and extracellular pH during periods of hypoxia in tumor cells.[17] Hypoxia has been implicated in the pathogenesis of RCC in the past, namely with the role of vascular endothelial growth factor (VEGF).[18] Bui and associates reported that 94% of their 321 tumor specimens stained for CA IX.[17] Upon detailed statistical analysis, the authors found that a cutoff of less than 85% staining implicated worsened survival.[17] Tumors with decreased CA IX expression were found to have the highest malignant potential and the highest propensity to metastasize. In fact, those patients with a higher percentage of CA IX staining also responded better to interleukin-2 (IL-2) immunotherapy.[17] The authors postulate that this type of information can potentially select out patients who would favorably respond to IL-2. For example, a recommendation for immunotherapy would be made in cases of high-risk localized RCC and low CA IX expression, a situation where currently, a diagnosis of localized RCC alone would rarely result in this recommendation.[17] In a separate study, Atkins and associates corroborated the results of the above study, showing that those with higher percentages of CA IX staining also responded more optimally to IL-2 immunotherapy.[19] If these findings hold true, this is a good example of the kind of specific prognostic knowledge that molecular markers can provide.

Ki-67 and silver-stained nucleolar organizer regions (AgNORs) have attained Category IIB status.[6] An increase in AgNOR proteins may signify an increased demand for ribosomal protein synthesis,[20] and in normal rapidly dividing cells, such as hepatocytes, a larger number of interphase AgNORs are observed.[20] Therefore, a high AgNOR quantity correlates with higher proliferative activity.[20] The theory is that aneuploid clones may contain more AgNOR regions

because of the need for increased ribosomal biogenesis in these rapidly dividing cells.[21] It is for these reasons that AgNORs are being intensively examined as prognostic factors. Pich and colleagues found that AgNOR quantity was independently significant for overall prognosis.[20] Also, those patients with lower levels of AgNORs had statistically improved survival than their counterparts with higher levels.[20] However, not all data have been consistent in showing AgNOR correlation with prognosis.[22] Yang and associates found that there were no survival differences between cohorts of patients with RCC with different AgNOR values. The authors concluded that they could not find prognostic value to AgNORs, unlike others.[22]

Ki-67 is a ubiquitous marker of cellular proliferation.[6] Its prognostic role appears to be in identifying clones of cells that are at higher propensity for active proliferation.[6] Some studies have shown its correlation with grade and survival in RCC.[23–25] Jochum and associates showed that MIB-1 staining, an antibody to Ki-67, was significantly lower in lower stage tumors and lower grade tumors.[23] Onda et al. showed a higher labeling index in patients who developed RCC recurrence compared to those who did not.[24] Rioux-Leclerq and colleagues found that Ki-67 immunostaining of RCC specimens was localized to the nucleus and from a prognostic standpoint, a 20% labeling index was the critical value. A labeling index of 20% or greater conferred independent statistical significance for poor outcome. A mean survival of 67 months was found in those patients with an index of less than 20% versus 42 months for those with an index of greater than 20% ($p < 0.00001$).[25] Incidentally, they also found a significant association with p53 also, with the same 20% cutoff labeling index applicable. Those patients with less than 20% p53 staining had a median survival of 61 months whereas those with greater than 20% p53 staining had a median survival of 34 months ($p < 0.0004$).[25] Such data could potentially be very helpful in identifying previously unidentifiable patients with localized RCC who are at greater risk for recurrence and metastasis. However, others have shown that Ki-67 did not offer any valuable prognostic information.[26] Gelb and associates found that higher Ki-67 expression did correlate with higher grade tumors, but that there was no independent prognostic value attributed to Ki-67 alone.[26] Therefore, more studies are needed to validate the use of Ki-67 in clinical practice.

Proliferating cell nuclear antigen (PCNA) is another molecular marker that holds promise. It also is an indicator of cell proliferative activity and therefore a potential marker for biological aggressiveness.[6] Onda et al. looked at the prognostic value of PCNA in association with Ki-67.[24] They found that PCNA levels tended to be higher in those patients who had RCC tumor recurrences compared with those did not have tumor recurrence.[24] Some authors have not found that PCNA provides prognostic information in RCC[25] while others have found it to be an independent prognostic factor predicting survival, with a higher PCNA index conferring poorer prognosis.[26] It was found that survival was significantly diminished in those patients whose tumors expressed greater than 5% of nuclei staining positive for PCNA. It was also found that PCNA immunostaining of the nucleus was an independent prognostic factor in those patients with Robson Stage 1 RCC.[26] Like many molecular factors, more studies and data are needed to elucidate the true value of PCNA in RCC.

p53 is a gene product that has been studied extensively in other genitourinary cancers, including transitional cell cancer. Normal p53 expression leads to cell cycle arrest and either DNA repair or apoptosis.[6] In cases where p53 is mutated, these normal processes are altered and can lead to tumorigenesis. p53's role in RCC has not been well characterized and the data are conflicting. One series showed that p53 expression did confer prognostic information.[27] Another study showed that p53 overexpression and a high mutation rate of the p53 gene seem to occur with sarcomatoid RCC, indicating a possible link with p53 and more aggressive histological behavior.[28] It was also found that the p53 gene was mutated at a high rate in those portions of the tumor that had undergone sarcomatoid transformation.[29,30] The authors concluded that p53 mutations may lead to sarcomatoid transformation of the tumor, which could lead to more aggressive biological behavior.[29–31] One study performed with microarray technology showed that p53 had prognostic significance in both univariate and multivariate analyses.[29] However, other series have not shown this association, with very minimal staining of RCC for p53. Gelb et al. found that only 2 out of 52 tumors stained positive for p53 protein expression, with statistical analysis confirming no prognostic significance.[26]

The overexpression of the Bcl-2 protein has been studied as a prognostic factor. It is postulated to inhibit apoptosis and therefore confer a survival advantage in those clones with the mutation, leading to neoplastic cellular behavior.[21] Skolarikos et al. found that although Bcl-2 protein expression was higher in RCC compared with normal renal tissue and aneuploid tumors had higher Bcl-2 expression than euploid tumors, and no prognostic significance was found with Bcl-2 expression.[32] More scientific research needs to be performed to accurately categorize this protein as important in predicting survival in a clinical setting.[21]

p21 is a target of p53 and an inhibitor of cyclin-dependent kinases,[21] which are implicated in the maintenance of the cell cycle and apoptotic processes. Because of its association with p53, it has been studied in relation to RCC. Shalitin et al. found that p21 could potentially be a tumor marker for RCC because changes in the level of serum p21 appears linked to the clinical course.[33] They showed that p21 protein was overexpressed in RCC compared to control normal kidney tissue.[33] In their series, two patients with elevated p21 levels after surgery were found to have distant metastatic disease and lower p21 levels overall seemed to correlate with a favorable prognosis. However, more studies and data are needed to validate this particular molecular marker.

In the production of new blood vessels that feed the growing tumor, neovascularization promotes growth of the tumor in the facilitation of nutrient and metabolite exchange in RCC.[21] In a study of intratumoral microvessel density as a measure of neovascularity, Yoshino and associates found that it was highly prognostic for overall survival.[34] In their series, the microvessel count was higher in patients with metastatic disease than in those who were disease free (p <0.004). Also, the survival was significantly less in patients with more than 30 microvessels per 200× field . On multivariate analysis, the only prognostic factor in patients with pathological stage T1–2 M0 disease was microvessel density.[34] However, in another study, MacLennan and Bostwick found that there was no association between microvessel density and cancer-specific survival.[35] They found no correlation between microvessel density and clinical stage, pathological stage, tumor grade, or cancer-specific survival.[33] Therefore, although intuitively speaking, this area of neovascularity and microvessel density seems promising as a measure of prognosis, it has yet to yield consistent results in clinical studies.

Clinical Signs and Symptoms

The classic triad of hematuria, flank pain, and a palpable mass causing symptomatic presentation of RCC is currently a rare entity. In contemporary practice, approximately 50% of the cases of RCC are discovered incidentally.[1] Not surprisingly, the presence of clinical symptoms or signs does confer a poorer prognosis than asymptomatic disease.[36] Several series in the literature have corroborated this. Pantuck and associates have described a significantly improved 5-year survival in those patients with incidentally diagnosed tumors (85.3%) versus those with clinically symptomatic RCC (62.5%).[37] Also, poor performance status or weight loss portends a poor prognosis.[36] Tsui and colleagues examined the effect of performance status as an independent factor for survival. They found that those patients with an ECOG performance status of 1 or greater were found to have a 5-year survival of 51% compared with a 81% 5-year survival in those with an ECOG status of 0.[38]

During physical examination, the presence of palpable disease indicating a large tumor[36] or palpable lymphadenopathy due to disseminated RCC portends a poor prognosis[36] as does the stigmata of vena cava involvement of tumor thrombus including lower extremity edema and right-sided or nonreducible varicocele. Kim and associates found that cachexia was an independent predictor of diminished survival.[39] The authors' definition of cachexia, which included hypoalbuminemia, weight loss, anorexia, or malaise, was found to be an independent prognostic factor on statistical analysis. Multivariate analysis revealed that cachexia was significantly associated with a lower cancer-specific survival.[39] Selli and colleagues also found that age and weight loss were prognostic factors for survival in those without metastatic disease.[40]

Sex

McNichols and associates describe a survival difference between men and women, with women having better survival, although women did not have a more favorable stage and grade than men.[41] These differences in survival were most apparent in pathological Stage I, Grade 1 tumors; in pathological Stage III, Grade 3 or 4 or in Stage IV tumors, there was no sex difference on survival.[41] In the UCLA Kidney Cancer Database, the ratio of male to female is 2.2:1, indicating that RCC is more common in men.[42] Green et al. also found that men had worse survival than women and also had more tumors of the worst nuclear grade, Grade 4.[43] However, Selli and colleagues found that the sex of the patient had no impact on survival.[40] There does not appear to be a unanimous consensus as to patient sex as a prognosticator for survival.

Laboratory Values

In a multivariate survival analysis, Motzer and colleagues found that abnormal laboratory values were prognostic factors in the survival in patients with RCC.[4] In their series, low Karnofsky performance status, low hemoglobin, high lactate dehydrogenase, and high corrected serum calcium were all prognostic factors predicting diminished survival.[4] With these factors in mind, Zisman and associates, also from UCLA, attempted to integrate multiple factors including conventional TNM stage, ECOG performance status, and the Fuhrman grade of the tumor into the UCLA Integrated Staging System (UISS). The authors found that their system, the UISS, did correlate with patient survival,[44] and has been validated in an international multicenter trial.[45] As mentioned previously, Kim and associates found that cachexia, defined as hypoalbuminemia, weight loss, anorexia, and malaise, conferred a poor prognosis in patients with pathological stage T1 RCC.[39] The patients with cachexia had a higher tumor grade, higher ECOG stage, and worse UISS than those without cachexia symptoms. Also, the disease-specific survival was significantly worse in those cachectic patients.[39] Boxer et al. also found weight loss and hyperhaptoglobinemia as predictive of patients living less than 2 years.[46] Lieber and associates found that the presence of weight loss, microhematuria, and fever portended a poor prognosis.[47]

The laboratory finding of hypercalcemia has been implicated as a poor prognostic factor in patients with RCC. Chasan et al. found that in their patient population of 160 with RCC, 27 had hypercalcemia and 24 of these 27 had Stage IV disease. The remaining three patients had Stage I and II RCC. From their study, it appears that the predilection for higher stage disease with hypercalcemia is clear. Also, the overall survival of all patients with hypercalcemia with Stage IV disease was on average only 87.3 days. Surprisingly, the authors did not find any differences in survival according to serum calcium level.[48]

Prognostic Nomograms and Algorithms

Zisman and colleagues from UCLA created a UISS in an attempt to optimize the current TNM staging system and add other prognostic factors into the equation, including performance status and Fuhrman tumor grade.[44] Their algorithm has been validated in an international multicenter, as previously mentioned.[45] However, the UISS has been criticized because it places patients in a low-risk, intermediate-risk, and high-risk category and does not make a prediction as to survival.[2] More recently, a prognostic nomogram has been created by Sorbellini and associates from Memorial Sloan Kettering Cancer Center (MSKCC). Their nomogram included multiple prognostic variables including pathological stage, Fuhrman grade, tumor size, the presence of necrosis, the presence of vascular invasion, and clinical presentation, whether it was incidental asymptomatic, locally symptomatic, or systemically symptomatic. These various prognostic factors were chosen because the authors felt they imparted important additional clinical information that would serve to better define the clinical behavior of each individual tumor. The nomogram is demonstrated in Fig. 5-1. The authors applied their nomogram to their database of approximately 700 patients and a concordance index of 0.82 was calculated.[49] Ultimately, the MSKCC nomogram does attempt to calculate a 5-year probability of freedom from recurrence, which is an advantage of it over the UISS. From the Mayo Clinic, Frank et al. created their own prognostic system, the size, stage, grade, and necrosis (SSIGN) score.[50] The variables in their system include 1997 TNM stage, tumor size, nuclear grade, histological tumor necrosis, sarcomatoid component, cystic architecture, multifocality, and surgical margin status. In their analysis of 1801 patients, they found that pathological stage, tumor size greater than 5 cm, nuclear grade, and tumor necrosis were associated with poor patient outcome on multivariate analysis.[50] The SSIGN score assigns an individual score to each prognostic variable and the final tally is plugged into the final algorithm, which determines estimated cancer-specific survival at years 1, 3, 5, 7, and 10 (Fig. 5-2 and Tables 5-4 and 5-5).[50]

Tumor Size and Stage

Currently, the prognosis of RCC can be surmised by a variety of means. First and foremost, the pathological staging and grading of the primary tumor leads to value in predicting outcomes. However, a criticism is that staging alone combines a heterogeneous group of patients together, so that the natural history and biological aggressiveness of each individual tumor can be hard to predict by staging alone.[3] Some tumors will inevitably behave more indolently than others, but we currently do not have an accurate method to determine which ones will and which ones will not.

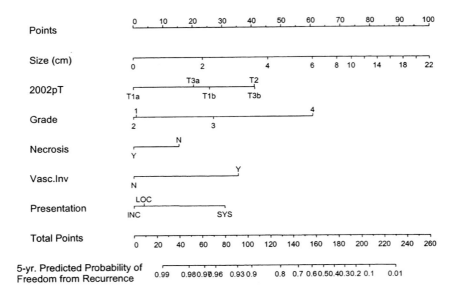

Indications for Physician: Locate the patient's tumor size on the Size axis. Draw a line upwards to the Points axis to determine how many points towards recurrence the patient receives for his symptoms. Repeat this process for the other axes, each time drawing straight upward to the Point axis. Sum the points achieved for each predictor and locate this sum on the Total Points axis. Draw a straight line down to find the patient's probability of remaining recurrence free for 5 years assuming he or she does not die of another cause first.
Instruction to the Patient: "Mr. X, if we had 100 men or women exactly like you, we would expect (predicted percentage from nomogram) to remain free of their disease 5 years following surgery, though recurrence after 5 years is still possible".

FIGURE 5-1. Nomogram of prognostic variables.

The size of tumors as well can be important in predicting prognosis. An early paper by Bell in 1938 found that tumors less than 3 cm in size had the lowest incidence of metastases.[51] Similarly, Fuhrman found that no RCC tumor in their cohort measuring 3 cm or less metastasized, whereas 86% of tumors 12 cm or greater metastasized.[52] Grignon et al. found that when a cutoff size of 5 cm was employed into

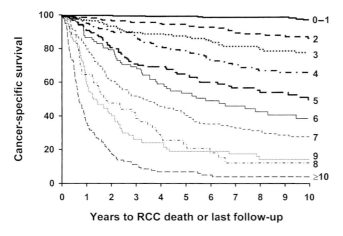

FIGURE 5-2. Clear cell SSICN score.

survival analysis, the survival difference between the two groups reached statistical significance.[15] Of note, the smallest tumor that caused patient death was only 2.7 cm in size.[15] Green and colleagues found that patients with a tumor size greater than 8 cm had significantly worse survival than those with tumor size smaller than 8 cm.[48] Others have found that patients with tumors less than 10 cm in size had a significantly better cancer-free survival than those with tumors greater than 10 cm in size. They also reported a 3 cm tumor having metastasized, which is somewhat alarming, given the low rate of metastasis historically of a tumor this size.[53]

Tumor staging systems, which have been modified as clinical data have further clarified outcomes, have been shown to impart important prognostic information.[37,54] Currently, the most widely used tumor staging is the TNM system. Although the accuracy of the current system is occasionally brought into question,[55,56] especially regarding the level of caval involvement and differences in survival, the TNM system will continue to be fine tuned as needed. For example, the recently proposed T1a and T1b cutoff reflects that RCC <4 cm in size are amenable to partial nephrectomy.[57] Most would agree that TNM staging is an integral contemporary prognosticator of RCC and cancer-free survival, despite its potential shortcomings.

TABLE 5-4. SSIGN score algorithm.[a]

Feature	Score
T Stage	
pT1	0
pT2	1
pT3a	2
pT3b	2
pT3c	2
pT4	0
N stage	
pNx	0
pN0	0
pN1	2
pN2	2
M stage	
pM0	0
pM1	4
Tumor size (cm)	
Less than 5	0
5 or greater	2
Nuclear grade	
1	0
2	0
3	1
4	3
Necrosis	
Absent	0
Present	2

[a] The scores in this table are added together and the total is used to determine survival using Table 5-5.

Since Robson described the modern radical nephrectomy, multiple studies have been performed to illustrate long-term survival after the procedure is completed. Bassil et al. found that the TNM staging system can accurately predict survival and prognosis in RCC.[58] Golimbu and associates showed that improved overall survival was correlated with lower stage disease.[59] Moch and colleagues showed that the 1997 pathologic T staging classification system significantly correlated with overall patient survival in their patient cohort with conventional clear cell RCC.[60] They also found that the presence of hematogeneous metastases, lymph node dissem-

inated disease, tumor necrosis, and sarcomatoid features was all associated with poor overall outcome.[60] Giuliani and associates found that higher pathological T stages were associated with an increased incidence of lymph node metastases and also distant metastases.[61] Selli and associates also found a strong correlation between pathological stage and overall survival.[40] It appears clear from the data above that survival is inversely correlated with higher stage disease.[54] Pathological stage as a prognostic factor appears to be relatively free of controversy.

The question of renal vein involvement and the impact of this finding on survival, however, is controversial. Some have argued that the presence of renal vein involvement uniformly predicts a poor outcome, while others have stated the opposite. Fuhrman and associates found no difference in survival between Stage I renal tumors that had renal vein involvement and those Stage I tumors without renal vein involvement.[52] Selli et al. found that renal vein involvement was not prognostic for a worse outcome.[40] Golimbu and colleagues found that there was no significant difference in 5-year survival whether renal vein involvement was either gross or microscopic. However, when 10-year survival was examined, there was a worse prognosis when gross renal vein involvement existed, when compared with microscopic renal vein involvement.[59] They also found that lymph node-positive disease conferred a poorer prognosis and when concomitant tumor extension into the renal vein and perinephric fat also existed, survival was even worse, with a 17% 5-year survival and a 5% 10-year survival.[59]

Lymph Node-Positive Disease

Bassil and associates found that lymph node-positive disease was prognostic for poor survival. They found only a 7% 5-year survival in their cohort with N+ disease.[58] Pantuck et al. found that the presence of positive lymph nodes in patients with metastatic disease portended a worse prognosis than in those patients with metastatic disease without lymph node involvement.[62] Survival was 20.4 months in their N0M1 cohort compared to 10.5 months in their N + M1 cohort

TABLE 5-5. Estimated cancer-specific survival following radical nephrectomy for clear cell renal cell carcinoma by SSIGN score.

SSIGN score	No. (%)	% Estimated cancer-specific survival (SE, No. at risk)				
		Year 1	Year 3	Year 5	Year 7	Year 10
0–1	402 (22.3)	100.0 (0.0, 378)	99.7 (0.3, 340)	99.4 (0.4, 303)	98.7 (0.6, 235)	97.1 (1.1, 162)
2	235 (13.0)	99.1 (0.6, 221)	95.9 (1.4, 191)	94.8 (1.5, 162)	90.3 (2.2, 131)	85.3 (2.9, 89)
3	199 (11.0)	97.4 (1.1, 185)	90.3 (2.2, 153)	87.8 (2.5, 127)	81.8 (3.1, 95)	77.9 (3.5, 62)
4	206 (11.4)	95.4 (1.5, 182)	87.1 (2.5, 147)	79.1 (3.1, 116)	70.8 (3.6, 86)	66.2 (3.9, 53)
5	153 (8.5)	91.1 (2.4, 131)	71.3 (3.8, 92)	65.4 (4.1, 70)	57.1 (4.5, 48)	50.0 (5.0, 33)
6	88 (4.9)	87.0 (3.7, 73)	69.8 (5.1, 55)	54.0 (5.6, 37)	46.4 (5.8, 30)	38.8 (6.0, 18)
7	200 (11.1)	80.3 (2.9, 152)	52.4 (3.7, 89)	41.0 (3.8, 61)	34.0 (3.7, 45)	28.1 (3.7, 27)
8	61 (3.4)	65.1 (6.1, 39)	38.9 (6.4, 21)	23.6 (5.8, 10)	12.7 (5.1, 4)	12.7 (5.1, 4)
9	100 (5.6)	60.5 (5.0, 57)	26.8 (4.7, 23)	19.6 (4.3, 14)	18.1 (4.2, 12)	14.8 (4.0, 8)
10 or greater	157 (8.7)	36.2 (4.0, 53)	11.9 (2.8, 14)	7.4 (2.4, 8)	4.6 (1.9, 5)	4.6 (1.9, 4)

($p < 0.002$). Another study showed very similar results, with a median 14.7-month survival in patients with N0M1 disease and a median 8.5 months in those with N + M1 disease.[63] In a paper from our institution, we found that patients with caval tumor thrombus and concomitant lymph node involvement or metastatic disease had a median survival of only 1.2 years, with no patient surviving beyond 4.8 years.[64] Skinner showed that if the tumor was confined to Gerota's fascia without regional lymph node involvement, in his series, 5- and 10-year survival was 55% and 43%, respectively.[65] In their series, however, if regional lymph nodes were involved in the tumor, there was a dramatic decrease in survival with 5- and 10-year survival at 16% and 8%. Also, if direct extension to contiguous visceral structures existed, 5- and 10-year survivals were dismal, each at 0%.[65]

Metastatic Disease

The presence of metastatic disease is an ominous clinical finding. Skinner et al. found that in their 77 patients with Robson Stage IV disease, the 5-year survival was 8% and the 10-year survival was 7%.[66] Selli and associates from Duke showed that the presence of metastatic disease greatly diminished overall survival. In fact, they found that the most important factor in predicting survival was the presence or absence of metastatic disease.[40] No patient with metastatic disease had a Grade 1 tumor, tying in the association between grade and stage. The authors found that 86% of those with no metastatic disease had either Grade 1 or 2 tumors and, conversely, of those with metastatic disease, 78% had either Grade 3 or 4 tumors. There was no difference in survival between those with soft tissue metastases or with bony metastases. Also, renal vein involvement, in their cohort, did not portend a worse prognosis in those with nonmetastatic RCC. Neither sex nor race had an impact on survival. Siminovitch and associates also found that 66 out of 71 patients with metastatic disease had died over a mean follow-up interval of 43 months.[67] They also found that there was no difference in survival dependent upon site of metastasis, whether lung, bone, liver, or a combination of sites was involved.[67] With regard to what factors could possibly improve prognosis in those with metastatic RCC, Maldazys and de Kernion found that a long time interval between nephrectomy and the onset of metastases, normal performance status, and pulmonary-only metastases improved survival in this cohort.[68]

Golimbu et al. in their analysis of their cohort with metastatic disease found that all, except the patients with a solitary metastasis to the contralateral kidney, treated by partial nephrectomy, had a uniformly poor prognosis.[59] Those with a solitary metastasis to the contralateral kidney only numbered five in total. Of these, three out of the five were alive at 60, 96, and 139 months postoperatively. The rest of the patients with distant metastases did poorly. Of the 88 patients with distant metastases to organs other than the contralateral kidney, only two survived more than 5 years.

The 28 patients with lung metastases had a mean survival of 11 months. Those 25 patients with bone metastases had an average survival of 14 months. The 11 patients with soft tissue and bone metastases had a mean survival of 12 months. The 28 patients with soft tissue metastases other than pulmonary metastases survived an average of 10 months.[59] No matter how one looks at the data, the presence of metastatic disease is an ominous prognostic sign and few would argue to the contrary.

Collecting System Involvement

With regards to collecting system invasion of RCC tumor, Uzzo and associates found that prognosis was determined upon the pathological stage of the tumor. In those tumors that were stage pT3 or greater, there was no difference in survival based on whether the tumor invaded the collecting system. However, in those lower stage tumors, less than pathological stage T3, which involved the collecting system, did confer a poorer prognosis.[69] In another study, Palapattu and colleagues found that like the above study, patients with collecting system involvement, especially those with lower stage tumors, had a significantly lower cancer-specific survival. Also, in multivariate statistical analysis, a 1.4 times greater risk for death was conferred in those with collecting system invasion.[70] Golimbu and associates also found that lack of collecting system invasion by RCC was significantly associated with a better overall prognosis.[59] Siminovitch et al. showed a sharply decreased survival in those with tumor invasion through the medulla and into the collecting system, with a 5-year survival diminishing from 82% to 58%.[67] On the other hand, McNichols et al. from the Mayo Clinic showed no significant difference in survival in patients of the same pathologic stage (Stage III), whether they had tumor invasion of the renal pelvis or not.[41] Overall, there is discrepancy as to the prognostic impact of collecting system invasion by tumor. The fact that higher stage tumors with collecting system invasion have a higher predilection to other aggressive features, such as larger size, invasion of perinephric fat, and lymph node involvement, makes it hard to make a sweeping statement about the prognostic value of collecting system invasion.[54]

Inferior Vena Cava Involvement

One of the characteristics of renal cell carcinoma is the ability of the tumor to extend into the venous outflow of the kidney via the renal vein and inferior vena cava. In most published studies, the incidence of this occurrence is approximately 4–10% of cases.[71,72] When RCC presents in this fashion, the management becomes tailored to the level of caval extension. No matter what the level of tumor thrombus extension, the management is strictly surgical.

Despite the presence of tumor thrombus, excellent 5- and 10-year survivals have been reported in the literature. If the tumor is surgically resectable and there are no lymph node metastases, survival at 5 years had been reported to be as high as 68%.[73] At our institution, we have shown a survival of 64% at 5 years and 57% 10-year survival in a cohort of 100 patients.[74] Sogani and associates reported a 50% survival in those patients with no evidence of metastasis at surgery over a mean duration of 93 months.[72]

Unresectable Caval Thrombus

Hatcher et al. performed a retrospective study that underscores the need for complete removal of tumor thrombus, including thrombus that invades the caval wall. In their series, they found that in those patients with free floating tumor thrombus that was completely removed with a primary tumor confined to Gerota's fascia, the survival was 69% at 5 years, compared to those patients with the tumor invading the caval wall, whose survival was 26% at 5 years. In those patients with caval wall extension of tumor, which was completely resected, their 5-year survival was 57%. Their surgical technique included utilizing frozen section analysis of the cava until a negative margin was obtained.[75] This study underscores other authors' findings that residual tumor thrombus will lead to greatly diminished survival. Neves and Zincke found a similar result. In those patients with incomplete thrombus removal, 5-year survival was 17.5% as opposed to a 68% 5-year survival when thrombus was completely removed.[73] The authors also found that the grade of tumor significantly affected survival with those with Grade 1 and 2 tumors doing significantly better than those with Grade 3 and 4 tumors (approximately 70% vs. 40% 5-year survival).[73] Skinner and colleagues also found that if a complete tumor resection was not possible, those patients uniformly did poorly, with only 8% survival at 1 year postoperatively.[76] These findings indicate that tumor thrombus that is not amenable to complete resection is a poor prognostic factor.

Level of Caval Involvement

Sosa and colleagues explored the significance of level of vena caval involvement in overall survival. In their series of 24 patients, they found that the 10 patients who had infrahepatic involvement had a 2-year survival of 80% and a mean survival of 61.4 months, whereas the 14 patients with thrombus to the level of the hepatic veins or above had a 2-year survival of 21% and a mean survival of 22.9 months suggesting a survival advantage to a lower level of thrombus involvement.[77] Other authors have not found a difference in survival based on the level of tumor thrombus.[78] At our institution, we examined the prognostic significance of tumor thrombus level in our cohort of 153 patients. We found no statistically significant survival differences dependent upon tumor thrombus level. The 10-year overall cancer specific survival was 30%, 19%, and 29% for level I, II, and III,

respectively ($p = 0.48$).[55] However, others have found a survival difference dependent upon level of tumor thrombus. Kim et al. found that in their patient cohort, those with T3c disease, a tumor extending above the diaphragm, had significantly worse survival than those with tumor involvement below the diaphragm.[79] They also found no difference in survival between patients with renal vein involvement of the tumor and those with a tumor extending below the diaphragm.[79] The question regarding a difference in survival based on tumor thrombus therefore remains unanswered and controversial.

Lymph Node-Positive Disease and Metastatic Tumor in Caval Thrombus

Skinner showed that if the tumor was confined to Gerota's fascia without regional lymph node involvement, in his series, 5- and 10-year survival was 55% and 43%, respectively.[65] In that series, however, if regional lymph nodes were involved in the tumor, there was a dramatic decrease in survival with 5- and 10-year survival at 16% and 8%. Also, if direct extension to contiguous visceral structures existed, 5- and 10-year survivals were dismal, each at 0%.[65] However, most large studies have demonstrated acceptable 5- and 10-year survival in such patients in the absence of metastatic disease. Despite a few studies in the literature that report modest survival with adjuvant immunotherapy for metastatic disease in such cases,[80] most other authors report uniformly dismal survival with metastatic disease.[64,81]

Tumor Grade

Because of the unpredictable behavior and histological appearance of RCC, Fuhrman and associates classified histological RCC into grades, dependent upon morphological parameters.[52] Their grading system is based solely upon nuclear features and has been shown to have prognostic significance.[52] In their original paper, Grade 1 tumors were characterized by small, round uniform nuclei with absent or inconspicuous nucleoli. Grade 2 tumors had larger nuclei than Grade 1, approximately 15 μm in size, with apparent irregularities in outline and nucleoli visible under high power. Grade 3 tumors had larger, approximately 20-μm nuclei, with an obvious irregularity in outline, and large nucleoli visible under low power. Grade 4 tumors have features similar to Grade 3 tumors and also bizarrely shaped, often multilobar nuclei and chromatin clumping.[52] Over time, the most widely utilized tumor grading system for RCC in North America has become the Fuhrman system.[36] Fuhrman's original paper demonstrated that their nuclear grading system was correlated with rate of metastatic disease, with higher grade tumors having a higher rate of metastases.[52] Fuhrman also found that the rate of metastases in Grade 1 tumors was significantly less than in Grade 2 tumors.[52] The authors found that nuclear grade was the most significant prognostic factor in predicting outcome in their patient cohort with Stage I RCC. Ultimately, they concluded that nuclear grading could expand on the limitations of staging as a prognostic factor, in stratifying survival in Stage I disease.[52]

Like many grading systems, the Fuhrman system does suffer from interobserver variability and lack of reproducibility.[36] The Fuhrman system is split into four grades[52] with a favorable prognosis assigned with lower grade tumors. However, the difficulty of assigning grades to RCC is reflected in the high interobserver variability and low reproducibility.[82] The level of interobserver agreement appears to be quite variable.[82] Also, the four-grade Fuhrman system may be suboptimal partly due to the fact that RCC is a heterogeneous tumor, composed of cells of different grades, rather than cells that all have the same grade.[82] Lang and colleagues found that a better level of agreement was achieved with a two-tiered grading system, where tumors were split into low grade (Grades 1–2) and high grade (Grades 3–4).[82] Part of the problem in a four-tiered grading system may be that the original system did not define the minimum proportion of the highest grade area that warranted assignment of this elevated grade to the tumor.[82] Conversely, some authors have shown a good interobserver agreement and concordance in Fuhrman grading.[83] Nevertheless, despite its shortcomings, many studies have shown grading to be a significant prognostic factor. Bretheau et al. found that nuclear grade was significantly correlated with tumor stage, synchronous metastases, lymph node involvement, renal vein involvement, tumor size, and perirenal fat involvment.[83] Selli and associates showed that the grade of the tumor was an important predictor of survival. Patients with low-grade RCC had a statistically significant increased survival over their counterparts with higher grade disease. They showed that 90% of patients with Grade 1 or Grade 2 tumors survived 5 years, but only 55% of those with Grade 3 and 33% of those with Grade 4 RCC survived 5 years.[40] Patients without metastatic disease also tended to have lower grade RCC than those with metastases. Skinner found that the prognostic factor that was most highly correlated with survival was pathological stage; however, grading was also correlated with survival, but not as closely as was stage. The authors speculated that the reason for this could be due to the overall heterogeneity of RCC, with a large variability in histological patterns and grades, even within a single specimen.[66] Giuliani and colleagues found that higher grade tumors were associated with more aggressive behavior, including an increased incidence of lymph node metastases and distant metastases.[61]

Sarcomatoid Renal Cell Carcinoma

Sarcomatoid RCC represents an aggressive variant of RCC. In Fuhrman's original series, spindle cell histology showed a high rate of metastatic disease.[52] In another large series, Mian and colleagues examined a cohort of 108 patients with sarcomatoid RCC. Their analysis revealed, not surprisingly, very

unfavorable findings with regard to overall survival. Median overall survival was only 9 months. Even those patients with localized disease had a median survival of only 17 months. A large number (89%) were symptomatic at presentation and metastatic disease was present in 77% at presentation. The most common symptoms were pain, hematuria, weight loss, and fatigue. Systemic therapy, including chemotherapy and immunotherapy, were largely ineffective. When prognostic factors specific to sarcomatoid RCC were analyzed, the authors found that survival was improved in those with clinically localized disease, a single metastatic site, and in those who had a partial response to systemic therapy.[84] Skinner and associates showed that pure spindle cell tumors had significantly decreased survival. Like Skinner,[66] Boxer et al. also found that the presence of fusiform (spindle-shaped, sarcomatoid) cells in the pathological specimen was strongly prognostic for a survival of less than 2 years.[46] Similarly, Medeiros and associates found a significantly adverse prognosis in those patients with spindle cell sarcomatoid RCC.[53] Others have illustrated that a histological predominance of pure clear and granular cells in the tumor correlated with improved survival and that those patients with mostly spindle cells and anaplastic elements usually died of their disease within 5 years.[59] They also found that with increasing pathological stage, the percentage of spindle cell tumors increased, conferring a poor prognosis.[59] The authors felt that considering their findings, those tumors composed of pure clear or granular well-differentiated cells conferred a good prognosis, whereas those tumors with predominantly spindle cell and anaplastic elements conferred a poor prognosis.

Nuclear Morphometry

Pound et al. examined nuclear morphometry as a prognosticator for RCC recurrence in clinically localized disease.[85] As mentioned previously, the rationale for improved prognostic factors in this group of patients is the approximately 30% of patients with clinically localized disease who develop metastatic disease and the difficulty in predicting who will and who will not develop metastases.[85] Pound found that ellipticity, which is calculated by measuring the ratio of the long and short axes of the nucleus, and chain code, which measures irregularities in the nuclear contour, when combined into an equation, were able to predict disease recurrence.[85] Carducci and colleagues, in a follow-up paper, found that nuclear morphometry again had prognostic significance.[86] Range of ellipticity of the nucleus was used to stratify patients into low-, moderate-, and high-risk groups for recurrence. The authors found that their method was statistically significant in predicting prognosis.[86]

Histology

RCC histology has been examined in the past for prognostic significance. Fuhrman found that clear cell RCC had a lower rate of metastases than granular and mixed cell tumors.[52] They also discovered that clear cell tumors were of a lower grade and that granular and mixed cell tumors were of a higher grade[52] and cells that are predominantly well differentiated are 93% clear cell, whereas those that are high grade are 100% mixed cell type.[52] The prognosis of those tumors that are not conventional clear cell type RCC also has been examined. Skinner found that the prognosis of pure clear cell tumors was only slightly better than that of pure granular cell or mixed granular cell and clear cell types.[66]

Papillary and chromophobe RCC as distinct histological entities have been described and Moch and associates examined the outcomes in those patients with papillary type RCC and with chromophobe type RCC.[60] They found that unlike their clear cell cohort, the presence of tumor necrosis in these patients did not confer a poor prognosis. Also, they did not make any conclusions as to whether there were any differences in survival between their patients with clear cell versus papillary RCC, but they did conclude that those with eosinophilic type papillary RCC presented with a higher histological grade and stage than those with the basophilic type papillary RCC. The authors found that survival in those patients with papillary RCC was influenced by tumor grade, stage, and whether there were sarcomatoid histological features. Conversely, Fuhrman found that their patient cohort with papillary RCC had a poor prognosis, with all developing metastatic disease. Of note, however, their cohort size was small, with four patients with purely papillary histology. Interestingly, though, those patients with a papillary pattern mixed with other patterns also had a relatively high rate of metastases as well.[52] Despite Fuhrman's findings, most today would ascribe an improved prognosis in those with papillary RCC compared to that of conventional clear cell RCC.[87,88] Mydlo and Bard concluded that papillary RCC is generally well differentiated, hypovascular, or avascular, is less invasive, and confers improved survival.[88] Mancilla-Jimenez et al. also found a generally favorable prognosis in papillary RCC, which was, stage for stage, better than for conventional clear cell RCC.[89] On a slightly different perspective, Renshaw discovered that in his analysis of chromophobe RCC, despite the general impression of a favorable prognosis, a surprising number of patients developed metastatic disease. On further examination, he found that those with concomitant chromophobe RCC and papillary RCC developed metastatic disease (n = 2).[90] Similarly, Medeiros et al. found that their patients with papillary RCC had a much worse prognosis than those with conventional clear cell RCC and that the prognosis with papillary RCC was independent of nuclear grade.[53] How this reflects upon the aggressiveness of papillary RCC is unclear, though it does cast some doubt on the contention that the diagnosis of papillary RCC also confers a favorable prognosis.

With regards to chromophobe RCC, as noted above, most authors believe that prognosis in these patients was better than for clear cell RCC, with chromophobe tumors presenting at a lower stage and improved 5-year survival. Also, chromophobe RCC was more common in female patients (61%).[60] In a separate study, Crotty and associates examined their institution's experience with chromophobe RCC.[91] They found that the overall prognosis was favorable and comparable to that of low-stage, low-grade conventional clear cell RCC. Most of their patients (86%) were Stage I. The authors stress that the chromophobe tumor does bear many histological similarities to oncocytoma and it is necessary to be vigilant therefore at time of diagnosis so as not to confuse the two entities.[91] Amin et al. found that chromophobe RCC had the best prognosis and clear cell RCC had the worst prognosis, with papillary RCC having an intermediate prognosis between that of chromophobe and clear cell.[92]

Collecting duct carcinoma carries with it an ominous prognosis. Also known as medullary carcinoma, it is a rare entity and comprises less than 1% of cases of all renal cell carcinomas.[37] It is thought to arise from the collecting ducts in the renal medullary pyramids, which are also known as the collecting ducts of Bellini.[93] The poor outcome of this subtype of RCC is well known and has been documented.[93–95] Collecting duct carcinoma occurs at a younger age than conventional clear cell RCC and patients have a predilection toward having metastatic disease at presentation, with 30–40% presenting with metastases.[93,96] Patients often have imaging studies that are suggestive of renal pelvis transitional cell carcinoma.[93] Patients often present symptomatically, with weight loss, fever, and anorexia—-all of which are a harbinger for metastatic disease.[93]

Renal medullary carcinoma also has a predilection for early metastasis as well and tends to strike young black males who are either sickle cell carriers or have sickle cell disease. The prognosis is dismal and neither chemotherapy nor immunotherapy appears to have any benefit. Tumors are usually metastatic at the time of diagnosis and in the series of Davis of 22 patients, no tumor was organ confined at nephrectomy. The mean duration of survival after surgery was only 15 weeks.[93–95] The connection between sickle cell disease and renal medullary carcinoma has led to a putative mechanism with sickling red blood cells causing chronic damage to renal papillary epithelium, leading to neoplastic change.[93]

Tumor Necrosis

Tumor necrosis in the primary RCC tumor has carried with it an ominous prognosis. In such instances of tumor necrosis, Amin and associates found that histological evidence of tumor necrosis was significant for poorer survival in multivariate analysis.[92] Likewise, Frank et al. found that in their analysis of 1801 patients, tumor necrosis was also associated with a doubled increased risk of cancer-specific mortality.[50] Similarly, Leibovich and colleagues on both univariate and multivariate analysis found that the presence of tumor necrosis predicted a poor prognosis in a large series of 727 patients with metastatic clear cell RCC.[97] Other studies have corroborated the poor prognosis that RCC tumor necrosis entails. Lam et al. compared the outcome of patients with and without RCC tumor necrosis and found that the patients with necrosis had a higher likelihood of higher stage disease, higher grade, lymph node-positive disease, greater tumor size, higher performance score, higher UISS category, and higher Ki-67 expression.[98] Those patients with necrosis also had a worse 5-year survival than those without necrosis (36% vs. 75%). Another study showed that the presence of tumor necrosis in conventional clear cell RCC, papillary RCC, and chromophobe RCC increased the risk ratio for death on both univariate and multivariate analyses.[99] Tumor necrosis appears to clearly define a subset of patients at risk for poor overall outcome.

Conclusions

RCC remains a heterogeneous disease with an often unpredictable and capricious disease course and prognosis. Despite multiple prognostic factors of value in predicting survival, there are numerous potential factors that could do much to more accurately define those patients at increased risk, especially in localized disease. As more research and studies are conducted, those factors, especially those that reflect the molecular biological behavior of RCC, will be able to predict and stratify, with increasing accuracy, the individual clinical course of this unpredictable disease.

References

1. Cohen HT, McGovern FJ. Renal cell carcinoma. N Engl J Med 353:23, 2477, 2005.
2. Lane BR, Kattan GW. Predicting outcomes in renal cell carcinoma. Curr Opin Urol 15, 289–297, 2005.
3. Van den Berg E, Dijkhuizen T, Oosterhuis JW, van Kessel AG, de Jong B, Storkel S. Cytogenetic classification of renal cell cancer. Cancer Genet Cytogenet 95, 103–107, 1997.
4. Motzer RJ, Mazumdar M, Bacik J, Berg W, Amsterdam A, Ferrara J. Survival and prognostic stratification of 670 patients with advanced renal cell carcinoma. J Clin Oncol 17(8), 2530–2540, 1999.
5. Zhou M, Rubin MA. Molecular markers for renal cell carcinoma: impact on diagnosis and treatment. Semin Urol Oncol 19(2), 80–87, 2001.
6. Bui MH, Zisman A, Pantuck AJ, Han KR, Wieder J, Belldegrun AS. Prognostic factors and molecular markers for renal cell carcinoma. Expert Rev Anticancer Ther 1(4), 565–575, 2001.
7. Srigley JR, Hutter RVP, Gelb AB, Henson DE, Kenney G, King BF, Raziuddin S, Pisansky TM. Current prognostic factors—renal cell carcinoma. Cancer 80, 981–986, 1997.
8. Carroll PR, Murthy VVS, Reuter V, Jhanwar S, Fair WR, Whitmore WF, Chaganti RSK. Abnormalities at chromosome region 3p12–14 characterize clear cell renal cell carcinoma. Cancer Genet Cytogenet 26, 253–259, 1987.
9. Yoshida MA, Ohyashiki K, Ochi H, Gibas Z, Pontes JE, Prout GR, Huben R, Sandberg AA. Cytogenetic studies of tumor tissue from patients with nonfamilial renal cell carcinoma. Cancer Res 46, 2139–2147, 1986.
10. Kovacs G, Erlandsson R, Boldog F, Ingvarsson S, Muller-Brechlin R, Klein G, Sumegi J. Consistent chromosome 3p deletion and loss of heterozygosity in renal cell carcinoma. Proc Natl Acad Sci USA 85, 1571–1575, 1988.
11. Speicher MR, Schoell B, du Manoir S, Schrock E, Ried T, Cremer T, Storkel S, Kovacs A, Kovacs G. Specific loss of chromosomes 1, 2, 6, 10, 13, 17, and 21 in chromophobe RCC revealed by comparative genomic hybridization. Am J Pathol 145(2), 356–364, 1994.
12. Chung BI, Malkowicz SB, Nguyen TB, Libertino JA, McGarvey TW. Expression of the proto-oncogene Axl in renal cell carcinoma. DNA Cell Biol 22(8), 533–540, 2003.
13. Bonsib SM. Risk and prognosis in renal neoplasms, a pathologist's perspective. Urol Clin NA 26(3), 643–660, 1999.
14. Abou-Rebyeh H, Borgmann V, Nagel R, Al-Abadi H. DNA ploidy is a valuable predictor for prognosis of patients with resected renal cell carcinoma. Cancer 92(9), 2280–2285, 2001.
15. Grignon DJ, Ayala AG, el-Naggar A, et al. Renal cell carcinoma: a clinicopathologic and DNA flow cytometric analysis of 103 cases. Cancer 64, 2133, 1989.
16. Lam JS, Shvarts O, Leppert JT, Figlin RA, Belldegrun AS. Renal cell carcinoma 2005: new frontiers in staging, prognostication, and targeted molecular therapy. J Urol 173, 1853–1862, 2005.
17. Bui MH, Selgson D, Han KR, Pantuck AJ, Dorey FJ, Huang Y, et al. Carbonic anhydrase IX is an independent predictor of survival in advanced renal clear cell carcinoma: implications for prognosis and therapy. Clin Cancer Res 9, 802, 2003.
18. Iliopoulos O, Levy AP, Jiang C, Kaelin WG, Goldberg MA. Negative regulation of hypoxia-inducible genes by the von Hippel-Lindau protein. Proc Natl Acad Sci USA 93, 10595–10599, 1996.
19. Atkins M, McDermott D, Mier J, Stanbridge E, Youmans A, Polivy A, et al. Carbonic anhydrase IX expression predicts for renal cell cancer patient response and survival to IL-2 therapy. Proc Am Soc Clin Oncol 23, 383, abstract 4512, 2004.
20. Pich A, Chiusa L, Margaria E. Prognostic relevance of AgNORs in tumor pathology. Micron 31(2), 133–141, 2000.
21. Gelb AB. Renal cell carcinoma: current prognostic factors. Cancer 80, 981–986, 1997.
22. Yang AH, Wang TY, Liu HC. Comparative study of the prognostic value of nuclear grade and silver binding nucleolar region in renal cell carcinoma. J Pathol 166(2), 157–161, 1992.
23. Joachum W, Schroder S, al-Taha R, et al. Prognostic significance of nuclear DNA content and proliferative activity in renal cell carcinoma. A clinicopathologic study of 58 patients using mitotic count, MIB-1 staining, and DNA cytophotometry. Cancer 77(3), 514–521, 1996.
24. Onda H, Yasuda M, Serizawa A, Osamura RY, Kawamura N. Clinical outcome in localized renal cell carcinomas related to immunoexpression of proliferating cell nuclear antigen, Ki-67 antigen and tumor size. Oncol Rep 6(5), 1039–1043, 1999.
25. Rioux-Leclerq N, Turlin B, Bansard J, et al. Value of immunohistochemical Ki-67 and p53 determinations as predictive factors of outcome in renal cell carcinoma. Urology 55(4), 501–505, 2000.

26. Gelb AB, Sudilovsky D, Wu CD, Weiss LM, Medeiros LJ. Appraisal of intratumoral microvessel density, MIB-1 score, DNA content, and p53 protein expression as prognostic indicators in patients with locally confined renal cell carcinoma. Cancer 80(9), 1768–1775, 1997.

27. Lehmann J, Retz M, Nurnberg N, Schnockel U, Raffenberg U, Krams M, Kellner U, Siemer S, Weicher-Jacobsen K, Stockle M. The superior prognostic value of humoral factors compared with molecular proliferation markers in renal cell carcinoma. Cancer 101, 1552–1562, 2004.

28. Morell-Quadreny L, Clar-Blanch F, Fenollosa-Enterna B, Perez-Bacete M, Martinez-Lorente A, Llombart-Bosch A. Proliferating cell nuclear antigen (PCNA) as a prognostic factor in renal cell carcinoma. Anticancer Res 18(1B), 677–682, 1998.

29. Moch H, Sauter G, Gasser TC, Buchholz N, Bubendorf L, Richter J, Jiang F, Dellas A, Mihatsch MJ. p53 protein expression but not mdm-2 protein expression is associated with rapid tumor cell proliferation and prognosis in renal cell carcinoma. Urol Res 25 Suppl 1, S25–30, 1997.

30. Oda H, Nakatsuru Y, Ishikawa T. Mutations of the p53 gene and p53 protein overexpression are associated with sarcomatoid transformation in renal cell carcinomas. Cancer Res 55(3), 658–662, 1995.

31. Shvarts O, Seligson D, Lam J, Shi T, Horvath S, Figlin R, Belldegrun A, Pantuck AJ. P53 is an independent predictor of tumor recurrence and progression after nephrectomy in patients with localized renal cell carcinoma. J Urol 173, 725–728, 2005.

32. Skolarikos A, Alivizatos G, Bamias A, Mitropoulos D, Ferakis N, Deliveliotis C, Dimopoulos M-A. Bcl-2 protein and DNA ploidy in renal cell carcinoma: do they affect patient prognosis? Int J Urol 12, 563–569, 2005.

33. Shalitin C, Epelbaum R, Moskovitz B, Segal R, Valansi C, Werner M, et al. Increased levels of a 21 kDa protein in the circulation of tumor-bearing protein. Cancer Detect Prev 18, 357–365, 1994.

34. Yoshino S, Kato M, Ohada K. Prognostic significance of microvessel count in low stage renal cell carcinoma. Int J Urol 2, 156–160, 1995.

35. MacLennan GT, Bostwick DG. Microvessel density in renal cell carcinoma: lack of prognostic significance. Urology 46(1), 27–30, 1995.

36. Kontak JA, Campbell SC. Prognostic factors in renal cell carcinoma. Urol Clin N Am 30, 467–480, 2003.

37. Pantuck AJ, Zisman A, Belldegrun AS. The changing natural history of renal cell carcinoma. J Urol 166, 1611–1623, 2001.

38. Tsui KH, Shvarts O, Smith RB, Figlin RA, deKernion JB, Belldegrun A. Prognostic factors for renal cell carcinoma: a multivariate analysis of 643 patients using the revised 1997 TNM staging criteria. J Urol 165, 1090–1095, 2000.

39. Kim HL, Han KR, Zisman A, Figlin RA, Belldegrun AS. Cachexia-like symptoms predict a worse prognosis in localized T1 renal cell carcinoma. J Urol 171, 1810–1813, 2004.

40. Selli C, Hinshaw WM, Woodard BH, et al. Stratification of risk factors in renal cell carcinoma. Cancer 52, 899, 1983.

41. McNichols DW, Segura JW, DeWeerd JH. Renal cell carcinoma: long term survival and late recurrences. J Urol 126, 17, 1981.

42. Pantuck AJ, Zisman A, Dorey F, Chao DH, Han KR, Said J, Gitlitz B, Belldegrun AS, Figlin RA. Renal cell carcinoma with retroperitoneal lymph nodes. Impact on survival and benefits of immunotherapy. Cancer 97(12), 2995–3002, 2003.

43. Green LK, Ayala AG, Ro JY, Swanson DA, Grignon DJ, Giacco GG, Guinee VF. Role of nuclear grading in Stage I renal cell carcinoma. Urology 35(5), 310, 1989.

44. Zisman A, Pantuck AJ, Dorey F, Said JW, Shvarts O, Quintana D, Gitlitz BJ, deKernion JB, Figlin RA, Belldegrun AS. Improved prognostication of renal cell carcinoma using an integrated staging system. J Clin Oncol 19, 1649–1657, 2001.

45. Patard JJ, Kim HL, Lam JS, Dorey FJ, et al. Use of the University of California Los Angeles Integrating Staging System to predict survival in renal cell carcinoma: an international multicenter study. J Clin Oncol 22, 3316–3322, 2004.

46. Boxer RJ, Waisman J, Lieber MM, Mampaso FM, Skinner DG. Renal carcinoma: computer analysis of 96 patients treated by nephrectomy. J Urol 122, 598–601, 1979.

47. Lieber MM, Tomera FM, Taylor WF, Farrow GM. Renal adeno-carcinoma in young adults: survival and variables affecting prognosis. J Urol 125, 164–168, 1981.

48. Chasan SA, Pothel LR, Huben RP. Management and prognostic significance of hypercalcemia in renal cell carcinoma. Urology 33(3), 167–170, 1989.

49. Sorbellini M, Kattan MW, Snyder ME, Reuter V, Motzer R, Goetzl M, McKiernan J, Russo P. A postoperative prognostic nomogram predicting recurrence for patients with conventional clear cell renal cell carcinoma. J Urol 173, 48–51, 2005.

50. Frank I, Blute ML, Cheville JC, Lohse CM, Weaver AL, Zincke H. An outcome prediction model for patients with clear cell renal cell carcinoma treated with radical nephrectomy based on tumor stage, size, grade, and necrosis: the SSIGN score. J Urol 168, 2395–2400, 2002.

51. Bell ET. A classification of renal tumors with observations on the frequency of the various types. J Urol 39, 238, 1938.

52. Fuhrman SA, Lasky LC, Limas C. Prognostic significance of morphologic parameters in renal cell carcinoma. Am J Pathol 6, 655, 1982.

53. Medeiros LJ, Gelb AB, Weiss LM. Renal cell carcinoma. Prognostic significance of morphologic parameters in 121 cases. Cancer 61, 1639–1651, 1988.

54. Thrasher JB, Paulson DB. Prognostic factors in renal cancer. Urol Clin NA 20, 247, 1993.

55. Moinzadeh A, Libertino JA. Prognostic significance of tumor thrombus level in patients with renal cell carcinoma and venous tumor thrombus extension. Is all T3b the same? J Urol 171, 598–601, 2004.

56. Kim HL, Zisman A, Han KR, Figlin RA, Belldegrun A. Prognostic significance of venous thrombus in renal cell carcinoma. Are renal vein and inferior vena cava involvement different? J Urol 171, 588–591, 2004.

57. Fergany AF, Hafez KS, Novick AC. Long term results of nephron sparing surgery for localized renal cell carcinoma: 10 year follow up. J Urol 163, 442, 2000.

58. Bassil B, Dorsetz DE, Prout GR. Validation of the tumor, nodes, and metastasis classification of renal cell carcinoma. J Urol 134, 450–454, 1985.

59. Golimbu M, Joshi P, Sperber A, Tessler A, Al-Askari S, Morales P. Renal cell carcinoma: survival and prognostic factors. Urology 27(4), 291–301, 1986.

60. Moch H, Gasser T, Amin MB, Torhorst J, Sauter G, Mihatsch MJ. Prognostic utility of the recently recommended histologic

classification and revised TNM staging system of renal cell carcinoma. Cancer 89(3), 604–614, 2000.

61. Giuliani L, Giberti C, Martorana G, Rovida S. Radical extensive surgery for renal cell carcinoma: long term results and prognostic factors. J Urol 143, 468–474, 1990.

62. Pantuck AJ, Zisman A, Dorey F, Chao DH, Han K, Said J, Gitlitz BJ, Figlin RA, Belldegrun AS. Renal cell carcinoma with retroperitoneal lymph nodes: role of lymph node dissection. J Urol 169, 2076–2083, 2003.

63. Vasselli JR, Yang JC, Linehan WM, White DE, Rosenberg SA, Walther MW. Lack of retroperitoneal lymphadenopathy predicts survival of patients with metastatic renal cell carcinoma. J Urol 166, 68–72, 2001.

64. Libertino JA, Zinman L, Watkins E. Long term results of resection of renal cell cancer with extension into inferior vena cava. J Urol 137, 21–24, 1987.

65. Skinner DG, Pfister RF, Colvin R. Extension of renal cell carcinoma into the vena cava: the rationale for aggressive surgical management. J Urol 107, 711, 1972.

66. Skinner DG, Vermilion CD, Colvin RB. The surgical management of renal cell carcinoma. J Urology 107, 705, 1972.

67. Siminovitch JM, Montie JE, Straffon RA. Prognostic indicators in renal adenocarcinoma. J Urol 130, 20, 1983.

68. Maldazys JD, de Kernion JB. Prognostic factors in metastatic renal carcinoma. J Urol 136, 376–379, 1986.

69. Uzzo RG, Cherullo EE, Myles J, Novick AC. Renal cell carcinoma invading the urinary collecting system: implications for staging. J Urol 167, 2392, 2002.

70. Palapattu GS, Pantuck AJ, Dorey F, Said JW, Figlin RA, Belldegrun AS. Collecting system invasion in renal cell carcinoma: impact on prognosis and future staging strategies. J Urol 170(3), 768–772; discussion 772, 2003.

71. Kearney GP, Waters WB, Klein LA, Richie JP, Gittes RF. Results of inferior vena cava resection for renal cell carcinoma. J Urol 125, 769, 1981.

72. Sogani PC, Herr HW, Rains MS, Whitmore WF. Renal cell carcinoma extending into inferior vena cava. J Urol 130, 660–663, 1983.

73. Neves RJ, Zincke H. Surgical treatment of renal cancer with vena cava extension. Br J Urol 59, 390–395, 1987.

74. Swierzewski DJ, Swierzewski MJ, Libertino JA. Radical nephrectomy in patients with renal cell carcinoma with venous, vena caval, and atrial extension. Am J Surg 168(2), 205–209, 1994.

75. Hatcher PA, Anderson EE, Paulson DF, Carson CC, Robertson JE. Surgical management and prognosis of renal cell carcinoma invading the vena cava. J Urol 145, 20–24, 1991.

76. Skinner DG, Pritchett TR, Lieskovsky G, Boyd SD, Stiles QR. Vena caval involvement by renal cell carcinoma. Ann Surg 210(3), 387–394, 1989.

77. Sosa RE, Muecke EC, Vaughan ED, McCarron JP. Renal cell carcinoma extending into the inferior vena cava: the prognostic significance of the level of vena caval involvement. J Urol 132, 1097–1100, 1984.

78. Nesbitt JC, Soltero ER, Cinney CPN, Walsh GL, Schrump DS, Swanson DA, Pisters LL, Willis KD, Putnam JB. Surgical management of renal cell carcinoma with inferior vena cava tumor thrombus. Ann Thorac Surg 63, 1592–1600, 1997.

79. Kim HL, Zisman A, Han KR, Figlin RA, Belldegrun A. Prognostic significance of venous thrombus in renal cell carcinoma. Are renal vein and inferior vena cava involvement different? J Urol 171, 588–591, 2004.

80. Naitoh J, Kaplan A, Dorey F, Figlin R, Belldegrun A. Metastatic renal cell carcinoma with concurrent inferior vena caval invasion: long-term survival after combination therapy with radical nephrectomy, vena caval thrombectomy, and postoperative immunotherapy. J Urol 162, 46–50, 1999.

81. Suggs WD, Smith RB, Dodson TF, Salam AA, Graham SD. Renal cell carcinoma with inferior vena caval involvement. J Vasc Surg 14, 413–418, 1991.

82. Lang H, Lindner V, de Fromont M, Molinie V, Letourneux H, Meyer N, Martin M, Jacqmin D. Multicenter determination of optimal interobserver agreement using the Fuhrman grading system for renal cell carcinoma. Cancer 103(3), 625–629, 2005.

83. Bretheau D, Lechevallier E, de Fromont M, Sault MC, Rampal M, Coulange C. Prognostic value of nuclear grade of renal cell carcinoma. Cancer; 76, 2543–2549, 1995.

84. Mian BM, Bhadkamkar N, Slaton JW, Pisters PWT, Daliani D, Swanson DA, Pisters LL. Prognostic factors and survival of patients with sarcomatoid renal cell carcinoma. J Urol 167, 65–70, 2002.

85. Pound CR, Partin AW, Epstein JI, Simons JW, Marshall FF. Nuclear morphometry accurately predicts recurrence in clinically localized renal cell carcinoma. Urology 42(3), 243–248, 1993.

86. Carducci MA, Piatadosi M, Pound CR, Epstein JI, Simons JW, Marshall FF, Partin AW. Nuclear morphometry adds significant prognostic information to stage and grade for renal cell carcinoma. Urology 53(1), 44–49, 1999.

87. Boczko S, Fromowitz FB, Bard RH. Papillary adenocarcinoma of kidney. A new perspective. Urology 14(5), 491–495, 1979.

88. Mydlo JH, Bard RH. Analysis of papillary renal adenocarcinoma. Urology 30(6), 529–534, 1987.

89. Mancilla-Jimenez R, Stanley RJ, Blath RA. Papillary renal cell carcinoma. A clinical, radiologic, and pathologic study of 34 cases. Cancer 38, 2469–2480, 1976.

90. Renshaw AA, Henske EP, Loughlin KR, Shapiro C, Weinberg DS. Aggressive variants of chromophobe renal cell carcinoma. Cancer 78(8), 1756–1761, 1996.

91. Crotty TB, Farrow GM, Lieber MM. Chromophobe cell renal carcinoma: clincopathological features of 50 cases. J Urol 154, 964–967, 1995.

92. Amin MB, Amin MB, Tamboli P, et al. Prognostic impact of histologic subtyping of adult renal epithelial neoplasms. Am J Surg Pathol 26(3), 281–291, 2002.

93. Srigley JR, Eble JN. Collecting duct carcinoma of kidney. Semin Diag Pathol 15(1), 54–67, 1998.

94. Kennedy SM, Merino MJ, Linehan WM, et al. Collecting duct carcinoma of the kidney. Hum Pathol 21, 449, 1990.

95. Davis CJ, Jr, Mostofi FK, Sesterhenn IA. Renal medullary carcinoma. The seventh sickle cell nephropathy. Am J Surg Pathol 19, 1, 1995.

96. Carter MD, Tha S, McLoughlin MG, Owen DA. Collecting duct carcinoma of the kidney: a case report and review of the literature. J Urol 147, 1096–1098, 1992.

97. Leibovich BC, Cheville JC, Lohse CM, Zincke H, Frank I, Kwon ED, Merchan JR, Blute ML. A scoring algorithm to predict survival for patients with metastatic clear cell renal cell carcinoma: a stratification tool for prospective clinical trials. J Urol 174, 1759–1763, 2005.

98. Lam JS, Shvarts O, Said JW, Pantuck AJ, Seligson DB, Aldridge ME, Bui MHT, Liu X, Horvath S, Figlin RA, Belldegrun AS. Clinicopathologic and molecular correlations of necrosis in the primary tumor of patients with renal cell carcinoma. Cancer 103, 2517–2525, 2005.

99. Sengupta S, Lohse CM, Leibovich BL, Frank I, Thomson RH, Webster WS, Zincke H, Blute ML, Chevile JC, Kwon ED. Histologic coagulative tumor necrosis as a prognostic indicator of renal cell carcinoma aggressiveness. Cancer 104, 511–520, 2005.

6
Diagnostic Tests

6a
Ultrasound in Diagnosis and Follow-Up of Renal Cell Cancer

Margot H. Wink, Johan S. Laméris, and Jean J.M.C.H. de la Rosette

Introduction

Computed tomography (CT) imaging is the gold standard in diagnosing a renal cell carcinoma. Nevertheless, most renal tumors are first detected during sonographic investigations and many aspects of the diagnosis, treatment, and follow-up of this disease require ultrasound. It offers additional information in selected ambiguous cases and when venous invasion is suspected. Furthermore, sonography can be used to guide minimally invasive treatment modalities.

Sonography is a widely available, inexpensive, and easy to apply imaging tool, which is often the first choice of investigation for diagnosis. Developments in ultrasound techniques have led to improved quality of images and new methods such as contrast-enhanced ultrasound are promising for the near future.

Technologies

Since the first medical use of ultrasound in the mid-1950s, sonography has evolved rapidly, from A mode to B mode, via Doppler techniques and three-dimensional (3D) images, to harmonic imaging and contrast-enhanced ultrasound. The value of these techniques in the detection, characterization, treatment, and follow-up of renal cell cancer will be discussed below.

Doppler

The Doppler principle, first used in 1954, is based on changes of the frequency of sound being reflected from a moving target. A duplex investigation shows the B-mode ultrasound image and conventional Doppler signals together. Color Doppler is a technique with which information about the direction of the flow can be provided, whereas power Doppler informs about the velocity of the blood flow and is more sensitive for the detection of flow.

Although mainly used in vascular imaging, Doppler techniques can increase the value of sonography in many other diagnostic investigations. Because tumor growth is associated with neovascularization and changes in perfusion, Doppler can improve the detection of malignancies. A separate classification for the characterization of small renal masses based on power Doppler findings was proposed in 1998.[1] For local staging of renal cell carcinomas, which is described below, some concluded that Doppler ultrasound is just as accurate as CT.[2,3] An example of Doppler imaging of a small renal tumor is shown in Fig. 6a-1C.

Harmonic Imaging

Harmonic imaging uses the echoes of harmonic instead of fundamental frequencies. It offers a better signal-to-noise ratio and displays fewer artifacts. Phase inversion tissue harmonic imaging is said to add crucial diagnostic information in the evaluation of renal lesions when compared to normal fundamental B-mode ultrasound.[4] Examples of a regular B-mode and a harmonic imaging image of a small renal tumor are shown in Fig. 6a-1A and B, respectively.

Contrast Enhanced Ultrasonography

In recent years, contrast-enhanced ultrasound has gained popularity. First used in echocardiography, it is now used in various fields of medicine. Microbubbles, small encapsulated gas bubbles smaller than erythrocytes, are used as a contrast agent. These bubbles resonate in an ultrasound field in a different way than the normal tissue does and thus send back different reflections. Because the bubbles remain stable inside the circulation, perfusion can be visualized.

The growth of tumors is associated with increased flow and altered perfusion patterns. This is why contrast-enhanced

(a)   (b)

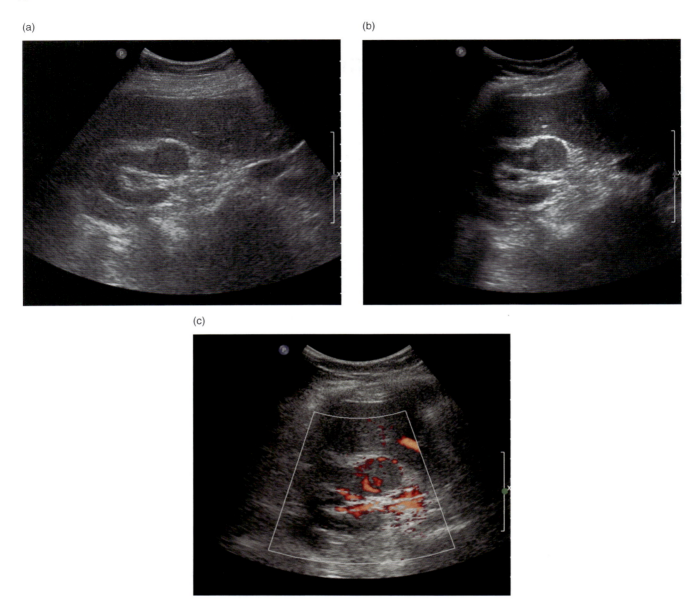

(c)

FIGURE 6a-1. (A) Regular B-mode ultrasound image of a small RCC. (B) The same renal mass, visualized with a harmonic imaging technique. (C) Power Doppler image of the small renal tumor.

ultrasound has been described for the detection and characterization of various tumors. The role of this new imaging modality in the diagnosis of renal cell carcinoma (RCC) will be described later in this chapter.

Other Techniques

Various other ultrasound techniques have been developed over time. Most of them, like 3D ultrasound, do not offer any additional value in the diagnosis of RCC. Computerized tissue characterization techniques are said to differentiate between angiomyolipomas and RCCs,[5,6] but are not widely in use.

Detection

One of the most apparent roles of sonography in renal cell cancer is tumor detection. The percentage of incidentally found renal cell cancers has risen from 7% in 1965 [7] to 61% in 1998.[8] Of these incidental findings, more than 80% are diagnosed by means of ultrasound.[9] The main limitation of sonography is the detection of small isoechoic intra-parenchymal masses. Masses larger than 1.5 cm can be detected with ultrasound; the sensitivity for lesions smaller than 3 cm is approximately 79%.[10]

Although some recent studies claim that coincidental tumors and symptomatic tumors share the same prognosis,[8] most reports agree that coincidentally discovered tumors are significantly smaller and of lower grade than symptomatic masses.[11,12] The incidental discovery of a tumor can be considered a good prognostic factor.[13–17] Nevertheless, in a recent report, screening for RCC using sonography did not lead to a shift in tumor grade or size as compared to tumors found by incident.[18] Screening for RCCs is useful in high risk groups. Conditions that predispose for renal tumors are described later.

In von Hippel–Lindau's disease multiple cysts, rarely larger than 3 cm in diameter, form in kidney and other organs. Besides these, in approximately 35% of the patients RCCs develop, which are bilateral in one-third of cases. Yearly ultrasound investigations of the kidneys are recommended from the age of 20. Tuberous sclerosis is an inherited neurocutaneous disorder that involves different organ systems and is associated with multiple benign neoplasms of the brain and skin and mainly cysts and angiomyolipomas in the kidney. Nevertheless, in 1–2% of these patients RCCs develop. Finally, acquired cystic disease of the kidney, which occurs in over 50% of all renal dialysis patients, is associated with RCC development in 4–5% of the patients. Hereditary factors for the development of RCC are described in detail in Chapter 7.

Characterization/Differential Diagnosis

Since RCC can present either as a cystic or a solid mass, the differential diagnosis of this tumor consists of both cystic and solid masses. The characterization of these two groups of renal masses will be described below.

Cystic Masses

The Bosniak classification was designed in 1986 for based on CT findings. It differentiates between the following four types of cystic lesions in the kidney.

Simple cysts can be accurately diagnosed on sonographic examinations. These masses are anechoic, sharply demarcated, and spherical. They have thin, smooth walls and a good through transmission of sound. The sonographic diagnosis of a simple cyst is 95–98% accurate.

Although the Bosniak classification is essentially used for interpretation of CT scans, it is useful for ultrasound (US) investigations as well. It can be applied to US when a typical Bosniak 1 or 2 lesion is observed. A class 1 lesion is a typical anechoic simple cyst and a class 2 cyst presents as an anechoic lesion with one or two thin septations or tiny calcifications, without a thickened wall. Thin septations occur in 5% of benign renal cysts, whereas the presence of thick septations is an indication for CT. Furthermore, 1–2% of simple cysts contain calcifications, often after a period of infection or bleeding. The addition of Doppler sonography

and power Doppler techniques does not preclude the need for CT or magnetic resonance (MR).[1,19] New techniques such as contrast-enhanced ultrasonography will be discussed below.

The main problem with this classification is differentiating between the mildly complicated Category II lesions, which are considered benign, from the slightly more complex Category III lesions that require histological diagnosis. This is why a subcategory 2F is introduced in the Bosniak classification. This represents class 2 lesions that require follow-up by means of imaging.

Bosniak 3 and 4 lesions can demonstrate small or large intracystic nodules, calcifications, thick septae, and thickened or irregular walls. Histological evaluation is necessary to exclude malignancy. For the diagnosis of a class 3/4 lesion, CT is necessary. Class 3 lesions need histological evaluation for diagnosis, because these cannot be distinguished from malignant lesions with imaging. This usually results in a radical or partial nephrectomy, unless clinically contraindicated. In selected cases an image-guided biopsy can be performed as is described in Chapter 6f. Class 4 lesions are clearly malignant masses with large cystic components, and should always be treated by radical removal. Some other benign, cystic masses that do not fulfill the characteristics of a simple cyst are listed below.

Parapelvic Cysts

Parapelvic cysts are usually of lymphatic origin and are located within the perirenal fat. They sometimes occur bilateral and are irregularly shaped.

Hemorrhagic Cysts

In case of an acute bleeding inside a cyst, the mass appears hyperechoic. The content of the mass confirms to the shape of the cyst. The image of a hemorrhagic cyst changes through resolving. Older hemorrhagic cysts can contain fluid debris and fibrinous membranes. Due to this, lack of enhancement behind the posterior wall exists; the through transmission of sound is decreased. Hemorrhagic cysts are difficult to distinguish from RCCs; repeated imaging after several months is advised. Hemorrhage is reported to occur in about 6% of renal cysts. However, because of increased diagnosis of simple cysts due to better imaging this percentage is probably lower.

Infected Cysts

Infected cysts can show internal echoes in complex patterns, thicker walls, debris or pus inside the cyst, and necrotic exudates. Reflectivity is increased and there is loss of sharp margination of the lesion. Diagnosis is mainly based on clinical symptoms and CT, cytology, and cultures. A resolving infected cystic lesion can be seen in Fig. 6a-2.

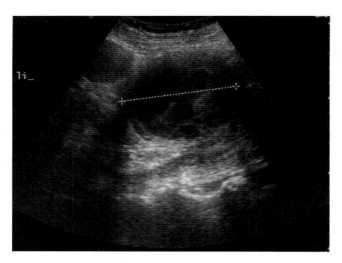

FIGURE 6a-2. Ultrasound image of a resolving infected cystic lesion in a patient with flank pain and fever. The cyst displays heterogeneous echoic contents in the B-mode ultrasound image. During Doppler investigation, no Doppler signal was detected in the cystic mass; during contrast-enhanced ultrasound no contrast signals were visualized in the mass, suggesting that no perfusion is present. This way, differentiation between benign and possibly malignant complex cysts might be possible.

Milk-of-Calcium Cyst

Milk cysts develop due to stasis of urine in calyceal diverticulas. Because of this, calcium carbonate crystallization occurs. Milk cysts are characterized by gravity-dependent, echogenic shadowy material in a renal cyst and acoustic shadowing behind the posterior wall. These cysts can be misinterpreted as a renal stone, but differentiation is possible using an upright plain abdominal X-ray. The milk cyst will demonstrate a "half-moon" image.

Cystic nephroma

Multilocular cystic nephromas are rare and completely benign. There are two peaks in incidence, one in childhood and one in middle age. Using ultrasound they look like multiple small cysts with hyperechoic septa in between. It can be difficult to differentiate these lesions from Bosniak class 3 cysts.

Solid Masses

It is essential to differentiate a renal cell carcinoma from a normal variant or pseudotumor and from one of the solid benign renal masses, as are described below. Around 85% of all solid masses are diagnosed as renal cell cancers. Ten percent of these lesions comprise other malignant masses, i.e., transitional cell cancers, sarcomas, lympho(blasto)mas, and metastases from other primary tumors. Only 5% of the solid renal masses are benign lesions, such as oncocytomas,

angiomyolipomas, and fibromas. The differential diagnostic criteria in sonographic investigations of solid renal masses are described below.

The appearance of renal cell cancer using ultrasound is miscellaneous. Lesions can demonstrate a hypo-, hyper-, or isoechoic appearance and can be either homogeneous or heterogeneous. Small lesions tend to be iso- or hyperechoic and homogeneous, whereas larger lesions mostly have a heterogeneous appearance. In these larger tumors, signs of necrosis can be observed, although these are hard to characterize with regular sonography. Figure 6a-3 shows a small histological proven RCC with a cystic and a solid component. RCCs with massive necrosis can mimic a Bosniak class 3 cystic mass. These lesions show a heterogeneous echoic image inside a thick walled mass, whereas a cystic lesion always exhibits an anechoic component.

The incidence of synchronous bilateral renal carcinomas is 3–5%; calcifications occur in 5–10% of solid tumors.

Various benign solid lesions can be observed in the renal parenchyma. It often is complicated, if not impossible, to differentiate these from RCCs. A selection of the most common benign solid lesions is discussed below.

Lesions Mimicking Solid Renal Tumors

Some hyperechoic cortical defects may mimic the appearance of a small RCC. These junctional parenchymal defects are usually connected to the renal sinus with a hyperechoic line

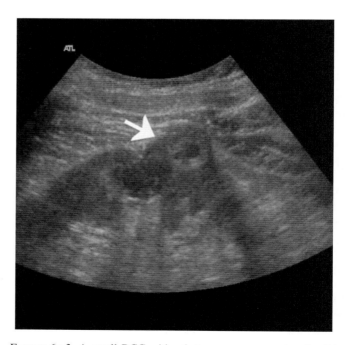

FIGURE 6a-3. A small RCC with a heterogeneous aspect and solid and cystic components. This patient underwent cryoablation of this mass during which biopsies were obtained. Histological evaluation showed an RCC.

and need no further evaluation. Furthermore, after partial nephrectomy, the postoperative defect can be filled with fatty tissue, which can simulate a tumor. Other benign variants that can imitate tumors are lobar dysmorphisms and fetal lobulations. Both these abnormalities show normal vascular patterns on Doppler investigations, but sometimes CT is necessary to exclude malignancy.

Angiomyolipoma

The appearance of an angiomyolipoma depends on the proportions of fat, smooth muscle, and thick-walled vascular tissue inside the mass. Typically, an angiomyolipoma is found during sonography as a small well-circumscribed, homogeneous, hyperechoic mass. An example of a typical angiomyolipoma is demonstrated in Fig. 6a-4. Posterior shadowing occurs in about 30%. However, angiomyolipomas can sometimes have an iso- or nonechogenic appearance. It is the most highly reflective of renal tumors, but this finding alone is not enough to make a diagnosis, since 32% of renal cell cancers are hyperechogenic. Jinzaki et al. describe the different vascular patterns as seen on power Doppler ultrasound bases on which a differentiation can be made between larger angiomyolipomas and renal carcinomas.[1] Nevertheless, in larger lesions, a CT scan is required to confirm the presence of fat inside the tumor. Hemorrhage and necrosis can be seen after a bleeding, but cystic areas due to necrosis and calcifications are not compatible with angiomyolipoma.

Oncocytoma

Oncocytomas originate from collecting duct cells and are considered benign. They can be seen as well-circumscribed

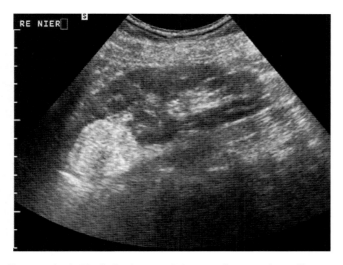

FIGURE 6a-4. Typical ultrasound image of an angiomyolipoma. Because of an elevated risk for hemorrhage in this patient she underwent selective embolization without complications.

solid lesions with homogeneous internal echoes of variable echogenicity with ultrasound. Differentiation with RCC is not possible with gray scale sonography. However, oncocytomas present with a typical vascularization pattern. In Doppler investigations a radial spoke wheel flow pattern around a central scar can be observed.

Multifocality, bilateralism, and metachronous tumors develop in approximately 4–6% of all cases. Early reports of metastatic oncocytomas are probably based on falsely diagnosed chromophobic RCCs. RCC coexists in 10–32% of oncocytoma cases.[20]

Contrast-Enhanced Ultrasound

Contrast-enhanced ultrasound has evolved and sensitivity for the detection of the contrast agent is still improving. In the early days, intravenous injection of microbubbles was used to enhance regular B-mode ultrasonography. The reflections of these intravascular bubbles, however, enhance the Doppler signal of blood flow as well. This is why power Doppler contrast-enhanced ultrasound provides extra information above Doppler ultrasound alone. In the characterization of renal masses it helps in differentiating between lesions mimicking tumors and real renal malignancies.[21,22]

The nonlinear behavior of microbubbles in an ultrasound field can be used to improve the sensitivity of contrast detection. Harmonic imaging techniques use this phenomenon with success. However, to visualize perfusion the signal reflected from the contrast agent should be isolated. Recent contrast-specific imaging techniques provide a contrast-only and tissue- only image simultaneously.[23] Examples of contrast-enhanced ultrasound images using this new technique are shown in Figs. 6a-5, 6a-6, and 6a-7. This technique has been described for use in renal ultrasonography for the first time by Nilsson.[24]

Harmonic imaging contrast-enhanced ultrasound was able to distinguish angiomyolipomas from renal cell cancers[25,26] and could identify pseudocapsules in the preoperative evaluation of RCCs.[27] Contrast-specific imaging has potential in the characterization of solid renal masses, because it enables visualization of different vascular patterns.[26,28] Furthermore, these techniques can be used in the evaluation of atypical cysts. The detection of contrast enhancement within the complex cyst is then equivalent to the existence of vessels, thus suspect for malignancy.[29,30] One of the future roles of contrast- enhanced ultrasound in the diagnostic process can be the discrimination between benign and potentially malignant atypical renal cysts, avoiding CT scans in some of the patients.[31,32] One advantage of this investigation is that the contrast agents are not nephrotoxic, thus renal impairment is not a contraindication. Furthermore, the real time evaluation, in which all the phases of contrast enhancement can be visualized, may add information in difficult diagnoses. The

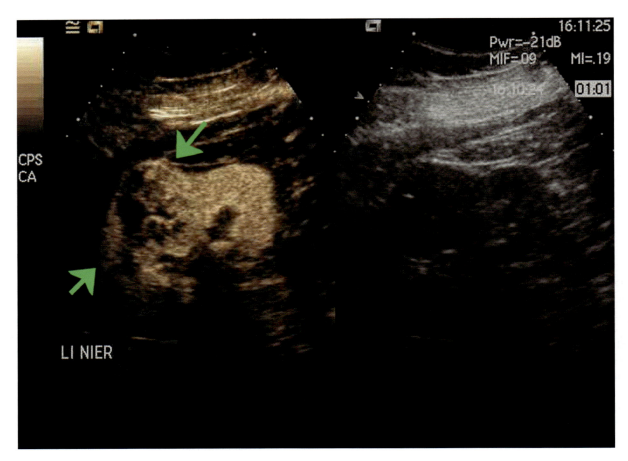

FIGURE 6a-5. Contrast enhanced ultrasound performed with a contrast pulse sequence imaging technique and Sonovue (Bracco) as a contrast agent. A histological proven RCC in the midsegment of a kidney. Note the inhomogeneous enhancement pattern compared to the renal parenchyma.

possible role of contrast ultrasound in the follow-up after treatment will be discussed below.

Staging

The stage of the tumors is determined by the size, ingrowth, lymph node involvement, and the presence of distant metastases. These features can all best be assessed on CT investigations. However, vascular involvement, which is an important finding in the preoperative assessment of a renal cell cancer, can be evaluated using different imaging modalities. The role of sonography will be described below.

The presence and extent of tumor thrombus are essential information in staging of RCC. A tumor thrombus can be visualized as a solid echoic mass within the lumen of the inferior caval vein. An example of an RCC with inferior caval vein involvement is shown in Fig. 6a-7. The upper limit of this thrombus, especially regarding the hepatic veins and the atrium, is a determination in the preoperative period with important consequences. Because extensive surgery is the mainstay of the treatment of these patients, the level of invasion is crucial for planning the operation. With color flow

Doppler the signals around the thrombus can be evaluated.[33] Contrast-enhanced ultrasound can possibly improve the detection of renal vein thrombosis.[24] Neovascularization inside the tumor thrombus can often be identified, differentiating it from normal bland thrombus. However, MRI has recently replaced all other imaging modalities in the precise detection of the cranial extension of the thrombi. Transesophageal ultrasound accurately predicts tumor thrombus level in 85%, compared to 90% in MRI and 75% in cavography,[34] but since the latter is an invasive procedure it is not routinely used in the preoperative work-up.

Nevertheless, during surgery, sonography is the only available imaging tool. Intraoperative monitoring of patients with tumor thrombi in the upper part of the inferior vena cava can be of great assistance.[35–38]

Guiding Treatment

Minimal invasive treatment options for RCCs are gaining popularity. These treatments, either under laparoscopic or percutaneous guidance, depend entirely on imaging

(a)   (b)

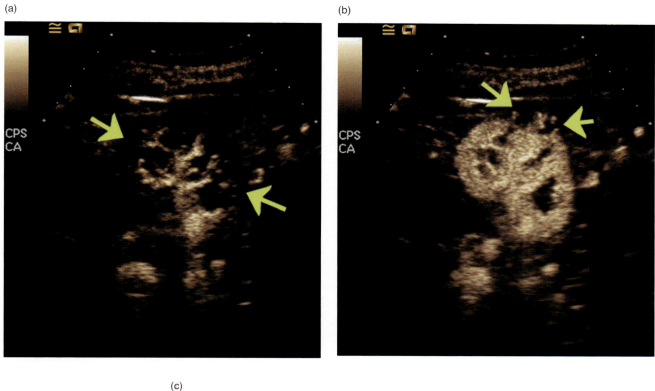

(c)

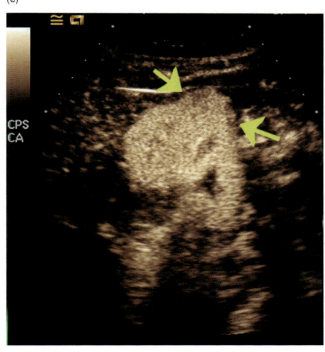

FIGURE 6a-6. Images from a contrast-enhanced ultrasound study performed with a contrast pulse sequence imaging technique and Sonovue (Bracco) as a contrast agent. On the right side of the image the regular B-mode tissue signal is displayed. On the left side of the illustrations the contrast-only image can be seen, in which all signals reflected from the tissue are annulled. The signals from this half of the image are the reflections of the microbubbles only. Right after a "burst," during which all microbubble contrast agents are destructed in the ultrasound field, a new influx of bubbles can be visualized. (A) First, the larger vasculature of the kidney becomes visible. The outline of the kidney is indicated with yellow arrows. (B) One second later, the renal parenchyma is completely filled with microbubbles and homogeneously enhanced. The small exophytic renal tumor is enhanced later and is less homogeneous than the parenchyma (arrows). (C) Several seconds later, the tumor (arrows) is completely enhanced and more difficult to distinguish from the parenchyma. The real time aspect of ultrasound is an important advantage of this imaging modality.

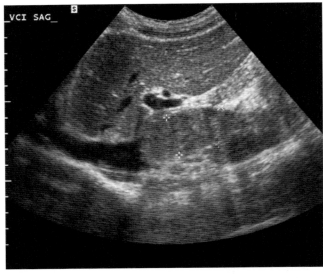

FIGURE 6a-7. Ultrasound image of inferior caval vein involvement in a young man with an RCC of 13 cm diameter. The thrombus did not reach the hepatic veins. Shortly after this investigation, various lymph node metastases were detected, which proved to be metastases of this RCC.

(a)

(b)

(c)

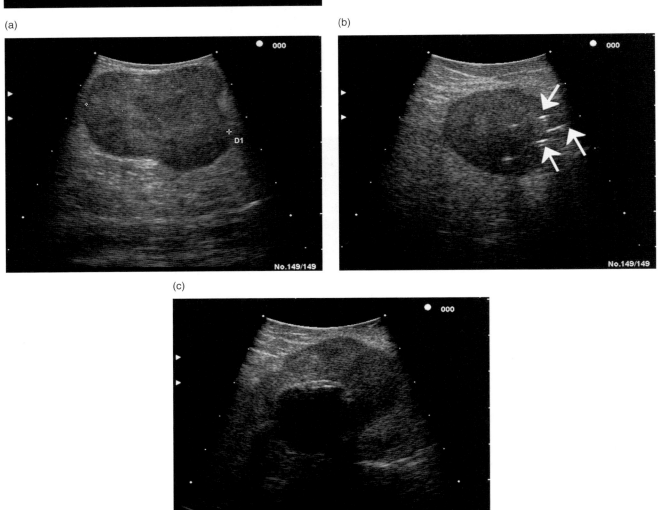

FIGURE 6a-8. Intraoperative ultrasound images of an RCC during laparoscopy assisted cryoablation of a renal tumor. Ultrasound, using a laparoscopic probe, can be used to localize the mass (**A**), to guide needle placement (arrows) (**B**), and to monitor the ablated area (ice-ball) directly after the ablation (**C**) .

because visualization of the tumor is required during the treatmen.[39] Intraoperative ultrasound examinations can guide the treatment and monitor the ablation as demonstrated in Fig. 6a-8.[40] As described in the ablation of liver tumors, the use of contrast can possibly improve the accuracy of intraoperative sonography in ablative therapies for RCC.[41] It is shown in porcine models that the lesions seen on contrast ultrasound evaluations correspond to regions of cell death in histological evaluation.[42,43] The extent of the ablation can be evaluated immediately after the procedure. This can reduce the need for repeated treatment sessions under anesthesia. [44]

Follow-up

Small lesions that do not require immediate surgery can be followed and measured with regular ultrasound. Patients suffering from polycystic kidney disease, von Hippel–Lindau disease, or tuberous sclerosis need to be screened for renal cancers. Sonography is the appropriate screening tool, reserving CT investigations for unclear cases and to confirm the diagnosis of a suspected tumor. Also after surgery for an RCC, ultrasound investigations can detect recurrences.

After nephron sparing surgery the mainstay of the follow-up is again imaging. After partial nephrectomy the pathology results will reveal the possible presence of tumor tissue in the remaining kidney. In ablation therapy, however, when the tumor is left *in situ*, it is essential to study the viability of the remaining tissue. Doppler ultrasound alone is not sensitive enough for capillary flow to exclude pathological perfusion. This is why the standard follow-up modality is CT or MRI. After administration of contrast, absence of perfusion can be objectified on ultrasound investigations. In the early assessment of patients who underwent radiofrequency ablation or cryoablation, contrast-enhanced ultrasound can visualize perfusion defects. This has been described for hepatic tumor ablations and recently for RCCs.[42,44,45] This way, residual tumor and early recurrences can possibly be detected.[46] However, accuracy depends on the vascular properties of the initial tumor. Patients with impaired renal function who underwent nephron sparing surgery for this reason can be, in addition to MRI, safely monitored with contrast-enhanced ultrasound.

References

1. Jinzaki M, Ohkuma K, Tanimoto A *et al*.: Small solid renal lesions: usefulness of power Doppler US. Radiology 209(2): 543–550, 1998.
2. Bos SD and Mensink HJ: Can duplex Doppler ultrasound replace computerized tomography in staging patients with renal cell carcinoma? Scand J Urol Nephrol 32(2): 87–91, 1998.
3. Kitamura H, Fujimoto H, Tobisu K *et al*.: Dynamic computed tomography and color Doppler ultrasound of renal parenchymal neoplasms: correlations with histopathological findings. Jpn J Clin Oncol 34(2): 78–81, 2004.
4. Schmidt T, Hohl C, Haage P *et al*.: Diagnostic accuracy of phase-inversion tissue harmonic imaging versus fundamental B-mode sonography in the evaluation of focal lesions of the kidney. AJR Am J Roentgenol 180(6): 1639–1647, 2003.
5. Sim JS, Seo CS, Kim SH *et al*.: Differentiation of small hyper-echoic renal cell carcinoma from angiomyolipoma: computer-aided tissue echo quantification. J Ultrasound Med 18(4): 261–264, 1999.
6. Taniguchi N, Itoh K, Nakamura S *et al*.: Differentiation of renal cell carcinomas from angiomyolipomas by ultrasonic frequency dependent attenuation. J Urol 157(4): 1242–1245, 1997.
7. Skinner DG, Colvin RB, Vermillion CD *et al*.: Diagnosis and management of renal cell carcinoma. A clinical and pathologic study of 309 cases. Cancer 28(5): 1165–1177, 1971.
8. Jayson M and Sanders H: Increased incidence of serendipitously discovered renal cell carcinoma. Urology 51(2): 203–205, 1998.
9. Siemer S, Uder M, Humke U *et al*.: [Value of ultrasound in early diagnosis of renal cell carcinoma]. Urologe A 39(2): 149–153, 2000.
10. Amendola MA, Bree RL, Pollack HM *et al*.: Small renal cell carcinomas: resolving a diagnostic dilemma. Radiology 166(3): 637–641, 1988.
11. Helenon O, Correas JM, Balleyguier C *et al*.: Ultrasound of renal tumors. Eur Radiol 11(10): 1890–1901, 2001.
12. Luciani LG, Cestari R, and Tallarigo C: Incidental renal cell carcinoma-age and stage characterization and clinical implications: study of 1092 patients (1982–1997). Urology 56(1): 58–62, 2000.
13. Ficarra V, Prayer-Galetti T, Novella G *et al*.: Incidental detection beyond pathological factors as prognostic predictor of renal cell carcinoma. Eur Urol 43(6): 663–669, 2003.
14. Ishikawa I, Honda R, Yamada Y *et al*.: Renal cell carcinoma detected by screening shows better patient survival than that detected following symptoms in dialysis patients. Ther Apher Dial 8(6): 468–473, 2004.
15. Patard JJ, Leray E, Rodriguez A *et al*.: Correlation between symptom graduation, tumor characteristics and survival in renal cell carcinoma. Eur Urol 44(2): 226–232, 2003.
16. Patard JJ, Leray E, Cindolo L *et al*.: Multi-institutional validation of a symptom based classification for renal cell carcinoma. J Urol 172(3): 858–862, 2004.
17. Patard JJ, Rodriguez A, Rioux-Leclercq N *et al*.: Prognostic significance of the mode of detection in renal tumours. BJU Int 90(4): 358–363, 2002.
18. Filipas D, Spix C, Schulz-Lampel D *et al*.: Screening for renal cell carcinoma using ultrasonography: a feasibility study. BJU Int 91(7): 595–599, 2003.
19. Kier R, Taylor KJ, Feyock AL *et al*.: Renal masses: characterization with Doppler US. Radiology 176(3): 703–707, 1990.
20. Dechet CB, Bostwick DG, Blute ML *et al*.: Renal oncocytoma: multifocality, bilateralism, metachronous tumor development and coexistent renal cell carcinoma. J Urol 162(1):40–42, 1999.
21. Ascenti G, Zimbaro G, Mazziotti S *et al*.: Usefulness of power Doppler and contrast-enhanced sonography in the differentiation of hyperechoic renal masses. Abdom Imaging 26(6): 654–660, 2001.

22. Ascenti G, Zimbaro G, Mazziotti S *et al.*: Contrast-enhanced power Doppler US in the diagnosis of renal pseudotumors. Eur Radiol 11(12): 2496–2499, 2001.

23. Phillips P and Gardner E: Contrast-agent detection and quantification. Eur Radiol 14(Suppl 8): 4–10, 2004.

24. Nilsson A: Contrast-enhanced ultrasound of the kidneys. Eur Radiol 14(Suppl 8): 104–109, 2004.

25. Quaia E, Siracusano S, Bertolotto M *et al.*: Characterization of renal tumours with pulse inversion harmonic imaging by intermittent high mechanical index technique: initial results. Eur Radiol 13(6): 1402–1412, 2003.

26. Siracusano S, Quaia E, Bertolotto M *et al.*: The application of ultrasound contrast agents in the characterization of renal tumors. J Urol 175: 1272–1273, 2004.

27. Ascenti G, Gaeta M, Magno C *et al.*: Contrast-enhanced second-harmonic sonography in the detection of pseudocapsule in renal cell carcinoma. AJR Am J Roentgenol 182(6): 1525–1530, 2004.

28. Thorelius L: Contrast-enhanced ultrasound for extrahepatic lesions: preliminary experience. Eur J Radiol 51(Suppl): S31–S38, 2004.

29. Nilsson A and Krause J: Targeted tumour biopsy under contrast-enhanced ultrasound guidance. Eur Radiol 13(Suppl 4): L239–L240, 2003.

30. Robbin ML, Lockhart ME, and Barr RG: Renal imaging with ultrasound contrast: current status. Radiol Clin North Am 41(5): 963–978, 2003.

31. Kim AY, Kim SH, Kim YJ *et al.*: Contrast-enhanced power Doppler sonography for the differentiation of cystic renal lesions: preliminary study. J Ultrasound Med 18(9): 581–588, 1999.

32. Correas JM, Claudon M, Tranquart F *et al.*: The kidney: imaging with microbubble contrast agents. Ultrasound Q 22(1): 53–66, 2006.

33. Bos SD and Mensink HJ: Can duplex Doppler ultrasound replace computerized tomography in staging patients with renal cell carcinoma? Scand J Urol Nephrol 32(2): 87–91, 1998.

34. Glazer A and Novick AC: Preoperative transesophageal echocardiography for assessment of vena caval tumor thrombi: a comparative study with venacavography and magnetic resonance imaging. Urology 49(1): 32–34, 1997.

35. Tomita Y, Kurumada S, Takahashi K *et al.*: Intraoperative transesophageal sonographic monitoring of tumor thrombus in the inferior vena cava during radical nephrectomy and thrombectomy for renal cell carcinoma. J Clin Ultrasound 31(5): 274–277, 2003.

36. Harkin CP, Roberts PF, Nelson RS *et al.*: Re-evaluation of renal cell carcinoma tumor thrombus extension by intraoperative transesophageal echocardiography. J Cardiothorac Vasc Anesth 14(2): 182–185, 2000.

37. Hsu TH, Jeffrey RB Jr, Chon C *et al.*: Laparoscopic radical nephrectomy incorporating intraoperative ultrasonography for renal cell carcinoma with renal vein tumor thrombus. Urology 61(6): 1246–1248, 2003.

38. Oikawa T, Shimazui T, Johraku A *et al.*: Intraoperative transesophageal echocardiography for inferior vena caval tumor thrombus in renal cell carcinoma. Int J Urol 11(4): 189–192, 2004.

39. Hinshaw JL and Lee FT Jr: Image-guided ablation of renal cell carcinoma. Magn Reson Imaging Clin N Am 12(3): 429–47, vi, 2004.

40. Remer EM, Hale JC, O'Malley CM *et al.*: Sonographic guidance of laparoscopic renal cryoablation. AJR Am J Roentgenol 174(6): 1595–1596, 2000.

41. Siosteen AK and Elvin A: Intra-operative uses of contrast-enhanced ultrasound. Eur Radiol 14(Suppl 8): 87–95, 2004.

42. Johnson DB, Duchene DA, Taylor GD *et al.*: Contrast-enhanced ultrasound evaluation of radiofrequency ablation of the kidney: reliable imaging of the thermolesion. J Endourol 19(2): 248–252, 2005.

43. Slabaugh TK, Machaidze Z, Hennigar R *et al.*: Monitoring radiofrequency renal lesions in real time using contrast-enhanced ultrasonography: a porcine model. J Endourol 19(5): 579–583, 2005.

44. Solbiati L, Tonolini M, and Cova L: Monitoring RF ablation. Eur Radiol 14(Suppl 8): 34–42, 2004.

45. Zhu Q, Shimizu T, Endo H *et al.*: Assessment of renal cell carcinoma after cryoablation using contrast-enhanced gray-scale ultrasound: a case series. Clin Imaging 29(2): 102–108, 2005.

46. Morimoto M, Nozawa A, Numata K *et al.*: Evaluation using contrast-enhanced harmonic gray scale sonography after radio frequency ablation of small hepatocellular carcinoma: sonographic-histopathologic correlation. J Ultrasound Med 24(3): 273–283, 2005.

6b
Computer Tomography in Renal Cell Cancer

Saffire S.K.S. Phoa

Introduction

Small renal cell cancers are increasingly detected incidentally by the widespread use of routine cross-sectional imaging and ultrasonography (US). Sonography may be sufficient to characterize an incidental renal finding as a simple cyst that requires no further follow-up. The sonographic criteria for a simple cyst are a sharply delineated anechoic lesion, with a clear backwall, that shows enhanced sound through transmission. One or two small (hairline) septations may be present in a simple cyst. Further computed tomography (CT) or magnetic resonance (MR) imaging is required for all solid lesons or if signs of a complicated cyst are detected by sonography, e.g., thickening or nodularity of the cyst wall or of a septa within the cyst, the presence of more than two septa, and the presence of large calcifications (Zagoria et al., 2004).

For the characterization and staging of renal lesions CT is most frequently used, because it is widely available and has a short examination time. MR may have some advantages over CT, e.g., the presence of a tumor capsule is better demonstrated by MR. Also MR and US are both superior to CT for the demonstration of thin septations within a cystic lesion. The presence of calcifications are better detected by CT (Yamashita et al., 2004; Sheth et al., 2001). Another advantage of CT may be a high spatial resolution and the capability of volume acquisitions and three-dimensional (3D) rendering. For patients with an allergy to iodine contrast media or severe impairment of renal function, MR is the method of choice.

Computed Tomography Technique

Spiral CT with a single intravenous (IV) contrast bolus technique and multiphase imaging of the kidney has been the standard for evaluating a renal mass of unknown origin. The importance of different phases of scanning has been well shown and its relevance for diagnosis and staging is discussed below (Sheth et al., 2001; Suh et al., 2003; Kopka et al., 1997; Macari and Bosniak, 1999; Goldman, 1998).

Some authors describe the use of a limited three-phase scan for known solid tumors.

Unenhanced Computed Tomography

The unenhanced images are used to detect stones or calcifications, which may be present in up to 30% of solid tumors. Also unenhanced images are needed to demonstrate the hyperdensity of a lesion (hyperdense cyst) and to determine whether there is enhancement of the lesion after contrast administration.

The Corticomedullary Phase 25–70 Seconds

The corticomedullary phase is early after IV contrast, with a delay of 25–70 seconds, and is also referred to as the arterial phase. During this phase the outer cortex and the renal arteries show the best enhancement. This phase has limited value for the detection of tumors and a centrally located lesion may easily be missed (Figs. 6b-1 and 6b-2) (Sheth et al., 2001; Kopka et al., 1997). However, an early enhancement pattern is useful to characterize the lesions (Fig. 6b-3). This phase may be omitted to limit radiation dose. On occasion a hypervascular tumor may be detectable only during this phase. Scanning of the liver during the early corticomedullary phase (arterial phase) may be helpful for the detection of hypervascular liver metastases.

The Nephrographic Phase 80–180 Seconds

This phase is optimal for the detection and characterization of lesions. A delay of 70–80 seconds is optimal for the evaluation of the renal vein and the suprarenal part of the inferior caval vein. The infrarenal part of the caval vein usually enhances later.

Delayed Phase >3–5 Minutes

Contrast excretion after 3–5 minutes allows visualization of the collecting system and demonstration of the relationship

(a)   (b)

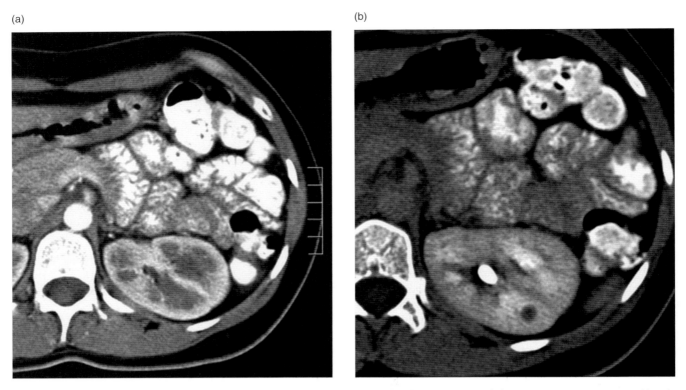

FIGURE 6b-1. (**A**) Corticomedullary phase; centrally located hypodense lesion (cyst) is not visible. (**B**) Delayed phase is most sensitive for the detection of lesions.

(a)   (b)

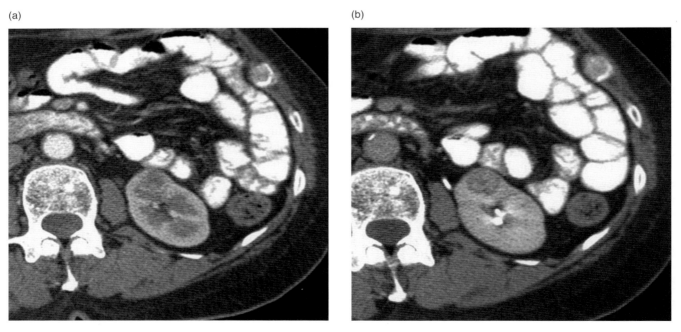

FIGURE 6b-2. (**A**) Corticomedullary phase poorly shows a hypodense solid lesion, compared to the parenchymal phase (**B**).

(a)

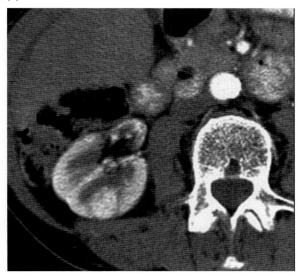

(b)

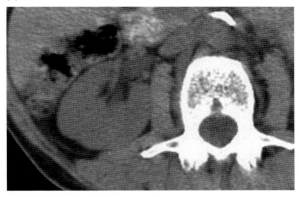

(c)

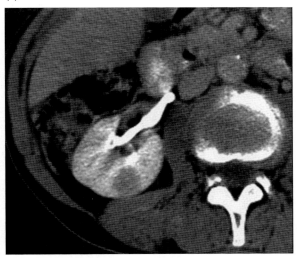

FIGURE 6b-3. (**A**) Corticomedullary phase; helps to characterize an enhancing lesion as solid. This would be difficult on delayed images and noncontrast images alone (**B, C**).

of the renal pelvis and the tumor. For the evaluation of the complete excretory system including the ureter and bladder a longer delay of approximately 7 minutes and the use of compression (CT urography or CT hydrography) are suggested (Kawashima et al., 2004).

The development of the multirow-detector CT has raised the standard of CT further. The 4-, 16-, and 64-row detectors allow rapid acquisition of up to 64 slices per rotation of the X-ray tube. Multiphase scanning with 1-mm slice collimation will become a routine protocol. From the obtained data, thicker slices may be reconstructed for reviewing. Thinner slice collimation allows superior reformatting of other nonaxial scan planes and of 3D rendering of arteries (Coll et al., 2000). The use of thin slices enables better detection and characterization of small lesions. In one study with 3-mm slice thickness and 1-mm overlapping reconstructions, CT detected 17% more lesions than with 5-mm slice reconstructions. For small lesions a better differentiation between cyst or solid tumor can be made.

However, finding a large number of small uncharacterized incidental renal lesions in routine examinations may also be regarded as a potential drawback of multirow CT (Jinzaki et al., 2004).

Solid Masses, Renal Cell Carcinoma

If a lesion has been detected in the kidney, CT is often performed for further characterization and staging. Density measurements, the demonstration of fat or calcifications, and enhancement patterns are all helpful in characterizing a mass as cystic or solid and in determining whether the lesion is potentially malignant.

Demonstration of Fat in a Lesion

If fat can be demonstrated in a tumor, this is regarded as sufficient proof of a benign lesion (angiomyolipoma) (Fig. 6b-4). In renal cell carcinoma (RCC) the presence of fat is very rare, although papillary RCCs have been described that contained minimal fat. In malignant tumors that contain small amounts of fat (Fig. 6b-5), usually other signs of malignancy, such as central necrosis, were found to be present (Lesavre et al., 2003).

CT may prove the presence of fat within a lesion, if the CT density on unenhanced scans is measured as lower than −10 HU (Hounsfield units). However, there are some restrictions. Thin collimation should be made used with

(a)   (b)

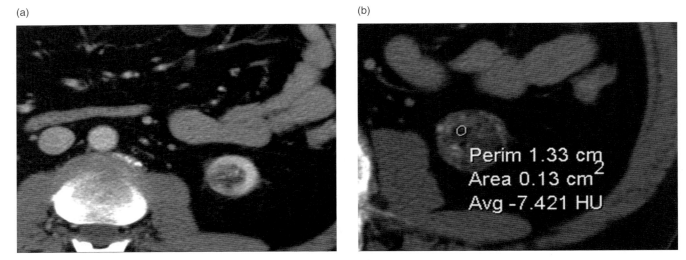

FIGURE 6b-4. (**A, B**) Angiomyolipoma; demonstration of fat on CT is regarded as sufficient for this diagnosis.

reconstruction of thin slices in order to prevent so-called volume averaging. If a thick CT slice is used, part of the normal tissue surrounding a lesion may be measured instead of the lesion itself. Second, for CT density measurements, proper calibration of the CT scanner is necessary using a phantom. This is rarely performed on a routine basis and some margin for error should be considered when CT density measurements are made (such as fat measurement or enhancement after IV contrast), e.g., use a density of <-10 HU as proof of fat density instead of a density of <0 HU. Third, in centrally located lesions the normal peripelvine fatty tissue may be mistaken for fat in the tumor (Fig. 6b-6) (Pereira et al., 2005).

Enhancement

Nearly 70% of RCCs are clear cell type tumors or so-called conventional RCC. This type of tumor usually shows strong enhancement after IV contrast. The enhancement is predominantly peripheral and the lesions show marked heterogeneity. On unenhanced CT the RCC may be isodense to slightly hypodense or hyperdense compared to normal parenchyma (Ruppert-Kohlmayr et al., 2004).

Heterogeneous enhancement is more common in the clear cell type and in papillary carcinoma than in chromophobe carcinoma. Kim et al. (2002) found marked heterogeneous enhancement in 68% of clear cell RCCs, in approximately

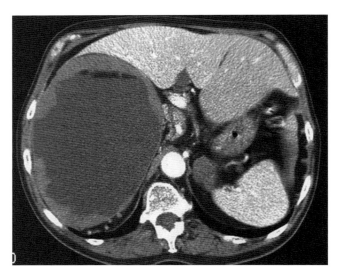

FIGURE 6b-5. Papillary cell carcinoma with small area of fat density. Papillary carcinoma may rarely contain some cholesterol crystals.

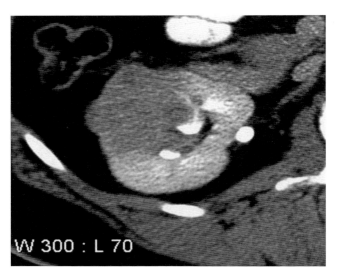

FIGURE 6b-6. Renal cell carcinoma, oncocytic type. Renal sinus fat should not be mistaken for fat inside the tumor.

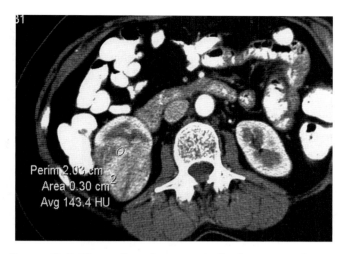

FIGURE 6b-7. Clear cell carcinoma, typically shows strong heterogenic contrast enhancement. The density of >140 HU excludes a chromophobe or papillary carcinoma.

50% of papillary RCCs and collecting duct tumors, and in approximately 25% of chromophobe RCCs (Figs. 6b-7 and 6b-8).

Also the degree of enhancement is much higher for clear cell type carcinoma than for other types of RCC (Kim et al., 2002). A density of >84 HU of a lesion in the nephrographic phase seemed optimal to differentiate tumor subtypes.

Calcifications

Calcifications are relatively rare in conventional RCC and occur in approximately 11% of clear cell tumors. Calcifications are more common in papillary carcinoma and in chromophobe carcinoma (32% and 38%, respectively, in one series).

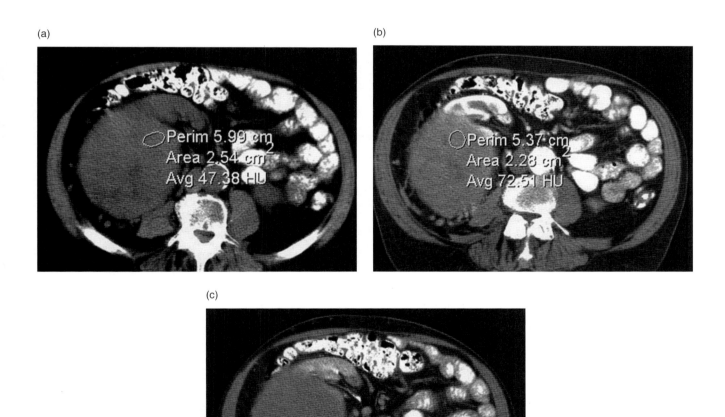

FIGURE 6b-8. (A–C) Plain film; nephrographic and parenchymal phase. Papillary carcinoma, typically shows moderate enhancement.

Hyperdense Cyst

If a lesion on CT shows enhancement of more than 12 HU, compared to the precontrast scan, the lesion can be regarded as a solid lesion (Figs. 6b-9 and 6b-10). A hyperdense cyst may be diagnosed when a homogeneous lesion is denser than 20 HU on the precontrast scan and when no enhancement after IV contrast injection or less enhancement than 12 HU is present (Figs. 6b-11, 6b-12, 6b-13, and 6b-14). On

(a)   (b)

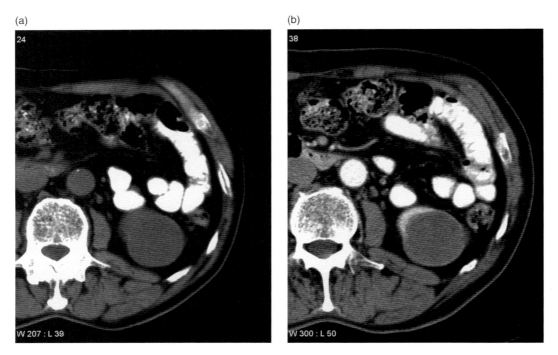

FIGURE 6b-9. (**A, B**) Low-density lesion, enhancement after contrast 15 HU. Solid renal cell carcinoma.

(a)   (b)

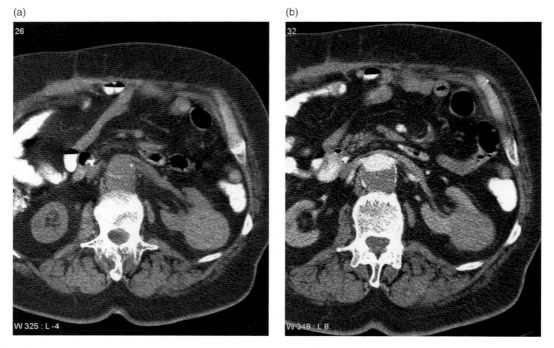

FIGURE 6b-10. (**A**) Precontrast scan shows a hyperdense lesion 45 HU. (**B**) Enhancement after contrast 15 HU. Thus a solid lesion is present. Pa: papillary carcinoma.

(a)

(b)

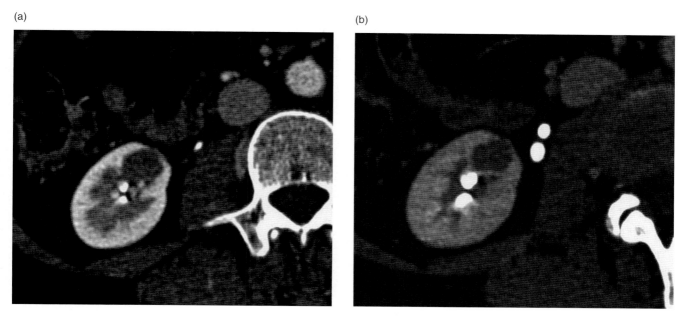

FIGURE 6b-11. (**A**) Corticomedullary and (**B**) delayed phase. Contrast enhancement <10 HU in a lesion, compatible with a cyst.

(a)

(b)

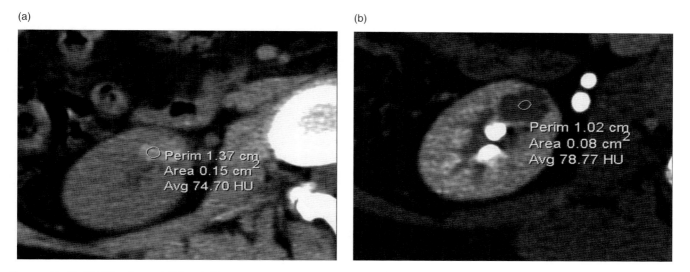

FIGURE 6b-12. (**A**) Unenhanced CT and (**B**) parenchymal phase. Hyperdense (hemorrhagic) cyst. Density measurements show the absence of contrast uptake in the lesion. Uptake of contrast would signify a solid lesion. The parenchymal phase alone would be insufficient to diagnose a hyperdense cystic lesion from a solid lesion. In general, a density of >70 HU on parenchymal images signifies a solid lesion.

(a)   (b)

(c)   (d)

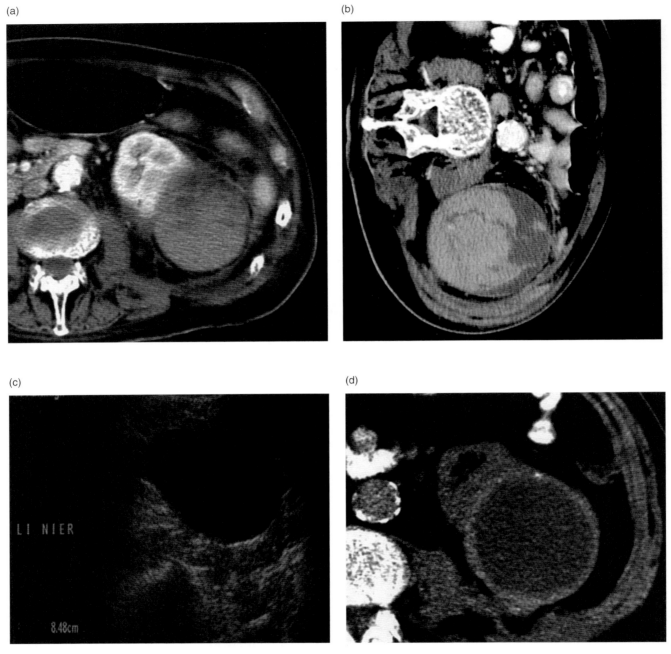

FIGURE 6b-13. (**A, B**) Nephrographic phase; shows a hyperdense lesion (73 HU) in a 67-year-old patient with acute flank pain and fever. On delayed scans (not shown) there are no signs of deenhancement. Dx: acute bleeding in a cyst. (**C**) Previous US showed a simple cyst. (**D**) Follow-up CT after 3 years: thick walled cyst, resorption of bleeding.

(a)   (b)

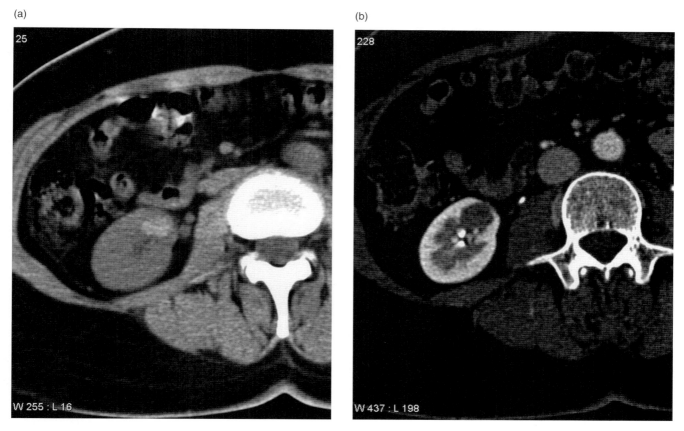

FIGURE 6b-14. (**A, B**) Hyperdense cyst; no enhancement after IV contrast. No follow-up is needed.

routine CT often only post IV contrast scans are made. A delayed scan after 15 minutes may then be obtained to demonstrate deenhancement or contrast wash-out of a lesion. Deenhancement of more than 15 HU confirms the presence of a solid lesion (Macari and Bosniak, 1999).

When scans of only a single, postcontrast phase are available a solid lesion may still be differentiated from a hyperdense cyst if the lesion has a density >70 HU. In a hyperdense cyst the density is due to bleeding in the cyst and the CT density of blood usually is lower than 70 HU. A density >70 is therefore likely to be due to tumor enhancement. If only postcontrast scans are available, small calcifications should not be mistaken for contrast enhancement.

Staging

Although the accuracy of CT for staging RCC has been reported to be high (91%) (Sheth et al., 2001), CT is still poor in defining whether the tumor is confined to within the renal capsule or whether the perinephric space has been invaded.

Even in small RCCs (<3 cm) the perinephric spread of the tumor is present in a high percentage (Hsu et al., 2004). However, the CT sign of stranding of the perinephric fatty tissue is unreliable for diagnosing a T3 stage tumor (Figs. 6b-15 and 6b-16). Only the demonstration of perinephric enhancing nodules is regarded as a reliable sign

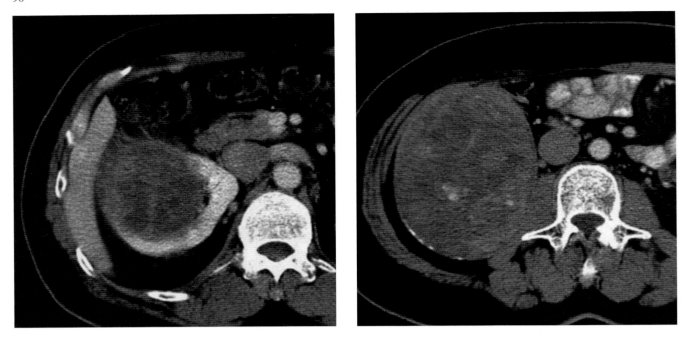

FIGURE 6b-15. False-positive perinephric stranding in a male patient (56 years old) with papillary carcinoma. At pathology pT2, there was no perirenal invasion. Note the slight calcifications in the tumor.

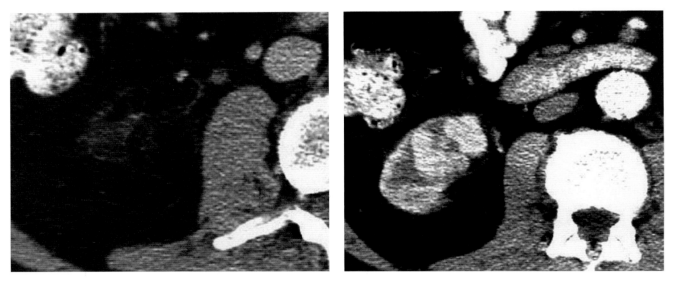

FIGURE 6b-16. Perinephric stranding caudal to the tumor. Pathology proven perinephric tumor spread.

for perinephric tumor spread. The sensitivity of this sign is relatively low (45%). The presence of perirenal tumor vessels is also an unreliable sign for diagnosing perinephric tumor spread.

Furthermore, CT has limited value in demonstrating the presence of a pseudocapsule surrounding the tumor. Such capsules are clearly better depicted by MRI. The presence of a pseudocapsule has been associated with limited tumors (T1, T2) with lower histological grading (Yamashita et al., 1996; Roy et al., 2005).

Venous Invasion

Thrombus in the renal vein or in the inferior vena cava (IVC) is reliably demonstrated by CT (Figs. 6b-17 and 6b-18). Some limitations arise in the right kidney where large tumors may easily compress and obscure the short right renal vein. Another pitfall may be poor enhancement of the infrarenal IVC, due to inflow effects of unopacified blood from the legs. For the detection of thrombus of the renal vein, multidetector CT has been found to be equivalent to MRI.

Renal Sinus Fat Invasion

In 50% of clear cell carcinomas renal sinus fat infiltration is found at pathology (Bonsib, 2005). Invasion of the renal sinus fat is understimated by CT. Studies that have compared CT findings with findings at pathology have found renal sinus invasion in 30% of tumers thought to be a T1 tumor at CT. Invasion of the renal sinus would mean a T3 stage and a worse prognosis for the patient (Fig. 6b-19).

In spite of the limitations of CT for staging, it is still very useful to guide treatment decisions, e.g., whether to locally treat the tumor. It was shown that in patients with a T1 stage

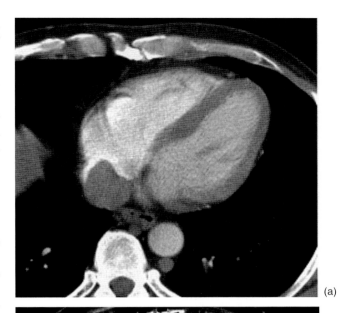
(a)

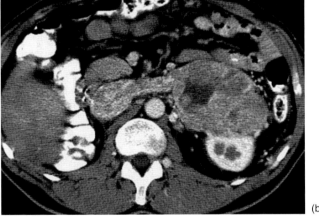
(b)

FIGURE 6b-18. (**A, B**) RCC with tumor thrombus in the renal vein, the inferior vena cava, and the right atrium. Note enhancement of tumor thrombus. Tumor stage T3c.

at CT, the prognosis was equal to the prognosis of patients who actually had a T3pa stage at pathology (renal sinus fat invasion undetected by CT) (Roberts et al., 2005).

Pseudocapsule

The presence of a pseudocapsule is associated with low-grade tumors and a better prognosis. In two-thirds of small RCCs (<4 cm) and in one-third of large RCCs (>7 cm) a pseudocapsule may be shown by MRI, using T2 weighted and postcontrast T1 weighted sequences. In a series comparing MRI with CT all pseudocapsules were visible on MRI, but no capsule was visible on CT (Yamashita et al., 1996). However, it is unclear whether the demonstration of a pseudocapsule

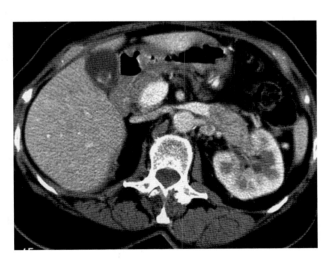

FIGURE 6b-17. RCC with renal vein invasion, stage T3b.

(a)

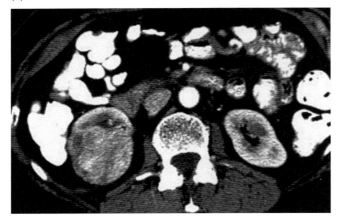

(b)

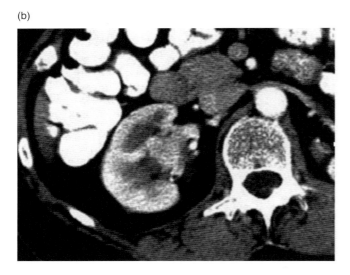

(c)

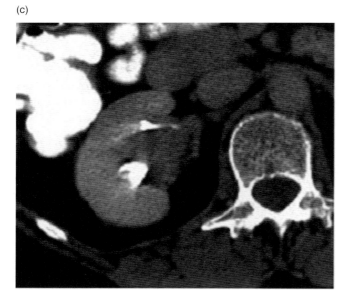

FIGURE 6b-19. (**A–C**) Clear cell carcinoma. Delayed phase (**c**) shows renal sinus fat invasion stage T3a.

influences the choice of therapy and whether an MRI should therefore be obtained in all these patients.

Cystic Lesions

The Bosniak classification to categorize cystic lesions by morphology has been very useful, although there are ongoing discussions on the treatment of lesions in several categories.

In simple cysts and in Bosniak 2 lesions no further follow-up is needed. These cysts may contain some thin septa or hairline calcifications. Complications in a simple cyst, like hemorrhage or infection, may lead to alterations in a cyst. Wall thickening, formation of septa, and enhancement of the wall or nodularity in a complicated cyst may be indistinguishable from a cystic RCC.

Bosniak has defined a type 2F lesion for which he recommended follow-up. These lesions showed "more than hairline" calcifications, a slightly thickened septum or slightly thickened walls of the cyst, enhancement of the wall, or the presence of an intrarenal cyst with a diameter >3 cm. His recommendations for follow-up were based on a retrospective study: two carcinomas were detected in 42 patients with type 2F cysts (mean follow-up of 5.8 years). In one patient the tumor was detected after 4 years (Israel and Bosniak, 2003).

Bosniak has recommended resection in all patients with type 3 cysts. These lesions have thickened (smooth or irregular) walls or septa that show contrast enhancement (Fig. 6b-20). Also multilocular lesions (more than two septa) are categorized as type 3 (Fig. 6b-21). Other authors recommend the use of histological biopsy in type 3 lesions. In one study biopsies taken in type 3 lesions proved malignancy in 60% of the cases. This may facilitate the decision to undergo a resection. Benign lesions were diagnosed in 40% of the cases, although follow-up in benign lesions was very short (1 year). Another drawback of this study was that it was retrospective (Harisinghani et al., 2003).

For type 2F and type 3 lesions most studies performed were retrospective and evidence for treatment policy is less solid. Unilocular cystic RCC is rare, but may be hard to recognize on CT. Slight enhancement of a lesion may be the key factor to differentiate a solid lesion from a hyperdense cyst or a cystic RCC from a type 2 cyst. When there is any doubt as to whether a lesion enhances other investigations (MR, biopsy) or follow-up studies are needed.

Differential Diagnosis of RCC

Although most solid renal tumors are RCC, other malignant tumors such as lymphoma, metastasis, and transitional cell carcinoma may present as a solid renal mass (Fig. 6b-22). A recent study of 2770 resected solid renal lesions showed that nearly 13% were benign. When stratified for size

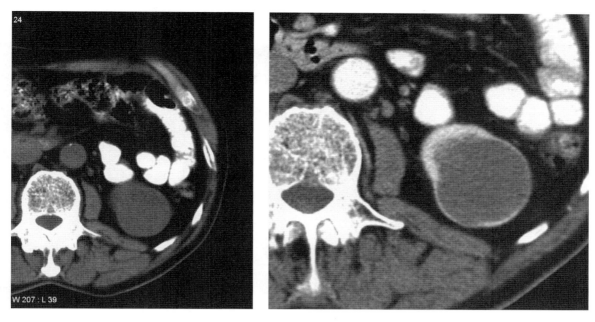

FIGURE 6b-20. Cystic lesion with enhancement of the cyst wall: renal cell carcinoma.

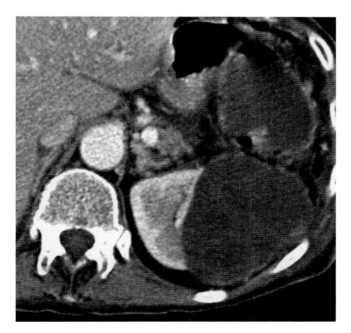

FIGURE 6b-21. Multiloculated cyst. Type 3 Bosniak. Cystic nephroma.

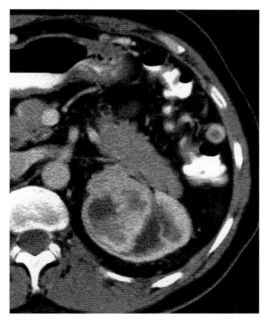

FIGURE 6b-22. Metastatic lesion to the kidney in a patient with previous ipsilateral adrenal pheochromocytoma.

(a)

(b)

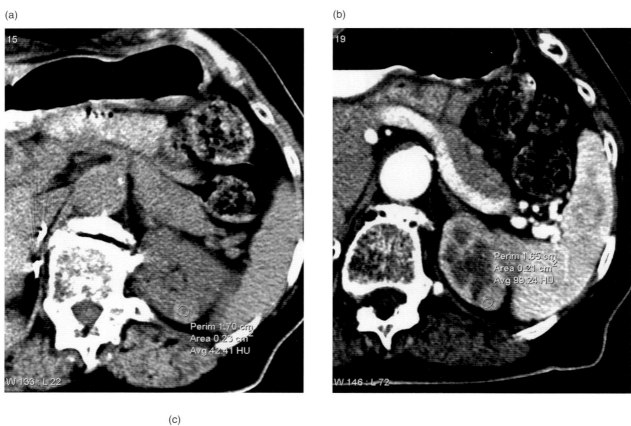

(c)

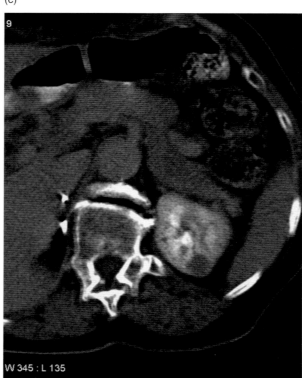

FIGURE 6b-23. (**A–C**) Hyperdense lesion on plain CT, appearing cystic on delayed images. Contrast CT (**b**) shows homogeneous enhancement of the lesion. PA: oncocytoma (partial volume artifact of the spleen).

25% of resected renal masses <3 cm were benign and 30% of the resected lesions <2 cm were benign (Frank et al., 2003). Most benign lesions were oncocytoma and angiomyolipoma.

Oncocytoma

This benign tumor usually is small and unilateral, though large tumors and bilateral oncocytoma have been reported. The tumor is homogeneous and shows uniform strong enhancement (Fig. 6b-23). A low-density, stellate, central or eccentric scar in the lesion is characteristic, and is present in approximately two-thirds of oncocytomas that are larger than 3 cm. Small oncocytomas rarely show a central scar (Weirich et al., 1998). Oncocytomas do not show cystic degeneration, central necrosis, or hemorrhage. Oncocytomas comprise 1–3% of renal neoplasms. However, in the subgroup of small solid renal lesions, supected carcinoma, that are amendable for local treatment, there may be a high percentage of oncocytomas. In one series of 52 indeterminate tumors that were treated conservatively (local surgery/cryosurgery/
radiofrequency ablation or follow-up), 23% of tumors were oncocytic at pathological examination of biopsies (Shah et al., 2005).

Angiomyolipoma

Angiomyolipomas (AMLs) are benign renal tumors, composed of fat, smooth muscle, and abnormal blood vessels. Demonstration of fat in the lesion by CT is sufficient to identify these lesions. There is a small subgroup of angiomyolipomas (5%) that contains minimal fat and therefore may mimic a RCC (Fig. 6b-24). These AMLs with minimal fat show a slight difference with RCC in attenuation (high for AML) and enhancement pattern (homogeneous, prolonged enhancement for AML). In a study comparing RCC and AML with minimal fat, none of the AMLs showed calcifications. In practice, the diagnosis of AML with minimal fat can be suggested only on the basis of multiphasic CT, and biopsy may be indicated to confirm the diagnosis (Kim et al., 2002).

In patients with tuberous sclerosis the development of multiple renal angiomyolipomas is common. This genetic disease is characterized by hamartomas in the skin, brain,

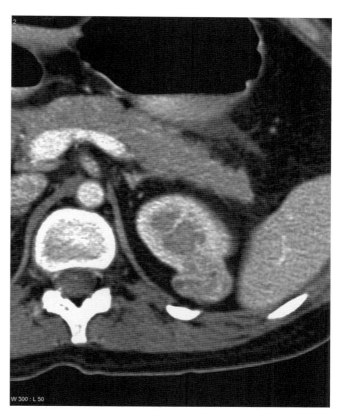

FIGURE 6b-24. Angiomyolipoma containing minimal fat. This may be indistinguishable from renal cell carcinoma.

and viscera. The classic triad consists of adenoma sebaceum (angiofibroma), cerebral sclerosis (tubers), and cardiac and renal tumors (Table 6b-1). These patients also have an increased risk of RCC of 1–2% and involvement of other organ systems (Fig. 6b-25) (Choyke et al.,2003).

von Hippel–Lindau Disease

Patients with this hereditary disease have an increased risk of developing an RCC. The lifetime risk for acquiring this tumor is estimated to be 28–45%. All carcinomas are of the clear cell type. Typically in young patients the kidneys show bilateral solid and cystic lesions (Fig. 6b-26). A variety of benign and malignant lesions may arise in several other organ systems (Table 6b-2) (Choyke et al., 2003).

Urothelial Cell Carcinoma

RCC located in the renal hilum may be difficult to differentiate from urothelial cell carcinoma. Especially in large tumors invading both the pyelum and renal parenchyma the origin of the mass will remain unclear. The demonstration

TABLE 6b-1. Tuberous sclerosis.

Cortical tubers, astrocytoma, brain
Hamartoma, skin, brain, retina, viscera
Rhabdomyoma, heart
Lymphangioleiomyomatosis, lung
Cysts, angiomyolipoma, kidney
Risk for renal cell carcinoma: 1–2%

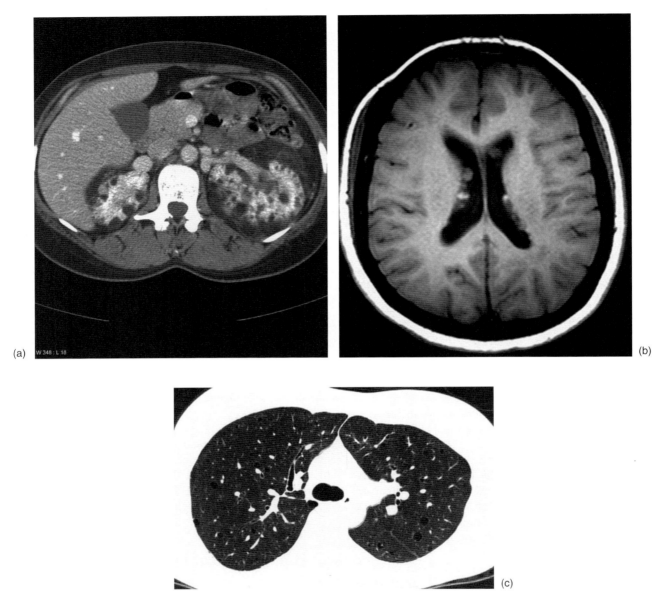

FIGURE 6b-25. (**A**) Multiple renal angiomyolipoma and RCC in a patient with tuberous sclerosis. (**B**) Brain tubers in tuberous sclerosis. (**C**) Lymphangioleiomatosis in a patient with tubereous sclerosis.

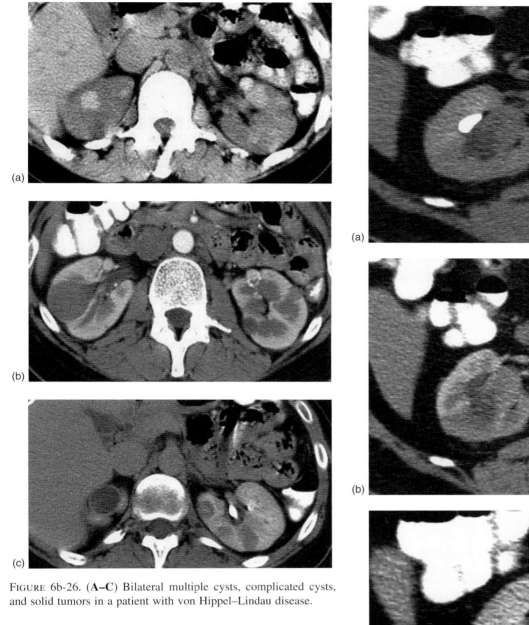

(a)

(b)

(c)

FIGURE 6b-26. (**A–C**) Bilateral multiple cysts, complicated cysts, and solid tumors in a patient with von Hippel–Lindau disease.

of pyelum invasion by the tumor is best shown on delayed images (Figs. 6b-27 and 6b-28). In small urothelial carcinomas CT can easily demonstrate the tumor origin in the pyelum.

TABLE 6b-2. von Hippel–Landau disease.

Autosomal dominant
Retinal angiomas
Cerebellar hemangioblastoma
Endolymphatic sac tumors
Epididymal cystadenoma
Pancreatic cysts, cystadenoma, neuroendocrine tumors
Pheochromocytoma (bilateral)
Renal cysts, clear cell carcinoma

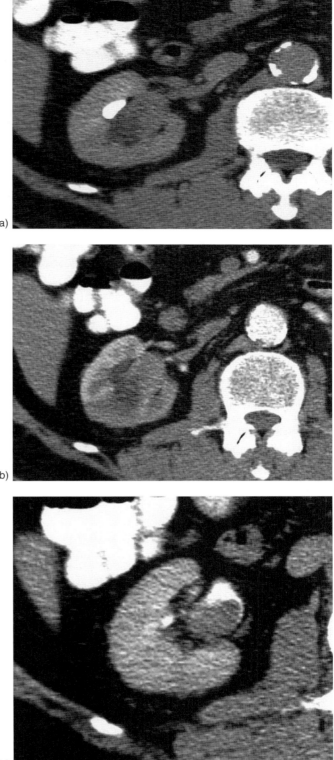

(a)

(b)

(c)

FIGURE 6b-27. (**A–C**) Central mass; delayed phase demonstrates pyelum invasion:urothelial cell carcinoma.

(a)   (b)

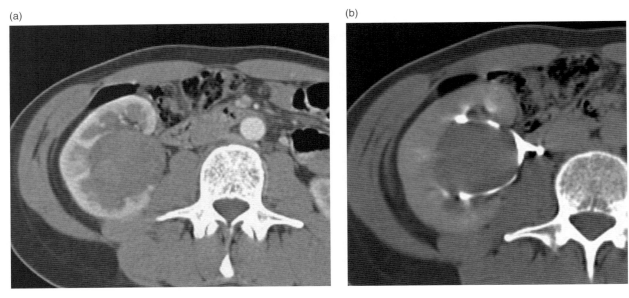

FIGURE 6b-28. Central mass; delayed phase shows compression of the pyelum: renal cell carcinoma.

References

Bonsib, S.M. "T2 clear cell renal cell carcinoma is a rare entity: a study of 120 clear cell renal cell carcinomas." *J. Urol.* 174.4 Pt 1 (2005): 1199–1202.

Choyke, P.L., et al. "Hereditary renal cancers." *Radiology* 226.1 (2003): 33–46.

Coll, D.M., et al. "Preoperative use of 3D volume rendering to demonstrate renal tumors and renal anatomy." *Radiographics* 20.2 (2000): 431–438.

Frank, I., et al. "Solid renal tumors: an analysis of pathological features related to tumor size." *J. Urol.* 170.6 Pt 1 (2003): 2217–2220.

Goldman, S.M. "Dual-phase helical CT of the kidney: value of the corticomedullary and nephrographic phase for evaluation of renal lesions and preoperative staging of renal cell carcinoma." *J. Urol.* 160.4 (1998): 1586–1587.

Harisinghani, M.G., et al. "Incidence of malignancy in complex cystic renal masses (Bosniak category III): should imaging-guided biopsy precede surgery?" *AJR Am. J. Roentgenol.* 180.3 (2003): 755–758.

Hsu, R.M., D.Y. Chan, and S.S. Siegelman. "Small renal cell carcinomas: correlation of size with tumor stage, nuclear grade, and histologic subtype." *AJR Am. J. Roentgenol.* 182.3 (2004): 551–557.

Israel, G.M. and M.A. Bosniak. "Follow-up CT of moderately complex cystic lesions of the kidney (Bosniak category IIF)." *AJR Am. J. Roentgenol.* 181.3 (2003): 627–633.

Jinzaki, M., et al. "Evaluation of small (</= 3 cm) renal masses with MDCT: benefits of thin overlapping reconstructions." *AJR Am. J. Roentgenol.* 183.1 (2004): 223–228.

Kawashima, A., et al. "CT urography." *Radiographics* 24 Suppl 1 (2004): S35–S54.

Kim, J.K., et al. "Differentiation of subtypes of renal cell carcinoma on helical CT scans." *AJR Am. J. Roentgenol.* 178.6 (2002): 1499–1506.

Kopka, L., et al. "Dual-phase helical CT of the kidney: value of the corticomedullary and nephrographic phase for evaluation of renal lesions and preoperative staging of renal cell carcinoma." *AJR Am. J. Roentgenol.* 169.6 (1997): 1573–1578.

Lesavre, A., et al. "CT of papillary renal cell carcinomas with cholesterol necrosis mimicking angiomyolipomas." *AJR Am. J. Roentgenol.* 181.1 (2003): 143–145.

Macari, M. and M.A. Bosniak. "Delayed CT to evaluate renal masses incidentally discovered at contrast-enhanced CT: demonstration of vascularity with deenhancement." *Radiology* 213.3 (1999): 674–680.

Pereira, J.M., et al. "CT and MR imaging of extrahepatic fatty masses of the abdomen and pelvis: techniques, diagnosis, differential diagnosis, and pitfalls." *Radiographics* 25.1 (2005): 69–85.

Roberts, W.W., et al. "Pathological stage does not alter the prognosis for renal lesions determined to be stage T1 by computerized tomography." *J. Urol.* 173.3 (2005): 713–715.

Roy, C., Sr., et al. "Significance of the pseudocapsule on MRI of renal neoplasms and its potential application for local staging: a retrospective study." *AJR Am. J. Roentgenol.* 184.1 (2005): 113–120.

Ruppert-Kohlmayr, A.J., et al. "Differentiation of renal clear cell carcinoma and renal papillary carcinoma using quantitative CT enhancement parameters." *AJR Am. J. Roentgenol.* 183.5 (2004): 1387–1391.

Shah, R.B., et al. "Image-guided biopsy in the evaluation of renal mass lesions in contemporary urologicalpractice: indications, adequacy, clinical impact, and limitations of the pathological diagnosis." *Hum. Pathol.* 36.12 (2005): 1309–1515.

Sheth, S., et al. "Current concepts in the diagnosis and management of renal cell carcinoma: role of multidetector CT and three-dimensional CT." *Radiographics* 21 Spec No (2001): S237–S254.

Suh, M., et al. "Distinction of renal cell carcinomas from high-attenuation renal cysts at portal venous phase contrast-enhanced CT." *Radiology* 228.2 (2003): 330–334.

Weirich, G., et al. "Familial renal oncocytoma: clinicopathological study of 5 families." *J. Urol.* 160.2 (1998): 335–340.

Yamashita, Y., et al. "Detection of pseudocapsule of renal cell carcinoma with MR imaging and CT." *AJR Am. J. Roentgenol.* 166.5 (1996): 1151–1155.

Zagoria, R.J., et al. "Percutaneous CT-guided radiofrequency ablation of renal neoplasms: factors influencing success." *AJR Am. J. Roentgenol.* 183.1 (2004): 201–207.

6c
Magnetic Resonance Imaging of Renal Cell Cancer

Els L.F. Nijs and Raymond H. Oyen

Introduction

Radiology has a key role in the detection and determination of management strategies in patients with renal cell carcinoma (RCC). With the widespread use of cross-sectional techniques, it is estimated that at least one-third of RCC is diagnosed incidentally (Leslie et al., 2003). Such tumors are smaller and generally of lower stage and lower grade, usually less biologically aggressive, and have a slow but variable rate of growth (Bosniak et al., 1995). Patients with incidentally discovered RCC have a more favorable prognosis than patients presenting with symptomatic RCC.

The radiological detection of a solid renal parenchymal mass without fat is virtually diagnostic for RCC. Indeed, RCC is the most common malignant, solid renal parenchymal neoplasm. The differential includes benign tumors, lymphoma, metastases, and various sarcomas.

Predominantly cystic RCCs comprise only a small portion of all cystic or cyst-like renal masses. The differentiation between a benign cyst or cyst-like lesion and a cystic RCC is important for appropriate patient management. The "Bosniak classification" is based on objective criteria for characterization of cystic renal masses (nonsurgical vs. surgical) and can serve as a practical guideline (Bosniak, 1997).

Although computed tomography (CT) has emerged as the procedure of choice for detecting and staging RCC, dedicated magnetic resonance imaging (MRI) is equally useful for renal lesion characterization, staging, and follow-up (Beer et al., 2006).

Magnetic Resonance Technique

Multiple studies have been reported in the late 1980s and in the 1990s to outline the value and the place of MRI versus existing modalities (e.g., ultrasound, CT, angiography) for the diagnosis and staging of renal mass lesions, in particular RCC. In the late 1980s, Fritzsche stated that MRI had several advantages compared to CT, based on the improved tissue contrast resolution and the multiplanar imaging capabilities (Fritzsche, 1989). MRI was found to be valuable for the determination of tumor origin, evaluation of vascular patency, evaluation of direct tumor extension into adjacent organs, and detection of lymph node metastases. Because of the widespread availability of CT, however, in practice MRI became accepted in selected patients only, i.e., to evaluate possible tumor thrombus in the renal vein and inferior vena cava (IVC) (Arlart et al., 1992). Indeed, MRI gradually replaced CT and substraction angiography for this indication. Contrast-enhanced dynamic MRI proved also to be useful for the diagnosis of small RCC in patients with impaired renal function or allergy to iodinated contrast material (Yamashita et al., 1995). MRI is theoretically ideal for screening purposes in patients with hereditary renal cancer, but is not widely recommended because of wide variations in quality and because of the expense (Choyke et al., 2003).

Although CT is widely accepted as the imaging modality of choice for the detection, characterization, and staging of renal mass lesions, MRI is reliable for preoperative characterization and staging of RCC (Ergen et al., 2004; Beer et al., 2006). In addition, Pretorius et al. (1999) found that dynamic and delayed postgadolinium images are particularly accurate in identifying the true-negative findings by correctly depicting that the perinephric fat (100%), the renal sinus fat (91%), and the renal collecting system (100%) were uninvolved by the tumor. It also became clear that the pseudocapsule of RCC could be reliably detected with MR (Huang et al., 1992), especially on T2-weighted images (Takahashi et al., 1996). The presence of a pseudocapsule indicates the absence of any perinephric fat invasion and therefore the tumor is more likely to be amenable to partial nephrectomy (Roy et al., 2005).

Many studies were performed to define a "state-of-the-art" MR study: several combinations of different sequences without or with intravenous injection of gadolinium were proposed on different field strength magnets. Some protocols are extensive, yet provide all essential information on renal vessels, renal lesions, renal parenchyma, the excretory system, adrenals, lymph nodes, and liver in a single examination (so called "one-stop-shopping"). These protocols kept on changing over the years, in accordance with the technical improvements in newer equipment. In the meantime, CT also made spectacular progress in the past decade. Multislice and multidetector CT has become as accurate in defining the extent of tumor thrombus as MRI (Hallscheidt et al., 2005; Lawrentschuk et al., 2005). The favorable evolution of CT and the limited access to MRI contribute to the reason why MRI has not been able to fully replace CT for the diagnosis and staging of RCC (Sheth et al., 2001), with only few institutional exceptions.

For the evaluation of a renal mass, a combination of T1- and T2-weighted sequences, without and with intravenous contrast administration, is essential for lesion characterization. The signal intensity of RCC varies along with the histological subtype of RCC. Nevertheless, there is some overlap between the features of these subtypes, and although experience makes it possible to optimize the diagnosis of RCC, the final histological diagnosis can be obtained only by percutaneous biopsy or surgery.

The evaluation of a renal parenchymal mass involves roughly two stages: (1) characterization of the renal mass lesion, i.e., whether the mass represents a surgical or a nonsurgical lesion, and (2) staging (Israel et al., 2005). In practice, the two stages are tightly interwoven, since some staging features may be indicative of the histological type or even subtype.

To achieve these goals at MRI, several sequences are required. The evaluation of a renal mass lesion includes turboflash T1-weighted images (T1WI) (the absence or presence of lesional hemorrhage) (Figs. 6c-1a and 6c-2a), T2-weighted images (T2WI) as the HASTE sequence (to detect intralesional necrosis) (Fig. 6c-1b), and opposed-phase chemical shift imaging (to demonstrate or exclude intralesional fat) (Fig. 6c-1c). An image section thickness of 5–8 mm is recommended. Fat-suppressed T1WI before and after administration during the corticomedullary phase (Fig. 6c-1d), the parenchymal phase (Fig. 6c-1e and f), and the excretory phase should be obtained and has more or less become standard for the evaluation of renal mass lesions. Most radiologists (and urologists) feel comfortable with these images since from a morphological point of view they closely resemble CT images, with which they have become familiar. The spatial orientation of the sequences may be tailored according to the location of the (main) lesion, in the axial, coronal, or sagittal plane. A lesion located in the pole of the kidney will be preferably scanned in the coronal plane; sagittal series are recommended when the lesion is located at the anterior or posterior surface of the kidney.

Scialpi et al. (2000) demonstrated that in the characterization of small renal lesions (<3 cm), quantitative analysis of signal intensity variations during dynamic contrast-enhanced MR imaging with fat suppression is essential, in particular in hypovascular lesions. The optimal percentage of enhancement threshold for distinguishing cysts from malignancies is 15% at images obtained 2–4 minutes after administration of gadolinium (Ho et al., 2002; Hecht et al., 2004).

Image substraction enables an accurate assessment of renal tumor enhancement, particularly in the setting of masses that are hyperintense on unenhanced MR images and should be performed to avoid false-negative quantitative results (Hecht et al., 2004).

A promising tool for future lesion characterization seems to be diffusion-weighted MR of renal mass lesions. Diffusion is a physical process based on the Brownian movement (and random movement of water molecules). With this technique information about the biophysical properties of tissues is obtained including cell organization and density, microstructure, and microcirculation. This information harbors the potential to differentiate between normal tissue and different renal tumors (Squillaci et al., 2004; Manenti et al., 2004).

Classification of Renal Cell Carcinoma

A new simplified classification of RCC was proposed by Union Internationale Contre le Cancer (UICC) and the American Joint Committee on Cancer in 1997. This classification is now widely used and is based on morphological and molecular characteristics and correlates well with prognosis (Moch et al., 2000; Amin et al., 2002; Cohen et al., 2005). There are five different subtypes of which the clear cell type (also referred to as the conventional RCC) is the most common, representing 70–85% of cases. The cells are characterized by their lipid and glycogen-rich cytoplasm. The papillary carcinoma (also referred to as the chromophylic subtype) is the second most common subtype representing approximately 10–15% of cases and generally has a better prognosis than clear cell RCC. The chromophobic subtype (2–4%) arises from the cortical collecting ducts. The collecting duct (Bellini duct) subtype (1%) arises from the medullary collecting duct. Finally there is a subgroup of yet undefined cancers, the unclassified type (4–5%).

The previously described sarcomatoid subtype is not considered a separate subgroup; it has become clear that this subtype may arise from other subtypes of RCC (clear cell, papillary, chromophobic, Bellini duct). Furthermore, there is a lack of convincing evidence of *de novo* development of sarcomatoid carcinoma. Anyhow, sarcomas constitute a heterogeneous subgroup with a poor prognosis.

Renal Cell Carcinoma of the Clear Cell Type or Classic/Conventional Renal Cell Carcinoma

The conventional or clear cell subtype is the most common subtype of malignant epithelial renal parenchymal tumors, representing at least 75% of cases. There is a male predominance (male/female ratio: 1.5–2/1). In the majority of cases clear cell RCC occurs sporadically and as a solitary tumor. In 4% of cases, however, there are multiple tumors in the same

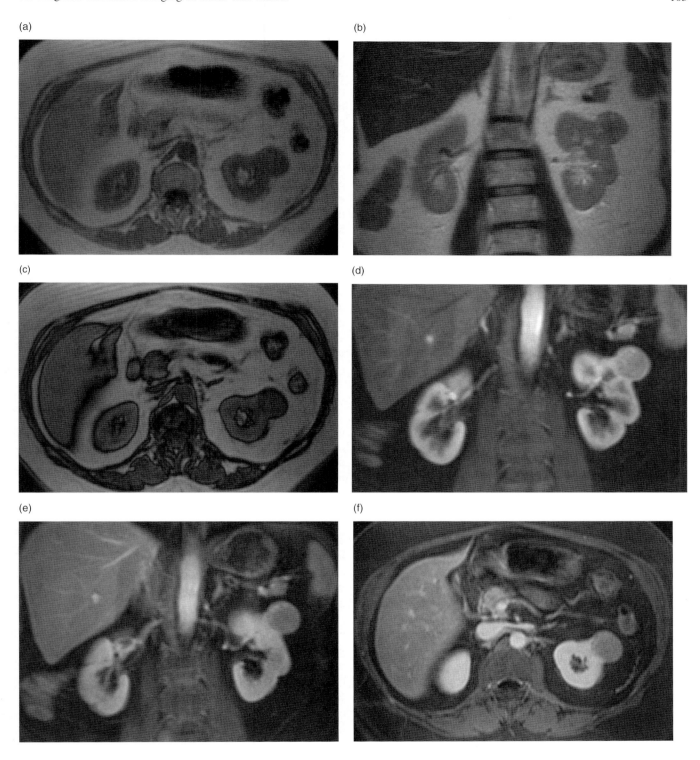

FIGURE 6c-1. (A) Clear cell RCC in a 62-year-old female. Axial T1WI: the mass in the left kidney is slightly hypointense compared to the normal renal cortex. (B) Out-of-phase image: small areas of signal loss compared with the in-phase images, indicating the presence of fat. (C) Coronal T2WI: slightly hypointense lesion with some hyperintense foci in the periphery, and protruding outside the normal renal contour (exophytic growth pattern) at the upper pole of the left kidney. Eccentric lesional necrosis is rather typical for a clear cell RCC. (D) Coronal T1WI, fat suppressed, and after the administration of IV gadolinium; corticomedullary phase: strong enhancement in the arterial phase. (E) Coronal T1WI, fat suppressed, and after the administration of IV gadolinium; parenchymal phase: quick wash-out in the venous phase. (F) Axial T1WI, fat suppressed, after the administration of IV gadolinium; late venous phase: the typical "crab sign" at the junction between the lesion and the renal cortex, indicating the renal origin of the lesion.

kidney, synchronous or metachronous (Prando et al., 2006). Bilateral tumors can be expected in approximately 0.5–3% of patients. The prevalence of RCC in patients with hereditary renal cancers as in von Hippel–Lindau disease is 35–38% . In these syndromes, RCC will present more often with multifocality and/or bilaterality (Choyke et al., 2003; Tattersall et al., 2002; Prando et al., 2006). Furthermore, these cancers may develop much earlier in life [mean patient age at discovery 37 years, or almost 20 years younger than for sporadic RCC (Tattersall et al., 2002)] and there is no sex predominance (Choyke et al., 2003).

RCC of the clear cell type is randomly distributed in the renal cortex; it is ball-shaped with exophytic growth (protruding outside the renal border) or almost complete intrarenal growth. In most instances the tumor is sharply demarcated from the surrounding normal parenchyma; however, a definite pseudocapsule depends on the nuclear grading: a pseudocapsule is more often present in well-differentiated lesions. Clear cell RCC may present as an infiltrating mass with preservation of the renal shape. In these cases the differential diagnosis includes infiltrating tumors such as urothelial carcinoma.

Areas of necrosis, hemorrhage, cystic degeneration, and coarse calcification can be expected. Distinct areas of fat may be observed, almost exclusively in association with extensive calcification. These coarse calcifications may be present in the periphery, near the center, or scattered throughout the mass. This contrasts with the benign angiomyolipoma, where calcifications are not likely to be seen.

These morphological features are translated at MRI. Clear cell RCCs are slightly hypointense on T1WI and slightly hyperintense on T2WI. A key feature is intralesional necrosis, typically in an eccentric location: necrosis extends asymmetrically to the periphery of the lesion usually at the opposite site of the implantation base in the renal parenchyma (Oyen et al., 1999). Necrosis is also seen in small lesions. Intralesional necrosis appears as a low signal on T1WI and a high signal on T2WI (Fig. 6c-2). Calcifications are difficult to appreciate on MRI. A pseudocapsule can be seen as a hypointense rim surrounding the lesion on T1WI and T2WI (Fig. 6c-3).

Typical of the clear cell subtype is the hypervascularity in the arterial or corticomedullary phase after the intravenous administration of gadolinium (Hricak et al., 1988). Only 20% will be isovascular or hypovascular compared to the renal cortex. Due to a fast wash-out, the tumor will become hypointense in the venous/parenchymal and excretory phase. Extension to the renal vein (Figs. 6c-4 and 6c-5), IVC, or adjacent structures is virtually pathognomonic for this subtype. Postcontrast evaluation is essential for lesion detection too, since small tumors may be difficult to detect on the precontrast images only (a similar signal intensity to renal parenchyma on both T1WI and T2WI) (Yamashita et al., 1995).

Chemical shift gradient-echo MR imaging (CSI) can detect area fat as signal loss on out-of-phase images as compared to in-phase images. An index to represent the signal loss was proposed by Yoshimitsu et al. (2004). A signal loss ratio (SLR) of more than 0.1 is significant, representing the presence of intravoxel fat. Tissues without fat have an SLR of about zero. Less than zero is due to focal susceptibility, i.e., hemosiderin deposition. A clear cell RCC is characterized by the presence of fat in the cytoplasm in the cells, which can be clearly demonstrated by this technique (Yoshimitsu et al., 2004). Metastases from clear cell RCC will demonstrate signal intensities similar to the primary tumor and thus may occasionally have signal loss on the out-of-phase images. Muram and Aisen (2003) described fatty metastatic lesions in the pleura/chest wall and liver in patients with a previous history of clear cell RCC. Caution is warranted in cases in which an adrenal mass is found in patients with clear cell RCC (Fig. 6c-6; the same patient as in Fig. 6c-1). In patients without known malignancy, the presence of fat in a small adrenal lesion favors the diagnosis of an adrenal adenoma, whereas in oncological patients this finding may be consistent with a fat-containing metastasis from a clear cell RCC (Shinozaki et al., 2001).

Approximately 10% of clear cell RCC are almost completely cystic, unilocular, or multilocular (Nassir et al., 2002; Prando et al., 2006). Cystic RCCs tend also to present as a solitary lesion, predominantly on the right side (75%) and in the interpolar region. Like its solid counterpart, there is a male-to-female ratio of 2:1. They usually present as rounded mass lesions.

Cystic RCC may be difficult to differentiate from benign neoplasms, especially from benign multilocular cystic nephroma. Additional features, such as focal mural thickening or protrusions, focal thickening at septations, gender, location, protrusion in the renal hilum, regional lymph nodes, and renal vein patency may contribute to lesion discrimination (Oyen et al., 2005). The differentiation between a benign cyst and a cystic RCC is important for therapeutic management. Bosniak proposed a CT-based classification system for cystic renal masses that can be used as a guideline in clinical practice (surgical lesion or not). This well-accepted classification system may be extrapolated for evaluation of renal lesions with MRI (Israel et al., 2004). In a study performed by Israel et al. (2004) the findings on CT and MR were similar in the majority of cases, but in some MRI was more sensitive in depicting additional septa, thickening of the wall, and/or septa or enhancement, which finally may lead to an upgraded Bosniak classification. Mural irregularity, mural masses, or nodules, increased mural thickness (>2 mm), and intense mural enhancement are all suggestive of malignancy (Balci et al., 1999) and require surgery (Hartman et al., 2004). These features indeed virtually exclude the radiological diagnosis of benign disease.

(a)

(b)

(c)

(d)

(e)

(f)

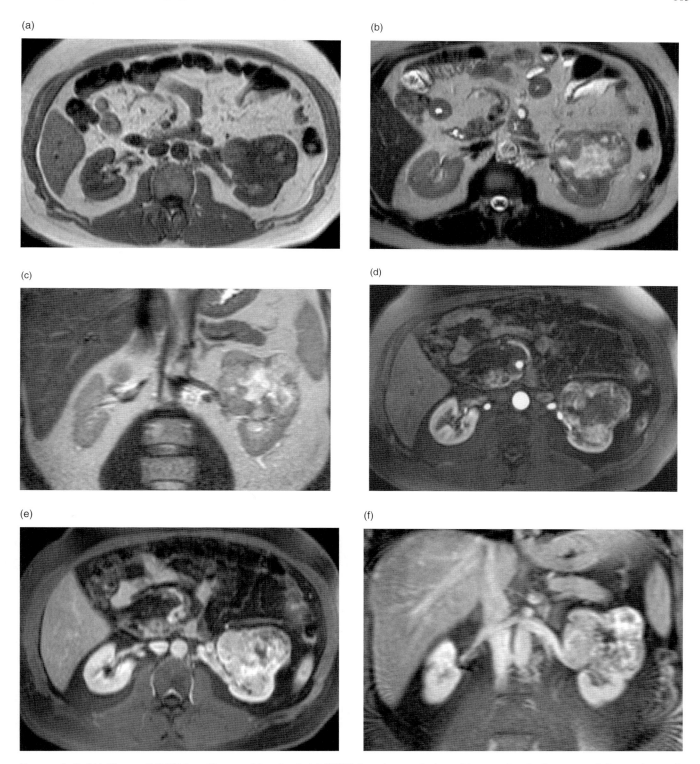

FIGURE 6c-2. (**A**) Clear cell RCC in a 42-year-old male. Axial T1WI: hypointense lesion with posterior displacement of the renal vascular pedicle. (**B**) Axial T2WI: bulky heterogeneous lesion in the left kidney. This lesion extends into the renal sinus. (**C**) Coronal T2WI: large tumor in the interpolar region extending into the upper calices of the kidney. This image suggests that the vascular pedicle of the kidney may be compromised by the tumor. (**D**) Axial T1WI, fat suppressed, after the administration of IV gadolinium: hypervascularity of the lesion in the arterial phase, mainly in the periphery. (**E**) Axial T1WI, fat suppressed, after the administration of IV gadolinium; arterial and venous phase: strong lesional enhancement. The hypointense areas correspond to the areas of necrosis. The main renal vein is patent. (**F**) Coronal T1WI, fat suppressed, after the administration of IV gadolinium. Confirmation of the patency of the main renal vein.

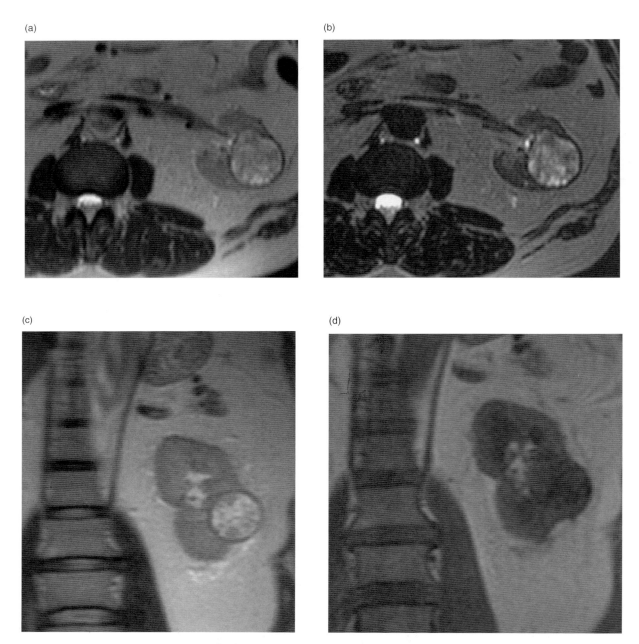

FIGURE 6c-3. (**A**) Clear cell RCC. Axial T2WI (short echo): well-defined rounded heterogeneously hyperintense lesion at the interpolar area of the left kidney, almost completely located in the cortex. The hypointense rim surrounding this lesion is consistent with a pseudocapsule, and is more likely in well-differentiated RCC. On pathology this lesion was a clear cell RCC, Fuhrman nuclear Grade II. (**B**) Axial T2WI (long echo). (**C**) Coronal T2WI: confirmation of the hypointense pseudocapsule surrounding the tumor. (**D**) Coronal T1WI: the tumor is a hypointense lesion compared to the normal renal cortex. (**E**) Axial T1WI, fat suppressed, after the administration of IV gadolinium: the arterial phase shows that the tumor enhances heterogeneously in the periphery. (**F**) Axial T1WI, fat suppressed, after the administration of IV gadolinium: strong lesional enhancement in the venous phase. (**G**) Axial T1WI, fat suppressed, after the administration of IV gadolinium: strong lesional enhance- ment in the excretory phase. The unenhancing areas of the tumor are consistent with necrosis. The renal vein is patent.

(e)

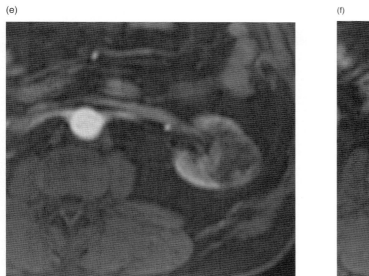

(f)

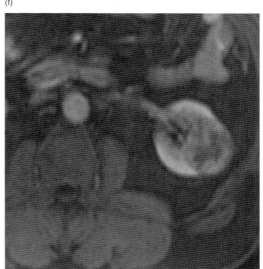

(g)

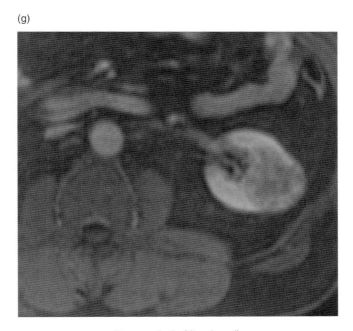

FIGURE 6c-3. (Continued)

(a)

(b)

(c)

(d)

(e)

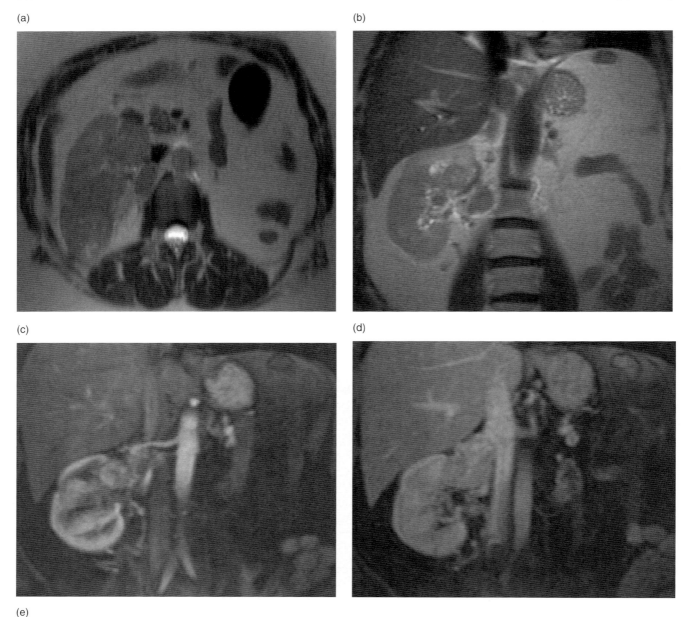

FIGURE 6c-4. (A) Clear cell RCC in a 62-year-old female. Axial T2WI: large almost isointense lesion at the posterior aspect of the right kidney, extending into the renal sinus, and probably to the main renal vein. This lesion is not well defined, but appears infiltrative. A well-defined rounded lesion with similar signal characteristics is seen posterior to the IVC, suggestive of lymph node metastases. (B) Coronal T2WI: enlarged lymph node is well observed. (C) Coronal T1WI, fat suppressed, after the administration of IV gadolinium: the arterial phase demonstrates the main renal artery, as well as a smaller additional renal artery. Enhancing tumor thrombus in the renal vein. (D) Coronal T1WI, fat suppressed, after the administration of IV gadolinium: the venous phase shows the tumor thrombus in the main renal vein extending up to the level of the junction with the IVC. (E) Axial T1WI, fat suppressed, after the administration of IV gadolinium: tumor and thrombus in the main renal vein.

Papillary/Chromophilic Renal Cell Carcinoma

Papillary carcinoma is the second most common malignant renal parenchymal neoplasm representing approximately 10–15% of RCC. There is a male predominance (2.5–5:1). The mean age is in the sixth decade, but with a wide age range.

In fact, there are two distinctive subgroups of papillary carcinoma. In one subgroup (type A, accounting for 75% of papillary cancers) the tumors are usually larger with a mixture of solid and cystic multinodules. The biological behavior is more aggressive. Lymph node metastases or distant soft tissue metastases may be the presenting symptom. Liver metastases or renal vein invasion are rare.

In the other subgroup (type B, accounting for approximately 25% of papillary carcinomas) the lesions are multiple in the same and/or contralateral kidney, frequently with one or two larger lesions (mother lesion) and multiple small lesions (daughter lesions), ranging in size from microscopic to subcentimetric lesions. The larger lesion (usually ±3 cm in diameter) grows exophytically with a partial extrarenal growth; the smaller lesions remain almost completely intracortical, or just slightly bulge from the renal surface. The smaller (microscopic) lesions remain undetected with imaging. In this subtype lymph node or distant metastases are rarely seen. The differential diagnosis includes anatomic variants, pseudotumors, cysts, and other tumors.

Papillary cancers are slightly hypointense (Fig. 6c-7) or isointense on T1WI (Figs. 6c-8 and 6c-9), with variable signal intensity on T2WI, and sometimes with hyperintense areas of necrosis (Figs. 6c-10 and 6c-11). This probably reflects different cytological variants (basophilic, eosinophilic, sarcomatoid) with different nuclear grades. In contrast to the clear cell subtype, these lesions are typically hypovascular in the corticomedullary phase or can be isovascular with wash-out in the venous phase. For differentiation from cysts, it is essential to quantify signal intensities on pre- and postcontrast series appropriately with similar parameters (the same plane of scanning, slice thickness, location, and voxel area). The optimal percentage of enhancement threshold for distinguishing cysts from malignancies is 15% 2–4 minutes after administration of gadolinium (Ho et al., 2002; Hecht et al., 2004). Image substraction enables accurate assessment of renal tumor enhancement, particularly in the setting of masses that are hyperintense on unenhanced MR images and should be performed to avoid false-negative quantitative results (Hecht et al., 2004). Calcification can be more frequently seen than in clear cell RCC. In type A these are usually punctiform and peripheral, yet calcifications remain difficult to appreciate on MRI.

T2*-weighted gradient-echo or echo-planar MR imaging can detect local susceptibility, for example, due to cytoplasmic or interstitial histiocytic hemosiderin deposition in papillary cell RCC. This focal susceptibility can also be demonstrated by CSI as excessive signal loss on in-phase images as compared to opposed-phase images (Yoshimitsu et al., 2004).

Hereditary papillary renal cancer type 1 (Choyke et al., 2003) tends to be hypovascular similar to the sporadic papillary RCC.

Chromophobe Cell Carcinoma

Chromophobe renal cell carcinoma is estimated to account for approximately 2–4% of all cases of RCC (Megumi et al., 1998; Kondo et al., 2004) (Fig. 6c-12). There seems to be two peak incidences: in the middle-aged female and in the older male (Verswijvel et al., 2004) with a median incidence in the sixth decade.

These tumors present as solitary masses, often located near the pole of the kidney and well circumscribed, but in contrast to the clear cell subtype, without evidence of extensive hemorrhage or necrosis (except in very large lesions).

There are two different variants microscopically. The typical variant consists of tumor cells with transparent cytoplasm showing a reticular or cloudy appearance. The eosinophilic variant is characterized by neoplastic cells containing eosinophilic cytoplasm with a perinuclear halo. Histochemical staining with Hale's colloidal iron stain demonstrates a distinctive positive cytoplasmic reaction in both types. The latter feature is seen in oncocytomas (Megumi et al., 1998) due to the presence of many vesicular structures inside the cytoplasm.

Since this is a rare tumor, typical imaging findings are not well defined. Kondo et al. (2004) retrospectively reviewed the images of seven patients with chromophobe carcinoma on MRI and found that none of the tumors was homogeneous on MRI. On T1WI the tumor was hypointense in one, isointense in five, and hyperintense in one, while on T2WI one tumor was hypointense, four were isointense, and two were hyperintense. All tumors were hypovascular to the renal medulla in the venous phase on contrast-enhanced dynamic MRI. In three patients with larger tumors (>7 cm) a spoke-wheel-like enhancement with a central scar was seen. Microscopically this correlated with thick vessels running along fibrous bands, which appeared to be strongly enhancing with gadolinium. A spoke-wheel-like enhancement, however, has been recognized as a characteristic finding of oncocytoma. Since several pathological features of chromophobe carcinoma correspond to those of oncocytoma (Weiss et al., 1995) similarities in imaging findings can be expected. Kondo et al. (2004) classified the tumors according to two different patterns. However, these did not correlate with the pathological variants (typical and eosinophilic) nor was there any relation with the clinical aspects of chromophobe tumors. The first pattern was characterized by tumors that demonstrated low density to isodensity in the corticomedullary phase during dynamic scanning. A spoke-wheel-like enhancement was observed in some patients. Pattern 2 was seen in tumors that demonstrated high density in the corticomedullary phase.

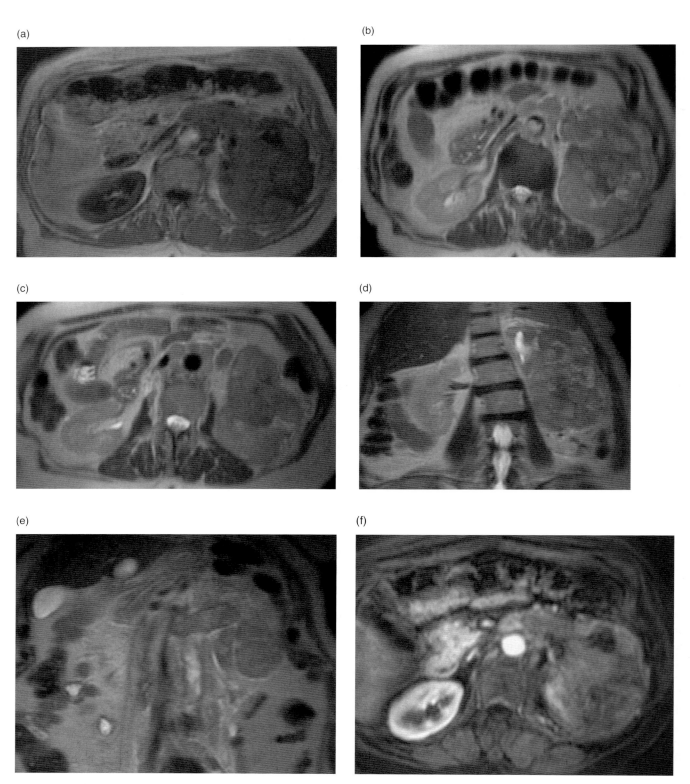

FIGURE 6c-5. (**A**) Clear cell RCC in a 75-year-old female. Axial T1WI: large tumor almost isointense with extension to the main renal vein. (**B**) Axial T2WI: heterogeneous mass lesion in the left kidney and multiple enlarged retroperitoneal lymph nodes. (**C**) Axial T2WI: heterogeneous mass lesion in the left kidney (lower level) and multiple enlarged retroperitoneal lymph nodes. (**D**) Coronal T2WI: bulky tumor infiltrating in the left kidney. (**E**)Coronal T2WI: the tumor extends into the main renal vein, and in the excretory system and the proximal ureter. (**F**) Axial T1WI, fat suppressed, after the administration of IV gadolinium: hypervascular tumor. (**G**) Axial T1WI, fat suppressed, after the administration of IV gadolinium: the late venous/excretory phase demonstrates the enhancing thrombus in the main renal vein. Note the eccentric areas of hypointensity in the tumor, indicating the eccentric intralesional necrosis. (**H**) Axial T1WI, fat suppressed, after the administration of IV gadolinium: the late venous/excretory phase demonstrates the enlarged retroperitoneal lymph nodes. Note the eccentric areas of hypointensity in the tumor, indicating the eccentric intralesional necrosis.

(g)

(h)

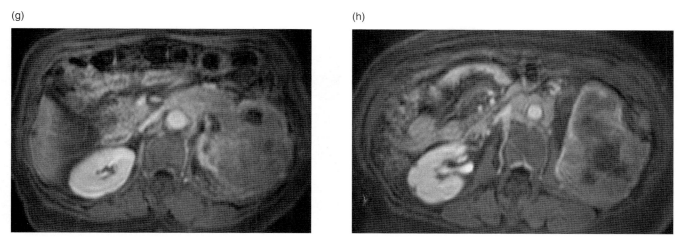

FIGURE 6c-5. (Continued)

(a)

(b)

(c)

(d)

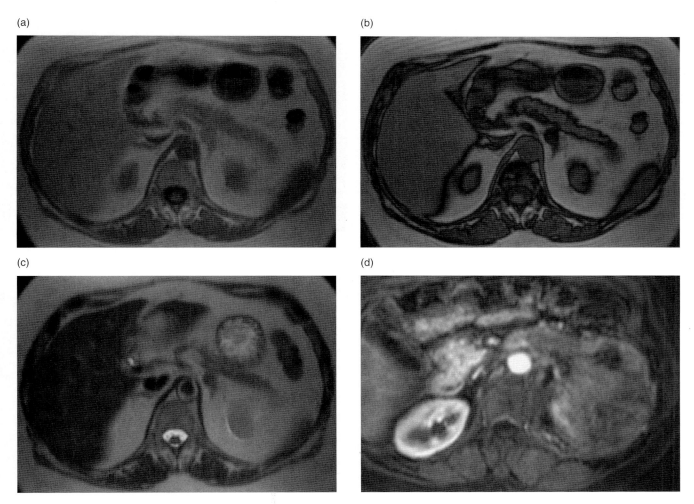

FIGURE 6c-6. (**A**) Axial T1WI: small hypointense nodule in the left adrenal gland. (**B**) Out-of-phase image: the adrenal lesion shows significant signal drop. Histologically proven fat-containing adrenal adenoma and not a fat-containing metastasis from the ipsilateral clear cell RCC. (**C**) Axial T2WI: shows that this lesion is hyperintense. (**D**) Axial T1WI, fat suppressed, after the administration of IV gadolinium: peripheral enhancement of the left adrenal nodule. In fact, these sequences are not contributional for adrenal lesion characterization.

(a)

(b)

(c)

(d)

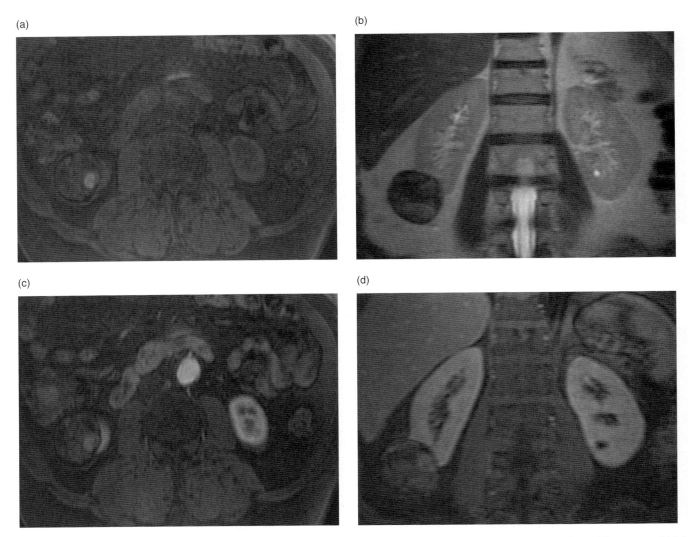

FIGURE 6c-7. (**A**) Papillary RCC in a 71-year-old male. Axial T1WI, fat suppressed: overall hypointense mass, but with an area of high signal intensity, indicating hemorrhage. (**B**) Coronal T2WI: well-defined rounded hypointense lesion with exophytic growth at the lower pole of the right kidney. (**C**) Axial T1WI, fat suppressed, after the administration of IV gadolinium: in the arterial phase the almost complete absence of contrast enhancement is shown. (**D**) Coronal T1WI, fat suppressed, after the administration of IV gadolinium: no obvious enhancement.

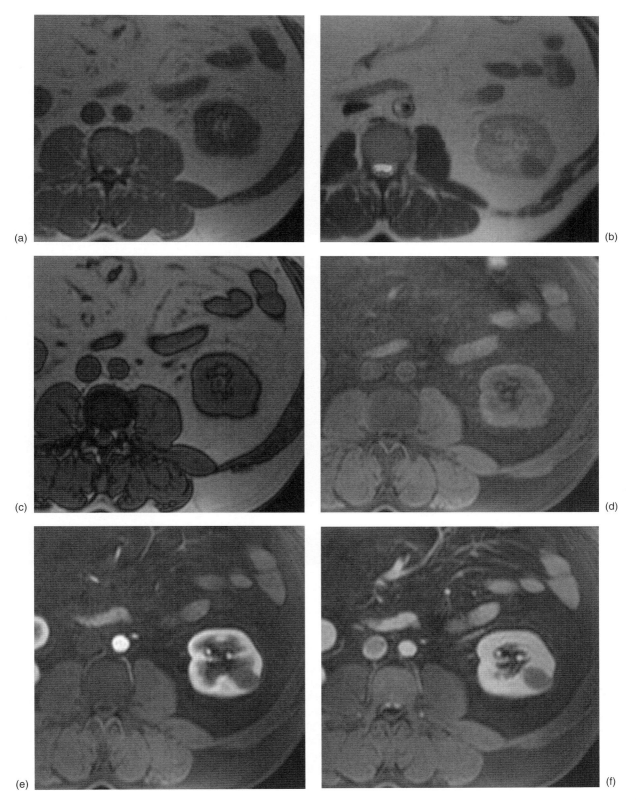

FIGURE 6c-8. (**A**) Papillary RCC in a 45-year-old male. Axial T1WI: no lesion is recognizable in the left kidney. (**B**) Axial T2WI: hypointense lesion intracortically in the posterolateral aspect of the left kidney. (**C**) Out-of-phase image: there is no significant signal loss compared to the in-phase image, indicating the absence of fat. (**D**) Axial T1WI, fat-suppressed: this lesion is completely isointense to the renal cortex. (**E**) Axial T1WI, fat suppressed, after the administration of IV gadolinium: the arterial phase shows only minimal contrast enhancement. (**F**) Axial T1WI, fat suppressed, after the administration of IV gadolinium: minimal contrast enhancement on the venous phase.

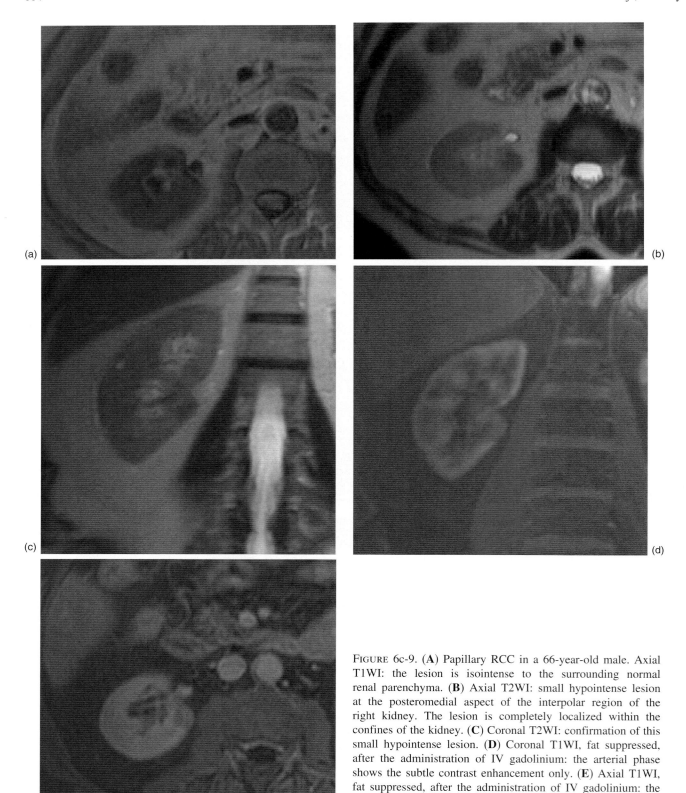

FIGURE 6c-9. (**A**) Papillary RCC in a 66-year-old male. Axial T1WI: the lesion is isointense to the surrounding normal renal parenchyma. (**B**) Axial T2WI: small hypointense lesion at the posteromedial aspect of the interpolar region of the right kidney. The lesion is completely localized within the confines of the kidney. (**C**) Coronal T2WI: confirmation of this small hypointense lesion. (**D**) Coronal T1WI, fat suppressed, after the administration of IV gadolinium: the arterial phase shows the subtle contrast enhancement only. (**E**) Axial T1WI, fat suppressed, after the administration of IV gadolinium: the venous phase confirms the lesional hypovascularity.

(a)

(b)

(c)

(d)

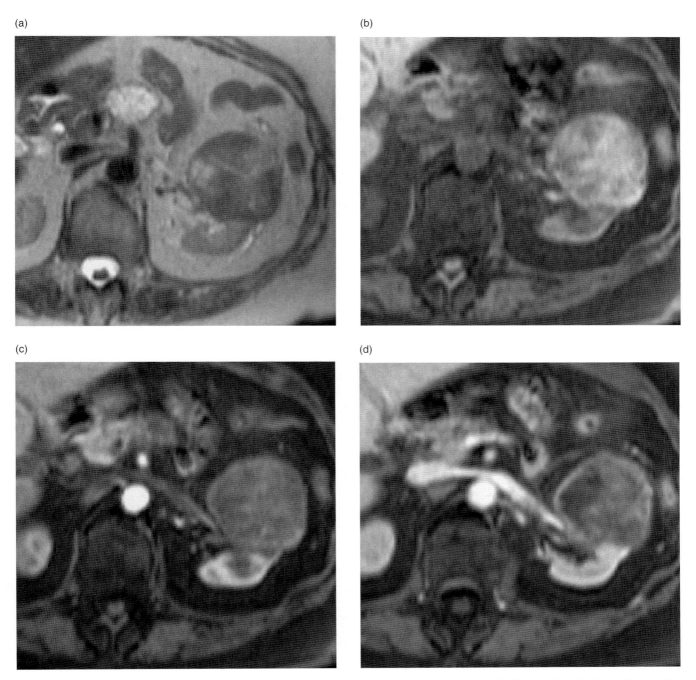

FIGURE 6c-10. (**A**) Papillary RCC in a 73-year-old female. Axial T2WI: ball-shaped tumor in the left kidney with mixed signal intensities: overall hypointensity with focal areas of high signal intensity. (**B**) Axial T1WI, fat suppressed: hyperintense tumor signal intensity in the interpolar region. (**C**) Axial T1WI, fat suppressed, after the administration of IV gadolinium: the arterial phase shows the hypovascular nature of the tumor. (**D**) Axial T1WI, fat suppressed, after the administration of IV gadolinium: the venous phase shows some enhancement of the tumor. The main renal vein is patent. In these cases, substraction may be indicated to objectify lesional enhancement.

(a)

(b)

(c)

(d)

(e)

(f)

(g)

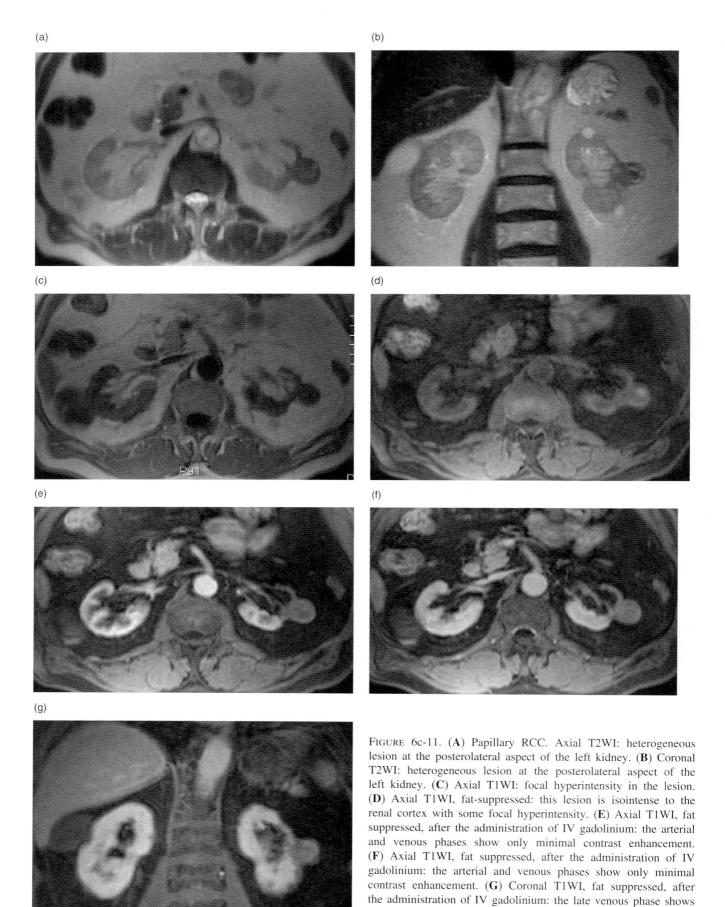

Figure 6c-11. (A) Papillary RCC. Axial T2WI: heterogeneous lesion at the posterolateral aspect of the left kidney. (B) Coronal T2WI: heterogeneous lesion at the posterolateral aspect of the left kidney. (C) Axial T1WI: focal hyperintensity in the lesion. (D) Axial T1WI, fat-suppressed: this lesion is isointense to the renal cortex with some focal hyperintensity. (E) Axial T1WI, fat suppressed, after the administration of IV gadolinium: the arterial and venous phases show only minimal contrast enhancement. (F) Axial T1WI, fat suppressed, after the administration of IV gadolinium: the arterial and venous phases show only minimal contrast enhancement. (G) Coronal T1WI, fat suppressed, after the administration of IV gadolinium: the late venous phase shows only minimal contrast enhancement. In these cases, appropriate measurement of substraction techniques is required to prove or to exclude lesional enhancement.

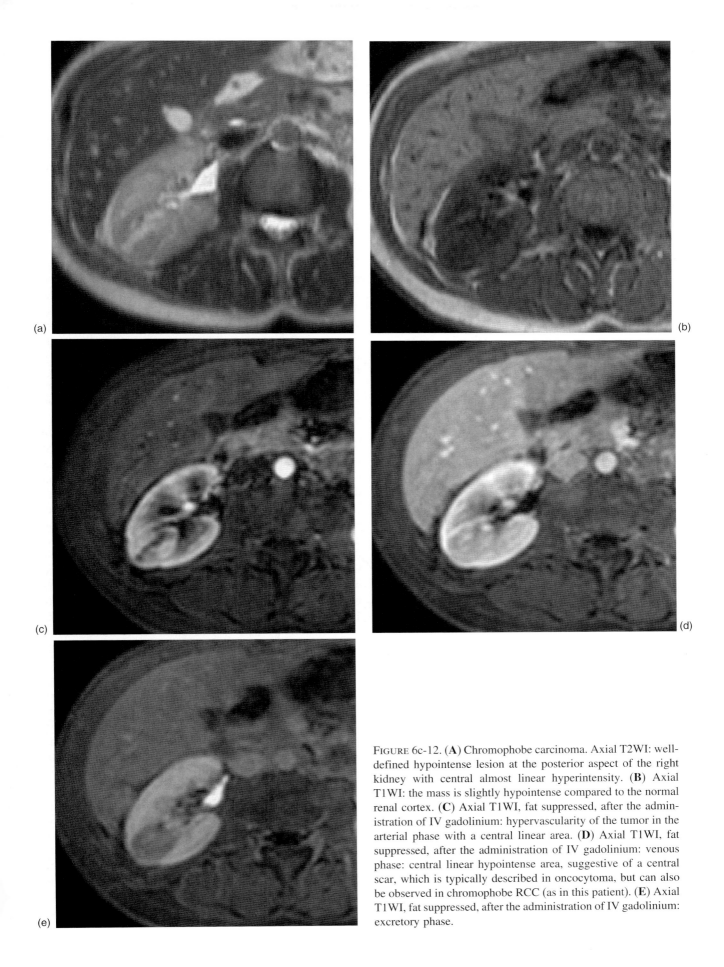

FIGURE 6c-12. (A) Chromophobe carcinoma. Axial T2WI: well-defined hypointense lesion at the posterior aspect of the right kidney with central almost linear hyperintensity. (B) Axial T1WI: the mass is slightly hypointense compared to the normal renal cortex. (C) Axial T1WI, fat suppressed, after the administration of IV gadolinium: hypervascularity of the tumor in the arterial phase with a central linear area. (D) Axial T1WI, fat suppressed, after the administration of IV gadolinium: venous phase: central linear hypointense area, suggestive of a central scar, which is typically described in oncocytoma, but can also be observed in chromophobe RCC (as in this patient). (E) Axial T1WI, fat suppressed, after the administration of IV gadolinium: excretory phase.

The radiological features of these tumors were very similar to those of clear cell renal carcinoma with an alveolar structure.

Collecting Duct Carcinoma (Bellini Duct Carcinoma)

Renal collecting duct carcinoma arises from distal collecting duct epithelium (Fig. 6c-13). This subtype seems to be more common in a younger population than the other RCC. The tumor is usually localized in the renal medulla with distortion of the pelvicaliceal system and typically infiltrating into the renal cortex with preservation of the normal renal contour (Prasad et al., 2005). In fact, renal collecting duct carcinoma displays characteristics similar to upper tract urothelial cell carcinoma (Pickardt et al., 2001; Orsola et al., 2004). Lymph node metastases are frequently present at the time of diagnosis and the prognosis is very poor.

The tumor is hypovascular after the administration of IV contrast. There may be central fluid-like areas due to extensive reactive desmoplatic fibrosis instead of necrosis as seen in the clear cell subtype.

A variant of collecting duct carcinoma, the so-called medullary carcinoma, has been identified in patients with sickle cell trait, which is also typically seen in a younger age group than the classic subtype (Blitman et al., 2005). This is a rare tumor and has only recently been described as a distinct pathological entity by Davis et al. (1995). It is located in the renal medulla, but frequently with satellite lesions in the renal cortex or adjacent peripelvic soft tissue. This is typically an infiltrating tumor with associated retroperitoneal lymphadenopathy and caliectasis (Blitman et al., 2005; Prasad et al., 2005). Hemorrhage as well as extensive necrosis can be seen.

Unclassified Carcinoma

Tumors in this category are histologically heterogeneous and most often of high grade (Amin et al., 2002), with high tumor, nodes, metastasis (TNM) stage and extremely poor survival. These tumors are also reported in patients treated for carcinomas during childhood. They contain an odd mixture of components, tumors with an unrecognizable architectural or cytological pattern or sarcomatoid carcinoma in which the original epithelium element cannot be identified or classified properly.

Sarcomatoid Carcinoma

Although not a definite subgroup these tumors may have distinct features. They are bulky masses at presentation. Lymph node, adrenal, or liver metastases are frequently present at the time of diagnosis. They appear very aggressive with invasion of adjacent organs (liver, spleen, pancreas, abdominal wall) and with "atypical" metastatic deposits.

On T1-weighted images, the solid component will be hypo- or isointense and on T2-weighted images it will be heterogeneous and predominantly isointense. They appear heterogeneously hypo- or hyperintense after intravenous administration of contrast. Typically there will be extensive necrosis in these lesions.

Staging: TNM

MRI can be helpful in determining the presence of adjacent organ invasion when this remains unclear after CT and ultrasound (US). A fat plane between the RCC and the adjacent organ is usually definitive in excluding direct organ invasion. However, alteration of the organ signal characteristics may be a consequence of organ compression rather than organ invasion, and therefore should be interpreted with care, in particular when appearing as a single abnormality.

Although RCC is common, a perinephric pattern of spread is seen only occasionally, typically in bulky tumors (Westphalen et al., 2004).

Venous tumor extension can be accurately depicted with multiplanar MRI. Standard spin-echo T1WI are well suited to demonstrate tumor thrombus as a relative intense mass compared to signal void of the flowing blood. Tumor thrombus appears as a hypointense filling defect on brightblood imaging by low-flip-angle gradient-echo sequences (Fig. 6c-14a–e). In addition, the evaluation of the tumor extension in the IVC is important for the surgical approach. Extension of the thrombus above the level of the hepatic veins warrants an intrathoracic approach with cardiopulmonary bypass. Contrast-enhanced series are required to differentiate between bland thrombus and tumor thrombus (Fig. 6c-14f and g; the same patient as in Fig. 6c-14a–e). This may be of importance since tumor thrombus is more likely to invade the vessel wall and thus partial resection may be required.

The detection of retroperitoneal lymph adenopathy is based on the size. Nodes larger than 1.5 cm (in short axis) are pathological. Based on the lymph node size it is not possible to differentiate metastatic lymphadenopathy from reactive lymph node hyperplasia. This is not uncommon with necrotic RCC and RCC with venous extension. Microscopic metastases in normal-sized lymph nodes cannot be excluded.

MR makes it possible to depict metastatic deposits in the liver and in the bone. The so-called "flow-void" sign refers to the presence of multiple dot-like or tubular structures with low signal intensity, which can be seen in osseous metastasis from RCC in the center or the periphery of the lesion. It correlates with dilated blood vessels or veins. The presence of the flow-void sign in musculoskeletal lesions may be helpful in diagnosing osseous metastasis from RCC. This can become

(a)   (b)

(c)   (d)

                          (e)

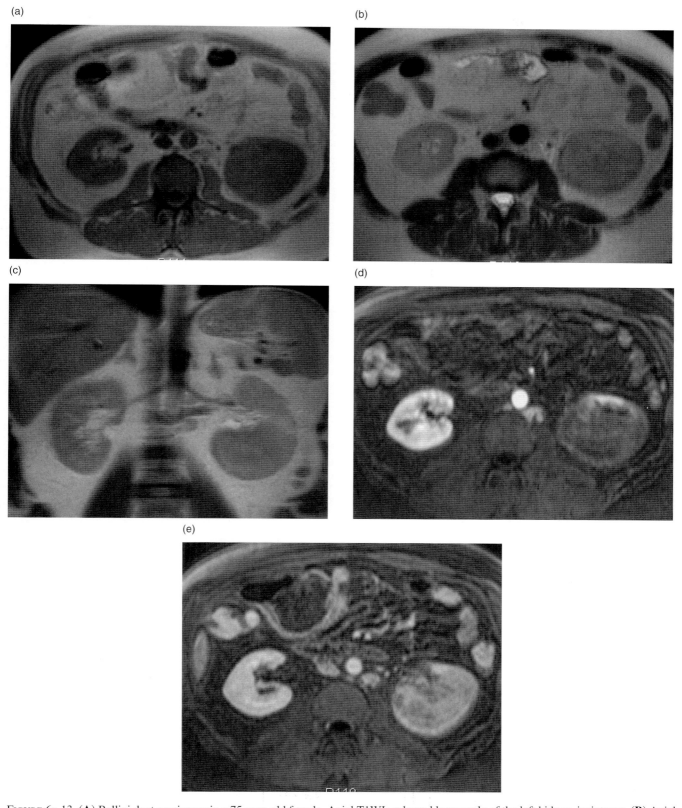

FIGURE 6c-13. (A) Bellini duct carcinoma in a 75-year-old female. Axial T1WI: enlarged lower pole of the left kidney, isointense. (B) Axial T2WI: enlarged lower pole of the left kidney, isointense. Obliteration of the renal sinus. (C) Coronal T2WI: enlarged lower pole of the left kidney, isointense. Obliteration of the renal sinus. (D) Axial T1WI, fat suppressed, after the administration of IV gadolinium: the arterial phase shows an infiltrative, hypovascular lesion at the lower pole of the left kidney. (E) Axial T1WI, fat suppressed, after the administration of IV gadolinium: persistent hypovascularity of the lower pole of the left kidney. Note the enlarged paraaortic lymph node.

(a)   (b)

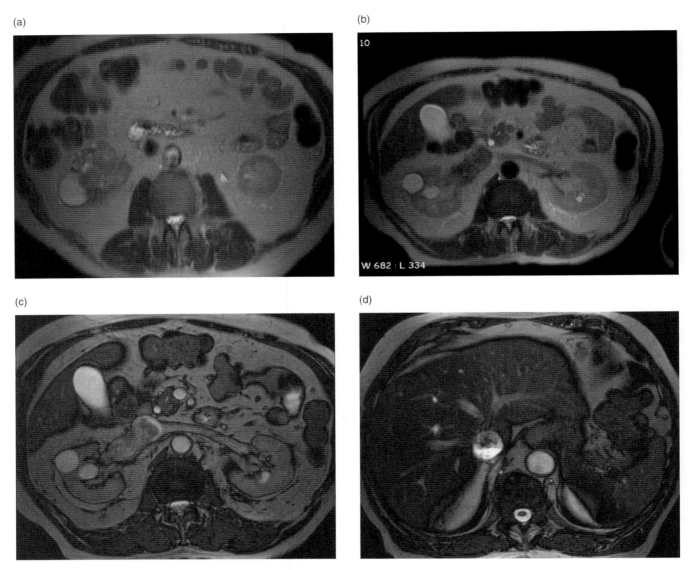

(c)   (d)

FIGURE 6c-14. (**A**) VCI extension in a 76-year-old male. Axial T2WI: isointense lesion in the lower pole of the right kidney with some small central areas of hyperintensity, consistent with RCC. (**B**) Axial T2WI: heterogeneous mass, with signal characteristics similar to the primary tumor, at the level of the right renal vein. (**C**) Axial true FISP image: enlarged right renal vein harboring a heterogeneous mass extending into the IVC, consistent with a tumor thrombus. (**D**) Axial true FISP image: extension of the thrombus up to the intrahepatic IVC just distal to the hepatic veins. (**E**) Coronal true FISP image: the extension of the thrombus is well observed. (**F**) Axial T1WI, fat suppressed, after the administration of IV gadolinium: enhancement of the tumor. (**G**) Axial T1WI, fat suppressed, after the administration of IV gadolinium: enhancement of the thrombus in the right renal vein, consistent with tumor thrombus, and contrary to a bland thrombus.

of interest since RCC can manifest first as an osseous metastasis from a clinically occult primary tumor (48% of patients with osse- ous involvement of RCC and 4% of all patients with RCC).

The development of comprehensive staging systems has led to the availability of better diagnostic and prognostic information for patients with RCC; the incorporation of molecular tumor markers into future staging systems is expected to revolutionize completely the approach to diagnosis and prognosis (Lam et al., 2005)

Recurrence

Renal cell cancer can recur at any time after nephrectomy (Ascenti et al., 2004) (Fig. 6c-15). Although most metastases from RCC appear within 1–2 years after nephrectomy, bone metastases can manifest more than 20 years after treatment without any other sign of interval relapses (Choi et al., 2003). McNichols et al. (1981) reported that 11% of patients developed metastases 10 or more years after nephrectomy, even with early stage disease. The most common sites of

(e)

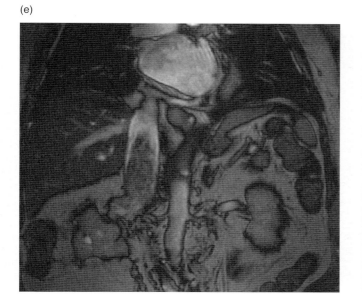

(f)

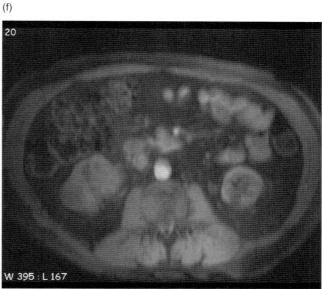

(g)

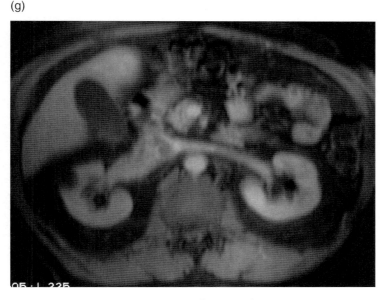

FIGURE 6c-14. (Continued)

tumor spread are the lung (50–60%), liver (30–40%), bone (30%), and brain (5%) (Kassabian et al., 2000).

Pancreatic metastases are rare in patients with RCC and can be found in 1.3–3.0% of patients in autopsy studies. About 100 cases have been described in the literature (Ascenti et al., 2004). On the other hand, RCC is the most common primary neoplasm known to metastasize to the pancreas (30% of metastatic pancreatic tumors) (Klein et al., 1998; Robbins et al., 1996). These pancreatic metastases have distinctive MR features: high signal intensity on T2-weighted images and diffuse enhancement in small lesions and rim enhancement in large lesions on corticomedullary phase postgadolinium images (Kelekis et al., 1996). In cases of suspected pancreatic

metastasis from clear cell renal carcinoma, chemical shift imaging can be used since some clear cell renal carcinomas contain intracellular lipid, which can be seen as signal loss on the out-of-phase images in comparison with the in-phase images (Carucci et al., 1999).

Imaging after Treatment

The standard therapy of choice for a primary RCC used to be a radical nephrectomy since Robson described this procedure as curative for patients with localized disease (Robson, 1963). More frequently, however, patients will be

(a)

(b)

(c)

(d)

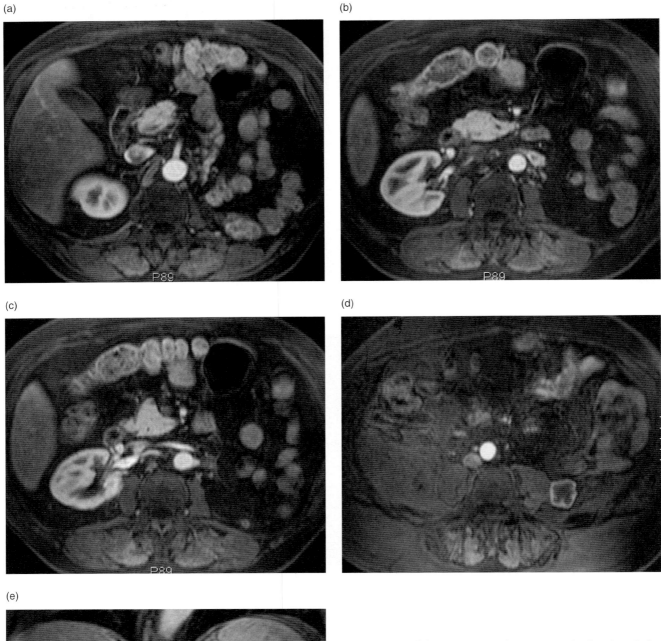

(e)

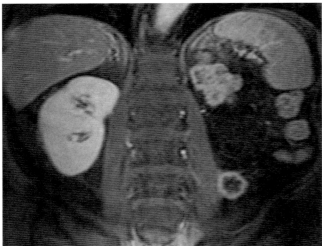

FIGURE 6C-15 (**A**) Axial T1WI, fat suppressed, after the administration of IV gadolinium: after radical nephrectomy for clear
cell RCC, Fuhrman Grade I. Infracentimetric enhancing nodule
adjacent to the posterior abdominal wall. (**B**) Axial T1WI, fat
suppressed, after the administration of IV gadolinium: after radical
nephrectomy for clear cell RCC, Fuhrman Grade I. Enhancing
nodule, paraaortic at the tip of the left renal vein. (**C**) Axial T1WI,
fat suppressed, after the administration of IV gadolinium: After
radical nephrectomy for clear cell RCC, Fuhrman Grade I. Nodule
of 1 cm diameter, enhancing at the posterior abdominal wall.
(**D**) Axial T1WI, fat suppressed, after the administration of IV
gadolinium: after radical nephrectomy for clear cell RCC, Fuhrman
Grade I. Central necrotic nodule of 2.5 cm diameter. (**E**) Coronal
T1WI, fat suppressed, after the administration of IV gadolinium:
after radical nephrectomy for clear cell RCC, Fuhrman Grade I.
Central necrotic nodule of 2.5 cm diameter.

treated with nephron-sparing therapies if possible, including partial nephrectomies, wedge resections, or tumorectomies. There is growing evidence that partial nephrectomy is as effective for Stage I and II RCC as radical nephrectomy. It is important that with this treatment option metastases to the ipsilateral adrenal gland are excluded.

New minimal invasive techniques are developing rapidly including imaging-guided radiofrequency thermal ablation, imaging-guided percutaneous renal cryosurgery, high intensity focused ultrasound, and microwave coagulation; although preliminary, these present promising results (Kagebayashi et al., 1995; Harada et al., 2001; Köhrmann et al., 2002; Farrell et al., 2003; Lewin et al., 2004; Boss et al., 2005; Gervais et al., 2005; Silverman et al., 2005). This implies that follow-up studies are required and that good criteria to differentiate between therapy-related changes and tumor recurrence need to be established. MR perfusion imaging can be applied for the assessment of completeness in the destruction of RCC by radiofrequency (RF) ablation (Boss et al., 2006).

Merkle et al. (2005) prospectively evaluated the changes seen on MR imaging after RF thermal ablation of RCC. They performed studies immediately after the procedure, and 2 weeks, 3 months, and 6 months after ablation including T2-weighted sequences and unenhanced and gadolinium-enhanced T1-weighted images. On T2-weighted images thermal ablation zones appear uniformly hypointense centrally with a hyperintense surrounding rim (Fig. 6c-16). On T1-weighted images they appear hyperintense (Fig. 6c-17). After the administration of gadolinium there is central hypointensity with thin rim enhancement, the so-called periablational enhancement. An increase in size of the thermal ablation zone was noted within the first 2 weeks, followed by involution on the remainder of the follow-up period. The residual tumor was best seen on unenhanced T2-weighted and gadolinium-enhanced T1-weighted images.

One disadvantage of all these newer techniques is that it is no longer possible to evaluate the entire tumor at pathology, so the diagnosis of malignancy depends solely on imaging and percutaneous biopsy (Silverman et al., 2006). In some clinical trials of percutaneous ablation in which imaging alone was used, the efficacy of ablation may be overestimated since benign tumors may have been included. If imaging cannot be used to diagnose a benign entity, patients should undergo a biopsy before the treatment session (Tuncali et al., 2004).

Medical therapies are generally offered for locally advanced or metastatic RCC. Much of the clinical experience is in patients with clear cell RCC. Because response rates are rather low, the need to identify new therapeutic agents is great (Cohen et al., 2005).

(a)   (b)

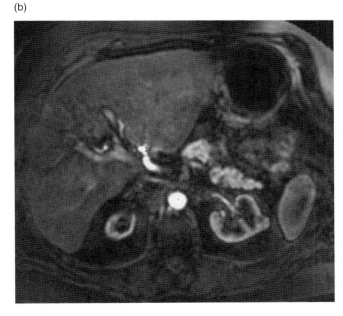

FIGURE 6c-16. (A) Clear cell RCC in a 61-year-old male before RF ablation. Axial T2WI: slightly hyperintense lesion, 14 mm diameter, in the interpolar area of the left kidney. (B) Axial T1WI, fat suppressed, after the administration of IV gadolinium: the arterial phase demonstrates obvious contrast enhancement. (C) Axial T1WI, fat suppressed, after the administration of IV gadolinium: the venous phase confirms the moderate lesional contrast enhancement. (D) Coronal T1WI, fat suppressed, after the administration of IV gadolinium: moderate lesional contrast enhancement. (E) Follow-up MR after RF ablation: axial T1WI: slightly hyperintense lesion in the interpolar area of the left kidney. (F) Axial T2WI: slightly hypointense lesion in the interpolar area of the left kidney. (G) Coronal T2WI: slightly hypointense lesion in the interpolar area of the left kidney. (H) Axial T2WI, fat suppressed, after the administration of IV gadolinium: the arterial phase demonstrates no lesional enhancement. (I) Coronal T1WI, fat suppressed, after the administration of IV gadolinium: the venous phase confirms the absence of lesional enhancement.

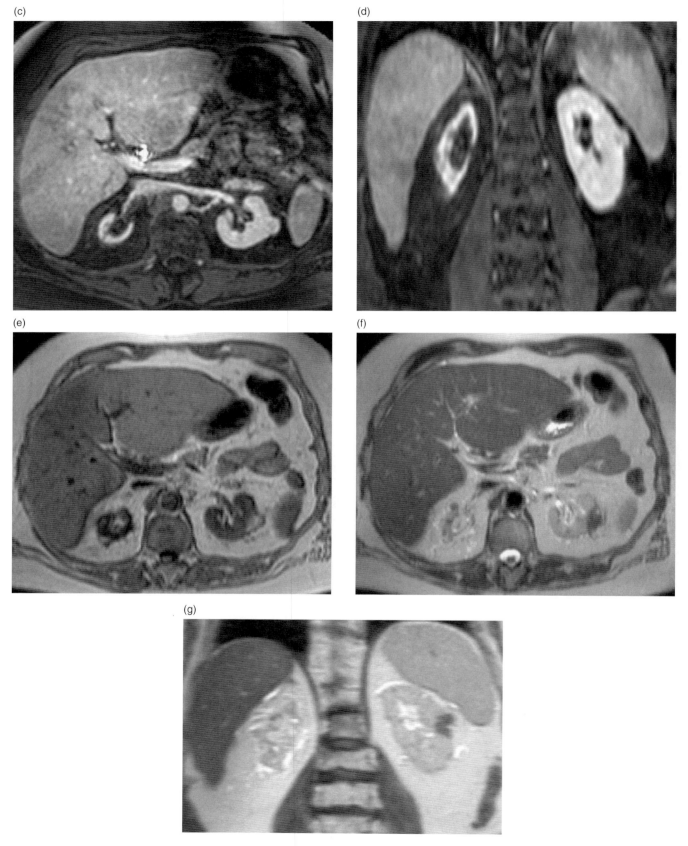

FIGURE 6c-16. (Continued)

(h)   (i)

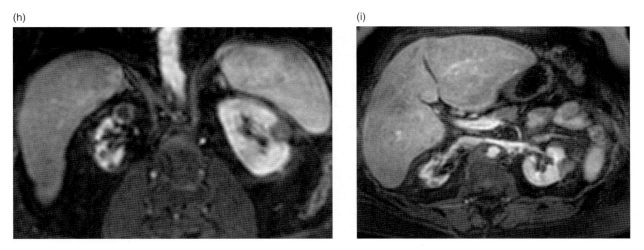

FIGURE 6c-16. (Continued)

(a)   (b)

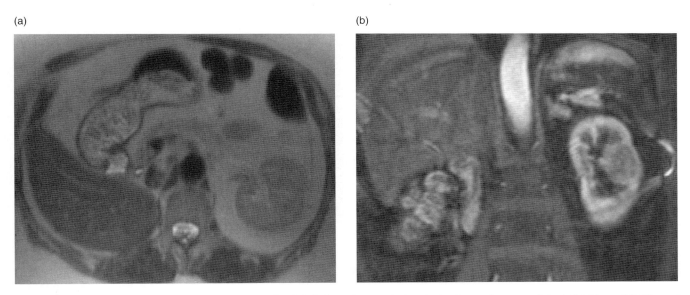

FIGURE 6c-17. (**A**) A 71-year-old female. Axial T2WI: slightly hyperintense lesion in the interpolar area of the left kidney. (**B**) Coronal T1WI, fat suppressed, after the administration of IV gadolinium: the arterial phase demonstrates obvious contrast enhancement. (**C**) Coronal T1WI, fat suppressed, after the administration of IV gadolinium: the venous phase confirms the moderate lesional contrast enhancement.(**D**) Sagittal T1WI, fat suppressed, after the administration of IV gadolinium: the venous phase confirms the moderate lesional contrast enhancement. (**E**) Follow-up MR after RF ablation. Axial T1WI: the tumor area is now hyperintense, consistent with hemorrhage. (**F**) Axial T2WI: follow-up after RF ablation: the lesion now appears hypointense. (**G**) Coronal T1WI: fat suppressed, after the administration of IV gadolinium: absence of contrast enhancement in the treated area indicating the absence of viable tumor. (**H**) Sagittal T1WI: fat suppressed, after the administration of IV gadolinium: no contrast enhancement in the treated area is seen.

(c)

(d)

(e)

(f)

(g)

(h)

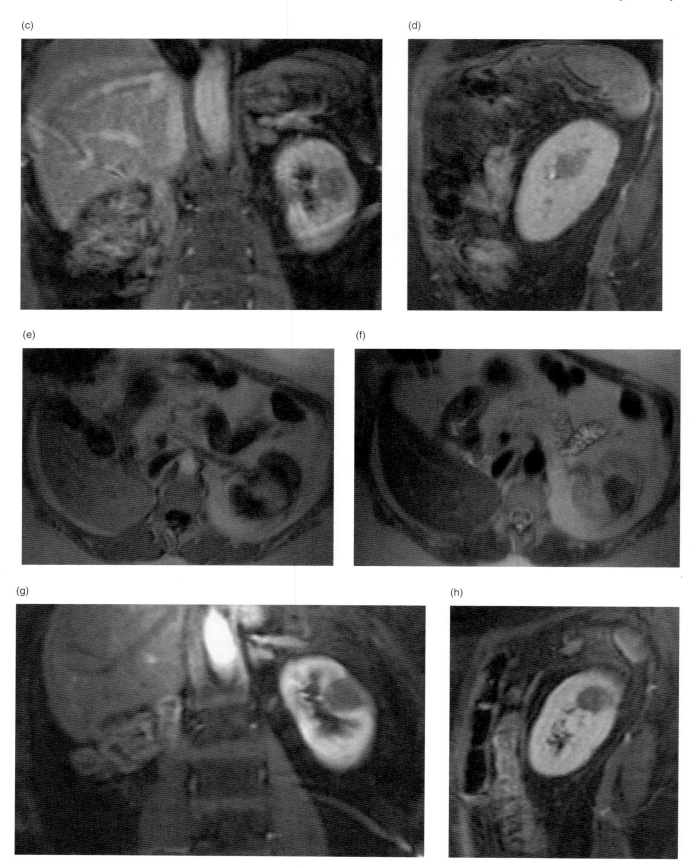

FIGURE 6c-17. (Continued)

6d
Angiography as a Diagnostic Tool in Renal Cell Carcinoma

Didier Jacqmin and Catherine Roy

Introduction

Before the advent of ultrasound, computed tomography (CT) scan, and magnetic resonance (MR) imaging techniques, the best tool for the diagnosis of renal masses before surgery was angiography. Since that time, the usefulness of angiography has dramatically decreased. In this chapter we will try to determine the actual role of this old technique in the diagnosis of renal cell carcinoma.

Angiography is not used routinely anymore. This is a consequence of the invasiveness of the technique and also the good quality of the images obtained by other means. Ultrasound, CT scan, and MRI have other advantages, making it possible to evaluate the lymph nodes and the surrounding organs as well as the kidney vessels.

Angiographic Aspects of Renal Cell Carcinoma

The typical angiographic pattern of renal cell carcinoma (RCC) is the presence of a hypervascularized mass with irregular vessels inside, tortuous, with an absence of normal tapering randomly distributed, variable in size, and unpredictable in branching (Fig. 6d-1).

Another typical aspect is the presence of arteriovenous shunts leading to an early opacification of the renal vein (Fig. 6d-2). In case of a huge tumor mass, aortography shows the full blood supply coming from the lumbar, adrenal, urétéral gonadal, and mesenteric arteries.

However, in approximately 20% of the cases the pattern of RCC is hypovascularization, which is mainly the case in the cystic forms of RCC.

Small tumors, even hypervascularized ones, can be missed by angiography. However, exceptional indications remain for the diagnosis of tiny medullary small tumors found with other imaging modalities.

In the 1980s, Amendola et al.[1] stated that CT scan and ultrasound (US) were both more sensitive than angiography for the detection of small RCC. Since that time many studies advocated CT as the method of choice for the diagnosis of renal tumors.[2–4]

The combination of US and CT is the most often used imaging approach. These two modalities are pertinent enough to supply all information needed for therapy.[5]

Differential Diagnosis

Oncocytoma

One of the challenges of the radiologist in identifying a tumor mass is the detection of a renal oncocytoma. Because of its benign behavior, its diagnosis preoperatively might induce a change in surgical strategy. Typically in this kind of tumor, there is a central stellate scar that is not always visible on CT, MRI, and US. The typical angiographic aspect is the so-called "spoke-wheel" pattern of vascularity. This is associated with the absence of venous shunt and vascular puddling. However, these characteristics are often not present in small and medium sized oncocytomas. Furthermore, this pattern has also been observed in cases of RCC.

An oncocytoma can be similar to a true RCC and vice versa on all imaging modalities, so there is no advantage in using angiography for the diagnosis of oncocytoma.

Angiomyolipoma

The key for the diagnosis of angiomyolipoma is the demonstration of fat inside of the renal mass. CT is the optimal imaging modality in this situation because of its sensitivity in the detection of small foci of fat. Even in cases of nonfatty or hemorrhagic angiomyolipomas, angiography cannot do better than CT (Fig. 6d-3).

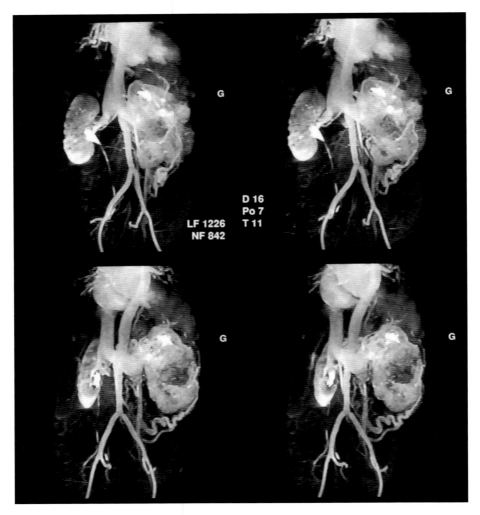

FIGURE 6d-1. MR angiography, MIP reconstruction, oblique view, venous phase. Large left kidney tumor with venous collateral circulation and large renal vein. Free vena cava.

Acquired Cystic Disease of the Kidney

This disease is characterized by the development of multiple renal cysts on native kidneys of patients with chronic renal failure on long-term hemodialysis. It is associated with atrophic kidneys. The major concern in this setting is the increased incidence of RCC seen more often than in patients with healtly kidneys. RCC associated with acquired cystic kidney disease (ACKD) is frequently multifocal and bilateral. Acquired cysts are often small and hypovascularized, with intracystic clots and fibrous tissue, both of which may mimic malignant disease on CT and US. Angiography is accurate in depicting tumors over 3 cm in diameter but is less accurate in detecting smaller tumors,[6] with a sensitivity inferior to that of both CT and US.

In conclusion, angiography was a good modality for the diagnosis of renal cell carcinoma but it has now been replaced by more sophisticated tools with better sensitivity.

Role of Vascular Imaging Procedure for Venous Involvement

In approximately 5% of the cases, RCC is associated with a tumoral thrombus in the inferior vena cava.

To plan the procedure, the surgeon needs to know the precise level of the thrombus. The key imaging procedure in the past was venacavography, which shows a filling defect inside the caval lumen. It also makes it possible to see the collateral veins (Fig. 6d-4).

Today, US and MRI provide even better information than venacavography. Furthermore, MRI is particularly useful in identifying the nature (blood clots or tumor) of the thrombus. Venacavography is still used in centers that do not have an MRI or helical CT scan.

When planning kidney-sparing surgery some surgeons like to have a road map of the arterial kidney supply.[7] However, it does not supply more information than can be obtained with a 3D angio CT or angio MR.[8]

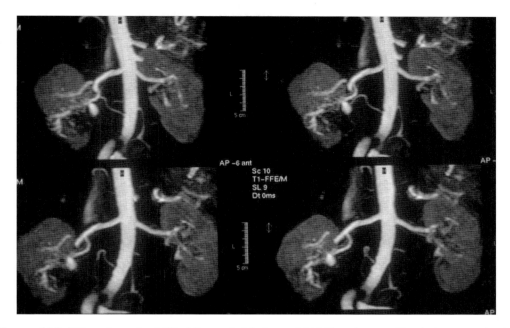

FIGURE 6d-2. MR angiography, MIP oblique arterial phase, right kidney tumor with arteriovenous shunt.

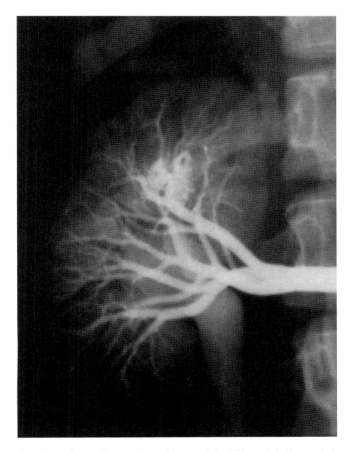

FIGURE 6d-3. Conventional arteriography, angiomyolipoma. No differential diagnosis is accurate with RCC.

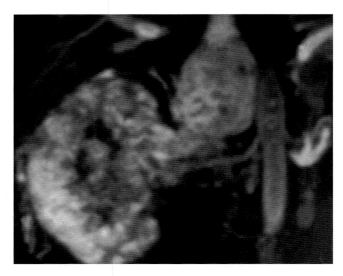

FIGURE 6d-4. MR angiography, frontal native image. Huge caval thrombus with right kidney tumor, arterial phase.

Preoperative Angiography

Arterial embolization was used by some urologists just before surgery or with a palliative intent.

Conclusions

Except for certain uncommon circumstances, angiography is no longer of value for the diagnosis of RCC. However, it still has an important role in interventional radiology.

References

1. Amendola MA, Bree RL, Pollack HM et al. (1988) Small renal cell carcinoma: resolving a diagnostic dilemma. Radiology 166: 637–641.
2. Frohmuller HG, Grups JW, Heller V (1987) Comparative value of ultrasonography, cumputerized tomography, angiography and excretory urography in the staging of renal cell carcinoma. J Urol 138: 482–484.
3. Veda T, Nishitani H, Kudo H (1988) Comparison of angiogrpahy and computed tomography using new morphologic criteria in staging of renal cell carcinoma. Urology 32: 439–464.
4. Weyman PJ, McClennan BL, Stanley RJ, Levitt RG, Saget SS (1980) Comparison of computed tomography and angiography in the evaluation of renal cell carcinoma. Radiology 133: 417–424.
5. Roy C, Tuchmann C, Morel M et al. (1999) Is there still a place for angiography in the management of renal mass lesions? Eur Radiol 9: 329–335.
6. Sasagawa I, Teresawa Y, Ishizaki et al. (1992) Comparison of ultrasonography, computerized tomography and angiography in dialysis patients with renal cell carcinoma. Urol Int 49: 206–210.
7. Sandhu C, Belli AM, Petel U (2003) Demonstration of renal arterial anatomy and tumor neovascularity for vascular mapping of renal cell carcinoma: the value of CO_2 angiography. Br J Radiol 76: 89–93.
8. Ueda T, Tobe T, Yamamoto S et al. (2004) Selective intra-arterial 3-dimensional computed tomography angiography for preoperative evaluation of nephron-sparing surgery. J Comput Assist Tomogr 4: 496–504.

6e
Positron Emission Tomography in Renal Cancer

Sarah K. Ceyssens and Luc Mortelmans

Introduction

Positron Emission Tomography

Positron emission tomography (PET) makes it possible to evaluate the biodistribution of small amounts of positron-emitting radiopharmaceuticals and is considered the most sensitive and specific technique for *in vivo* imaging of metabolic pathways and receptor–ligand interactions in tissues.[1] PET uses radioisotopes of natural elements: oxygen-15, carbon-11, nitrogen-13, and fluorine-18. Because of their resemblance to naturally occurring molecules in the human body, these radioisotopes can be incorporated into physiological compounds without disturbing their characteristics ("physiological labeling").

Positron-emitting isotopes such as fluorine-18 (^{18}F) have an excess of protons and are therefore unstable. They decay by emission of a positron, which is the positively charged antiparticle of the electron. This positron travels a short distance through a substance until it is annihilated with an electron. This annihilation generates a pair of photons that travel in nearly opposite directions (180°) with an energy of 511 keV each (Fig. 6e-1)

The PET camera consists of a ring of detectors coupled to a coincidence circuit. The incoming photon interacts with the detector and is converted to visible light. This light is transformed and amplified to an electric current using photomultiplier tubes. A coincidence circuit is coupled to the detectors/photomultipliers and determines if two photons are detected almost simultaneously, i.e., within a predefined time window (6–12 nsec). If so, we know that somewhere along the line connecting these two detectors the annihilation took place. Since the PET camera consists of a ring of detectors, it is possible to generate a map of the distribution of the positron-emitting isotope throughout the body. Once all data are acquired, a tomographic reconstruction can be made.

^{18}Fluorodeoxyglucose

The tracer most commonly used is fluorine-18-labeled 2-fluoro-2-deoxy-D-glucose, [^{18}F]FDG. This is a D-glucose molecule in which a hydroxyl group in the 2-position is replaced by a positron-emitting ^{18}F.

Several decades ago, Warburg et al.[2] described the higher rate of glucose metabolism in cancer cells compared to nonmalignant tissue. After malignant transformation, there is an increased expression of epithelial glucose transporter proteins and an upregulation of hexokinase activity. After intravenous injection, [^{18}F]FDG undergoes the same uptake as glucose. Once in the cell, it is rapidly phosphorylated to [^{18}F]FDG-6-phosphate, which in contrast to glucose-6-phosphate is not a substrate for the glucosephosphate isomerase, since FDG lacks a hydroxyl group in position-2, and therefore cannot be converted to the fructose analogue. As most tumors have a low phosphatase activity, the negatively charged [^{18}F]FDG-6-phosphate will accumulate in the cell, resulting in so-called "metabolic trapping" (Fig. 6e-2). It has been demonstrated that increased FDG uptake by malignant cells, although a function of the proliferative activity, is mainly related to the number of viable tumor cells.[3] However, increased FDG uptake is not specific for cancer cells, but is also seen in neutrophils, eosinophils, macrophages, and proliferating fibroblasts, to a degree sometimes more marked than in malignant cells.[4] Therefore, an increased FDG uptake can also be seen in some inflammatory conditions, being the most common cause of a false-positive FDG signal.[5]

[^{18}F]FDG PET: General Clinical Applications

Although in the 1980s, PET scans were mainly used in research focusing on neuroscience and cardiology, advances in molecular biology and important improvements in technology showed that PET was a promising new technique in the imaging and management of the oncologic patient. Since PET relies on the detection of metabolic alterations observed in cancer cells, these examinations yield data independently of structural features as provided by computed tomography (CT) and magnetic resonance imaging (MRI),

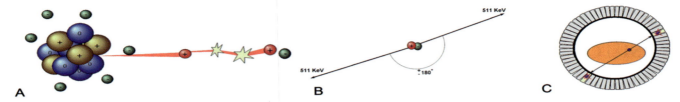

FIGURE 6e-1. ^{18}F decays by emitting a positron (**A**). This positron is annihilated with an electron, with the generation of a pair of photons of 511 keV that travel in nearly opposite directions (**B**). These photons can be detected by detector pairs installed in a PET camera (**C**).

and therefore allow detection or monitoring of specific perturbations that are not associated with or that precede the anatomical changes.

Numerous articles have been published about the use of [^{18}F]FDG-PET in neoplasms of the brain, head and neck, and lung, as well as in colorectal cancer, ovarian cancer, lymphoma, and melanoma.[6–8] The use of PET in urological malignancies, however, is still not clearly defined.[9] We reviewed the literature to determine the role of PET in renal cell cancer (RCC).

Primary Detection of Renal Cell Cancer

Since Wahl and co-workers reported FDG uptake in renal cancer in 1991,[10] several studies have been published, albeit nearly all limited in size and presenting conflicting results (see Table 6e-1). Kang et al. found that the role of [^{18}F]FDG PET in the detection of RCC was rather limited by low sensitivity (60%). These results were thought to be mainly a consequence of the increased background activity of healthy renal tissue and the renal excretion of [^{18}F]FDG,[11] both factors also resulting in the unreliability of the standardized uptake value

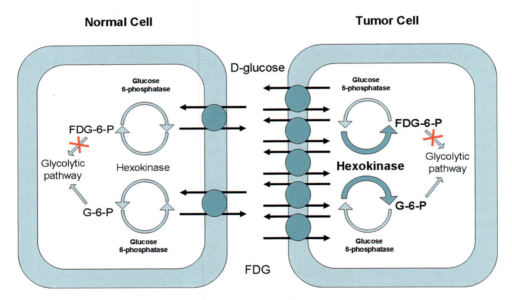

FIGURE 6e-2. FDG metabolism in normal cells and cancer cells.

TABLE 6e-1. Primary detection of renal cell carcinoma.

Study	Number of patients	Number of studies	Size of the lesions (visualized)	Size of the lesions (nonvisualized)	Sensitivity		Specificity		Accuracy	
					PET	CT	PET	CT	PET	CT
Kang[11]	66	90			60%	92%	100%	100%		
Aide[13]		53	7.75 ± 3 cm	4.25 ± 2.3 cm	47%	97%	80%	0/5 benign lesions	51%	83%
Ramdave[14]	17								94%	94%
Goldberg[15]		10		90%	100%					

PPV, positive predictive value; NPV, negative predictive value; PET, positron emission tomography; CT, computed tomography.

(SUV, a method to quantify tracer concentration) in renal cancer.[12] Another study, performed by Aide and co-workers, showed a high rate of false-negative results even in larger tumors, leading to a low sensitivity (47%).[13]

However, these findings were in conflict with the results of several previous studies: Ramdave et al. evaluated [18F]FDG PET in 17 patients with known or suspected primary renal tumors, showing PET and CT having a similar accuracy (94%).[14] In a study by Goldberg et al., an increased FDG uptake was observed in 9 of 10 solid neoplasms investigated.[15] [18F]FDG PET may be useful not only in RCC, but even in the case of Wilms tumor.[16]

The efficacy of [18F]FDG PET in detecting malignant tumors of the kidney may be limited by the increased background activity of healthy renal tissue and the renal excretion of [18F]FDG.[11] Nevertheless, other factors might be involved since some large tumors with extrarenal development are not always visualized or show only slight [18F]FDG uptake. Bachor and co-workers investigated the staging of renal cell cancer by [18F]FDG PET, showing a correct diagnosis in 20 of 26 patients with RCC and a false-negative result in the remaining 6 patients. Activity on PET scan was compared to histology on surgical specimens, revealing that diagnostic accuracy depended on the degree to which the tumors were differentiated.[17] Miyauchi et al. observed a correlation between positive PET findings at the primary tumor site and higher tumor grades, with respect to higher glucose transporter 1 (GLUT-1) intensity,[18] though these results could not be confirmed by other studies.[19] The relationship between blood flow and glucose metabolism has also been investigated, suggesting that the glucose supply is in excess of glucose demand and/or consumption, and that the blood flow and glucose metabolism appeared uncoupled in renal cell cancer.[20] Yet to date, the true reason for the inconsistent nature of FDG uptake is still not known.

Although showing diverse results concerning sensitivity, most of these studies demonstrated a superior specificity of [18F]FDG PET, results suggesting [18F]FDG PET might have a role as a problem-solving tool in patients with equivocal findings on conventional imaging. Only a few studies report false-positive PET results. In the study of Bachor et al. mentioned above, a false-positive PET result was obtained in an angiomyolipoma, a pericytoma, and a pheochromocytoma.[18] An increased FDG uptake can also be seen in some inflammatory conditions, since increased FDG uptake is not specific for cancer cells, but is also seen in neutrophils, eosinophils, macrophages, and proliferating fibroblasts.[4]

[18F]FDG PET in Lymph Node Staging

In addition to the detection of the primary tumor, another benefit of [18F]FDG PET in RCC may lie in lymph node staging, since conventional imaging techniques rely on size criteria, although even normal sized lymph nodes can contain tumor cells and nonspecific enlargement of lymph nodes can be present. In the aforementioned studies of Kang, Ramdave, and Bachor, lymph node status was also evaluated. Kang found a sensitivity of 75% and a specificity of 100% for [18F]FDG PET for the detection of retroperitoneal lymph node metastasis, compared to 92.6% and 98.1%, respectively, for abdominal CT,[11] while in the study of Ramdave there were two cases of regional lymph node involvement detected on [18F]FDG PET but not on CT.[14] Bachor found that lymph node staging was judged true positive in three patients and true negative in 25 patients; there were no false-negative PET findings.[17] Although preliminary results seem promising, further studies are necessary to determine the true place of [18F]FDG PET in lymph node staging in this setting.

Figure 6e-3 shows [18F]FDG PET with an increased uptake in the primary renal tumor and a moderate uptake in a paraaortic lymph node.

[18F]FDG PET in Recurrent and Metastatic Disease

In the abovementioned study of Ramdave et al., another eight patients with suspected local recurrence and/or metastatic disease were evaluated. [18F]FDG PET was more accurate in detecting local recurrence and distant metastases and in differentiating recurrence from radiation necrosis, compared to CT (diagnostic accuracy of 100% and 88%, respectively).[14] However, the study of Aide et al.[13] did not show any advantage of [18F]FDG PET over CT for the characterization of renal masses; the study suggests that PET is an efficient tool for the detection of distant metastasis in renal cancer (diagnostic accuracy of 94% for FDG PET and 89% for CT).[13]

The main conclusion of the various studies dedicated to the evaluation of [18F]FDG PET in recurrent and/or metastatic disease (see Table 6e-2) is that although a negative PET study in this setting cannot rule out disseminated disease, especially small metastatic lesions, a positive PET scan should be considered as highly suspicious for local recurrence or metastases, as a result of the high positive predictive value of the test.[21–23] However, because of the limited anatomic information, PET cannot replace the need for CT in these patients. Therefore [18F]FDG PET should be seen as an imaging modality complementary to anatomic imaging techniques and an aid in deciding on the need for biopsy in selected situations. Figure 6e–3 shows increased [18F]FDG uptake in lung metastasis.

There are also reports of [18F]FDG PET showing a higher sensitivity and a better accuracy than bone scintigraphy in detecting bone metastases in patients with renal cell carcinoma (in the study of Wu et al.: a diagnostic sensitivity of 100% versus 77.5% and an accuracy of 100% versus 59.6%, respectively).[24, 25]

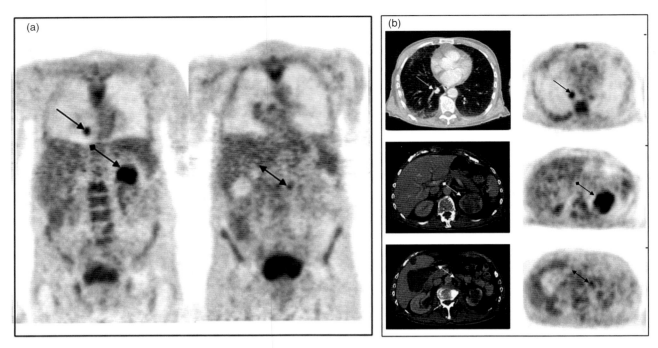

FIGURE 6e-3. [18F]FDG PET and correlating CT images showing an increased [18F]FDG uptake in the primary renal tumor ($\rightarrow$), a moderate uptake in a paraaortic lymph node ($\leftrightarrow$), and an increased uptake in the right lung: metastasis ($\rightarrow$) (**A** : coronal slides [18F]FDG PET; **B**: transverse CT images and correlating [18F]FDG PET slides).

Future Aspects

The range of biological processes that can be studied with PET has rapidly expanded. Depending on the biological function of interest to the investigators, a specific tracer can be chosen: e.g., [18F]FDG (glucose metabolism), [18F]FLT (cell proliferation), [18F]FMISO (hypoxia), [13N]ammonia (blood flow), [11C]acetate (oxidative metabolism and lipid synthesis), and [11C]methionine (amino acid uptake and protein synthesis). Carbon-11-acetate has to date been tested in only small groups of patients with RCC, although the first results do suggest a potential clinical application. In contrast to the uptake of

carbon-11-acetate by the myocardium providing an indirect noninvasive measurement of regional oxygen utilization, uptake of the tracer in tumor cells is related to lipid synthesis, which reflects the high growth activity of neoplasms.[26] The tracer is cleared from the renal parenchyma without urinary excretion, which makes it a very attractive tracer for the study of urological malignancies.[27] Shreve et al. investigated the use of carbon-11-acetate PET imaging in 18 patients, using dynamic PET imaging of the kidneys after bolus injection of the tracer. They found that renal cell carcinoma demonstrated a similar rapid tracer uptake and high target-to-background ratio, but a substantially reduced clearance rate compared to normal and nonneoplastic renal tissue, allowing differentiation between

TABLE 6e-2. Recurrent and metastatic disease.

Study		Number of patients	Number of studies	Sensitivity		Specificity		Accuracy	
				PET	CT	PET	CT	PET	CT
Kang[11]		66	90						
	Locoregional lymph node metastases and/or recurrence			75%	93%	100%	98%		
	Distant metastases (lung)			75%	91%	97%	73%		
	Distant metastases (bone)			77%	94%	100%	87%		
Aide[13]	Distant metastases	53						94%	89%
Ramdave[14]	Local recurrence and/or distant metastases	8						100%	88%
Jadvar[21]	Local recurrence and/or distant metastases	25	71%	75%	94%	33%	72%		
Majhail[22]	Distant metastases	24	64%	100%	100%				
Safaei[23]	Restaging	36	87%	100%			89%		
Wu[24]	Distant metastases (bone)	18	100%				100%		

PPV, positive predictive value; NPV, negative predictive value; PET, positron emission tomography; CT, computed tomography.

renal cell carcinoma and nonneoplastic tissue.[28] It should be mentioned, however, that only a small group of patients was examined and that further studies are needed to determine the true place of carbon-11-acetate PET imaging in patients with RCC.

Another fascinating development is the introduction of combined PET-CT cameras, which allow acquisition of PET images and CT images in one single examination. With the patient position remaining unchanged, an accurate coregistration of the images can be obtained, leading to an improved lesion localization, especially in lesions on PET not showing any anatomic abnormality on CT, unexpected metastatic lesions detected on PET, and in lesions on PET obscured by CT artifacts. On the other hand, the CT component may detect non-FDG avid tumors or lesions located in organs with physiological FDG uptake.[29-31] CT offers excellent anatomical resolution and tissue differentiation, increasing specificity, and decreasing interpretative pitfalls, e.g., abnormal FDG uptake in inflammatory conditions such as xanthogranulomatous pyelonephritis.[32] By merging the metabolic information of PET and the anatomical information of CT in one single procedure, this technique not only increases confidence and reduces equivocal interpretations, thus improving diagnostic accuracy, it also provides information on surgery and radiation therapy planning and can guide biopsies. Fast, low-noise attenuation correction from the CT component will also speed up the PET component.

There is also a renewed interest in radioimmunoscintigraphy (RIS) using positron emitters (immuno-PET) for the analysis of tumors. However, the development of immuno-PET is still in an early phase, mainly because the short half-life of the most commonly used positron emitters does not match the relatively slow pharmacokinetics of radiolabeled monoclonal antibodies (mAbs) *in vivo*. This is in contrast to positron emitters like ^{89}Zr and ^{124}I with a half-life of 78 and 100 hours, respectively. Brouwers et al. showed that ^{89}Zr-labeled mAb cG250 can be used for immuno-PET of RCC in nude rats and that even relatively small tumors of approximately 100 mg could be visualised. ^{89}Zr-Df-cG250 could improve the detection of metastases in RCC in patients, but further studies have to be done.[33]

Conclusions

In the primary detection of RCC, the main role of [^{18}F]FDG PET seems to be problem solving in patients with equivocal findings on conventional imaging, classifying indeterminate renal masses as well as a residual mass in the renal fossa following nephrectomy. Preliminary results also seem to be in favor of [^{18}F]FDG PET for the detection of retroperitoneal lymph node metastasis. With regard to recurrent or metastatic disease, it should be mentioned that although a negative [^{18}F]FDG PET study in this setting cannot rule out disseminated disease, a positive PET scan should be considered as highly suspicious for local recurrence or metastases, as a result of the high positive predictive value of the test.

Because of limited anatomic information, PET cannot replace CT in the staging and follow-up of these patients. As the combination of these two imaging modalities (PET-CT) has proven value in many other areas in oncology, there is no doubt that staging and restaging of RCC will also gain from this technique. The advantages of this latter technique in combination with future, more tumor-specific radiopharmaceuticals may enhance both sensitivity and specificity for the diagnosis of RCC.

References

1 Jones T. The imaging science of positron emission tomography. Eur J Nucl Med 1996; 23: 807–813.

2 Warburg O, Posener K, Negelein E. The metabolism of the carcinoma cell. In: Warburg O, ed. The Metabolism of Tumors. New York, Richard R. Smith, Inc, 1931, 29–169.

3 Higashi K, Clavo AC, Wahl RL. In vitro assessment of 2-fluoro-2-deoxy-D-glucose, L-methionine and thymidine as agents to monitor the early response of a human adenocarcinoma cell line to radiotherapy. J Nucl Med 1993; 34: 773–779.

4 Kubota R, Yamada S, Kubota K, et al. Intratumoural distribution of fluorine-18-fluorodeoxyglucose in vivo: high accumulation in macrophages and granulation tissues studied by microautoradiography. J Nucl Med 1992; 33: 1972–1980.

5 Yamada S, Kubota K, Kubota R, et al. High accumulation of fluorine-18-fluorodeoxyglucose in turpentine-induced inflammatory tissue. J Nucl Med 1995; 36: 1301–1306.

6 Conti PS, Lilien DL, Hawley K, et al. PET and (18F)-FDG in oncology: a clinical update. Nucl Med Biol 1996; 23: 717–735.

7 Weber WA, Avril N, Schwaiger M. Relevance of positron emission tomography (PET) in oncology. Strahlenther Onkol 1999; 175: 356–373.

8 Reske SN, Kotzerke J. FDG-PET for clinical use. Results of the 3rd German Interdisciplinary Consensus Conference, "onko-PET III," 21 July and 19 September 2000. Eur J Nucl Med 2001; 28: 1707–1023.

9 Gambhir SS, Czernin J, Schwimmer J, et al. A tabulated summary of the FDG PET literature. J Nucl Med 2001; 42: 15.

10 Wahl RL, Harney J, Hutchins G, et al. Imaging of renal cancer using positron emission tomography with 2-deoxy-2-(18F)-fluoro-D-glucose: pilot animal and human studies. J Urol 1991; 146: 1470.

11 Kang DE, White RL, Zuger JH, et al. Clinical use of fluorodeoxyglucose F18 positron emission tomography for detection of renal cell carcinoma. J Urol 2004; 171: 1806–1809.

12 Zhuang H, Duarte PS, Pourdehnad M, et al. Standardized uptake value as an unreliable index of renal disease on fluorodeoxyglucose PET imaging. Clin Nucl Med 2000; 25(5): 358–360.

13 Aide N, Bensadoun H, Bottet P, et al. Inaccuracy of 18F-FDG PET for characterisation of suspicious renal masses. J Nucl Med 2003; 44 (5 Suppl): 397P.

14 Ramdave S, Thomas GW, Berlandieri SU, et al. Clinical role of F-18 fluorodeoxyglucose positron emission tomography for detection and management of renal cell carcinoma. J Urol 2001; 166(3): 825–830.

15 Goldberg MA, Mayo-Smith WW, Papanicolaou N. FDG PET characterization of renal masses: preliminary experience. Clin Radiol 1997; 52(7): 510–515.

16 Shulkin BL, Chang E, Strouse PJ, et al. PET FDG studies of Wilms tumors. J Pediatr Hematol Oncol 1997; 19(4): 334–338.

17 Bachor R, Kotzerke J, Gottfried HW, et al. Positron emission tomography in diagnosis of renal cell carcinoma. Urologe A 1996; 35(2): 146–150.

18 Miyauchi T, Brown RS, Grossman HB, et al. Correlation between visualisation of primary renal cancer by FDG-PET and histopathological findings. J Nucl Med 1996; 37 (Suppl): 64P.

19 Miyakita H, Tokunaga M, Onda H, et al. Significance of 18F-fluorodeoxyglucose positron emission tomography (FDG-PET) for detection of renal cell carcinoma and immunohistochemical glucose transporter 1 (GLUT-1) expression in the cancer. Int J Urol 2002; 9(1): 15–18.

20 Sundaram SK, Carrasquillo JA, Carson JM, et al. Relationship between blood flow and FDG metabolism in renal cell cancer: implications for therapy? J Nucl Med 2003; 44 (5 Suppl): 82P.

21 Jadvar H, Kherbache HM, Pinski JK, Conti PS. Diagnostic role of [^{18}F]FDG positron emission tomography in restaging renal cell carcinoma. Clin Nephrol 2003; 60: 395–400.

22 Majhail NS, Urbain JL, Albani JM, et al. F-18 fluorodeoxy-glucose positron emission tomography in the evaluation of distant metastases of renal cell carcinoma. J Clin Oncol 2003;21: 3995–4000.

23 Safaei A, Figlin R, Hoh CK, et al. The usefulness of F-18 deoxyglucose whole-body positron emission tomography (PET) for re-staging of renal cell cancer. Clin Nephrol 2002; 57(1): 56–62.

24 Wu HC, Yen RF, Shen YY, et al. Comparing whole body 18F-2-deoxyglucose positron emission tomography and technetium-99m methylene diphosphate bone scan to detect bone metastases in patients with renal cell carcinomas—a preliminary report. J Cancer Res Clin Oncol 2002; 128 (9): 503–506.

25 Seto E, Segall GM, Terris MK. Positron emission tomography detection of osseous metastases of renal cell carcinoma not identified on bone scan. Urology 2000; 55(2): 286.

26 Yoshimoto M, Waki A, Yonekura Y, et al. Characterization of acetate metabolism in tumor cells in relation to cell proliferation: acetate metabolism in tumor cells. Nucl Med Biol. 2001; 28(2): 117–122.

27 Seltzer MA, Jahan SA, Sparks R, et al. Radiation dose estimates in humans for (11)C-acetate whole-body PET. J Nucl Med. 2004; 45(7): 1233–1236.

28 Shreve P, Chiao PC, Humes HD, et al. Carbon-11-acetate PET imaging in renal disease. J Nucl Med 1995; 36 (9): 1595–1601.

29 Blodgett TD, Casagranda B, Townsend DW, Meltzer CC. Issues, controversies, and clinical utility of combined PET/CT imaging: what is the interpreting physician facing? Am J Roentgenol 2005; 184 (5 Suppl): S138–145.

30 Wechalekar K, Sharma B, Cook G. PET/CT in oncology—a major advance. Clin Radiol 2005; 60(11): 1143–1155.

31 Even-Sapir E, Lerman H, et al. The presentation of malignant tumours and pre-malignant lesions incidentally found on PET-CT. Eur J Nucl Med Mol Imaging 2006; 33(5): 541–552.

32 Swingle CA, Baumgarten DA, Schuster DM. Xanthogranulo-matous pyelonephritis characterized on PET/CT. Clin Nucl Med 2005; 30(11): 728–729.

33 Brouwers A, Verel I, Van Eerd J, et al. PET Radioimmunoscintig-raphy of renal cell cancer using ^{89}Zr-labeled cG250 monoclonal antibody in nude rats. Cancer Biother Radiopharm 2004; 19: 155–163.

6f
Biopsies and Cytological Punctures

Intan P.E.D. Kümmerlin and Fiebo J.W. Ten Kate

Introduction

Since the increased use of computerized tomography (CT) and ultrasonography (US), the incidental finding of renal masses has increased. In 1970 approximately 10% of renal cell tumors were discovered incidentally, compared to 61% in 1998 (Jayson, 1998). Moreover, unpublished data from the European Organization for Research and Treatment of Cancer (EORTC) study 30904 (H. van Poppel, 2005, unpublished work), comparing radical surgery to elective kidney-sparing surgery for low stage renal cell carcinoma (RCC), showed that the incidence of small (≤ 4.0 cm) renal tumors is rising. Furthermore, data from the study of Dechet et al. (1999) showed that if lesions are ≤ 4.0 cm, the incidence of benign masses is 22%. Although 22% of the tumors ≤ 4.0 cm are benign, surgery is the treatment of choice, because the growth rate of small tumors is variable and small tumors can have certain histopathological features that predict rapid progression and have a poor prognosis (Kato, 2004; Rendon, 2000). Still, nearly 25% of patients have an unnecessary radical or partial nephrectomy, which results in significant overtreatment. A preoperative diagnosis to differentiate between malignant and benign renal masses is warranted. In addition, different therapy options renewed interest in a preoperative diagnosis. Among the procedures to obtain a preoperative diagnosis, percutaneous fine needle aspiration (FNA) and Tru-Cut Biopsy (TCB) are the most plausible. FNA and TCB play a limited role in the diagnosis and treatment of renal masses. Limited studies are performed to study the accuracy, sensitivity, and specificity and positive and negative predictive value of FNA and TCB. Most studies were performed on patients with metastases or contraindications to nephrectomy. These studies, often dealing with a small number of patients, contain several limitations. One of the most important limitations is that not all biopsies were compared to the gold standard, the surgery specimen. The published studies report varying rates of sensitivity and specificity in determining the exact nature of the renal masses. Furthermore, needle tract seeding (Abe,1992; Denton, 1990; Gibbons, 1997; Kiser, 1986; Slywotzky, 1994;Wolf, 1998), associated morbidity (Campbell et al., 1997: Herts, 1995), and

low specificity (Campbell et al., 1997; Dechet et al., 2003; Goethuys, 1996) are considered major drawbacks and therefore FNA and TCB are not recommended (Campbell et al., 1997; Goethuys, 1996;Novick, 2002). They should be used to establish a diagnosis of RCC in patients mentioned below (see "Current practical applications").

Both FNA and TCB are performed under radiological (US or CT) guidance. In addition to the percutaneous route, other routes reported in the literature are transurethral placement of an aspiration catheter into the renal mass (Leal, 1992) and transvenous biopsies of RCC invading the renal vein and inferior vena cava (Coel, 1975;Wendth, 1976), but these methods are very unusual. For that reason, only percutaneous FNA and TCB will be discussed in this chapter. Current practical applications (indications, procedures, and complications), diagnostic accuracy, the possibility of subclassification, and grading of RCC in FNA and TCB will be mentioned.

Current Practical Applications

Indications

FNA and TCB can be important in the following four specific situations:

1. In patients with a presumed malignant lesion who may not be a candidate for resection, such as patients with unresectable primary lesions and patients with metastatic diseases.
2. In radiographically indeterminate lesions.
3. In patients for whom partial rather than radical nephrectomy may be a preferred alternative treatment.
4. In patients who will receive targeted therapy.

Of these four indications, the first one is the least controversial and most well defined. In patients with high stage renal lesions or who cannot tolerate surgery for other medical reasons, FNA or TCB could establish the diagnosis for RCC and adjuvant therapy can be instituted.

The possibility of the renal mass being a metastasis could have a significant impact on clinical management, although the majority of patients with renal masses in the setting of a clinically localized nonrenal malignancy will not have metastatic disease to the kidney (Sanchez-Ortiz, 2004).

FNA and TCB can also be important in the nature of indeterminate renal masses. Unfortunately, TCB and FNA yield a low specificity (Campbell, 1997; Dechet, 2003; Goethuys, 1996) (see below), which is necessary to exclude the benign tumors from partial or radical nephrectomy.

TCB and FNA can also be important in patients for whom partial rather than radical nephrectomy may be a preferred alternative treatment. Patients with bilateral disease and patients with impaired renal function might benefit from retaining renal function as much as possible.

Finally, several new agents have been developed for targeted therapies, such as angiogenesis inhibitors (Hampton, 2006). These target the vascular endothelial growth factor receptor, which is the primary angiogenesis inducer in clear cell RCC (Ferrara, 2003). For these patients, FNA or TCB could be an aid in the selection of patients eligible for this therapy.

lower exposure to radiation, and it is accurate and relatively inexpensive. A disadvantage of US is that it depends on the expertise of the person using it. CT is a very good alternative because it has an advantage due to clear visualization of the kidneys. A dedicated (thin-slice) renal CT is the most important radiographic test for delineating the nature of a renal mass (Novick, 2002).

A part of the material is nondiagnostic, due to an inadequate amount of cells or tissue obtained by biopsy or puncture, which could be a cause for false-negative results (Wood, 1999). It is thought that for FNA, the addition of a CT-guided core biopsy should substantially increase the diagnostic accuracy and avoid false-negative biopsy results (Richter, 2000). Insufficient material can be partly explained by the central necrosis of the tumor and cystic changes, which are more common in large tumors. Due to this central necrosis, biopsies or punctures should not be taken in the center of (large) tumors. Not only necrotic tissue, but also blood and normal kidney tissue are examples of nondiagnostic material or false-negative results.

Procedure

Both procedures are performed with needles from 17 up to 22 gauge. The effect of needle size on the biopsy is mentioned in the work of Rybicki et al. (2003): they recommend using fine needles for percutaneous biopsies and reserving the use of thicker needles for selected cases. FNA is mostly performed with a 22-gauge needle and TCB with an 18-gauge needle (see Table 6f-1), which is thicker but has a higher diagnostic yield (Johnson, 2001). Although no major complications are stated in the literature concerning needle size, needle size should be considered.

As mentioned earlier, FNA and TCB are performed under US or CT guidance. There is no agreement on which imaging modality is best to perform FNA or TCB. The study of Rybicki et al. (2003) shows that imaging modality affected neither the sensitivity nor the negative predictive value. There are several studies in which US is compared to CT in the evaluation of renal masses (la-Palma, 1990; Riccabona, 1990; Spahn, 2001). Both imaging modalities provide good visualization and both have their advantages and disadvantages. Because of this both techniques are complementary, even in small renal masses (Jamis-Dow, 1996). The advantages of US are the fact that it is real time, it is noninvasive, it has

Complications

Complications of FNA or TCB include bleeding, pneumothorax, infection, arteriovenous fistula, urinoma, tumor seeding along the needle tract, and death, although the last two complications are very uncommon. Tumor location, operator skills, and the number of biopsy or puncture attempts will influence the complication rates. However, it must be emphasized that renal biopsies or punctures are not routinely performed and that the risk may be underestimated. As a consequence, the complications of FNA or TCB are rarely mentioned and never reviewed.

Although uncommon, death and needle tract seeding are the complications most feared. To determine the incidence of mortality rates and needle tract seeding for renal tumors, a review of complications of percutaneous abdominal fine-needle biopsy revealed mortality rates of 0.031% and needle tract seeding of <0.009% (Smith, 1991). The indication to perform biopsies is more common among nephrologists. The complications are thus more often described for biopsies performed with nephrological diseases. Complications for these biopsies are theoretically similar to TCB, although needle tract seeding will not occur. Bleeding is the primary complication of renal biopsy. The incidence of bleeding

TABLE 6f-1. Differences between FNA and TCB.[a]

	FNA	TCB
Retrieval rate (Torp-Pedersen, 1991)	97.8%	79.1%
Needle size	22-18 gauge (usually 22)	20-18 gauge (usually 18)
Immunohistochemistry	Limited possibilities	Good possibilities
Material amount (e.g., ancillary tests)	↓	↑
Complications	↓	↑
Histological architecture	No	Yes

[a]FNA, fine needle aspiration; TCB, Tru-Cut biopsies.

complications differs in relation to the severity of bleeding (microscopic hematuria to decrease in hemoglobin level) and is connected to the skill of the operator.

Although complications are rare, it has been shown that there are lower complication rates when using finer needles for biopsies (Cozens, 1992). This difference is not as clear in the kidney as it is for the liver. There is a preference for 18-gauge needles for TCB and a thinner 22-gauge needle for FNA. It is therefore thought that FNA yields a lower complication rate than TCB (see Table 6f-1).

Fine Needle Aspiration

The site of puncture plays a smaller role in FNA, because FNAs are taken through aspiration, which is preceded by loosening the tumor cells by moving the needle up and down. With this technique, tumor cells from different directions can be obtained. Although theoretically enough material should be obtained by this technique, it is not always the case in the clinical setting. In the study of Campbell et al. (1997), where they evaluated small renal masses, the failure to obtain sufficient diagnostic material is not explained by necrosis, because this is not common in small tumors. Up to 60% of their punctures had an insufficient amount of material for pathological analysis. It could be the result of the hard consistency of the tumor, which makes it very difficult to aspirate the material. In general, approximately 30% of the punctures are nondiagnostic and repeated punctures are not always helpful.

The outcome of FNA depends on many factors, such as the quality and amount of material and the skill and knowledge of the professionals involved in the process of obtaining, preparing, and interpreting the puncture. Aspiration cytology of the kidneys has limitations and pitfalls (Zardawi, 1999), which will be discussed below.

Wolf (1998) summarized several published reports of percutaneous fine needle aspiration or biopsy of renal masses. The sensitivity and specificity were 90% and 92%, respectively. The positive predictive value was 96%, but the negative predictive value was only 80%. This is a high degree of inaccuracy for the prediction of a benign tumor in most settings. A negative result of the biopsy should thus be viewed with caution. To minimize the risk for the patient, surgery remains the best option to rule out cancer. FNA and TCB are therefore of limited value for patients with small renal tumors. The studies of Campbell et al. 1997 and Brierly et al. (2000) determined the accuracy and clinical utility of FNA for small, solid renal masses. They concluded that the diagnostic yield of FNA for small, solid renal masses appears to be too low to justify the potential morbidity of the procedure. However, FNA in large renal masses has a good sensitivity rate. However, most of these lesions are diagnosed by good quality imaging and FNA provides no additional contribution.

Not all urologists agree with the statements above and believe that FNA is a safe and accurate diagnostic procedure, even for complex cystic renal masses (Harisinghani, 2003; Richter, 2000; Truong, 1999; Wood, 1999). Wood et al. (1999) suggest that false-negative biopsies may be caused by insufficient material. The addition of a CT-guided core biopsy should substantially increase the diagnostic accuracy and avoid false-negative biopsies (Lang, 2002).

To improve the diagnostic accuracy of FNA, several ancillary tests including special stains, immunochemistry, electron microscopy, and image analysis are available to differentiate between benign and malignant lesions. But the availability of tissue with FNA is more limited in contrast to TCB. Hence, TCB can occasionally offer additional information by extra ancillary tests (see Table 6f–1).

Cytologically, oncocytomas are sometimes difficult to differentiate from chromophobe renal cell carcinoma and special types of clear cell renal cell carcinoma (Liu, 2001). The cellular compounds can easily be mistaken for malignant and they can have dispersed cytological features. Careful attention to cytoplasmic and nuclear features makes it possible to distinguish between chromophobe and renal oncocytoma in cytological preparations (Granter, 1997; Wiatrowska, 1999). See Figs. 6f-1A and 6f-2 for examples of an FNA from an oncocytoma.

The value of FNA for diagnosing angiomyolipoma is limited because the diagnosis can easily be made radiographically and it is often straightforward. When the can be difficult (Granter, 1999). Angiomyolipoma may have alarming features, such as cytological atypia and increased mitotic activity. Diagnosis can also be difficult when not all three elements are present (mature adipose tissue, spindled or round smooth muscle cells, and vessels) and, therefore, misdiagnosing angiomyolipomas remains a pitfall in renal FNA. Moreover, puncture of an angiomatous part of the tumor can provoke hemorrhage. Another potential pitfall for a false-positive diagnosis of malignant renal tumor is a repair-like reaction, as in primary glomerular disease with renal scarring. See Figs. 6f-3A and B, and 6f-4 for examples of an FNA from an angiomyolipoma.

In addition to the distinction between malignant and benign, the subclassification of RCC is of importance because it can have prognostic and therapeutic implications. The study of Renshaw et al. (1997) shows a high overall accuracy in distinguishing subtypes of RCC in FNA.

The cells in FNA from a clear cell RCC can generally be well distinguished from normal renal cells. There can be diagnostic confusion with other subtypes, like papillary and chromophobe RCC. See Figs. 6f-5A and 6f-6 for examples of an FNA from a clear cell RCC.

Papillary RCCs are easily recognized on FNA when they are arranged in papillary groups. Papillary RCC FNA cannot always be easily distinguished from clear cell RCC FNA, especially in high grade tumors (Granter, 1998; Renshaw, 1997). Nuclear grooves, mostly present in papillary RCC, can also be present in clear cell RCC. See Figs. 6f-7 and 6f-8 for examples of an FNA from papillary RCC.

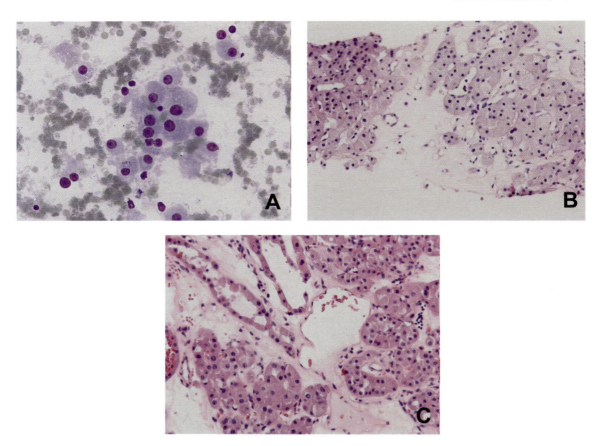

FIGURE 6f-1. Oncocytoma. (**A**) FNA showing epithelial groups of cells with homogeneous cytoplasm without vacuolization and a round nucleus of different diameter (Giemsa stain, ×32). (**B**) TCB (hematoxylin and eosin stain, ×16). For text see **C**. (**C**) Nephrectomy specimen showing a tumor with solid fields of cells with ground-glass-like appearance within the eosinophilic ground substance (hematoxylin and eosin stain, ×16).

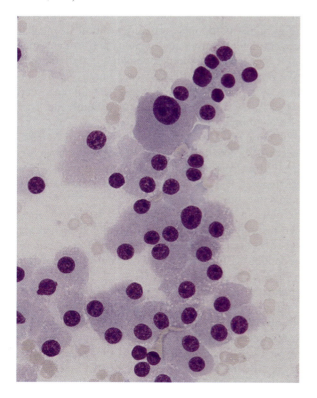

FIGURE 6f-2. Oncocytoma, characterized by isolated cells or occasional small groups of cells with abundant, eosinophilic, granular cytoplasm, well-demarcated borders, occasional binucleation, and bland round nuclei with inconspicuous nucleoli.

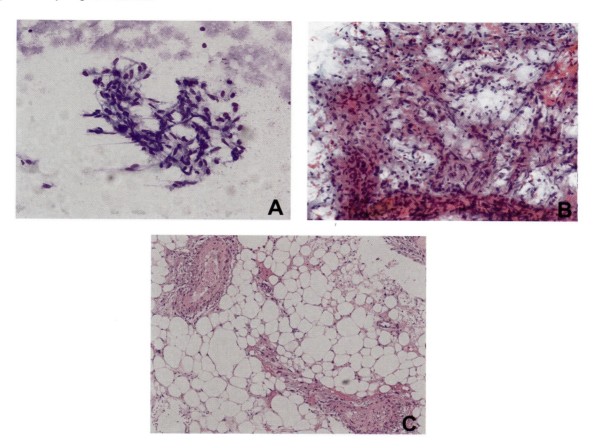

FIGURE 6f-3. Angiomyolipoma. (**A**) FNA showing clusters of spindle cells, without nuclear polymorphism (Giemsa stain, ×16). (**B**) FNA; note the vascular structures (Papanicolaou stain, ×16). (**C**) Nephrectomy specimen showing mature fatty tissue, irregular areas of myocytes and some thick walled vessels (hematoxylin and eosin stain, ×6).

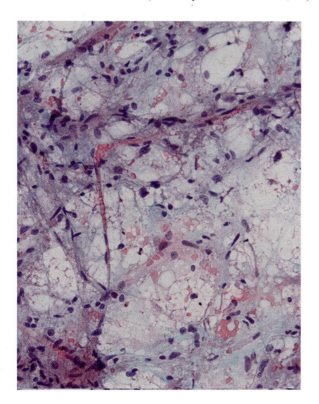

FIGURE 6f-4. Angiomyolipoma, characterized by spindle or round smooth muscle cells, mature adipose tissue, branching vascular structures, and macrophages.

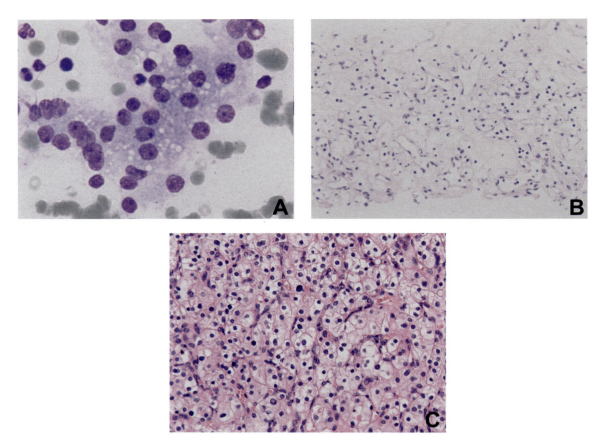

FIGURE 6f-5. Clear cell RCC. (**A**) FNA showing clusters of epithelial cells with round smooth nuclei and small vacuoles in the cytoplasm (Giemsa stain, ×64). (**B**) TCB (hematoxylin and eosin stain, ×13). For text see **C**. (**C**) Nephrectomy specimen showing a tumor with trabecular growth pattern. The tumor cells are well demarcated with an optical clear cytoplasm caused by an accumulation of glycogen and they have a lymphocyte-like small nucleus. In between the tumor cells, a sinusoidal vascular pattern is seen (hematoxylin and eosin stain, ×25).

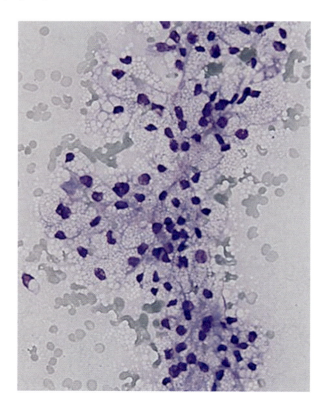

FIGURE 6f-6. Clear cell RCC is highly cellular and is characterized by large groups or isolated cells, abundant cytoplasm, eosinophilic inclusions in the cytoplasm, a low nuclear/cytoplasmic ratio, a centrally or eccentrically located round to slightly irregular nucleus, a sometimes prominent nucleolus, and basal membrane material.

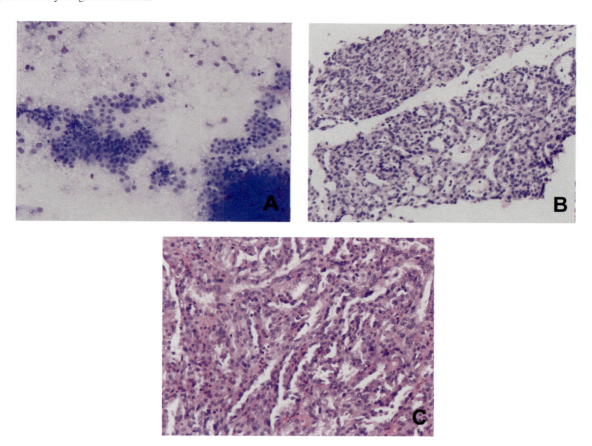

FIGURE 6f-7. Papillary RCC. (**A**) FNA showing papillary sheets and three-dimensional groups of epithelial cells with small round nuclei (Giemsa stain, ×16). (**B**) TCB showing a tumor with a papillary and acinar growth pattern (hematoxylin and eosin stain, ×16). (**C**) Nephrectomy specimen showing a typical papillary growth pattern of small tumor cells (hematoxylin and eosin stain, ×16).

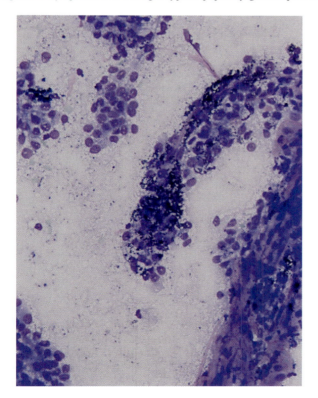

FIGURE 6f-8. Papillary RCC involves papillary groups that resemble spherules. It is characterized by bland nuclei, sometimes with grooves, histiocytes, hemosiderin, and occasionally by psammoma bodies.

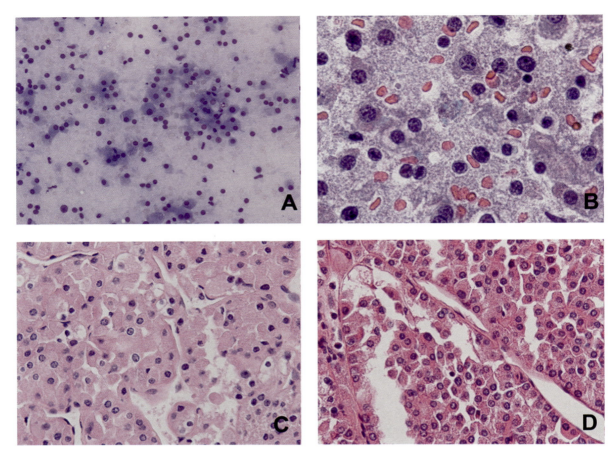

FIGURE 6f-9. Chromophobe RCC. (A) FNA. The tumor is composed of epithelial cells with a homogeneous eosinophilic cytoplasm and nuclei with round contours (Giemsa stain, ×16). (B) The Papanicolaou stain (×64) shows azurophilic granules. (C) TCB. (hematoxylin and eosin stain, ×32). For text see D. (D) Nephrectomy specimen showing sheets of well demarcated and slightly atypical cells with a homogenous eosinophilic cytoplasm (hematoxylin and eosin stain, ×32).

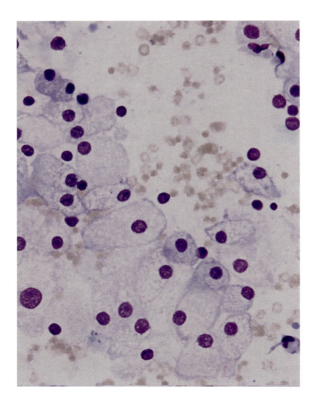

FIGURE 6f-10. Chromophobe RCC is very cellular and involves groups and isolated cells. It is characterized by frequent binucleation, variations in nuclear size and outline, nuclear vacuoles, a perinuclear halo, a coarse chromatin pattern, abundant fluffy granular cytoplasm, and a prominent cell border.

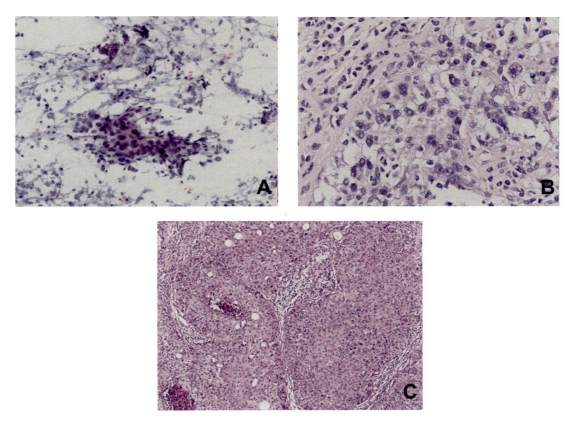

FIGURE 6f-11. Urothelial cell carcinoma. (**A**) FNA showing large sheets of polymorphic cells with irregular dark nuclei (Papanicolaou stain, ×16). (**B**) TCB showing irregular nuclei with prominent nucleoli (hematoxylin and eosin stain, ×32). (**C**) Nephrectomy specimen (hematoxylin and eosin stain, ×6). For text see **B**.

The differentiation of a chromophobe RCC from a clear cell RCC and oncocytomas is sometimes problematic. See Figs. 6f-9A and B and 6f-10 for examples of an FNA from a chromophobe RCC.

Collecting duct carcinomas are very rare. The features in FNA are infrequently described and will not be discussed in this chapter.

The distinction between a renal cell tumor and urothelial tumor of the kidney is not always obvious on a radiological imaging modality. To discuss FNA and TCB of tumors other than RCC goes beyond the scope of this chapter, but examples of an urothelial cell carcinoma can be seen in Figs. 6f-11 and 6f-12.

The study of Young et al. (2002) reviewed the performance of participating pathologists in making patient diagnoses with FNA specimens, with particular interest in the false neoplastic diagnoses (both benign and malignant neoplasms) that were submitted for benign aspirates containing only normal cellular components. They showed that the false neoplastic rate for a renal mass was highest and they concluded that normal cellular elements are a significant pitfall for overinterpretation of FNA specimens. This study again illustrates the difficulty in the interpretation of FNA specimens and questions the use of FNA in clinical practice.

Nuclear grading according to the Fuhrman classification is considered an important prognostic factor (Fuhrman, 1982). Al Nazer et al. (2000) attempted in their study to grade cases of RCC on smears obtained from preoperative FNA. They concluded that grading of RCC can be reliably achieved in FNA material. First, it should be remembered that the reproducibility of the Fuhrman system appears to be moderate (Al-Aynati, 2003;Lang 2005). Second, diagnosing the tumor is of greater importance than its grading.

Biopsies of cystic lesions continue to be a difficult issue. FNA of cysts (aspiration of the cystic fluid) for cytological evaluation was often performed in the past (Novick, 2002). However, this technique is frequently nondiagnostic and of limited value (Renshaw, 1997) because negative cytology does not exclude RCC (Hayakawa, 1996). Moreover, because FNA or TCB may leave some footprints, radiologists prefer that complex cystic masses are not being aspirated or that biopsies are performed.

In summary, FNA can provide important information in selected cases, especially to prove malignancy. However, the overall low specificity makes FNA an unusable tool in those cases in which preoperative diagnosis would be preferable, namely the indeterminate (small) renal tumors.

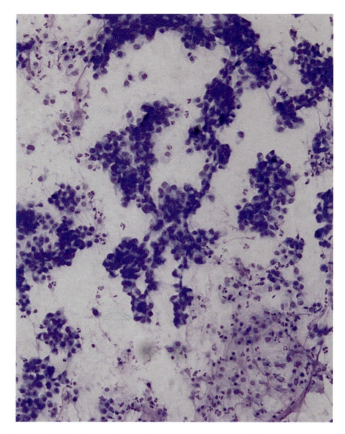

FIGURE 6f-12. Urothelial cell carcinoma is very cellular and involves groups and isolated cells and sometimes papillary structures. It is characterized by large polymorphic nuclei, variable hyperchromasia and a coarse chromatin pattern, prominent nucleoli, and sometimes spindle cells.

Tru-Cut Biopsies

Core biopsies submitted for histological analysis are thought to be more informative than cytological punctures, but in the series by Torp-Pedersen et al. (1991) and Dechet et al. (2003) the accuracy of core biopsies did not improve over FNA. In comparison to FNA, TCB have the advantage of maintained mutual cellular cohesion, providing a picture of the tumor comparable to that found in the routine histological evaluation of tumor slides from operated specimens (see Table 6f–1). However, because many renal cell masses have an inhomogeneous composition with the formation of cysts, bleeding, and central scarring, receiving a nonrepresentative, nondiagnostic tissue sample is a substantial problem. In larger inhomogeneous tumors, FNA has an advantage over TCB by reaching a greater extent of the tumor. In general, smaller tumors have a more homogeneous make-up and the chance of obtaining a diagnostic representative sample is higher. But in the case of a small tumor, it is more difficult to generate a biopsy of the tumor. It depends on the skills and experience of the person performing the biopsy.

For examples of TCB from renal tumors, see Figs. 6f-1B to 6f-7B, 6f-9C, and 6f-11B.

Overall, in adequately performing TCB, the possibility for ancillary studies is more extensive than FNA, which results in TCB having an advantage over FNA.

Conclusions

Radiological imaging allows a better assessment of renal masses and therefore an increasing percentage of renal lesions is found incidentally. FNA and TCB do not contribute to the diagnosis of malignancy in large renal masses, because radiological imaging is nearly always diagnostic. With small lesions, where FNA and TCB should serve as a diagnostic tool, the high incidence of false-negative biopsies in patients with renal masses and the lack of accordance in the literature prevent both techniques from being reliable diagnostic tools that can help in the routine management of patients with suspicious indeterminant renal masses. They are therefore of limited value.

References

Abe M, Saitoh M. Selective renal tumour biopsy under ultrasonic guidance. Br J Urol 1992;70:7–11.

Al Nazer M, Mourad WA. Successful grading of renal-cell carcinoma in fine-needle aspirates. Diagn Cytopathol 2000;22:223–226.

Al-Aynati M, Chen V, Salama S et al. Interobserver and intraobserver variability using the Fuhrman grading system for renal cell carcinoma. Arch Pathol Lab Med 2003;127:593–596.

Brierly RD, Thomas PJ, Harrison NW et al. Evaluation of fine-needle aspiration cytology for renal masses. BJU Int 2000;85: 14–18.

Campbell SC, Novick AC, Herts B et al. Prospective evaluation of fine needle aspiration of small, solid renal masses: accuracy and morbidity. Urology 1997;50:25–29.

Coel MN, Chalmers J. Percutaneous catheter transcaval tumor biopsy. Radiology 1975;116:222.

Cozens NJ, Murchison JT, Allan PL et al. Conventional 15 G needle technique for renal biopsy compared with ultrasound-guided spring-loaded 18 G needle biopsy. Br J Radiol 1992;65:594–597.

Dechet CB, Sebo T, Farrow G et al. Prospective analysis of intra-operative frozen needle biopsy of solid renal masses in adults. J Urol 1999;162:1282–1284.

Dechet CB, Zincke H, Sebo TJ et al. Prospective analysis of computerized tomography and needle biopsy with permanent sectioning to determine the nature of solid renal masses in adults. J Urol 2003;169:71–74.

Denton KJ, Cotton DW, Nakielny RA et al. Secondary tumour deposits in needle biopsy tracks: an underestimated risk? J Clin Pathol 1990;43:83.

Ferrara N, Gerber HP, LeCouter J. The biology of VEGF and its receptors. Nat Med 2003;9:669–676.

Fuhrman SA, Lasky LC, Limas C. Prognostic significance of morphologic parameters in renal cell carcinoma. Am J Surg Pathol 1982;6:655–663.

Gibbons RP, Bush WH Jr, Burnett LL. Needle tract seeding following aspiration of renal cell carcinoma. J Urol 1977;118:865–867.

Goethuys H, Van PH, Oyen R et al. The case against fine-needle aspiration cytology for small solid kidney tumors. Eur Urol 1996;29:284–287.

Granter SR, Renshaw AA. Fine-needle aspiration of chromophobe renal cell carcinoma. Analysis of six cases. Cancer 1997;81: 122–128.

Granter SR, Perez-Atayde AR, Renshaw AA. Cytologic analysis of papillary renal cell carcinoma. Cancer 1998;84:303–308.

Granter SR, Renshaw AA. Cytologic analysis of renal angiomyolipoma: a comparison of radiologically classic and challenging cases. Cancer 1999;87:135–140.

Hampton T. Trials probe new agents for kidney cancer. JAMA 2006;296:155–157.

Harisinghani MG, Maher MM, Gervais DA et al. Incidence of malignancy in complex cystic renal masses (Bosniak category III): should imaging-guided biopsy precede surgery? AJR Am J Roentgenol 2003;180:755–758.

Hayakawa M, Hatano T, Tsuji A et al. Patients with renal cysts associated with renal cell carcinoma and the clinical implications of cyst puncture: a study of 223 cases. Urology 1996;47: 643–646.

Herts BR, Baker ME. The current role of percutaneous biopsy in the evaluation of renal masses. Semin Urol Oncol 1995;13: 254–261.

Jamis-Dow CA, Choyke PL, Jennings SB et al. Small (< or = 3-cm) renal masses: detection with CT versus US and pathologic correlation. Radiology 1996;198:785–788.

Jayson M, Sanders H. Increased incidence of serendipitously discovered renal cell carcinoma. Urology 1998;51:203–205.

Johnson PT, Nazarian LN, Feld RI et al. Sonographically guided renal mass biopsy: indications and efficacy. J Ultrasound Med 2001;20:749–753.

Kato M, Suzuki T, Suzuki Y et al. Natural history of small renal cell carcinoma: evaluation of growth rate, histological grade, cell proliferation and apoptosis. J Urol 2004;172:863–866.

Kiser GC, Totonchy M, Barry JM. Needle tract seeding after percutaneous renal adenocarcinoma aspiration. J Urol 1986;136: 1292–1293.

la-Palma L, Pozzi-Mucelli R. Problematic renal masses in ultrasonography and computed tomography. Clin Imaging 1990;14:83–98.

Lang EK, Macchia RJ, Gayle B et al. CT-guided biopsy of indeterminate renal cystic masses (Bosniak 3 and 2F): accuracy and impact on clinical management. Eur Radiol 2002;12:2518–2524.

Lang H, Lindner V, de FM et al. Multicenter determination of optimal interobserver agreement using the Fuhrman grading system for renal cell carcinoma: assessment of 241 patients with >15-year follow-up. Cancer 2005;103: 625–629.

Leal JJ. A new procedure for biopsy of a solid renal mass: transurethral approach under fluoroscopic control. J Urol 1992;148:98–100.

Liu J, Fanning CV. Can renal oncocytomas be distinguished from renal cell carcinoma on fine-needle aspiration specimens? A study

of conventional smears in conjunction with ancillary studies. Cancer 2001;93:390–397.

Novick A, Campbell S. Renal tumors. In Walsh P, Retik A, Vaughan E et al. (Eds). Campbell's Urology. W.B. Saunders, Philadelphia, 2002, 2675–2678.

Rendon RA, Stanietzky N, Panzarella T et al. The natural history of small renal masses. J Urol 2000;164:1143–1147.

Renshaw AA, Granter SR, Cibas ES. Fine-needle aspiration of the adult kidney. Cancer 1997;81:71–88.

Renshaw AA, Lee KR, Madge R et al. Accuracy of fine needle aspiration in distinguishing subtypes of renal cell carcinoma. Acta Cytol 1997;41:987–994.

Riccabona M, Szolar D, Preidler K et al. Renal masses—evaluation by amplitude coded colour Doppler sonography and multiphasic contrast-enhanced CT. Acta Radiol 1999;40: 457–461.

Richter F, Kasabian NG, Irwin RJ Jr et al. Accuracy of diagnosis by guided biopsy of renal mass lesions classified indeterminate by imaging studies. Urology 2000;55:348–352.

Rybicki FJ, Shu KM, Cibas ES et al. Percutaneous biopsy of renal masses: sensitivity and negative predictive value stratified by clinical setting and size of masses. AJR Am J Roentgenol 2003;180:1281–1287.

Sanchez-Ortiz RF, Madsen LT, Bermejo CE et al. A renal mass in the setting of a nonrenal malignancy: when is a renal tumor biopsy appropriate? Cancer 2004;101:2195–2201.

Slywotzky C, Maya M. Needle tract seeding of transitional cell carcinoma following fine-needle aspiration of a renal mass. Abdom Imaging 1994;19:174–176.

Smith EH. Complications of percutaneous abdominal fine-needle biopsy. Review. Radiology 1991;178:253–258.

Spahn M, Portillo FJ, Michel MS et al. Color duplex sonography vs. computed tomography: accuracy in the preoperative evaluation of renal cell carcinoma. Eur Urol 2001;40:337–342.

Torp-Pedersen S, Juul N, Larsen T et al. US-guided fine needle biopsy of solid renal masses—comparison of histology and cytology. Scand J Urol Nephrol Suppl 1991;137:41–43.

Truong LD, Todd TD, Dhurandhar B et al. Fine-needle aspiration of renal masses in adults: analysis of results and diagnostic problems in 108 cases. Diagn Cytopathol 1999;20:339–349.

Wendth AJ Jr, Garlick WB, Pantoja GE et al. Transcatheter biopsy of renal carcinoma invading the inferior vena cava. J Urol 1976;115:331–332.

Wiatrowska BA, Zakowski MF. Fine-needle aspiration biopsy of chromophobe renal cell carcinoma and oncocytoma: comparison of cytomorphologic features. Cancer 1999;87:161–167.

Wolf JS Jr. Evaluation and management of solid and cystic renal masses. J Urol 1998;159:1120–1133.

Wood BJ, Khan MA, McGovern F et al. Imaging guided biopsy of renal masses: indications, accuracy and impact on clinical management. J Urol 1999;161:1470–1474.

Young NA, Mody DR, Davey DD. Misinterpretation of normal cellular elements in fine-needle aspiration biopsy specimens: observations from the College of American Pathologists Interlaboratory Comparison Program in Non-Gynecologic Cytopathology. Arch Pathol Lab Med 2002;126:670–675.

Zardawi IM. Renal fine needle aspiration cytology. Acta Cytol 1999;43:184–190.

7
Hereditary Factors

7a
von Hippel–Lindau Disease

Martijn P. Lolkema and Emile E. Voest

Introduction

The development of renal cell carcinoma has been associated with a number of hereditary cancer syndromes. These syndromes usually lead to the development of multiple bilateral tumors in the kidney at a relatively young age and are therefore a major diagnostic and therapeutic challenge. The different syndromes that lead to kidney tumors are summarized in Table 7a-1 together with the genes that are commonly affected in individuals suffering from these diseases. Tumor hereditary syndromes involving the kidney lead to different types of kidney cancer (Table 7a-1) and this heterogeneity reflects the different nature of functional aberrancies in these syndromes.[1] Apart from being a clinically important entity these hereditary cancer syndromes can help us decipher the etiology of different forms of kidney cancer and are therefore important in the understanding of sporadic forms of kidney cancer. Here we will discuss the von Hippel–Lindau (VHL) tumor suppressor syndrome because the function of this tumor suppressor gene has been widely studied and it is the only tumor suppressor positively associated with the development of sporadic renal cell carcinomas (Table 7a-1). Moreover, the inactivation of the *VHL* tumor suppressor gene shows a remarkable correlation with the development of sporadic clear cell renal cell carcinoma (ccRCC) but not with other renal kidney tumor types. Different studies have addressed this issue and 60–70% of the sporadic ccRCC samples that have been tested revealed the presence of inactivating mutations of *VHL* or epigenetic silencing through promotor methylation.[2] Although multiple malignant tumors have been described in association with the VHL syndrome, until now there has been no convincing evidence for a direct role for *VHL* mutations in the development of other sporadic malignancies except for pheochromocytoma.[3] This suggests that ccRCC has a unique etiology that is closely linked to the function of the *VHL* gene product. In this chapter we will try to describe the clinical problems of the VHL patients and elucidate the current knowledge about the mechanism of tumor suppression by *VHL*.

von Hippel–Lindau Syndrome: Clinical Characteristics

The German ophthalmologist Dr. Eugen von Hippel, who described the ocular angiomas, and the Swedish pathologist Dr. Arven Lindau, who first described the cerebellar haemangiomas, defined a hereditary syndrome now known as the von Hippel–Lindau syndrome. The description by Dr. Arven Lindau included a systematic compilation of all other published cases, including those of von Hippel, and described changes in different abdominal organs. Patients suffering from the VHL syndrome develop multiple problems as shown in Fig. 7a-1 In 1988 the position of the gene involved in VHL disease was mapped to the short arm of chromosome 3[4] and in 1993 the *VHL* gene was identified and sequenced.[5–7] The most frequently occurring abnormalities are hemangioblastomas in the retina and central nervous system (CNS), ccRCC, pheochromocytomas, pancreatic cysts and tumors, and cystic lesions in various visceral organs.[8] Less well known and less frequent complications of VHL disease are epididymal cystadenoma in men,[9] broad ligament cystadenoma in women, and endolymphatic sac tumors.

Hemangioblastomas

The onset of tumorigenesis in patients suffering from VHL disease differs for the various tumors. Retinal hemangioblastomas, which are benign vascularized lesions, may be seen even in early childhood. The mean age of occurrence in a large French study comprising 103 VHL patients with ocular manifestations was 24.4 years (range: 6–51 years) and visual impairment correlated directly and only with the number of lesions that developed.[10] This complication of VHL disease is often the first manifestation and can be the sole symptom. Retinal hemangiomas should be treated using laser coagulation and warrant frequent ophthalmological controls, as treatment is most effective in early stages of the disease.[11,12] CNS hemangioblastomas represent a similar benign vascular tumor, however, the localization of the tumor differs. The most frequent localization is in the cerebellum and tumors

TABLE 7a-1. Known hereditary renal tumor syndromes.

Syndrome	Chromosome locus	Gene associated with syndrome	Predominant renal tumor type	Other renal tumor types	Frequency of gene mutations in sporadic tumors
Von Hippel–Lindau	3p26	*VHL*	Clear cell	Cysts	60–70% reviewed in Kim and Kaelin[2]
Tuberous sclerosis	9q34	*hamartin*	Angiomyolipoma	Cysts, papillary chromophobe carcinoma	None detected so far
	16p13	*tuberin*			
Hereditary papillary renal cancer	7q34	*HGF receptor*	Papillary type 1	None	None detected so far
Hereditary leiomyoma renal cell carcinoma	1q42-43	*Fumarate hydratase*	Papillary type 2	None	None detected so far
Birt–Hogg–Dubé	17p11.2	*BHD*[79]	Chromophobe	Clear cell, papillary oncocytic neoplasm, oncocytoma	No gene known
Hereditary renal oncocytoma	Unknown	Unknown	Oncocytoma	None	No gene known
Translocation from chromosome 3	To chromosome 2, 6, 8, or 11	Unknown	Clear cell	None	No gene known
Lynch type 2	2p16	*MSH*	Transitional cell carcinoma of renal pelvis	None	None detected so far
	3p31	*MLH1*			Two kidney cancer cell lines and tumors[80]
Medullary carcinoma of the kidney	11p	Unknown	Medullary carcinoma	None	No gene known

Source: Adapted from Choyke et al.[1]

are less frequently found in the brainstem and the spinal cord. In very rare cases these tumors have been found in the lumbosacral nerve roots and supratentorial. Similar to the occurrence of retinal hemangioblastomas these lesions may develop in young individuals with a peak incidence around 33 years (range: 9–78 years).[11–17] The main morbidity of CNS hemangioblastoma is related to the increased pressure on adjacent normal neuronal tissue often leading to neurological symptoms accompanied by increased intracranial pressure. Neurosurgical removal of the tumor is the only effective treatment option to date; less invasive methods such as stereotactic radiotherapy have been tried, however these methods have not yet been firmly established, lacking sufficient long-term follow-up data.[16,18–21]

Clear Cell Renal Cell Carcinoma and Renal Cysts

The second most frequent tumor occurring in VHL patients is ccRCC. This tumor is characterized by its typical histology with cells interspersed with thin-walled blood vessels; most cells are filled with lipids, cholesterol, or glycogen and stain positively on PAS staining (Fig. 7a-2). In 25–60% of the patients suffering from VHL disease ccRCC develops with

a mean onset of 39 years (range: 16–67 years).[8] This is considerably earlier as compared to the sporadic occurrence of ccRCC, which peaks at 64 years (range: 24–89 years).[22] In patients suffering from VHL disease bilateral, multiple, often-cystic lesions develop during their lifetime. Apart from multi-focal ccRCC lesions, VHL disease is characterized by the increased frequency of cystic lesions in the kidney. Both the cysts and the ccRCC have been shown to behave according to the Knudson-two-hit model for tumor suppressor genes with the inactivation of the second wild-type allele of the *VHL* gene, so-called loss of heterozygosity (LOH).[23–25] A question that remains to be resolved is whether the cysts in VHL disease are preneoplastic lesions. In favor of this hypothesis is the fact that the tumors that are associated with VHL disease are often macroscopically cystic or multilobulated and both are associated with the inactivation of both *VHL* alleles. However, unlike polyps in the colon, renal cysts that are sporadic or occur in the context of other genetic disorders causing polycystic kidney disease have never been associated with the development of renal tumors. These conflicting arguments and the absence of good animal models to study the progression of renal cysts into tumors leave this an open question. In VHL disease the occurrence of simple cysts in the kidney does not require therapy; however, complex cysts

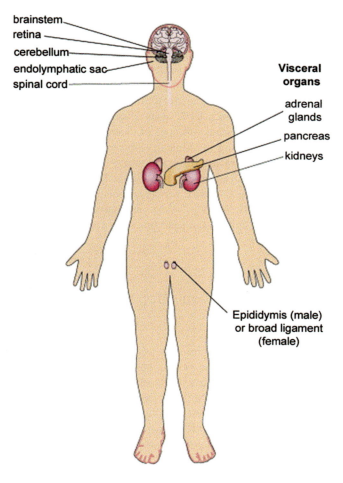

brainstem
retina
cerebellum
endolymphatic sac
spinal cord

Visceral organs

adrenal glands

pancreas

kidneys

Epididymis (male) or broad ligament (female)

Adjusted from (8)

FIGURE 7a-1. Different tumors associated with von Hippel–Lindau disease.

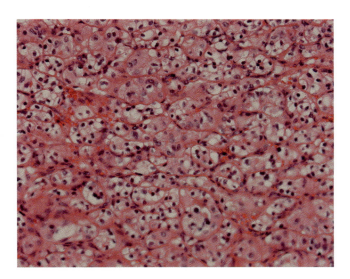

FIGURE 7a-2. Typical histology of a clear cell renal cell carcinoma associated with the inactivation of von Hippel–Lindau tumor suppressor gene. (Image supplied by P. van der Groep, Department of Pathology, University Medical Center, Utrecht).

and solid masses do require attention. The general recommendation for the follow-up of these more complex lesions is to use computer-assisted tomography (CAT) scans or magnetic resonance imaging (MRI) scans every 6–12 months to measure whether these lesions grow. A recent study has evaluated the chances of metastasizing ccRCC as a function of the size of the original lesion and found that no metastases occurred derived from lesions with a diameter of less than 3 cm.[26] Therefore it was suggested that the resection of these lesions can be considered as soon as they grow beyond 3 cm; however, this can be done safely only if there is a rigorous follow-up of the lesions. Resection of growing lesions measuring 2–3 cm could be considered to avoid any metastasis. This observation suggests that the ccRCC that is associated with VHL disease is not a very aggressive metastasizing tumor and this might be true in a similar way for sporadic tumors associated with functional inactivation of the *VHL* gene. In particular, Stage I–III tumors with *VHL* mutations seem to have a better prognosis than those without *VHL* mutations.[27,28] The bilateral and frequent occurrence of kidney tumors in VHL patients obviates the need for nephron-sparing therapy, as renal insufficiency would easily result from radical surgical removal. The recent literature has shown that sporadic clear cell renal cell tumors can safely be removed through the use of nephron-sparing surgery.[29,30] The natural history of kidney involvement in VHL disease provides a strong argument to perform nephron-sparing surgery in selected cases with an emphasis on the preservation of kidney function.[31]

Pheochromocytoma

Pheochromocytomas arise in about 10–20% of VHL patients with a median age of presentation of 30 years (range: 5–58 years) and this tumor can be the sole presentation in VHL patients.[8] Sporadic pheochromocytomas are associated in some cases with the inactivation of the *VHL* gene.[3] It appears that pheochromocytoma is the second tumor associated with both the germ line inactivation of the *VHL* gene and the sporadic inactivation, although this association is much weaker than in ccRCC. Other genes involved in the development of endocrine tumors such as the *RET* oncogene and *MEN2* tumor suppressor gene are also associated with the development of pheochromocytoma. Therefore this tumor is less specific for VHL disease. Pheochromocytoma is an endocrine tumor of the adrenal gland that produces either adrenaline or noradrenaline and is malignant in only 5% of all cases. The main clinical symptoms are related to the excess of adrenergic stimulation: weight loss, tachycardia, hypertension, palpitations, headaches, episodic sweating, pallor, and nausea. There are no specific precautions that need to be taken in treating VHL patients with this disease other than the normal diagnostic and therapeutic protocols for sporadic pheochromocytomas. However, clinicians treating VHL patients should be aware of the possible presence of this tumor.

Pancreatic Neuroendocrine Tumors and Cysts

Another organ, the pancreas, is less frequently involved in VHL disease but with better and more adequate follow-up and treatment of other complications it is becoming more important in the clinical management of patients. Pancreatic neuroendocrine tumors arise in 8–17% of patients with VHL disease with a higher rate of cystic disease comparable to the manifestation in the kidney.[8] Resection of these tumors can be performed on the basis of the size of the tumors and their localization. In the pancreatic head region tumors exceed 2 cm and in the tail exceed 3 cm.[32,33]

Genotype–Phenotype Correlation in von Hippel–Lindau Disease

According to the specific mutations that have been found in different families VHL disease can be classified into different subtypes. The first major subclassification, type 1 vs. type 2, can be separated based on the risk of developing pheochromocytomas. Patients suffering from type 1 disease have an increased risk of developing hemangioblastomas and ccRCC; however, they do not develop pheochromocytomas. Type 2 VHL disease patients do develop pheochromocytomas and these patients can be further subclassified into type 2A/2B and 2C according to their risk of developing hemangioblastoma and ccRCC (Table 7a-2). This correlation of the different mutations found in the VHL gene with different clinical manifestations of the disease makes it important to always perform genetic counseling and molecular diagnostics to obtain a proper diagnosis.[34] Although different mutations lead to different clinical manifestations, the type of mutation

differs only for the type 2C subgroup. In this group 94% of the mutations found are missense mutations (Fig. 7a-3). The different mutations that have been found and analyzed for their subtype of disease will improve patient care as they will focus attention on those manifestations of VHL disease that are most important. For pancreatic involvement and sporadic tumors associated with VHL disease there has not been any association with certain subtypes of disease.

Apart from being a clinically important phenomenon, the classification of the different subtypes of VHL disease reveals a potentially important clue into the pathogenesis of this disease. The complex genotype–phenotype correlation as found in VHL disease seems rare among other genetic syndromes and hints to multiple functions for the VHL tumor suppressor gene.

Function of the von Hippel–Lindau Protein

The function of the VHL protein has been widely studied and has contributed enormously to a better understanding of the pathology of VHL disease. Early clinical observation hinted at the involvement of the VHL gene in the aberrant generation of blood vessels. All the tumors associated with the biallellic inactivation of VHL resulted in well-vascularized, angiogenic lesions with very similar histological phenotypes. Now VHL is known to play a role in the physiological response to oxygen tension in all multicellular organisms tested to date. Apart from its role in regulating the response to oxygen tension, multiple other functions have been ascribed to the VHL tumor suppressor gene in an effort to explain the complex genotype–phenotype correlations.

TABLE 7a-2. Different phenotypes of von Hippel–Lindau disease, clinical manifestations, and mutations.[a]

Type	Hemangioblastoma	ccRCC	Pheochromocytoma	Typical mutation VHL gene
Type 1	High	High	Low	ΔVHL Δ exon 2 76 Δ Phe Ser 65 Trp Leu 158 Pro Leu 188 Gln Asn 78 Ser Tyr 112 His
Type 2A	High	Low	High	Tyr 98 His[81]
Type 2B	High	High	High	Arg 167 Gln Gln 195 Ser
Type 2C	Absent	Absent	High	Val 84 Leu Leu 188 Val Ser 80 Gln

Source: Adapted from Clifford et al.[82]
[a]ccRCC, clear cell renal cell carcinoma; VHL, von Hippel–Lindau.

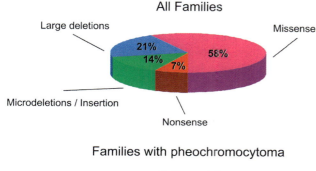

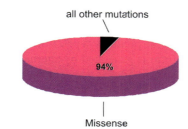

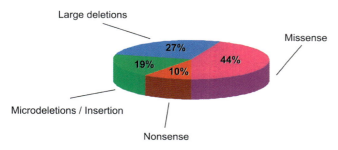

FIGURE 7a-3. Distribution of different kind of mutations associated with the different subtypes of VHL disease.

Mechanism of von Hippel–Lindau: Its Role in Oxygen Sensing

The best-known function for VHL is its role in the oxygen sensing pathway. A wide variety of symptoms associated with VHL disease and ccRCC suggested the existence of a correlation between the function of VHL and the adaptive response to oxygen deprivation. Increased angiogenesis through the accumulation of vascular endothelial growth factor (VEGF), an important cytokine in angiogenesis,[35–37] and polycythemia due to overproduction of erythropoietin (EPO) are the most important examples.[38,39] Showing an accumulation of hypoxia-inducible factor (HIF) in cells devoid of *VHL* established the link between VHL and HIF.[40] HIF is a key transcription factor involved in the adaptive response to decreased oxygen tension: it is known to stimulate the expression of multiple genes involved in the expression of genes necessary for angiogenesis, anerobic metabolism, cell migration, and cell cycle apoptosis.[41,42] The functional HIF protein complex consists of two subunits: an α- and a β-subunit. The α-subunit is regulated and

inherently unstable in *VHL*-proficient cells whereas the β-subunit is ubiquitously expressed and can be found in the nucleus under almost all circumstances. The complex of an α- with a β-subunit is necessary for the stimulation of hypoxia-induced transcription.[43] The next important finding was that HIF-α could be hydroxylated and that this posttranslational modification is essential for its interaction with the VHL gene product under normoxic conditions. Under hypoxic conditions HIF-α could no longer be hydroxylated and was therefore no longer recognized by VHL.[44,45] Once HIF-α is recognized by VHL it is polyubiquitinated and targeted to the proteasome for destruction.[46] The first insight into the molecular mechanism of oxygen-dependent hydroxylation required for VHL–HIF interaction came from a landmark study in the model organism *Caenorhabditis elegans*. Genetic defects in the genes encoding for VHL and so-called prolyl hydroxylases (PHD) gave similar phenotypes.[47] This genetic insight now paved the way for the elucidation of a simple but elegant mechanism for the biological oxygen sensor. Multiple lines of evidence showed that HIF-α was subject to PHD-mediated hydroxylation under normoxic conditions. This enzymatic reaction requires the presence of iron, 2-oxoglutarate, PHD, and most importantly oxygen. This complex interaction of proteins results in a direct oxygen sensor as the absence of oxygen results in the inherent stabilization of HIF-α allowing it to mediate its function as a transcription factor (Fig. 7a-4).[48]

The elucidation of the hypoxia response pathway as described above has led to the first attempts at targeted therapy. For the treatment of ocular hemangioblastomas the first successful trial using an anti-VEGFR small molecule tyrosine kinase inhibitor has been performed.[49] Moreover, for

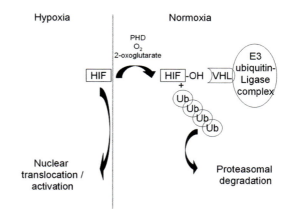

FIGURE 7a-4. The mechanism of hypoxic activation of HIF. At the left side HIF is translated and directly transported into the nucleus to activate gene transcription of genes needed in hypoxic environments. At the right side the mechanism leading to the efficient and swift breakdown of HIF during normoxia is depicted. HIF, hypoxia inducible factor; PHD, prolylhydroxylase; Ub, ubiquitin; VHL, von Hippel–Lindau protein.

the treatment of ccRCC a number of clinical trials testing anti-VEGF strategies and broad-spectrum tyrosine kinase inhibitors blocking the pathways activated by the hypoxia response have been performed and show remarkable responses.[50–52] ccRCC has been a notoriously treatment-resistant tumor type for which therapy targeting the derailed hypoxia response could develop into an effective antitumor therapy.

Role for Hypoxia-Inducible Factor Regulation in Renal Tumorigenesis

Multiple studies have shown increased HIF expression among various tumors such as breast, colon, head and neck, and cervix.[53,54] Moreover in breast cancer the patient prognosis seems to correlate with the expression of HIF.[55,56] Therefore it seems plausible that HIF plays a prominent role in the development of RCC. To establish whether indeed HIF causes renal tumorigenesis different groups have performed experiments trying to determine whether HIF is necessary and sufficient for the development of ccRCC. Collectively, these articles suggest that HIF2α and not HIF1α is the main effector of tumorigenesis upon loss of functional VHL. The first two studies addressed whether overexpressed stabilized HIF can counteract tumor suppression by VHL. The model they used is a xenograft of 786-O VHL-deficient ccRCC cells genetically engineered to reexpress functional VHL. These cells were subsequently engineered to express HIF2α with a point mutation in the amino acid crucial for the oxygen-dependent prolylhydroxylation.[57] These cells were able to override VHL-mediated tumor suppression. However, similar experiments using HIF1α did not result in a similar abolition of VHL-mediated tumor suppression.[58] Although these studies suggest a role for HIF2α, they do not address the more physiologically relevant question of whether the suppression of endogenous HIF2α would be sufficient to abrogate tumor development in these patient-derived RCC cells. This question was addressed using HIF2α RNAi; this is a method to suppress the endogenous expression of proteins using small fragments of complementary RNA.[59] These data indeed support an oncogenic role for HIF2α.[60,61] These experimental data do not, however, exclude further tumor suppressor functions for *VHL*. The *in vivo* experiments described in these papers were terminated after 8–10 weeks, whereas recent experiments demonstrate that beyond this time point 786-O cells engineered to express a mutant *VHL* that is still capable of controlling HIF levels fails to suppress tumor formation.[62] So although HIF seems to be important for the development of ccRCC it might not be the entire story.

Acidic Domain: A Functional Region in the von Hippel–Lindau Gene?

A major advancement in the knowledge about the *VHL* gene function came from the elucidation of the crystal structure of VHL with the other members of the E3 ubiquitin ligase complex and the refinement of this structure with the peptide containing the hydroxyproline of HIF that is essential for its binding to VHL (Fig. 7a-5).[63–65] This crystal structure showed that there are two very well-conserved amino acids in the VHL protein, a serine at position 111 and a histidine at position 115, that are essential in the binding of VHL to HIF. These amino acids form hydrogen bonds with the hydroxyproline of HIF1α and are essential for the recognition of HIF1α. This region in the *VHL* gene that is important lies within the second exon and is part of a so-called β-sheet structure. The third exon forms an α-helical structure important for the binding of VHL to its direct binding partner: Elongin C. However, the VHL gene produces two different gene products: a p30 isoform and a p19 isoform. The p19 isoform is generated by alternative translation initiation at amino acid 54 and does not comprise the N-terminal acidic domain.[66–68] Both the p30 and p19 isoforms were shown to suppress tumor formation in nude mice and both are fully capable of recognizing HIFα subunits and target them to the proteasome.[7,67,68] The N-terminal acidic domain is not included in the crystal structure of the VHL protein because it was technically hard to determine its configuration.[63] However, this region does not seem to be indifferent for the function of VHL as a tumor suppressor protein. Careful analysis of the known mutations in the acidic domain of VHL reveals the presence of tumor-associated mutations that are predicted to affect only the generation of a proper p30 isoform and not the proper generation of the p19 isoform. Furthermore, recently phosphorylation of the acidic domain of VHL by CK2 was shown to be important for the development of xenografts in nude mice.[62] Therefore the acidic domain might play a role in an additional mechanism of *VHL*-mediated tumor suppression.

Fibronectin Binding: An Important Characteristic of von Hippel–Lindau Disease

The first described HIF-independent function for VHL was its binding to the extracellular matrix protein fibronectin and

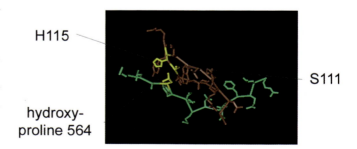

FIGURE 7a-5. Structural basis of the recognition of the hydroxyproline at position 564(P564) of hypoxia-inducible factor (HIF) by the von Hippel–Lindau tumor suppressor protein (VHL). Both S111 and H115 form hydrogen bridges with the hydroxyproline as revealed by the crystal structure of the complex between VHL and the HIF peptide that contains the hydroxylated P564.

consequently the proper deposition of a fibronectin matrix.[69] The fibronectin-binding capacity of VHL is closely linked to the development of VHL disease and unlike the HIF-binding capacity of VHL, seems to be disrupted in all of the disease-associated mutations tested to date, including the mutations associated with type 2C disease, which are known not to be deficient in HIF binding.[70] The mechanism by which VHL influences the proper deposition of a fibronectin matrix is unknown; however, there are multiple levels of fibronectin regulation by VHL. First, VHL positively regulates the transcription of the gene encoding fibronectin, *FN1*, in an HIF-independent manner.[71] Second, phosphorylation of the N-terminal acidic domain of VHL mediates the engagement and/or disengagement of fibronectin.[62] Third, modification of VHL by the ubiquitin-like molecule NEDD8 (neddylation) is linked to fibronectin binding, where the inhibition of VHL neddylation prohibited fibronectin binding.[72] Thus, fibronectin deposition by VHL seems to be a highly regulated process and it is unique to the p30 isoform, as the p19 isoform does not bind fibronectin.[66] Fibronectin deposition may be a crucial function of the tumor suppressive function of *VHL* and might account for part of the complex genotype–phenotype correlation in VHL disease.

Other Hypoxia-Inducible Factor Independent von Hippel–Lindau Functions

A number of other targets for the VHL-E3 ligase complex have been suggested: Jade-1, VDU-1/2, and atypical PKC.[73–76] However, only one group has described each of these new targets and whether they are important in tumorigenesis remains to be shown. So whereas the specificity of the interaction between VHL and HIF is striking, there are possibly other targets for this particular ubiquitin E3 ligase complex.

Recently a role for VHL has been described in stabilizing microtubules.[77,78] In a number of tumor cells the misbalance of microtubule dynamics has been reported. Microtubule dynamics is potentially important in regulating chromosomal stability and other cellular processes such as migration and polarity. This function is E3 ligase independent and seems to depend upon the binding of VHL to microtubules. Strikingly this function seems to be impaired, especially in type 2A disease-associated mutants.[77] However, these novel functions for VHL need to be further solidified before their role in tumorigenesis can be assessed.

Conclusions

VHL disease is a hereditary syndrome with multiple tumor phenotypes. The treatment of patients suffering from this disease depends on the early detection of the associated tumors and the development of functional sparing therapy as the occurrence of multiple lesions in the lifetime of patients

suffering from this disease is probable. The elucidation of the molecular mechanism in which VHL is involved has led to the understanding that VHL plays a pivotal role in the physiological response to oxygen tension. Debate exists about other molecular functions of VHL; however, clinical data suggest other functions for VHL. Future research into the role of VHL in ccRCC will probably contribute to our knowledge of how ccRCC develops and and hopefully aid in developing rational targeted therapies.

References

1. Choyke, P. L., Glenn, G. M., Walther, M. M., Zbar, B., and Linehan, W. M. (2003) *Radiology* **226**(1), 33–46.
2. Kim, W. Y., and Kaelin, W. G. (2004) *J Clin Oncol* **22**(24), 4991–5004.
3. Dannenberg, H., De Krijger, R. R., van der Harst, E., Abbou, M., Y, I. J., Komminoth, P., and Dinjens, W. N. (2003) *Int J Cancer* **105**(2), 190–195.
4. Seizinger, B. R., Smith, D. I., Filling-Katz, M. R., Neumann, H., Green, J. S., Choyke, P. L., Anderson, K. M., Freiman, R. N., Klauck, S. M., Whaley, J., et al. (1991) *Proc Natl Acad Sci USA* **88**(7), 2864–2868.
5. Latif, F., Tory, K., Gnarra, J., Yao, M., Duh, F. M., Orcutt, M. L., Stackhouse, T., Kuzmin, I., Modi, W., Geil, L., and et al. (1993) *Science* **260**(5112), 1317–1320.
6. Renbaum, P., Duh, F. M., Latif, F., Zbar, B., Lerman, M. I., and Kuzmin, I. (1996) *Hum Genet* **98**(6), 666–671.
7. Iliopoulos, O., Kibel, A., Gray, S., and Kaelin, W. G., Jr. (1995) *Nat Med* **1**(8), 822–826.
8. Lonser, R. R., Glenn, G. M., Walther, M., Chew, E. Y., Libutti, S. K., Linehan, W. M., and Oldfield, E. H. (2003) *Lancet* **361**(9374), 2059–2067.
9. Choyke, P. L., Glenn, G. M., Wagner, J. P., Lubensky, I. A., Thakore, K., Zbar, B., Linehan, W. M., and Walther, M. M. (1997) *Urology* **49**(6), 926–931.
10. Dollfus, H., Massin, P., Taupin, P., Nemeth, C., Amara, S., Giraud, S., Beroud, C., Dureau, P., Gaudric, A., Landais, P., and Richard, S. (2002) *Invest Ophthalmol Vis Sci* **43**(9), 3067–3074.
11. Schmidt, D., Natt, E., and Neumann, H. P. (2000) *Eur J Med Res* **5**(2), 47–58.
12. Wittebol-Post, D., Hes, F. J., and Lips, C. J. (1998) *J Intern Med* **243**(6), 555–561.
13. Richard, S., Campello, C., Taillandier, L., Parker, F., and Resche, F. (1998) *J Intern Med* **243**(6), 547–553.
14. Maddock, I. R., Moran, A., Maher, E. R., Teare, M. D., Norman, A., Payne, S. J., Whitehouse, R., Dodd, C., Lavin, M., Hartley, N., Super, M., and Evans, D. G. (1996) *J Med Genet* **33**(2), 120–127.
15. Lamiell, J. M., Salazar, F. G., and Hsia, Y. E. (1989) *Medicine (Baltimore)* **68**(1), 1–29.
16. Weil, R. J., Lonser, R. R., DeVroom, H. L., Wanebo, J. E., and Oldfield, E. H. (2003) *J Neurosurg* **98**(1), 95–105.
17. Richard, S., David, P., Marsot-Dupuch, K., Giraud, S., Beroud, C., and Resche, F. (2000) *Neurosurg Rev* **23**(1), 1–22; discussion 23–24.
18. Lonser, R. R., Weil, R. J., Wanebo, J. E., DeVroom, H. L., and Oldfield, E. H. (2003) *J Neurosurg* **98**(1), 106–116.

19. Wanebo, J. E., Lonser, R. R., Glenn, G. M., and Oldfield, E. H. (2003) *J Neurosurg* **98**(1), 82–94.

20. Rajaraman, C., Rowe, J. G., Walton, L., Malik, I., Radatz, M., and Kemeny, A. A. (2004) *Br J Neurosurg* **18**(4), 338–342.

21. Chang, S. D., Meisel, J. A., Hancock, S. L., Martin, D. P., McManus, M., and Adler, J. R., Jr. (1998) *Neurosurgery* **43**(1), 28–34; discussion 34–35.

22. Bani-Hani, A. H., Leibovich, B. C., Lohse, C. M., Cheville, J. C., Zincke, H., and Blute, M. L. (2005) *J Urol* **173**(2), 391–394.

23. Prowse, A. H., Webster, A. R., Richards, F. M., Richard, S., Olschwang, S., Resche, F., Affara, N. A., and Maher, E. R. (1997) *Am J Hum Genet* **60**(4), 765–771.

24. Gnarra, J. R., Tory, K., Weng, Y., Schmidt, L., Wei, M. H., Li, H., Latif, F., Liu, S., Chen, F., Duh, F. M., et al. (1994) *Nat Genet* **7**(1), 85–90.

25. Crossey, P. A., Foster, K., Richards, F. M., Phipps, M. E., Latif, F., Tory, K., Jones, M. H., Bentley, E., Kumar, R., Lerman, M. I., et al. (1994) *Hum Genet* **93**(1), 53–58.

26. Duffey, B. G., Choyke, P. L., Glenn, G., Grubb, R. L., Venzon, D., Linehan, W. M., and Walther, M. M. (2004) *J Urol* **172**(1), 63–65.

27. Yao, M., Yoshida, M., Kishida, T., Nakaigawa, N., Baba, M., Kobayashi, K., Miura, T., Moriyama, M., Nagashima, Y., Nakatani, Y., Kubota, Y., and Kondo, K. (2002) *J Natl Cancer Inst* **94**(20), 1569–1575.

28. Kim, J. H., Jung, C. W., Cho, Y. H., Lee, J., Lee, S. H., Kim, H. Y., Park, J., Park, J. O., Kim, K., Kim, W. S., Park, Y. S., Im, Y. H., Kang, W. K., and Park, K. (2005) *Oncol Rep* **13**(5), 859–864.

29. Krejci, K. G., Blute, M. L., Cheville, J. C., Sebo, T. J., Lohse, C. M., and Zincke, H. (2003) *Urology* **62**(4), 641–646.

30. Ghavamian, R., Cheville, J. C., Lohse, C. M., Weaver, A. L., Zincke, H., and Blute, M. L. (2002) *J Urol* **168**(2), 454–459.

31. Los, M., Links, T. P., Lenders, J. W., and Voest, E. E. (2000) *Ned Tijdschr Geneeskd* **144**(11), 497–501.

32. Libutti, S. K., Choyke, P. L., Alexander, H. R., Glenn, G., Bartlett, D. L., Zbar, B., Lubensky, I., McKee, S. A., Maher, E. R., Linehan, W. M., and Walther, M. M. (2000) *Surgery* **128**(6), 1022–1027; discussion 1027–1028.

33. Libutti, S. K., Choyke, P. L., Bartlett, D. L., Vargas, H., Walther, M., Lubensky, I., Glenn, G., Linehan, W. M., and Alexander, H. R. (1998) *Surgery* **124**(6), 1153–1159.

34. Lips, C. J., Hoppener, J. W., Van Nesselrooij, B. P., and Van der Luijt, R. B. (2005) *J Intern Med* **257**(1), 69–77.

35. Los, M., Aarsman, C. J., Terpstra, L., Wittebol-Post, D., Lips, C. J., Blijham, G. H., and Voest, E. E. (1997) *Ann Oncol* **8**(10), 1015–1022.

36. Stratmann, R., Krieg, M., Haas, R., and Plate, K. H. (1997) *J Neuropathol Exp Neurol* **56**(11), 1242–1252.

37. Siemeister, G., Weindel, K., Mohrs, K., Barleon, B., Martiny-Baron, G., and Marme, D. (1996) *Cancer Res* **56**(10), 2299–2301.

38. Wiesener, M. S., Seyfarth, M., Warnecke, C., Jurgensen, J. S., Rosenberger, C., Morgan, N. V., Maher, E. R., Frei, U., and Eckardt, K. U. (2002) *Blood* **99**(10), 3562–3565.

39. Marshall, F. F., and Walsh, P. C. (1977) *J Urol* **117**(4), 439–440.

40. Maxwell, P. H., Wiesener, M. S., Chang, G. W., Clifford, S. C., Vaux, E. C., Cockman, M. E., Wykoff, C. C., Pugh, C. W., Maher, E. R., and Ratcliffe, P. J. (1999) *Nature* **399**(6733), 271–275.

41. Greijer, A., van der Groep, P., Kemming, D., Shvarts, A., Semenza, G., Meijer, G., van de Wiel, M., Belien, J., van Diest, P., and van der Wall, E. (2005) *J Pathol* **286**(3), 291–304.

42. Ruas, J. L., and Poellinger, L. (2005) *Semin Cell Dev Biol* **16**, 564–574.

43. Wang, G. L., and Semenza, G. L. (1995) *J Biol Chem* **270**(3), 1230–1237.

44. Jaakkola, P., Mole, D. R., Tian, Y. M., Wilson, M. I., Gielbert, J., Gaskell, S. J., Kriegsheim, A., Hebestreit, H. F., Mukherji, M., Schofield, C. J., Maxwell, P. H., Pugh, C. W., and Ratcliffe, P. J. (2001) *Science* **292**(5516), 468–472.

45. Ivan, M., Kondo, K., Yang, H., Kim, W., Valiando, J., Ohh, M., Salic, A., Asara, J. M., Lane, W. S., and Kaelin, W. G., Jr. (2001) *Science* **292**(5516), 464–468.

46. Ohh, M., Park, C. W., Ivan, M., Hoffman, M. A., Kim, T. Y., Huang, L. E., Pavletich, N., Chau, V., and Kaelin, W. G. (2000) *Nat Cell Biol* **2**(7), 423–427.

47. Epstein, A. C., Gleadle, J. M., McNeill, L. A., Hewitson, K. S., O'Rourke, J., Mole, D. R., Mukherji, M., Metzen, E., Wilson, M. I., Dhanda, A., Tian, Y. M., Masson, N., Hamilton, D. L., Jaakkola, P., Barstead, R., Hodgkin, J., Maxwell, P. H., Pugh, C. W., Schofield, C. J., and Ratcliffe, P. J. (2001) *Cell* **107**(1), 43–54.

48. Semenza, G. L. (2004) *Physiology (Bethesda)* **19**, 176–182.

49. Aiello, L. P., George, D. J., Cahill, M. T., Wong, J. S., Cavallerano, J., Hannah, A. L., and Kaelin, W. G., Jr. (2002) *Ophthalmology* **109**(9), 1745–1751.

50. Motzer, R. J., Michaelson, M. D., Redman, B. G., Hudes, G. R., Wilding, G., Figlin, R. A., Ginsberg, M. S., Kim, S. T., Baum, C. M., DePrimo, S. E., Li, J. Z., Bello, C. L., Theuer, C. P., George, D. J., and Rini, B. I. (2006) *J Clin Oncol* **24**(1), 16–24.

51. Patel, P. H., Chaganti, R. S., and Motzer, R. J. (2006) *Br J Cancer* **94**(5), 614–619.

52. Rini, B. I., Halabi, S., Taylor, J., Small, E. J., and Schilsky, R. L. (2004) *Clin Cancer Res* **10**(8), 2584–2586.

53. Jubb, A. M., Pham, T. Q., Hanby, A. M., Frantz, G. D., Peale, F. V., Wu, T. D., Koeppen, H. W., and Hillan, K. J. (2004) *J Clin Pathol* **57**(5), 504–512.

54. Talks, K. L., Turley, H., Gatter, K. C., Maxwell, P. H., Pugh, C. W., Ratcliffe, P. J., and Harris, A. L. (2000) *Am J Pathol* **157**(2), 411–421.

55. Bos, R., van der Groep, P., Greijer, A. E., Shvarts, A., Meijer, S., Pinedo, H. M., Semenza, G. L., van Diest, P. J., and van der Wall, E. (2003) *Cancer* **97**(6), 1573–1581.

56. Vleugel, M. M., Greijer, A. E., Shvarts, A., van der Groep, P., van Berkel, M., Aarbodem, Y., van Tinteren, H., Harris, A. L., van Diest, P. J., and van der Wall, E. (2005) *J Clin Pathol* **58**(2), 172–177.

57. Kondo, K., Klco, J., Nakamura, E., Lechpammer, M., and Kaelin, W. G., Jr. (2002) *Cancer Cell* **1**(3), 237–246.

58. Maranchie, J. K., Vasselli, J. R., Riss, J., Bonifacino, J. S., Linehan, W. M., and Klausner, R. D. (2002) *Cancer Cell* **1**(3), 247–255.

59. Agami, R. (2002) *Curr Opin Chem Biol* **6**(6), 829–834.

60. Kondo, K., Kim, W. Y., Lechpammer, M., and Kaelin, W. G., Jr. (2003) *PLoS Biol* **1**(3), E83.

61. Zimmer, M., Doucette, D., Siddiqui, N., and Iliopoulos, O. (2004) *Mol Cancer Res* **2**(2), 89–95.

62. Lolkema, M. P., Gervais, M. L., Snijckers, C. M., Hill, R. P., Giles, R. H., Voest, E. E., and Ohh, M. (2005) *J Biol Chem* **280**(23), 22205–22211.

63. Stebbins, C. E., Kaelin, W. G., Jr., and Pavletich, N. P. (1999) *Science* **284**(5413), 455–461.

64. Min, J. H., Yang, H., Ivan, M., Gertler, F., Kaelin, W. G., Jr., and Pavletich, N. P. (2002) *Science* **296**(5574), 1886–1889.

65. Hon, W. C., Wilson, M. I., Harlos, K., Claridge, T. D., Schofield, C. J., Pugh, C. W., Maxwell, P. H., Ratcliffe, P. J., Stuart, D. I., and Jones, E. Y. (2002) *Nature* **417**(6892), 975–978.

66. Iliopoulos, O., Ohh, M., and Kaelin, W. G., Jr. (1998) *Proc Natl Acad Sci USA* **95**(20), 11661–11666.

67. Schoenfeld. A., Davidowitz, E. J., and Burk, R. D. (1998) *Proc Natl Acad Sci USA* **95**(15), 8817–8822.

68. Blankenship, C., Naglich, J. G., Whaley, J. M., Seizinger, B., and Kley, N. (1999) *Oncogene* **18**(8), 1529–1535.

69. Ohh, M., Yauch, R. L., Lonergan, K. M., Whaley, J. M., Stemmer-Rachamimov, A. O., Louis, D. N., Gavin, B. J., Kley, N., Kaelin, W. G., Jr., and Iliopoulos, O. (1998) *Mol Cell* **1**(7), 959–968.

70. Hoffman, M. A., Ohh, M., Yang, H., Klco, J. M., Ivan, M., and Kaelin, W. G., Jr. (2001) *Hum Mol Genet* **10**(10), 1019–1027.

71. Bluyssen, H. A., Lolkema, M. P., van Beest, M., Boone, M., Snijckers, C. M., Los, M., Gebbink, M. F., Braam, B., Holstege, F. C., Giles, R. H., and Voest, E. E. (2004) *FEBS Lett* **556**(1–3), 137–142.

72. Stickle, N. H., Chung, J., Klco, J. M., Hill, R. P., Kaelin, W. G., Jr., and Ohh, M. (2004) *Mol Cell Biol* **24**(8), 3251–3261.

73. Zhou, M. I., Wang, H., Foy, R. L., Ross, J. J., and Cohen, H. T. (2004) *Cancer Res* **64**(4), 1278–1286.

74. Li, Z., Na, X., Wang, D., Schoen, S. R., Messing, E. M., and Wu, G. (2002) *J Biol Chem* **277**(7), 4656–4662.

75. Li, Z., Wang, D., Na, X., Schoen, S. R., Messing, E. M., and Wu, G. (2002) *Biochem Biophys Res Commun* **294**(3), 700–709.

76. Okuda, H., Hirai, S., Takaki, Y., Kamada, M., Baba, M., Sakai, N., Kishida, T., Kaneko, S., Yao, M., Ohno, S., and Shuin, T. (1999) *Biochem Biophys Res Commun* **263**(2), 491–497.

77. Hergovich, A., Lisztwan, J., Barry, R., Ballschmieter, P., and Krek, W. (2003) *Nat Cell Biol* **5**(1), 64–70.

78. Lolkema, M. P., Mehra, N., Jorna, A. S., van Beest, M., Giles, R. H., and Voest, E. E. (2004) *Exp Cell Res* **301**(2), 139–146.

79. Nickerson, M. L., Warren, M. B., Toro, J. R., Matrosova, V., Glenn, G., Turner, M. L., Duray, P., Merino, M., Choyke, P., Pavlovich, C. P., Sharma, N., Walther, M., Munroe, D., Hill, R., Maher, E., Greenberg, C., Lerman, M. I., Linehan, W. M., Zbar, B., and Schmidt, L. S. (2002) *Cancer Cell* **2**(2), 157–164.

80. Leach, F. S., Koh, M., Sharma, K., McWilliams, G., Talifero-Smith, L., Codd, A., Olea, R., and Elbahloul, O. (2002) *Cancer Biol Ther* **1**(5), 530–536.

81. Brauch, H., Kishida, T., Glavac, D., Chen, F., Pausch, F., Hofler, H., Latif, F., Lerman, M. I., Zbar, B., and Neumann, H. P. (1995) *Hum Genet* **95**(5), 551–556.

82. Clifford, S. C., Cockman, M. E., Smallwood, A. C., Mole, D. R., Woodward, E. R., Maxwell, P. H., Ratcliffe, P. J., and Maher, E. R. (2001) *Hum Mol Genet* **10**(10), 1029–1038.

7b
Genetic Counseling for Inherited Forms of Kidney Cancer

Peter Hulick, Gayun Chan-Smutko, Michael Zimmer, and Othon Iliopoulos

Introduction

Inherited forms of renal cancer are transmitted through germline mutations. Germline mutations in genes associated with inherited renal cancer may predispose affected individuals not only to renal cell carcinoma (RCC) but also to lesions and symptoms of specific tissues, depending on the affected gene. The family medical history of the patient presenting with RCC may be suggestive of an inherited form. In the most classic examples of hereditary RCC, several members of the family across two or more generations developed kidney cancer, often with an early age of onset. In other cases, the family history will appear noncontributory. The clinical question of whether a patient harbors a genetic predisposition to RCC, therefore, may be raised either because of the occurrence of RCC in the family or because of the coexistence of RCC with other symptoms or lesions that indicate a germline mutation.

In this chapter, we will describe the clinical presentation of inherited forms of RCC and the germline mutations associated with them. We will provide a working approach for the evaluation of hereditary RCC and genetic testing for underlining germline mutations. We will also discuss prenatal counseling and the possibility of a noncontributory family history. The reader is encouraged to refer to the Online Mendelian Inheritance in Man (OMIM) for a detailed and continuously updated description of the diseases and their molecular defects.

RCCs are histologically heterogeneous. The majority of noninherited (sporadic) tumors consist of clear cell carcinoma (75%). The rest are papillary carcinoma (15%), chromophobe (5%), and oncocytomas (5%).[1] Inherited forms of kidney cancer are usually of the same histology and correspond to specific mutations, with the notable exception of the Birt–Hogg–Dube disease. This observation provides a strong diagnostic framework for describing the specific diseases.

Familial Clear Cell Renal Cell Carcinoma

von Hippel–Lindau Disease (OMIM 193300)

This disease is discussed in detail in Chapter 7a of this book. We highlight here some features of the disease that integrate with the differential diagnostics of inherited kidney cancers. Melmon and Rosen compiled the first clinical criteria for von Hippel–Lindau (VHL) disease.[2] However, cloning of the VHL susceptibility gene[3] and the availability of genetic testing have led to a revision of the "classic" clinical criteria.

Clinical Manifestations

This is a disease of almost complete penetrance; almost every individual who harbors a germline mutation will develop some lesion(s) of the disease by the sixth decade of life. Typically signs and symptoms develop during the second to third decade of life.

VHL-associated lesions include clear cell cancer exclusively of clear cell histology. No other histological type of RCC has been reported so far in VHL patients. Extrarenal lesions include central nervous system (CNS) hemangioblastomas (HB), mostly in the cerebellum, spine, and retina, pheochromocytoma, papillary cystadenomas and endocrine tumors of the pancreas, cystadenomas of the epididymis and the middle ear, as well as cysts in the pancreas, the kidneys, and the epididymis.

The clinical presentation of VHL disease clusters in two phenotypes.[4–6] Type 1 patients develop HB and RCC but not pheochromocytoma. In contrast, type 2 patients are at risk for pheochromocytoma and are subdivided in three subtypes. Type 2A are at low risk for RCC and type 2B are at high risk for RCC. Type 2C patients present as familial pheochromocytoma only without development of RCC or HB. Germline mutations in the VHL gene consist of large or small deletions, nonsense mutations, missense mutations, or silencing of the gene by methylation. Mutations that result in total protein deletion or unfolding lead to type 1 disease, whereas missense mutations present with pheochromocytoma.

The expressivity of the disease may vary significantly among individuals with the same germline mutation. In some cases, young patients present with multiple foci of hemangioblastoma in areas difficult to treat with surgery or radiation and/or multiple renal cancers. Individuals harboring the same mutation may run a much milder course or may be identified later in life through incidental findings during imaging. As an example, we established the diagnosis of VHL disease in a 52-year-old asymptomatic male with negative family history, referred to us with a single pancreatic cyst and a single cerebellar hemangioblastoma.

Diagnostic Considerations

The criteria to refer a patient for evaluation and testing for VHL disease that we use in the Massachusetts General Hospital VHL Clinic are listed in Table 7b-1. Molecular diagnosis of the disease is made by sequencing the entire gene for point mutations and evaluation of the presence of one or both copies of the gene by Northern blot analysis. The test has an almost 100% sensitivity and specificity in laboratories with professional licensing for the test.[7]

TABLE 7b-1. Criteria for referral to a VHL clinic (Massachusetts General Hospital).

1. Any blood relative of an individual diagnosed with VHL disease.
2. Individuals with one VHL-associated lesion[a] **and** a positive FH of VHL-associated lesion(s)
3. Any individual with **two** VHL-associated lesions
4. Individual with any of the following:

HB diagnosed in a <30-year-old patient with two or more CNS HBs (any age of diagnosis) and one HB + RCC or PHE or pancreatic neuroendocrine tumor

Clear cell RCC diagnosed in a < 40-year-old patient
Bilateral and/or multiple clear cell RCC
Clear cell RCC with a positive FH

PHEO diagnosed in a <40-year-old patient
Bilateral and/or multiple PHEO
PHEO with a positive FH

More than one pancreatic serous cystadenoma
More than one pancreatic neuroendocrine tumor
Multiple pancreatic cysts + any VHL-associated lesion

Endolymphatic sac tumor (ELST)
Epididymal papillary cystadenoma

[a]von Hippel–Lindau (VHL)-associated lesions: hemangioblastoma (HB), clear cell renal carcinoma (RCC), pheochromocytoma (PHEO), endolymphatic sac tumor (ELST), epididymal papillary cystadenoma, pancreatic serous cystadenomas, pancreatic neuroendocrine tumors. FH, family history; CNS, central nervous system.

Tuberous Sclerosis Complex (TSC1, OMIM 191100 and TSC2, OMIM 191092)

There are two genes corresponding to the disease: the TSC1 gene (OMIM 191100) maps to chromosome 9q34[8] and TSC2 (OMIM 191092) to chromosome 16p13.3.[9] The clinical manifestations deriving from mutations in either gene are the same, although TSC1-associated disease may have a milder clinical course.[10]

Clinical Manifestations

Major and minor diagnostic criteria for clinical diagnosis of TSC have been compiled and recently revised.[11, 12] TSC patients develop predominantly nonmalignant, hamartomatous lesions in the CNS (including the retina), kidneys, skin, lungs, and heart (Table 7b-1).

Cortical tubers, calcified subependymal nodules, and subependymal giant cell astrocytomas are CNS lesions characteristic of TSC and constitute part of the major diagnostic criteria.[11] These lesions have a characteristic radiological appearance on brain magnetic resonance imaging (MRI) and cause epilepsy, partial seizures (60% of TSC patients), or learning disabilities. Giant cell astrocytomas may obstruct normal cerebrospinal fluid (CSF) flow and cause symptoms and signs of increased intracranial pressure. Single or multiple retinal hamartomas occur in approximately 50% of TSC patients and are often asymptomatic.[13] The typical lesion is called a mulberry tumor, a gray/yellowish lesion with a characteristic surface resembling a mulberry. Flat, discolored retinal hamartomas also occur. Retinal detachment may occur, although this problem is not as frequent as in VHL patients.

The most common kidney lesions in patients with TSC are benign angiomyolipomas. They occur in 70–80% of adults and are possibly the most common TSC lesion. They are usually multiple and bilateral. They grow with age and become symptomatic later in life, causing discomfort, pain, and hematuria, often resulting from intratumoric hemorrhage.[14] Malignant angiomyolipomas, although much less frequent than the hamartomatous ones, do occur.[15] Radiological differentiation between the two entities is of paramount importance since malignant angiomyolipomas need to be treated surgically. An additional diagnostic dilemma for the physician who follows the TSC patient is the occurrence of clear cell renal carcinoma. Lastly, TSC patients may develop oncocytoma. MRI is the method of choice for the differential diagnosis between the various kidney tumors, although computed tomography (CT) gives very characteristic lesions in case of angiomyolipomas. Multiple and bilateral renal cysts displaying atypical and hyperplastic epithelium are common in TSC patients. The TSC2 gene is adjacent to the PKD1 gene. Large germline deletions accompanying both genes have been reported to result in a clinical picture of polycystic kidney disease (PKD) with features of TSC as angiomyolipomas, termed the "continuous TSC/PKD syndrome."[16]

Skin lesions resulting from TSC include hypomelanotic macules, shagreen patches, and facial angiofibromas.[17] All three, along with the presence of nontraumatic ungual or periungual fibromas, constitute major clinical criteria for the presence of the disease. Cardiac rhabdomyomas, single or multiple, may occur. Lesion onset clusters to early in life or around puberty. Childhood rhabdomyomas tend to regress spontaneously, but the ones around puberty persist and may cause arrythmias. Lung function is also affected in patients with TSC. Patients, particularly females, may develop lymphangiomyomatosis that may lead to spontaneous pneumothorax and/or respiratory insufficiency.[18] Other lung lesions include micronodular hyperplasia and lung tumors.

Diagnostic Considerations

Lesions of TSC can be classified as major or minor, depending on their specificity for TSC. Clinical diagnostic criteria comprise a combination of major and/or minor features as listed in Table 7b-2.

The TSC2 gene consists of 42 exons and encodes a 5.5-kb mRNA.[8] The gene is expressed in all adult human tissue examined so far. Rat,[19] mouse,[20] and *Drosophila* [21,22]

TABLE 7b-2. Diagnostic criteria for tuberous sclerosis complex (TSC).

Major features
  Facial angiofibromas or forehead plaque
  Nontraumatic ungual or periungual fibroma
  Hypomelanotic macules (three or more)
  Shagreen patch (connective tissue nevus)
  Multiple retinal nodular hamartomas
  Cortical tuber[a]
  Subependymal nodule
Subependymal giant cell astrocytoma
Cardiac rhabdomyoma, single or multiple
Lymphangiomyomatosis[b]
Renal angiomyolipoma[b]

Minor features
  Multiple, randomly distributed pits in dental enamel
  Hamartomatous rectal polyps[c]
  Bone cysts
  Cerebral white matter radial migration lines[a]
  Gingival fibromas
  Nonrenal hamartoma[c]
  Retinal achromic patch
  Confetti skin lesions
  Multiple renal cysts[c]

Definite TSC: Two major features **or** one major + one minor feature
Probable TSC: One major + one minor feature
Suspect TSC: One major feature **or** two or more minor features

Source: Adapted from Roach et al.[12]
[a]When cortical tuber and radial migration lines occur together they should be counted as one rather than two features of TSC.
[b]When lymphangiomyomatosis and angiomyolipoma are present, other features of TSC should also be present before a definitive diagnosis is made.
[c]Histological confirmation is suggested.

homologues of TSC2 have been cloned. The TSC1 gene consists of 23 exons and encodes an 8.6-kb mRNA.

TSC germline mutations can be traced to the parents in approximately one-third of all TSC patients.[23] The rest constitute *de novo* mutations. Evidence exists that a small percentage of *de novo* mutations can actually be attributed to parent mosaicism.[24,25] Germline TSC2 mutations involve large and small intragenic deletions, nonsense mutations resulting in a truncated protein, and missense mutations to a lesser extent. In the case of contiguous TSC/PKD1 syndrome, large germline deletions inactivate both genes.[26] The majority of characterized TSC1 mutations are predicted to result in a truncated protein.[10]

Patients with *de novo* TSC mutations are more likely to harbor a germline mutation in the TSC2 gene.[23] In contrast, TSC1 mutations are encountered with higher frequency in familial cases, where the mutation can be traced to one of the parents. It is possible, though, that these differences are due to ascertainment bias: TSC2 mutations result in a more severe disease phenotype, especially mental retardation, compared to that from TSC1 mutations.[27,28] It is therefore possible that TSC2 mutation carriers might have a reduced reproductive fitness.

Functions of TSC1 and TSC2 Proteins

The TSC2 gene encodes for a 1807 amino acid protein (tuberin) that migrates with an apparent molecular weight of approximately 200 kDa[8] while the TSC1 gene encodes for a 1164 amino acid protein (130 kDa, hamartin). Tuberin and hamartin form a heterodimeric complex *in vitro* and *in vivo* that mediates the downstream action of these proteins.[29]

TSC2 and TSC1 are tumor suppressor genes. Mice in which both alleles of Tsc2 were inactivated die as embryos. Heterozygous $Tsc2^{+/-}$ mice (one copy of the gene has been inactivated) survive to develop multiple and bilateral renal cystadenomas, liver hemangiomas, and lung adenomas.[30,31] $Tsc1^{+/-}$ heterozygous mice develop a similar pattern of neoplasms,[32] indicating that TSC1/TSC2 proteins have markedly overlapping functions and act as a heterodimer in the same signal transduction pathway.

TSC-associated tumors display loss of heterozygosity (LOH) in the TSC1 or TSC2 locus.[33–35] Sporadic counterparts of TSC-associated tumors, in particular renal angiomyolipomas and pulmonary lymphangiomas, also display LOH in the TSC1 or TSC2 locus.[36,37] Reintroduction of wild-type but not mutant tuberin in $TSC2^{-/-}$ cell lines inhibits their growth *in vitro* and suppresses tumor formation in the nude mouse xenograft assay.[38] These genetic and biological data indicate that TSC1/2 are tumor suppressor genes and that inactivation of both alleles is necessary for tumor formation.

The TSC1/TSC2 heterodimer inhibits Rheb and through this action inhibits mTOR, and thereby negatively regulates cell growth.[39–41] Activation of phosphatidylinositol-3'-kinase (PI3K) leads to phosphorylation and activation of Akt/PKB.[42] Akt phosphorylates TSC2, which inhibits binding to its heterodimeric partner, TSC1, and becomes unstable. Genetic experiments in *Drosophila* and biochemical experiments in mammalian TSC1 or $TSC2^{-/-}$ cells indicate that loss of TSC protein results in constitutively active TOR.[21,22] Of direct clinical importance is that these observations suggest rapamycin may be a drug of choice for TSC1/2 tumors that are characterized by constitutive TOR upregulation. The reader is referred to scholarly reviews of the signaling interplay between activation of PI3K, Akt, TSC, and mTOR.[43]

Constitutive Translocations Involving Chromosome 3p

Germline balanced translocations occur at a relatively low frequency in some cases of familial clear cell RCC. These translocations typically involve the short or long arm of chromosome 3 and either chromosome 6, 2, or 8 as follows: (1) t(3;6)(q13;q25)[44] and t(3;6)(q12;q15), (2) t(2;3) (q35;q21),[45,46] (3) t(2;3) (q33;q21),[47] and (4) t(3;8) (p14;q34).[48]

The mechanism(s) linking the translocation with malignant transformation are currently under investigation. One explanation invokes loss of the derivative chromosome bearing the short arm of chromosome 3 (der3) in tumors and therefore loss of one copy of the VHL gene, while the other allele was reported mutated in several studies.[48–50] An alternative explanation predicts that the translocation disrupts genes spanning the specific area. Breaks in the chromosome 3p14 region disrupt the FHIT (fragile histidine triad) gene that encodes for an Ap3A hydrolase.[51,52] Mice with germline deletion of the FHIT gene have an increased incidence of carcinogen-induced tumors (53). The chromosome 8q24 region encompasses the gene TRC8, which is disrupted by the translocations involving this area[54] and TRC8 mutations have been detected in RCC.[54] Although the function of TRC8 is not established, its similarity with patched (PTCH) raises the possibility that it is involved in hedgehog signaling. The 2q33 area and the 3q21 area encode for the genes deleted in renal cancer 1 (DIRC1) and DIRC2, respectively. The function of these genes is currently under investigation with regards to RCC.[55,56] In summary, the various models proposed as explanations of 3p translocation-associated RCC require further experimental testing but, at a clinical level, detection of these cytogenetic abnormalities may help to evaluate an inherited predisposition to RCC.

Supernumerary Nipple Syndrome

An association between polymastia and renal carcinoma has been reported in which a Hungarian family has been described with both renal carcinoma and polymastia.[57] Although a molecular genetic analysis for this family is not yet available, it has been hypothesized that developmental abnormalities affecting the urogenital tract predispose to RCC and also cause supernumerary nipples.[58]

Familial Renal Cell Carcinoma with Papillary Histology

Papillary carcinoma comprises approximately 10% of the sporadic RCC tumors.[1] Tumors are classified as papillary when >75% of the tumor mass consists of papillary components. Histologically and clinically papillary cancers are subdivided into type 1 and type 2.[1,59] There is evidence that type 1 tumors have a better clinical prognosis than type 2 tumors and familial predispositions to either type exist. Sporadic papillary RCC are characterized by trisomy of chromosomes 7, 16, and 17 and loss of the Y chromosome.

Hereditary Papillary Renal Cell Carcinoma Type 1 (OMIM 1447000)

Clinical and Diagnostic Considerations

Family members with Hereditary Papillary Renal Cell Carcinoma Type 1 (HPRCC-1) develop multiple and bilateral papillary type 1 RCC at a much younger age than those with sporadic papillary RCC and the disease is inherited in an autosomal dominant fashion. The frequency of HPRCC type 1 is estimated at 1 in one million.[60] Linkage analysis mapped the gene responsible for HPRCC 1 to chromosome 7q31–q34[61] and later studies identified it as the c-MET protooncogene. Approximately 80% of the families presenting with the phenotype of the disease harbor germline mutations in c-MET.[61] As in sporadic papillary RCC tumors, several HPRCC type 1 tumors manifest trisomy of chromosome 7, with the duplicated chromosome 7 also harboring a mutation of the c-MET protooncogene.[62] No extrarenal clinical manifestations have been described in the HPRCC type 1 patients so far.

Functions of the c-MET Protooncogene

The c-MET protooncogene consists of 21 exons.[63] It is expressed in several adult tissues including the kidney. MET encodes for a 1390 amino acid precursor protein, which is cleaved into α and β chains. The chains are linked by a disulfide bond and form the tyrosine kinase transmembrane c-met receptor.[64] Hepatocyte growth factor/scatter factor (HGF/SF) is the ligand of the c-met receptor.[65] The intracellular part of the receptor has a catalytic domain and a C-terminal "multidocking domain." Ligand-induced dimerization activates the receptor through transphosphorylation of specific tyrosine residues of the catalytic domain.[66] This in turn leads to a second autophosphorylation step of specific tyrosine residues at the "docking" domain. The phosphorylated docking domain interacts with SH2 domain-containing proteins,[67] resulting in activation of the PI3K, Grb2/Sos/Ras, Src, and phospholipase C gamma (PLCγ) pathways. HPRC type 1-associated germline mutations map to the catalytic site of the receptor and are predicted to promote phosphory-lation of the critical tyrosines.[61] c-MET receptor activation in epithelial cells results in (1) increased proliferation, (2) increased motility, (3) increased metastatic potential, and (4) polarization and tubule formation. Activation of the Ras pathway appears necessary and sufficient for proliferation. Activation of PI3K appears responsible only for increased motility. Activation of both pathways is necessary for acqui-sition of an invasive and metastatic phenotype.[68]

Of particular interest for renal carcinogenesis is the obser-vation that c-met and VHL signaling pathways intersect via VHL-mediated regulation of HIF function. Hypoxia and loss-of-VHL-mediated activation of HIF results in upregulation and therefore promotion of the transforming potential of the c-MET receptor.[69] Stimulation of VHL$^{-/-}$ cells with HGF/SF promotes scattering and stable reintroduction of pVHL in these cells markedly decreases the effect of HGF/SF.[69]

Hereditary Leiomyomatosis with Renal Cell Carcinoma (OMIM 150800)

Clinical Considerations

Patients with Hereditary Leiomyomatosis with Renal Cell Carcinoma (HLRCC) disease develop leiomyomas of the skin and uterus (fibroids) and RCCs with the character-istic papillary type 2 histology.[70] Leiomyomas derive from the smooth muscle cells of the organs in which the tumors develop. The disease is autosomal dominant with variable expressivity and the tumors appear around the second or third decade of life. The majority of the patients will develop cutaneous leiomyomas and the overwhelming majority of the women will develop uterine fibroids at an early age. Documented cases of HLRCC without skin leiomyomas exist and this is therefore not a criterion for exclusion. Renal tumors occurring in the HLRCC do not present with the typical multifocal and bilateral pattern that is the hallmark of VHL disease. They may be single and the clinical course appears aggressive. It is therefore not recommended that these tumors be observed until they reach a certain size, as is the case in VHL patients. The frequency of RCC varies among different series, ranging from 6% to 60%.

Functions of the Gene Responsible for Hereditary Leiomyomatosis with Renal Cell Carcinoma

The gene responsible for HLRCC had been mapped by linkage analysis to chromosome 1q42.3-45[70,71] and identified as the Kreb's cycle enzyme fumarase hydratase (FH).[72] Most of the mutations identified so far are missense mutations, but small deletions, insertions, and nonsense mutations have been reported and are predicted to lead to loss-of-FH function.[73] Molecular analysis has shown that the wild-type allele is lost in the HLRCC-associated tumors, indicating that FH acts as a tumor suppressor gene. Lymphoblastoid cell lines from affected individuals had marked reduction in FH enzymatic

activity, due to the germline mutation in one allele. Tumors harboring LOH had no FH activity.

FH catalyzes the hydration of fumarate to malate. Loss of FH activity increases fumarate and, subsequently, succinate concentrations. Succinate diffuses into the cytoplasm and competes with 2-oxoglutarate for binding to EGLN, a cellular 2-oxoglutarate oxygenase that regulates hydroxylation of specific hypoxia-inducible factor (HIF) proline residues (see the previous section on the regulation of HIF in VHL disease). The result of succinate build-up in the cytoplasm is the inhibition of EGLN and subsequent stabilization of HIF.[74,75] This may provide an explanation of how loss-of-FH function results in cellular transformation. Whether HIF is critical for the maintenance of FH-related tumors remains to be determined.

HPRCC Associated with Papillary Thyroid Cancer

Families with papillary RCC and papillary thyroid carcinoma have been described.[76] The c-MET gene is not mutated in these cases. The gene responsible for the syndrome is currently unknown.

Familial Oncocytoma

Birt–Hogg–Dube Syndrome (OMIM 135150)
Clinical Manifestations

Birt, Hogg, and Dube first described an inherited dermato-logical condition characterized by multiple fibrofolliculomas, trichodiscomas, and acrochordons in individuals >25 years old.[77] Patients with Birt–Hogg–Dube (BHD) are at high risk of developing these skin lesions, renal tumors, and sponta-neous pneumothorax. Fibrofolliculomas and trichodiscomas are benign hamartomatous tumors of the skin originating from cellular elements at the base of the hair follicle.[78] Clini-cally they are almost indistinguishable and present as multiple yellowish or skin-colored papules of the face (including oral mucosa), neck, scalp, and upper trunk. Acrochordons have a "skin tag" more than "papular" appearance, but are most likely histological variants of fibrofolliculomas and trichodis-comas. Lipomas and collagenomas are less characteristic, but they have been described in BHD patients.

Members of families affected with BHD syndrome may develop multiple and bilateral renal neoplasms.[79,80] In contrast to other inherited diseases of predisposition to kidney tumor, BHD disease predisposes individuals to tumors of more than one histological type, which may coexist in the same individual. In 17 affected individuals of a Swedish pedigree, two cases of renal cancer were diagnosed: one tumor had mixed clear cell and papillary elements and the second was a chromophobe RCC.[81] Toro et al. examined 152 patients from 49 families. Two of these families had renal oncocytomas and the third had papillary carcinoma.[79]

In a recent review of a large cohort of BHD families the predominant histology of renal tumors was chromophobe RCC, followed by chromophobe/oncocytic hybrids and, less frequently, clear or papillary type.[82]

In addition to skin and renal lesions BHD patients have lung cysts and suffer from spontaneous pneumothorax.[82] Colonic polyps and the possibility of colon cancer, although initially reported as part of the syndrome, are not currently considered part of the disease.[82]

Diagnostic Considerations and the Birt–Hogg–Dube Protein

The BHD gene maps to chromosome 17p11.2 [81,83] and has been cloned.[84] The gene is composed of 13 exons and encodes a 754 amino acid protein of currently unknown function. Germline mutations are mainly nonsense mutations leading to frameshift and early protein truncation and intragenic or larger deletions. No point mutations linked to an inherited syndrome have been reported so far. Initial studies indicate that the BHD protein is a 57-kDa phosphoprotein that localizes to the nucleus and the cytoplasm and has no motif indicating its function (our observation).

Familial Renal Oncocytoma

Sporadic and familial oncocytomas of the kidney are mostly nonmetastatic benign tumors. Microscopically, they consist of foci of epithelial cells with densely eosinophilic cytoplasm. Electron microscopy studies show a characteristic abundance of mitochondria that "fill" the cytoplasm.[1] A clear report of familiar predisposition to oncocytoma was provided by Weinrich et al. who described five nuclear families with multiple members affected with renal oncocytomas.[85] On subsequent clinical reevaluation they noted that three of these five families manifested skin lesions compatible with BHD syndrome (see above). It is therefore likely that several of the previously reported familial renal oncocytomas represent cases of BHD syndrome, although non-BHD-associated renal oncocytoma may exist. Cytogenetic analysis of sporadic tumors classifies oncocytomas as those characterized by either loss of chromosome 1p or those harboring one of the reported somatic reciprocal translocations: t(9;11) involving 11q13, t(9;11)(p23;q23), t(5;11)(q35;13), or t(1;12)(p36;q13).[86]

Evaluation for Inherited Renal Cancer

Patients are usually referred to genetic counseling and testing because of a positive family history for RCC, multifocal RCC, the occurrence of the disease in young age, and/or the presence of extrarenal lesions associated with a specific inheritable form of kidney cancer. Any of these reasons, if appropriately evaluated and documented, may justify genetic testing.

Family History

In general, the documented occurrence of kidney cancer in two or more members of the family at least in two successive generations raises the possibility of an inherited form of RCC. Interpretation of the family history is dependent upon documentation of the following: (1) pathology reports confirming tumor histology, (2) age of onset of the tumor in the index case and the family members, (3) bilateral disease in family members, (4) multiple primaries in family members, (5) multiple members of family affected, (6) occurrence of the disease in more than one generation, (7) extrarenal pathology, and (8) potential environmental exposure.

Documentation of a four-generation family medical history provides an invaluable tool for the evaluation of inherited disease. The family history can be documented in the form of a pedigree, which is a representation of the family medical history and biological relationships using standardized symbols.[87] The advantages of such a method include efficiency in documentation, visual aid for diagnosis and evaluation of mode of inheritance, evaluating testing strategies and identifying at-risk family members, and serving as a visual aid in explaining basic genetics concepts to the patient.

Although this is a typical presentation, the absence of family history does not rule out the possibility of inheritable kidney cancer. Several factors may explain a noncontributory family history despite the presence of a genetic predisposition. For example, a patient may harbor a *de novo* mutation, which is a mutation that occurred spontaneously during gametogenesis in one of the parents. Alternatively, one of the parents may harbor germline mosaicism. In this case, the precursor cells of the gametes are composed of two (or more) different cell lines: one with the wild-type allele and the other with the mutant allele. It is often difficult to distinguish between *de novo* mutation and germline mosaicism given that in both instances the patient will harbor a constitutive mutation and both parents will often test negative for the mutation in the peripheral blood cells.

For many genetic conditions, reduced penetrance and variable expressivity are possible contributors to a negative family history. This can be confirmed only in cases in which a pathogenic mutation is identified in the index patient and other at-risk family members are present for genetic testing. In examples of reduced penetrance and variable expressivity, a parent will test positive for the mutation but does not demonstrate clinically apparent symptoms of the disease. It is important to note that penetrance is an "all-or-nothing" concept. A condition is said to have reduced penetrance when some individuals carrying a mutation do not express any features of the expected phenotype. With variable expressivity it is the degree of clinical severity that differs within a family. Finally, it is appropriate to give thoughtful consideration of nonpaternity or adoption as additional possibilities. Thus, while the family history may not assist in making a genetic diagnosis, it does not rule out a hereditary cause.

Multifocal Disease

The typical presentation consists of multifocal synchronous or metachronous tumor foci. This is not necessary, though, and the metachronous presentation can be evaluated only in retrospect. Patients treated for localized, sporadic (noninheritable) RCC are at risk for either distant metastasis or local recurrence. They also run a definite risk of developing a second primary tumor in the contralateral kidney over at least a period of 10 years (metachronous lesion). Inherited forms presenting metachronously have a shorter interval between the first and second lesion than the sporadic form.

Extrarenal Lesions and Corresponding Symptoms

Typically, extrarenal lesions are present in the referred patient (Table 7b-3). It is possible, though, that they manifest only in other family members affected by the disease. Their presence therefore has to be considered in the context of the whole family and uncovered through a careful family history and reference to medical documentation.

For VHL patients these lesions include hemangioblastomas of the CNS, including the retina, pheochromocytomas, pancreatic lesions (cysts, neuroendocrine tumors, papillary cystadenoma), adnexal and epididymal cysts or papillary cystadenomas, and extralymphatic sac tumors of the middle ear. Symptoms corresponding to these lesions may provide clues regarding the presence of an inherited form.

It is worth emphasizing that the availability of genetic testing expanded our appreciation of the diverse phenotypic combinations of the disease as well as the fact that the disease may have very mild clinical manifestations.

Patients with HPRC type 2 provide a personal or family history of skin and/or uterine leiomyomas. In contrast, HPRCC type 1 is currently thought to be restricted to the kidneys exclusively.

Patients with BHD disease may have the characteristic folliculomatous lesions and/or a personal and family history of spontaneous pneumothorax.

Genetic Counseling Process

Genetic counseling is a communication process through which the genetics professional provides information and psychosocial support to individuals/families with an established or suspected diagnosis of a hereditary condition. The overall goal is to empower the individual/family with the necessary knowledge to make informed choices. The following is an overview of the essential components of the genetics consult in the setting of the hereditary renal carcinoma clinic and is not intended to be a comprehensive tutorial.

Family History

A complete and accurate multigenerational family medical history (as detailed above) is essential to the visit.

TABLE 7b-3. Molecular genetics of kidney cancer.[a]

Inherited renal cancer	Gene	Renal lesion	CNS	Skin	Other features
von Hippel–Lindau	VHL	Clear cell	Hemangioblastoma		Pheochromocytoma, papillary cystadenoma, pancreatic and renal cysts, islet cell tumor
Tuberous sclerosis complex	TSC1, TSC2	Angiomyolipoma, clear cell, cysts	Cortical tuber, calcified subependymal nodule, subependymal giant cell astrocytoma, retinal hamartoma	Hypomelanotic macule, shagreen patch, and facial angiofibroma	Cardiac rhabdomyoma, micronodular hyperplasia, lung tumor
Familial clear cell RCC	Constitutional translocation 3p	Clear cell			
Hereditary papillary RCC type 1	c-MET	Papillary type 1			
Hereditary leiomyomatosis with RCC	FH	Papillary type 2		Cutaneous leiomyoma	Uterine leiomyoma
HPRCC with PTC	Unknown	Papillary			Papillary thyroid carcinoma
Birt–Hogg–Dube	BHD	Chromophobe, oncocytoma, papillary, clear, or a mixed histology		Fibrofolliculoma, trichodiscoma, acrochordon, lipoma, collagenoma	Spontaneous pneumothorax, lung cysts

[a]CNS, central nervous system; VHL, von Hippel–Lindau; RCC, renal cell carcinoma; PTC, papillary thyroid carcinoma.

Risk Assessment

This includes making the differential diagnosis and evaluation of the family history for mode of inheritance. The individual with a personal history of RCC is the most informative person to whom genetic testing should be offered first. In most cases this is the index patient; however, in our experience some individuals present to the clinic with a family history of RCC alone and they themselves do not have a cancer diagnosis. A negative genetic test result is inconclusive and uninformative for an unaffected individual unless a family member who is at higher probability of having the disease is tested first and a mutation is identified.

Risk Communication and Basic Cancer Genetics Concepts

Each individual interprets and understands risk numbers and figures differently according to a variety of factors such as their age, ethnocultural background, occupation, and education level. By initially seeking out what information the patient hopes to gain from the consultation, the health care practitioner can use these goals to guide the consult. From the patient education standpoint, the pedigree is a useful tool for demonstrating concepts such as autosomal dominant inheritance and variable expressivity and for showing which family members are at risk. Additionally, genetics professionals often use visual aids and drawings to describe a "gene" and explain the differences and similarities between tumorigenesis in sporadic and inherited cases (i.e., Knudson's two-hit hypothesis).

Risks, Benefits, and Limitations of Genetic Testing

The individual being offered genetic testing must understand the risks, benefits, and limitations of genetic testing in order to make an informed choice to pursue or decline testing. The primary risk is that of genetic discrimination, defined for these purposes as the use of genetic information to deny insurance coverage or employment. In the area of health insurance discrimination, the opportunity for group health insurers to deny coverage or change rates and coverage based on genetic information is greatly limited, due to existing federal and state antidiscrimination legislation (an updated report on the status of federal and state genetic nondiscrimination legislation can be found at www.genome.gov/PolicyEthics/). Few states have legislation limiting life or long-term care insurance discrimination, therefore patients need to be aware of this prior to genetic testing. This is of particular concern for presymptomatic family members of a mutation carrier, and the option of obtaining a policy prior to testing should be raised.

The benefits of genetic testing from the patient and family perspective include confirmation of a clinical diagnosis and the ability to offer screening to at-risk family members. A negative test result may provide patients with some relief that their renal cancer was unlikely to be part of a known hereditary syndrome. When a familial mutation is identified, a negative result in a relative puts the individual at a general population risk for RCC.

The current landscape of genetic testing provides limited power in predicting disease phenotype in that there is a paucity of data on genotype/phenotype correlations. Furthermore, an identified germline mutation does not predict when a patient may develop a tumor, if at all. A negative genetic test result in an affected individual carries limitations as well. A negative result (when no one in the family has previously tested positive) can be explained by one of three reasons: (1) the individual does not have the condition in question, (2) the individual has the condition based on clinical diagnostic criteria but represents a somatic mosaic,[1] or (3) the individual and the individual's family demonstrate familial clustering of RCC but the causative gene has not yet been elucidated.

Psychosocial Assessment and Support

The genetic counseling interview process brings up a multitude of issues for the patient that extend beyond the disease alone. The patient brings to the interview his or her sense of self as an individual, as a member of a family, as a parent, as a spouse, and as a member of society. Risk perception is influenced by personal experience and cultural, ethnic, and religious background. A lack of awareness of these factors poses a barrier to effective risk communication on the part of the healthcare practitioner. The techniques employed in psychosocial genetic counseling are beyond the scope of this chapter.[88,89] However, the reader is encouraged to keep in mind that each patient possesses different emotional reactions to cancer risk and different coping strategies. Each patient is endowed with different emotional resources for dealing with new information, whether it is a new cancer diagnosis, genetic test result, or the concept of inherited predisposition. Asking a patient "how are you coping with [your diagnosis or this information]?" can often be revealing. The patient's reply may simply indicate that a misunderstanding of the information has taken place, or that additional mental health or social support may be indicated. Probing into the patients' current health behavior practices and beliefs about their cancer risk permits insight into the potential impact the information may have on their health behavior. By integrating social work, psychiatry, or psychology specialties to the multidisciplinary health care team, the genetic counselor and physician can provide patients and their families with a myriad of resources to which they can turn for support or information.

Preconception Genetic Counseling

Prospective parents planning or carrying a pregnancy at risk for an inherited RCC condition such as VHL or TSC face different options for learning the carrier status of the fetus. The couple may choose not to know until after the child is born. Alternatively, a couple may choose prenatal diagnosis, utilizing a sample obtained by amniocentesis or chorionic villus sampling. Some couples who choose prenatal diagnosis wish to know the carrier status prior to birth in order to prepare, while others may elect to terminate a pregnancy if the fetus is affected.

Prospective parents should also be provided with information about reproductive technologies that greatly lower their risk of having a child with an inherited cancer predisposition syndrome, such as sperm or oocyte donation (depending on which parent is affected) and preimplantation genetic diagnosis. Preimplantation genetic diagnosis (PGD) involves testing embryos fertilized *in vitro* for the familial VHL mutation, usually on a single cell of a blastocyst, and selecting unaffected embryos for implantation. PGD has been performed for highly penetrant conditions with early age of onset such as VHL, familial adenomatous polyposis coli (FAP), and Li-Fraumeni syndrome (LFS).[90,91] The various reproductive options available to prospective parents require thoughtful discussion and genetic counseling. In our clinical experience, few couples elect to have prenatal testing or assisted reproductive technology for inherited cancer predisposition due to factors such as cost or based on their personal ethical beliefs. Furthermore, in our experience, couples who have effective coping skills and well-managed disease tend to decline preconception testing services; the reasons for this observation remain to be studied.

Conclusions

Patients suspected of being genetically predisposed to RCC should be referred to specialized centers for genetic counseling and evaluation. A negative family history does not preclude germline mutations predisposing to the disease. Detection of germline mutations in such patients will allow surveillance for RCC and extrarenal tumors as well as evaluation of their siblings. Their cancers bear molecular hallmarks that in the near future result in therapies targeted to the specific genetic events leading to carcinogenesis. For example, loss-of-VHL function leads to constitutive activation of HIF and its downstream targets vascular endothelial growth factor (VEGF), platelet-derived growth factor (PDGF), and transforming growth factor-α (TGF-α) and its receptor epidermal growth factor receptor (EGFR). Pleiotropic small molecule inhibitors of these receptors are under development and they may provide specific and potent avenues for treatment and/or prevention of tumors in these high-risk individuals. Similarly, c-met inhibitors are being developed and it is conceivable that they will be used in the treatment and/or prevention of HPRCC type 1.

Lastly, the individual genetic background in which these germline mutations are embedded may play a significant role in the expressivity and penetrance of the disease. Genome-wide profiling of the genetic background is becoming feasible and may lead to identification of genetic modifiers/cofactors with an important role in the natural history of the disease.

References

1. Reuter, V. E. and Presti, J. C. Contemporary approach to the classification of renal epithelial tumors, Semin Oncol 27: 124–137, 2000.
2. Melmon, K. and Rosen, S. Lindau's disease, Am J Med. 36: 595–617, 1964.
3. Latif, F., Tory, K., Gnarra, J., Yao, M., Duh, F.-M., Orcutt, M. L., Stackhouse, T., Kuzmin, I., Modi, W., Geil, L., Schmidt, L., Zhou, F., Li, H., Wei, M. H., Chen, F., Glenn, G., Choyke, P., Walther, M. M., Weng, Y., Duan, D.-S. R., Dean, M., Glavac, D., Richards, F. M., Crossey, P. A., Ferguson-Smith, M. A., Pasiler, D. L., Chumakov, I., Cohen, D., Chinault, A. C., Maher, E. R., Linehan, W. M., Zbar, B., and Lerman, M. I. Identification of the von Hippel-Lindau disease tumor suppressor gene, Science. 260: 1317–1320, 1993.
4. Chen, F., Kishida, T., Yao, M., Hustad, T., Glavac, D., Dean, M., Gnarra, J. R., Orcutt, M. L., Duh, F. M., Glenn, G., Green, J., Hsia, Y. E., Lamiell, J., Ming, H. W., Schmidt, L., Kalman, T., Kuzmin, I., Stackhouse, T., Latif, F., Linehan, W. M., Lerman, M., and Zbar, B. Germline mutations in the von Hippel-Lindau disease tumor suppressor gene: correlations with phenotype, Hum Mutat 5: 66–75, 1995.
5. Crossey, P. A., Richards, F. M., Foster, K., Green, J. S., Prowse, A., Latif, F., Lerman, M. I., Zbar, B., Affara, N. A., Ferguson-Smith, M. A., and Maher, E. R. Identification of intragenic mutations in the von Hippel-Lindau disease tumor suppressor gene and correlation with disease phenotype, Hum Mol Gen 3: 1303–1308, 1994.
6. Maher, E., Webster, A., Richards, F., Green, J., Crossey, P., Payne, S., and Moore, A. Phenotypic expression in von Hippel-Lindau disease: correlations with germline VHL gene mutations, J Med Genet 33: 328–332, 1996.
7. Stolle, C., Glenn, G., Zbar, B., Humphrey, J., Choyke, P., Walther, M., Pack, S., Hurley, K., Andrey, C., Klausner, R., and Linehan, W. Improved detection of germline mutations in the von Hippel-Lindau disease tumor suppressor gene., Hum Mutat 12: 417–423, 1998.
8. European Consortium on Tuberous Sclerosis: Identification and characterization of the tuberous sclerosis gene on chromosome 16, Cell. 75: 1305–1315, 1993.
9. van Slegtenhorst, E. A. Identification of the tuberous sclerosis gene TSC1 on chromosome 9q34, Science. 277: 805–808, 1997.
10. Niida, Y., Lawrence-Smith, N., Banwell, A., Hammer, E., Lewis, J., Beauchamp, R. L., Sims, K., Ramesh, V., and Ozelius, L. Analysis of both TSC1 and TSC2 for germline mutations in 126 unrelated patients with tuberous sclerosis, Hum Mutat. 14: 412–422, 1999.

11. Roach, E. S., Gomez, M. R., and Northurp, H. Tuberous sclerosis complex consensus conference: revised clinical diagnostic criteria, J Child Neurol. 13: 624–628, 1988.

12. Roach, E. S., DiMario, F. J., and Northurp, H. Tuberous Sclerosis Consensus Conference: recommendations for diagnostic evaluation, J Child Neurol. 14: 401–407, 1998.

13. Zimmer-Galler, I. E. and Robertson, D. M. Long-term observation of retinal lesions in tuberous sclerosis, Am J Ophthalmol. 119: 318–324, 1995.

14. Ewalt, D. H., Sheffield, E., Sparagana, S. P., Delgado, M. R., and Roach, E. S. Renal lesion growth in children with tuberous sclerosis complex, J Urol. 160(1): 141–145, 1998.

15. Al-Saleem, T., Wessner, L. L., Scheithauer, B. W., Patterson, K., Roach, E. S., Dreyer, S. J., Fujikawa, K., Bjornsson, J., Bernstein, J., and Henske, E. P. Malignant tumors of the kidney, brain, and soft tissues in children and young adults with the tuberous sclerosis complex, Cancer. 83: 2208–2216, 1998.

16. Martignoni, G., Bonetti, F., Pea, M., Tardanico, R., Brunelli, M., and Eble, J. N. Renal disease in adults with TSC2/PKD1 contiguous gene syndrome, Am J Surg Pathol. 26: 198–205, 2002.

17. Siegel, D. H. and Howard, R. Molecular advances in genetic skin diseases, Curr Opin Pediatr. 14: 419–425, 2002.

18. Pacheco-Rodriguez, G., Kristof, A. S., Stevens, L. A., Zhang, Y., Crooks, D., and Moss, J. Giles F. Filley Lecture: Genetics and gene expression in lymphangioleiomyomatosis, Chest. 121: 56S–60S, 2002.

19. Yeung, R. S., Xiao, G.-H., Jin, F., Lee, W.-C., Testa, J. R., and Knudson, A. G. Predisposition to renal carcinoma in the Eker rat is determined by germ-line mutation of the tuberous sclerosis 2 (TSC2) gene, Proc Natl Acad Sci USA. 91: 11413–11416, 1994.

20. Rennebeck, G., Kleymenova, E. V., Anderson, R., Yeung, R. S., Artzt, K., and Walker, C. L. Loss of function of the tuberous sclerosis 2 tumor suppressor gene results in embryonic lethality characterized by disrupted neuroepithelial growth and development, Proc Natl Acad Sci USA. 95: 15629–15634, 1998.

21. Ito, N. and Rubin, G. M. Gigas, a Drosophila homolog of tuberous sclerosis gene product-2, regulates the cell cycle, Cell. 96: 529–539, 1999.

22. Tapon, N., Ito, N., Dickson, B. J., Treisman, J. E., and Hariharan, I. K. The Drosophila tuberous sclerosis complex gene homologs restrict cell growth and cell proliferation, Cell. 105: 345–355, 2001.

23. MacCollin, M. and Kwiatkowski, D. Molecular genetic aspects of the phakomatoses: tuberous sclerosis complex and neurofibromatosis 1, Curr Opin Neurol. 14: 163–169, 2001.

24. Kwiatkowska, J., Wigowska-Sowinska, J., Napierala, D., Slomski, R., and Kwiatkowski, D. J. Mosaicism in tuberous sclerosis as a potential cause of the failure of molecular diagnosis, N Engl J Med. 340: 703–707, 1999.

25. Rose, V. M., Au, K. S., Pollom, G., Roach, E. S., Prashner, H. R., and Northrup, H. Germ-line mosaicism in tuberous sclerosis: how common? Am J Hum Genet. 64: 986–992, 1999.

26. Brook-Carter, P. T., Peral, B., Ward, C., et al. Deletion of the TSC2 and PKD1 gene associated with severe infantile polycystic kidney disease—-A contiguous gene syndrome, Nat Genet. 8: 328–332, 1994.

27. Dabora, S. L., Jozwiak, S., Franz, D. N., Roberts, P. S., Nieto, A., Chung, J., Choy, Y. S., Reeve, M. P., Thiele, E., Egelhoff, J. C., Kasprzyk-Obara, J., Domanska-Pakiela, D., and Kwiatkowski, D. J. Mutational analysis in a cohort of 224 tuberous sclerosis patients indicates increased severity of TSC2, compared with TSC1, disease in multiple organs, Am J Hum Genet. 68: 64–80, 2001.

28. Langkau, N., Martin, N., Brandt, R., Zugge, K., Quast, S., Wiegele, G., Jauch, A., Rehm, M., Kuhl, A., Mack-Vette, r. M., Zimmerhackl, B., and Janssen, B. TSC1 and TSC2 mutations in tuberous sclerosis, the associated phenotypes and a model to explain observed TSC1/ TSC2 frequency ratios, Eur J Pediatr. 161: 393–402, 2002.

29. Van Slegtenhorst, M., Nellist, M., Nagelkerken, B., Cheadle, J., Snell, R., van den Ouweland, A., Reuser, A., Sampson, J. P., Halley, D., and Sluijs, P. Interaction between hamartin and tuberin, TSC1 and TSC2 gene products, Hum Mol Genet. 7: 1053–1057, 1998.

30. Kobayashi, T., Minowa, O., Kuno, J., Mitani, H., Hino, O., and Noda, T. Renal carcinogenesis, hepatic hemangiomatosis, and embryonic lethality caused by a germ-line Tsc2 mutation in mice, Cancer Res. 59: 1206–1211, 1999.

31. Onda, H., Lueck, A., Marks, P. W., Warren, H. B., and Kwiatkowski, D. J. Tsc2(+/-) mice develop tumors in multiple sites that express gelsolin and are influenced by genetic background, J Clin Invest. 104: 687–695, 1999.

32. Kobayashi, T., Minowa, O., Sugitani, Y., Takai, S., Mitani, H., Kobayashi, E., Noda, T., and Hino, O. A germ-line Tsc1 mutation causes tumor development and embryonic lethality that are similar, but not identical to, those caused by Tsc2 mutation in mice, Proc Natl Acad Sci USA. 98: 8762–8767, 2001.

33. Green, A. J., Smith, M., and Yates, J. R. W. Loss of heterozygosity on chromosome 16p13.3 in hamartomas from tuberous sclerosis patients, Nat Genet. 6: 192–196, 1994.

34. Sepp, T., Yates, J. R., and Green, A. J. Loss of heterozygosity in tuberous sclerosis hamartomas, J Med Genet. 33: 962–964, 1996.

35. Henske, E. P., Neumann, H. P., Scheithauer, B. W., Herbst, E. W., Short, M. P., and Kwiatkowski, D. J. Loss of heterozygosity in the tuberous sclerosis (TSC2) region of chromosome band 16p13 occurs in sporadic as well as TSC-associated renal angiomyolipomas, Gene Chromosomes Cancer. 13: 295–298, 1995.

36. Carsillo, T., Astrinidis, A., and Henske, E. P. Mutations in the tuberous sclerosis complex gene TSC2 are a cause of sporadic pulmonary lymphangioleiomyomatosis, Proc Natl Acad Sci USA. 97: 6085–6090, 2000.

37. Henske, E. P., Neumann, H. P., Scheithauer, B. W., Herbst, E. W., Short, M. P., and Kwiatkowski, D. J. Loss of heterozygosity in the tuberous sclerosis (TSC2) region of chromosome band 16p13 occurs in sporadic as well as TSC-associated renal angiomyolipomas, Genes Chromosomes Cancer. 13: 295–298, 1995.

38. Jin, F., Wienecke, R., Xiao, G. H., Maize, J. C., DeClue, J. E., and Yeung, R. S. Suppression of tumorigenicity by the wild-type tuberous sclerosis 2 (Tsc2) gene and its C-terminal region., Proc Natl Acad Sci USA. 93: 9154–9159, 1996.

39. Potter, C. J., Pedraza, L. G., and Xu, T. Akt regulates growth by directly phosphorylating Tsc2, Nat Cell Biol. 4: 658–665, 2002.

40. Gao, X., Zhang, Y., Arrazola, P., Hino, O., Kobayashi, T., Yeung, R. S., Ru, B., and Pan, D. Tsc tumour suppressor proteins antagonize amino-acid-TOR signalling, Nat Cell Biol. 4: 699–704, 2002.

41. Inoki, K., Li, Y., Zhu, T., Wu, J., and Guan, K. L. TSC2 is phosphorylated and inhibited by Akt and suppresses mTOR signalling, Nat Cell Biol. 4: 648–657, 2002.

42. Manning, B. D., Tee, A. R., Logsdon, M. N., Blenis, J., and Cantley, L. C. Identification of the tuberous sclerosis complex-2 tumor suppressor gene product tuberin as a target of the phosphoinositide 3-kinase/akt pathway, Mol Cell. 10: 151–162, 2002.

43. Hay, N. The Akt-mTOR tango and its relevance to cancer, Cancer Cell. 8: 179–183, 2005.

44. Kovacs, G., Brusa, P., and De Riese, W. Tissue-specific expression of a constitutional 3;6 translocation: development of multiple bilateral renal-cell carcinomas, Int J Cancer. 43: 422–427, 1989.

45. Bodmer, D., Eleveld, M. J., Ligtenberg. M. J., Weterman, M. A., Janssen, B. A., Smeets, D. F., de Wit, P. E., van den Berg, A., van den Berg, E., Koolen, M. I., and Geurts van Kessel, A. An alternative route for multistep tumorigenesis in a novel case of hereditary renal cell cancer and a t(2;3)(q35;q21) chromosome translocation, Am J Hum Genet. 62(6): 1475–1483, 1998.

46. Bodmer, D., Eleveld, M., Ligtenberg, M., Weterman, M., van der Meijden, A., Koolen, M., Hulsbergen-van der Kaa, C., Smits A, S. D., and Geurts van Kessel, A. Cytogenetic and molecular analysis of early stage renal cell carcinomas in a family with a translocation (2;3)(q35;q21), Cancer Genet Cytogenet. 134: 6–12, 2002.

47. Podolski, J., Byrski, T., Zajaczek, S., Druck, T., Zimonjic, D. B., Popescu, N. C., Kata, G., Borowka, A., Gronwald, J., Lubinski, J., and Huebne, R. K. Characterization of a familial RCC-associated t(2;3)(q33;q21) chromosome translocation, J Hum Genet. 46: 685–693, 2001.

48. Li, F. P., Decker, H. J., Zbar, B., Stanton, V. P., Kovacs, G., Seizinger, B. R., Aburatani, H., Sandberg, A. A., Berg, S., Hosoe, S., et al. Clinical and genetic studies of renal cell carcinomas in a family with a constitutional chromosome 3;8 translocation, Ann Intern Med. 118: 106–111, 1993.

49. Schmidt, L., Li, F., Brown, R. S., Berg, S., Chen, F., Wei, M. H., Tory, K., Lerman, M. I., and Zbar, B. Mechanism of tumorigenesis of renal carcinomas associated with the constitutional chromosome 3;8 translocation, Cancer J Sci Am. 1: 191, 1995.

50. Eleveld, M. J., Bodmer, D., Merkx, G., Siepman, A., Sprenger, S. H., Weterman, M. A., Ligtenberg, M. J., Kamp, J., Stapper, W., Jeuken, J. W., Smeets, D., Smits, A., and Geurts Van Kessel, A. Molecular analysis of a familial case of renal cell cancer and a t(3;6)(q12;q15), Genes Chromosomes Cancer. 31: 23–32, 2001.

51. Ohta, M., Inoue, H., Cotticelli, M. G., Kastury, K., Baffa, R., Palazzo, J., Siprashvili, Z., Mori, M., McCue, P., Druck T, et al. The FHIT gene, spanning the chromosome 3p14.2 fragile site and renal carcinoma-associated t(3;8) breakpoint, is abnormal in digestive tract cancers, Cell. 84: 587–597, 1996.

52. Siprashvili, Z., Sozzi, G., Barnes, L. D., McCue, P., Robinson, A. K., Eryomin, V., Sard, L., Tagliabue, E., Greco, A., Fusetti, L., Schwartz, G., Pierotti, M. A., Croce, C. M., and Huebner, K. Replacement of Fhit in cancer

cells suppresses tumorigenicity, Proc Natl Acad Sci USA. 94: 13771–13776, 1997.

53. Fong, L. Y., Fidanza, V., Zanesi, N., Lock, L. F., Siracusa, L. D., Mancini, R., Siprashvili, Z., Ottey, M., Martin, S. E., Druck, T., McCue, P., Croce, C. M., and Huebner, K. Muir-Torre-like syndrome in Fhit-deficient mice, Proc Natl Acad Sci USA. 97: 4742–4747, 2000.

54. Gemmill, R. M., West, J. D., Boldog, F., Tanaka, N., Robinson, L. J., Smith, D. I., Li, F., and Drabkin, H. A. The hereditary renal cell carcinoma 3;8 translocation fuses FHIT to a patched-related gene, TRC8, Proc Natl Acad Sci USA. 95: 9572–9577, 1998.

55. Druck, T., Podolski, J., Byrski, T., Wyrwicz, L., Zajaczek, S., Kata, G., Borowka, A., Lubinski, J., and Huebner, K. The DIRC1 gene at chromosome 2q33 spans a familial RCC-associated t(2;3)(q33;q21) chromosome translocation, J Hum Genet. 46: 583–589, 2001.

56. Bodmer, D., Eleveld, M., Kater-Baats, E., Janssen, I., Janssen, B., Weterman, M., Schoenmaker, E., Nickerson, M., Linehan, M., Zbar, B., and van Kessel, A. G. Disruption of a novel MFS transporter gene, DIRC2, by a familial renal cell carcinoma-associated t(2;3)(q35;q21), Hum Mol Genet. 11(6): 641–649, 2002.

57. Goedert, J. J., McKeen, E. A., and Fraumeni, J. F. Polymastia and renal adenocarcinoma, Ann Intern Med. 95: 182–184, 1981.

58. Mehes, K. Familial association of supernumerary nipple with renal cancer, Cancer Genet Cytogenet. 86: 129–130, 1996.

59. Zbar, B. and Lerman, M. Inherited carcinomas of the kidney, Adv Cancer Res. 75: 163–201, 1998.

60. Zbar, B. Inherited epithelial tumors of the kidney: old and new disease, Semin Cancer Biol. 10: 313–318, 2000.

61. Schmidt, L., Duh, F. M., Chen, F., Kishida, T., Glenn, G., Choyke, P., Scherer, S. W., Zhuang, Z., Lubensky, I., Dean, M., Allikmets, R., Chidambaram, A., Bergerheim, U. R., Feltis, J. T., Casadevall, C., Zamarron, A., Bernues, M., Richard, S., Lips, C. J., Walther, M. M., Tsui, L. C., Geil, L., Orcutt, M. L., Stackhouse, T., and Zbar, B. Germline and somatic mutations in the tyrosine kinase domain of the MET proto-oncogene in papillary renal carcinomas, Nat Genet. 16: 68–73, 1997.

62. Zhuang, Z., Park, W. S., Pack, S., Schmidt, L., Vortmeyer, A. O., Pak, E., Pham, T., Weil, R. J., Candidus, S., Lubensky, I. A., Linehan, W. M., Zbar, B., and Weirich, G. Trisomy 7-harbouring non-random duplication of the mutant MET allele in hereditary papillary renal carcinomas, Nat Genet. 20(1): 66–69, 1998.

63. Duh, F. M., Scherer, S. W., Tsui, L. C., Lerman, M. I., Zbar, B., and Schmidt, L. Gene structure of the human MET proto-oncogene, Oncogene. 15: 1583–1586, 1997.

64. Bardelli, A., Ponzetto, C., and Comoglio, P. M. Identification of functional domains in the hepatocyte growth factor and its receptor by molecular engineering, J Biotechnol. 37: 109–122, 1994.

65. Bottaro, D. P., Rubin, J. S., Faletto, D. L., Chan, A. M., Kmiecik, T. E., Vande Woude, G. F., and Aaronson, S. A. Identification of the hepatocyte growth factor receptor as the c-met proto-oncogene product, Science. 251: 802–804, 1991.

66. Ponzetto, C., Bardelli, A., Zhen, Z., Maina, F., dalla Zonca, P., Giordano, S., Graziani, A., Panayotou, G., and Comoglio, P. M. A multifunctional docking site mediates signaling and

transformation by the hepatocyte growth factor/scatter factor receptor family, Cell. 77: 261–271, 1994.

67. Naldini, L., Vigna, E., Ferracini, R., Longati, P., Gandino, L., Prat, M., and Comoglio, P. M. The tyrosine kinase encoded by the MET proto-oncogene is activated by autophosphorylation, Mol Cell Biol. 4: 1793–1803, 1991.

68. Giordano, S., Zhen, Z., Medico, E., Gaudino, G., Galimi, F., and Comoglio, P. M. Transfer of mitogenic and invasive response to scatter factor/hepatocyte growth factor by transfection of human MET protooncogene, Proc Natl Acad Sci USA. 90: 649–653, 1993.

69. Koochekpour, S., Jeffers, M., Wang, P. H., Gong, C., Taylor, G. A., Roessler, L. M., Stearman, R., Vasselli, J. R., Stetler-Stevenson, W. G., Kaelin, W. G., Linehan, W. M., Klausner, R. D., Gnarra, J. R., and Vande Woude, G. F. The von Hippel-Lindau tumor suppressor gene inhibits hepatocyte growth factor/scatter factor-induced invasion and branching morphogenesis in renal carcinoma cells, Mol Cell Biol. 19: 5902–5912, 1999.

70. Launonen, V., Vierimaa, O., Kiuru, M., Isola, J., Roth, S., Pukkala, E., Sistonen, P., Herva, R., and Aaltonen, L. A. Inherited susceptibility to uterine leiomyomas and renal cell cancer, Proc Natl Acad Sci USA. 98: 3387–3392, 2001.

71. Alam, N. A., Bevan, S., Churchman, M., et al. Localization of a gene (MCUL1) for multiple cutaneous leiomyomata and uterine fibroids to chromosome 1q42.3-q43, Am J Hum Genet. 68: 1264–1269, 2001.

72. Consortium, T. M. L. Germline mutations in FH predispose to dominantly inherited uterine fibroids, skin leiomyomata and papillary renal cell cancer, Nat Genet. 30: 306–310, 2002.

73. Alam, N. A., Olpin, S., and Leigh, I. M. Fumarate hydratase mutations and predisposition to cutaneous leiomyomas, uterine leiomyomas and renal cancer, Br J Dermatol. 153(1): 11–17, 2005.

74. Isaacs, J. S., Jung, Y. J., Mole, D. R., Lee, S., Torres-Cabala, C., Chung, Y. L., Merino, M., Trepel, J., Zbar, B., Toro, J., Ratcliffe, P. J., Linehan, W. M., and Neckers, L. HIF overexpression correlates with biallelic loss of fumarate hydratase in renal cancer: novel role of fumarate in regulation of HIF stability, Cancer Cell. 8: 143–153, 2005.

75. Selak, M. A., Armour, S. M., MacKenzie, E. D., Boulahbel, H., Watson, D. G., Mansfield, K. D., Pan, Y., Simon, M. C., Thompson, C., and Gottlieb, E. Succinate links TCA cycle dysfunction to oncogenesis by inhibiting HIF-alpha prolyl hydroxylase, Cancer Cell. 7: 77–85, 2005.

76. Malchoff, C. D., Sarfarazi, M., Tendler, B., Forouhar, F., Whalen, G., Joshi, V., Arnold, A., and Malchoff, D. M. Papillary thyroid carcinoma associated with papillary renal neoplasia: genetic linkage analysis of a distinct heritable tumor syndrome, J Clin Endocrinol Metab. 85: 1758–1764, 2000.

77. Birt, A. R., Hogg, G. R., and Dube, W. J. Hereditary multiple fibrofolliculomas with trichodiscomas and acrochordons, Arch Dermatol. 113: 1674–1677, 1977.

78. Scalvenzi, M., Argenziano, G., Sammarco, E., and Delfino, M. Hereditary multiple fibrofolliculomas, trichodiscomas and acrochordons: syndrome of Birt-Hogg-Dube, J Eur Acad Dermatol Venereol. 11: 45–47, 1998.

79. Toro, J. R., Glenn, G., Duray, P., Darling, T., Weirich, G., Zbar, B., Linehan, M., and Turner, M. L. Birt-Hogg-Dube syndrome: a novel marker of kidney neoplasia, Arch Dermatol. 135: 1195–1202, 1999.

80. Roth, J. S., Rabinowitz, A. D., Benson, M., and Grossman, M. E. Bilateral renal cell carcinoma in the Birt-Hogg-Dube syndrome, J Am Acad Dermatol. 29: 1055–1056, 1993.

81. Khoo, S. K., Bradley, M., Wong, F. K., Hedblad, M. A., Nordenskjold, M., and Teh, B. T. Birt-Hogg-Dube syndrome: mapping of a novel hereditary neoplasia gene to chromosome 17p12-q11.2, Oncogene. 20: 5239–5242, 2001.

82. Zbar, B., Alvord, W. G., Glenn, G., Turner, M., Pavlovich, C. P., Schmidt, L., Walther, M., Choyke, P., Weirich, G., Hewitt, S. M., Duray, P., Gabril, F., Greenberg, C., Merino, M. J., Toro, J., and Linehan, W. M. Risk of renal and colonic neoplasms and spontaneous pneumothorax in the Birt-Hogg-Dube syndrome, Cancer Epidemiol Biomarkers Prev. 11: 393–400, 2002.

83. Schmidt, L. S., Warren, M. B., Nickerson, M. L., Weirich, G., Matrosova, V., Toro, J. R., Turner, M. L., Duray, P., Merino, M., Hewitt, S., Pavlovich, C. P., Glenn, G., Greenberg, C. R., Linehan, W. M., and Zbar, B. Birt-Hogg-Dube syndrome, a genodermatosis associated with spontaneous pneumothorax and kidney neoplasia, maps to chromosome 17p11.2, Am J Hum Genet. 69: 876–882, 2001.

84. Nickerson, M. L., Warren, M. B., Toro, J. R., Matrosova, V., Glenn, G., Turner, M. L., Duray, P., Merino, M., Choyke, P., Pavlovich, C. P., Sharma, N., Walther, M., Munroe, D., Hill, R., Maher, E., Greenberg, C., Lerman, M. I., Linehan, W. M., Zbar, B., and Schmidt, L. S. Mutations in a novel gene lead to kidney tumors, lung wall defects, and benign tumors of the hair follicle in patients with the Birt-Hogg-Dube syndrome, Cancer Cell. 2: 157–164, 2002.

85. Weirich, G., Glenn, G., Junke, R. K., Merino, M., Storkel, S., Lubensky, I., Choyke, P., Pack, S., Amin, M., Walther, M. M., Lineha, W. M., and Zbar, B. Familial renal oncocytoma: clinicopathological study of 5 families, J Urol. 160: 335–340, 1998.

86. Leroy, X., Leteurtre, E., Mahe, P. H., Gosselin, B., Delobel, B., and Croquette, M. F. Renal oncocytoma with a novel chromosomal rearrangement, der(13)t(13;16)(p11;p11), associated with a renal cell carcinoma, J Clin Pathol. 55: 157–158, 2002.

87. Bennett, R. L., Steinhaus, K. A., Uhrich, S. B., O'Sullivan, C. K., Resta, R. G., Lochner-Doyle, D., Markel, D. S., Vincent, V., and Hamanishi, J. Recommendations for standardized human pedigree nomenclature. Pedigree Standardization Task Force of the National Society of Genetic Counselors, Am J Hum Genet. 56: 745–752, 1995.

88. Trepanier, A., Ahrens, M., McKinnon, W., Peters, J., Stopfer, J., Grumet, S. C., et al. Genetic cancer risk assessment and counseling: recommendations of the national society of genetic counselors, J Genet Couns. 13: 83–114, 2004.

89. Weil, J. E. Psychosocial Genetic Counseling. Oxford University Press, New York, 2002.

90. Simpson, J. L., Carson, S. A., and Cisneros, P. Preimplantation genetic diagnosis (PGD) heritable neoplasia, J Natl Cancer Inst Monogr. 34: 87–90, 2005.

91. Rechitsky, S., Verlinsky, O., Chistokhina, A., Sharapova, T., Ozen, S., Masciangelo, C., Kuliev, A., and Verlinsky, Y. Preimplantation genetic diagnosis for cancer predisposition, Reprod Biomed Online. 5: 148–155, 2002.

8
Surgery

8a
Open Radical Nephrectomy for Localized Renal Cell Carcinoma

Sreenivas N. Vemulapalli and Jean B. deKernion

Introduction

The incidence of renal cell carcinoma is rising. An estimated 30,000 cases were diagnosed in the United States in 2005.[1] The use of modern imaging techniques has led to earlier detection and an increase in incidentally found renal masses. Technological advancements have revolutionized the surgical management of renal masses through laparoscopic and other minimally invasive modalities. However, patients continue to present with renal masses that are not amenable to these techniques and require traditional open surgery. Multiple references are available describing the numerous incisions for nephrectomy. In this chapter, we discuss incisions that we have found to be quite useful in open nephrectomy and currently in use at The University of California–Los Angeles (UCLA).

History

Robson described the general principles of radical nephrectomy in 1963.[2] He recommended early vascular control of the renal vessels to minimize tumor embolization, en bloc excision of Gerota's fascia with the kidney and adrenal gland, as well as an extensive lymph node dissection (LND). Currently, the need for LND[3] and adrenalectomy[4,5] has been challenged, most notably in clinically localized disease. However, early vascular control and removal of the kidney within Gerota's fascia remain central oncological principles in radical nephrectomy.

The editors and authors thank Michelle Moeck for preparation of the medical art for this chapter.

Preoperative Evaluation

All patients who are discovered to have a renal mass require a thorough preoperative evaluation to determine their ability to tolerate surgical intervention. This includes a history and physical examination with special attention to the cardiac and respiratory status of the patient. At a minimum, patients require an electrocardiogram and chest radiograph. Should suspicion of cardiopulmonary disease exist, a cardiac stress test and consultation with appropriate specialists are warranted. Aggressive medical intervention is warranted preoperatively to maximize positive outcomes during and after surgery. In addition, measurement of contralateral renal function is essential in patients with known medical renal disease, hypertension, diabetes, and other comorbidities that may affect kidney function (see Table 8a-1). A nuclear renal scan is a useful modality to evaluate differential renal function. Consultation with a nephrologist is sought when concern exists regarding the contralateral kidney's ability to sustain adequate renal function.

Assessment of the extent of local and metastatic disease is essential in planning for the type of operative exposure and in determining the role of nephrectomy and need for adjuvant therapies after surgery (see Table 8a-2). Computed tomography (CT) and magnetic resonance imaging (MRI) are utilized for the evaluation of the primary tumor, renal vein, and vena caval involvement and for the presence of metastatic disease. Cytoreductive nephrectomy[6,7] has been shown to offer some survival benefit in patients with metastatic disease, especially in those with symptoms or who are candidates for immunotherapy. However, patients must demonstrate good preoperative performance status to benefit. Careful consideration must be given prior to performing cytoreductive nephrectomy, as not all patients should be offered this therapy.

We currently use CT scan as our primary imaging technique. MRI is obtained when there is a suspicion of renal vein or vena caval tumor thrombus involvement. While duplex vascular ultrasound has also had good results in determining the extent of tumor thrombus, MRI offers the additional benefit of anatomic visualization.

TABLE 8a-1. Preoperative laboratory assessment for patients undergoing nephrectomy.

Laboratory evaluation
Complete blood count with platelets
Complete chemistry panel
Liver function panel (AST, ALT, ALK-P)
Blood type and crossmatch
Coagulation panel (PT, PTT, INR)
Urinalysis and culture

TABLE 8a-2. Preoperative radiological assessment for patients undergoing nephrectomy.

Radiological imaging
Minimal required
Chest radiograph
CT scan of abdomen and pelvis
Optional
CT scan of chest—when chest radiograph is suspicious
MRI of abdomen—if suspicion of renal vein/vena caval thrombus
Bone scan—if suspicion of metastatic disease
MRI of brain—if suspicion for metastatic disease
Nuclear renal scan—if concern over renal function

Preoperative Preparation

Patients undergo a bowel preparation the day prior to surgery that includes a clear liquid diet and use of a cathartic agent to enhance emptying of the bowel. Caution must be employed when using any hypertonic solution in patients with poor baseline renal function to prevent hyperphosphatemia or other potentially dangerous electrolyte abnormalities. Patients are asked to cease all anticoagulants at least 7 days prior to surgery. Prevention of perioperative deep venous thrombosis is achieved with the use of a thromboembolic (TED) hose and a sequential compression device (SCD) that is instituted prior to induction of anesthesia. Prior to incision, patients are administered a cephalosporin intravenous antibiotic for prophylaxis of wound infection. A nasogastric tube is placed after endotracheal intubation and in some patients is left in place overnight.

Surgical Incisions and Operative Exposure

Each surgical incision for radical nephrectomy has certain advantages and disadvantages. Some incisions utilize an extraperitoneal exposure while others are transperitoneal. The appropriate choice of incision for a given patient is governed by several factors including size of tumor, presence of tumor thrombus, prior surgical history, and patient body habitus.

Anterior Eleventh Rib Exposure

This incision is quite similar to a flank incision in positioning of the patient, operative exposure and extraperitoneal approach. However, it also offers the benefits of a smaller incision, obviates the need for rib removal, and minimizes the risk of pneumothorax. Drawbacks of the incision include the inability to examine intraperitoneal contents and slightly decreased exposure of the hilar vessels when compared to a transperitoneal approach. At UCLA, we routinely perform partial nephrectomies with this incision as it allows the surgeon to examine and operate on the kidney at skin level. It is also a valuable incision for small to moderate sized tumors that require radical nephrectomy and are not amenable to laparoscopic nephrectomy. In addition, patients have less pain than with a standard flank or transperitoneal incision.

After induction of general anesthesia and appropriate monitor placement, a Foley catheter is placed. The patient is placed in a semiflank torque position with the operative side and torso rotated medially 45° off the table, while the hips and lower extremities remain in a supine position (Fig. 8a-1A and B). The anterior superior iliac spine is placed just below the inferior aspect of the kidney rest. This allows for maximal exposure in the operative area after the table is maximally flexed and the kidney rest is elevated. The table is placed into a mild Trendelenburg position to keep the patient parallel to the floor. An axillary roll is placed as well as a posterior role to maintain the flank position. All extremities and pressure points are carefully padded and protected. The upper extremity, ipsilateral to the tumor, is placed onto a padded aeroplane arm board. The contralateral upper extremity is placed on a standard arm board. The patient is secured into position with the use of wide adhesive tape. The operative area is shaved and prepared with the agent of choice.

The ribs are palpated and identified. A marking pen is used to outline ribs 10, 11, and 12. A straight incision is made from the tip of rib 11 toward a mark 1 cm above the umbilicus (Fig. 8a-1A). The length of the incision is tailored individually for the patient's body habitus and size of tumor. Dissection is carried through the external oblique and internal oblique muscles laterally. The medial extent of the incision extends to the lateral aspect of the ipsilateral rectus muscle (Fig. 8a-1C and D). Should a larger incision be necessary, the rectus fascia can be opened and rectus muscle divided also.

The authors prefer to remain extraperitoneal with this exposure. The transversus abdominis muscle overlies the peritoneum and must be opened while the peritoneum is dissected off posteriorly to remain extraperitoneal. The cut edges of the internal oblique muscle are grasped with Alice clamps at the lateral edge of the incision and the transversus abdominis fascia is dissected off the posterior abdominal wall both inferiorly and superiorly. A handheld Richardson retractor allows for elevation of the anterior abdominal wall as a sponge stick or Kittner is utilized for mobilization of the peritoneum (Fig. 8a-1E and F). The transversus is incised taking care to not open the peritoneum.

A self-retaining Buchwalter retractor is utilized to maintain exposure. Moistened laparotomy sponges are used to protect soft tissues from retractor damage. Blunt dissection is used to mobilize the peritoneum medially off of Gerota's fascia. With adequate mobilization, the renal hilum becomes visible. Additional retractors are carefully placed to hold the peritoneum medially (Fig. 8a-1G). In right nephrectomy, the second portion of the duodenum can be visualized and retracted medially.

Closure is performed with Looped 0-PDS suture to reapproximate the internal oblique and rectus muscles. Interrupted 0 Vicryl sutures are used to reapproximate the external oblique fascia. Marcaine (0.5%) is infiltrated into the muscle, subcutaneous tissues, and along rib 11 medially for postoperative analgesia. The skin can be closed with subcuticular closure or staples.

Anterior Subcostal Incision

This is a transperitoneal incision that offers the advantages of intraperitoneal content examination, excellent access to the upper pole and adrenal gland, as well as good exposure of the renal hilum. It is possible to perform this as an extraperitoneal surgery; however, the above advantages are lost and we prefer the anterior rib 11 exposure when attempting to remain extraperitoneal. There is less risk of pleurotomy and pneumothorax than seen in the standard flank incision. Potential disadvantages include prolonged ileus or delayed small bowel obstruction secondary to adhesion formation from manipulation of the bowel.

After adequate induction of general anesthesia and appropriate monitor placement the patient is positioned with the anterior superior iliac spine at the level of the kidney rest. The patient is maintained in the supine position; however, a small roll can be placed behind the patient on the operative side, rotating the patient slightly. The table is flexed slightly to help open up the operative area. A Foley catheter is inserted. A marking pen is used to delineate the costal margin. An incision is made two fingerbreadths from the costal margin, starting from the anterior axillary line and extending medially through the ipsilateral rectus (Fig. 8a-2A).

Should increased exposure be necessary, the incision can be lengthened, extending through the contralateral rectus muscle or even further into a chevron incision (Fig. 8a-3). After incision of the anterior fascia, dissection is carried through the external oblique, internal oblique, transverse abdominal, and rectus muscles (Fig. 8a-2B and C). Cautery is utilized to incise the muscles and excellent hemostasis is essential to prevent delayed bleeding and hematoma formation. The remaining posterior rectus sheath is carefully incised in the midline in the direction of the original incision

exposing the peritoneum (Fig. 8a-2D). After entering the peritoneum in the midline it is incised toward the lateral extent of the incision. The ligamentum teres is doubly ligated and incised to allow for maximal exposure.

The peritoneum is visually and manually examined to evaluate for metastatic disease. The retroperitoneum and perinephric space are entered by mobilizing the colon with incision of the white line of Toldt while retracting the colon medially (Fig. 8a-2E). The assistant utilizes a handheld Richardson retractor to lift the anterior abdominal wall improving access to the White line. After mobilization of the colon, a self-retaining Buchwalter retractor is placed.

In right nephrectomy, the hepatic flexure of the colon is mobilized to minimize the risk of hepatic capsular tear and to improve visualization of the upper pole and adrenal gland. The hepatorenal ligament is also incised to allow the upper pole of the kidney to fall away from the liver. The Falciform ligament is also incised to allow the liver to be retracted without injury. The second portion of the duodenum lies directly anterior to the renal hilum, renal pelvis, and ureteropelvic junction (Fig. 8a-2F) and is mobilized medially as well. Great care must be taken to prevent inadvertent injury with risk of possible duodenal leak. The inferior vena cava is seen after mobilization of the duodenum and serves as the primary landmark to begin renal hilar dissection (Fig. 8a-2G and H). Left nephrectomy requires incision of the splenocolic attachments to free the splenic flexure of the colon. The aorta can be palpated to determine the medial extent of the required exposure.

Closure of the incision is performed with looped 0-PDS to reapproximate the rectus and internal oblique muscles. The external oblique fascia is reapproximated using interrupted 0-Vicryl sutures. The incision is infiltrated with 0.5% Marcaine and the skin is closed with subcuticular closure or staples.

Chevron Incision

The chevron incision is similar to the subcostal incision. It is performed as described earlier with incision from the anterior axillary line through the ipsilateral rectus approximately two fingerbreadths from the costal margin. However, it is extended through the contralateral rectus to the anterior axillary line (Fig. 8a-3). Once again, after entering the peritoneum, mobilization of the colon is performed to enter the retroperitoneum and access the great vessels and kidney. This incision provides excellent exposure in very large tumors and in cases that require renal vein and inferior vena caval thrombectomy as well as hepatic mobilization.

Thoracoabdominal Incision

The thoracoabdominal incision provides excellent operative exposure and is especially useful in cases of large upper pole tumors. Other advantages include access to the lung

(a)

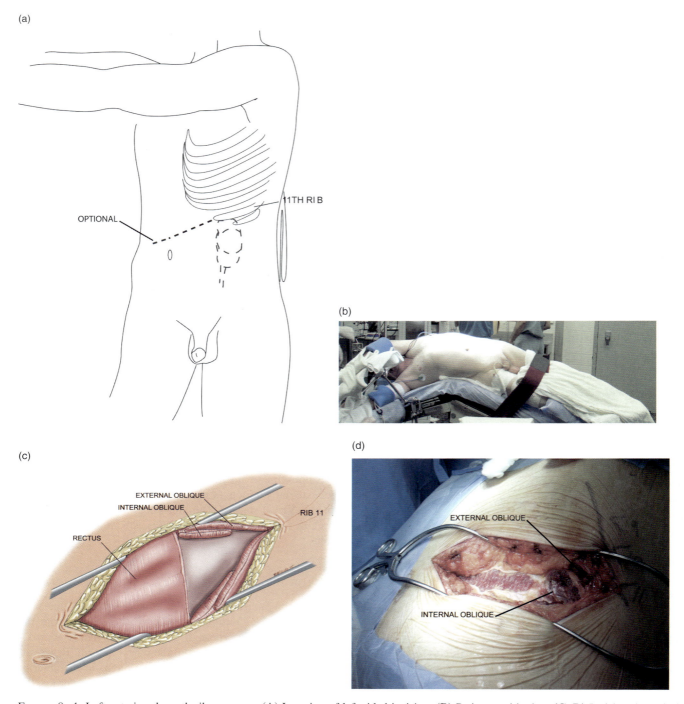

(b)

(c)

(d)

FIGURE 8a-1. Left anterior eleventh rib exposure. (**A**) Location of left-sided incision. (**B**) Patient positioning. (**C, D**) Incision through the external and internal oblique; the rectus can also be incised for increased exposure. (**E, F**) Mobilization of the peritoneum to expose the retroperitoneum. (**G**) Extraperitoneal exposure of the renal hilum.

parenchyma for biopsy or excision of lung lesions. The incision also allows for hepatic mobilization in cases of vena caval thrombus. Disadvantages include the need for postoperative chest tube drainage, longer operative time, and increased pain.

The patient is placed in a torque, a semiflank position with the operative side rotated medially 30° with a blanket roll. The pelvis and lower extremities are maintained in a relatively supine position. The ipsilateral upper extremity is placed on an aeroplane arm board and the contralateral arm

(e)

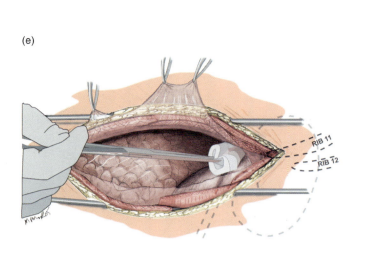

(f)

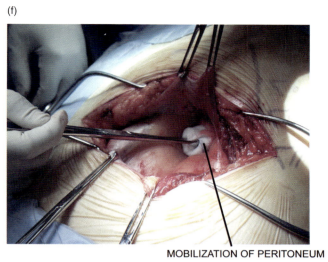

MOBILIZATION OF PERITONEUM

(g)

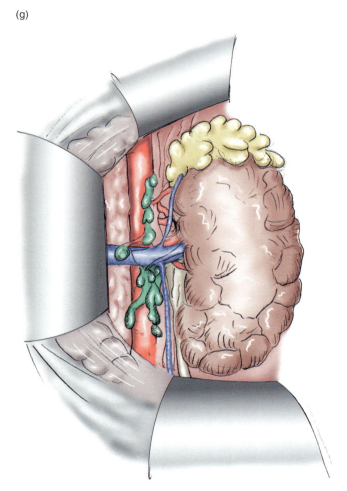

FIGURE 8a-1. (Continued)

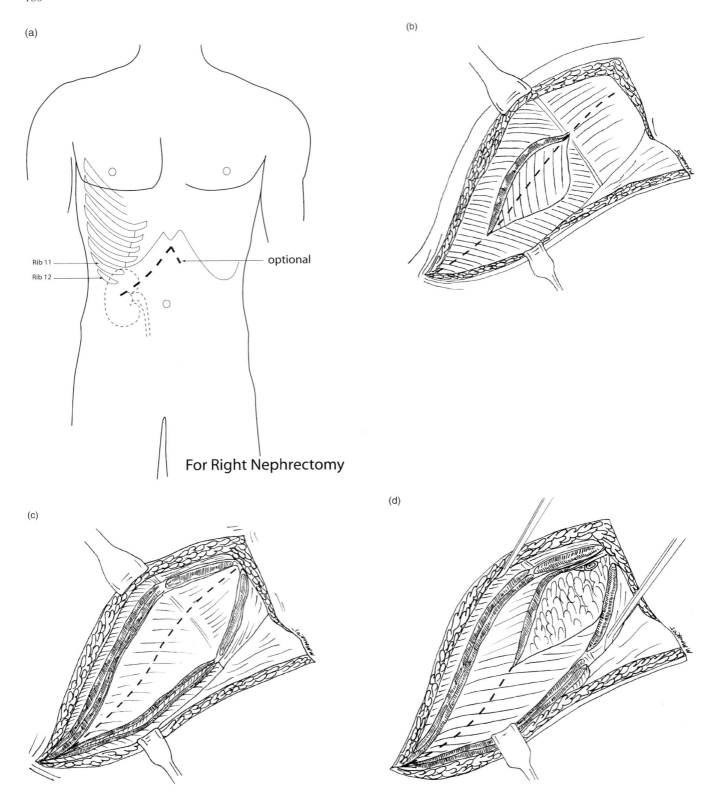

FIGURE 8a-2. Right-sided anterior subcostal incision. (**A**) Location of right-sided incision. (**B**) Partially incised external oblique; the dashed line represents the direction of incision through the rectus and internal oblique. (**C**) Incised external and internal obliques and rectus with intact posterior sheath. (**D**) Incision of the posterior sheath and peritoneum. (**E**) Incision of the White line of Toldt with mobilization of the colon. (**F**) Anatomic relation of intraperitoneal contents to kidneys. (**G, H**) Exposed kidney and retroperitoneum.

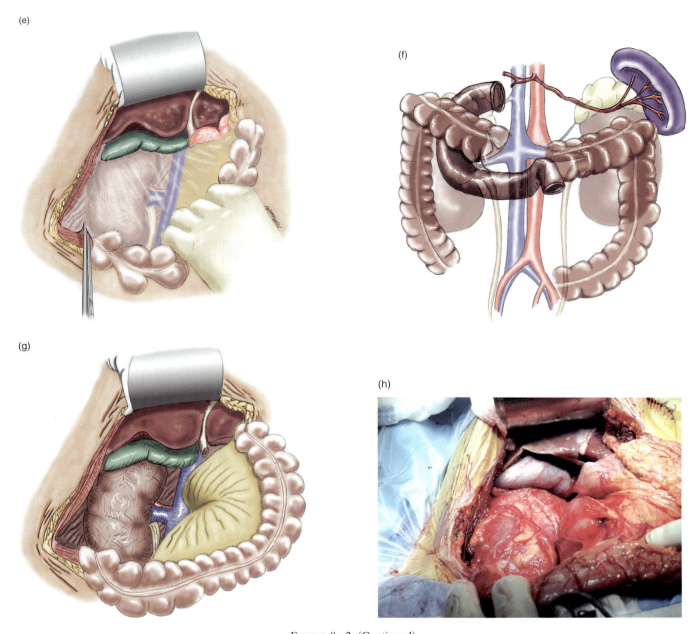

(e)

(f)

(g)

(h)

FIGURE 8a-2. (Continued)

on a standard arm board. All extremities are carefully padded and the patient is secured in position with wide adhesive tape.

The incision can be made in any intercostal space; however, we generally make the incision above rib 9 or 10, extending from the posterior axillary line laterally through the costal margin extending to the contralateral rectus (Fig. 8a-4A and B). For left-sided tumor, with vena caval thrombus, a right thoracoabdominal incision is extended into a left subcostal incision (see Fig. 8a-4B). Dissection is continued through the latissimus dorsi and external oblique laterally (Fig. 8a-4C). The rectus fascia and muscle are incised medially. The internal oblique is then incised. Once the

intercostal muscles are visualized they are incised with cautery, taking care to incise at the superior aspect of the rib to prevent inadvertent injury to the intercostal nerve and vessels, which travel at the inferior aspect of the rib. The costal cartilage is divided with a curved scissor to allow for maximal retraction of the ribs (Fig. 8a-4D). Blunt dissection is used to open the costovertebral ligament posteriorly, allowing for free retraction of the rib. We do not resect a rib, since it is not necessary for exposure, and may result in larger flank defects.

After incision of the intercostal muscles and opening of the pleura, the diaphragm is visualized. The diaphragm is incised from its anteromedial attachment to the chest wall to

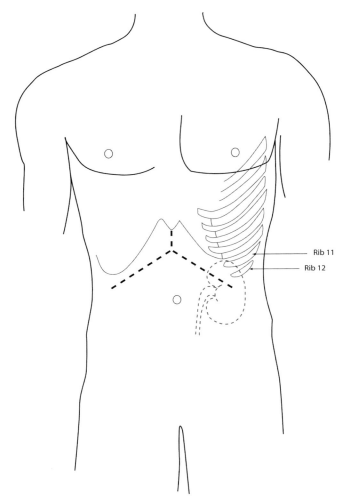

Rib 11

Rib 12

FIGURE 8a-3. Chevron incision.

its posterior aspect in a curved fashion to prevent injury to the phrenic nerve (Fig. 8a-4E). We elect to enter the peritoneum with this incision rather than remain extraperitoneal as it gives us the ability to examine intraperitoneal contents and decreases operative time (Fig. 8a-4F). Once the exposure has been achieved, the colon is mobilized as described earlier in the anterior subcostal incision (see Fig. 8a-2E and G).

Closure of the thoracoabdominal incision requires reapproximation of the diaphragm. Interrupted 2-0 Vicryl sutures are used for this, ensuring that the knots are toward the peritoneum rather than the intrapleural space to prevent lung irritation. A 20 French chest tube is placed from one rib below the posterior aspect of the incision, taking care to ensure the chest tube does not travel through the peritoneum. The ribs are reapproximated with 0-PDS suture encompassing both the ribs and overlying muscle. A #2 Vicryl suture is used to reapproximate the costal cartilage. Marcaine (0.5%) is infiltrated along the rib above and below the incision to block the intercostal nerves for postoperative analgesia. The muscle and subcutaneous

tissues are infiltrated as well. The skin is reapproximated with staples. The chest tube is removed within 24 hours, after the chest radiograph demonstrates resolution of any pneumothorax.

Nephrectomy

After exposure of the renal hilum and kidney has been achieved by any of the incisions discussed here, removal of the kidney is performed. En bloc resection of the kidney and Gerota's fascia is performed after early ligation of the renal arterial supply followed by ligation of the renal vein. An understanding of the vasculature of the right and left kidneys and their differences is essential.

The right renal vein is quite short given its proximity to the inferior vena cava. It is rare to encounter a lumbar vein draining directly into the renal vein, however, this is possible and care must be taken when dissecting posteriorly to the right renal vein. The right gonadal vein generally drains into the vena cava but can drain into the right renal vein as well. The right renal artery generally arises from a superior position on the aorta than the left renal artery and passes behind the vena cava on its course to the right kidney. The right renal artery can be ligated lateral to the vena cava (Fig. 8a-5A and B); however, in cases of large right-sided tumors it may be beneficial to dissect the artery medial to the vena cava and perform ligation there (Fig. 8a-5C and D). The artery is posterior to the renal vein and anterior to the renal pelvis and ureter on both sides.

The left renal vein is quite long, travels anteriorly to the aorta, and often has lumbar veins draining into it. Caution must be used when dissecting posterior to the left renal vein to avoid troublesome bleeding from inadvertent injury to lumbar veins. In addition, the left adrenal vein emerges from the superior aspect and the left gonadal vein from the inferior aspect of the left renal vein (Fig. 8a-6A). We routinely ligate the gonadal and adrenal veins when performing left-sided nephrectomy (Fig. 8a-6B). This allows clearer access to the left renal vein and left renal artery posteriorly.

Multiple anatomic vascular variations are possible, the most common being the presence of multiple arteries. Preoperative imaging may not clearly elucidate the actual number of arteries. Once the renal artery is ligated, examination of the turgor of the kidney can be a clue to the presence of additional arteries. However, this may be difficult in large tumors and careful dissection to ensure all arteries have been ligated is essential.

The kidney and perinephric fat contained within Gerota's fascia are separated from the paranephric fat overlying the psoas muscle posteriorly and the liver or spleen superiorly using surgical clips and cautery to maintain hemostasis (Fig. 8a-5E). On the right side the hepatorenal attachments should be incised carefully to prevent hepatic capsular tear and bleeding. A completed right nephrectomy with hilar

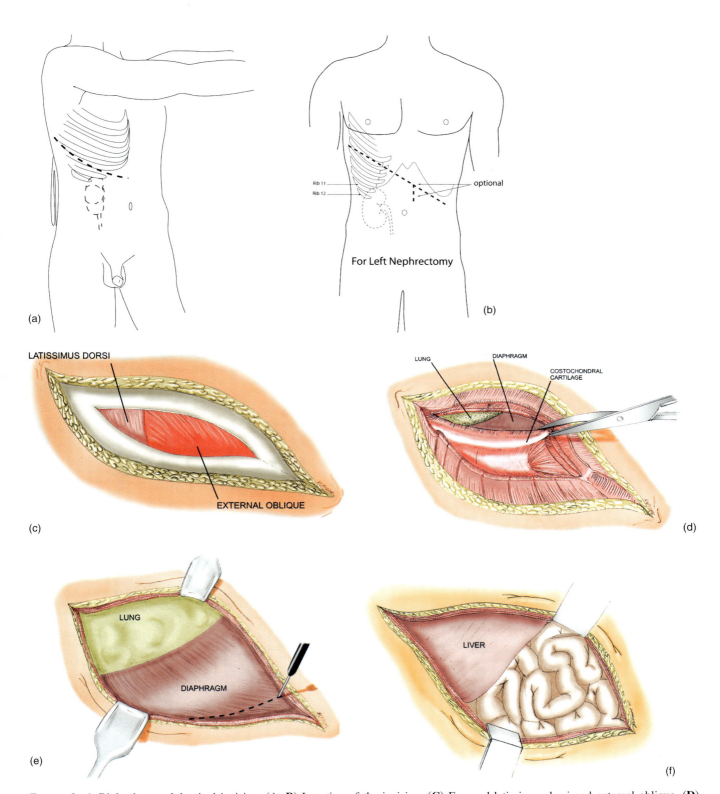

FIGURE 8a-4. Right thoracoabdominal incision. (**A, B**) Location of the incision. (**C**) Exposed latissimus dorsi and external oblique. (**D**) Incision of the costal cartilage. (**E**) Curved incision through the diaphragm. (**F**) Opened peritoneum. (Visual reference provided with permission of Andrew C. Novick, MD, Chairman, Glickman Urological Institute, Cleveland Clinic Foundation from Marshall's Textbook of Operative Urology.)

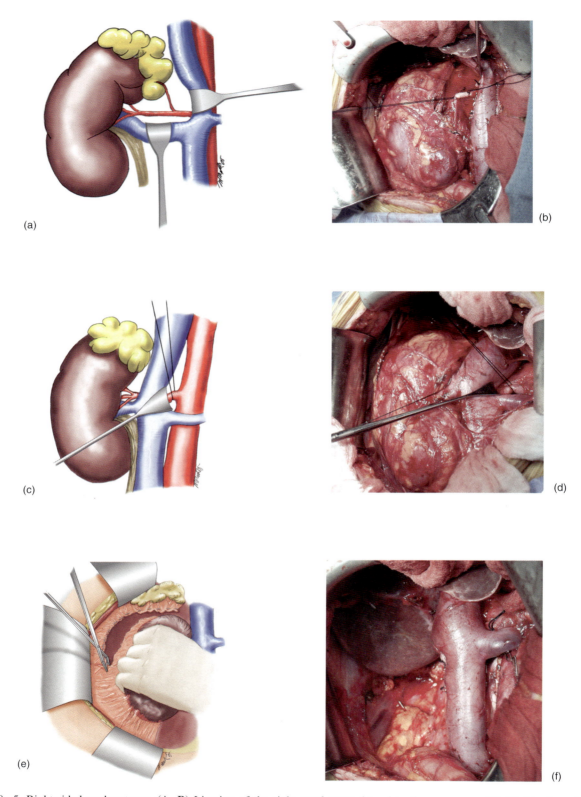

FIGURE 8a-5. Right-sided nephrectomy. (**A, B**) Ligation of the right renal artery lateral to the vena cava. (**C, D**) Ligation of the right renal artery medial to the vena cava. (**E**) Removal of the kidney within Gerota's fascia from the retroperitoneum with adrenal sparing. (**F**) Completed right nephrectomy and hilar lymphadenectomy.

(a)

(b)

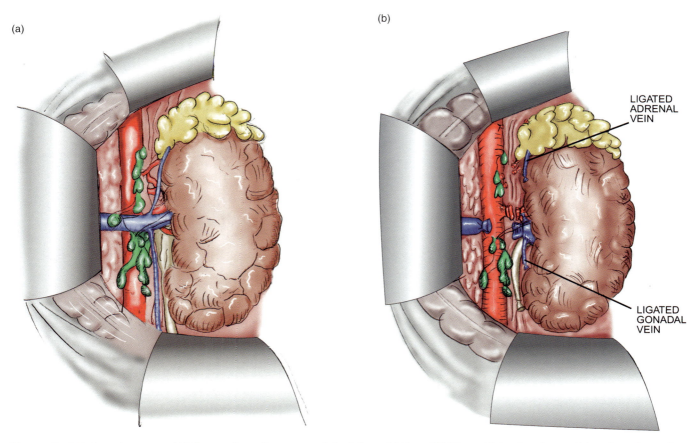

LIGATED
ADRENAL
VEIN

LIGATED
GONADAL
VEIN

FIGURE 8a-6. Left nephrectomy. (**A**) Extraperitoneal exposure of the left renal hilum. (**B**) Ligated left adrenal, gonadal, and renal vessels.

lymph node dissection is shown in Fig. 8a-5F. The ureter is doubly ligated with a surgical clip or suture and transected.

Need for Adrenalectomy and Lymph Node Dissection

With the advent of improved imaging techniques including CT and MRI scans, adrenal metastases are usually seen preoperatively.[5] In patients who require adjuvant immunotherapy for metastatic disease, preservation of adrenal function is of the utmost importance to prevent adrenal insufficiency. We routinely attempt to preserve the ipsilateral adrenal gland. An adrenalectomy is performed when one or more of the following criteria are met. Preoperative imaging demonstrates likely metastasis to the adrenal and in cases of large upper pole renal tumors where direct extension is likely or adrenal sparing is challenging given the tumor size.

Robson[2] advocated an extensive LND involving all of the nodes anterior and posterior to the great vessels from the crus of the diaphragm to the aortic bifurcation. Much controversy currently exists regarding the role of LND in renal cell carcinoma.[3] LND clearly improves our staging of disease;

however, whether extended LND provides a survival benefit is still unclear.

We routinely perform a hilar lymphadenectomy for staging purposes. On the right side this involves the lymph nodes overlying and just superior to the right renal vein. We extend medially to remove the interaortocaval nodes and inferiorly to the origin of the gonadal vein (Fig. 8a-7A and B). Left-sided hilar lymphadenectomy involves tissue overlying the left renal vein and the lateral half of the aorta (Fig. 8a-7C and D). In cases of bulky lymphadenopathy with a high suspicion of metastatic disease or cytoreductive nephrectomy with known metastatic disease, an extended lymph node dissection is performed to remove all bulky nodes.

Complications of Radical Nephrectomy

There are several complications associated with radical nephrectomy. Knowledge of the surgical anatomy and meticulous surgical technique are critical to prevent them. However, they may still occur and an understanding of their management is essential.

The complications can be subdivided into groups including pulmonary, vascular, and abdominal. The risks vary based on

(a)

(b)

(c)

(d)

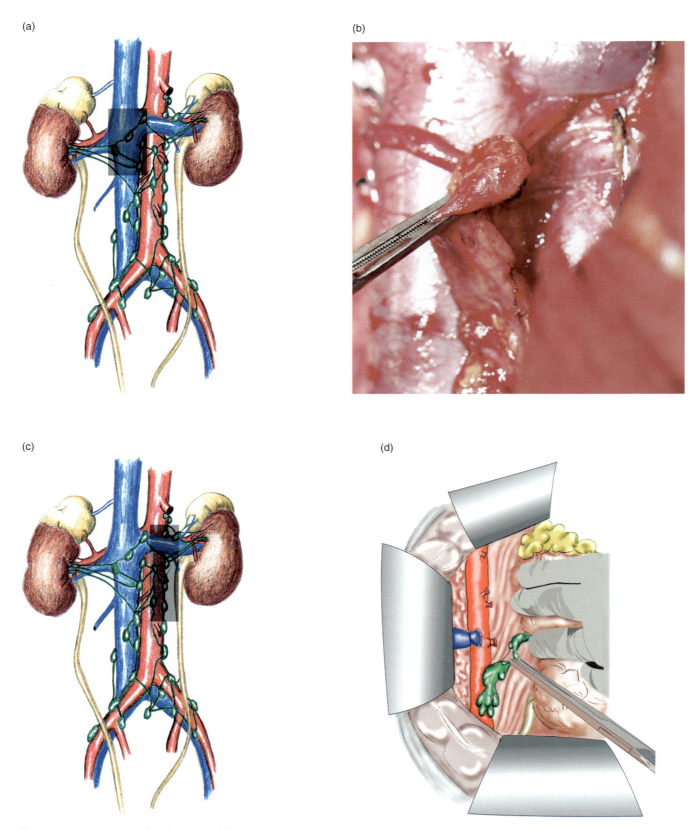

FIGURE 8a-7. Lymph node dissection. (**A**) Limits of right-sided dissection. (**B**) Removal of interaortocaval nodes during right-sided dissection. (**C**) Limits of left-sided dissection. (**D**) Removal of periaortic nodes.

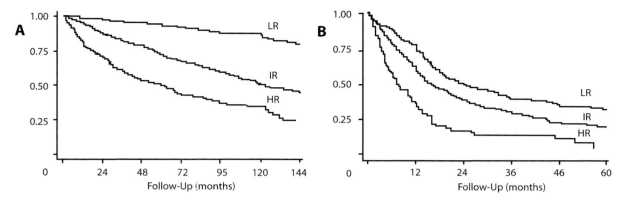

FIGURE 8a-8. Kaplan–Meier survival estimates according to University of California Los Angeles Integrated Staging system in 3119 (**A**) and 1083 (**B**) patients with localized and metastatic disease. LR, low risk; IR, intermediate risk; HR, high risk. (From Patard et al.,[12] with permission of the author. Reprinted with permission from the American Society of Clinical Oncology.)

surgical exposure, location of the kidney, stage of disease, and medical comorbidities.

Pulmonary complications include postoperative atelectasis, which can be treated with aggressive pulmonary therapy including incentive spirometry, the use of inhaled bronchodilators, and chest percussion with postural drainage when warranted. If extensive lymph node dissection is performed, careful dissection to prevent injury to the crus of the diaphragm is necessary. The risk of pulmonary complication is higher in thoracoabdominal exposures, which necessitate the use of chest tubes. Careful reapproximation of the diaphragm is necessary to prevent postoperative pneumothorax. A postoperative chest radiograph is necessary to ensure proper placement of the chest tube as well as resolution of pneumothorax. In cases in which the lung fails to reexpand with a properly functioning chest tube, bronchoscopy is warranted.

Vascular complications can be anticipated and prevented with attention to anatomy and surgical technique. During right-sided dissection the vena cava serves as an anatomic landmark. The short right adrenal vein can be injured and cause troublesome bleeding. The assistant can retract the right lobe of the liver as the inferior vena cava is retracted medially with a curved vein retractor to identify the right adrenal vein, which should be ligated in cases requiring adrenalectomy. Some surgeons advocate routine ligation of the right gonadal vessels to prevent inadvertent injury. It is our practice to do this with large tumors that bring the vessels into the operative field. When right-sided lymphadenectomy is performed attention must be given to the lumbar vessels that drain into the vena cava at each vertebral level. When injury to the lumbar vessels is encountered, Allis clamps can be utilized to control the bleeding vessels, and then they are ligated with 3-0 silk ties or vascular suture ligature. Vena caval injuries can be managed in a similar fashion and closed with 5-0 vascular suture. During left-sided nephrectomy, the left renal vein may have lumbar vessels entering posteriorly and injury can be managed similarly. At the completion of nephrectomy, careful examination of the ligated renal hilar

vessels is performed to ensure that all vessels have been controlled adequately.

Abdominal complications include injury to any abdominal structures, most notably the liver, spleen, and pancreas. Careful transection of the hepatorenal and splenorenal ligaments is essential during mobilization of the kidney to prevent capsular tear of the liver and spleen. Should capsular tear occur, management can include reapproximation of the capsule, application of a thrombogenic agent, and/or argon beam coagulation. In cases of severe uncontrollable splenic bleeding, splenectomy may be necessary. These patients should be treated with pneumococcal vaccine postoperatively. In cases of undetected pancreatic injury, postoperative symptoms may include prolonged ileus with elevated serum amylase, alkaline drainage from the wound, or retroperitoneal fluid collection on radiological imaging. Management includes institution of parenteral nutrition, bowel rest, and percutaneous drainage for persistent fistula.

Outcomes of Radical Nephrectomy

Multiple systems for outcome stratification in renal cell carcinoma (RCC) have been created.[8,9] The University of California at Los Angeles Integrated Staging System (UISS)[10] was developed to better stratify patient outcomes in both localized and metastatic RCC. The UISS utilizes TNM stage,[11] Fuhrman grade, and Eastern Cooperative Oncology Group (ECOG) performance status to group patients with RCC into low-, intermediate-, and high-risk groups.

Patard et al.[12] reported on the use of the UISS in a multicenter study that included 4202 patients from 8 international academic centers. For localized RCC (3119 patients), see Fig. 8a-8A; the 5-year survival rates were 92%, 67%, and 44% for low-, intermediate-, and high-risk groups, respectively. For metastatic RCC (1083 patients), see Fig. 8a-8B; the 3-year survival rates were 37%, 23%, and 12% for low-, intermediate-, and high-risk groups, respectively.

We currently utilize the UISS in our practice at UCLA. Future improvements in outcome prognostic models may rely on the development of biomarkers for RCC, further refinement of the TNM [11] staging system, and the incorporation of patient outcomes with emerging targeted therapies for metastatic RCC.

Conclusions

The emergence of minimally invasive techniques for the management of clinically localized renal tumors has revolutionized the management of the renal mass. However, open radical nephrectomy remains an important tool when the patient cannot undergo less invasive therapies. The surgical exposures discussed here have been very useful and remain the incisions of choice at UCLA. Lymphadenectomy remains a useful staging tool and further study is necessary to determine if any survival benefit is achieved. The majority of patients can undergo an adrenal sparing procedure; however, should any concern exist based on criteria discussed above, an adrenalectomy should be performed.

The UISS and other RCC prognostic models have been useful in counseling patients and further refinement of these models will improve their accuracy.

References

1. Jemal A, Murray T, Samuels A, et al. Cancer statistics, 2003. CA Cancer J Clin 2003;53:5–26.
2. Robson CJ. Radical nephrectomy for renal cell carcinoma. J Urol 1963;89:37.
3. Phillips CK, Taneja SS. The role of lymphadenectomy in the surgical management of renal cell carcinoma. Urol Oncol 2004;22(3):214–223.
4. Kobayashi T, Nakamura E, Yamamoto S, et al. Low incidence of ipsilateral adrenal involvement and recurrences in patients with renal cell carcinoma undergoing radical nephrectomy: a retrospective analysis of 393 patients. Urology 2003;62(1):40–45.
5. Tsui KH, Shvarts O, Barbaric Z, et al. Is adrenalectomy a necessary component of radical nephrectomy? UCLA experience with 511 radical nephrectomies. J Urol 2000;163(2):437–441.
6. Mickisch GH, Garin A, van Poppel H, et al. Radical nephrectomy plus interferon-alfa-based immunotherapy compared with interferon alfa alone in metastatic renal-cell carcinoma: a randomized trial. Lancet 2001;358:966–970.
7. Flanigan RC, Salmon SE, Blumenstein BA, et al. Nephrectomy followed by interferon alfa-2b compared with interferon alfa 2-b alone for metastatic renal-cell cancer. N Engl J Med 2001;345:1655–1659.
8. Kattan MW, Reuter V, Motzer RJ, et al. A postoperative prognostic nomogram for renal cell carcinoma. J Urol 2001; 166:63–67.
9. Frank I, Blute ML, Cheville JC, et al. An outcome prediction model for patients with clear cell renal cell carcinoma treated with radical nephrectomy based on tumor stage, size, grade and necrosis: The SSIGN score. J Urol 2002;168:2395–2400.
10. Zisman A, Pantuck AJ, Dorey F, et al. Improved prognostication of renal cell carcinoma using an integrated staging system. J Clin Oncol 2001;19(6):1649–1657.
11. Guinan P, Sobin LH, Algaba F, et al. TNM staging of renal cell carcinoma: Workgroup No. 3–Union International Contre le Cancer (UICC) and the American Joint Committee on Cancer (AJCC). Cancer 1997;80:992–993.
12. Patard JJ, Kim HL, Lam JS, et al. Use of the University of California Los Angeles integrated staging system to predict survival in renal cell carcinoma: an international multicenter study. J Clin Oncol 2004;22:16:3316–3322.

8b
Radical Nephrectomy, Laparoscopic Transperitoneal

Yi-Hsiu Huang and Allen W. Chiu

Introduction

Open radical nephrectomy is traditionally performed as described by Robson et al. in 1969.[1] The surgical principles are early ligation of the renal artery and vein, en bloc removal of the kidney with the upper third of the ureter and the perirenal fat embedded within Gerota's fascia, removal of the ipsilateral adrenal gland, and regional renal hilar lymphadenectomy. However, the morbidity associated with open surgery (severe postoperative wound pain, lengthy hospitalization and convalescence) can be significant. The laparoscopic approach is an elegant alternative for many open procedures because it has the advantages of minimally invasive surgery. The first laparoscopic nephrectomy was performed in 1990 by Clayman et al. at Washington University.[2] Since then, the laparoscopic approach for renal pathology has gained popularity worldwide. Rapid advances and refinement in laparoscopic instruments together with growing experience have made this technique the standard of care in many centers worldwide for the treatment of renal neoplasms. The procedure can be performed by a transperitoneal or retroperitoneal approach. We will elaborate on the transperitoneal approach.

Indications and Contraindications

The indications for laparoscopic radical nephrectomy are similar to those of open surgery. Although there are some difficulties when dealing with advanced stage or large size renal cell carcinoma (RCC), the operation is successfully performed in experienced hands, with excellent results.[3,4] The size of RCC is no longer considered a limitation for laparoscopic nephrectomy by experienced laparoscopists.[4]

Laparoscopic surgery has some relative contraindications: chronic obstructive pulmonary disease (COPD), emphysema, heart failure, morbid obesity, extensive prior abdominal surgery, ascites, etc. A relative contraindication specific for laparoscopic radical nephrectomy is a level I renal vein thrombosis. However, Desai et al. have successfully performed laparoscopic radical nephrectomy in patients with RCC associated with level I renal vein thrombosis.[5] Extension of the tumor thrombus into the inferior vena cava (IVC) is a contraindication for laparoscopic radical nephrectomy.

Operation Technique

Preoperative Evaluation and Preparation

The preoperative evaluation for patients with RCC includes ultrasonography, computerized tomography (CT) scanning, and magnetic resonance imaging (MRI). Metastatic evaluation consists of chest X-ray, abdominal sonography or CT scanning, and bone scan. If renal vein or IVC tumor thrombus is suspected, MRI or angiography is mandatory. Assessment of the pulmonary function and arterial blood gas analysis should be done in patients with impaired pulmonary function. Patients with cardiac problems require echocardiography and/or cardiac functional studies.

Before surgery an informed consent including the risk of laparoscopic radical nephrectomy and the possibility of conversion to open surgery should be read and signed by the patient. Bowel preparation can be given if so desired by the surgeon.

Patient Positioning

The patient positioning for transperitoneal laparoscopic radical nephrectomy is a modified lateral decubitus position with the kidney bridge mildly elevated. The shoulder, buttocks, flank, and bony prominence should be carefully padded. Wide cloth tape is used to fix the patient securely in place (Fig. 8b-1).

Some surgeons are used to a full flank position, which would allow the colon to get out of the way by itself. There

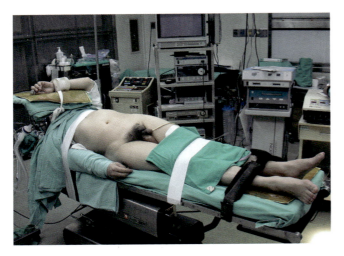

FIGURE 8b-1. The patient is placed in a modified lateral decubitus position with the kidney bridge mildly elevated. The shoulder, buttocks, flank, and bony prominence should be carefully padded. Wide cloth tape is used to fix the patient securely in place.

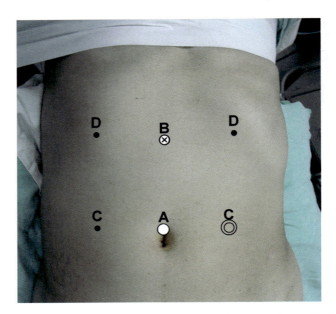

FIGURE 8b-2. Trocar placement for laparoscopic radical nephrectomy. (**A**) A 10-mm trocar for the camera at the umbilicus. (**B**) A 5-mm (for left side) or 12-mm (for right side) trocar in the midline between the umbilicus and the xiphoid process. (**C**) A 5-mm (for right side) or 12-mm (for left side) trocar lateral to the rectus muscle at the level of the umbilicus. (**D**) A 5-mm trocar for retraction or to assist in dissection if needed.

might be some difficulties in creating pneumoperitoneum in such positioning, however.

Trocar Placement

Pneumoperitoneum can be achieved by blind puncture with the Veress needle or by open introduction of the first trocar (Hasson cannula technique). Insufflation is done with CO_2, until an abdominal pressure of 15 mm Hg is reached (12 mm Hg in infants). Care should be taken in patients with a history of prior abdominal surgery in order to prevent an access-related bowel or vascular injury. The Hasson cannula technique may be used in such patients to prevent bowel injury.

A four-trocar technique is usually employed (Fig. 8b-2). The first trocar, i.e., the Veress needle insertion site, is usually placed at the umbilicus with a 10-mm trocar for the 0 or 30° camera. A 5-mm (for left side) or 12-mm (for right side) trocar is inserted in the midline between the umbilicus and the xiphoid process. A 5-mm (for right side) or 12-mm (for left side) trocar is placed lateral to the rectus muscle at the level of the umbilicus. Another 5-mm trocar may be placed for retraction or assistance with dissection if needed. In cases of morbid obesity, the trocar position should be moved laterally and upward.

Operative Procedure

Mobilization of the Colon

For a right nephrectomy, the peritoneal incision is started at the white line of Toldt and continued toward the hepatic flexure. The incision then runs transversely along the undersurface of the liver until the vena cava is encountered. The ascending colon is mobilized and reflected medially. An avascular plane between the anterior surface of Gerota's fascia and the posterior surface of the mesocolon can be identified. The duodenum will be seen and it can be bluntly dissected medially until the anterior aspect of the inferior vena cava is exposed (Kocher maneuver).

For a left nephrectomy, a similar procedure is performed to reflect the descending colon. The splenic flexure, splenorenal fascial attachment should be divided to avoid laceration of the spleen, and to facilitate the mobilization of the colon for better exposure of the renal hilum. The pancreas lies anterior to the renal hilum and can be bluntly dissected medially. Dissection of this plane should not be too deep and too medial to avoid pancreas injury.

Dissection of the Ureter

The white line of Toldt can be incised as low as the level of the iliac vessels. The ureter can be identified cephalad and anterior to the common iliac artery. It is usually located medial to the psoas muscle in the retroperitoneal fat. The gonadal vein accompanies the ureter. The ureter is elevated and retracted laterally. The dissection of the ureter is continued proximally to approach the renal hilum. The right gonadal vein should be secured and divided to open the plane between the ureter and the vena cava. The left gonadal vein can be used as a marker to identify the left renal vein. The gonadal vein is preferably ligated not too close to the renal vein.

Mobilization of the Lower Pole and Dissection of the Renal Hilum

While the dissection is carried along the ureter proximally until the level of the ureteropelvic junction, the lower pole of the kidney should be mobilized to facilitate dissection of the renal hilum. The kidney can be elevated with a retractor and the attachments between the Gerota's fascia and side wall are divided.

With gentle lateral retraction of the kidney, the renal hilum can easily be dissected. On the right side, as the dissection goes along the ureter and vena cava proximally after division of the gonadal vein, the renal vein is usually identified. The adrenal vein lies cephalad to the renal vein. On the left side, we follow the gonadal vein to reach its junction with the renal vein. The gonadal vein is then secured and divided at a distance about 2 cm from the junction with the renal vein. This will prevent interference with later placement of the Endo-GIA vascular stapler on the renal vein. The lumbar vein, which is usually located inferior to the renal vein, may be found and has to be controlled carefully. The left adrenal vein, located on the superior edge of the renal vein, should be dissected out, too.

After mobilization of the lower pole and dissection of the renal vein, the renal artery can easily be caught behind the renal vein. The renal artery should be circumferentially dissected, clipped with multiple 9-mm or 11-mm clips, and transected, leaving at least three clips on the aorta side. The Endo-GIA may be needed in case of a large artery.

After dividing the renal artery, the renal vein is transected with an Endo-GIA vascular stapler. On the left side, if the adrenal gland is to be left, the Endo-GIA should be placed distal to the adrenal vein. If the adrenal gland is to be removed with the specimen, the Endo-GIA should be placed proximal to the adrenal vein.

Dissection of the Upper Pole and the Adrenal Gland

After controlling the renal hilar vessels, the remaining attachments of the kidney are the upper pole and the adrenal gland. The upper margin of the dissection depends on whether the adrenal gland has to be removed. If this is the case the adrenal vein has to be dissected and transected and the dissection goes cephalad to the adrenal gland. The short right adrenal vein drains directly into the vena cava and the left adrenal vein drains into the left renal vein. The attachment of the upper pole can be divided with electrocautery or an ultrasonic dissector. The specimen is completely free after dissection of the upper pole. The ureter is then dissected as low as possible, secured with clips, and divided.

Extraction of the Specimen

The specimen can be removed in two different ways, depending on the surgeon's preference: either remove it intact or morcellate it. If it is to be removed intact, an Endocatch bag (Autosuture, Norwalk, CT) is suggested. It is a self-opening transparent sack and the specimen can be put into the opening easily with one grasper. The entrapped specimen can be removed through an extended incision at one of the port sites, a lower midline incision, or a Pfannenstiel incision. If the specimen is to be morcellated, a Lapsac (Cook Urological, Spencer, IN) should be used. It is a double layer impermeable Nylon bag. After the specimen is put into the bag, morcellation is performed with a mechanical clamp or electrical tissue morcellator. Although the risk of cancer spillage during morcellation is always present, no such instance has yet been reported.

Intact specimen extraction is preferable for several reasons. It enables the accurate study of the surgical margins and pathological staging of the tumor, which is paramount for the prognosis and follow-up protocol. It does not appear to increase incisional morbidity either. Mean specimen weights, analgesic requirements, duration of hospital stay, and convalescence are similar for intact extraction and morcellation.[6]

Operative Results

Laparoscopic radical nephrectomy is intended to duplicate the excellent results of open surgery. The worldwide experience gives an operative time of 3–5 hours, an average blood loss of 100–300 ml, a conversion rate to open surgery of 0–8.5%, and a complication rate of 8–34%.[7] Several reports comparing laparoscopic radical nephrectomy to open surgery have been published (Table 8b-1).

In 1998, Cadeddu et al. presented the multiinstitutional experience of 157 patients receiving a laparoscopic radical nephrectomy for clinically localized RCC.[8] During a mean follow-up of 19.2 months (range 1–72), there was no local or distant recurrence. The 5-year actuarial disease-free rate was 91%. In 2001, Chan et al. reported their experience on 67 patients with clinically localized RCC undergoing laparoscopic radical nephrectomy. They compared these results with 54 patients who underwent an open nephrectomy.[9] They adopted the transperitoneal approach in 66 patients and morcellated 40 specimens before extraction. The mean tumor size (5.1 cm vs. 5.4 cm) and the mean blood loss (289 ml vs. 309 ml) showed no significant difference. The mean operative time of laparoscopic radical nephrectomy (256 minutes) was significantly longer than that of open radical nephrectomy (193 minutes). Noticeably, there was a significant difference between the operative time of the first 34 and last 33 laparoscopic radical nephrectomies (289 minutes vs. 222 minutes). The hospital stay was shorter in the laparoscopic group (3.8 days vs. 7.2 days). At a mean follow-up of 35.6 months, there was no local or distant tumor recurrence. The 5-year disease-free survival rate for the laparoscopic group vs. the

TABLE 8b-1. Worldwide reports of laparoscopic radical nephrectomy.[a]

Author	Number of patients	Technique	Surgical approach	Mean tumorsize, cm	Follow-upmonths	5-year disease-free survival (%)	5-year recurrence-free survival (%)	Overall survival(%)
Cadeddu et al.[8]	157	LRN	18 Retro 139 Trans	NA	19.2 (mean)	91	NA	NA
Chan et al.[9]	67	LRN	NA	5.1	36.5 (mean)	95	NA	86
	54	ORN		5.4	44 (mean)	86	NA	75
Gill et al.[10]	100	LRN	73 Retro 27 Trans	5.1	16.1 (mean)	NA	NA	NA
Ono et al.[11]	103	LRN	18 Retro 85 Trans	3.1	29 (median)	95	NA	95
	46	ORN		3.3	39 (median)	90	NA	97
Portis et al.[12]	64	LRN	12 Retro 52 Trans	4.3	54 (median)	98	92	81
	49	ORN		6.2	69 (median)	92	91	89

[a] Retro, retroperitoneal; Trans, transperitoneal; NA, not available; LRN, laparoscopic radical nephrectomy; ORN, open radical nephrectomy.

open group was 95% and 86%, respectively. This difference was not statistically significant.

Gill and associates reviewed their single surgeon, single center experience with an initial 100 laparoscopic radical nephrectomies in 2001.[10] They used a retroperitoneal approach in 73 patients and a transperitoneal approach in 27 patients. Comparison was also made with 40 contemporary open procedures. The mean tumor size was 5.1 cm, the mean operative time was 2.8 hours, the blood loss was 212 ml, and the hospital stay was 1.6 days. There were two conversions. The complication rate was 14%. At a mean follow-up of 16.1 months, there was no local recurrence, but there were two distant metastases. All surgical margins were negative for tumor. There was no significant difference in the preoperative radiological and postoperative histopathological parameters between the open and the laparoscopic group.

Ono and colleagues reviewed their experience with laparoscopic radical nephrectomy in patients with a renal tumor less than 5 cm.[11] Of the 149 patients, 103 were treated laparoscopically and 46 underwent open surgery. The median follow-up was 29 months (range 3–95 months) for the laparoscopic patients. There was no port site seeding but one local recurrence and three metastasis. The 5-year disease-free and patient survival rates were 95.1%, and 95.0%, respectively. Of the 46 patients who received open surgery, 44 were followed from 11 to 101 months (median 39). The 5-year disease-free and patient survival rates were 89.7% and 95.6%, respectively.

In 2002, Portis et al. reported the long-term results of three centers that performed laparoscopic radical nephrectomy for 64 patients with clinical T1, T2 RCC before 1996.[12]

Sixty-nine patients with RCC treated with open radical nephrectomy were compared with this group. A transperitoneal approach was used in 52 patients and retroperitoneal approach in 12 patients. The specimens were removed intact in 39; 25 were morcellated. At a median follow-up of 54 months (range 0–94 months) in the laparoscopic group and 69 months (range 8–114 months) in the open group, the Kaplan–Meier 5-year recurrence-free survival rate was 92% and 91%, the 5-years cancer specific survival was 98% and 92%, and the nonspecific survival was 81% and 89% for the two groups, respectively. The long-term oncological effectiveness was equivalent in the two groups.

Conclusions

It has been more than 10 years since the initial laparoscopic nephrectomy was reported by Clayman et al.[2] With the improvement of laparoscopic instruments and techniques, the worldwide experience has grown and matured rapidly. Currently, there are at least 6000 patients with RCC who have been treated with a laparoscopic radical nephrectomy. The long-term oncological results are comparable to those of open surgery. The gold standard in treating organ-confined RCC has shifted from open radical nephrectomy to laparoscopic radical nephrectomy in patients for whom nephron-sparing surgery is not possible. The place of laparoscopy in advanced stage disease is less clear at the moment.

References

1. Robson CJ, Churchill BM, Anderson W: The results of radical nephrectomy for renal cell carcinoma. J Urol, 101: 297–301, 1969.
2. Clayman RV, Kavoussi LR, Soper NJ, Dierks SM, Meretyk S, Darcy MD, Roemer FD, Pingleton ED, Thomson PG, Long SR: Laparoscopic nephrectomy: initial case report. J Urol, 146: 278–282, 1991.
3. Walther MM, Lune JC, Libutti SK, Linehan WM: Laparoscopic cytoreductive nephrectomy as preparation for administration of systemic interleukin-2 in the treatment of metastatic renal cell carcinoma: a pilot study. Urology, 53: 496–501, 1999.
4. Steinberg AP, Finelli A, Desai MM, Abreu SC, Ramani AP, Spaliviero M, Rybicki L, Kaouk JH, Novick AC, Gill IS: Laparoscopic radical nephrectomy for large (greater than 7cm, T2) renal tumors. J Urol, 172: 2172–2176, 2004.

5. Desai MM, Gill IS, Ramani AP, Matin SF, Kaouk JH, Campero JM: Laparoscopic radical nephrectomy for cancer with level I renal vein involvement. J Urol, 169: 487–491, 2003.

6. Novick AC: Laparoscopic radical nephrectomy: specimen extraction. BJU Int, 95(Suppl 2):32–33, 2005.

7. Ono Y, Hattori R, Gotoh M, Yoshino Y, Yoshikawa Y, Kamihira O: Laparoscopic radical nephrectomy for renal cell carcinoma: the standard of care already? Curr Opin Urol, 15: 75–78, 2005.

8. Cadeddu JA, Ono Y, Clayman RV, Barrett PH, Janetschek G, Fentie DD, Mcdougall EM, Moore RG, Kinukawa T, Elbahnasy AM, Nelson JB, Kavoussi LR. Laparoscopic nephrectomy for renal cell cancer: evaluation of efficacy and safety: a multicenter experience. Urology, 52: 773–777, 1998.

9. Chan DY, Cadeddu JA, Jarrett TW, Marshall FF, Kavoussi LR. Laparoscopic radical nephrectomy: cancer control for renal cell carcinoma. J Urol, 166: 2095–2100, 2001.

10. Gill IS, Meraney AM, Schweizer DK, Savage SS, Hobart MG, Sung GT, Nelson D, Novick AC. Laparoscopic radical nephrectomy in 100 patients. A single center experience from the United States. Cancer, 92: 1843–1855, 2001.

11. Ono Y, Kinukawa T, Hattori R, Gotoh M, Kamihira O, Ohshima S. The long-term outcome of laparoscopic radical nephrectomy for small renal cell carcinoma. J Urol, 165: 1867–1870, 2001.

12. Portis AJ, Yan Y, Landman J, Chen C, Barrett PH, Fentie DD, Ono Y, Mcdougall EM, Clayman RV. Long-term followup after laparoscopic radical nephrectomy. J Urol, 167: 1257–1262, 2002.

8c
Retroperitoneoscopic Radical Nephrectomy

Dogu Teber, Ali S. Gözen, Tibet Erdogru, Marto Sugiono, Michael Schulze, and Jens Rassweiler

Introduction

The reported worldwide steady increase in the incidence of renal cell carcinomas might undoubtedly be a result of the increasing availability of ultrasonography and computer tomography. Because more incidental renal tumors are diagnosed, the profile of patients seeking treatment for renal carcinoma has changed. As a result, different treatment strategies (i.e., high-intensity focus ultrasound, radiofrequency ablation, cryotherapy, radical and partial surgery, laparoscopy) have emerged. Nevertheless, surgical removal is still considered to be the treatment of choice in the management of renal cell carcinoma. During the past decade, however, open surgery has increasingly been replaced by the laparoscopic approach.

Clayman et al. pioneered laparoscopic nephrectomy when they removed a renal oncocytoma in 1990.[10] Almost 1 year later Coptcoat et al. used the same technique for a T2 renal cell carcinoma.[11] In 1992, Chiu et al. reported on laparoscopic nephroureterectomy for malignant disease.[8] These techniques have since developed into one of the most innovative and successful challenges to the conventional gold standard open approach and is currently the preferred option in many urology centers, particularly for T1 tumors (TNM staging, UICC 2002).[1]

It was not until 1992 that Gaur described an atraumatic balloon dilatation technique to expand the retroperitoneum that retroperitoneoscopy became a truly viable approach to treat urological pathology.[16] In 1993, the first series of retroperitoneoscopic nephrectomies was published in the literature with promising perioperative and postoperative results.[16, 24]

Numerous experiences reported worldwide have demonstrated very good surgical and perioperative results with retroperitoneoscopic access that are at least comparable to open surgery,[37] with many results having even better outcomes. In addition, a few published series with long-term follow-up has shown similar oncological results compared to the open counterpart.[14, 37] However, the technique demands adequate surgical skills in laparoscopic urological surgery and

its development will require the implementation of efficient training programs for future generations of urologists.

The basic oncological surgical principles applied for open surgery are exactly the same for laparoscopic surgery. Similarly, the criteria used for diagnosis, staging, follow-up, and general management are identical.

The objective of this communication is therefore to focus more on the technical aspects of surgery than on the disease itself, presenting a review of the current state of laparoscopic retroperitoneal radical nephrectomy and a description of the surgical technique.

Indications

The indications for a retroperitoneoscopic radical nephrectomy were initially limited to renal tumors smaller than 7 cm. With growing experience the laparoscopic repertoire has expanded to patients with non-organ-confined renal cell carcinoma and invasion of the renal vein. Regarding tumor stage, T1, T2, and T3a-b tumors have all been treated successfully through retroperitoneoscopy.[12, 36, 38, 42]

A relative contraindication is the presence of intense perirenal fibrosis secondary to xanthogranulomatous pyelonephritis or genitourinary tuberculosis. Recent open surgery of the retroperitoneum, percutaneous renal surgery, or renal biopsy does not exclude the retroperitoneoscopic approach.[15, 39, 40]

Retroperitoneal Approach

Patient Preparation

All patients receive preoperative preparations similar to those undergoing open surgery (including informed consent and bowel preparation). Prior to the procedure, a nasogastric tube and urinary catheter are inserted. Under general anesthesia, the patient is placed in the traditional lateral flank position. The table flexed to elevate the uppermost flank and then turned to a more oblique position (Fig 8c-1).

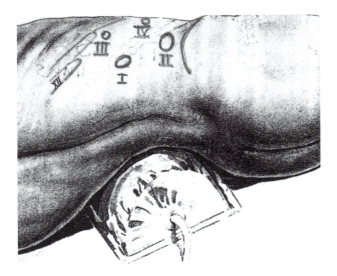

FIGURE 8c-1. Lateral flank position and trocar insertion.

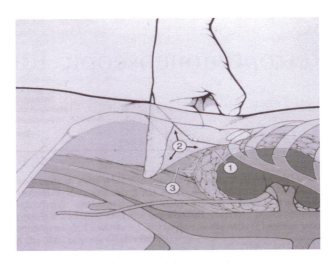

FIGURE 8c-3. Finger dissection of the retroperitoneal space between the lumbodorsal aponeurosis and Gerota's fascia. (1) Perirenal fat; (2) retroperitoneal space; (3) Gerota's fascia.

Access to the Retroperitoneum

A 15- to 18-mm incision is made in the "muscle-free" triangle between the lateral edges of the musculus latissimus dorsi and musculus obliquus externus (Fig 8c-2). A canal down to the

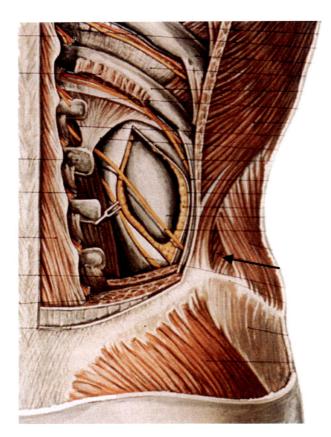

FIGURE 8c-2. "Muscle-free" triangle between M. latissimus dorsi and M. obliquus externus (←).

retroperitoneal space is then created by blunt dissection and then dilated with the index finger, which dissects the plane between the lumbodorsal aponeurosis and Gerota's fascia by pushing the peritoneum medially to create space for the placement of other trocars (Fig 8c-3).

Alternatively, the creation of the retroperitoneal space can be done with commercially available balloon trocars or self-made balloon dilators.

Placement of Secondary Trocars

The next two trocars are placed under direct palpation lateral to the index finger, which is introduced via the primary access.[44] To avoid injury to the surgeon's finger, the canal needs to be dilated using forceps (Fig 8c-4): Port II (11 mm) for the right hand of the surgeon (use of endo-shears and endo-clip applicator) and Port III (5 mm) for the

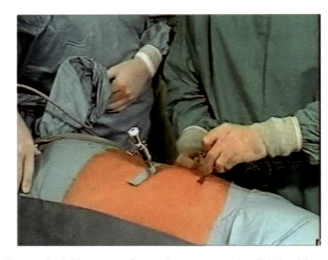

FIGURE 8c-4. Placement of secondary trocars under digital guidance.

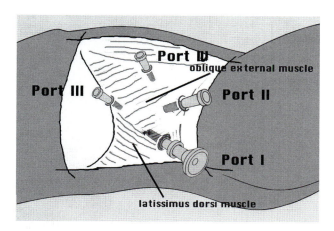

FIGURE 8c-5. Position of trocars, right nephrectomy.

left hand of the surgeon (use of endo-dissect).The trocar site of Port I is then closed with a mattress suture around the sheath to avoid gas leakage and is connected to the CO_2-insufflator to establish a pneumoretroperitoneum (12 mm Hg, 3.5 liters/min).

If necessary, another 5-mm trocar (Port IV) is inserted medially to the edge of the peritoneum under endoscopic view to aid in retraction of the kidney during the dissection (Fig 8c-5). As in the open procedure, the surgeon and the camera-assistant stand on the dorsal side of the patient.

Early Control of the Hilar Vessels

The first step in the retroperitoneal approach is a generous horizontal incision of Gerota's fascia to expose the psoas muscle (Fig 8c-6) up to the diaphragm by blunt and sharp dissection. The carbon dioxide insufflation allows retraction of the peritoneum and exposes all other anatomic landmarks. These are the lumbar ureter, spermatic/ovarian vein, and the lower pole of the kidney.[18,44] It is important for the correct

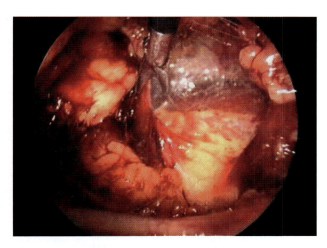

FIGURE 8c-6. Incision of Gerota's fascia and exposure of the psoas muscle.

orientation in the retroperitoneum that the camera always visualizes the psoas muscle absolutely horizontally. A search for vascular pulsations is initiated. Undulating pulsations are characteristic of the inferior vena cava while sharp well-defined pulsations reveal the location of the fat-covered renal artery. The kidney should then be retracted anterolaterally, placing the renal hilum on traction. Alternatively, the ureter can be followed cranially and the surface of the kidney identified and traced medially to its hilum. The renal hilum can be accessed by gentle progression toward the pulsations. This is followed by the dissection of the renal artery using a right-angle forceps. The renal artery is clipped and transected, followed by isolation of the renal vein. Early control of the renal hilum is one of the main advantages of the retroperitoneal approach. Once the vessels are identified and dissected, the clipping and transection are done following the principles of open surgery and starting with the artery (Fig 8c-7).

There are a number of different ligating systems, including the Lapro-Clip® (Tyco-Braun, Ethicon), an absorbable single ligating clip, the Challenger®-titanium-clip (Aesculap), the nonabsorbable lockable plastic Hem-o-lok-clips® (Wick), or the EndoGIA® endoscopic stapling device (Tyco), particularly used for the vein. In most occasions, we prefer titanium clips for the artery (three clips on the stay side) and the Lapro-Clip for the renal vein. We prefer an endoscopic stapler only for larger renal veins (Fig 8c-8). Dissection of the renal vessels is carried out bimanually with endo-shears, -dissector, and right-angle clamp.

Dissection of the Kidney and Ureter

After controlling the hilar vessels, the kidney is freed. The ureter and gonadal vein are dissected, identified, and transected (Fig 8c-9 and 8c-10). When indicated, the adrenal gland is taken en bloc with the specimen, requiring clipping of the adrenal vessels.

Removal of Specimen

Several methods of specimen retrieval have been described.

Morcellation

To extract the specimen, an organ bag (i.e., LapSac) is inserted[41] and pulled out through Port I with the kidney entrapped inside. For morcellation of the specimen, the initial incision is enlarged to 25–30 mm (Fig 8c-11) However, the disadvantages of this technique in terms of potential compromise of oncological safety and loss of histopathological information must be taken into consideration. As such, a mechanical liquidizer, aspirator, or morcellator device is not used for removal of the specimen.[34,41]

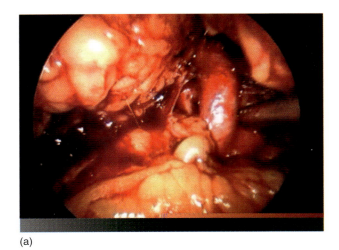

(a)

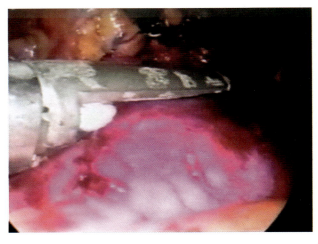

FIGURE 8c-8. Transection of the renal vein with the EndoGIA® stapling device (Tyco).

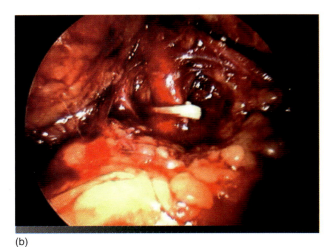

(b)

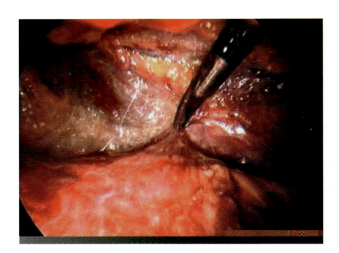

FIGURE 8c-9. Dissection of the medial part of the kidney.

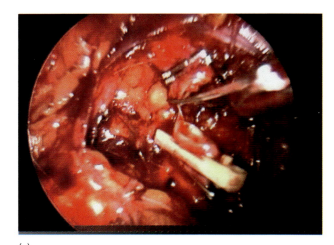

(c)

FIGURE 8c-7. (A) Dissection of the renal artery. (B) Clipping of the artery with the lapro clip (Tyco-Braun). (C) Transection of the renal artery.

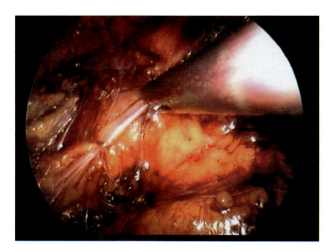

FIGURE 8c-10. Clipping of the ureter before dissection.

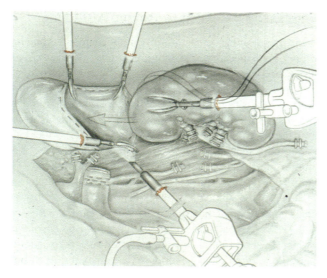

FIGURE 8c-11. Specimen and adequate organ bag.

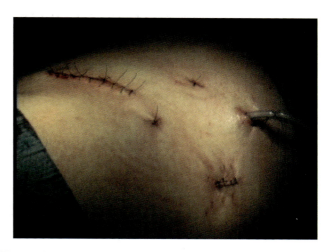

FIGURE 8c-12. Muscle splitting retroperitoneal incision in the lower abdomen for en bloc removal of the specimen (postoperative picture).

Digital Fragmentation

After the Endo-dissector pulls the drawstring thereby closing the bag, the trocar sleeve is removed and the neck of the bag is pulled out over the surface of the abdomen (via Port II for the right kidney and Port III for the left side). The port site is further incised (20 mm) and covered with an adhesive drape making forceps removal of fatty tissue and digital fragmentation of the kidney into three to five pieces possible. This is done very carefully to distinguish between fatty capsule, normal renal tissue, and renal tumor, which was sent separately for histopathological analysis.

Complete Organ Removal

En bloc removal of the specimen is performed via a muscle-splitting retroperitoneal incision in the lower abdomen (Fig 8c-12).

This access can also be used for a hand-assisted laparoscopic approach, particularly toward the end of the procedure. Alternatively, Matins et al. described a modified Pfannenstiel incision with a transverse skin incision (5 cm) over the symphysis pubis and a vertical incision (5 cm) in the anterior rectus fascia near the lateral aspect of the ipsilateral rectus muscle to enable specimen retrieval.[28]

Finally, before all trocars are removed the renal fossa has to be inspected after reducing the pressure to 5 mm Hg to reveal any bleeding. A drainage is used through Port I to permit drainage of fluid, which may reveal postoperative bleeding. The enlarged incision (for organ removal) is closed with fascia and skin suture. All other port incisions are sutured subcutaneously and intracutaneously or covered with adhesive strips.

Single Center Experience with Laparoscopic Radical Nephrectomy

Since 1992, we have performed 100 laparoscopic radical nephrectomies in 98 patients (58 male, 40 female) The retroperitoneal route was used in 80 cases and the transperitoneal route in 20 cases. Seventy-two percent were pT1 tumors, 13% pT2 and 12% pT3, including three with renal oncocytoma and two cases of bilateral renal cell carcinomas in patients on renal dialysis (Table 8c-1).

TABLE 8c-1. Single center experience with laparoscopic radical nephrectomy.

Parameter	Patient numbers ($n = 100$)
Histology and stage	
Renal cell carcinoma	72
pT1	
pT2	13
pT3a	9
pT3b	3
Oncocytoma	3
Perioperative data	
Specimen retrieval Morcellation	28
Intact	72
Complications Intraoperative bleeding	2
Pulmonary embolism	1
Ileal stenosis	1
Secondary bleeding	1
Follow-up Mean time	75 months (range 36–85 months)
Disease-specific deaths	6 (6%)
Deaths from other causes	2 (2%)
Overall survival (5 years)	92 (92%)
Disease-specific survival (5 years)	94 (94%)
pT1/pT2	96 (96%)
pT3	75 (75%)

Perioperative Data

The mean operating time was 135 (90–410) minutes, with no difference between the transperitoneal and retroperitoneal groups. Mean blood loss was 140 ml (range 100–700 ml) and there was no conversion to open surgery despite two cases of significant intraoperative bleeding. One of these was from the spleen and was managed by laparoscopic tamponading using hemostatic gauze (Tachotamp®, Ethicon, Norderstedt). The other patient bled from a port site postoperatively and required a transcutaneous stitch. He later developed a stenosis at the terminal ileum possibly related to the aforementioned suture, but was treated successfully by segmental ileal resection.

Other major complications included one pulmonary embolism (PE) managed conservatively and another requiring reintervention for secondary bleeding postoperatively. The mean postoperative hospital stay was 7 (4–16) days, although the policy of the German health insurance system is partly responsible for this.

Pathology

The mean tumor size was 5.1 cm (range 0.5–8) with upper, central, and lower pole tumors occurring in 34%, 43%, and 23% of patients, respectively. The surgical margins were negative in all cases.

Follow-up Data

At a mean follow up of 75 months (36–85 months), no port-site metastasis was observed. One patient with a pT2G2 tumor developed a local recurrence and bone metastases 4 years later and died 56 months after the procedure. Another five patients with pT1G3 ($n=1$), pT2G3 ($n=1$), pT3aG3 ($n=2$), and pT3b ($n=1$) tumor developed pulmonary and bony metastases and died 34 months after surgery. The cumulative overall disease-free survival rate after 5 years was 94%, revealing 96% for pT1/pT2 and 75% for pT3 tumors (Table 8c-1).

Complications and Their Management in Laparoscopic Retroperitoneal Radical Nephrectomy

The complications unique to laparoscopy include those related to patient positioning, access (insertion of trocars, creation of the pneumoretroperitoneum), and the anatomical dissection. Documented complications were vascular (1.7%) and visceral (0.25%) injuries followed by complications of healing and infection.[4,32]

Complications Related to Patient Positioning

Patient positioning is of utmost importance to preclude postoperative neurological complications. Neuromuscular injuries are rare, but contribute significantly to patients' morbidity. All body prominences should be padded in order to minimize positional pressure, especially on the axilla, legs, and arms.[19] In a multicenter study with 1651 patients undergoing urological laparoscopic procedures a 2.7% incidence of neuromuscular injuries was reported. These were more common during upper retroperitoneal procedures (3.1%) than in pelvic laparoscopy (1.5%). Rhabdomyolysis occurred in 0.4% of the patients who underwent upper retroperitoneal laparoscopy. In particular, those with small body habitus or obese patients are at risk. It should be considered postoperatively in cases of extensive muscle pain and low urine output. Treatment is supportive, consisting of volume expansion, alkalinization, and diuretics. In cases of acute renal failure a nephrology consultation and dialysis may be required.

Complications Related to Access

The retroperitoneoscopic access is rarely associated with complications during trocar insertion, especially if it is done under manual guidance with or without the help of a balloon dilator. This allows the peritoneum to be pushed away before inserting the trocar. When using a balloon care must be taken at the stage of placement. Placements in the abdominal wall musculature may result in severe abdominal wall hemorrhage and postoperative hernia.[18,25]

Either with a balloon dilator or during blunt finger dissection it is of importance to avoid a peritoneal tear when inserting the ports. If a tear occurs, the retroperitoneal space narrows and the preoperative exposure of the working area is compromised. This problem can be managed by inserting another trocar to retract the peritoneum or by inserting an intravenous cannula into the peritoneum to vent the CO_2 and reduce the intraperitoneal pressure. Another option is widening the tear intentionally to equalize the pressure.[25]

One of the typical problems of retroperitoneoscopy is the development of a subcutaneous emphysema caused by the leakage of CO_2 from the port sites.

Retroperitoneally insufflated CO_2 can dissect along the natural musculofascial planes up to the neck and allow CO_2 to enter the superior mediastinum and apical pleural space. This complication was reported in five patients (2.5%) during 200 retroperitoneoscopies but resolved spontaneously within 24 hours.[40] There are only casuistic reports in the literature after CO_2 entry into the pleural cavity, resulting in a formation of a pneumothorax that needed further intervention.[2,25]

To avoid this problem only small incisions should be made without creating any plane between skin, subcutaneous tissue, and muscle. Sutures should be placed through all layers of the abdominal wall to fix the port cannula.[25]

Complications During Dissection

Vascular and bowel injuries constitute most of the major complications encountered during retroperitoneoscopic surgery.

In a recent analysis of retroperitoneoscopic procedures, the incidences of vascular and bowel complications were 1.7% and 0.25%, respectively.[32]

Injuries of minor vascular structures (gonadal vessels, lumbar vessels) can be successfully managed laparoscopically.

Increasing the pressure to 20 mm Hg also helps to tamponade small bleeding vessels. This can help the surgeon to gain some time before the final control of the bleeding.

Injuries of vascular structures mostly require conversion to open surgery.

This should be optimally managed by definite steps, which include laparoscopic assistance until the abdomen is opened. Most important before opening the patient is to tamponade the bleeding by a grasping forceps, which can also serve as a guide for the surgeon to identify the injury in the open setting. The skin, subcutaneous fat, and muscles can be incised directly over the laparoscope, which can be torqued toward the abdominal wall.[19,43,45]

A meticulous complete dissection of the renal hilum is crucial. The renal artery should be clearly separated from the renal vein.

This avoids complications such as that reported by McAllister et al.[29] in which the vena cava was transected during retroperitoneoscopic nephrectomy. In the published two cases of this group the vena cava was misidentified as the renal vein.

Other vascular injuries may occur during the simultaneous ligation of the artery and vein with a GIA stapler in order to gain time. It may result in acute bleeding or a delayed arteriovenous fistula and is recommended only in very selected cases. It is essential to inspect the operative site with the pressure reduced to 5 mm Hg to reveal any venous bleedings.

Although the rate of bowel injuries is low in the published literature, when choosing a retroperitoneal access, the intraperitoneal visceral structures are in the immediate vicinity covered only by a thin peritoneal membrane. The fact that intraperitoneal structures are out of direct sight is undoubtedly a positive aspect of retroperitoneoscopy. But this can also elevate the potential risk for bowel injuries, especially if monopolar coagulation near the peritoneum is used for the ventral mobilization of the kidney.[19,21] This should be kept in mind during mobilization of the kidney in the small retroperitoneal space. Sharp or thermal injuries to other retroperitoneal visceral structures, such as the pancreas, ascending colon, and descending colon, are reported with low incidence in the literature.

In summary, laparoscopic retroperitoneoscopic nephrectomy for the treatment of renal cell carcinoma can be performed with acceptable morbidity.

Complications that are unique to laparoscopy exist, but they decrease with growing experience. Rassweiler et al. report that the incidence of complications decreases after approximately 30–50 procedures.[40,46,47] The increased experience not only avoids the incidence of complications but also changes the approach to their management. Most complications could be solved laparoscopically in the recent literature.[13] This is reflected by the decreasing incidence of conversion rates from 28% to almost zero in current studies.[5,13,20,39]

Discussion

Laparoscopic radical nephrectomy has largely overtaken traditional surgery in many centers (Tables 8c-2 and 8c-3). Beyond the discussion of access (retroperitoneal or transperitoneal) the review of the literature documents the perioperative benefits of laparoscopy.

In a multicenter study, Ono et al.[36] compared 103 patients operated by laparoscopy (85 transperitoneal and 18 retroperitoneal) with 46 operated by the classic open procedure. The mean blood loss was 254 ml vs. 465 ml, with a transfusion rate of 5% vs. 9%, respectively, for the two groups (Tables 8c-2 and 8c-3).

Gill et al.[21] compared retrospectively 34 patients operated laparoscopically using a retroperitoneal approach with 34 patients who underwent traditional open methods. They found a mean blood loss of 97.4 ml versus 295.1 ml and a complication rate of 13% vs. 24% in comparable cases (Table 8c-2).

The mean operating time initially reported to be in the range of 240 minutes decreased in recent publications to 150 minutes (Tables 8c-2 and 8c-3). We made the same observation, emphasizing the importance of the learning curve to achieve comparable or better operating times than the open approach.[14,21,22] A major key to that problem is that the same experienced laparoscopic team treats all cases. Dunn et al. reported a decrease in the operating time by nearly 50% comparing the first 10 and the last 10 patients who underwent a laparoscopic radical nephrectomy in the same institution.[14]

As far as the duration of the hospital stay was concerned, different authors described a significant advantage of laparoscopy: Gill et al.[21] 1.4 vs. 5.8 days, Abbou et al.[1] 4.8 vs. 9.7 days.

The comparison of complication rate, length of hospital stay, blood loss, and a decreasing operating time confirms significantly lower perioperative morbidity (Table 8c-2).

More than 10 years after its first description, the technique of retroperitoneal laparoscopic radical nephrectomy has been standardized fulfilling the principles of a nontouch minimally invasive urooncological surgery. Various series have proposed the retroperitoneal approach, advocating the advantage of earlier control of the renal artery and the reduced need of dissection (i.e., deflection of the colon).[1,20,40]

TABLE 8c-2. Laparoscopic (Lap) versus open (Op) radical nephrectomy: review of the literature.

Criteria	Abbou[1]		Ono[36]		Gill[21]		Jeschke[23]	
	Lap	Op	Lap	Op	Lap	Op	Lap	Op
Patients (n)	29	29	103	46	34	34	31	34
Tumor size (cm)	5.7	3.1	3.3	5.0	6.1	3.8	5.7	4.1
OR time (minutes)	121	282	198	186	174	125	145	145
Blood loss (ml)	285	254	465	98	370	n.a.	n.a	100
Complication (%)	27	n.a.	n.a	13	24	n.a.	n.a	7
Hospital stay (days)	9.7	n.a.	n.a.	1.4	5.8	6.8	11.5	4.8
Follow-up (months)	13	29	39	10	29	n.a.	n.a.	15

TABLE 8c-3. Worldwide experience of laparoscopic radical nephrectomy: perioperative data.

(a) Overall combined transperitoneal and retroperitoneal radical nephrectomy data

Author	Patients (n)	Operative time (hours)	Blood loss (ml)	Complication rate		Conversion	Hospital stay (days)
				Minor	Major		
Barrett[3]	72	2.9	–	3%	8%	8%	4.4
Abbou[1]	29	2.4	100	8%	3.4%	4.8	
Dunn[14]	60	5.5	172	34%	3%	1.6%	3.4
Ono[36]	103	4.7	254	3%	10%	3.4%	–
Chan[7]	67	4.2	289	15%	1.5%	3.8	
Gill[21]	100	2.8	212	11%	3%	2%	1.6
Janetschek[22]	121	2.4	154	5%	4%	0%	6.1
Rassweiler[a]	100	2.2	135	5.0%		0%	7

[a]Present series.

(b) Results of radical nephrectomy in the literature: categorized into transperitoneal and retroperitoneal groups

Author	Year	Total patients	Operative time (hours)	Blood loss (ml)	Complications (%)		Open conversation (%)
					Minor	Major	
Transperitoneal							
Barrett et al.[3]	1998	72	2.9	–	3	8	8
Ono et al.[36]	1999	60	5.2	255	5	8	3
Dunn et al.[14]	1999	61	5.5	172	48	5	–
Janetschek[22]	2000	73	2.4	170	8	4	4
Nambirajan[35]	2004	20	3,0	179	10	0	0
Desai[13]	2005	50	3.4	180	6	3	0
Rassweiler[a]	2005	20	2,7	200	3	1	0
Retroperitoneal							
Ono[36]	1999	14	4.9	285	7	7	0
Abbou[1]	1999	29	2.4	100			0
Nambirajan[35]	2004	20	3,2	208	0	5	
Desai[13]	2005	52	2.5	242	2	4	0
Rassweiler[a]	2005	80	2,0	120	2	0	0

[a] Present series.

In two prospective randomized comparisons of transperitoneal versus retroperitoneal radical nephrectomies Nambirajan et al.[35] and Desai et al.[13] indicated no statistical difference in the overall operative morbidity. Both approaches were similar in terms of blood loss, intraoperative and postoperative complications, length of hospital stay, and analgesia requirements. Nevertheless, it is remarkable that the retroperitoneal group, compared to the transperitoneal approach, was associated with a shorter total OR time (150 vs. 270 minutes, $p = 0.001$), quicker time to control the renal artery (34 vs. 91 minutes, $p <0.0001$), and quicker control of the renal vein (45 vs. 98 minutes, $p <0.0001$; Table 8c-3b).

The reproducibility of the procedure has been documented in multicenter studies,[5,39] as well as in a review of the

TABLE 8c-4. Worldwide experience with laparoscopic radical nephrectomy: oncological aspects.

Author	Patient (n)	Specimen removal	pT stage	Surgical margin	Follow-up (months)	Recurrenceport site/local/distant (%)	5-year survival
Janetschek[22]	73	Intact	T1–T3a	Negative	13.3	0/0/ 0	n.a.
Abbou[1]	41	Intact	T1–T3b	Negative	24.7	0/2/0	n.a.
Ono[36]	103	Morcellated and intact	–	–	29	0/1/3	92%
Chan[7]	67	Morcellated and intact	T1–T3b	Negative	35.7	0/0/3	n.a.
Gill[20]	100	Intact	T1–T3b	Negative	16.1	0/0/2	n.a.
Portis[37]	64	Morcellated and intact	T1–T3b	Negative	54	0/1/2	
Rassweiler[a]	100	Morcellated and intact	T1–T3b	Negative	75	0/2/4	92%

[a]Present series.

literature. The complication rate is acceptable and still decreasing; the operative time exceeds that of open surgery (140–150 minutes) by about 60–100 minutes. The retrieval of the specimen is accomplished mostly by a small incision after entrapment in an organ bag rather than by morcellation.

This incision has been used earlier during the procedure to perform hand-assisted laparoscopy. This would speed up the procedure and reduce the learning curve.[3,46,47] According to our own early experience, we could reduce the operative time by about 60 minutes.[40,46,47] However, standardization of the use of hand assistance proved to be very difficult, particularly because the surgeon has to insert different hands for left- and right-sided radical nephrectomies. With the interest of a standard training program of laparoscopy and retroperitoneoscopy in urology, we feel that hand assistance should be limited to manage problematic situations only.

Much more important than technical feasibility of the retroperitoneoscopic radical nephrectomy is the long-term outcome (Table 8c-4). It has to be noted that all studies limited the range of indications to clinical stage T1. However, as in our series, histopathology also revealed pT3 tumors among the treated cases.[5,12,30,31,42] This has to be taken into consideration when discussing the long-term results. The overall 5-year disease-free survival rates are excellent ranging between 89% and 96%. The published long-term follow-up by Portis et al. in 2002 (mean follow-up 5 years) confers equivalent long-term results to the traditional open technique.[37] Our own 5-year experience confirms these results (Table 8c-1).

Even after open surgery of clinical T1 tumors, local recurrence as well as distant metastases have been observed.[27,33,34] It must be emphasized that until now, after more than 2000 documented cases, only three port site metastases have been documented (all related to advanced diseases) following laparoscopic radical nephrectomy for renal cell cancer.[3,6] The need for intact specimen removal is still discussed controversially, although there is no difference in morbidity and oncological outcome as reported recently.[9,26] Therefore morcellation can be safely done without compromising survival,[17] although the risk of understaging the tumor on preoperative computed tomography (CT) scan must be borne in mind.

In conclusion, despite some technical modifications by the different groups, retroperitoneoscopic radical nephrectomy can be regarded as a standardized and safe procedure. We are now able to perform an oncologically adequate procedure, with negative tumor margins achieved in all cases. Ideal indications are small tumors (T1) that are not candidates for nephron-sparing surgery. The complication rates are acceptable and still decreasing. The long-term results are excellent and are similar to the results of open surgery.

References

1. Abbou CC, Cicco A, Gasman D et al. Retroperitoneal laparoscopic versus open radical nephrectomy. J Urol 1999;161:1776–1780.
2. Abreu SC, Sharp DS, Ramani AP et al. Thoracic complications during urological laparoscopy. J Urol 2004;171:1451–1455.
3. Barrett PH, Fentie DD, Taranger L. Laparoscopic radical nephrectomy with morcellation for renal cell carcinoma: The Saskatoon experience. Urology 1998;52:23–28.
4. Bishoff JT, Allaf ME, Kirkels W et al. Laparoscopic bowel injury: incidence and clinical presentation. J Urol 1999;161:887–891.
5. Cadeddu JA, Ono Y, Clayman RV et al. Laparoscopic nephrectomy for renal cell cancer: evaluation of efficacy and safety: a multicenter experience. Urology 1998;52:773–777.
6. Castilho LN, Fugita OEH, Mitre AI et al. Port site tumor recurrences of renal cell carcinoma after videolaparoscopic radical nephrectomy. J Urol 2001;165:519.
7. Chan DY, Cadeddu JA, Jarret TW et al. Laparoscopic radical nephrectomy: cancer control for renal cell carcinoma. J Urol 2001;166:2095–2100.
8. Chiu AW, Chen MT, Huang WJS et al. Laparoscopic nephroureterectomy and endoscopic incision of bladder cuff. Min Inv Ther 1992;1:299–303.
9. Cicco A, Salomon L, Hoznek H et al. Carcinological risks and retroperitoneal laparoscopy. Eur Urol 2000;38:606–612.
10. Clayman RV, Kavoussi LR, Soper NJ et al. Laparoscopic nephrectomy: initial case report. J Urol 1991;146:278–282.
11. Coptcoat MJ, Ison KT, Wickham JEA. Endoscopic tissue liquidization and surgical aspiration. J Endourol 1988;2: 321–329.
12. Desai MM, Gill IS, Ramani AP et al. Laparoscopic radical nephrectomy for cancer with level I renal vein involvement. J Urol 2003;169:487–491.

13. Desai MM, Strzempkowski B, Matin SF *et al.* Prospective randomized comparison of transperitoneal versus retroperitoneal laparoscopic radical nephrectomy. *J Urol* 2005;173: 38–41.

14. Dunn MD, Portis AJ, Shalhav AL *et al.* Laparoscopic versus open radical nephrectomy: a 9-year experience. *J Urol* 2000;164:1153–1159.

15. Fahlenkamp D, Rassweiler J, Fornara P *et al.* Complications of laparoscopic procedures in urology: experience with 2,407 procedures at 4 German centers. *J Urol* 1999;162:765–770.

16. Gaur DD, Agarwal DK, Purohit KC. Retroperitoneal laparoscopic nephrectomy: initial case report. *J Urol* 1993;149: 103–105.

17. Gettman MT, Napper C, Spark-Corwin T *et al.* Laparoscopic radical nephrectomy: prospective assessment of impact of intact versus fragmented specimen removal on postoperative quality of life. *J Endure* 2002;1:23–25.

18. Gill IS, Rassweiler JJ. Retroperitoneoscopic renal surgery: our approach. *Urology* 1999;54:734–738.

19. Gill IS, Kaposi LR, Clayman RV *et al.* Complications of laparoscopic nephrectomy in 185 patients: a multi-institutional review. *J Urol* 1995;154:479–483.

20. Gill IS, Meaner AM, Schweitzer DK et al.: Laparoscopic radical nephrectomy in 100 patients. *Cancer* 2001;92:1843–1855.

21. Gill IS, Schweizer D, Hobart MG *et al.* Retroperitoneal laparoscopic radical nephrectomy: the Cleveland Clinic experience. *J Urol* 2000;163:1665–1670.

22. Janetschek G, Jeschke K, Pechel R *et al.* Laparoscopic surgery for stage T1 renal cell carcinoma: radical nephrectomy and wedge resection. *Eur Urol* 2000;38:131–138.

23. Jeschke K, Wakonig J, Winzely M *et al.* Laparoscopic radical nephrectomy: overcoming the main problems. *BJU* 2000;85:163–165.

24. Kerbl K, Figenshau RS, Clayman RV *et al.* Retroperitoneal laparoscopic nephrectomy: laboratory and clinical experience. *J Endourol* 1993;7:23–26.

25. Kumar M, Kumar R, Hemal AK *et al.* Complications of retroperitoneoscopic surgery at one centre. *BJU Int* 2001;87:607–612.

26. Landman J, Lento P, Hassen W *et al.* Feasibility of pathological evaluation of morcellated kidneys after radical nephrectomy. *J Urol* 2001;164:2086–2089.

27. Levy DA, Slaton JW, Swanson DA *et al.* Stage specific guidelines for survival after radical nephrectomy for local renal cell carcinoma. *J Urol* 1998;159:1163–1167.

28. Matin SF, Gill IS. Modified Pfannenstiel incision for intact specimen extraction after retroperitoneoscopic renal surgery. *Urology* 2003;61:830–832.

29. McAllister M, Bhayani SB, Ong A *et al.* Vena caval transection during retroperitoneoscopic nephrectomy: report of the complication and review of the literature. *J Urol* 2004;172:183–185.

30. McDougall EM, Clayman RV, Elashry OM *et al.* Laparoscopic nephroureterectomy for upper tract transitional cell cancer: Washington University experience. *J Urol* 1995;154:975–980.

31. McDougall EM, Clayman RV, Elashry OM *et al.* Laparoscopic radical nephrectomy for renal tumor: The Washington University experience. *J Urol* 1996;155:1180–1185.

32. Meraney AM, Samee AA, Gill IS. Vascular and bowel complications during retroperitoneal laparoscopic surgery. *J Urol* 2002;168:1941–1944.

33. Mickisch G, Tschada R, Rassweiler J *et al.* Das lokale Rezidiv nach Nierentumoroperation. *Akt Urol* 1990;21:77–81.

34. Moch H, Gasser TC, Urrejola C *et al.* Metastastic behavior of renal cell cancer: an analysis of 871 autopsies. *J Urol* 1997;157:66 A (abstract no. 254).

35. Nambirajan T, Jeschke S, Al-Zahrani H *et al.* Prospective, randomized controlled study: transperitoneal laparoscopic versus retroperitoneoscopic radical nephrectomy. *Urology* 2004;64:919–924.

36. Ono Y, Kinukawa T, Hattori R *et al.* The long term outcome of laparoscopic nephrectomy for small renal cell carcinoma. *J Urol* 2001;165:1867–1870.

37. Portis AJ, Yan Y, Landman J *et al.* Long-term follow-up after laparoscopic radical nephrectomy. *J Urol* 2002;167:1257–1262.

38. Rassweiler J, Coptcoat MJ. Laparoscopic surgery of the kidney and adrenal gland. In: Janetschek G, Rassweiler J, Griffith D (eds.): *Laparoscopic Surgery in Urology.* 1996; Thieme, Stuttgart and New York, pp. 139–155.

39. Rassweiler J, Fornara P, Weber M *et al.* Laparoscopic nephrectomy: the experience of the laparoscopic working group of the German Urological Association. *J Urol* 1998;160: 18–21.

40. Rassweiler J, Seemann O, Frede T *et al.* Retroperitoneoscopy: experience with 200 cases. *J Urol* 1998;160:1265–1269.

41. Rassweiler J, Stock C, Frede T *et al.* Organ retrieval systems for endoscopic nephrectomy: a comparative study. *J Endourol* 1998;12:325–333.

42. Savage SJ, Gill IS. Laparoscopic radical nephrectomy for renal cell carcinoma in a patient with level I renal vein tumor thrombus. *J Urol* 2000;163:1243–1244.

43. Simon SD, Castle EP, Ferrigni RG *et al.* Complications of laparoscopic nephrectomy: the Mayo clinic experience. *J Urol* 2004;171:1447–1450.

44. Sung GT, Gill IS. Anatomic landmarks and time management during retroperitoneoscopic radical nephrectomy. *J Endourol* 2002;16:165–169.

45. Swanson DA, Borges PM. Complications of transabdominal radical nephrectomy for renal cell carcinoma. *J Urol* 1983;129:704–707.

46. Tschada RK, Henkel TO, Seemann O *et al.* First experiences with laparoscopic radical nephrectomy. *J Endourol* 1994;8:S80 (abstract no. P1–68).

47. Tschada RK, Rassweiler JJ, Schmeller N *et al.* Laparoscopic radical nephrectomy—the German experience. *J Urol* 1995;153:479 A (abstract no. 1003).

48. Wolf S, Moon TD, Madisom WI *et al.* Hand-assisted laparoscopic nephrectomy: comparison to standard laparoscopic nephrectomy. *J Urol* 1998;160:22–27.

8d
Radical Nephrectomy: Lymph Node Dissection

Alexander Roosen, Elmar W. Gerharz, and Hubertus Riedmiller

Introduction

When Alice E. Parker[26] of Denver injected Baum's modification of Gerota's Prussian blue dye into the renal parenchyma of stillborn fetuses and adult cadavers in 1934 to study "*the main posterior lymph channels of the abdomen and their connections with the lymphatics of the genitourinary system*" she provided the anatomical basis for a debate that started several decades later and has continued for nearly half a century now: Although retroperitoneal lymph node dissection (LND) may provide more accurate pathological staging in the surgical management of renal cell cancer (RCC), the independent value of extended LND for all patients with RCC remains a highly controversial issue among urologists. While Robson's original description of radical nephrectomy (RN) as the "gold standard" in the curative treatment of localized RCC included excision of the perinephric tissue, adrenalectomy, and "complete regional" lymphadenectomy (from the diaphragm to the aortic bifurcation),[30] the therapeutic efficacy of the latter has been questioned repeatedly over time. Given the strong prognostic value of nodal status, one might expect a consensus for routine LND for this malignancy. In reality, RCC is the opposite extreme of testes cancer, where the pattern of lymphatic spread tends to be reliable, a beneficial effect of LND is proven, and the indications for LND are well defined.

Significant advances in the diagnosis, staging, and treatment of patients with RCC during the past 20 years have not only resulted in improved survival of a select group of patients and an overall change in the natural history of the disease, but also altered the philosophical framework for the discussion regarding LND.[20,28] Therefore, the role of LND must be critically reappraised in light of the steady increase in incidental detection of asymptomatic renal masses, the consecutive stage migration, and the shift toward nephron-sparing surgery (NSS) and minimally invasive tissue ablative technology.

Potential benefits to performing LND at the time of RN include more accurate pathological staging, removal of micrometastases, a lower risk of positive margins due to a more extensive dissection of perinephric tissue (leading to a lower risk of local recurrence), reduction of locoregional complications, cure in a select group of patients with metastatic disease limited to the resected nodes, and improved likelihood of a favorable response to systemic therapy in the setting of cytoreduction in advanced disease.[20]

The two subsequent key questions are whether there is any clinically relevant benefit of knowing lymph node metastasis (*diagnostic value*) and of the removal of lymph node metastasis (*therapeutic value*).

This chapter examines the current indications and scope of LND in the surgical treatment of patients with RCC.

Evidence-Based Medicine

"A formal lymph node dissection is a valuable diagnostic tool (staging); however, therapeutic efficacy is unproven." This short but concise statement from the European Association of Urology (EAU) "Guidelines on renal cell cancer"[22] clearly reflects the notion that the existing data regarding LND in the surgical management of RCC is rather extensive but generally of poor quality. Only **one** prospective randomized trial exists in the field achieving an evidence level better that III (European Organization for the Research and Treatment of Cancer Genitourinary Group, protocol 30881). However, the study has not yet matured sufficiently to guide clinical decision making.[5] All other investigations are retrospective in nature with the well-known weaknesses of this approach including unknown confounding factors, missing data, and selection bias. Most case series were single institutional, with extremely heterogeneous study cohorts and changing surgical concepts and staging modalities within the study period.

However, there are two major obstacles to a meaningful analysis of the available historic data, making comparison between different studies difficult, if not impossible. First, different tumour classifications have been used over time. Until the 1990s Robson's staging criteria were the most commonly applied system.[30] In this system renal vein thrombus and regional lymph node metastases were grouped in the same stage interfering with accurate risk stratification of data from that period. It was then gradually replaced by the TNM system.[2] In 1997, the TNM system was revised with a new definition of T1 and T2 stages.[35] As the TNM classification allows a more accurate description of lymph node involvement, contemporary studies may provide more valid information regarding the management of node-positive disease.

Second, LND in the setting of RCC is far from being a standardized procedure, resulting in a confusing terminology. Without an explanatory adjective the term as such is next to useless. Authors have used *limited, confined, Hilary, regional, extended regional, extended, complete, full, systematic,* and *facultative* in a variable fashion to specify the extent of their LND. While the lack of standardized template-based dissections must be seen as a deficiency, the data from the National Surveillance, Epidemiology, and End Results database may at least be representative of the actual clinical practice.[19] This study draws from a large population base with different surgeons adopting different surgical techniques and embracing individual definitions of LND for RCC. Thus, a crucial prerequisite of performing randomized multicenter trials of LND in the future is a universally agreed upon definition of lymphadenectomy ensuring that the quality of dissection can be reliably reproduced.

Retroperitoneal Lymphatic Anatomy and Metastatic Spread

Parker studied the main posterior lymph channels of the abdomen. She demonstrated that the lymph drainage of normal renal parenchyma proceeded along three main vertical parallel lymphatic columns (left lateral lumbar, interaortocaval, lateral caval) (Figs. 8d-1 and 8d-2) functionally linked together by preaortic, postaortic, precaval, postcaval, and sacral promontory groups of lymph nodes. While the right kidney drained to the precaval, postcaval, and interaortocaval nodes, primary sites of drainage for the left kidney were the paraaortic, preaortic, and postaortic nodes. Although these lymphatic routes were consistently observed in most specimens, many unexpected bypasses were noted.[26]

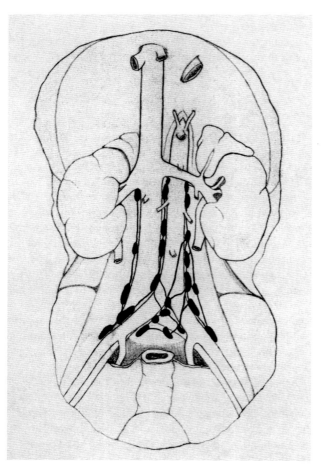

FIGURE 8d-1. Semidiagram that shows corresponding vertical right and left lateral lumbar lymph channels. In the original nomenclature, the right lateral lumbar channels were named interaorticocaval and lateral caval lymph channels. (From Parker, 1935.)

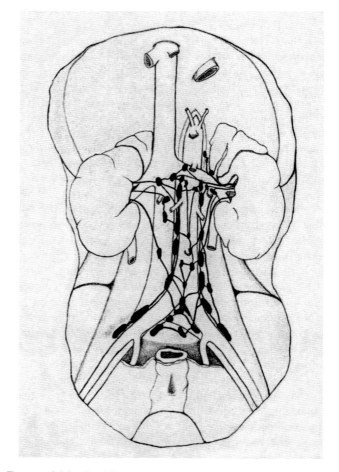

FIGURE 8d-2. Semidiagram that shows the left lateral lumbar and interaorticocaval lymph channels and the preaortic, precaval, and sacral promontory groups of lymph nodes. (From: Parker, 1935.)

While studies of normal anatomy are critical in understanding the physiological lymphatic drainage, malignant disease may distort topography significantly, establishing patterns of metastasis that are virtually unpredictable. The latter may explain the occasionally striking discrepancies between Parker's classic study and the distribution of metastases in patients with RCC.[16] As RCC is a highly vascularized solid tumor with the potential to induce angiogenesis and collateral circulation, this may interfere significantly with lymph drainage. When locally advanced tumors invade the perinephric fat, the situation may be completely changed, because there is access to a different drainage system.[28]

The interindividually highly variable distribution pattern of lymph node metastases in RCC has been well documented in numerous surgical and autopsy series. Giuliani et al. studied 200 patients with RCC who had undergone RN and complete regional LND. Hilar nodes were involved in only 33% of all patients with lymph node metastasis. In right-sided tumors, most lymph node metastases were found in the interaortocaval lymph channels (46%). In left-sided RCC, there was an equal distribution of metastases among hilar, postaortic, and paraaortic nodes (40% in each location).[13] Saitoh et al. proved that distant metastasis can occur in the absence of positive regional lymph nodes. In the majority of patients with metastases to one organ only the lymph nodes were skipped altogether, reflecting the significance of hematogenous spread in RCC: only 21 of 148 patients with solitary distant metastasis involved lymph nodes.[31] More important than the poor negative predictive value of hilar or regional LND in the estimation of disease progression is the fact that many patients with positive lymph nodes have bloodborne metastases. Johnson and Hellsten reported 554 cases of RCC that had been diagnosed at autopsy between 1958 and 1982. Distant metastases were revealed in 119 cases (21.5%), including 31 (5.6%) with solitary metastases. Lymphogenous dissemination was detected in 80 cases of which 75 had additional, mostly multifocal metastatic spread. Consequently, lymph node metastases confined to the paracaval and/or paraaortic lymph nodes were noted in only five cases (0.9%). The authors concluded that the therapeutic effect of extensive retroperitoneal LND in association with RN seemed to be low.[18]

Incidence of Lymph Node Metastasis

The overall risk of lymph node metastasis is approximately 20%, ranging from less than 5% to more than 50% in clinical and autopsy series.[24,31,34] The striking disparity in incidence is likely multifactorial. The risk of lymph node involvement varies greatly depending upon patient selection; primary tumor stage and size, renal vein involvement, the presence of metastases, clinical presentation (symptomatic vs. asymptomatic), and extent of LND performed.[28]

In their attempt to develop a protocol for the selective use of extended LND Blute et al.[6] determined the *primary pathological features* of clear cell RCC that are predictive of positive regional lymph nodes at RN. They studied 1652 patients who underwent RN for unilateral pM0 sporadic RCC between 1970 and 2000. A multivariate logistic regression model was used to determine the pathological features of the primary tumor that were associated with positive regional lymph nodes at RN. There were 887 (54%) patients with no positive nodes (pN0), 57 (3%) with one positive node (pN1), 11 (1%) with two or more positive nodes (pN2), and 697 (42%) who did not have any lymph nodes dissected (pNx). Nuclear grade 3 or 4, the presence of a sarcomatoid component, tumor size 10 cm or greater, tumor stage pT3 or pT4, and histological tumor necrosis were significantly associated with positive regional lymph nodes in a multivariate setting. These features can be used to identify candidates for extended lymph node dissection at the time of RN. For example, only 6 (0.6%) of the 1031 patients with none or one of these features had positive lymph nodes at RN compared with 62 (10%) of the 621 patients with at least two of these features.

There is a correlation between the incidence of lymph node metastasis and the *extent of LND*. While the rate of lymph node metastasis was reported as low as 5–8.8% when hilar or regional LND was perfomed,[24,33] formal extended LND increased the yield to 38%.[32] Sigel et al. compared different retroperitoneal LND techniques, reporting positive lymph nodes in 4% of patients undergoing translumbar nephrectomy without LND, in 14% of patients undergoing transperitoneal nephrectomy without LND, and in 38% of patients undergoing transperitoneal nephrectomy with LND.[32] Herrlinger et al.[15] observed a 7.5% difference in lymph node involvement between complete lymph node dissection and facultative dissection for gross disease.

Terrone et al. showed that the *number of removed lymph nodes* correlated directly with the likelihood of lymph node metastasis. In a subset of patients with clinically organ-confined disease, patients with less than 13 nodes recovered had a 3.4% risk of being staged node positive, whereas patients with more than 13 nodes recovered had a 10.5% risk of lymph node involvement.[37]

The incidence of lymph node metastases increases with the *stage of the tumor*. Giuliani et al. found a 6% incidence of lymph node involvement in tumors confined to the kidney, a 46.4% incidence in locally advanced tumors, a 61.9% incidence in patients with distant metastases, and a 66.6% incidence in patients with both vascular infiltration and distant metastases.[13] In the contemporary UCLA series, 28% of 661 individuals undergoing RN were found to have lymph node metastases. The likelihood of isolated lymph node involvement increased with local tumor stage staging from 2% among T1M0 patients to 3% among T2M0 patients to 20% among T3/4M0 patients (1997 UICC TNM classification).[25]

Prognostic Value of Lymph Node Metastasis in Renal Cell Cancer

Although the value of LND in treating RCC is debated, there is no doubt as to its prognostic role. Lymph node metastasis is well established as an adverse prognostic factor for RCC.[14,20,22] Life expectancy decreases considerably when lymph node metastases are present, with overall 5- and 10-year survival rates of 5–30% and 0–5%, respectively. Nodal involvement not only has a negative impact on the prognosis for patients with otherwise confined disease, but also for patients with distant metastases. In these cases, lymph node metastases are associated with a 2-fold reduction in median survival rates.[5]

Staging

The value of LND cannot be discussed without a thorough consideration of noninvasive staging.[3] In older series using axial computed tomography (CT) scans, the identification of lymph node metastases remained a significant problem since the limiting size was 10 mm.[36] Waters and Richie[39] reported that 30% of patients with "node only" disease (pN+ M0) had microscopic involvement. Studer et al.[36] demonstrated that only 42% of patients with enlarged nodes in preoperative CT had histologically proven metastases, while the incidence of false-negative results was 4.1%. The false-positive rate (58%) was mainly due to inflammatory changes and/or follicular hyperplasia. New technologies such as high-resolution multi-detector CT (MDCT) with thin collimation and multiplanar reformatting might result in a diagnostic improvement, as shown by Catalano et al.[8] Using MDCT, all patients with synchronous lymphadenopathy at the time of RN were identified; the false-positive rate due to reactive hyperplasia was reduced to 6.3%. However, these data have to be confirmed in larger series before MDCT can be recommended as a standard preoperative imaging technique for the clinical staging of RCC. Although the superiority of MRI in the detection of lymph node involvement was suggested in early reports,[11] the role of MRI in the assessment of regional lymph nodes has not been evaluated in large clinical series so that no final recommendation can be made.

Adjuvant Therapy

When assessing lymph node dissection in the staging of RCC, it must be noted that, to date, there is no efficacious adjuvant therapy available for high-risk disease. The use of interleukin-2 (IL-2) in completely resected Tx, N1-2, M0 patients is controversial, but as randomized data failed to show a survival advantage in the adjuvant setting,[1,10] the application of IL-2 in the absence of measurable disease is questionable. Therefore, the presence of lymph node metastases in the absence of distant metastases will likely provide prognostic information or allow risk stratification only in the setting of clinical trials.

Complications

The risk of complications is related to the individual surgeon's skills, experience, and familiarity with retroperitoneal LND, the extent of LND, the extent of lymph node metastasis, and the distortion of the normal anatomy by the disease. Specific LND-related intraoperative complications involve vascular and bowel injuries as well as hepatic and splenic tears.[40] Acute and delayed postoperative complications include lower extremity edema, deep vein thrombosis, hemorrhage, renal failure, adrenal insufficiency, chylous ascites, prolonged ileus, and ischemic colitis.[28]

In the UCLA series, there were no statistically significant differences between patients who did and those who did not undergo LND regarding procedure time, estimated blood loss, transfusion requirements, perioperative complication rates, or length of hospital stay. These observations were basically confirmed by Carmignani et al.[7] and Blom et al. in their prospective randomized Phase III EORTC trial.[5] Surprisingly, Herrlinger et al.[15] observed a lower mortality in patients undergoing extended LND when compared to patients undergoing RN only.

Available data suggest that LND in and of itself does not add significant morbidity and mortality to RN.

Organ-Confined Disease

Since the accuracy of preoperative staging [magnetic resonance imaging (MRI), CT] has improved over the past decades with excellent sensitivity, imaging has become a clinically relevant and reliable alternative to surgical exploration in the $T_{any}N0M0$ scenario. The American College of Radiology considers CT "very appropriate" in the detection of lymph node metastases in patients with RCC.[9] Only 3% of patients whose regional lymph nodes were judged to be negative in CT had histologically proven metastases in the corresponding surgical specimens.[5,24] This clearly demonstrates the limited additional value of (extended) LND in the detection of occult lymphatic disease.

However, the more intriguing question is whether detection and removal of occult lymph nodes (micrometastases) improve the oncological outcome in terms of a survival benefit. Retrospective data in the older literature suggest that there is a decrease in local recurrence for patients who undergo RN plus LND (2.5–8%) versus RN alone (11%).[21,30] However, these studies were performed prior to the widespread use of modern imaging technology and many of these patients were likely understaged. In more recent series, local recurrences are rare even when LND is not performed. Itano et al. reported that an isolated local recurrence occurred in only 1.8% of 1737 patients who underwent RN for T1-3N0M0 RCC.[17] Rassweiler et al. reported a local recurrence rate of 2.2% following laparoscopic RN for localized RCC.[29] At UCLA, the local recurrence rate is approximately 2.8% following RN, and there is no significant difference when patients with and without LND are compared.[25] Similarly, data from the NSS literature demonstrate that the incidence of local recurrence following NSS is generally <3%.[4]

The impact of LND on survival was addressed in several retrospective studies. When comparing complete regional LND to facultative LND, Herrlinger et al. reported an increase in survival rate of patients with pT1-2N0M0 RCC from 81.3% to 91.6% and from 54% to 80.2% after 5 and 10 years, respectively. In patients with pT3aN0M0 tumors survival rate increased from 54.5% to 76% and from 41.2% to 58.2% after 5 and 10 years when RN had been combined with complete LND.[15] The UCLA group detected lymph node metastases in only 10 of 238 clinical N0M0 patients by performing LND. The survival of 257 clinical N0M0 without LND was the same as for the lymphadenectomy group.[25] Among 49 patients without clinical suspicion of nodal disease, Minervini et al. found metastatic spread in 2%. The 5-year survival rate was the same for those patients who had undergone dissection and for those who had not (78% vs. 79%).[24] Similarly, Siminovitch et al.[33] failed to demonstrate statistically significant differences in terms of 2- and 5-year disease-free survival rate when comparing hilar, regional, or extended LND.

The only prospective randomized Phase III trial comparing patients with clinically localized, resectable renal tumors undergoing standardized retroperitoneal LND plus RN with a group not undergoing LND is being conducted by the EORTC (protocol 30881).[5] Of the 772 randomized patients, 3.3% had positive nodes. The overall 5-year survival rate was 82%. Minimal morbidity was associated with LND, but no demonstrable benefit was reported. The final analysis is pending maturation of the survival data, as only 17% of the patients have reached the study endpoint (either progression or death).

Contemporary series suggest that the true incidence of isolated lymph node metastases in clinically localized disease is small, and the location of such metastases is unpredictable. Although anecdotal data exist to both support and refute the value of LND in this setting, the majority of studies suggest that in locally confined disease, regional or extended LND is of no therapeutic benefit. Until randomized data prove the routine use of LND, this procedure should be avoided in these patients. Since T3–4 primary tumors carry a slightly higher risk of lymph node metastases, lymph node dissection may be appropriate in these individuals to increase staging accuracy, especially in clinical trials of adjuvant therapies.

Lymph Node Involvement Without Distant Metastases

In N+M0 ("node only") disease, the primary goal of LND, at least in theory, is complete resection of diseased tissue and cure. However, the proportion of patients that has lymph node involvement only is rather small (4.2–10%) and many patients have occult distant metastatic disease.[13,18,25]

Twenty-five years ago, Peters and Brown[27] compared N+M0 patients undergoing RN and extended LND to patients undergoing RN only. They found an increased survival rate after LND both after 1 year (87.5% vs. 56.5%) and after 5 years (43.75 vs. 25.69%). Ten years later, Giuliani et al. reported a similar survival rate of 52% 5 years after "radical extensive surgery" at the University of Genoa for N+M0 disease in a series of 200 consecutive patients with RCC. Only 10% had positive nodes without distant metastases and/or venous spread of the tumor.[13] When comparing systematic extended to optional LND (removal of grossly involved nodes and nodes for staging purposes only) in the same clinical setting, Herrlinger et al. found significantly higher survival rates only within the first 3 years of follow-up. After 4 and 5 years, the advantage lost its significance.[15] In a series of 328 patients with RCC operated by radical transabdominal nephrectomy with regional LND, survival of the pN+M0 V0 patients was 53.20% at 5 years, 39.10% at 10 years, and 16% at 15 and 20 years. Giberti et al. explained the low impact of nodal involvement on survival by the completeness of lymphadenectomy.

Joslyn et al. recently examined a subset of patients (n = 4453) from the SEER (Surveillance, Epidemiology, and End Results) database who had undergone RN. They identified 876 patients with regional disease who had undergone RN. Regional disease was defined as neoplasms that have extended beyond the limits of the kidney and/or into the regional lymph nodes by the way of the lymphatic system.[19] An inverse correlation was found between the likelihood of cancer-specific survival and the number of nodes examined. Aggressive LND did not affect the likelihood of survival. This was in part explained by the positive correlation between the extent of LND and the presence of positive nodes (i.e., the more aggressive the LND, the greater the number of positive nodes discovered).

As responses to systemic therapy are poor in individuals with lymph node metastases only, and LND does not seem to increase overall surgical morbidity, dissection of all gross nodal disease may be considered under these particular circumstances, as it may impact favorably on the prognosis.

Advanced Disease

While the management of metastatic RCC has historically been mainly surgical, contemporary approaches often incorporate systemic immunotherapy. Cytoreductive surgery prior to immunotherapy appears to confer a survival advantage, but only a subset of patients is suitable for this treatment regimen. Selection of such individuals for surgery relies upon careful assessment of performance status, comorbidities, burden of retroperitoneal disease, and resectability.[28] Primary immunotherapy followed by surgical removal of the tumor in partial responders is an alternative treatment strategy, which has not yet been evaluated in randomized trials. As immunotherapy develops further, the precise timing and role of surgery in multimodality treatment will need to be carefully assessed.

The value of LND in this scenario ($T_{any}N_{any}M+$) is even less well defined than in localized and node only disease. In 1980, Peters and Brown[27] published a study retrospectively comparing 148 patients with lymph node and distant metastases who underwent either RN with regional LND ($n = 23$), RN only ($n = 36$), or no surgery at all ($n = 89$). One-year survival was 81% vs. 47.7% vs. 32.3% and 5-year survival 28.9% vs. 9.1% vs. 11.4%, suggesting a survival benefit in the first group.

The more recent series assess the value of LND in the setting of cytoreduction before systemic immunotherapy. In a retrospective analysis of all patients undergoing cytoreductive nephrectomy at the National Cancer Institute between 1985 and 1996 ($n = 154$), Vasselli et al.[38] observed a close association of lymph node involvement and shorter survival. There were 82 patients with metastatic RCC and no preoperative retroperitoneal lymphadenopathy who survived longer (median 14.7 months) than the 72 with lymphadenopathy (median 8.5 months, $p = 0.0004$). After complete resection of the affected lymph nodes survival was similar to patients without lymphadenopathy. Although LND did not appear to enhance the response to IL-2, the authors suggested a therapeutic role for resection of gross disease.

In a recent analysis of the contemporary UCLA series, Pantuck et al.[38] compared the survival of 129 patients (43 N+M0; 86 N+M+) undergoing either cytoreductive nephrectomy alone ($n = 17$) or in combination with LND ($n = 112$) prior to systemic immunotherapy. They demonstrated that the survival of patients with metastatic disease undergoing cytoreductive nephrectomy was significantly better (approximately 5 months) if simultaneous LND had been performed. There was also a trend toward a higher likelihood of response to systemic immunotherapy among individuals who underwent LND at the time of RN.

In the recent analysis of the SEER database[19] see above), nodal debulking did not affect the probability of cancer-specific survival in patients with distant disease. However, one of the limitations posed by using the SEER data is the lack of information regarding adjuvant immunotherapy.

In patients with positive lymph nodes LND can be associated with improved survival when it is performed in carefully selected patients undergoing cytoreductive nephrectomy and postoperative immunotherapy. As the intent of resection is not curative in this setting, dissection of only grossly enlarged lymph nodes would appear most appropriate.

Conclusions

While LND is an integral part in the therapy of most urological malignancies, there is currently no accepted standard for managing lymph nodes at the time of RN. Decision making is hampered by the lack of high-quality clinical data. While the literature on this issue is rather extensive, there is only one prospective randomized trial with the final analysis still pending. The decision to proceed with LND should be dependent upon the likelihood of lymph node metastases along with the potential clinical relevance of lymph node involvement, balanced against the increase in perioperative risk and the potential prolongation of recovery in the individual case.

With adequate preoperative imaging, the occurrence of unsuspected lymph node involvement will be rare in patients with localized RCC. As formal LND is unlikely to lower the risk of local recurrence or improve survival in this setting it should be avoided outside of clinical trials.

Given the high false-positive rate associated with CT and MRI, LND may be useful for accurately staging patients when lymph nodes are enlarged preoperatively and adjuvant treatment is considered. However, it should be understood that the absence of regional nodal disease by no means rules out the involvement of distant lymph node chains or even occult organ metastases.

Only in a small subset of patients with renal cell cancer regional lymph nodes is affected without clinical evidence of distant metastasis. These patients may potentially be cured by LND and aggressive resection of gross nodal disease with curative intent may be considered in otherwise healthy individuals.

In patients with both nodal and distant metastases, resection of visible gross disease may improve the likelihood of a favorable response to systemic disease.

Therapeutic extended lymphadenectomy in the absence of known lymphadenopathy should be avoided in the absence of randomized data indicating a survival advantage.

References

1. Atzpodien J and the German Cooperative Renal Carcinoma Chemo-Immunotherapy Trials Group (DGCIN) (2005) Adjuvant treatment with interleukin-2- and interferon-alpha2a-based chemoimmunotherapy in renal cell carcinoma post tumour nephrectomy: results of a prospectively randomised trial of the German Cooperative Renal Carcinoma Chemo-Immunotherapy Trials Group. Br J Cancer 92:843–846.
2. Bassil B, Dosoretz DE, Prout GR (1985) Validation of the tumor, nodes and metastasis classification of renal cell carcinoma. J Urol 134:450–454.
3. Bechtold RE, Zagoria RJ (1997) Imaging approach to staging of renal cell carcinoma. Urol Clin N Am 24:507–522.
4. Belldegrun A, Tsui KH, DeKernion JB, Smith RB (1999) Efficacy of nephron-sparing surgery for renal cell carcinoma: analysis based on the new 1997 tumor-node-metastasis staging system. J Clin Oncol 17:2868–2875.

5. Blom JHM, van Poppel H, Marechal JM, Jacqmin D, Sylvester R, Schroeder FH, de Prijck L (1999) Radical nephrectomy with and without lymph node dissection: preliminary results of EORTC randomized phase III protocol 30881. Eur Urol 36:570–575.

6. Blute ML, Leibovich BC, Cheville JC, Lohse CM, Zincke H (2004) A protocol for performing extended lymph node dissection using primary tumor pathological features for patients treated with radical nephrectomy for clear cell renal cell carcinoma. J Urol 172:465–469.

7. Carmignani G, Belgrano E, Puppo P, et al. Lymphadenectomy in renal cancer. Cancer of Prostate and Kidney. Plenum Press: New York, 1983, pp. 645–650.

8. Catalano C, Fraioli F, Laghi A, Napoli A, Pediconi F, Danti M, Passarillo R (2003) High-resolution multidetector CT in the preoperative evaluation of patients with renal cell carcinoma. Am J Roentgenol 180:1271–1277.

9. Choyke PL, Amis ES, Bigongiari LR, Bluth EI, Bush WH, Fritzsche P, Holder L, Newhouse JH, Sandler CM, Segal AJ, Resnick MI, Rutsky EA (2000) Renal cell carcinoma staging. American College of Radiology ACR Appropriateness Criteria. Radiology 215 (supplement):721–725.

10. Clark JI, Atkins MB, Urba WJ (2003) Adjuvant high-dose bolus interleukin-2 for patients with high-risk renal cell carcinoma: a cytokine working group randomized trial. J Clin Oncol 21:3133–3140.

11. Constantinides C, Recker F, Bruehlmann W, Von Schultheiss G, Goebel M, Zollikofer C, Jaeger P, Hauri D (1991) Accuracy of magnetic resonance imaging compared to computerized tomography and renal selected angiography in preoperative staging renal cell carcinoma. Urol Int 47:181–185.

12. Giberti C, Oneto F, Martorana G, Rovida S, Carmignani G (1997) Radical nephrectomy for renal cell carcinoma: long-term results and prognostic factors on a series of 328 cases. Eur Urol 31:40–48.

13. Giuliani L, Giberti C, Martorana G, Rovida S (1990) Radical extensive surgery for renal cell carcinoma: long-term results and prognostic factors. J Urol 143:468–473; discussion 473–474.

14. Golimbu M, Joshi P, SperberA, Tessler A, Al-Askari S, Morales P (1986) Renal cell carcinoma: survival and prognostic factors. Urology 27:291–301.

15. Herrlinger A, Schrott KM, Schott G, Sigel A (1991) What are the benefits of extended dissection of the regional renal lymph nodes in the therapy of renal cell carcinoma? J Urol 146: 1224–1227.

16. Hülten L, Rosenkrantz T, Seeman L, Wahlquist L, Ahren C (1969) Occurrence and localisation of lymph node metastases in renal cell carcinoma. A lymphographic and histopathological investigation in connection with nephrectomy. Scand J Urol Nephrol 3:129–130.

17. Itano NB, Blute ML, Spotts B, Zincke H (2000) Outcome of isolated renal cell carcinoma fossa recurrence after nephrectomy. J Urol 164:322–325.

18. Johnson JA, Hellsten S (1997) Lymphatogenous spread of renal cell carcinoma: an autopsy study. J Urol 157:450–453.

19. Joslyn SA, Sirintrapun SJ, Konety BR (2005) Impact of lymphadenectomy and nodal burden in renal cell carcinoma: retrospective analysis of the National Surveillance, Epidemiology, and End Results database. Urology 65:675–680.

20. Lam JS, Shvarts O, Pantuck AJ (2004) Changing concepts in the surgical management of renal cell carcinoma. Eur Urol 45:692–705.

21. Marshall FF (2005) Lymphadenectomy for renal cell carcinoma. BJU Int 95 (supplement 2):34.

22. Mickisch G, Carballido J, Hellsten S, Schulze H, Mensink H; European Association of Urology (2001) Guidelines on renal cell cancer. Eur Urol 40:252–255.

23. Mickisch GH, Garin A, van Poppel H, de Prijck L, Sylvester R (2001) European Organisation for Research and Treatment of Cancer (EORTC) Genitourinary Group: Radical nephrectomy plus interferon-alfa-based immunotherapy compared with interferon alfa alone in metastatic renal-cell carcinoma: a randomised trial. Lancet 358:966–970.

24. Minervini A, Lilas L, Morelli G, Traversi C, Battaglia S, Cristofani R, Minervini R (2001) Regional lymph node dissection in the treatment of renal cell carcinoma: is it useful in patients with no suspected adenopathy before or during surgery? BJU Int 88:169–172.

25. Pantuck AJ, Zisman A, Dorey F, Chao DH, Han K, Said J, Belldegrun AS, Figlin RA (2003) Renal cell carcinoma with retroperitoneal lymph nodes: role of lymph node dissection. J Urol 169:2067–2083.

26. Parker AE (1935) Studies on the main posterior lymph channels of the abdomen and their connections with the lymphatics of the genito-urinary system. Am J Anat 56:409–442.

27. Peters P, Brown GL (1980) The role of lymphadenectomy in the management of renal cell carcinoma. Urol Clin N Am 7: 705–709.

28. Phillips CK, Taneja SS (2004) The role of lymphadenectomy in the surgical management of renal cell carcinoma. Urol Oncol 22:214–224.

29. Rassweiler J, Tsivian A, Kumar AV, Lymberakis C, Schulze M, Seemann O (2003) Oncological safety of laparoscopic surgery for urological malignancy: experience with more than 1000 operations. J Urol 169:2072–2075.

30. Robson CJ, Churchill BM, Anderson W (1969) The results of radical nephrectomy for renal cell carcinoma. J Urol 101: 297–301.

31. Saitoh H, Nakayama M, Nakamura K, Satoh T (1982) Distant metastases of renal adenocarcinoma in nephrectomized cases. J Urol 127:1092–1095.

32. Sigel A, Chlepas S, Schrott KM, Hermanek P (1981) Die Operation des Nieren-tumors. Chirurg 52:545–553.

33. Siminovitch JP, Montie JE, Straffon RA (1982) Lymphadenectomy in renal adenocarcinoma. J Urol 127: 1090–1091.

34. Skinner DG, Vermillion CD, Colvin RB (1972) The surgical management of renal cell carcinoma. J Urol 107: 705–710.

35. Sobin LH, Wittekind CH, editors. International Union Against Cancer (UICC). TNM Classification of Malignant Tumors, 5th ed. New York: 1997:180–182.

36. Studer UE, Scherz S, Scheidegger J, Kraft R, Sonntag R, Ackermann D, Zingg EJ (1990) Enlargement of regional lymph nodes in renal cell carcinoma is often not due to metastases. J Urol 144:243–245.

37. Terrone C, Guercio S, De Luca S, Poggio M, Castelli E, Scoffone E (2003) The number of lymph nodes examined and staging accuracy in renal cell carcinoma. BJU Int 91: 37–40.

38. Vasselli JR, Yang JC, Linehan WM, White DE, Rosenberg SA, Walther MM (2001) Lack of retroperitoneal lymphadenopathy predicts survival of patients with metastatic renal cell carcinoma. J Urol 166:68–72.

39. Waters WB, Richie JP (1979) Aggressive surgical approach to renal cell carcinoma. Review of 130 cases. J Urol 122: 306–309.

40. Wood DP (1991) Role of lymphadenectomy in renal cell carcinoma. Urol Clin N Am 18:421–426.

41. Zisman A, Pantuck AJ, Belldegrun AS. Lymph Node Dissection in Renal and Adrenal Tumors: Biology and Management. New York: Oxford University Press, 2003, p. 318.

8e
Nephron-Sparing Surgery: Partial Nephrectomy Open

Frank Steinbach, Fred Schuster, and Ernst P. Allhoff

Introduction

Epithelial tumors of the kidney account for approximately 3% off all solid neoplasms with an incidence roughly equal to that of all forms of leukemia combined.[17] Adenocarcinoma or renal cell carcinoma (RCC) represents nearly 85% of newly diagnosed renal malignancies with a steady rise in RCC rates.[13]

Surgery still remains the cornerstone of treatment for RCC. The classic concept of wide excision of the tumor-bearing kidney outside of Gerota's fascia, to include the perirenal fat and ipsilateral adrenal gland, was the traditional surgical approach in the management of this tumor for over a half a century. This technique removes the primary tumor with a wide surgical margin and most patients have another healthy contralateral kidney.[35]

However, the appearance of RCC has undergone a considerable change during the past two decades. Interestingly, small and mostly asymptomatic renal tumors are detected incidentally by means of modern imaging techniques, such as ultrasound, computerized tomography (CT), and magnetic resonance imaging (MRI) during the investigation of other complaints and diseases.[42] Incidental tumors carry a better prognosis than do symptomatic tumors of the same stage and size.[23] Therefore, RCC surgery has evolved in recent years toward a trend of kidney sparing and minimal invasive techniques. Vincenz Czerny is credited with being the first surgeon to perform deliberate partial resection of a renal tumor in 1887.[11] The technique of nephron sparing-surgery (NSS) has now advanced from experimental surgery reserved for high-risk patients with a solitary kidney to a procedure commonly employed in the elective treatment of properly selected patients even in the presence of a normal contralateral kidney.

Partial nephrectomy has been stimulated by several factors, including advances in renal imaging and the widespread use of these noninvasive imaging techniques, improved surgical techniques with methods to prevent ischemic renal injury and to determine surgical margins, better postoperative management, and excellent long-term cancer-free survival data.[30] Furthermore, a greater rationale for partial nephrectomy may exist given the increased longevity of patients. In our daily practice and in most reports in the literature NSS is a treatment option for selected patients that can be performed safely, with low morbidity, preservation of renal function, low local recurrence rates, and high patient satisfaction.

Current Indications

Acceptable indications for NSS fall into three categories, including absolute or imperative, relative, and elective indications.

Imperative indications for NSS include circumstances in which radical nephrectomy would render the patient anephric with subsequent immediate need for dialysis. Even in the current era of dialysis, the morbidity of an anephric state is considerable high, particularly in the elderly. These imperative indications include RCC involving an anatomically or functionally solitary kidney due to unilateral renal agenesis, previous contralateral nephrectomy, or irreversible impairment of contralateral renal function due to a benign disease. Furthermore, patients with synchronous bilateral renal tumors have an absolute indication for NSS. In this situation an attempt should be made to preserve as much functioning parenchyma as possible. However, the desire to spare renal parenchyma does not supersede the primary goal of the operation, that is, to remove the RCC completely. In patients with synchronous bilateral RCCs preservation of renal parenchyma involves a bilateral nephron-sparing approach when feasible, usually as a staged procedure with the less involved side done first.[43] When NSS is impossible on one kidney due to tumor size or location, initial NSS is performed on the less involved kidney, followed by contralateral radical nephrectomy as a separate procedure. In most cases this sequence obviates the need for a temporary dialysis in the immediate postoperative period after the NSS.

Relative indications are those in which the opposite kidney has a preexisting renal disease or is at substantial risk for future compromise. These relative indications include patients with mild-to-moderate renal insufficiency, a history of calculous disease, chronic pyelonephritis, vesicoureteral reflux, uretropelvic junction obstruction, and renal artery stenosis. Furthermore, patients who have a risk of future renal function deterioration due to medical diseases such as diabetes mellitus, hypertension, and other causes of glomerulopathy or nephrosclerosis are also included in this category.[28] Patients with underlying genetic syndromes predisposing to bilateral disease and multifocality, such as von Hippel–Lindau disease, are also considered candidates for NSS due to the high likelihood of subsequent lesions developing in the remaining renal parenchyma. Especially in patients with von Hippel–Lindau disease RCCs often develop at a younger age and usually are multifocal and bilateral.[38]

In patients with a relative indication for NSS the benefits and risks should be individually assessed in the context of the overall clinical situation, including comorbidities, patient age, and risk of disease progression.

The early 1980s marked the beginning of the era of *elective indications* for NSS for RCC. For the next 2 decades this indication was controversial in the urological community. Several studies have now clarified the role of NSS in patients with a localized unilateral RCC and a normal contralateral kidney. Based on the existing data, the generally accepted indication is a single, small tumor ($\leq$4 cm), located peripherally and easily amenable to resection.[2,8,12,18,21,22,34,39] In this clinical situation NSS is equally effective as radical nephrectomy in terms of overall and cancer-specific survival. More recent data further suggest that elective NSS may be appropriate for carefully selected patients with RCC between 4 and 7 cm.[20]

Preoperative Preparation

Candidates for NSS for renal malignancy should not have locally extensive or metastatic disease and be medically able to withstand the anesthetic and surgery. The preoperative evaluation consists of a detailed history and physical examination and standard laboratory work involving serum creatinine determination, liver function tests, and urinalysis to screen for preoperative proteinuria. A nephrologist is consulted if a patient is at high risk for postoperative hemodialysis.

To rule out locally extensive or metastatic disease several imaging examinations are performed, including abdominal sonography (a 3.5-MHz probe is most commonly used), abdominal CT, as well as possible bone scan and chest CT depending on the clinical circumstances. CT should be performed before and after administration of intravenous contrast material and in sections thin enough to avoid volume averaging, particularly in the presence of small lesions. Contrast-enhanced CT images are also useful for planning the site and extent of planned tumor resection, for determining the proximity to the renal hilum and collecting system. Advances in helical CT and computer technology now allow the creation of high-quality 3D images of the involved kidney, which integrate the essential information from conventional 2D CT, angiography, venography, and excretory urography into a single preoperative radiographic testing.[5] Thus, more extensive and invasive imaging studies such as conventional renal angiography and MRI are performed only occasionally.

We usually perform radionuclide imaging only in circumstances with a relative or absolute indication for NSS and in patients with synchronous bilateral RCC to document that the remaining partial renal unit after NSS is functioning well before proceeding with contralateral nephrectomy.

Preoperative attention to a sufficient hydration is essential. We usually hydrate the patient intravenously (1.5–2 liters Ringers lactate) the night before surgery in a carefully monitored setting. We routinely do not offer the opportunity for autologous blood donation for these patients because the need for postoperative transfusion is uncommon. Finally, the urine should be cultured preoperatively and any bacterial infection aggressively treated with antibiotics.

Operative Technique

In the majority of patients undergoing NSS for renal malignancies, the tumor excision is performed *in situ* by wedge or segmental resection obtaining a thin margin of adjacent normal parenchyma. Extracorporeal conservative surgery with autotransplantation of the kidney is required only in rare cases with an imperative indication and exceptionally large and anatomically challenging tumors.[44] Several modifications of technique over the past years have resulted in improved technical outcomes. The basic surgical principles of NSS are early vascular control, avoidance of ischemic renal damage, complete tumor excision with negative surgical margins, precise closure of the renal collecting system, careful hemostasis, and closure or coverage of the renal defect with adjacent fat, peritoneum, or a hemostatic vlies.[32]

The patient is placed in a standard flank position and secured to the table (Fig. 8e-1) A cephalosporin is administered for antibiotic coverage. We usually favor a supracostal extraperitoneal flank incision over the 12th or 11th rib for almost all of these operations (Fig. 8e-2). The level of incision is determined by the position of the kidney in relation to the ribs as seen on preoperative radiographic studies and by the position and size of the tumor. Rib resection is avoided because it may increase postoperative pain, sometimes in a

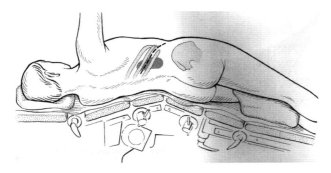

FIGURE 8e-1. The patient is placed in a standard flank position and secured to the table with a vacuum mattress.

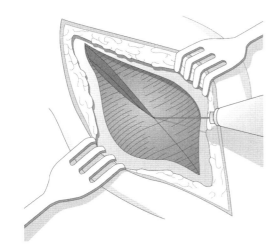

FIGURE 8e-2. The kidney is exposed by a supracostal extraperitoneal flank incision over the 12th or 11th rib.

chronic fashion. This extraperitoneal flank approach allows the urologist to operate on the mobilized kidney almost at skin level and provide excellent access to the renal vessels.

The incision is deepened through the three abdominal muscle layers and the intercostal musculature. The transversus abdominis muscle is sharply incised directly medial to the tip of the rib and the underlying peritoneum is bluntly swept away from the overlying musculature. After incising the remainder of the transversus abdominis muscle, the retroperitoneal space is entered and the pleura parietalis is bluntly dissected away from the thoracal wall. A Finochetto rip retractor is placed, providing excellent deep exposure of the surgical field.

The kidney is approached posterolaterally and the Gerota's fascia is incised from the upper to the lower pole. Inferiorly the ureter is identified and tagged with a vessel loop. After opening Gerota's fascia, the kidney is freed from the surrounding fatty tissue. Only the tissue lying directly on the surface of the tumor is left and removed later along with the tumor. The surface of the kidney is then carefully evaluated

for small second tumors that may occasionally be missed by the radiographic studies.

With rare exceptions, every NSS should commence with identification, dissection, and control of the renal artery and vein. The latter is achieved by placing vessel loops or Rumel tourniquets. In small, peripheral renal tumors without deep involvement of renal parenchyma, it is not necessary to occlude the renal artery. However, in our opinion NSS is most effectively and safely performed after temporary occlusion of the renal artery. Furthermore, in patients with large or centrally located tumors it is helpful to occlude the renal vein temporarily to minimize intraoperative bleeding from major venous branches. In most cases a temporary vascular occlusion is useful for decreasing bleeding and renal tissue turgor. In order to minimize the risk of intrarenal thrombosis we heparinize the patient systemically with 3000 IE heparin before clamping the renal vessels. To prevent ischemic renal damage the patient is vigorously hydrated and 250 ml mannitol is given intravenously 10 minutes before arterial occlusion. After the main renal artery is occluded, the kidney is surrounded by an intestinal bag (a plastic bag with a drawstring) and surface hypothermia is instituted with a sterilized slush saline solution poured into the wound and around the kidney. Surface cooling of the kidney allows as much as 3 hours of safe ischemia without permanent renal damage.[31] An important caveat with this method of surface cooling is to keep the entire kidney covered with the ice slush for 10 minutes before commencing the tumor resection. This amount of time is necessary to obtain a kidney temperature that optimizes *in situ* parenchymal preservation.

The renal capsule is sharply incised leaving a 0.5–0.7 cm margin of normal-appearing parenchyma beyond the visual limits of the tumor. A scissor or neurosurgical brain elevator is used bluntly to separate the lesion from the surrounding normal parenchyma (Fig 8e-3). Renal vessels encountered are directly suture ligated with 5/0 PDS before division adjacent to the specimen parenchyma. The advantage of such an approach is excellent hemostasis and minimization of the risk of accidentally ligating large renal arteries running deep in the tumor bed. The specimen consists of the tumor circumscribed by a rim of normal-appearing parenchyma and abundant perinephric fatty tissue overlying the tumor. The entire specimen is sent to frozen section examination to confirm the absence of residual cancer at the surgical margin. It is unusual that the frozen section examination demonstrates a positive surgical margin but, if it does, additional renal tissue must be excised in patients with an imperative indication or a radical nephrectomy is indicated in patients with an elective indication for NSS. Recently, Sutherland and co-workers demonstrated that only a minimal margin of 2–5 mm must be removed during NSS for low stage RCC to be safe.[41]

In patients with a tumor deep in the renal parenchyma, a centrally located lesion or a tumor not visable on the renal

(a)

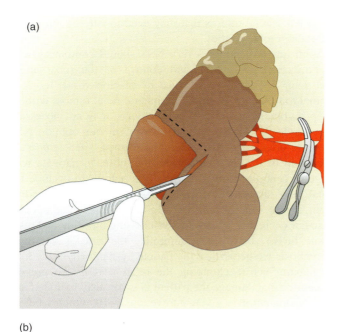

(b)

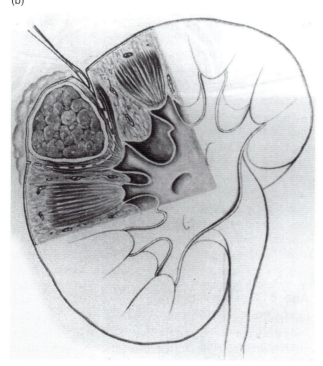

FIGURE 8e-3. (**A, B**) The renal capsule is sharply incised leaving a 0.5–0.7 cm margin of normal-appearing parenchyma beyond the visual limits of the tumor. A scissor or neurosurgical brain elevator is used bluntly to separate the lesion from the surrounding normal parenchyma.

surface, intraoperative ultrasonography (7.5 MHz probe most commonly used) is an important technique, by providing accurate intrarenal localization of the tumor and thereby enabling its precise removal with a surrounding margin of normal tissue.[3]

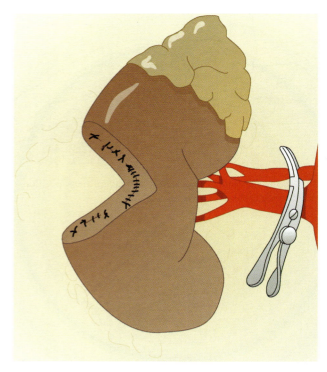

FIGURE 8e-4. After excision of the tumor, transected blood vessels on the tumor bed are secured with figure-of-eight 5/0 PDS sutures. Watertight closure of collecting system injuries with fine absorbable sutures is essential to prevent a urinary fistual formation in the postoperative period.

After excision of the tumor, transected blood vessels on the tumor bed are secured with figure-of-eight 5/0 PDS sutures (Fig. 8e-4). When the renal sinus is exposed, larger blood vessels require direct repair, taking care to maintain the patency of large bifurcation vessels.

Watertight closure of collecting system injuries with fine absorbable sutures is essential to prevent a urinary fistual formation in the postoperative period. We repair collecting system defects under direct vision with interrupted or continuous 5/0 PDS sutures. In patients with major reconstruction of the collecting system a 6 Fr. ureteral stent in combination with a suprapubic cystostomy should be placed for prophylaxis.

Additional hemostasis can be achieved with electrocautery or the argon beam coagulator, a powerful tissue coagulator that works well through a relatively wet or sanguineous tissue surface. However, care should be taken to avoid thermal destruction of previously placed sutures or injury to the collecting system. A further important hemostatic measure is a piece of a thrombin-soaked Gelfoam (e.g., Tachosil) that is laid directly into the partial nephrectomy defect.

Whenever possible, the kidney should be closed on itself by approximating the transected cortical margins with a continuous 3/0 PDS suture (Fig. 8e-5). This is the best method to achieve satisfactory hemostasis and avoid postoperative urinary fistula formation. If this is done, there must

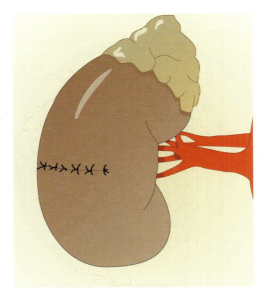

FIGURE 8e-5. Whenever possible, the kidney should be closed on itself by approximating the transected cortical margins with a continuous 3/0 PDS suture.

be no significant angulation or kinking of blood vessels supplying the kidney. Alternatively, a portion of perirenal fat or a peritoneal flap may be inserted into the base of the renal defect and sutured to the parenchymal margins with continuous 4/0 PDS sutures (Fig. 8e-6).

After closure or coverage of the renal defect, the renal vessels are unclamped and the circulation to the kidney is restored. Following removal of the vascular clamp, the entire kidney is wrapped for 10 minutes with warm towels. The

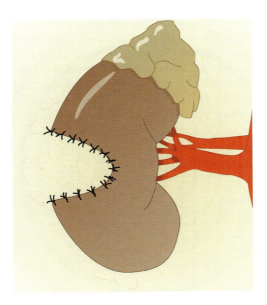

FIGURE 8e-6. Alternatively, a portion of perirenal fat or a peritoneal flap may be inserted into the base of the renal defect and sutured to the parenchymal margins with continuous 4/0 PDS sutures.

kidney is fixed by reapproximating Gerota's fascia with 4/0 vicryl sutures. Regional lymphadenectomy is not performed routinely. However, enlarged or suspicious-looking lymph nodes should be removed and sent for frozen section analysis before initiating the renal tumor resection.

A closed 24 Fr. drainage system is placed in the retroperitoneal space outside Gerota's fascia and the flank and abdominal musculature is closed in two layers.

During the extended postoperative period, patients are routinely evaluated with serum creatinine measurements, urinalysis to excluded bacterial infection, and renal sonography. The retroperitoneal drain is always left in place for at least 5 days, and an ureteral stent should be removed at the earliest 1 month after surgery.

Complications

Open NSS for RCCs is an established and safe technique. In our institution this operation is performed by chief residents under the supervision of a board-certified urologist.

An early series of NSS described a significant risk of complications, including acute and chronic renal failure, urinary fistula, and hemorrhage.[4,7] In contemporary series the incidence of postoperative complications after NSS continues to decrease, most likely secondary to improved surgical experience, patient selection, better perioperative care and an increased prevalence of incidentally discovered smaller tumors.[37] Corman et al. compared the morbidity and mortality of patients undergoing either radical or partial nephrectomy.[6] For 512 patients who underwent NSS and 1373 patients who underwent radical nephrectomy there were no statistically significant differences in the rates of postoperative acute renal failure, progressive renal failure, transfusion, prolonged ileus, urinary tract infection, deep wound infection, or length of hospitalization. The unadjusted 30-day mortality rate was 2% and 1.6% for patients undergoing radical nephrectomy and NSS, respectively ($p = 0.58$). Table 8e-1 summarizes the frequency of common complications observed after NSS in several large series.

Urinary fistula is the most common complication after NSS. The diagnosis is made when persistent drainage demonstrates elevated creatinine levels. To prevent a retroperitoneal urinoma a prolonged urine drainage (2 weeks) with an insertion of a ureteral stent (6 Fr.) and a suprapubic catheter is the treatment of choice.

The risk of acute renal failure after NSS has been reported to range from 0% to 15%. Risk factors for postoperative acute renal failure include imperative indication for NSS, tumor size greater than 7 cm, excision of more than 50% of the parenchyma, and ischemia time greater than 60 minutes.[28]

Bleeding after NSS may be acute or delayed. In the immediate postoperative period surgical reexploration is in our opinion the best method to save the renal remnant. In

TABLE 8e-1. Complications of nephron-sparing surgery.

Study	No. patients	No. urinary leaks (%)	No. acute or chronic renal failure (%)	No. postoperative bleeding (%)	No. reoperation (%)	No. infection/ abscess (%)	No. Deaths (%)
Lerner[21]	169	3 (1.8)	0	0	–	–	1 (0.5)
Morgan[27]	104	1 (0.9)	–	1 (0.9)	–	–	2 (1.9)
Steinbach[40]	140	3 (2.1)	1 (0.7)	2 (1.4)	2 (1.4)	–	2 (1.4)
Moll[26]	164	11 (6.7)	–	6 (3.7)	1 (0.6)	–	–
Filipas[9]	180	3 (1.5)	0	4 (2.4)	–	5 (2.8)	0
Belldegrun[1]	146	2 (1.4)	–	3 (2)	3 (2)	–	3 (2)
Marszalek[24]	129	–	0	4 (3.1)	2 (1.5)	–	0
Lau[18]	164	3 (1.8)	0	2 (1.2)	1 (0.6)	2 (1.2)	0
Ghavamian[10]	76	2 (3.2)	8 (12.7)	1 (1.1)	7 (11.1)	2 (3.0)	0
Duque[7]	64	6 (9.1)	10 (15)	3 (4.5)	2 (3)	–	0
Campbell[4]	259	45 (17.4)	19 (7.3)	6 (2.3)	8 (3.1)	11 (4.2)	4 (1.5)

patients with delayed bleeding after NSS a radiological intervention with selective arterial embolization of the bleeding renal vessel is indicated.

However, careful intraoperative attention to hemostasis and precise reconstruction of the renal calical system are mandatory to avoid these complications.

Clinical Results of Open Nephron-Sparing Surgery

The technical success rate with NSS for RCC is excellent, and several large studies with extended follow-up data have reported cancer-specific survival rates comparable to those obtained after radical nephrectomy (Table 8e-2). Cancer-specific survival rates are lower in patients with an imperative compared with an elective indication for NSS secondary to increased age, tumor size, stage, and overall decreased health. Ghavamian et al. reported the outcome of 76 patients who underwent NSS for RCC in a solitary kidney. The cancer-specific survival rates at 5 and 10 years were 81% and 64%, respectively.[10] Similarly, Fergany from the Cleveland Clinic reviewed 107 patients of whom 90% had an imperative

indication for NSS. The cancer specific survival rate for this cohort was 88% and 73% at 5 and 10 years, respectively.[8] Long-term preservation of renal function was achieved in 93% of these patients. Important negative predictors of survival included high tumor grade, high tumor stage, bilateral disease, and tumors larger than 4 cm in diameter.[29]

Elective NSS in patients with a normal contralateral kidney has been shown to have excellent cancer-specific survival rates ranging from 89% to 100% (Table 8e-3). The mean tumor size in most of these series is less than 4 cm. NSS is now the therapeutic approach of choice in patients who have a single, small (less than 4 cm) RCC and a normal contralateral kidney. However, careful selection of the patient seems essential in deriving such good results in cancer control.

The major disadvantage of NSS for RCC is the risk of postoperative local tumor recurrence in the operated kidney. Local recurrence following NSS may be secondary to incomplete resection of the primary tumor, unrecognized synchronous lesions, or the subsequent development of a metachronous lesion. High rates of multicentric tumors have been described in several diseases, including von Hippel–Lindau syndrome, acquired renal cystic disease, and hereditary papillary RCC.[38] The incidence of multifocality in sporadic cases of RCC, however, is much lower, and the

TABLE 8e-2. Studies comparing cancer-specific survival in radical versus partial nephrectomy.[a]

Author	No. of patients undergoing RN/NSS	Median follow-up (months)	RN	NSS
McKiernan, 2002[25]	173/117	26	99	96
Lee, 2000[19]	183/79	40	95	95
Lau, 2000[18]	164/164	47	97	98
Belldegrun, 1999[1]	125/108	74	91	98
Lerner, 1996[21]	209/185	52	89	89
Butler, 1995[2]	42/46	48	97	100

Source: Adapted from Filipas et al.[9]

[a]RN, Radical nephrectomy; NSS, nephron-sparing surgery.

TABLE 8e-3. Results of elective nephron-sparing surgery.

Author	Year	Patients	5-year survival(%)	Local recurrence (%)
Steinbach[40]	1992	72	94.4	2.7
Moll[26]	1993	98	100	1
Butler[2]	1995	46	100	2.2
Lerner[21]	1996	54	92	5.6
Van Poppel[34]	1998	51	98	0
Herr[12]	1999	70	97.5	1.5
Belldegrun[1]	1999	63	100	3.2
Filipas[9]	2000	180	98	1.6
Lau[18]	2000	164	98	1.7
Kural[16]	2003	76	98	0
Leibovich[20]	2004	91	98.3	5.4

biological behavior of these secondary lesions is not well characterized. In a prospective analysis from the Mayo Clinic the incidence of true unknown multifocality (at the time of surgery) was 6%, corresponding roughly to the local recurrence rates reported in several studies (Table 8e-3).[15] With proper patient selection, the use of preoperative modern imaging methods, and a thorough inspection of the entire surface of the kidney at the time of surgery the risk of local tumor recurrence can be further minimized.[14]

RCC with concomitant systemic disease engaging the renal parenchyma, hereditary RCC, and patients with RCC in a solitary kidney or a malfunctioning contralateral kidney. Furthermore, long-term survival and local tumor control are excellent in patients with a small unilateral RCC and a normal contralateral kidney after open NSS. These results indicate that NSS is an effective treatment for localized RCC, providing both long-term tumor control and preservation of renal function.

Long-Term Renal Function after Open Nephron-Sparing Surgery

Lau et al. and McKiernan et al. have directly compared radical nephrectomy and NSS and have demonstrated a statistically significant decreased risk of chronic renal failure among patients undergoing NSS.[18,25]

In an earlier report from the Cleveland Clinic, Novick et al. reported a statistically significant association between proteinuria and the development of renal failure after NSS.[33] Data from this study revealed that patients with a greater than 50% loss of functional renal parenchyma are at an increased risk for proteinuria, glomerulopathy, and progressive renal failure. In a recent report from the same institution the long-term renal function after open NSS in 400 patients with a solitary kidney was evaluated.[36] On long-term follow-up 268 (67%) patients showed an insignificant change in their creatinine levels, and only 12 (3%) patients developed end-stage renal disease requiring hemodialysis or renal transplantation.

These data demonstrate that with open NSS a long-term preservation of renal function is possible, without the need for dialysis in the majority of cases.

Conclusions

Open NSS has proved to be a safe and effective treatment modality in patients with an RCC. NSS is the standard surgical method in patients with bilateral RCC, unilateral

References

1. Belldegrun A, Tsui KH, deKernion JB, et al. Efficacy of nephron-sparing surgery for RCC: analysis based on the new 1997 tumor-node-metastasis staging system. J Clin Oncol 1999; 17: 968–997.
2. Bulter BP, Novick AC, Miller DP, et al. Management of small unilateral RCCs: radical versus nephron-sparing surgery. Urology 1995; 45: 34–40.
3. Campbell SC, Fichtner J, Steinbach F, et al. Intraoperative evaluation of RCC: a prospective study of the role of ultrasonography and histopathological frozen sections. J Urol 1996; 155: 1191–1195.
4. Campbell SC, Novick AC, Streem SB, et al. Complications of NSS for renal tumors. J Urol 1994; 151: 1177–1180.
5. Coll DM, Uzzo RG, Herts BR, et al. 3-Dimensional volume rendered computerized tomography for preoperative evaluation and intraoperative treatment of patients undergoing NSS. J Urol 1999; 161: 1097–1102.
6. Corman JM, Penson DF, Hur K, et al. Comparison of complications after radical and partial nephrectomy: results from the National Veterans Administration Surgical Quality Improvement Program. BJU Int 2000; 86: 782–789.
7. Duque JL, Loughlin KR, O'Leary MP, et al. Partial nephrectomy: alternative treatment for selected patients with RCC. Urology 1998; 52: 584–590.
8. Fergany AF, Hafez KS, Novick AC. Long-term results of nephron-sparing surgery for localized RCC: 10-year followup. J Urol 2000; 163(2): 442–445.
9. Filipas D, Fichtner J, Spix C, et al. Nephron-sparing surgery of RCC with a normal opposite kidney: long-term outcome in 180 patients. Urology 2000; 56: 387–392.

10. Ghavamian R, Cheville JC, Lohse CM, et al. RCC in the solitary kidney: an analysis of complications and outcome after NSS. J. Urol 2002; 168: 454–459.

11. Herr HW. A history of partial nephrectomy for renal tumors. J Urol 2005; 173: 705–708.

12. Herr HW. Partial nephrectomy for unilateral renal carcinoma and a normal contralateral kidney: 10-year followup. J Urol 1999; 161: 33–34.

13. Hock LM, Lynch J, Balaji KC. Increasing incidence of all stages of kidney cancer in the last 2 decades in the United States: an analysis of surveillance, epidemiology and end results program data. J Urol 2002; 167: 57–60.

14. Huang GJ, Israel G, Berman, et al. Preoperative renal tumor evaluation by three-dimensional magnetic resonance imaging: staging and detection of multifocality. Urology 2004; 64: 453–457.

15. Kletscher BA, Qian J, Bostwick DG, et al. Prospective analysis of multifocality in RCC: influence of histopathological pattern, grade, number, size, volume and deoxyribonucleic acid ploidy. J Urol 1995; 153: 904–906.

16. Kural AR, Demirkesen O, Onal B, et al. Outcome of nephron-sparing surgery: elective versus imperative indications. Urol Int 2003; 71: 190–196.

17. Landis SH, Murray T, Bolden S et al. Cancer statistics. CA Cancer J Clin 1999; 49(1): 8–31.

18. Lau WK, Blute ML, Weaver AL, et al. Matched comparison of radical nephrectomy vs nephron-sparing surgery in patients with unilateral RCC and a normal contralateral kidney. Mayo Clin Proc 2000; 75: 1236–1242.

19. Lee CT, Katz J, Shi W, et al. Surgical management of renal tumors 4 cm or less in a contemporary cohort. J Urol 2000; 163: 730–736.

20. Leibovich BC, Blute ML, Cheville JC, et al. NSS for appropriately selected RCC between 4 and 7 cm results in outcome similar to radical nephrectomy. J Urol 2004; 171: 1066–1070.

21. Lerner SE, Hawkins CA, Blute ML, et al. Disease outcome in patients with low stage RCC treated with nephron-sparing or radical surgery. J Urol 1996; 155: 1868–1873.

22. Licht MR, Novick AC. Nephron-sparing surgery for RCC. J Urol 1993; 149: 1–7.

23. Licht MR, Novick AC, Goormastic M. NSS in incidental versus suspected RCC. J Urol 1994; 152(1): 39–42.

24. Marszalek M, Ponholzer A, Brössner C, et al. Elective open nephron-sparing surgery for renal masses: single-center experience with 129 consecutive patients. Urology 2004; 64: 38–42.

25. McKiernan J, Simmons R, Katz J, et al. Natural history of chronic renal insufficiency after partial and radical nephrectomy. Urology 2002; 59: 816–820.

26. Moll V, Becht E and Ziegler, M. Kidney preserving surgery in renal cell tumors: indications, techniques and results in 152 patients. J Urol 1993; 150: 319–323.

27. Morgan WR, Zincke H: Progression and survival after renal-conserving surgery for RCC: experience in 104 patients and extended followup. J Urol 1990; 144: 852–857.

28. Nieder AM, Taneja SS. The role of partial nephrectomy for RCC in contemporary practice. Urol Clin N Am 2003; 30: 529–542.

29. Novick AC. Laparoscopic and partial nephrectomy. Clin Cancer Res 2004; 10: 6322–6327.

30. Novick AC. Nephron-sparing surgery for RCC. Annu Rev Med 2002; 53: 393–407.

31. Novick AC. Renal hypothermia: in vivo and ex vivo. Urol Clin North Am 1983; 10: 637–644.

32. Novick AC. Surgery of the kidney. In: Walsh P, editor. Campbell's Urology, Vol IV, 8th ed. Philadelphia: Saunders, 2002: 3571–3613.

33. Novick AC, Gephardt G, Guz B, et al. Long-term follow-up after partial removal of a solitary kidney. N Engl J Med 1991; 325: 1058–1062.

34. van Poppel H, Bamelis B, Oyen R, et al. Partial nephrectomy for RCC can achieve long term tumor control. J Urol 1998; 160: 674.

35. Robson CJ. Radical nephrectomy for RCC. J Urol 1963; 89: 37–42.

36. Saad IR, Woo LL, Fergany AF, et al. Long-term renal function after partial nephrectomy in patients with solitary kidney. J Urol 2005; 173: 360 (suppl.).

37. Shekarriz B, Upadhyay J, Shekarriz H, et al. Comparison of costs and complications of radical and partial nephrectomy for treatment of localized RCC. Urology 2002; 59: 211–215.

38. Steinbach F. Arbeit von Hippel Lindau.

39. Steinbach F, Stöckle M, Hohenfellner R. Clinical experience with nephron-sparing surgery in the presence of a normal contralateral kidney. Semin Urol Oncol 1995; 13: 288–291.

40. Steinbach F, Stöckle M, Müller SC, et al. Conservative surgery of renal cell tumors in 140 patients: 21 years of experience. J Urol 1992; 148: 24–30.

41. Sutherland SE, Resnick MI, Maclennan GT, et al. Does the size of the surgical margin in partial nephrectomy for renal cell cancer really matter? J Urol 2002; 167: 61–64.

42. Tosaka A, Ohya K, Yamada K, et al. Incidence and properties of renal masses and asymptomatic RCC detected by abdominal ultrasonography. J Urol 1990; 144(5): 1097–1099.

43. Uzzo RG, Novick AC. NSS for renal tumors: indications, techniques and outcomes. J Urol 2001; 166: 6–18.

44. Wickham JE. Conservative renal surgery for adenocarcinomas: the place of bench surgery. Br J Urol 1975; 47: 25–36.

8f
Nephron-Sparing Surgery: Laparoscopic Partial Nephrectomy

Georges-Pascal Haber, Jose R. Colombo Jr., and Inderbir S. Gill

Introduction

With the widespread use of contemporary imaging techniques, small renal tumors are now being diagnosed with increased frequency. As a result, the application of nephron-sparing techniques has increased in contemporary patients with renal cancer. Partial nephrectomy allows excision of the renal tumor completely and remains the standard technique for nephron-sparing surgery.[1] Open partial nephrectomy offers long-term oncological outcomes equivalent to that of radical nephrectomy and long-term preservation of renal function in selected patients with a small renal tumor.[2]

With increasing experience in laparoscopic reconstructive and oncological procedures, significant interest has centered worldwide on laparoscopic partial nephrectomy (LPN).[3] LPN has emerged as a viable alternative to open partial nephrectomy while minimizing patient morbidity. The technique of LPN is now refined and standardized, duplicating established principles of open partial nephrectomy.[4]

Initially, LPN was limited to patients with a small, superficial, solitary, peripheral, exophytic tumor. Advances in laparoscopic skills and technology have allowed efficacious achievement of renal hilar vascular control, renal hypothermia, tumor excision, caliceal suture repair, and hemostatic parenchymal suture repair. As result, the indications for LPN have been expanded to include larger, central, hilar, and infiltrating tumors.

The experience with laparoscopic partial nephrectomy in the Cleveland Clinic now exceeds 550 cases. In this chapter, the current technique for LPN is detailed, including technical tips, results, and complications.

Equipment

The basic set includes a Veress needle, blunt-tip 5- and 10/12-mm trocar/ports, two small atraumatic bowel graspers, a Maryland grasper, an Alice grasper, "J-hook" electrocautery, a titanium clip applier, 10-mm Weck clips and applier, and 10-mm right-angle and bulldog clamps. Only equipment useful for performing LPN is discussed in this section. The Stryker suction is used, as it has a smooth, blunt, rounded gently beveled tip that allows atraumatic dissection around the hilum and provides good suction/irrigation of the partial nephrectomy bed. A Satinsky vascular clamp is used for hilar clamping in the transperitoneal access. FloSeal (Baxter, Deerfield, IL) is used routinely as a hemostatic agent, with a reusable metal laparoscopic applicator. A CT-1 needle 2-0 vicryl and a CTX needle 0-vicryl are used for parenchymal reconstruction. Two straight 5-mm Ethicon needle drivers are used for suturing.

Technique

Patient Preparation

Precise imaging using a 3-mm sections computed tomography (CT) scan with volume rendered three-dimensional (3D) video reconstruction is performed prior to the operation. This CT scan provides information regarding tumor size, location, parenchymal infiltration, and relation to the collecting system, and defines the renal vasculature, with details on the number, location, spatial interrelationships of vessels, and any congenital vascular anomalies. Arteriography is typically reserved for patients with suspected concomitant renovascular disease or a large tumor requiring angioinfarction. In the afternoon before surgery, the patient takes two bottles (296 ml/bottle) of magnesium citrate.

The choice of the laparoscopic approach is dictated by the location and the technical complexity of the renal mass. In general, the transperitoneal approach provides more working space and excellent suturing angles when reconstructing the partial nephrectomy defect. On the CT scan, a straight line is drawn from the renal hilum to the lateral border of the kidney. All anterior tumors or tumors transgressing this line are preferentially approached transperitoneally. Tumors posterior to this line are approached retroperitoneoscopically. As such, anterior, anterolateral, and lateral tumors are preferentially approached transperitoneally. Posterior, posteromedial, and posterolateral tumors are approached retroperitoneoscopically.

Positioning

After general anesthesia, cystoscopy is performed, and a 5 Fr. open-ended ureteral catheter is positioned in the ipsilateral renal pelvis over a guidewire. A sterile intravenous extension tubing is attached to the ureteral catheter for intraoperative retrograde dilute methylene blue injection. Similar to laparoscopic radical nephrectomy, the patient is placed in a 45°–60° flank position for the transperitoneal approach and a 90° lateral position for the retroperitoneal approach.

Port Placement

During the transperitoneal approach, pneumoperitoneum is obtained by the Veress needle technique. A four or five port approach is used. The primary port (10/12 mm) is placed lateral to the rectus muscle at the level of the umbilicus. The next port is placed lateral to the rectus muscle and just inferior to the costochondral margin. On the right side, this subcostal 10/12-mm trocar is used to facilitate the passage of suture needles for the right-handed surgeon. On the left side, this subcostal port can be a 5-mm port. The reverse arrangement would be used by a left-handed surgeon. A 10/12-mm port for the laparoscope is placed 3 cm inferior and medial to the subcostal port. A 5-mm port is inserted in approximately the mid-axillary line in the vicinity of the rib 11 to permit countertraction laterally during renal hilar dissection. Additionally,

a grasping instrument inserted through this port can hold the knot of the renorraphy stitches during parenchymal repair to prevent slippage. Finally, a 10/12-mm port is placed in the suprapubic area lateral to the rectus muscle for the Satinsky vascular clamp (Fig. 8f-1).

During the retroperitoneal approach, the first port is placed at the tip of the rib 12. The retroperitoneal space is created with balloon expansion and a 10-mm blunt-tip balloon port is placed. A second, anterior port (10 mm) is inserted two to three fingerbreadths cephalad to the anterior–superior iliac spine. The third, posterior port (10/12 mm) is placed in the costovertebral angle, under rib 12 and lateral to the erector spinae muscle. A 5-mm port is inserted approximately 3–4 cm superior to the anterior 10/12-mm anterior port and is used to grasp the knot of the renorraphy stitches. An extra 10/12-mm port can also be used if a Satinsky vascular clamp is desired; this port is placed in the iliac fossa just anterior to the inferior superior iliac spine (Fig. 8f-2).

Hilar and Kidney Dissection

This operative strategy consists of three steps: (1) hilar dissection, (2) mobilization of kidney, and then (3) tumor resection. On the right side, the liver is retracted anteriorly. On the left side, the spleen and pancreas are reflected medially. On either side, the colon is mobilized. The kidney is dissected using a standard technique. The ureter and gonadal vein packet are identified and retracted anteriorly off the psoas muscle. The renal vein is dissected enough to appreciate its precise location and clearly visualize its anterior surface. Individual dissection of the renal artery and renal vein is unnecessary for adequate clamping and may cause arterial vasospasm, increase the risk of vascular injury, and increase

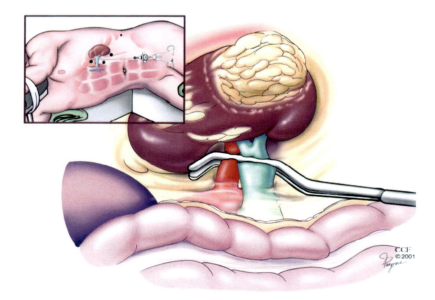

FIGURE 8f-1. Transperitoneal laparoscopic partial nephrectomy. Laparoscopic Satinsky clamp is used to obtain en bloc of renal hilum. Inset shows port arrangement. (Adapted from Rassweiler et al.[3])

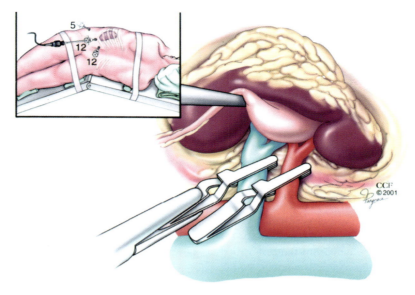

FIGURE 8f-2. Retroperitoneal laparoscopic partial nephrectomy. Because of the limited space in the retroperitoneum, the renal vessels are dissected individually to facilitate application of laparoscopic bulldog clamps on the renal artery and renal vein. Inset shows a three-port retroperitoneal approach. (Adapted from Rassweiler et al.[3])

the operating time. Superior to the renal hilum, the adrenal gland is dissected off the medial aspect of the kidney, which is then mobilized anteriorly off the psoas muscle. These maneuvers allow the Satinsky vascular clamp to be deployed safely across the en bloc renal hilum. The kidney is mobilized within Gerota's fascia and defatted. This allows the kidney to be mobile, may expose other satellite tumors, permits intraoperative ultrasound, and facilitates resection and suturing angles. Perirenal fat over the tumor is maintained to permit adequate staging for potential stage pT3a tumors and to serve as a handle during tumor resection.

Ultrasonography

Intraoperative flexible laparoscopic ultrasonography is performed with a 7-MHz probe to facilitate planning of the tumor resection. The information obtained includes the size of the tumor, the depth of infiltration, the relation of the tumor to the pelvicaliceal system, and any small synchronous lesions missed on the preoperative imaging. With real-time ultrasonographic guidance, the tumor is circumferentially delineated using a cautery J-hook. An adequate margin of renal parenchyma around the tumor is confirmed with ultrasonography prior to initiating resection.

Hilar Clamping

The bloodless operative field with clear visibility achieved by en bloc hilar clamping with a Satinsky clamp is essential for a technically precise tumor excision, precise pelvicalyceal suture repair, and precise parenchymal closure. As a nephron-protective measure, 12.5 g of mannitol is given intravenously 30 minutes prior to clamping. The Satinsky clamp must be

placed medial to the ureter and renal pelvis, thus avoiding crush injury of these structures. Additionally the Satinsky clamp should be opened fully and advanced such that the jaw of the clamp facing the surgeon is anterior to the renal vein, while the posterior jaw hugs the psoas muscle (Fig. 8f-1). Thus, the renal artery and renal vein are included in the clamp jaws along with some hilar fat, which cushions the renal vessels against clamp injury. A time clock is started to monitor the duration of warm ischemia. During the retroperitoneal approach, the jaw of the clamp facing the surgeon would be posterior to the renal artery. The other jaw must be anatomically anterior enough to safely include the renal vein. Additionally, there must be enough separation of the kidney from the peritoneum to avoid peritoneal entry with the clamp. If the small retroperitoneal working space does not allow the placement of a Satinsky clamp, each vascular structure is circumferentially mobilized and individual bulldog clamps can be placed on the renal artery and renal vein separately (Fig. 8f-2).

Renal Hypothermia

When the anticipated duration of warm ischemia time is greater than 30 minutes, renal hypothermia should be used.[5] The technique of hypothermia used by the authors duplicates the open partial nephrectomy surface cooling technique of the kidney.[6] Finely crushed ice slurry is preloaded into 30-ml syringes, whose nozzle end has been cut off. An Endocatch-II bag (U.S. Surgical, Norwalk, CT) is placed around the mobilized kidney, whose drawstring is cinched down around the intact renal hilum, thus completely entrapping the kidney. The renal hilum is clamped with a Satinsky clamp. The bottom of the bag is retrieved through a 12-mm port site and

600–750 ml of ice slush is delivered rapidly via the 30-ml modified syringes. Typically, 4–7 minutes is required to fill the bag. After allowing 10 minutes for achievement of core renal cooling, the bag is incised, the ice crystals removed from the vicinity of the tumor, and partial nephrectomy is completed.[7]

Tumor Resection

Once the hilum is clamped, the J-hook monopolar electrocautery device is used to incise deeply the renal capsule along the previously scored line of resection. Parenchymal incision and tumor resection are performed using heavier reusable scissors, the jaws of which are larger than those of the disposable scissors. The tumor is excised in a medial-to-lateral direction. The tumor is elevated from the tumor bed by placing countertraction with the suction cannula, which also simultaneously aspirates the blood, thereby maintaining a clear operative field. If achievement of an adequate margin requires entry into the collecting system, the calyx or renal pelvis is divided sharply without electrocautery. The magnification afforded by the laparoscope, combined with the bloodless field and ultrasound guidance, ensures that the line of parenchymal resection maintains approximately a 0.5 cm margin of healthy tissue around the tumor. The specimen is placed in an Endocatch bag and positioned within the abdomen away from the operative field in preparation for subsequent intact extraction. Targeted excisional biopsies of the tumor bed may be sent for frozen section in case of suspicion regarding margin status.

Pelvicaliceal Repair and Parenchymal Hemostasis

The collecting system is suture repaired with a running 2-0 Vicryl on a CT-1 needle. The water tightness of the caliceal repair is confirmed by repeat retrograde injection of dilute methylene blue. Only a small injection is needed for this confirmation; forceful repeated injections can actually create a leak. Any large parenchymal vessels can be closed with a specific figure-of-eight suture using 2-0 Vicryl on a CT-1 needle. Renal parenchymal repair is performed with 1-0 Polyglactin on a GS-25 needle. The needle should be well loaded on the needle holder and its intrarenal passage well planned to prevent multiple passages, minimizing possible puncture injury to intrarenal vessels. The needle is inserted approximately 1–1.5 cm away from the resection edge. Three to five interrupted sutures are placed over a preprepared oxidized cellulose Surgicel bolster (Johnson & Johnson, New Brunswick, NJ) that has been positioned over the cut surface of the kidney. A Hem-o-Lok clip (Weck Closure System, Research Triangle Park, NC) is secured on the suture to prevent it from pulling through. Biological hemostatic gelatin-matrix-thrombin tissue sealant FloSeal (Baxter Healthcare, Deerfield, IL) is applied to the cut renal

parenchymal surface underneath the bolster. Another Hem-o-Lok clip is applied to the suture flush with the opposite renal surface, compressing the kidney. The suture is then tightly tied across the bolster, maintaining adequate parenchymal compression.

Unclamping

Mannitol (12.5 g) and furosemide (10–20 mg) are given intravenously prior to unclamping, with the aim of promoting diuresis and minimizing the sequelae of revascularization injury-induced cell swelling and free-radical release. The hilum is unclamped and the Satinsky clamp is opened but not yet removed. Once hemostasis from the parenchymal closure is confirmed, the Satinsky clamp is slowly and carefully removed under direct vision. The en bloc specimen is extracted in an EndoCatch bag. The abdomen is reinspected after 5–10 minutes of zero pneumoperitoneum to ensure adequate hemostasis. A Jackson-Pratt drain is left in patients in whom pelvicaliceal repair is performed.

During the retroperitoneal approach and in case of individual bulldog clamp use, the bulldog clamp is removed from the renal vein initially, followed by the artery. A Penrose drain is left when pelvicaliceal repair is performed.

Postoperative Care

The patient is advised to allow 24 hours of strict bed rest, followed by gradual mobilization. The ureteral and Foley catheters are removed on the morning of postoperative day 2 as the patient begins ambulation. The perirenal drain is maintained for at least 3–5 days and removed when the drainage is less than 50 ml per day for 3 consecutive days. Following discharge from the hospital, the patient is advised to maintain restricted activity for 2 weeks. Physical activity is inadvisable in the early postoperative period. An MAG-3 radionuclide scan is performed at 1 month to evaluate renal function and assess pelvicaliceal system integrity. In patients with pathologically confirmed renal cancer, a follow-up CT scan and chest X-ray are obtained at 6 months. Subsequent oncological surveillance is as per the individual pathological tumor stage.

Outcomes

Overall Results

More than 550 laparoscopic partial nephrectomies have been performed in the authors' institution since 1999. The mean age of the patients was 58 years and the mean tumor size was 2.9 cm (0.5–10.3 cm). The transperitoneal approach was employed in 65% of the cases. Tumors were greater than 3 cm in size in 31% of the cases, 5% of the patients had a tumor in a solitary kidney, 40% had a central tumor, 54% had a peripheral tumor, and 6% had a hilar tumor. The mean warm ischemia time was 32 minutes. Indication for surgery was elective in 46%, relative in 26%, and absolute in 28%. Renal cell carcinoma was confirmed on pathology in 75% of the tumors.[8]

Comparison of Transperitoneal versus Retroperitoneal Approach

Comparing the transperitoneal approach with the retroperitoneal approach for LPN, the transperitoneal approach was associated with a significantly longer operative time (3.5 vs. 2.9 hours, $p < 0.001$) and longer hospital stay (2.9 vs. 2.2 days, $p < 0.01$). Blood loss, perioperative complications, postoperative functional outcomes, and histological outcomes were comparable.[9] As mentioned above, the approaches differed primarily by a technique of hilar control since en bloc hilar control was achieved with a Satinsky clamp during transperitoneal LPN, while during the retroperitoneal approach individual control of the renal artery and vein was obtained with two bulldog clamps.

Impact of Warm Ischemia

The impact of warm ischemia time on renal function after LPN was evaluated in a series with 179 patients. In these patients, the mean warm ischemia time was 31 minutes (4–55 minutes) and the function of the operated kidney was reduced by a mean of 29%, accordingly to renal scintilography, corresponding to the amount of parenchyma excised. No significant change in renal function was related to duration of warm ischemia, age, and/or baseline serum creatinine. Impaired renal function and advanced age increased the risk of postoperative kidney dysfunction, especially when the warm ischemia time was longer than 30 minutes.[10]

Comparison of Central versus Peripheral Tumor

Comparing LPN for central tumors (154 patients) to LPN for peripheral tumor (209 patients), the patients with central tumors presented larger tumor size (3.0 vs. 2.4 cm, $p < 0.001$), larger specimens (43 vs. 22 g, $p < 0.001$), longer warm ischemia time (33.5 vs. 30 minutes, $p < 0.001$), longer operative time (3.5 vs. 3 hours, $p = 0.008$), longer hospital stay (2.8 vs. 2.4 days, $p < 0.001$), and a higher early postoperative complication rate (6% vs. 2%, $p = 0.05$). Although these differences were significant, we did not observe any clinical difference in outcomes between the groups. The intraoperative and late complication rates were not significantly different between the two groups. The median postoperative serum creatinine was similar (1.2 vs. 1.1 mg/dl) and there was no difference in compromised surgical margin rate (0.8% vs. 0.7%, $p = 0.5$).[11]

For tumors in physical contact with the renal vascular pedicle (hilar tumors), the data on LPN in 25 patients showed a mean tumor size of 3.7 cm, mean warm ischemia of 36.4 minutes, and mean blood loss of 231 ml. There was no open conversion in this series and no kidney was lost. All patients had negative surgical margins.[12]

Laparoscopic Partial Nephrectomy in Solitary Kidney

In a series with 22 patients with solitary kidney, the median tumor size was 3 cm (1.4–8.3) and warm ischemia time was 29 minutes (14–55 minutes). The median preoperative and postoperative serum creatinine was 1.1 (0.8–2.1) and 1.5 mg/dl (0.8–3.3), respectively (increasing of 33%). The median preoperative and postoperative glomerular filtration rate was 67.5 and 50 ml/minute/1.73m^2, respectively (decreasing of 27%). This variation in renal function was proportional to the median amount of parenchyma excised (23%). Temporary kidney replacement therapy for 3 weeks was required in one patient (4.5%) following a heminephrectomy.[13]

Comparison of Laparoscopic versus Open Partial Nephrectomy

In the study with 200 partial nephrectomies (100 LPN and 100 open partial nephrectomy), the median surgical time was 3 vs. 3.9 hours ($p < 0.001$), the estimated blood loss was 125 vs. 250 ml ($p < 0.001$), and the mean warm ischemia time was 28 vs. 18 minutes ($p < 0.001$). The group with the minimally invasive approach required less postoperative analgesia and had a shorter hospital stay and quicker convalescence. The intraoperative complication rate was higher in the laparoscopic group (5% vs. 0%; $p = 0.02$) and the postoperative complications were similar (9% vs. 14%; $p = 0.27$). Functional outcomes were similar in both groups. Three patients in the laparoscopic group had a positive surgical margin compared to none in the open groups (3% vs. 0%, $p < 0.1$).

Oncological Outcomes

Mid-term oncological outcomes are now available. A series with 100 patients, each with 3 years of minimum follow-up, with an overall survival of 86% and cancer-specific survival of 100%, was reported.[15] The data on 50 patients with 5 years of follow-up indicate an overall and cancer-specific survival of 84% and 100%, respectively.[16]

In a multiinstitutional study with 511 LPN performed, nine positive parenchymal margins were identified on the final pathology. Of these, two patients underwent radical nephrectomy and seven were under surveillance. After a mean follow-up of 32 months, one patient with a $pT_1N_0M_0$ clear cell carcinoma tumor developed a metastatic disease 10 months after the LPN.[17]

Complications

In the initial 200 patients undergoing LPN for renal mass, the complication rate was 33% (urological 18%, other 15%). This included hemorrhage in 9.5%, urine leakage in 4.5%, and open conversion in 1%, with no perioperative mortality [17] (Table 8f-1). Biologic hemostatic sealants have been used in open and laparoscopic partial nephrectomy, improving the risk of postoperative hemorrhage. In a recent study with 100 patients, the use of gelatin matrix thrombin sealant Floseal® (Baxter Healthcare, Deerfield, IL) decreased the postoperative hemorrhagic rate to 3.2% and urine leak to less than 1.5%, similar to open partial nephrectomy[19] (Table 8f-2). This hemostatic agent was approved by the Food and Drug Administration in 1999 and is composed of glutaraldehyde cross-linked fibers derived from bovine collagen. The gelatin granules swell on contact with blood, creating a physical plug that mechanically controls the bleeding.

TABLE 8f-1. Intraoperative, postoperative, and delayed complications in 200 laparoscopic partial nephrectomies.

Complications	Number (%)
Intraoperative	11 (5.5%)
Bleeding	8 (4%)
Bowel injury	1 (0.5%)
Resected ureter	1 (0.5%)
Pleural injury	1 (0.5%)
Convert to open	0
Postoperative	24 (12%)
Pulmonary	7 (3.5%)
Cardiovascular	5 (2.5%)
Bleeding	4 (4%)
Renal insufficiency	3 (1.5%)
Urine leakage	2 (1%)
Gastrointestinal	2 (1%)
Gluteal fasciotomy	1 (0.5%)
Delayed	31 (15.5%)
Bleeding	9 (4.5%)
Urine leakage	7 (3.5%)
Infection	7 (3.5%)
Renal insufficiency	1 (0.5%)
Other	5 (2.5%)

Source: Adapted from Permpongkosol et al.[17]

TABLE 8f-2. Complications of laparoscopic partial nephrectomy: no Floseal vs. with Floseal.

	No Floseal ($n = 68$)	With Floseal ($n = 63$)	p-value
Hemorrhage	11.8%	3.2%	0.08
Urine leak	5.9%	1.5%	0.12
Overall complications	36.8%	16%	0.008

Source: Adapted from Gill et al.[7]

Costs

In the retrospective financial analysis with 30 partial nephrectomies with uncomplicated perioperative course (15 LPN vs. 15 open partial nephrectomies), the LPN was associated with 20% greater intraoperative costs ($p < 0.001$) and 55% less postoperative costs ($p < 0.001$). The overall hospital costs was 15% lower in LPN ($p = 0.002$).[20]

Future Directions

Hemorrhage and urinary leak are still the major complications of open and LPN. Biological sealants are available for adjuvant hemostasis and collecting system closure. New technologies such as laser and hydro-jet have been clinically investigated and are promising techniques for performing LPN without hilar control.

Conclusions

Laparoscopic partial nephrectomy is a technically challenging procedure, reserved for those surgeons with adequate prior laparoscopic experience. It is the only form of minimally invasive treatment for small renal tumors that duplicates the open technique. It should be employed in selected patients who are candidates for nephron-sparing surgery. At the Cleveland Clinic, LPN is now being performed for complex and infiltrating tumors in patients who are candidates for nephron-sparing surgery. Complications and long-term oncological and renal functional outcomes are equivalent to those of open partial nephrectomy.

References

1. Licht MR, Novick AC. Nephron sparing surgery for renal cell carcinoma. J Urol 1993; 149: 1–7.
2. Fergany AF, Hafez KS, Novick AC. Long-term results of nephron sparing surgery for localized renal cell carcinoma: 10-year followup. J Urol 2000; 163: 442–445.
3. Rassweiler JJ, Abbou C, Janetschek G, Jeschke K. Laparoscopic partial nephrectomy. The European experience. Urol Clin North Am. 2000; 27: 721–736.
4. Gill IS, Desai MM, Kaouk JH, Meraney AM, Murphy DP, Sung GT, et al. Laparoscopic partial nephrectomy for renal tumor: duplicating open surgical techniques. J Urol 2002; 167: 469–467.
5. Ward JP. Determination of the optimum temperature for regional renal hypothermia during temporary renal ischemia. Br J Urol 1975; 47: 17–24.
6. Novick AC. Renal hypothermia: in vivo and ex vivo. Urol Clin North Am 1983; 10:637–644.
7. Gill IS, Abreu SC, Desai MM, Steinberg AP, Ramani AP, Ng C, et al. Laparoscopic ice slush renal hypothermia for partial nephrectomy: the initial experience. J Urol 2003; 170: 52–56.

8. Haber G P, Gill I S. Laparoscopic partial nephrectomy: contemporary technique and outcomes. Eur Urol 2006; 20: 660–665.

9. Ng CS, Gill IS, Ramani AP, Steinberg AP, Spaliviero M, Abreu SC, et al. Transperitoneal versus retroperitoneal laparoscopic partial nephrectomy: patient selection and perioperative outcomes. J Urol 2005; 174: 846–849.

10. Desai MM, Gill IS, Ramani AP, Spaliviero M, Rybicki L, Kaouk JH. The impact of warm ischaemia on renal function after laparoscopic partial nephrectomy. BJU Int 2005; 95: 377–383.

11. Frank I, Colombo JR Jr, Rubinstein M, Desai M, Kaouk J, Gill IS. Laparoscopic partial nephrectomy for centrally located renal tumors. J Urol 2006; 175; 849–852.

12. Gill IS, Colombo JR, Jr., Frank I, Moinzadeh A, Kaouk J, Desai M. Laparoscopic partial nephrectomy for hilar tumors. J Urol 2005; 174: 850–853.

13. Gill IS, Colombo JR, Jr., Moinzadeh A, Finelli A, Ukimura O, Tucker K, et al. Laparoscopic partial nephrectomy in solitary kidney. J Urol 2006; 175: 454–458.

14. Gill IS, Matin SF, Desai MM, Kaouk JH, Steinberg A, Mascha E, et al. Comparative analysis of laparoscopic versus open partial nephrectomy for renal tumors in 200 patients. J Urol 2003; 170: 64–68.

15. Moinzadeh A, Gill IS, Finelli A, Kaouk J, Desai M. Laparoscopic partial nephrectomy: 3-year followup. J Urol 2006; 175: 459–462.

16. Lane B, Gill IS. Five year oncological outcomes of laparoscopic partial nephrectomy. J Urol 2007; 177: 70–74.

17. Permpongkosol S, Colombo JR Jr, Gill IS, Kavoussi LR. Positive surgical parenchymal margins after laparoscopic partial nephrectomy for renal cell carcinoma: oncologic outcomes. J Urol 2006; 176: 2401–2404.

18. Ramani AP, Desai MM, Steinberg AP, Ng CS, Abreu SC, Kaouk JH, Finelli A, Novick AC, Gill IS. Complications of laparoscopic partial nephrectomy in 200 cases. J Urol 2005; 173: 42–47.

19. Gill IS, Ramani AP, Spaliviero M, Xu M, Finelli A, Kaouk JH, et al. Improved hemostasis during laparoscopic partial nephrectomy using gelatin matrix thrombin sealant. Urology 2005; 65: 463–466.

20. Steinberg AP, Desai MM, Gill IS: Financial analysis of laparoscopic versus open partial nephrectomy. J Endourol 2002; 16(suppl 1): 158.

8g
How Much Margin to Spare in Partial Nephrectomy

Hein P.A. van Poppel and Raf van Reusel

Introduction

Nephron-sparing surgery (NSS) has undergone an enormous shift from absolute, imperative indications to elective indications, in the presence of a normal contralateral kidney. While it is obvious that complete excision is mandatory, the size of the margin remains debated.

On the basis of retrospective analyses, it appears that a normal tissue margin of just 1 mm or more may be adequate to prevent local recurrence from renal cell carcinoma. The margin status is more important than the margin size.

How Much Margin to Spare in Partial Nephrectomy?

Nephron-Sparing Surgery in Historical Perspective

The history of renal surgery had an inauspicious beginning when a whole kidney (Walcott, 1861) and a part of a kidney (Spiegelberg, 1867) were mistakenly removed during operations for liver cysts. The two patients died.

In 1869 Simon successfully performed the first planned nephrectomy to cure a urinary fistula. Largely forgotten although is that a year later in 1870 he also performed the first deliberate partial nephrectomy for hydronephrosis.[1]

Partial nephrectomy for excising renal lesions dates back as far as 1884, when Wells described a technique for removing a perirenal fibrolipoma.[2] In 1887, Czerny was the first to perform a partial nephrectomy as therapy for renal malignancy.[3] Excessive morbidity limited its application at that time.

In 1950 Vermooten described how conservative surgery for certain renal tumors had to be performed. One of the issues was that a margin of at least 1 cm of healthy renal parenchyma had to be resected together with the tumor.[4]

The role of partial nephrectomy was subsequently challenged by Robson who stated that early ligation of the renal vessels decreased the risk of hematological spread. Radical nephrectomy was thus defined with removal of the perinephric fat and excision of all regional lymph nodes.[5]

Since that time, radical nephrectomy has remained the standard against which all other forms of surgical treatment for renal cell carcinoma were compared.

A second interest for NSS renal cell carcinoma could date back to the late 1960s and early 1970s when discussion was stimulated by papers showing tumor-free survival rates after partial nephrectomy comparable to those after radical nephrectomy.[6]

In early series of partial nephrectomy for renal cancer, this was done in high-risk cases in which NSS was the only alternative to renal replacement therapy.

An excellent tumor-free survival rate after partial nephrectomy for renal cell carcinoma of a solitary or single functioning kidney was reported for the first time by Grabstald and Aviles in 1968. They performed 30 partial nephrectomies and concluded that this approach was feasible since 23 of their patients had a long-term tumor-free survival.[7]

The subsequent review of Schiff in 1979 confirmed a 78% cancer-free survival rate in 62 patients with absolute indications for NSS.[8]

In 1980 Jacobs et al. noted a significantly improved survival rate after NSS when comparing the results of bilateral partial nephrectomy versus bilateral total nephrectomy and dialysis for bilateral synchronous renal cell carcinoma.[9]

This marked the beginning of the era of elective NSS for renal tumors. Well encapsulated tumors proved to be amenable for simple tumorectomy and for other small renal tumors, the urologist tried to avoid radical nephrectomy in order to spare as much healthy parenchyma as possible (Fig. 8g-1).

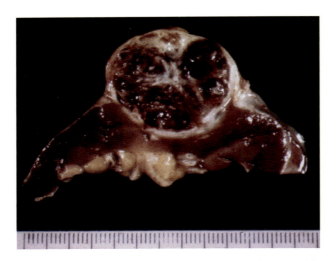

FIGURE 8g-1. Cystic clear cell renal cell carcinoma with a firm pseudocapsule that would have been perfectly amenable to enucleation.

From Imperative to Elective Nephron-Sparing Surgery

Meanwhile, NSS has been subject to an evolution from imperative to elective indications.

NSS was initially indicated for solitary kidney or bilateral tumors. It was, however, suggested that low-grade, low-stage tumors, that might not need a 1-cm margin to be cured, can be treated as well in those with normal contralateral kidneys. The number of such tumors has increased in recent years due to the increased use of noninvasive radiological imaging techniques, especially ultrasound and computed tomography (CT) scan. A 1-cm margin in these patients may require the sacrifice of more healthy renal parenchyma than necessary to guarantee oncological cure.

Although the long-term functional advantage of NSS when there is a normal contralateral kidney remains to be definitively shown, the benefit of maximal nephron preservation might include a decreased risk of progression to chronic renal insufficiency and end-stage renal disease.

In recent studies patients who had a radical nephrectomy were compared to patients who underwent elective NSS. Both groups were well matched for age, tumor size, preoperative serum creatinine level, and year of surgery. Although the authors identified no significant difference in cancer-free survival, they showed that at 10 years, renal insufficiency (defined as an increase in serum creatinine above 20 mg/liter) was significantly different between the groups, occurring in 12.4% of radical nephrectomy cases compared to only 2.3% of partial nephrectomy cases.[10]

Similarly, McKiernan et al. found that the chance of progression to renal insufficiency was significantly higher after radical nephrectomy.[11]

In both groups, differences in functional renal reserve were obviously responsible for these findings.

Local Recurrence after Conservative Surgery

The major disadvantage of this type of surgery remains the risk of local recurrence. The results of partial nephrectomy for small renal cell carcinoma, however, are excellent and local recurrences have been reported to occur in less than 1% of cases.

In 1992 an extensive patient series from Mainz, Germany, about 72 cases of elective NSS for renal cell carcinoma was reported. No patient had a local recurrence after a mean follow-up of 40 months.[12]

One year later, another German center published results of 105 cases of NSS for renal cell carcinoma with a normal contralateral kidney. None of the patients had a local recurrence or developed metastatic disease.[13]

Another European centre reported on 76 patients who underwent NSS for renal cell carcinoma from 1981 to 1996. Fifty-one of these patients had a normal contralateral kidney. With a mean follow-up of 75 months no local recurrence was noted, although three patients developed systemic disease.[14]

In a report from the Mayo clinic in 1996, no difference in cancer-specific survival or progression-free intervals at 5 or 10 years was found in patients who underwent radical nephrectomy versus NSS. Tumor size and stage were the primary determinants of outcome in the two treatment groups.[15]

An Italian prospective study randomly assigned 19 patients to NSS and 21 to radical nephrectomy. After a mean follow-up of 70 months there were no significantly important differences in cancer-specific survival between the two groups.[16]

Barbalias et al. compared radical nephrectomy with NSS in 89 patients with sporadic, localized, asymptomatic renal masses less than 5 cm in diameter and observed no difference in disease-specific survival at a mean follow-up of 59 months.[17]

Butler et al. compared NSS with radical nephrectomy in patients who presented with a single renal cell carcinoma of 4 cm or less and a normal contralateral kidney. The pathological stage was low (pT1 or pT2) in 90% of the lesions and 5-year cancer-free survival did not differ in the groups.[18]

A study from the Cleveland Clinic in 1999 evaluated the impact of tumor size on patient survival and tumor recurrence after NSS for localized renal cell carcinoma. A total of 485 patients were stratified based on size criteria, including cutoffs of less than 2.5 cm, 2.5–4 cm, 4–7 cm, and more than 7 cm. The findings showed a significantly lower recurrence rate and significantly improved survival after NSS for tumors of 4 cm or less compared to those of more than 4 cm.[19]

A long-term follow-up study from the same institute published data after 10 years of experience with NSS for renal cell carcinoma. It became clear that the mean time to recurrence was related to the tumor stage. For stage T1a tumors (< 4 cm) there was a 4% recurrence rate with a mean time to recurrence of 70 months. Stage T1b tumors (4–7 cm) had a remarkably high recurrence rate of 33% with a mean time to recurrence of 47 months. T2 tumors (>7 cm) had a local recurrence in 20% of cases after a mean time of 91 months, and finally stage T3a tumors recurred locally in 53% of the patients with a mean recurrence time of 57 months. Interestingly enough, a complete tumor resection was carried out in all patients and this was confirmed by pathological examination. The 5-year cause-specific survival rate was 84%. At 10 years the cause-specific survival was 73%. Of the patients 26% died from metastatic disease. Long-term preservation of renal function was achieved in 93% of patients. Cause-specific survival for patients with tumors of <4 cm was 98% at 5 years and 92% at 10 years, regardless of the indication of partial nephrectomy.

These data suggest that important negative predictors of survival include high tumor grade, high tumor stage, and tumors of >4 cm.[20]

The largest review ever included more than 1800 cases of NSS for renal cell carcinoma. The authors concluded that the overall risk for tumor recurrence lies between 0% and 10%. The risk is clearly the lowest in patients who underwent NSS for the T1a low stage lesions of 4 cm or less.[21]

Based on these findings a subclassification for organ-confined stage T1 tumors has been proposed to distinguish those 4 cm or less (T1a) from those more than 4 cm (stage T1b).

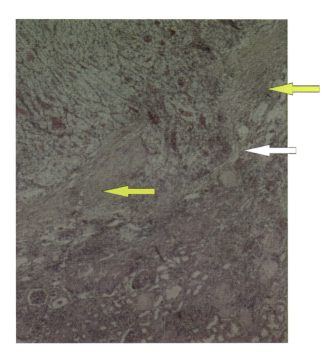

FIGURE 8g-2. Renal cell carcinoma (top)—-perforation (white arrow) of pseudocapsule (yellow arrows).

Multifocality and Margin Status

Tumor recurrence after NSS may be due to the presence of undetected, unrecognizable or occult multifocal lesions or to the development of a new primary or a metastatic focus of renal cell carcinoma in the renal remnant. This is then defined as "kidney recurrence."[22] Besides a higher multifocality rate in papillary renal cell carcinoma, multifocality seems to be more frequent in patients with germ line mutations such as von Hippel–Lindau disease[23] and in patients with larger tumors, especially tumors that extended beyond the renal capsule.[24] In the large series report from the Cleveland clinic, multifocal disease occurred in approximately 5% of cases.[21]

A true "local recurrence" results from incomplete resection of the primary tumor or from tumor invasion beyond the pseudocapsule when the margin is not resected wide enough.[22,25,26]

While most renal cell carcinomas have a rather solid intact pseudocapsule (Fig. 8g-1), FIG 8g-1some, often smaller, tumors have no pseudocapsule or present with an incomplete pseudocapsule, so that an attempt at enucleation can result in a positive section margin that might lead to local recurrence (Figs. 8g-2, 8g-3 and 8g-4).

It is widely accepted that tumor excision with a surrounding margin of normal parenchyma is the safest approach to ensure no residual tumor in the renal remnant. However, the optimal margin size remains a subject of debate.

In most series the authors have performed either a wedge resection in healthy parenchyma, an enucleoresection where tumor is resected with a rim of just a few millimeters of normal tissue, or finally even a pure enucleation relying on

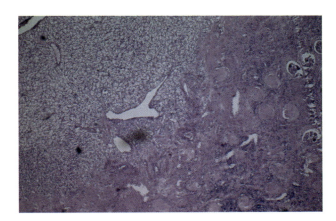

FIGURE 8g-3. Clear cell type renal cell carcinoma without any pseudocapsule.

the presence of an intact pseudocapsule (Fig. 8g-5). This can be easily done in peripherally located exophytic tumors and could be more challenging in centrally located tumors.

Although central or peripheral tumor localization within the renal parenchyma is a relevant technical consideration for nephron-sparing approaches, it has no important role for determining cancer-specific outcome and does not appear to mitigate the excellent results of NSS for small solitary unilateral lesions.[27,28]

Reports from some expert centers advocate verifying intra-operatively the absence of malignancy in the remaining portion of the kidney by frozen-section examinations of the specimen or random biopsy examinations from the specimens

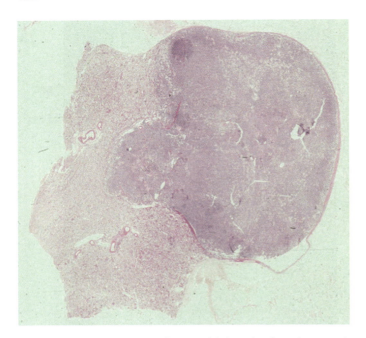

FIGURE 8g-4. Renal cell carcinoma with invasion into the normal renal parenchyma.

from the renal margin of excision.[29] The problem with intra-operatively frozen section is that false-positive and false-negative results can be obtained.

Pitfalls in the evaluation of frozen section specimens in NSS have been described, emphasizing the difficulty of distinguishing crushed tubules and detached atypical cells from really malignant cells. Benign renal tubules can be mistaken for neoplastic ones and damaged minifragments of renal parenchyma with freeze artifacts can make the interpretation by the pathologist extremely difficult.[30] This means that a positive pathological report would indicate a possibly unnecessary more extensive resection or radical nephrectomy.

On the other hand, the meaning of a negative frozen section is not equally unambiguous. Reports on partial nephrectomy cases where the frozen section of the margins was negative while the definitive margin was positive have been published.

A multicenter study was conducted in which disease progression, margin status, and the shortest distance of normal parenchyma around the tumor in the final pathological specimen were analyzed. The authors showed that only a minority (28%) of patients with a positive margin on final pathological examination developed a local recurrence during a mean follow-up of 60 months (range 5–124). The mean tumor size was 3.0 cm (range 0.9–11.0 cm). Out of 67 cases, 7 patients were found to have a positive margin. One patient died of metastatic disease, one was alive with systemic recurrence, and five patients had no evidence of disease after follow-up.[31] No higher recurrence rate was noticed in patients with positive margins on definitive pathology and salvage nephrectomy performed in some of them could not find residual tumor in the remnant kidney.[32]

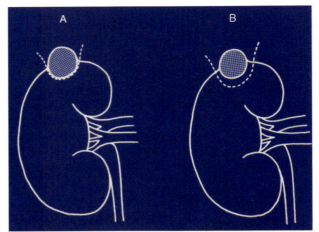

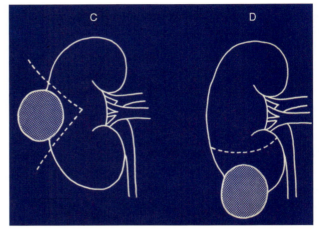

FIGURE 8g-5. (A) Pure enucleation relying on the intact tumoral pseudocapsule. (B) Enucleoresection or excavation with a rim of healthy parenchyma. (C) Wedge resection. (D) Polar nephrectomy.

A recently published clinical pathological study reports on 301 partial nephrectomies with the routine use of frozen section analysis. The frozen section found two positive tumor margins (0.7%) and in both the tumor was centrally located. In the subsequent immediate radical nephrectomy, no residual tumor was found. Parafin section disclosed positive margins in four other cases (1.3%) and only one of these underwent radical nephrectomy for local recurrence after 9 months, while the three others remained tumor free at 2, 5, and 10 years. The authors concluded that frozen section analysis during NSS has minimal clinical significance.[33]

Therefore, the relevance of intraoperative assessment of the surgical margins (and even the definitive pathology of the margin status) remains doubtful. It has never been demonstrated that biopsy of the tumor bed may decrease the positive margin rate. Moreover, it is technically not easy to perform and if extensive biopsies are taken, it may increase the risk of complications.

Therefore, recommendation of biopsy of the tumor bed seems to be more a consequence of a consolidated surgical tradition than an evidence-based suggestion, at least for renal cell carcinoma.[34]

Margin Size

While it is obvious that complete excision is mandatory, the size of the margin remains debated.

From at least a 1-cm margin of normal parenchyma around the tumor in the beginning of NSS, more recently it was suggested that a safe excision necessitates a margin of 5 mm (Fig. 8g-6).

Long-term results of partial nephrectomy were presented, leaving no more than a 5-mm rim of normal parenchyma around the tumor at resection for unilateral renal cell carcinoma in 70 patients with a normal contralateral kidney. No local recurrence was reported, but two patients, however, died of metastatic disease.[35]

When NSS is performed for a small renal cell carcinoma, a 10- or even a 5-mm margin may still be too large. However, enucleation alone would not be sufficient due to significant risk of incomplete excision.

A more recent retrospective analysis shows, however, that a resection margin of just 1 mm or more may be perfectly adequate to prevent local recurrences from renal cell carcinoma.[32] The same study noted disease progression in 18% of patients with a negative margin distance of less than 1 mm after NSS. Of 11 patients with a negative margin distance less than 1 mm, nine were recurrence free, one had simultaneous local and pulmonary relapse, and the other had pulmonary recurrence only. The remainder of the study (49 patients) had negative margins greater than 1 mm. All of them were alive without evidence of disease at the last follow-up.

Castilla et al. published in 2002 a review of the resection margins, tumor size, TNM stage, and Fuhrman nuclear grade in 69 patients who underwent NSS surgery for renal cell

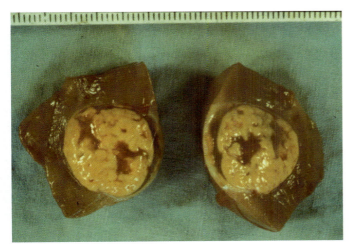

FIGURE 8g-6. Small papillary renal cell carcinoma (18 mm diameter) with very tiny pseudocapsule treated by enucleoresection with a safe 4-mm margin.

carcinoma between 1976 and 1988.[36] The mean postoperative follow-up was 102 months. The goal of this study was to determine whether these parameters were associated with disease progression after NSS (defined as local tumor recurrence or metastasis). TNM stage and Fuhrman nuclear grade correlated with disease progression. Patients with T1–T2 tumors had less disease progression than did patients with T3 tumors ($p < 0.001$). Disease progression also worsened with Fuhrman nuclear grade ($p < 0.001$). Tumor size did even so correlate with disease progression ($p < 0.001$).

The conclusion was that the width of the resection margin did not correlate with long-term disease progression ($p = 0.98$) and that a histological tumor-free margin is sufficient to achieve complete local excision of renal cell cancer.[36]

These findings were confirmed by another publication in the same year. A total of 44 patients who had a median follow-up of 49 months after NSS for renal cell carcinoma were studied. The mean tumor size was 3.22 cm. Three patients had positive surgical margins on the final pathological report. The mean and median size of the negative margins was 0.25 and 0.2 cm with a range from 0.05–0.7 cm. None of the patients with negative parenchymal margins after NSS for stages T1–T2 N0M0 renal cell carcinoma had a local recurrence at the resection site.[37]

In 2004 Puppo et al. reviewed the records of 94 patients who underwent NSS for renal cell carcinoma leaving around the tumor a thin layer of grossly normal parenchyma and adjacent perinephric fat.[34] The patients were followed up by blood examination, ultrasound, and CT scan every 6 months during the first 2 years and then annually afterward. The pathological stage was T1a in 84 cases, T1b in 4 cases, and T3a in 3 cases. The surgical margins were negative in all patients. The mean and median shortest distance from tumor to inked healthy tissue margin was 2.4 and 1.9 mm, respectively. The median follow-up was 59 months (range 10–128). One pT3a patient developed metastatic disease and died 2 years after surgery. The other patients had no local recurrence. The 5-year cancer-specific survival and 5-year disease-free survival were 98.9%. They concluded that enucleoresection of small renal tumors leaving only a minimal rim of grossly normal renal parenchyma (in this study a mean shortest distance of 2.4 mm between the tumor and the inked healthy tissue) is a safe and is a reliable procedure that can be adopted without significantly increasing the oncological risk.[34]

A prospective study of 82 radical nephrectomy specimens for T1 renal cell carcinoma of 4 cm or less was reported recently. Of tumors 30% had no intact pseudocapsule (cf. Fig. 8g-2). In 20% of cases there was positive cancerous growth beyond the pseudocapsule with invasion into the normal parenchyma in 12.5%, venous invasion in 2.5%, and satellite tumors in 5%. The mean distance between the primary tumor and the extrapseudocapsular lesion was 1.5 mm.[38]

Therefore it seems that the margin status is the most important issue and not the margin size. Pure enucleation, however, should be further discouraged because of the risk of incomplete resection in patients other than those with von Hippel–Lindau disease who have multiple low-stage, low-grade encapsulated tumors in both kidneys with a high risk of tumor recurrence in other locations in the kidney. On the other hand, leaving a margin of healthy parenchyma of 0.5 cm or more as advocated in the beginning of the experience with NSS for renal cell carcinoma means the sacrifice or more normal tissue than necessary.

Recent long-term data support the role of NSS, leaving less than 0.5 cm of normal parenchyma as an appropriate oncological procedure in properly selected patients. A rim of normal tissue should surround the tumor in elective kidney-sparing surgery. Enucleoresection remains the resection technique of choice.

The use of routine frozen section is not advocated.[39]

Partial nephrectomy is becoming the standard for the treatment of renal cell carcinoma less than 4 cm in size. Further expansion of the indications of partial nephrectomy can be expected.[40]

Careful patient selection and application of oncological principles are important to guarantee a successful nephron-sparing resection of renal cell carcinoma.

References

1. Herr, H.W. (2005) A history of partial nephrectomy for renal tumors. *J. Urol.*, 173:705–708.
2. Wells, S. (1884) Successful removal of two solid circumrenal tumors. *Br. Med. J.*, 1:758.
3. Herczel, E. (1890) Uber nierenextirpation. *Bietr. Klinich Chirur.g*, 6:485.
4. Vermooten, V. (1950) Indications for conservative surgery in certain renal tumors: a study based on the growth pattern of the clear cell carcinoma. *J. Urol.*, 64:200–202.
5. Robson, C.J., Churchill, B.M., Anderson, W. (1969) The results of radical nephrectomy for renal cell carcinoma. *J. Urol.*, 101:297.
6. Wickham, J.E. (1975) Conservative renal surgery for adenocarcinoma: the place of bench surgery. *Br. J. Urol.*, 47:25.
7. Grabstald, H., Aviles, E. (1968) Renal cell cancer in the solitary or sole-functioning kidney. *Cancer*, 22:973–987.
8. Schiff, M., Bagley, D.H., Lytton, B. (1979) Treatment of solitary and bilateral renal carcinomas. *J. Urol.*, 121:581.
9. Jacobs, S.C., Berg, S.I., Lawson, R.K. (1980) Synchronous bilateral renal cell carcinoma: total surgical excision. *Cancer*, 46:2341–2345.
10. Lau, W., Blute, M.L., Zincke, H. (2000) Matched comparison of radical nephrectomy versus elective nephron-sparing surgery for renal cell carcinoma: evidence for increased renal failure rate on long term follow-up (> 10years). *J. Urol.*, suppl, 163:153, abstract 681.
11. McKiernan, J., Yossepowitch, O., Kattan, M.W., Simmons, R., Motzer, R.J., Reuter, V.E., Russo P. (2000) Partial nephrectomy for renal cortical tumors: pathological findings and impact on outcome. *Urology*, 60:1003.
12. Steinbach, F., Stockle, M., Muller, S.C., Thuroff, J.W., Melchior, S.W., Stein, R. et al. (1992) Conservative surgery

13. Moll, V., Becht, E., Ziegler, M. (1993) Kidney preserving surgery in renal cell tumors: indications, techniques and results in 152 patients. *J. Urol.*, 150:319–323.
14. Van Poppel, H., Barmelis, B., Oyen, R., Baert, L. (1998) Partial nephrectomy for renal cell carcinoma can achieve long-term tumor control. *J. Urol.*, 160:674–678.
15. Lerner, S.E., Hawkins, C.A., Blute, M.L. et al. (1996) Disease outcome in patients with low stage renal cell carcinoma treated with nephron-sparing or radical surgery. *J. Urol.*, 155:1868.
16. D'Armiento, M., Damiano, R., Feleppa, B. et al. (1997) Elective conservative surgery for renal cell carcinoma versus radical nephrectomy: a prospective study. *Br. J. Urol.*, 79:15.
17. Barbalias, G.A., Liatsikos, E.N., Tsintavis, A., et al. (1999) Adenocarcinoma of the kidney: nephron-sparing approach versus radical nephrectomy. *J. Surg. Oncol.*, 72:156.
18. Butler, B.P., Novick, A.C., Miller, D.P. (1995) Management of small unilateral renal cell carcinomas: radical versus nephron-sparing surgery. *Urology*, 45:34.
19. Hafez, K.S., Novick, A.C., Campbell, N.C. (1997) Patterns of tumor recurrence and guidelines for follow-up after nephron-sparing surgery for sporadic renal cell carcinoma. *J. Urol.*, 157:2067.
20. Fergany, A.F., Hafez, K.S., Novick, A.C. (2000) Long term results of nephron sparing surgery for localized renal cell carcinoma: 10 year follow-up. *J. Urol.*, 163:442–445.
21. Uzzo, R.G., Novick, A.C. (2001) Nephron sparing surgery for renal tumors: indications, techniques and outcomes. *J. Urol.*, 166:6–18.
22. Van Poppel, H. (2003) Partial nephrectomy: the standard approach for small renal cell carcinoma. *Curr.t Opin. Urol.*, 13:431–432.
23. Zbar, B. (1995) Von Hippel-Lindau disease and sporadic renal cell carcinoma. *Cancer Surv.*, 25:219–232.
24. Whang, M., O'Toole, K., Bixon, R., Brunetti, J., Ikeguchi, E., Olsson, C.A. et al. (1995) The incidence of multifocal renal cell carcinoma in patients who are candidates for partial nephrectomy. *J. Urol.*, 154:968–970.
25. Rosenthal, C.L., Kraft, R., Zingg, E.J. (1984) Organ-preserving surgery in renal cell carcinoma; tumor enucleation versus partial kidney resection. *Eur. Urol.*, 10:222–228.
26. Marshall, F.F., Taxy, J.B., Fishman, E.K., Chang, R. (1986) The feasibility of surgical enucleation for renal cell carcinoma. *J. Urol.*, 135:231–234.
27. Hafez, K.S., Novick, A.C., Butler, B.P. (1998) Management of small solitary unilateral renal cell carcinomas: impact of central versus peripheral tumor localisation. *J. Urol.*, 159:1156.
28. Black, P., Filipas, D., Hohenfellner, R. (2000) Nephron-sparing surgery for central renal tumors: experience with 33 cases, *J. Urol.*, 163:737.
29. Novick, A.C. (2002) Nephron-sparing surgery for renal cell carcinoma. *Annu. Rev. Med.*, 53:393–407.
30. McHale, T., Malkowicz, S.B., Tomaszewski, J.E., Genega, E.M. (2002) Potential pitfalls in the frozen section evaluation of parenchymal margins in nephron-sparing surgery. *Am. J. Clin. Pathol.*, 118:903–910.
31. Piper, N.Y., Bishoff, J.T., Magee, C., Haffron, J.M., Flanigan, R.C., Mintiens A, Van Poppel et al. (2001) Is a 1-cm

margin necessary during nephron-sparing surgery for renal cell carcinoma? *Urology*, 58:849–852.

32. Zigeuner, R., Quehenberger, F., Pummer, K. *et al.* (2003) Long-term results of nephron-sparing surgery for renal cell carcinoma in 114 patients: risk factors for progressive disease. *BJU Int.*, 92: 567–571.

33. Duvdevani, M., Laufer, M., Kastin, A., Mor, Y., Nadu, A., Hanani, J., Nativ, O., Ramon, J. (2005) Is frozen section analysis in nephron sparing surgery necessary? A clinicopathological study in 301 cases. *J. Urol.*, 173:385–387.

34. Puppo, P., Introini, C., Calvi, P., Naselli, A. (2004), Long term results of excision of small renal cancer surrounded by a minimal layer of grossly normal parenchyma; review of 94 cases. *Eur. Urol.*, 46:477–481.

35. Herr, H.W. (1999) Partial nephrectomy for unilateral renal cell carcinoma and a normal contralateral kidney: 10 year follow-up. *J. Urol.*, 161:33–34.

36. Castilla, E.A., Liou, L.S., Abrahams, N.A., Fergany, A., Rybicki, L.A., Myles, J. et al. (2002) Prognostic importance of resection margin width after nephron-sparing surgery for renal cell carcinoma. *Urology*, 60;993–997.

37. Sutherland, S.E., Resnick, M.I., Maclennan, G.T., Goldman, H.B. (2002) Does the size of the surgical margin in partial nephrectomy for renal cell cancer really matter? *J. Urol.*, 167:61–64.

38. Li, Q.L., Guan, H.W., Zhang, Q.P., Zhang, L.Z., Wang, F.P., Liu, Y.J. (2003) Optimal margin in nephron-sparing surgery for renal cell carcinoma 4cm or less. *Eur. Urol.*, 44: 448–451.

39. Van Poppel, H. (2004) The optimal margins in nephron sparing surgery. *Curr. Opin. Urol.*, 14:227–228.

40. Van Poppel, H. (2004) Conservative vs radical surgery for renal cell carcinoma. *BJU Int.*, 94:766–768.

8h
Advanced Tumors: Tumor Thrombus

Ziya Kirkali and Can Öbek

Introduction

One of the well-established features of renal cell carcinoma (RCC) is its propensity for growth intraluminally into the renal venous circulation, and cephalic propagation in the inferior vena cava (IVC). Involvement of the IVC is detected in 4–10% of newly diagnosed patients.[13,43,46,54,73,81,91] Approximately 50% of IVC thrombi are infrahepatic, 40% intrahepatic, and 10% intraatrial in location. IVC involvement is more common on the right-sided than on the left-sided RCCs. Although intravascular growth implies a worsened biological behavior of the tumor, the presence of tumor thrombus apparently does not ultimately affect the long-term prognosis; however, it has a significant impact on surgical management. Tumor thrombectomy in the IVC improves the prognosis, including those in whom the tumor thrombus extends far into the vessel. In contrast, if only nephrectomy is performed, the prognosis is poor and almost all patients die within a year.[106] Therefore, an aggressive approach to resection has been advocated for several decades and has remained the mainstay of treatment.[81,104] Historically, extensive propagation of thrombus above the hepatic veins was deemed incurable. The constant improvements in radiological imaging methods, perioperative care, anesthesiology, and specifically surgical techniques have changed the fate of these patients. Safer surgical removal of these tumors can now be offered to patients with RCC with venous involvement with survival rates of up to 68% at 5 years.[117]

History

As with any other advanced surgical procedure, the management of patients with RCC involving the IVC has evolved with the cumulative efforts and contributions of many physicians and surgeons over more than a century. It is important to briefly recall the historical landmarks concerning the management of this clinical condition to fully comprehend the current status.

IVC involvement was first described in 1688 by Blancardus.[122] In a review of previous reports of IVC occlusion, Pleasants reported that 16% were due to a neoplasm.[126] Berg, in 1923, described venacavotomy for the extraction of tumor thrombi at the time of nephrectomy.[61] In 1932, Walters and Priestly described controlling the venacavotomy defect with a rubber-covered Doyen clamp and suturing.[82] They noted a temporary increase in lower extremity edema and menstrual flow following ligation of the infrarenal vena cava. Despite these sporadic cases, extension into the IVC was synonymous with incurable disease at that time. The operative mortality was too high, the preoperative assessment of the presence and/or extent of tumor thrombus was not possible, and there was a lack of a staging system. Robson was the first to define a staging system for RCC.[96] He embraced the method of approaching most radical nephrectomies through a thoracoabdominal incision. With this approach, he was able to control the renal pedicle before excessive manipulation of the kidney, remove the kidney with intact Gerota's fascia, and have adequate exposure to the IVC. Later, a patient who survived for 12 years after undergoing a nephrectomy for RCC extending into the inferior vena cava was mentioned by Belt in a personal communication to Kaufmann.[53] In 1961, Clarke performed resection of the IVC with a right nephrectomy and tumor thrombus. He indicated the importance of the development of collateral venous circulation of the left kidney, as a consequence of slow vena cava obstruction.[18] In 1970, Marshall et al. discussed their experience with four patients.[73] They reported pulmonary embolism, even after taking precautions and placing tourniquets above and below the caval thrombus before extraction. More importantly, they reported utilization of cardiopulmonary bypass (CPB) in an effort to remove a suprahepatic IVC tumor thrombus. This was the first case of extracorporeal circulation without a pump, hypothermia, or cardiac arrest. In one of their patients, the contralateral renal vein was occluded during IVC occlusion from above and below the thrombus. This resulted in postoperative renal failure, making the authors think that clamping the renal artery, a technique previously described by Heaney et al.,[44] would have been better. They described occlusion of the IVC within the pericardium and aortic cross-clamping below the diaphragm to avoid pooling of blood within the portal system and lower extremities. The first report of atrial thrombus removal was described by Ardekani in 1971.[3] The preoperative diagnosis was an atrial myxoma, which postoperatively was discovered to be a thrombus extension of an RCC.[3] Skinner *et al.* reported their results on 11 patients and strongly argued that "venous invasion does not indicate an unusually aggressive RCC" and stated that the outcome for these patients was "considerably better than reported."[103] They emphasized the importance of preoperative angiographic evaluation of the thrombus along with attaining control of the IVC or right atrium proximal to the thrombus to avoid intraoperative embolization. In 1975, Freed and Gliedman described a technique using a Foley catheter to extract the thrombus through a cavotomy.[31] The method was associated with a substantial surge of blood during removal of the tumor thrombus, which was believed to aid in cleaning the remaining thrombus. A Pringle maneuver, initially described in 1908,[93] was first used during the resection of the RCC with IVC involvement by Abdelsayed *et al.* in 1978.[1] Preoperative angioinfarction was first suggested by Schefft *et al.*[100] In 1980, Clayman *et al.* referred to a technique of liver mobilization, in which the liver is rotated to the left side of the abdomen to expose the retrohepatic IVC.[19] This technique was originally described by Langenbuch in 1894.[59] They also described two simple yet important and practical tests to evaluate the functional potential of the remaining renal units in cases in which caval resection or renal vein ligation was necessary. With the IVC clamped above the thrombus, pressure in the unaffected renal vein can be determined. A pressure greater than 40 mm Hg would suggest renal congestion, proteinuria, and potential renal failure. The second test is performed after clamping the involved kidney. After the intravenous administration of 5 ml of indigo carmine, blue dyed urine should be visible within 12 minutes. If IVC clamping results in unfavorable hypertension, and/or the dye test is negative, renoportal anastomosis or autotransplantation of the remaining kidney should be considered. In 1980, Novick and Cosgrove reported their approach to the removal of thrombus from the right atrium.[84] An important technical point highlighted was kidney mobilization prior to CPB, thus avoiding heparin during radical nephrectomy in an effort to reduce blood loss. Careful retroperitoneal hemostasis was also achieved before CPB. In 1983, Vaislic *et al.* advocated CPB and deep hypothermic arrest in the management of tumor thrombus reaching the right atrium.[123] Marshall *et al.*, in 1984, described their technique using hypothermia, cardiac arrest, and temporary exsanguination in combination with CPB.[71] This technique allowed for a bloodless working field. The use of a vena caval umbrella filter to prevent intraoperative emboli was advocated by Giuliani *et al.*[35] Fiberoptic examination of the IVC was described by Hartman in 1989.[42] Transesophageal echocardiography was depicted as an accurate imaging technique to

determine the extent of thrombus by Treiger *et al.*[119] In 1994, Marsh and Lange reported their practice of applying liver transplant techniques to difficult upper abdominal urological cases.[68] Further application of liver transplant techniques was advocated by Ciancio *et al.*, who described the piggyback technique as well as the conventional technique of liver mobilization through a modified cruciate incision for gaining access to the retrohepatic IVC.[17] An RCC with renal vein thrombus was successfully removed laparoscopically in 1996 by McDougall *et al.* and in 2000 by Savage and Gill.[66,99]

Assessment of Venous Extension

Identification of the presence and extent of tumor thrombus associated with RCC is essential for proper staging and planning surgical strategy. Renal venous extension occurs more frequently with cancer of the right kidney and with relatively larger (>5 cm) tumors. Renal vein enlargement does not necessarily indicate tumor thrombus; it may be a consequence of increased blood flow from a hypervascular tumor. On the other hand, renal vein thrombosis may occur from either tumor or bland thrombus and may not result in venous enlargement.

Ultrasonography is an easy and noninvasive method that has been used extensively to evaluate venous extension. The cephalad extent can be clearly seen with this imaging modality. The overall accuracy is in the range of 60–100%.[47] The major shortcomings of ultrasonography are operator dependency and loss of dynamic information from real time to static images. The presence of bowel gas or obesity may also preclude accurate visualization of the IVC.[47,124]

Computed tomography (CT) scanning usually detects gross renal vein and IVC involvement (Fig. 8h-1); however, it is not accurate in delineating the cephalad extent of a thrombus[39] In a series of 431 consecutive patients, the sensitivity of magnetic resonance imaging (MRI) (90%) for detecting an IVC thrombus was superior to that of either CT (79%) or conventional sonography (68%).[51] MRI is a noninvasive and accurate modality for demonstrating both the presence and the distal extent of vena caval involvement, and thus has become the preferred diagnostic imaging approach. Axial, coronal, and sagittal images can be obtained (Fig. 8h-2).[39,90] Gadolinium-enhanced scanning may help to differentiate between tumor thrombus and bland thrombus.[90] A limitation to the current vena caval imaging modality is the inability to differentiate extrinsic vena caval compression from invasion of the vena cava wall.

Renal arteriography may prove to be a useful preoperative imaging study to define distinct arteriolization of a tumor thrombus. This is detected in 35–40% of cases, and in such patients preoperative embolization of the kidney often results in shrinkage of the thrombus facilitating surgical removal. For patients who require treatment with CPB and

(a)

(b)

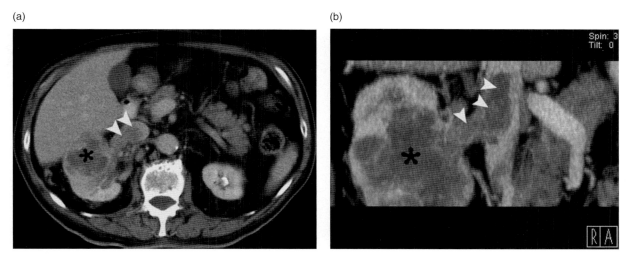

FIGURE 8h-1. Axial (**A**) and coronal (**B**) computerized tomography images demonstrating a right-sided renal mass (asterisk) and a hypodense tumor thrombus (arrows) extending through the renal vein into the vena cava.

(a)

(b)

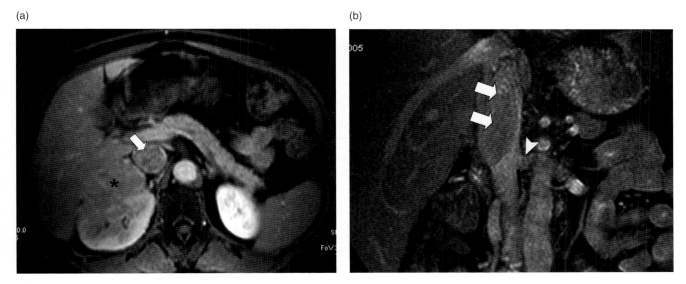

FIGURE 8h-2. (**A**) Axial, contrast-enhanced, T1-weighted image showing the enhanced tumor thrombus (arrow) in the inferior vena cava. The renal cell carcinoma (asterisk) is depicted on the anterior surface of the right kidney. (**B**) Coronal true FISP T2 weighted MR image showing tumor thrombus (arrows) in the inferior vena cava. Note that the left renal vein (arrowhead) is intact, and the lumen of the inferior vena cava is partially patent.

deep hypothermic circulatory arrest, an extensive preoperative evaluation of coronary and carotid arteries has been recommended.[83,86] When present, obstructing lesions of these arteries can be treated either preoperatively or simultaneously during CPB.[5,83] Successful coronary artery bypass grafting or carotid endarterectomy has been reported during the cooling or rewarming phase of the operation.[5,83]

Contrast inferior venacavography, once the gold standard for the imaging of these patients, is rarely used today. It is generally accurate in delineating the extent of the thrombus. When visualization of the upper extent of the tumor is troublesome, or there is complete obstruction, superior venacavography is usually performed.[65] Venacavography is

relatively invasive and it falls short of delineating the cephalic extent of the thrombus, particularly when there is caval occlusion (Fig. 8h-3). It is generally reserved for cases in which the MRI results are unequivocal or MRI is contraindicated (e.g., patients with pacemakers, claustrophobia, certain intracerebral vascular clips, cochlear implants, or intraocular foreign bodies).[83]

Real time transesophageal echocardiography, although invasive, is a useful tool for both preoperative, and more importantly intraoperative, surveillance of RCC with caval extension. During surgery it aids the surgeon in depicting the extent of the thrombus and thus placing the vascular clamp exactly above the thrombus, diagnosing an intraoperative

(a)   (b)

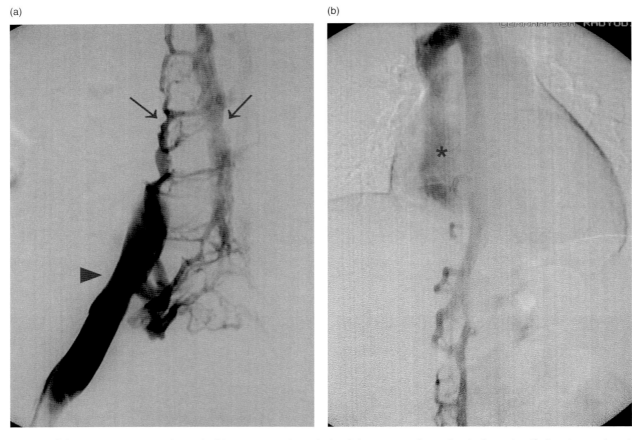

FIGURE 8h-3. (**A**) Vena cavogram performed with a puncture through the right common femoral vein (arrowhead) showing total occlusion of the inferior vena cava starting from the level of the fifth lumbar vertebra. Venous drainage is carried out through the paravertebral venous plexus (arrows). (**B**) Paravertebral venous channels join the azygos system at the level of the tenth thoracic vertebra, and venous flow reaches the superior vena cava and right atrium (asterisk) via the azygos vein.

pulmonary embolism immediately, and evaluating a residual thrombus after resection. Transesophageal echocardiography may also help with the placement of pulmonary artery catheters and assess left ventricular function.[119]

Clinical Findings

Tumor thrombus in the IVC will usually produce symptoms if it causes obstruction. Even in the presence of gradual obstruction, collateral veins may protect venous return, and thus the patient may be symptom free. The most common sign of impaired venous return is the presence of dilated superficial collateral veins on the lower abdomen with cephalad flow.[75] Lower extremity edema, penile or scrotal edema, varicocele, flank pain, thrombosed hemorrhoids, proteinuria, and micro-hematuria are some of the other symptoms and signs that may result from impaired venous return.[80] Varicocele has been reported in up to 30–40% of patients.[104] The acute onset of varicocele in a middle-aged man should raise the suspicion of obstructed venous flow. Flank pain was reported to be present in 14% of patients in the Mayo Clinic series.[11]

Pulmonary embolus is a life-threatening event that may be associated with IVC obstruction at any level. The typical clinical findings of a tumor or clot embolism are an acute increase in central venous or pulmonary artery pressure in the absence of air embolism. Budd–Chiari syndrome, or hepatic venous outflow obstruction, is a rare disorder resulting from the occlusion of the major hepatic veins or the suprahepatic IVC. It classically presents with the triad of hepatomegaly, right hypochondrial pain, and ascites.[16,67]

Classification

The operative technique is dictated by the extent of the tumor thrombus. Therefore, it is of the utmost importance to clearly determine and classify the extent of IVC involvement. Various classification systems have been proposed and used.[6,61,82,94,110] In all of these classification systems, the major important steps of thrombus propagation have been considered as exceeding the renal vein and reaching the IVC, reaching to or above the hepatic veins, and finally passing the diaphragmatic level and getting into the right atrium.

In the Mayo classification system there are four stages, or levels, of thrombus determined by the cephalad extent.[82] These levels influence the choice of the surgical incision and technique used for the surgical procedure. Level 1 refers to a tumor thrombus either at the entry of the renal vein or within the IVC less than 2 cm from the confluence of the renal vein and the IVC. Level 2 thrombus extends within the IVC more than 2 cm above the confluence of the renal vein and IVC, but still remains below the hepatic veins. Level 3 thrombus involves the intrahepatic IVC. The size of the thrombus ranges from a narrow tail that extends into the IVC to one that fills the lumen and enlarges the IVC. Level 4 thrombus extends above the diaphragm or into the right atrium.

Surgical Treatment

Anatomic Implications

For a better understanding, it may be useful to divide the IVC into three sections: the lower IVC (common iliac to renal vein), middle IVC (renal to hepatic veins), and upper IVC (hepatic veins to right atrium).[75] The right renal vein is shorter in length. Generally the right gonadal vein empties directly into the IVC, whereas the left gonadal vein drains into the left renal vein. There are two or more right main hepatic veins and one left main hepatic vein, which anastomose cephalad to the smaller, usually right-sided, minor hepatic veins.[64] Minor veins of the caudate lobe are highly variable and are not clearly depicted.

When the IVC is obstructed, collateral veins become an important means of venous return (Fig. 8h-3). Due to the anatomic differences between the right and left renal anatomy, collateral venous return also differs. The capsular and ureteral veins are the only potential collateral vessels on the right side, compared to a larger number of potential collaterals on the left: adrenal, inferior phrenic, gonadal, ureteral, capsular, and lumbars.[2, 19] The ascending lumbar vein is the major collateral pathway between the lower half of the body and the heart.[19] Together with the intercostal veins, the ascending lumbar veins form the hemizygous system on the left and the azygous on the right.[19] The ascending lumbar vein usually drains the left kidney via the lumbar veins; however, such drainage is usually not present for the right kidney. This anatomical difference has implications during surgery as will be discussed later.

Acute suprarenal obstruction of the IVC results in bilateral renal vein thrombosis, massive infarction, perirenal hemorrhage, and death.[75] However, in the presence of gradual obstruction, collateral vessels develop.[75] When IVC is partially occluded, collateral channels do not develop, and this is a more problematic situation. These patients are usually less symptomatic, leading to delayed diagnosis, and when performing a right nephrectomy, ligation of the left renal vein may result in some degree of loss in renal function.[64] In case of left nephrectomy, venous drainage from the right kidney needs to be sustained.

Preoperative Preparation

Prevention of Tumor Embolus

One of the feared potential complications of surgery for IVC tumor thrombus is pulmonary embolism. Although the embolus is usually from the thrombus itself (i.e., not a blood embolus), preoperative anticoagulation has been suggested. This may be in the form of intravenous heparin, subcutaneous heparin, or low-molecular-weight heparin.[94, 104] However, the physician should be cognizant of the fact that there are other factors potentially affecting the coagulation status of these patients. Obstruction of the hepatic veins may have a negative impact on coagulation factors.[104] Moreover, CPB is well known to cause platelet dysfunction.[80] We usually do not use routine anticoagulant treatment except in certain circumstances such as thrombocytosis (as a neoplastic syndrome), chronic obstructive lung disease, and a history of thromboembolism and thrombophlebitis.

Placement of a Suprarenal Inferior Vena Cava Filter

Prevention of tumor thrombus pulmonary embolus is a major issue. Although it is very rare, the result is catastrophic. Placement of a suprarenal IVC filter has been advocated as a means of preventing embolus.[50, 125] Cancer patients usually have a hypercoagulable state, and thus a tendency to develop recurrent thrombosis, when a permanent filter is placed. However, a temporary suprarenal IVC filter placed via the jugular vein is easy to insert and retrieve, has minimal morbidity, and does not carry the long-term risks of a permanent filter (Fig. 8h-4). The filter may be safely removed up to 2 weeks after surgery. Jibiki et al. also described plication of the IVC by inserting 3-0 polyprolene sutures in its suprahepatic or retrohepatic segment in an effort to prevent pulmonary embolus.[50]

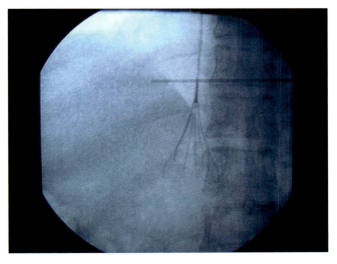

FIGURE 8h-4. Temporary suprarenal IVC filter placed via the jugular vein.

Preoperative Tumor Embolization

Several centers advocate performing renal arterial embolization for more extensive tumor thrombi that occlude the IVC, or extend above the hepatic veins.[116] In such cases renal arteriography is performed prior to surgery. Large caval thrombi often demonstrate hypervascularity with distinct arterial supply from the renal artery. When this finding is observed, embolization is usually performed 48–72 hours before definitive surgery. The potential advantages of embolization include tumor and thrombus shrinkage, reduced potential for bleeding, facilitation of surgical dissection, and improvement of liver function in cases with hepatic vein occlusion.[81,86,114] The procedure is usually well tolerated. Some patients experience flank pain, fever, and occasional ileus.[116] In view of the risk of ileus, bowel preparation may be performed prior to embolization.[116] We do not routinely use tumor embolization.

Incisions

A number of incisions have been favored by different surgeons and are illustrated in Fig. 8h-5. These mainly include thoracoabdominal, midline abdominal, and subcostal incisions with or without a sternotomy. A right thoracoabdominal incision has been extensively used. Some proposed that an RCC operation with a thrombus of the IVC is mainly an IVC operation, and thus a right thoracoabdominal access is required.[117] Despite its popularity, the thoracoabdominal approach has several disadvantages. It requires rib resection and entrance into the pleural cavity. It is associated with substantial pain as well as postoperative wound and pulmonary complications. A midline transabdominal incision may be associated with less pain[56] and helps the surgeon to avoid laterally placed collaterals and engorged intercostal

veins.[104] The exposure of the infrahepatic IVC may be inferior to the right thoracoabdominal incision. The anterior midline incision is one of the preferred incisions for left-sided tumors, since the dissection has to be performed in both the left and right sides of the abdomen and retroperitoneum. The bilateral subcostal incision has also been widely used, and has been suggested to be helpful for left-sided large tumors.[80] A subcostal incision appears to be associated with less pain and fewer pulmonary complications than a midline incision.[32] A bilateral subcostal incision with a cephalad T extension is used in liver transplantation[107,109] and occasionally for major urological cases.[10,41,58,85,118,121] Liver transplant recipients tolerate this incision well. Rib resection and entrance into the pleural cavity are obviated with this approach.

Minimal Inferior Vena Cava Extension

There are some basic steps that are valid in the majority of RCC cases with an IVC thrombus. After the abdomen is entered, the first step is mobilization of the colon medially. The renal artery is divided as early as possible in an effort to facilitate surgical removal of both the kidney and the thrombus. Accessory arteries must be carefully sought, and if found, tied and cut to minimize bleeding. The kidney is fully mobilized with an intact Gerota's fascia with the only attachment being the renal vein. Importantly, care should be taken to avoid extensive manipulation of the renal vein and vena cava during the initial dissection, until a clamp is placed on the IVC above the tumor thrombus to avoid dislodgement and dissemination of tumor emboli.

If the tumor involves only the renal vein, or is a small protruding tongue into the IVC, the thrombus can usually be milked proximally into the renal vein far enough to allow placement of a vascular clamp incorporating the renal vein

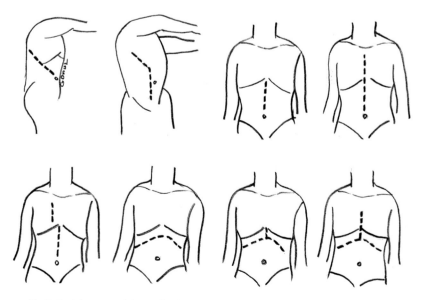

FIGURE 8h-5. Incisions used for radical nephrectomy with vena caval tumor thrombectomy.

and a portion of the IVC.[7] The kidney and the thrombus in the renal vein can be removed intact by excising distal to the clamp, while obviating the need to clamp the left renal vein, IVC, or lumbar veins.

Infrahepatic Inferior Vena Caval Involvement

When the thrombus extends into the vena cava, safe removal requires control of IVC on all sides prior to cavotomy (Figs. 8h-6 and 8h-7). The vena cava needs to be completely dissected from surrounding structures both above and below the renal vein. The contralateral renal vein should also be mobilized. Adequate control of IVC above the thrombus is critical. Care should be taken to control the collateral veins, since they may cause troublesome bleeding. The right adrenal vein should be ligated and divided. The hepatic veins to the caudate lobe can be secured and divided in an effort to free the IVC from the caudate lobe. This gains an extra 2–3 cm of additional IVC.[72] These veins can be variable in number. The infrarenal vena cava is then secured below the thrombus with a Satinsky clamp or Rummel tourniquet. The contralateral renal vein is also occluded. Some suggest clamping of the renal artery to avoid the risk of hemorrhagic infarct; nevertheless, renal artery clamping carries the inherent risk of warm ischemia.[94] If the surgeon elects to control the renal artery, administration of 20 mg of intravenous mannitol is recommended.[94] Finally, in preparation for cavotomy, the superior IVC is secured above the tumor thrombus with a clamp or DeWeese clip. This is followed by a circumferential incision at the junction of the involved renal vein and IVC creating a longitudinal cavotomy. Generally the thrombus is not fixed to the wall of the IVC and gentle traction on the kidney allows for removal of both the kidney and the tumor thrombus (Figs. 8h-6, 8h-7, and 8h-8). Once the specimen is freed, the suprarenal IVC clamp may be temporarily released with the application of positive pulmonary pressure to ensure complete removal of the thrombus. Intraoperative transesophageal echocardiography would be the optimal method to confirm complete thrombus removal, if there is any doubt. Upon completion of thrombus removal, the cavotomy incision is repaired with a continuous suture with the patient preferably in the Trendelenburg position. Just before the closure is completed, the distal IVC clamp may be released to fill the vena cava and decrease the risk of air embolus.

Intrahepatic or Suprahepatic Inferior Vena Cava Involvement

In patients with a tumor thrombus extending into the intrahepatic or suprahepatic IVC, surgery is more extensive and technically challenging. Attaining adequate exposure may be

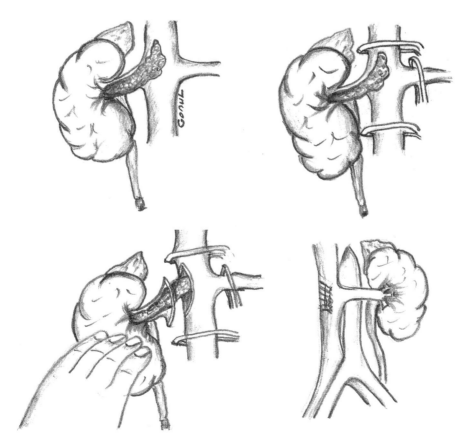

FIGURE 8h-6. Radical nephrectomy with removal of infrahepatic tumor thrombus.

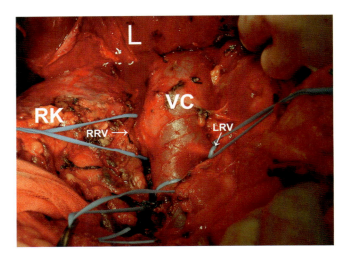

FIGURE 8h-7. Right radical nephrectomy with vena cava thrombectomy. Tumor thrombus fills the entire renal vein and the lumen of the inferior vena cava up to and beyond the hepatic veins. Safe removal requires control of IVC on all sides prior to cavotomy. Tourniquets are placed around both renal veins and the inferior vena cava below the thrombus. L, liver; RK, right kidney; RRV, right renal vein; LRV, left renal vein; VC, vena cava.

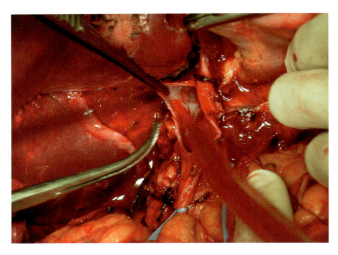

FIGURE 8h-8. The tumor and the thrombus depicted in Fig. 8h–8 are removed. Note the normal caliber and empty lumen of the inferior vena cava following thrombus removal.

more cumbersome for left-sided tumors. Simple reflection of the left colon may not be enough to expose the IVC on the right and the tumor on the left. Novick suggests transposing the mobilized left kidney anteriorly through a window in the mesentery of the left colon while leaving the left renal vein attached.[83] If a tumor thrombus is extending into the intrahepatic or suprahepatic IVC, subdiaphragmatic control of the IVC becomes necessary. Several different techniques have been described to safely overcome this difficult clinical problem.

Suprahepatic or supradiaphragmatic occlusion of the IVC may have profound impact on lowering systemic

blood pressure. Patients who have developed adequate collateral venous flow may tolerate this without developing hypotension. However, various other techniques may be necessary for some patients.

Venovenous bypass techniques and devices have been used to maintain a normotensive state as well as working in a bloodless field.[4,12,30,73,95] Cavoatrial or cavobrachial bypass systems with or without a pump have been described. These systems can be used with and without anticoagulation, allow patients to be warmed during the procedure, and may be converted to CPB as required.[49] When utilizing a cavoatrial shunt, the intrapericardial vena cava, infrarenal vena cava, and the opposite renal vein are temporarily occluded.[12,30] This is followed by inserting cannulas into the right atrium and infrarenal IVC. The cannulas are connected to a pump, which ensures adequate flow from the IVC to the heart (Fig. 8h-9).

To decrease hepatic venous congestion and backbleeding from major hepatic veins, temporary occlusion of the porta hepatis (hepatic artery, portal vein, and the common bile duct)

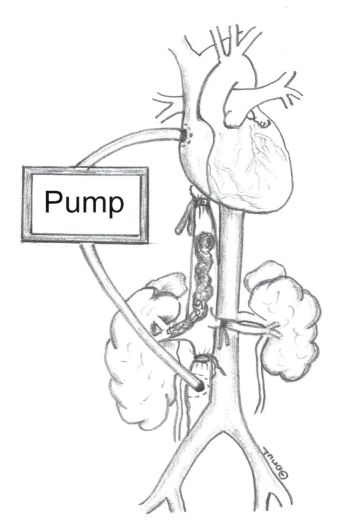

FIGURE 8h-9. Venovenous bypass for removal of a supradiaphragmatic vena caval thrombus.

has been advocated, as described by Pringle in 1908.[93] This maneuver controls the venous bleeding and can be safely carried out for 30 minutes. When the Pringle maneuver fails to control venous outflow adequately, the superior mesenteric artery may be temporarily occluded simultaneously with the Pringle maneuver, or the aorta may be cross-clamped (above the celiac axis).[104] Supraceliac aortic clamping creates a state of normothermic circulatory arrest, and has been successfully used to achieve a normotensive state while the suprahepatic IVC is occluded.[23] This maneuver, however, carries the potential risks of acute renal tubular necrosis, hypoxic liver injury, and paraplegia.[23]

With the employment of these additional measures to create a relatively bloodless field, an intrahepatic tumor thrombus can be removed through a cavotomy incision. Usage of a Fogarty vascular catheter or Foley urethral catheter to blindly extract the thrombus from higher levels in the vena cava has been described. The catheters are advanced up to the upper clamped IVC, inflated, and drawn to the opening in the IVC.[31] However, blunt thrombectomy with a balloon catheter is associated with IVC injury, pulmonary embolism, and residual tumor on the IVC wall.[120] Therefore, we do not advocate its routine use.

The management of patients with a complex supradiaphragmatic or right atrial thrombus remains even more challenging. Some centers prefer CPB with deep hypothermic arrest in these situations.[37,70–73,86] Proponents of CPB with deep hypothermic arrest advocate its use because of some advantages over other techniques. Unlike other techniques, extensive dissection and mobilization of the suprarenal IVC are not necessary with this approach. There is no need for occlusion of the porta hepatis, ligation of multiple lumbar veins, or aortic cross-clamping to prevent hemorrhage. It allows for direct visual inspection of the entire vena caval lumen in a completely bloodless field. An atriotomy can be performed easily. The risk of sudden massive hemorrhage or distal tumor thrombus embolization is decreased.

The Cleveland Clinic group has reported their extensive experience with this technique with excellent long-term cancer-free survival data.[77] Their technique will be briefly described here. A bilateral subcostal incision is combined with a median sternotomy. Intraoperative monitoring is undertaken via an arterial line, central venous pressure catheter, and a pulmonary artery catheter. Precise retroperitoneal hemostasis is very important before the initiation of CPB because of the risk of severe bleeding related to systemic heparinization. The heart and great vessels are exposed through the median sternotomy. Following heparinization, cannulas are placed into the ascending aorta and right atrium, and CPB is initiated. When the heart fibrillates, the aorta is clamped, and a crystalloid cardioplegic solution is infused. Under circulatory arrest, deep hypothermia is begun by decreasing the arterial inflow temperature to as low as 10°C. The patient's head and abdomen are packed in ice. A core temperature of 18–20°C is reached within 15–30 minutes.

Flow through the perfusion machine is then discontinued, and 95% of the patient's blood is drained into the pump (exsanguination). Hypothermic circulatory arrest can safely be maintained for up to 40–60 minutes without risking cerebral ischemia.[77] During this period, the surgeon can work in an essentially bloodless field. When the tumor extends into the right atrium, the atrium is opened in addition to a cavotomy. The tumor thrombus is removed intact with the kidney when possible. When this is not possible due to thrombus friability or its adherence to the caval wall, piecemeal removal of the thrombus from above and below may be required. Under deep hypothermic circulatory arrest, the surgeon has the luxury of inspecting the entire lumen of the vena cava directly to make sure that the thrombus is removed in its entirety. Moreover, the lumen of the major hepatic veins can also be inspected for retained tumor thrombus. Once thrombus removal is complete, the vena cavotomy is closed with a 5-0 vascular suture along with closure of the right atrium. Rewarming of the patient is initiated next and is continued until a core temperature of 37° is reached. CPB is then terminated. Protamine sulfate is administered to reverse the heparin. There are some disadvantages to using CPB. It may be associated with platelet dysfunction; furthermore, when combined with systemic heparinization, there is a risk of significant coagulopathy with bleeding, which is especially problematic in the setting of extensive retroperitoneal dissection.[104]

Nesbitt et al. indicated that even some intraatrial tumor thrombus could be resected without CPB.[81] Their maneuver is to gently palpate the tumor at the cavoatrial junction and manipulate the tumor into the suprahepatic IVC. A vascular cross-clamp is then applied across the IVC and cavotomy is performed.[81] As in our practice, they concurred with others that CPB with or without deep hypothermic circulatory arrest is not required in patients with minimal atrial or suprahepatic IVC involvement or with intrahepatic IVC extension.[60,81,104,108]

Ciancio et al. transferred their expertise with liver transplant techniques to patients with IVC thrombus, with the intention of avoiding CPB or venovenous bypass and sternotomy or thoracotomy.[17] A bilateral subcostal incision in combination with a midline incision up to the xyphoid process is used (triradiate incision). The liver is fully mobilized except for the hepatic veins and porta hepatis and gradually rolled to the left side or elevated (Fig. 8h-10). When there is a mobile thrombus at the cava atrial junction, or even within the atrium, the central diaphragm tendon is dissected off of the adventitia of the suprahepatic IVC. This piggyback exposure allows the tumor to be milked down below a vascular clamp placed on the suprahepatic IVC. This approach has a number of advantages. Sternotomy or opening in the diaphragm to control the intrapericardial IVC is avoided, resulting in decreased access, pulmonary complications, and the need for chest tube drainage. Coagulopathy and adverse neurological outcome associated with CPB may be avoided.[108] This exposure also minimizes the duration of vena cava cross-clamping. After a

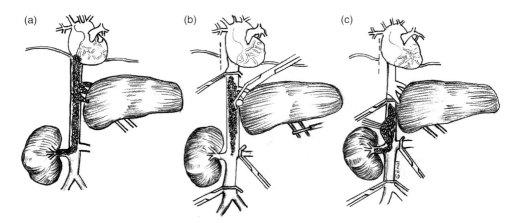

FIGURE 8h-10. (**A**) A patient with a level 4 tumor thrombus is illustrated. The liver is mobilized and dissected off the inferior vena cava. This dissection enables easy access to the retrohepatic vena cava. (**B**) The diaphragm is dissected off the suprahepatic inferior vena cava. The porta hepatis, major hepatic vein, contralateral renal vein, and distal vena cava are controlled with clamps. An intraatrial tumor thrombus is milked down and a vascular clamp is placed proximal to the thrombus. (**C**) The thrombus is removed through a cavotomy.

thrombus is drawn down below the level of the hepatic veins, the upper clamp may be repositioned to restore hepatic venous drainage and release the Pringle maneuver. When a thrombus is small and nonocclusive, placing a curved vascular clamp at the cavotomy site enables repair. The remaining renal vein is unclamped and this minimizes renal ischemia. It has been suggested that the role of CPB in patients with a bulky intraatrial thrombus is self-evident; however, those with a minimal atrial thrombus or one that terminates at a level between the major hepatic veins and diaphragm may not require cardiopulmonary and/or complete hypothermic arrest. Ciancio *et al.* do, however, concur with others that all retrohepatic and suprahepatic vena caval thrombi should be managed in an environment in which bypass infrastructure and cardiothoracic surgical expertise are immediately available.[17,110] Gallucci *et al.* confirmed these favorable results by using liver harvesting technique for isolation of the IVC from the liver as a safe and effective maneuver.[33]

Using a cell-saving device may conserve blood loss from lumbar and hepatic veins until the thrombus is fragmented.[81] Although this device potentially may disseminate the tumor, no evidence exists that shed cells from the tumor thrombus have an impact on survival.[78,108]

Inferior Vena Cava Resection

Invasion of the IVC wall by a tumor is usually rare, and unfortunately cannot be accurately detected by any of the current imaging modalities. Although the invasion generally is limited to the renal ostium, it can occur anywhere along the IVC.[7] Invasion of the IVC further complicates surgery. However, it is not necessarily an ominous prognosticator, if the involved section can be completely resected. Survival is markedly improved in patients with negative surgical margins.[43] On the other hand, incomplete resection has a dismal prognosis, with patients experiencing a survival rate

similar to patients with metastatic disease.[43] Resection of the involved portion of the vena cava is a solution. When the tumor-bearing kidney is on the right side, it is generally possible to rely on the collateral venous drainage and ligate the renal vein. A simple test has been described to test the adequacy of venous drainage from the normal kidney.[7,19] Dyed urine should appear within 12 minutes after intravenous administration of methylene blue or indigo carmine, with the artery and/or ureter of the tumor-bearing kidney occluded. When the test reveals inadequate drainage, or the involved kidney is on the left, some form of drainage must be established. The normal renal vein, or cuff of IVC, may be anastomosed to the portal vein either directly or via an intervening saphenous vein graft.[80] Postoperative thrombosis of the vena cava will be prevented, if the lumen is not compromised by more than 50% at the time of caval reconstruction.[70] Another alternative is to replace the IVC with a graft.[20,22,24,52,88,97,98] Total replacement of the IVC with a polytetrafluoroethylene (PTFE) graft was first reported by Sarti in 1970.[98] Okada *et al.* reported long-term patency after IVC replacement with an expanded PTFE tubular graft in four patients with tumor thrombi from RCC.[89] Long-term patency rates are inferior with grafts in the venous system compared to the arterial system, mainly due to thrombosis, and hence requires anticoagulant or antiplatelet therapy.[89] An alternative to prosthetic material is the use of autologous pericardium or saphenous vein patches. Autologous material potentially has a lower thrombosis rate and higher resistance to infection than prosthetic material.[69]

Laparoscopic Approach

RCC with associated tumor thrombus has traditionally been approached with open surgery due to the necessity for wide exposure, meticulous dissection, and secure vascular control of the vena cava. The presence of a tumor thrombus may be considered a relative contraindication to laparoscopic radical nephrectomy. However, several centers have reported successful laparoscopic management of renal cancer with an IVC thrombus.

A number of case reports have demonstrated the feasibility of laparoscopic radical nephrectomy for patients with level I tumor thrombus.[48,66,99,112] In a series of eight patients, Desai et al. reported on laparoscopic treatment of level I renal vein thrombus.[26] Seven were successfully treated with the laparoscopic approach, while conversion to open surgery was required in one patient. The operative technique is similar to that of classical laparoscopic radical nephectomy. The renal vein is fully mobilized toward the IVC to allow adequate room for proximal placement of the vascular stapling device. The tumor thrombus can often be clearly seen within the noncollapsing segment of the renal vein.[28] As in open surgery, care is taken not to manipulate the thrombus. Intraoperative ultrasonography would be optimal in both delineating the size and extent of the thrombus and aiding in controlled positioning of the vascular stapler proximal to the tumor thrombus.[48] Desai et al. suggest using the stapler device for "milking" the tumor thrombus toward the renal vein allowing an adequate uninvolved vein for stapler placement and division.[26]

Disanto et al. reported on retroperitoneal laparoscopic radical nephrectomy for RCC with infrahepatic vena caval thrombus in one patient.[27] Their approach involves performing the preliminary stages and the steps involving the deep tissues with laparoscopy (i.e., isolating the kidney, clipping and severing the renal artery, isolating the IVC, positioning the vessel loops above and below the thrombus, and dissecting the ureter), whereas the more delicate steps (incising the IVC, removing the thrombus, applying hemostatic forceps, extracting the kidney and the thrombus, and suturing the IVC) are performed under direct vision, in open surgery, through a small incision. The investigators favor the retroperitoneal approach and state that it affords easier access to the IVC than the transperitoneal approach, since it is not necessary to rotate the liver or mobilize the colon and duodenum.

Recently, a level 2 IVC thrombus was developed in a porcine model and treated successfully with laparoscopic caval thrombectomy.[29] Moreover, simulated tumor thrombus extending into the right atrium was successfully managed laparoscopically in a calf model.[74] This required the simultaneous work of two teams together with both a laparoscopic and thoracoscopic approach, using deep hypothermic circulatory arrest and CPB. Tumor thrombi in both the IVC and the right atrium were entirely removed in six calves, and all six animals were rewarmed and successfully taken off CPB.

We believe that laparoscopy may play an increasing role in the management of RCC patients with caval involvement in the future. The role of laparoscopy in the management of kidney cancer patients is expanding rapidly, and we look forward to the transfer of the successful management with level 2–4 thrombus in animal models to humans.

Complications

Radical nephrectomy with removal of thrombus from the IVC may be associated with major perioperative morbidity (11–71.4%) and mortality (3.4 – 16%).[8,60,62,78,81,82,87,94,104,106,111] As expected, these figures change according to the cephalic extension of the thrombus with a lower risk for infrahepatic caval thrombosis.

One of the major perioperative complications is blood loss. Blood replacement has been reported to range between 3 and 70 units.[86,104] The average blood loss is higher with the higher level of IVC involvement, and is higher for left-sided tumors, probably due to increased development of collateral veins. Skinner et al. reported a higher rate of blood loss in patients with extensive collaterals (6664 versus 5466 ml).[104] The most common postoperative complications are sepsis (30%), retroperitoneal hemorrhage (23%), and hepatic dysfunction (11%).[72,86,104] In a large contemporary series of cytoreductive nephrectomy, Goetzl et al. observed that patients with a thrombus were significantly more likely to have a complication ($p = 0.008$).[38]

Thus, this type of surgery usually has serious complications and a significant mortality rate. Therefore, it should be done in experienced centers by experienced surgeons. These centers must have well-furnished cardiovascular departments and intensive care units.

Prognosis

Many authors have demonstrated that long-term survival can be achieved in patients who suffer from RCC associated with a tumor thrombus into the IVC.[73,103] Postoperative survival rates range between 32 and 64% in patients with nonmetastatic disease and according to most published data, do not appear to be any different from those estimated for patients with renal vein involvement only.[36,37,78,82,104]

Adverse prognostic features for patients with RCC-associated thrombi include perinephric tumor extension,[45,94] lymph node metastasis,[14,43,46] distant metastasis,[14,21,43,100] incomplete tumor or thrombus excision,[43,82,104] and tumor invasion of the caval wall.[43] Controversy exists regarding possible adverse prognostic association with higher-level thrombi. This is confounded by the findings that patients with more extensive thrombus propagation tend to have tumors of higher grade and more advanced local stage.

Some reports have shown decreased survival in patients with tumor thrombus in the IVC, in particular, with higher cephalad extent.[5,94,104,106] Sosa et al. reported a 2-year survival rate of 80% in patients with retrohepatic IVC thrombus compared with only 21% in those with suprahepatic thrombus.[106] Skinner et al. found that the thrombus level was an important prognosticator and noted a 5-year survival rate of 35% for level 1, 18% for level 2, and 0% for level 3 patients.[104] Other studies have not identified IVC tumor thrombus level as a negative prognostic indicator.[34, 37, 95] Glazer and Novick reviewed 18 patients with IVC thrombus extending into the right atrium and concluded that their long-term survival was not significantly different from that of patients with infrahepatic or retrohepatic IVC thrombi.[37] The overall and cancer-specific 5-year survival rates were 57% and 60%, respectively. Survival was significantly improved in patients without renal capsular penetration, compared to those with perinephric fat involvement (58.1 versus 19.7 months). Bissada et al. reported that patients with infrahepatic, intrahepatic, and intracardiac tumor extension were alive with no evidence of disease at 52%, 43%, and 38%, respectively (no statistically significant difference).[9] Hatcher et al. indicated that prognosis was determined by pathological stage or the presence or absence of vena caval wall invasion, rather than the level of extension.[43] Tsuji et al. reported that the level of thrombus did not influence survival; however, a statistically significant correlation was noted between surgical staging and survival. The presence of lymph node metastasis was a particularly high-risk factor for disease-specific mortality.[120] Moinzadeh and Libertino recently reviewed their experience with 153 patients in 30 years.[76] They found that a higher level of thrombus was not associated with an increased spread of tumor in perinephric fat, lymph nodes, or distant metastasis. Although there was a trend toward decreased cancer-specific survival at 5 years with a higher extent of thrombus, this failed to reach statistical significance (52%, 39%, and 29% for levels 1, 2, and 3, respectively). Another observation was that patients with renal vein thrombus appeared to have better survival at 10 years compared to patients with tumor thrombus in the IVC (66% versus 29%). Kim et al. addressed the same question and found somewhat confounding results.[55] In their experience with 226 patients, disease-specific survival was similar for patients with renal vein involvement and IVC involvement below the diaphragm. However, patients with IVC involvement above the diaphragm had a significantly worse survival rate even after controlling for Fuhrman grade and Eastern Cooperative Oncology Group performance status.

Metastatic Renal Cell Carcinoma with Concurrent Thrombus

One-third of patients with an IVC thrombus will also have one or more metastatic lesions.[63, 102] When preliminary evaluation reveals distant metastasis, palliative surgery may still have a role for relieving the vena caval syndrome or other significant symptoms such as intractable edema, cardiac dysfunction, abdominal pain, or hematuria associated with the primary tumor.[49, 72, 86] With the advances in immunotherapy with agents such as interferon or interleukin, control of distant metastases in patients with RCC extending into the IVC can be achieved; thus survival of these patients may improve,

if aggressive surgery including tumor thrombectomy is combined with immunotherapy.

Bissada et al. noted a high perioperative mortality in patients with metastatic RCC with IVC involvement (33% versus 2% in patients without metastasis).[9] Of the four surviving patients who underwent radical nephrectomy, the 3-year survival rate was 25% (one patient with limited pulmonary metastases). Others have demonstrated that long-term disease-free survival can be achieved by the combination of radical nephrectomy, cava thrombectomy, and postoperative immunotherapy in selected patients with metastatic disease.[79] Naitoh et al. reported on a series of 30 patients.[79] Eighty percent of patients were able to complete adjuvant immunotherapy after surgery. An actuarial overall 5-year survival rate of 17% was achieved. Those with isolated pulmonary metastases and low-grade disease had a better prognosis with 5-year survival rates of 43% and 52%, respectively.[79, 92] In the M.D. Anderson Cancer Center experience, 10 of 13 patients who were symptomatic before surgery had complete palliation of their symptoms 3 months after surgery, and 8 of 12 patients who were followed for at least 1 year were alive with either no evidence of disease or with stable disease.[105]

In a large series of 207 patients with RCC and tumor thrombus, Zisman et al. reported that patients with tumor thrombus had a higher rate of metastasis at diagnosis than those without tumor thrombus (63% versus 25%).[127] However, the overall survival of patients with IVC thrombus was similar regardless of metastatic status. Patients with M1 disease and thrombus who underwent surgery had a significantly better response to immunotherapy than those treated nonoperatively. Moreover, immunotherapy after cytoreductive nephrectomy was associated with a similar response rate in thrombus and nonthrombus cases. In patients with renal vein thrombus and metastasis at presentation, surgical extirpation and immunotherapy achieved the longest survival. In patients with IVC thrombus and metastasis at presentation, the longest survival was achieved by surgical extirpation with or without immunotherapy. Thus, the investigators concluded that the combination of cytoreductive surgery and immunotherapy has an important role in patients with renal vein thrombus and a potential role in those with IVC thrombus. They concurred with others that patients with lung only metastases benefited most from cytoreductive surgery and immunotherapy, although the difference did not reach statistical significance.

Conclusions

One of the well-established features of RCC carcinoma is its potential for intraluminal growth into the renal venous circulation and cephalic propagation in the IVC. Although intravascular growth implies a worsened biological behavior of the tumor, the presence of tumor thrombus per se does not ultimately affect long-term prognosis with proper management. Surgical treatment remains the only curative treatment option for these patients, with removal of the thrombus along with radical nephrectomy.

Surgical management depends on the cranial extent of the thrombus. Levels 1 and 2 thrombi are managed by proximal and distal control of the vena cava and the control of the contralateral renal vein. Thrombus propagation up to or beyond the hepatic veins adds considerable complexity to surgery, specifically in cases with supradiaphragmatic or right atrial involvement. Once deemed incurable, with the improvements in surgical techniques and perioperative care, safe surgical removal of these tumors can now be offered to these patients with survival rates of over 50% at 5 years. One of the major determinants of long-term disease-free survival is complete removal of the thrombus.

The optimal surgical technique for patients with tumor thrombus at or beyond the entrance of the hepatic veins remains controversial. Some centers prefer CPB with or without deep hypothermic arrest in these situations, while others try to avoid this technique. Despite the choice of the surgical team, it should be emphasized that this type of surgery may have serious complications and a significant mortality rate. Therefore, it should be performed in experienced centers by experienced surgeons. These centers must have well-furnished cardiovascular departments and intensive care units.

For patients with metastatic RCC with a tumor thrombus, the combination of cytoreductive surgery and immunotherapy seems to have an important role. Evidence suggests that patients with low-grade disease and/or lung-only metastases benefit most from cytoreductive surgery and immunotherapy.

References

1. Abdelsayed MA, Bissada NK, Finkbeiner AE, et al. Renal tumors involving the vena cava: plan for management. *J Urol* 1978;120:153–155.
2. Anson BJ, Caldwell EW, Pick JW, et al. The blood supply of the kidney, suprarenal gland and associated structure. *Surg Gynecol Obstet* 1947;83:313–320.
3. Ardekani RG, Hunter JA, Thomson A. Hidden hydronephroma simulating right atrial tumor. *Ann Thorac Surg* 1971;11:371–375.
4. Baumgartner F, Scott R, Zane R, et al. Modified venovenous bypass technique for resection of renal and adrenal carcinoma with involvement of the inferior vena cava. *Eur J Surg* 1996;162:59–62.
5. Belis JA, Kandzari SJ. Five year survival following excision of renal cell carcinoma extending into inferior vena cava. *Urology* 1990;3:228.
6. Belis JA, Pae WE, Rohner TJ, et al. Cardiovascular evaluation before circulatory arrest and removal of vena caval extension of renal carcinoma. *J Urol* 1989;141:1302–1307.
7. Bihrle L, Libertino JA. Renal cell cancer with extension into the vena cava. In: DeKernion BJ, Pavone-MacAluso M,

eds. *Tumors of the Kidney.* Baltimore: Williams & Wilkins, 1986:111–123.
8. Bintz M, Cogbill TH, Klein AS. Surgical management of renal cell carcinoma involving the inferior vena cava. *J Vasc Surg* 1987;6:566–571.
9. Bissada NK, Yakout HH, Babanouri A, et al. Long-term experience with management of renal cell carcinoma involving the inferior vena cava. *Urology* 2003;61:89–92.
10. Bloom LS, Libertino JA. Surgical management of Cushing's syndrome. *Urol Clin N Am* 1989;16:547.
11. Blute ML, Zincke H. Surgical management of renal cell carcinoma with intracaval involvement. *AUA Update Series* 1994;17:134–139.
12. Burt M. Inferior vena caval involvement by renal cell carcinoma: use of venovenous bypass adjunct during resection. *Urol Clin N Am* 1991;18:437.
13. Casanova GA, Zingg EJ. Inferior vena caval tumor extension in renal cell carcinoma. *Urol Int* 1991;47:216.
14. Cherrie RJ, Goldman DG, Lindner A, et al. Prognostic implications of vena caval extension of renal cell carcinoma. *J Urol* 1982;128:910–912.
15. Choyke PL. Detection and staging of renal cancer. *Magn Reson Imaging Clin N Am* 1997;5:29–47.
16. Ciancio G, Soloway M. Renal cell carcinoma invading the hepatic veins. *Cancer* 2001;92:1836–1842.
17. Ciancio G, Hawke C, Soloway M. The use of liver transplant techniques to aid in the surgical management of urological tumors. *J Urol* 2000;164:665–672.
18. Clarke CD. Survival after excision of a kidney, segmental resection of the vena cava, and division of the opposite renal vein. *Lancet* 1961;2:1015–1016.
19. Clayman RV, Gonzalez R, Fraley EE. Renal cell cancer invading the inferior vena cava: clinical review and anatomical approach. *J Urol* 1980;123:157–163.
20. Cochran JL, Noble MG, Weigel JW, et al. Inferior vena cava replacement after resection of left renal tumor in canine model. *Urology* 1984;24:262–267.
21. Cole AT, Julian WA, Fried FA. Aggressive surgery for renal cell carcinoma with vena cava tumor thrombus. *Urology* 1975;6:227–229.
22. Crawford ES, DeBakey ME. Wide excision including involved aorta and vena cava and replacement with aortic homograft for retroperitoneal malignant tumors. Report of two cases. *Cancer* 1956;9:1085–1091.
23. Cummings KB, Li WI, Ryan JA, et al. Intraoperative management of renal cell cancer with supradiaphragmatic caval extension. *J Urol* 1979;122:829–832.
24. Dale WA, Harris J, Terry RB. Polytetrafluoroethylene reconstruction of the inferior vena cava. *Surgery* 1984;95:625–630.
25. Delis S, Dervenis C, Lytras D, et al. Liver transplantation techniques with preservation of the natural venovenous bypass: effect on surgical resection of renal cell carcinoma invading the inferior vena cava. *World J Surg* 2004;28:614–619.
26. Desai MM, Gill IS, Ramani AP, et al. Laparoscopic radical nephrectomy for cancer with level I renal vein involvement. *J Urol* 2003;169:487–491.
27. Disanto V, Pansadoro V, Portoghese F, et al. Retroperitoneal laparoscopic radical nephrectomy for renal cell carcinoma with infrahepatic vena caval thrombus. *Eur Urol* 2005;47:352–356.

28. Fenn NJ, Gill I. The expanding indications for laparoscopic radical nephrectomy. *BJU Int* 204;94:761–765.

29. Fergany AF, Gill IS, Schweizer DK, *et al.* Laparoscopic radical nephrectomy with level II vena caval thrombectomy: survival porcine model. *J Urol* 2002;168:2629–2631.

30. Foster RS, Mahomed Y, Bihrle RR, *et al.* Use of caval-atrial shunt for resection of a caval tumor thrombus in renal cell carcinoma. *J Urol* 1988;140:1370–1371.

31. Freed FZ, Gliedman ML. The removal of renal carcinoma thrombus extending into the right atrium. *J Urol* 1975;113:163–165.

32. Garcia-Valdecasas JC, Almenara R, Cabrer C, *et al.* Subcostal incision versus midline laparotomy in gallstone surgery: a prospective and randomized trial. *Br J Surg* 1988;75:473.

33. Galluci M, Borzomati D, Flamia G, *et al.* Liver harvesting surgical technique for the treatment of retro-hepatic caval thrombosis concomitant to renal cell carcinoma: perioperative and long-term results in 15 patients without mortality. *Eur Urol* 2004;45:194–202.

34. Gettman MT, Christopher BW, Blute ML, *et al.* Primary surgical treatment for renal cell carcinoma with renal vein, vena cava or atrial extension: identification of variables, including patient co-morbidity, which portend poor outcome. *J Urol* 2001; suppl., 165:158 (abstract 648).

35. Giuliani L, Giberti C, Martorana G, *et al.* Surgical management of renal cell carcinoma with vena cava tumor thrombus. *Eur Urol* 1986;12:145.

36. Giuliani L, Giberti C, Martorana G, *et al.* Radical extensive surgery for renal cell carcinoma: long term results and prognostic factors. *J Urol* 1990;143:468–474.

37. Glazer AA, Novick AC: Long-term follow-up after surgical treatment for renal cell carcinoma extending into the right atrium. *J Urol* 1996;155:448–450.

38. Goetzl MA, Goluboff ET, Murphy AM, *et al.* A contemporary evaluation of cytoreductive nephrectomy with tumor thrombus: morbidity and long term survival. *Urol Oncol* 2004;22:182–187.

39. Goldfarb DA, Novick AC, Lorig R, *et al.* Magnetic resonance imaging for assessment of vena caval tumor thrombi: a comparative study with venacavography and computerized tomography scanning. *J Urol* 1990;144:1100–1104.

40. Goncharenko V, Gerlock AJ Jr, Kadir S, *et al.* Incidence and distribution of venous extension in 70 hypernephromas. *AJR AM J Roentgenol* 1979;133:263–265.

41. Guz BV, Straffon RA, Novick AC. Operative approaches to the adrenal gland. *Urol Clin N Am* 1989;16:527.

42. Hartman AR, Zelen J, Mason RA, *et al.* Fiberoptic examination of the inferior vena cava during circulatory arrest for complete removal of renal cell carcinoma thrombus. *Surgery* 1990;107:695.

43. Hatcher PA, Anderson EE, Paulson DF, *et al.* Surgical management and prognosis of renal cell carcinoma invading the vena cava. *J Urol* 1991;145:20–24.

44. Heaney JP, Stanton WK, Halbert DS, *et al.* An improved technique for vascular isolation of the liver: experimental study and case reports. *Ann Surg* 1966;163:237.

45. Heney NM, Nocks BN. The influence of perinephric fat involvement on survival in patients with renal cell carcinoma extending into the vena cava. *J Urol* 1982;128:18–20.

46. Hoehn W, Hermanek P. Invasion of veins in renal cell carcinoma—frequency, correlation, and prognosis. *Eur Urol* 1983;9:276–280.

47. Horan JJ, Robertson CN, Choyke PL, *et al.* The detection of renal cell carcinoma into the renal vein and inferior vena cava : a prospective comparison of venography and magnetic resonance imaging. *J Urol* 1989;142:943–948.

48. Hsu THS, Jeffrey RB Jr, Chon C, *et al.* Laparoscopic radical nephrectomy incorporating intraoperative ultrasonography for renal cell carcinoma with renal vein tumor thrombus. *Urology* 2003;61:1246–1248.

49. Janosko EO, Powell CS, Spence PA, *et al.* Surgical management of renal cell carcinoma with extensive intra-caval involvement using a venous bypass system suitable for rapid conversion to cardiopulmonary bypass. *J Urol* 1991;145: 555–557.

50. Jibiki M, Iwai T, Inoue Y, *et al.* Surgical strategy for treating renal cell carcinoma with thrombus extending into the inferior vena cava. *J Vasc Surg* 2004;39:829–835.

51. Kallman DA, King BF, Hattery RR, *et al.* Renal vein and inferior vena tumor thrombus in renal cell carcinoma: CT, US, MRI, and vena cavography. *J Comput Assist Tomogr* 1992;16:240–247.

52. Katz NM, Spence IJ, Wallace RB. Reconstruction of the inferior vena cava with polytetrafluoroethylene tube graft after resection for hypernephroma of the right kidney. *J Thorac Cardiovasc Surg* 1984;87:791–797.

53. Kaufman JJ, Burke DE, Goodwin WE. Abdominal venography in urological diagnosis. *J Urol* 1956;75:160–168.

54. Kearney GP, Waters WB, Klein LA, *et al.* Results of IVC resection for renal cell carcinoma. *J Urol* 1981;125:769–773.

55. Kim HL, Zisman A, Han K, *et al.* Prognostic significance of venous thrombus in renal cell carcinoma. Are renal vein and inferior vena cava involvement different? *J Urol* 2004;171:588–591.

56. Kirkali Z, Van Poppel H, Tuzel E, *et al.* A prospective survey of surgical approaches in clinically localized renal cell carcinoma–A preliminary attempt at surgical quality control. *UroOncology* 2002:2(4):169–174.

57. Komatsu H, Yoh T, Murakami K, *et al.* Renal cell carcinoma with intracaval tumor thrombus extending to the diaphragm: ultrasonography and surgical management. *J Urol* 1985;134:122–125.

58. Komatsu H, Shirashu N, Takei K, *et al.* Right adrenal pheochromocytoma with anterolateral displacement of the inferior vena cava: skin incision and approach. *J Urol* 1987;137:477.

59. Langenbuch C. Chirurgie der leber und gallenblasse. *Dtsche Chir* 1894;45C:1.

60. Langenburg SE, Blackbourne LH, Sperling JW, *et al.* Management of renal tumors involving the inferior vena cava. *J Vasc Surg* 1994;20:385–388.

61. Libertino JA. Renal cell cancer with extension into the vena cava. In: McDougal WS, ed. *Rob and Smiths Operative Surgery: Urology.* London: Butterworths, 1986:127.

62. Libertino JA, Zinman L, Watkins E Jr. Long term results of resection of renal cell cancer with extension into inferior vena cava. *J Urol* 1987;137:21–24.

63. Lokich JJ, Harrison JH. Renal cell carcinoma: natural history and chemotherapeutic experience. *J Urol* 1975;114:371–374.

64. McCullough DL, Gittes RF. Vena cava resection for renal cell carcinoma. *J Urol* 1974;112:162–167.

65. McCullough DL, Talner LB. Inferior vena cava extension of renal carcinoma: a lost cause? Roentgenography and pathologic findings in surgical patients. *AJR AM Roentgenol* 1974;121:819–826.

66. McDougall EM, Clayman RV, Elashry OM. Laparoscopic radical nephrectomy for renal tumor: the Washington University experience. *J Urol* 1996;155:1180.

67. Mahmoud AEA, Elias E. New approaches to Budd-Chiari syndrome. *J Gastroenterol Hepatol* 1996;11:1121–1123.

68. Marsh CL, Lange PH. Application of liver transplant and organ procurement techniques to difficult upper abdominal urological cases. *J Urol* 1994;151:1652–1656.

69. Marshall FF, Reitz BA. Supradiaphragmatic renal cell carcinoma tumor thrombus: indication for vena caval reconstruction with pericardium. *J Urol* 1985;133:266–268.

70. Marshall FF, Reitz BA. Technique for removal of renal cell carcinoma with suprahepatic vena caval tumor thrombus. *Urol Clin N Am* 1986;13:551–557.

71. Marshall FF, Dietrick DD, Diamond DA. A new technique for management of renal cell carcinoma involving the right atrium: hypothermia and cardiac arrest. *J Urol* 1984;131:103.

72. Marshall FF, Dietrick DD, Baumgartner WA, *et al*. Surgical management of renal cell carcinoma with intracaval neoplastic extension above the hepatic veins. *J Urol* 1988;139:1166–1172.

73. Marshall VF, Midleton RG, Holswade GR, *et al*. Surgery for renal cell carcinoma in the vena cava. *J Urol* 1970;103:414–420.

74. Meraney AM, Gill IS, Desai MM, *et al*. Laparoscopic inferior vena cava and right atrial thrombectomy utilizing deep hypothermic circulatory arrest. *J Endourol* 2003;17:275–282.

75. Missal ME, Robinson JA, Tatum RW. Inferior vena cava obstruction. Clinical manifestation, diagnostic methods, and related problems. *Ann Intern Med* 1965;62:133–161.

76. Moinzadeh A, Libertino JA. Prognostic significance of tumor thrombus level in patients with renal cell carcinoma and venous tumor thrombus extension. Is all T3b the same? *J Urol* 2004;171:598–601.

77. Montie JE, Jackson CL, Cosgrove DM, *et al*. Resection of large inferior vena caval thrombi from renal cell carcinoma with the use of circulatory arrest. *J Urol* 1988;139:25–28.

78. Montie JE, El Ammar R, Pontes JE, *et al*. Renal cell carcinoma with inferior vena cava tumor thrombi. *Surg Gynecol Obstet* 1991;173:107–115.

79. Naitoh J, Kaplan A, Dorey F, *et al*. Metastatic renal cell carcinoma with concurrent inferior vena caval invasion: long-term survival after combination therapy with radical nephrectomy, vena caval thrombectomy and postoperative immunotherapy. *J Urol* 1999;162:46–50.

80. Nelson JB and Marshal FF. Surgical treatment of locally advanced renal cell carcinoma. In: Vogelzang NJ, Scardino PT, Shipley WU, Coffey DS, eds. *Comprehensive Textbook of Genitourinary Oncology*. Philadelphia: Lippincott Williams & Wilkins, 2000:183–201.

81. Nesbitt JC, Soltero ER, Dinney CPN, *et al*. Surgical management of renal cell carcinoma with inferior vena cava tumor thrombus. *Ann Thorac Surg* 1997;63:1592–1600.

82. Neves RJ, Zincke H. Surgical treatment of renal cancer with vena cava extension. *Br J Urol* 1987;59:390–395.

83. Novick AC, Campbell SC. Renal Tumors. In: Walsh PC, Retik AB, Vaughan ED, Wein AJ, eds. *Campbell's Urology*. Philadelphia: Saunders, 2002:2672–2731.

84. Novick AC, Cosgrove DM. Surgical approach for removal of renal cell carcinoma extending into the vena cava and the right atrium. *J Urol* 1980;123:947–950.

85. Novick AC, Streem SB, Pontes JE. *Stewarts Operative Urology*. Baltimore: Williams & Wilkins, 1989:88–104.

86. Novick AC, Kaye MC, Cosgrove DM, *et al*. Experience with cardiopulmonary bypass and hypothermic arrest in the management of retroperitoneal tumors with large vena cava thrombi. *Ann Surg* 1990;212:472–477.

87. O'Donohoe MK, Flanagan F, Fitzpatrick JM, *et al*. Surgical approach to inferior vena caval extension of renal carcinoma. *Br J Urol* 1987;60:492–496.

88. Okada Y, Kumada K, Habuchi T, *et al*. Total replacement of the suprarenal inferior vena cava with an expanded polytetrafluoroethylene tube graft in 2 patients with tumor thrombi from renal cell carcinoma. *J Urol* 1989;141:111–114.

89. Okada Y, Kumada K, Terachi T, *et al*. Long-term follow-up of patients with tumor thrombi from renal cell carcinoma and total replacement of the inferior vena cava using an expanded polytetrafluoroethylene tubular graft. *J Urol* 1996;155:444.

90. Oto A, Hertz BR, Remer EM, *et al*. Inferior vena cava tumor thrombus in renal cell carcinoma: staging by MR imaging impact on surgical treatment. *AJR Am J Roentgenol* 1998;171:1619–1624.

91. Pagano F, Bianco D, Artibani M, *et al*. Renal cell carcinoma with extension into the inferior vena cava: problems in diagnosis, staging, and treatment. *Eur Urol* 1992;22:200.

92. Pantuck AJ, Zisman A, Beldgrum AS. The challenging natural history of renal cell carcinoma. *J Urol* 2001;166:1611–1623.

93. Pringle JH. Notes on the arrest of the hepatic hemorrhage due to trauma. *Ann Surg* 1908;48:541–549.

94. Pritchett TR, Lieskovsky G, Skinner DG. Extension of renal cell carcinoma into the vena cava: clinical review and surgical approach. *J Urol* 1986;135:460–464.

95. Rivas LF, Brown AH, Neal DE. Venous bypass and filtration during nephrectomy for renal cell carcinoma with tumor thrombus in the retrohepatic cava. *Br J Urol* 1991;68:208–211.

96. Robson CJ. Radical nephrectomy for renal cell carcinoma. *J Urol* 1963;89:37.

97. Sakaguchi S, Hishiki S, Nakamura S, *et al*. Extension incision for renal carcinoma including invaded vena cava and right lobe of liver. *Urology* 1992;39:285–288.

98. Sarti L. Total prosthetic transplantation of the inferior vena cava with venous drainage restoration of the remaining kidney on the graft successfully performed on a child with Wilms' tumor. *Surgery* 1970;67:851–855.

99. Savage SJ and Gill I. Laparoscopic radical nephrectomy for renal cell carcinoma in a patient with level I renal vein thrombus. *J Urol* 2000;163:1243–1244.

100. Scheff P, Novick AC, Straffon RA, *et al*. Surgery for renal cell carcinoma extending into the inferior vena cava. *J Urol* 1978;120:28–31.

101. Sigman DB, Hasnain JU, Del Pizo JJ, *et al*. Real-time transesophageal echocardiography for intraoperative surveillance

of patients with renal cell carcinoma and vena caval extension undergoing radical nephrectomy. *J Urol* 1999;161:36–38.

102. Skinner DG, Colvin RB, Vermillion CD, *et al*. Diagnosis and management of renal cell carcinoma: a clinical and pathologic study 309 cases. *Cancer* 1971;28:1165–1177.

103. Skinner DG, Pfister RF, Colvin RB. Extension of renal cell cancer into the vena cava: the rationale for aggressive surgical removal. *J Urol* 1971;107:711–716.

104. Skinner DG, Pritchett TR, Lieskovsky G, *et al*. Vena caval involvement by renal cell carcinoma. Surgical resection provides meaningful long-term survival. *Ann Surg* 1989;210:387–394.

105. Slaton JW, Balbay MD, Levy DA, *et al*. Nephrectomy and vena caval thrombectomy in patients with metastatic renal cell carcinoma. *Urology* 1997;50:673–677.

106. Sosa RE, Muecke EC, Vaughan ED Jr, *et al*. Renal carcinoma extending into the inferior vena cava: the prognostic significance of the level of vena caval involvement. *J Urol* 1984;132:1097–1100.

107. Starzl TE, Iwatsuki S, Esquivel CO, *et al*. Refinements in the surgical technique of liver transplantation. *Sem Liver Dis* 1985;5:349.

108. Stewart JR, Carey JA, McDougal WS, *et al*. Cavoatrial tumor thrombectomy using cardiopulmonary bypass without circulatory arrest. *Ann Thorac Surg* 1991;51:717.

109. Stieber AC. Hepatic transplantation with the aid of the iron intern retractor. *Am J Surg* 1990;160:330.

110. Stief CG, Schafers HJ, Kuczyk M, *et al*. Renal cell carcinoma with intracaval neoplastic extension: stratification and surgical technique. *World J Urol* 1995;13:166.

111. Suggs WD, Smith RB III, Dodson TF, *et al*. Renal cell carcinoma with inferior vena caval involvement. *J Vasc Surg* 1991;14:413–418.

112. Sundaram CP, Rehman J, Landman J, *et al*. Hand assisted laparoscopic radical nephrectomy for renal cell carcinoma with inferior vena caval thrombus. *J Urol* 2002;168:176–179.

113. Swanson DA, Walace S, Johnson DE. The role of embolization and nephrectomy in the treatment of metastatic renal carcinoma. *J Urol* 1980;7:719–730.

114. Swanson DA, Johnson DE, von Eschenbach AC, *et al*. Angioinfarction plus nephrectomy for metastatic renal cell carcinoma: an update. *J Urol* 1983;130:449–452.

115. Svensson L, Cawford ES, Hess K, *et al*. Deep hypothermia with circulatory arrest. *J Thorac Cardiovasc Surg* 1993;106:19–28.

116. Sweeney P, Wood CG, Pisters LL, *et al*. Surgical management of renal cell carcinoma associated with complex inferior vena caval thrombi. *Urol Oncol* 2003;21:327–333.

117. Swierzewski DJ, Swierzewski MJ, Libertino JA. Radical nephrectomy in patients with renal cell carcinoma with venous, vena caval, and atrial extension. *Am J Surg* 1994;168:205–209.

118. Thomalla JV, Friend PJ. Modified cruciate incision for transabdominal radical nephrectomy. *J Urol* 1991;145:1245.

119. Treiger BFG, Humphrey LS, Peterson SL, *et al*. Transesophageal echocardiography in renal cell carcinoma: an accurate diagnostic technique for intracaval neoplastic extension. *J Urol* 1991;145:1138.

120. Tsuji Y, Goto A, Hara I, *et al*. Renal cell carcinoma with extension of tumor thrombus into the vena cava: surgical strategy and prognosis. *J Vasc Surg* 2001;33:789–796.

121. Turini D, Selli C, Barbanti G, *et al*. Removal of renal cell carcinoma extending to the supradiaphragmatic vena cava with the aid of cardiopulmonary bypass. *Urol Int* 1986;41:303.

122. Vaidya A, Ciancio G, Soloway MS. Surgical techniques for treating renal neoplasm invading the inferior vena cava. *J Urol* 2003;169:435–444.

123. Vaislic C, Puel P, Grondin P, *et al*. Surgical resection of neoplastic thrombosis in the inferior vena cava by neoplasms of renal-adrenal tract. *Vasc Surg* 1983;September-October:322.

124. Webb JAW, Murray A, Barry PR, *et al*. The accuracy and limitations of ultrasound in the assessment of venous extension in renal cell carcinoma. *Br J Urol* 1987;60:14–17.

125. Wellons E, Rosenthal D, Schobor T, *et al*. Renal cell carcinoma invading the inferior vena cava: use of a "temporary" vena cava filter to prevent tumor emboli during nephrectomy. *Urology* 2004;63(2):380–382.

126. Wilkinson CJ, Kimovec MA, Uejima T. Cardiopulmonary bypass in patients with malignant renal neoplasms. *Br J Anesth* 1986;58:461.

127. Zisman A, Wieder JA, Pantuck AJ, *et al*. Renal cell carcinoma with tumor thrombus extension: biology, role of nephrectomy and response to immunotherapy. *J Urol* 2003;169:909–916.

8i
Complicated Tumors: Bench Surgery

Gerald H.J. Mickisch

Introduction and Objective

Undoubtedly, with the increasing availability of ultrasonography and computer tomography (CT) scanning, incidental renal tumors are more frequently diagnosed. Therefore, the cohort of patients that seeks treatment for renal cell carcinoma (RCC) has dramatically changed over the past 25 years, and the question arises as to whether this alteration should also translate into different approaches to surgical treatment strategies.

An organ-sparing resection, sometimes called "partial nephrectomy" of a malignant tumor, is the most flagrant violation of Robsons' concepts of a "radical" tumor nephrectomy.[10] Here, the surgeon deliberately opens Gerota's fascia, frees the kidney from surrounding fatty tissue, and resects the tumor only. The techniques applied in various series[3] range from tumor excision over truly "partial" nephrectomy to *ex vivo* (bench) surgery. Nevertheless, from a theoretical point of view, the tumor dissection must be performed within a safe rim of healthy parenchyma guided by intraoperative frozen section analysis to avoid margin positivity responsible for local recurrence.

Indications for nephron-sparing surgery evolved out of necessity when malignancy was detected in a solitary kidney, or in the setting of bilateral cancer or diminished renal function. Results were reasonable with a mean recurrence rate of 7.5%.[8] More recently, in a review article about a single-center study with 500 patients,[6] preservation of kidney function was achieved in 489 patients (98%), exhibiting a cancer-specific 5-year survival rate of 93%. Recurrent RCC developed postoperatively in 39 of 473 patients (8,2%); 13 of these patients (2.7%) were diagnosed with a local recurrence in the remnant kidney while 26 developed metastatic disease.

Local recurrence was reported in three cases in a review article[8] incorporating 388 cases of elective nephron-sparing operations from 11 centers, which comprised two local recurrences in two cases and metachronous recurrence elsewhere in the kidney in one case. At a mean follow-up of 31–75 months, the local recurrence rate amounted to 0.8%, which is 10 times lower then after a mandatory indication for kidney-sparing operations. Appropriate patient selection is partly responsible for this excellent outcome. There is consensus that in addition to the size of the primary tumor, the feasibility of a radical resection in terms of the anatomical localization of the cancerous mass is critical.[9] In most series, elective indications are reserved for tumors $\leq 4\,cm$ in diameter.

In a few cases of a solitary kidney and an organ-confined albeit extensive or centrally located RCC, organ-sparing approaches are warranted, but technically not feasible *in situ* for a safe tumor resection without compromising the remaining kidney function. In those exceptional cases, bench surgery followed by autotransplantation may be indicated. This surgically challenging procedure should be regarded as the last resort, and may render acceptable results when strict selection criteria, multidisciplinary teamwork structures, and adequate quality control measures are applied. These conditions are best met in the context of "A Center Of Excellence" using defined protocols for inclusion and therapeutic outcome measurements.

Materials and Methods

We report on a prospective series of 34 cases of bench surgery followed by autotransplantation for complex RCC. The surgical procedure was performed by a multidisciplinary team consisting of a nephrologist specializing in hemodialysis, a transplant surgeon familiar with kidney transplantation procedures, and a urological surgeon specializing in oncological urology, who served as a team leader (G.H.J.M.). All patients were unanimously attested by the whole team to have an imperative indication for this operation, and were considered to be suitable surgical candidates. Informed consent was obtained after discussing possible alternative strategies such as a tumor nephrectomy followed by hemodialysis and a kidney transplantation in the follow-up period. Institutional ethical committees were duly informed on our treatment protocol and approved enrollment, treatment, and follow-up criteria.

Results

All tumors were invariably RCCs. In 30 cases a clear cell type, in three cases a papillary type, and in one case a chromophobe type carcinoma was diagnosed at histopathological examination. All cases were considered preoperatively by imaging procedures as "organ-confined" (Figs. 8i-1, 8i-2), whereas definitive pathology revealed a tumor stage ranging from pT1 to pT3a, always pN0, and M0 (UICC classification, 2002 edition) (Fig 8i-3). In two patients (see above), we did not carry out the autotransplantation. In one case we detected an unsuspected tumor-positive lymph node at frozen section analysis, and in the other case, one out of three resected

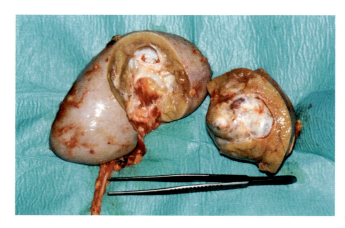

FIGURE 8i-3. Tumor resection: organ-confined, albeit extensive disease.

tumors was a Bellini duct type carcinoma. Because of the highly aggressive nature of this tumor entity, we did not dare to retransplant the kidney.

The reason for this kind of complex surgery was always an imperative indication, namely 33 solitary kidneys (25 large central masses and 8 bilateral tumors). In one patient with multiple bilateral tumors, a tumor nephrectomy on one side, and bench surgery with autotransplantation on the other side, was executed in two sessions. Patient age ranged from 31 to 70 years with a median age of 47 years. Preoperative creatinine levels varied from 59 to 221 μM (median 102 μM, normal range < 150 μM).

Surgical techniques generally followed the principles of a Robson type[10] radical nephrectomy using a modified Giuliani (anterior flank) incision.[2] In cases with an absent/dysfunctional contralateral adrenal gland, the ipsilateral adrenal gland was preserved in the case of undetectable tumor invasion. In addition, some kidney transplantation features were included such as resecting long vascular sleeves (Fig 8i-4) and heparinization as well as

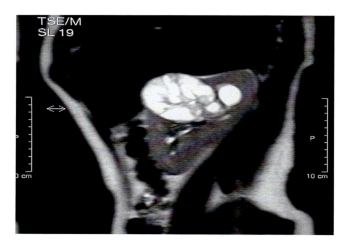

FIGURE 8i-1. Imaging procedures: MRI.

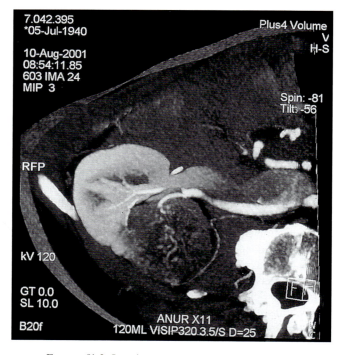

FIGURE 8i-2. Imaging procedures. CT angiography.

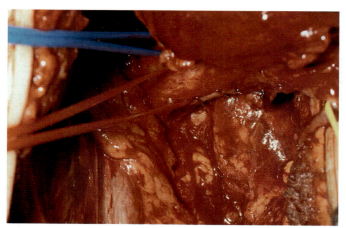

FIGURE 8i-4. Resection of tumor-bearing kidney.

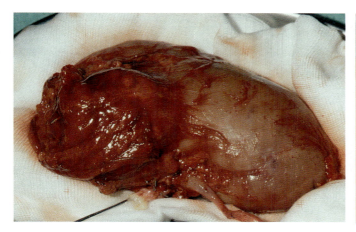

FIGURE 8i-5. Cooling on crushed ice and flushing by ice-cold solution.

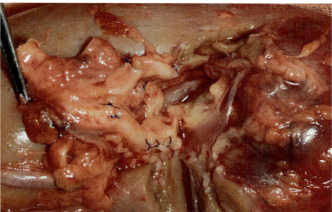

FIGURE 8i-7. Reconstruction of the caliceal system and the venous and arterial bloodstream.

induction of osmotic diuresis by mannitol prior to clamping the renal artery. The resected kidney was placed immediately on crushed ice (sterile working bench) and flushed with EURO-Collins solution at 4°C (Fig 8i-5). The kidney specimen was freed from all adjacent fatty tissues, and the tumor was resected radically (Fig 8i-6) using magnifying glasses or a surgical microscope. Multiple frozen sections were analyzed to ensure radicality. Following renal reconstruction (Fig 8i-7), an autotransplantation to the fossa illiaca was performed. Ureteric anastomosis was done either by formal antirefluxive implantation to the bladder (Fig 8i-8) or by ureteroureterostomy to the remnant ureteric stump.

Overall, surgical time (from incision to final wound closure) extended from 320 to 560 minutes (median 380 minutes) and total blood loss as calculated from anesthesiology charts varied from 170 to 620 ml with a median of 330 ml. Postoperative serum creatinine levels ranged from 71 to 239 μM (median 147 μM, normal range < 150 μM).

Surgical complications were few, but significant: one perioperative death after 5 days due to myocardial infarction, one

kidney lost due to transplantation failure, and one patient on hemodialysis for 3 weeks until complete functional recovery.

Oncologically, we noted, after a relatively short follow-up period of 2.4 years (median), one patient with distant metastasis and one patient with a recurrent tumor in his kidney after 13 months which may be a true local recurrence or a secondary tumor. This situation was salvaged by nephrectomy of the autotransplant.

Discussion

The first successful kidney transplantation was performed on December 23, 1954, and the surgical pioneer, Dr. M.E. Murray, received the Nobel Prize in 1990. To circumvent inherent immunological problems identical twins were the first patients to benefit from this revolutionary progress in surgical medicine, and graft survival extended to 11 months.

Currently, a 60–80% 5-year allogeneic graft survival is standard practice for kidney transplantation in Europe.

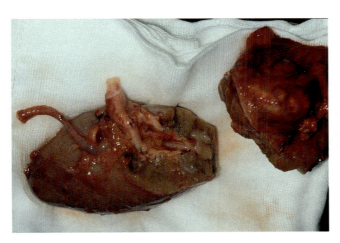

FIGURE 8i-6. Radical tumor resection.

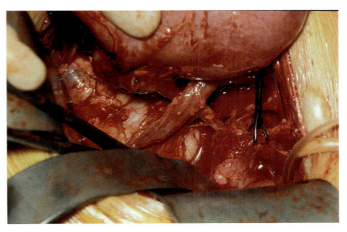

FIGURE 8i-8. Autotransplantation to fossa iliaca.

In the 1960s, the medical community experienced increasing numbers of bench surgery with kidney autotransplantations, which were often done for chronic benign diseases (chronic kidney failure) and a few RCCs. In the 1970s, peak incidences of this type of complex surgery were described, and RCC became an established indication. [1] In the 1980s there were decreasing numbers of this technique, parallel to the increasing availability of hemodialysis,[5] and in the 1990s, only a few case reports appeared advocating this surgical challenge.[7,11]

Nevertheless, in the past few years, there has been a remarkable revival of interest in bench surgery followed by autotransplantation. Several reasons may have contributed to this development. First and probably most important, there is a critical shortage of kidney donations suitable for transplantation, and tumor patients are not a priority for transplant centers. Hence, the alternative strategy for complex RCC to simply nephrectomize the patient and transplant a donor kidney at a later stage, while bridging the waiting period by hemodialysis has been seriously hampered by long and cumbersome waiting lists. In addition, hemodialysis has been proven to reduce the quality of life significantly, has a proper morbidity and mortality, and is expensive.

When critically appraising our personal experience consisting of 21 cases from 1992 to 2000 and of 34 prospective cases (this series) from 2001 to 2005, bench surgery and autotransplantation for complex cases of RCC are feasible and probably cost effective. There is a clear need for strict inclusion criteria such as an imperative indication and organ-confined (hence surgically curable disease) stages, a multidisciplinary team approach, a suitable infrastructure, and experience in major surgical procedures. If these criteria are met, bench surgery followed by autotransplantation hasagain

become a valuable last resort, is apparently safe, and has been increasingly requested.

References

1. Bellinger MF, Koontz WW Jr, Smith MJ. Renal cell carcinoma: twenty years of experience. *Va Med* 1979;106:819–824.
2. Giberti C, Schenone M. Giulianis's method of anterior-lateral transabdominal muscle splitting and nerve preservation for kidney tumors. *Prog Urol* 1999;9:562–566.
3. Hafez KS, Novick AC, Butler B. Management of small, solitary, unilateral renal cell carcinomas: Impact of central versus peripheral tumor location. *J Urol* 1998;159:1156–1160.
4. Mickisch GH. New trends in the treatment of renal cancer. *Akt Urol* 1994;25:77–83.
5. Montie JE. "Bench surgery" for renal cell carcinoma: a proper niche. *Mayo Clin Proc* 1992;67:701–702.
6. Novick AC. Nephron-sparing surgery for renal cell carcinoma. *Br J Urol* 1998;82:321–324.
7. Petritsch PH, Gruber H, Colombo T, Rauchenwald M, Breinl E, Ratschek M, Vilits P. Indications and results of ex vivo surgery of the kidney. *Wien Klin Wochenschr* 1995; 107:731–735.
8. Poppel v H, Baert L. Elective conservative surgery for renal cell carcinoma. *AUA Update Series* 1994;13:246–258.
9. Poppel v H, Bamelis B, Oyen R, Baert L. Partial nephrectomy for renal cell carcinoma can achieve long-term tumor control. *J Urol* 1998;160:674–678.
10. Robson CJ. Radical nephrectomy for renal cell carcinoma. *J Urol* 1963;89:37–42.
11. Stormont TJ, Bilhartz DL, Zincke H. Pitfalls of "bench surgery" and autotransplantation for renal cell carcinoma. *Mayo Clin Proc* 1992;67:621–628.

8j
Advanced Disease: Nonpulmonary Metastases

Bryan B. Voelzke and Robert C. Flanigan

Introduction

Epidemiology

In 2005 Jemal et al., estimated that there would be 36,160 new cases of cancer and 12,660 deaths in the United States from cancer located in the kidney and renal pelvis. This computes to approximately 2.6% new cases and 2.2% deaths among projected cancers in United States men and women in 2005. Despite the apparent low incidence of renal cell carcinoma (RCC), an analysis of United States Surveillance, Epidemiology, and End Results (SEER) data has shown an increase in the incidence of local, regional, and distant RCC from 1973 to 1998 (Hock et al., 2002). In another review of SEER data, RCC was found to have increased 2.3% annually from 1975 to 1995, with similar increases noted in all stages of presentation (Chow et al., 1999).

Presentation and Review of Treatment Options

These numbers are likely a result in the increased use of radiographic imaging modalities, which has led to many asymptomatic renal tumors being incidentally diagnosed earlier in their natural history, along with more advanced tumors presenting with a diverse set of symptoms. As a result, many physicians have been forced to change their view of RCC as the "radiologist's tumor" in contradistinction to its prior association as the "internist's tumor," due to RCC's paraneoplastic effects. For example, in 1971 approximately 10% of renal tumors were diagnosed radiographically (Skinner et al., 1971), as compared to a retrospective study from 1998 that found 61% of initially presenting RCCs being discovered via radiographic imaging (Jayson and Sanders 1998).

The classic triad of hematuria, abdominal pain, and flank pain is noteworthy for its uncommon occurrence, being present in only 10% of initial RCC diagnoses. Most patients with metastatic RCC at presentation will have no symptoms (Kierney et al., 1994; O'Dea et al., 1978); however, symptoms from metastatic sites at initial presentation will primarily depend upon the location of metastasis. Kavolius et al., (1998) performed a large retrospective study of 231 patients with metastatic RCC and found that the majority of patients had pulmonary metastasis ($n = 158$, 57%). Of the pulmonary cohort, only 10% were symptomatic. Likewise, patients with metastasis to the skin, lymph nodes, salivary glands, and thyroid gland were also generally asymptomatic. Bone ($n = 53$) and brain metastases ($n = 21$), the second and fourth most common metastatic sites in this series, more often presented symptomatically with 96% and 79% of these patients having symptoms, respectively.

From a review of SEER data from 1986 to 1998 in nine tumor registries representing 14% of the U.S. population, the percentages of patients presenting with localized, regional, and metastatic RCC were 54%, 21%, and 25%, respectively (Hock et al., 2002). As mentioned above, the increased use of radiographic imaging has yielded a higher number of patients who were diagnosed incidentally with clinically confined tumors. The cure rates of those with advanced or metastatic RCC is very poor, with a median survival time of 6–10 months without treatment (Flanigan et al.,2003; Kavolius et al.,1998). With the dismal outcomes associated with metastatic RCC, additional therapeutic options such as hormonal therapy, chemotherapy, and radiation therapy have been studied. All of these treatment strategies have been failures and are not considered acceptable treatment options (Montie et al., 1977; Motzer and Russo 2000; Onufrey and Mohiuddin 1985; Vis 2002; Yagoda 1990). In the case of chemotherapy, factors thought to be responsible for this poor response are multidrug resistance and intratumoral heterogeneity.

Immunotherapy with interleukin (IL)-2 and/or interferon (IFN)-α rarely produces a response rate in excess of 10–20% for advanced RCC, thus prompting physicians to reevaluate the use of surgery (Motzer and Russo 2000). Prior to the use of immunotherapy, nephrectomy as the sole treatment for advanced RCC was studied and rejected due to poor survival rates. However, later retrospective studies evaluating the role of combined nephrectomy and immunotherapy renewed interest in the potential use of nephrectomy in select patient populations (Walther et al., 1993). As a result, prospective studies of nephrectomy and adjuvant immunotherapy were conducted and confirmed the survival benefit of this treatment option for patients with advanced RCC (Flanigan et al., 2001; Mickisch et al., 2001). Surgical resection of solitary or limited metastatic disease has also become a credible management option as demonstrated by prolonged survival in select patient populations (Kavolius et al., 1998; Kierney et al., 1994). No current surgical management option for metastatic RCC has been defined as a gold standard treatment strategy, as there are important prognostic factors that influence physician decisions. However, the following surgical options are currently useful: nephrectomy combined with metasta-sectomy for curative intent, cytoreductive nephrectomy prior to systemic therapy, nephrectomy and/or metastasectomy to consolidate partial responses to systemic therapy, and nephrectomy as a component of adoptive immunotherapy protocols. Each surgical indication will be discussed in this chapter along with advanced surgical techniques.

Prognostic Factors

As mentioned above, the prognosis for metastatic RCC is grim with limited long-term survival. As such, prognostic factors have been developed to identify which patients will benefit from therapy for metastatic RCC. The following prognostic factors correlate with length of survival: perfor-mance status, sites of metastasis, total burden of disease, metastasis-free interval (> 2 months), pathological stage, tumor grade, and cell type. Other possible prognostic factors are tumor size, age, race, sex, and associated paraneoplastic syndromes. Of these factors, node (N) and metastasis (M) status from the TNM staging system are considered the most powerful prognostic factors predicting for survival. Perfor-mance status also strongly correlates with the outcomes for advanced RCC by reflecting the state of debilitation and ability to tolerate aggressive therapeutic treatment regimens. Median survival for patients with excellent performance status ranges from 10 to 20 months, while those with poor performance status can expect a median survival of only 2–5 months (Ljungberg et al., 2000; Masuda et al., 1997; Motzer et al., 1999). As mentioned above, total disease burden is a prognostic factor that can predict survival. In a retrospective review by Pantuck and colleagues, 322 patients with N0M1 and N+M1 disease underwent nephrectomy and a significant response to adjuvant immunotherapy was seen only in the N0M1 cohort (Pantuck et al., Pantuck et al.,). In this study, lymph node involvement (N+M0) was a strong predictor of failure; however, performance status and primary tumor grade were more powerful predictors of outcome. Pantuck postulated that patients who experience early lymph node involvement have an immune dysfunction that prevents the primary tumor site from controlling the spread of the tumor. Perhaps this explains the higher tumor grades, higher undif-ferentiated pathology, and larger tumor size that are often associated with lymphadenopathy.

Biochemical markers and immunohistochemical analyses are also being evaluated for their potential role in helping physicians predict pretherapy prognosis and survival. After reporting on a worse prognosis of patients with decreased expression of carbonic anhydrase IX in nephrectomy specimens (Bui et al., 2003), Bui performed additional studies with carbonic anhydrase IX (low staining = favorable) and Ki-67 (high staining = favorable) after nephrectomy in a retrospective setting and found that both param-eters allowed stratification of risk groups and predicted survival (Bui et al., 2004). Recently, Atkins expanded upon these encouraging reports of carbonic anhydrase IX by Bui. Upon retrospective review of patients with a response to IL-2-based immunotherapy, Atkins found that high expression of carbonic anhydrase IX (> 85%) correlated with improved outcomes with IL-2-based immunotherapy (Atkins et al., 2004). C-reactive protein (CRP) levels in patients with metastatic RCC have been studied with mixed results. In a small, retrospective study Fujikawa noted that 25 patients with elevated CRP levels prenephrectomy demonstrated enhanced serum immunosuppressive acidic protein and natural killer cell activity in the recovery period (Fujikawa et al., 2000). In a more recent and larger retrospective study, Casamassima studied CRP, fibrinogen, albumin, elevated sedimentation rate (ESR), lactate dehydrogenase, and total lymphocytes in patients with metastatic RCC under-going cytoreductive nephrectomy and IL-2 (Casamassima et al.,). These laboratory results were correlated with known prognostic factors that predicted for survival, and upon multivariate analysis, only CRP and disease-free interval > 12 months were associated with improved survival. Interestingly, a lower pretreatment CRP correlated with better survival and better prognosis. Lower pretreatment fibrinogen and albumin were also associated with better survival. Finally, postoperative azotemia after cytoreductive nephrectomy has also proven to be associated with a statisti-cally improved survival over patients who do not demonstrate azotemia after nephrectomy (17-month vs. 4-month survival) (Gatenby et al., 2002).

Radical Nephrectomy: Locally Advanced Disease

Preoperative Preparation

The most important factor for the rational use of nephrectomy with advanced disease is patient selection. Risk factors to consider at the time of nephrectomy for advanced disease will be covered later in this chapter under "Cytoreductive Nephrectomy" and will not be repeated in this section. All patients undergoing cytoreductive nephrectomy should have an appropriate preoperative evaluation for metastatic spread including a basic metabolic profile (including liver function tests), complete blood count, chest X-ray, abdominal computed tomography (CT) scan, and a bone scan if clinical bone pain or elevated alkaline phosphatase is present. A head

CT should also be ordered if symptoms of metastatic spread to the brain are clinically suspected. Three-dimensional CT reconstruction can also prove useful if knowledge of arterial and/or venous anatomy is required for complex RCC cases with venous extension. Lastly, if the patient presented with gross or microscopic hematuria, complete evaluation of the urinary tract with upper tract imaging and cystoscopy should be performed preoperatively.

The surgeon should be aware of the surgical approach to be utilized. The flank and thoracoabdominal incision often involves removal of a rib and/or transection of muscles used for respiration leading to patient discomfort and possible respiratory impairment in the postoperative period. This can increase the morbidity of the operation by placing the patient at risk for nosocomial respiratory infections. As such, a cautious review of smoking history and any associated pulmonary impairment should be noted and a different approach for nephrectomy used when possible to maximize patient recovery. Consultation with a pulmonologist to evaluate pulmonary function tests and arterial blood gas measurement may be required prior to surgery if any ventilatory problems are anticipated. Furthermore, the surgeon should be mindful of vertebral disc disease when the flank position is used for nephrectomy. Finally, venous return can be impaired from the flank position and lead to hypotension and ensuing cardiac impairment. From our experience with the flank position and the associated problems that may occur, we will observe the patient after positioning and periodically speak with our anesthesia colleagues during the case to ensure that cardiopulmonary status is stable. If the patient is not an appropriate candidate for either of these approaches, an alternative approach should be implemented.

Magnetic resonance imaging (MRI) is the imaging modality of choice to determine the extent of renal vein or inferior vena cava (IVC) tumor thrombus. Tumor thrombus should be suspected when there is lower extremity edema, pulmonary embolism, right atrial mass, nonfunction of the affected kidney, varicocele, dilated superficial veins, or proteinuria. Transesophageal echocardiography and transabdominal color Doppler ultrasonography can also be useful adjuncts when venous thrombus extension is suspected. IVC venography may also be implemented when the above choices are inconclusive (Novick 2002). Preoperative renal embolization should be considered when substantial collateralization of the arterial supply feeding the renal tumor is observed. Embolization of the tumor helps to shrink the tumor (and in some cases the IVC thrombus) thus making operative resection more feasible; however, the surgeon must be cognizant of possible postinfarction syndrome, which has viral-like symptoms of fever, chills, and nausea. As cautioned by Novick, when adjunctive cardiopulmonary bypass with deep hypothermic circulatory arrest is planned due to extensive IVC thrombus extension, a preoperative angiogram should be performed to determine if simultaneous cardiac bypass grafting will be needed (Novick 2002).

Radical Nephrectomy: Advanced Issues

Vena Caval Thrombectomy

Approximately 30% of patients with RCC will present with metastatic disease, and of these, 4–25% will be associated with venous tumor thrombosis (Slaton et al., 1997; Zisman et al., 2002). Venous thrombosis extension can be staged according to three levels: level I, below the hepatic veins; level II, at or above the hepatic veins but below the diaphragm; and level III, above the diaphragm. Preoperative evaluation should determine the cephalad extent of tumor thrombus in anticipation of the surgical approach and possible additional therapy (i.e., coronary angiography if supradiaphragmatic, intracardiac). CT scanning and ultrasound are useful to define the caudal extent of tumor thrombus; however, they have been shown to be inconclusive in defining the cephalad extent (Goldfarb et al., 1990). MRI has been shown to be the gold standard study to define the cephalad extent of the tumor thrombus and has largely replaced the invasive option, IVC venography. This later study should be reserved for equivocal MRI results or when MRI is contraindicated. Renal embolization should be considered if venous tumor thrombus is present to rule out hypervascularity of the tumor. This will serve to shrink the tumor and help alleviate bleeding and morbidity during the operation. At the time of surgery, central venous monitoring with possible Swan–Ganz catheterization should be considered in anticipation of intravascular fluid shifts from blood loss. Finally, consultation with a hepatic surgeon or vascular surgeon may be necessary for difficult cases. Regarding the surgical approach, a modified flank or bilateral subcostal incision provides excellent exposure for nephrectomy and resection of level I thrombus, with a thoracoabdominal approach reserved for large upper pole tumors. Level II or III tumors can be approached with a bilateral subcostal incision for the abdominal approach and a median sternotomy for the supradiaphragmatic portion of the case, if necessary.

Up to one-third of patients with vena cava tumor thrombus will also have distant metastatic disease. Studies have shown that those with tumor thrombus and metastasis fare worse than those with tumor thrombus and nonmetastatic RCC (Naitoh et al., 1999; Skinner et al., 1971; Slaton et al., 1997). As shown in Table 8j-1, the 5-year survival rates of patients with nonmetastatic RCC with thrombus invading the vena cava varied from 27 to 72%, while patients with metastatic RCC and tumor thrombus fared worse with 5-year survival rates of 12.5–19.6%. Some reports have expressed concern that metastasis is a contraindication for nephrectomy and thrombectomy, indicating that these patients tend to progress rapidly and/or respond poorly to immunotherapy (Bennett et al., 1995; Franklin et al., 1996; Hatcher et al., 1991; Skinner et al., 1989). However, a contrary opinion has been expressed by others who report the benefits of cytoreductive nephrectomy with or without thrombectomy when performed

TABLE 8j-1. Five-year survival for inferior vena cava thrombus in nonmetastatic and metastatic RCC.

Reference	Number of patients with nonmetastatic renal cellcarcinoma	Survival	Number of patients with metastatic RCC	Survival
Neves and Zincke (1987)	36	68%	18	12.5%
Skinner et al. (1989)	53	40%	N/A	N/A
Hatcher et al. (1991)	27	69%	8	13.0%
Swierzewski et al. (1994)	72	64%	28	19.6%

Source: Adapted from Slaton et al. (1997).

with additional therapeutic measures, such as metastasectomy or adjuvant immunotherapy (Flanigan et al., 2001; Mickisch et al., 2001; Rackley et al., 1994; Walther et al., 1993). Several authors have also shown that there is no difference in survival when comparing outcomes in those with and without tumor thrombus in the renal vein or IVC (Ficarra et al., Ficarra et al.,; Goetzl et al., 2004).

Additional concern has been expressed over the morbidity and mortality of nephrectomy with thrombectomy. Zisman and colleagues reviewed their data at UCLA from 1989 through 2000 in 254 patients with gross venous tumor thrombosis who were scheduled to receive unilateral cytoreductive nephrectomy (Zisman et al., 2002). Eighty-one percent ($n = 207$) were deemed eligible or consented to surgery. Thirty-seven percent (77/207) had nonmetastatic RCC, while 63% (130/207) had metastatic RCC. The surgical outcomes were compared to 607 patients who presented with localized RCC and no tumor thrombus. The majority of patients in both groups received a flank or thoracoabdominal incision (> 90% in both groups). The mean operative time was longer when metastatic RCC was present ($p < 0.05$); however, there was no difference in hospital stay. Mortality was higher in the group with tumor thrombus (3.1% vs. 0.8%). In regard to morbidity, higher blood loss and transfusion requirements were found to be present in those with tumor thrombus. There was no difference in blood loss or transfusion requirement when metastatic and nonmetastatic operations were compared.

Postoperative complications in the IVC thrombus group were separated to early (< 24 hours) and late. The early complications were myocardial infarction, myocardial ischemia, cardiac arrhythmia, cerebral vascular accident, pneumothorax, adult respiratory distress syndrome, hypertension, hemodynamic instability, and lower extremity edema. Late complications were most evident in the IVC thrombus group with atrial tumor involvement (5/39 patients) and consisted of pulmonary emboli, retroperitoneal hematoma, pneumothorax, arrhythmia, and chylous leakage. Lastly and most importantly, the percentage of those completing a full course of immunotherapy (59%, 61%, and 60%, respectively) and mean time to immunotherapy (2.0, 2.1, and 2.1 months, respectively) was not different among those with renal vein extension, IVC extension, or localized tumor without tumor thrombus.

Infrahepatic Tumor Thrombus (Level I)

When dealing with venous thrombi, it is important to obtain venous control cephalad to the tumor thrombus to avoid embolization of the thrombus. Patients without intraabdominal tumor thrombi can safely tolerate temporary occlusion of the IVC. After incision and reflection of the colon medially, the renal vasculature should be isolated with vessel loops and the kidney mobilized outside of Gerota's fascia leaving only the renal artery and vein. After ligating the renal artery, the renal vein should be dissected free of the surrounding structures with care to avoid injury to the posterior lumbar veins. The contralateral renal vein should also be mobilized if clamping of the infrahepatic IVC is planned (especially on the left side), as this will prevent embolization of tumor thrombus to the contralateral kidney. Figure 8j-1 provides information for the order of clamping of the vessels when complete IVC isolation is required: (1) renal artery(s), (2) subhepatic vena cava, (3) distal vena cava cephalad to bifurcation, (4) left renal vein, and (5) porta hepatis (control is not necessary for infrahepatic thrombus).

For small tumors confined to the renal vein, a Satinsky vascular clamp should be placed distal to the thrombus at the entrance to the IVC, and an incision around the renal vein and potentially IVC should be performed with an ample cuff of vein (Fig. 8j-2). If a small thrombus is present in the IVC, the clamp can be placed around the thrombus, partially occluding the IVC. At times, the thrombus can be freely milked back into the renal vein to allow less clamping and resection of the IVC. After thrombus removal, the IVC should be closed with running 5-0 vascular suture, preferably in two layers. Most commonly, tumor thrombi are not adherent to the IVC; however, if adherence to the venous wall exists, excision of a portion of the IVC wall will be necessary. Up to 50% of the wall can be resected without affecting venous flow. A venous graft may be necessary if a > 50% reduction in circumference exists after resection.

In large tumors with IVC thrombus, extensive venous collateralization often has developed as a result of long-standing occlusion of the IVC. Either kidney can be expected to do well after resection of the infrarenal IVC; however, this is not true if the suprarenal IVC is resected. The left kidney will do well in this situation as long as venous collaterals from the left gonadal and left suprarenal vein are left intact. The right kidney will not survive if the suprarenal IVC is removed.

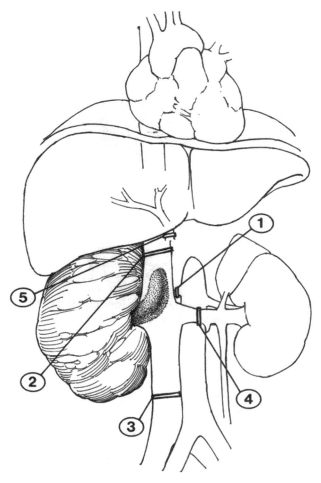

FIGURE 8j-1. Infrahepatic RCC: order of clamping (1–5). (Reproduced with permission from Hinman et al., 1998.)

In this circumstance, preserving a tumor-free strip of IVC, which can be augmented with a patch, anastomosing the right kidney to the splenic, portal, or inferior mesenteric vein via an interposition graft, or autotransplanting the kidney to the pelvis via the iliac veins can be performed (Novick, 2002).

Intrahepatic or Suprahepatic Tumor Thrombus (Levels II and III)

The same principles of vascular clamping in the abdomen are important; however, the presence of the liver can make immediate clamping proximal to infrahepatic tumor thrombi challenging, necessitating a thoracic exposure for better proximal venous control. When high-level II or level III thrombus is present, a bilateral subcostal incision is made to allow easy access to the renal vasculature and IVC with a median sternotomy incision for the thoracic portion of the case. After obtaining vascular control, the kidney is completely dissected free except for the involved renal vein.

Infrahepatic tumors may or may not require cardiopulmonary bypass or hypothermic cardiac arrest; however,

suprahepatic tumors will almost always involve these techniques, even if an intraatrial thrombus does not exist. After mobilizing the kidney, the liver should be mobilized from the diaphragm by cutting the hepatic, triangular, and coronary ligaments. Traction can then be applied to the liver to allow visualization of inferior hepatic veins and upper lumbar veins that must be ligated and divided. After the thrombus is isolated proximally, the patient should be placed in a Trendelenburg position to prevent an air embolus in anticipation of opening the IVC. For right-sided tumors, Fig. 8j-3 gives instructions for vascular occlusion. The vessels should be ligated in the following order: (1) cross-clamp the aorta—-optional (minimize to 30 minutes to avoid ischemia to the spinal cord, bowel, and left kidney), (2) cephalad vena cava in the pericardial sac, (3) caudal vena cava, (4) atraumatically porta hepatis, and (5) left renal vein (Hinman, 1998). At this point, the vena cava should be opened with fine scissors and the tumor excised. A freely mobile clot can be retracted in a manner similar to how vascular surgeons remove peripheral arterial clots with a Fogarty catheter. In this case, a 20-French Foley is passed cephalad to the thrombus and then inflated and withdrawn to remove the clot (Fig. 8j-4). Copious irrigation with sterile water should be performed after removal of the thrombus. If the thrombus is adherent to the vena cava wall, cardiopulmonary bypass with deep hypothermic arrest to allow removal in a bloodless field and/or to minimize potential warm ischemia from prolonged clamping of the aorta should be performed. After removal of the clot, the clamps should be removed in reverse order of their placement. For left renal tumors, Hinman recommends clamping in the following order (Fig. 8j-5): (1) left renal artery, (2) proximal aorta—optional, (3) cephalad intrapericardial vena cava, (4) caudal vena cava, (5) right renal vein with the ability to secure the right renal artery (poorer collateral right venous circulation), and (6) porta hepatis (Hinman, 1998). The cavotomy should be closed with running 5-0 vascular sutures, which are oversewn for a two-layered closure.

Suprahepatic tumors are best resected with cardiopulmonary bypass with hypothermic circulatory arrest, and readers are directed to this technique originally described by Marshall and colleagues (Marshall et al., 1984; Marshall and Reitz 1986). This technique should also be considered for infrahepatic tumors, so as to avoid extensive retrohepatic dissection that can be accompanied by potentially massive retroperitoneal bleeding. As a result of limited retrohepatic dissection and the ability to bypass sequential clamping of the aorta, caudal IVC, and porta hepatis, potentially massive retroperitoneal bleeding may be averted.

Finally, a longer period of cold ischemia time (60 minutes) is allowed, in comparison to the shorter warm ischemia time (30 minutes) allowed by sequential clamping. As mentioned previously, cardiac bypass grafting can also be employed while under cardiopulmonary bypass. Risks of cardiopulmonary bypass with circulatory arrest include cerebral

(a)

(b)

(c)

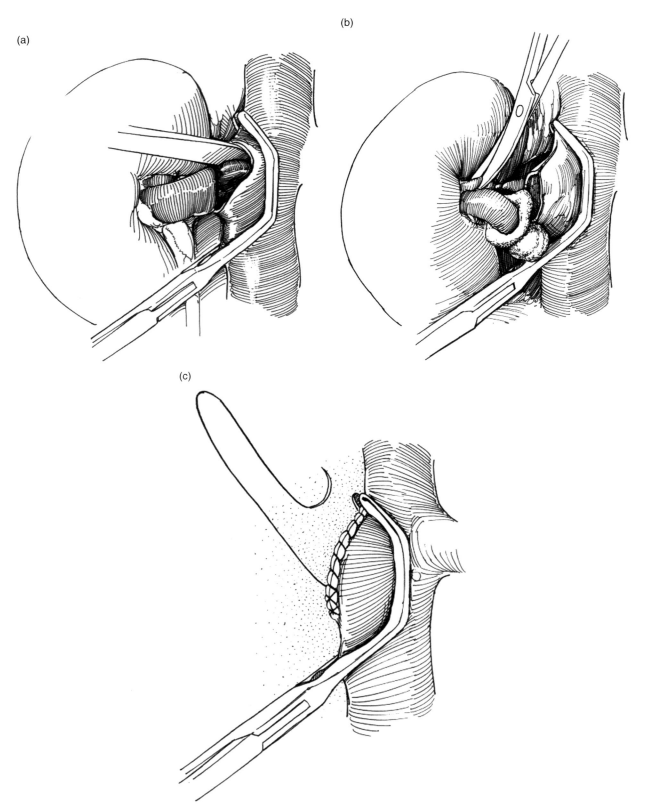

FIGURE 8j-2. (**A–C**) Management of tumors involving the renal vein with and without extension to the IVC. (Reproduced with permission from Hinman et al., 1998.)

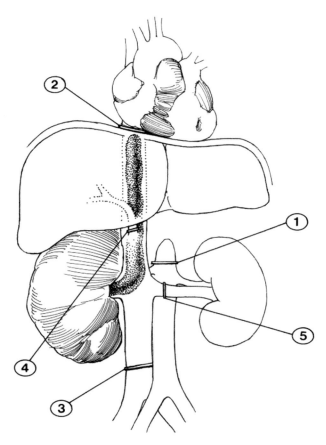

FIGURE 8j-3. Intrahepatic/suprahepatic RCC: order of clamping for right-sided tumors (1–5). (Reproduced with permission from Hinman et al., 1998.)

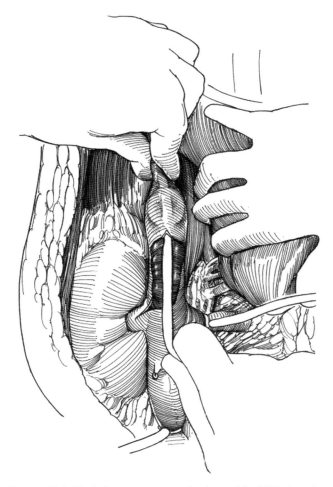

FIGURE 8j-4. Technique to manage freely mobile IVC thrombus. (Reproduced with permission from Hinman et al., 1998.)

ischemic insult, neurological insult, and coagulopathy. A series by Novick and colleagues detailing 43 patients undergoing deep hypothermic arrest demonstrated that this approach was safe and effective with no ischemic neurological complications or perioperative tumor embolization events (Novick et al., 1990).

Operative Complications

Perioperative complications can include injury to the spleen, pancreas, liver, and gastrointestinal system from contiguous tumor spread or unintended injury. Splenic injuries may require splenectomy, and injury to the pancreas, usually at the tail during resection of left-sided tumors, can be managed by partial resection. Hepatic tears can often be managed by application of hemostatic agents or sutures. If a gastrointestinal injury is suspected, the small and large bowel should be repaired appropriately. Chest tubes should be used for flank incisions that enter the thoracic space, and the pleural closure should be tested by submersion in water to check for air bubbles prior to wound closure. Chest radiographs should also be obtained in the recovery room when the chest pleura is entered or if suspicion of pneumothorax is high (i.e.,

central line placement, difficult upper pole mass) to evaluate for chest tube placement.

Air embolism is a serious intraoperative complication that should be prevented by proper clamping and sequential removal. Early and gentle control of the cephalad vena cava should be done to prevent embolism of the tumor or clot with a high suspicion of this complication if intraoperative respiratory distress develops. If so, thoracotomy with pulmonary arteriotomy to retrieve the clot should be performed expeditiously. As mentioned earlier, transarterial embolization is often considered prior to radical nephrectomy (RNx) due to extensive vascular collateralization of the tumor. Despite the introduction of ethanol to replace gel-foam, postinfarction syndrome (fever, pain, nausea for ~36 hours) is still reported, albeit at a lower rate than noted previously (Lanigan et al., 1992; Wells et al., 1983). Inadvertent embolization of peripheral vessels or erroneous infarction of the small bowel and other surrounding organs is a rare but feared complication that urologist should be cognizant of following embolization (Lammer et al., 1985).

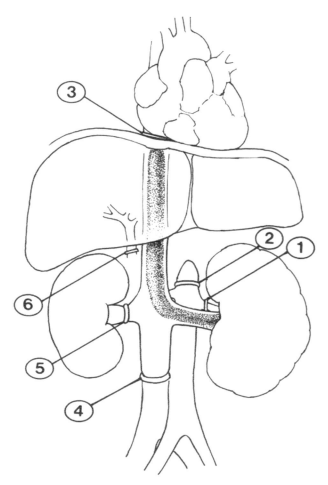

FIGURE 8j-5. Intrahepatic/suprahepatic RCC: order of clamping for left-sided tumors (1–5). (Reproduced with permission from Hinman et al., 1998.)

Massive retroperitoneal bleeding can be a troublesome complication, and an appropriate knowledge of how to manage this complication is a necessity. Initial management of massive bleeding should include direct pressure and use of additional suction devices to allow location of the bleeding source. Direct pressure will also allow the anesthesiologist to stabilize the patient. Severe venous bleeding from lumbar veins (that can shear from aggressive traction on the vena cava or renal vein) and from injuries to the short right adrenal vein and right gonadal vein can be avoided by an understanding of their propensity to bleed when injury occurs. The short lumbar vein can often retract into the psoas muscle after avulsion and become difficult to locate or control. Figure-of-eight sutures into the psoas muscle overlying the suspected shorn lumbar vein can be attempted in this circumstance. Placement of a vascular clamp should be used to control any tears in the vena cava or renal vein with appropriate suturing to close the defect.

Postoperative complications to be considered include acute renal insufficiency, deep venous thrombosis, and/or

pulmonary embolism, atelectasis with possible nosocomial pneumonia, and bleeding. Renal insufficiency usually results from venous ligation and should improve as collaterals develop. Due to poor right renal vein collaterals, ligation of the right renal vein can lead to permanent renal failure.

Nephrectomy Options for Advanced Disease

Nephrectomy with Metastasectomy for Curative Intent

Several series have demonstrated the potential benefit for complete surgical resection of all tumor burden, including removal of both the primary renal mass as well as metastatic deposits in carefully selected patients with minimal volume metastatic RCC. Five-year survival data when nephrectomy and simultaneous or subsequent metastasectomy were performed has ranged from 16% to 69% (Table 8j-2) (Kavolius et al., 1998). In one of the largest series, Kavolius retrospectively evaluated the value of aggressive metastasectomy in 278 patients treated at the Memorial Sloan-Kettering Cancer Center from 1980 to 1993 (Kavolius et al., 1998). Of these 278 patients, 141 were treated with curative surgery (curative resection defined as resection of all gross tumor), 70 patients underwent noncurative surgery, and 67 patients were treated nonsurgically. There was a statistically significant difference in 5-year overall survival data (44% curative vs. 14% noncurative) after curative resection of metastasis, and there was no significant difference in survival rates if curative resection was the initial ($n = 110$; 43%) or the second ($n = 62$; 46%) or third ($n = 22$; 44%) curative resection of metastasis. Favorable predictors of survival were a disease-free interval > 12 months after nephrectomy, solitary presentation of metastasis, metachronous presentation of recurrence, and curative resection of the first metastasis. Unfortunately, solitary presentation of metastatic RCC is uncommon and comprises only 2–5% of all patients diagnosed with metastatic RCC (Novick and Campbell 2002). The survival advantage for solitary versus multiple metastasis at the time of metastasectomy has been corroborated by additional studies (Swanson, 2004; O'Dea et al., 1978); however, a study of metastasectomy in 101 Dutch patients by van der Poel did not find an advantage for resection of solitary metastasis when compared to those with nonsolitary metastases (van der Poel et al., 1999). Concerning the location of the metastasis, Kavolius and colleagues demonstrated that a solitary pulmonary presentation was most favorable with a 54% 5-year survival compared to a 44% 5-year survival for the group as a whole (Kavolius et al., 1998). These data are consistent with other studies, which also found the pulmonary-only location to fare best when metastasectomy was performed (Kierney et al., 1994; Tolia and Whitmore, 1975; van der

TABLE 8j-2. Five-year survival of patients with metastatic renal cell carcinoma after metastasectomy.

Reference	Number of patients	5-year survival (%)
Middleton (1967)	59	34
Skinner et al. (1971)	41	29
Tolia and Whitmore (1975)	17	35
Klugo et al. (1977)	10	50
O'Dea et al. (1978)	44	16
deKernion et al. (1978)	20	25
McNichols et al. (1981)	13	69
Jett et al. (1983)	44	27
Dernevik et al. (1985)	33	21
Kierney et al. (1994)	36	31
Kavolius et al. (1998)	141	44

Source: Adapted from Kavolius et al. (1998).

Poel et al., 1999). A total of 179 patients with apparent solitary lesions were treated surgically at the M.D. Anderson Cancer Center, and the survival outcomes based upon location were reported (Swanson, 2004). As expected, pulmonary metastases were most favorable; however, it is important to understand the data for survival at other sites. Five-year survival rates were as follows: 56% pulmonary, 28% skin, 20% visceral organs, 18% appendicular bone, 13% brain, and 9% for axial bones.

When dealing with multiple metastases, surgery should be considered in select scenarios. High nuclear grade (especially tumors with sarcomatoid features), synchronous metastasis, a short disease-free interval after nephrectomy (< 12 months), poor performance status, and involvement of multiple organs with metastasis portend a more dismal prognosis (deKernion et al., 1978; Skinner et al., 1971). Consequently, urologists should perform careful selection of patients with multiple RCC metastases.

Adrenal

Ipsilateral adrenalectomy at the time of radical nephrectomy (RNx) has been a controversial topic for organ-confined RCC. However, most would agree that concomitant adrenalectomy during RNx for locally advanced or metastatic RCC is less controversial due to the risk of adrenal involvement and the poor overall prognosis for locally advanced or metastatic RCC despite concomitant adrenalectomy. Adrenal metastasis from the kidney may be due to either direct invasion from the primary renal tumor or hematogenous spread. Recently three large series, in which RNx and ipsilateral adrenalectomy were performed for pT1–pT4 RCC, found the incidence of adrenal involvement to be 3.1–7.1% (Moudouni et al., 2003; Paul et al., 2001; Siemer et al., 2004). In the study by Siemer, 1635 patients with pT1–pT4 RCC underwent RNx and ipsilateral adrenalectomy ($n=1010$) or RNx alone ($n=635$). Both groups contained an equal number of patients with nodal and metastatic disease (9.4%, 14.5% in the RNx + adrenalectomy group vs. 9.1%, 13.6% in the RNx alone group). In this study,

although adrenalectomy was chosen independent of preoperative criteria, cancer-specific survival rates were similar (75% vs. 73% for adrenalectomy vs. no adrenalectomy). In this series, more than two-thirds of the adrenal metastatic tumors were associated with either stage ≥pT3a disease and/or multifocal renal tumors. Interestingly, the false-negative rate for radiological detection of adrenal tumors was 23.3%, with all of these tumors > 4 cm in size. Given these results, the authors concluded that ipsilateral adrenalectomy should be offered for renal tumors > 4 cm or locally advanced RCC (≥ pT3 stage). This suggestion is in concordance with the other series referenced above, which also found renal tumor size and stage to be important criteria to assess for ipsilateral adrenalectomy. In addition, 5-year survival rates were better for solitary adrenal tumors than multiple metastatic tumors (61% vs. 19.6%, $p < 0.05$). Renal vein involvement was not assessed in this study, and no significance for adrenal involvement was noted when intrarenal tumor location was stratified (19.6% upper, 14.2% middle, and 17.9% lower pole tumors with adrenal metastasis).

In a similar study, 511 patients at the University of California–Los Angeles (UCLA) underwent RNx and ipsilateral adrenalectomy and were studied for possible prognostic indicators for adrenal involvement (Tsui et al., 2000). A larger percentage of this cohort had locally advanced RCC (68%) compared to the above studies, and additional prognostic factors predicting adrenal involvement were presented. In contrast to Siemer and colleagues, the UCLA group found an association between upper pole location and local adrenal invasion (58.4% of adrenal involvement), while middle and lower pole renal tumors involved the adrenal less often (4% and 7%, respectively). Although the numbers were small, there was a higher preponderance for renal vein thrombus involvement for left-sided adrenal metastasis (8/12 left and 2/9 right), which could be related to the common drainage of the left adrenal gland into the left renal vein. The authors concluded that upper pole and multifocal renal tumors, high clinical stage, and renal vein involvement should lead clinicians to perform ipsilateral adrenalectomy, even if preoperative CT scans do not demonstrate adrenal involvement.

Contralateral adrenal involvement by RCC is a more unusual phenomenon than ipsilateral involvement, and far fewer cases have been reported in the literature. The reported incidence in one autopsy study of 424 patients found an incidence of 0.7% (Saitoh et al., 1982). A recent study found only 56 cases in the literature of contralateral adrenal metastasis (Lau et al., 2003). There was an equal presentation of synchronous ($n=24$) and metachronous ($n=32$) presentations, and neither mode of presentation had an impact on cancer survival. The longest reported interval from primary RNx to detection was 23 years (range 0.3–14.3 years). The fact that adrenal lesions can be functionally and anatomically silent may contribute to latent presentation. The etiology of contralateral adrenal involvement is puzzling;

however, one theory is that the adrenal tissue may have a particular susceptibility to circulating renal cancer cells. After diagnosis of the adrenal lesion, the diagnostic strategy can be challenging. Consideration of a possible primary adrenal carcinoma, adrenal cortical adenoma, or metastasis from another location should be considered. A common distinction between RCC metastasis and other adrenal tumors or adenomas is their hypervascularity, which could prove helpful for radiographic studies with intravenous contrast; however, this particular characteristic can also make CT-guided needle biopsy challenging and morbid. Consequently, surgical excision and histopathological analysis are the most accurate means of diagnosis.

In summary, isolated adrenal metastasis fares better than adrenal metastasis with multiple concomitant metastasis; however, solitary adrenal lesions are uncommon. Pending the patient's performance status, surgical excision should be performed since these patients with complete excision will have longer survival. Lastly, an upper pole lesion, multiple intrarenal tumors, advanced clinical TNM stage, and renal vein involvement should lead clinicians to perform ipsilateral adrenalectomy when RNx is performed even if preoperative imaging is inconclusive.

Bone

From two large studies involving advanced RCC, osseous metastasis was present in 19–26% of patients with metastasis. Among those with solitary metastasis, an osseous lesion was present in only 5.3% (Kavolius et al., 1998; Motzer et al., 1999). Osseous metastasis can be especially debilitating due to the chance of pathologialc fracture, intractable pain, impaired mobility, nerve root compression, and hypercalcemia. In addition, the hypervascular nature of osseous lesions necessitates preoperative angiography or embolization to reduce morbidity. Treatment can be either curative (wide local excision) or palliative (marginal excision), with most palliative procedures performed for pain control or impending pathological fracture. Radiation therapy is another means to achieve palliation; however, it does not have an impact on survival. Chemotherapy has traditionally had no role in the management of osseous lesions from RCC (Kollender et al., 2000).

Although most reports of osseous metastasis are small, prognostic factors for enhanced survival have been proposed. A report from the Massachusetts General Hospital with 54 patients is notable for having follow-up data 10 years after surgery (Althausen et al., 1997). A long disease-free interval from RNx to first metastasis ($p < 0.0007$) and appendicular (vs. axial) location ($p < 0.008$) significantly correlated with enhanced survival. As expected, solitary metastasis, despite its low incidence, was another important prognostic factor. The 5- and 10-year survival outcomes were 55% and 39%, which are notably higher than other reports, which have reported 5-year survival between 0% and 13% (deKernion

et al., 1978; Middleton , 1967; Skinner et al., 1971). Selection bias and the utilization of aggressive surgical excision in a favorable patient cohort likely are likely related to longer survival.

Brain

Brain metastasis from RCC has been reported to occur between 4% and 17%, with treatment options consisting of surgical resection, stereotactic radiosurgery, whole-brain radiation, and symptomatic medical management with corticosteroids (Sheehan et al., 2003). In a report of 709 patients with brain metastasis, renal cell lesions comprised 50 (7%) of the histological lesions (Wronski et al., 1996). In this retrospective study of 50 patients with RCC brain metastasis, patients lived an average of 12.6 months after craniotomy. The majority of patients (47/50) presented symptomatically with headache, neurological deficit, or seizure. The tumors also generally presented in a metachronous fashion (40/50 patients) at a median of 17 months after diagnosis of the primary renal tumor; however, no difference in survival was noticed when compared to synchronous presentation. Important prognostic factors predicting improved survival were a supratentorial location of the lesion and lack of neurological deficit prior to craniotomy.

Radiosurgery has gained appeal for the treatment of RCC brain lesions due to the well-demarcated shape on CT/MRI, thus making the procedure amenable. Furthermore, the low morbidity and the ability to treat one or multiple brain lesions in one session are attractive. Survival rates have not matched the outcomes of craniotomy. In a review of 69 patients undergoing gamma knife radiosurgery, survival after the procedure was only 6 months (Sheehan et al., 2003). Seven patients received adjuvant fractionated radiation as boost therapy; however, there was no advantage in survival. Whole brain radiation therapy (WBRT) for metastatic RCC has typically been reserved for patients with unresectable brain lesions, multiple lesions, or patients who are not surgical candidates secondary to poor performance status. In a series of 119 patients receiving WBRT for RCC lesions of the brain, the overall median survival was poor at 4.4 months (Wronski et al., 1997). The larger number of patients in this retrospective study allowed evaluation of solitary vs. multiple metastasis outcomes and found only a 2-month advantage for solitary lesions (multiple lesions 3.0 months; solitary lesion 4.4 months). A lack of distant metastasis and tumor diameter < 2 cm were also significant prognostic parameters ($p < 0.05$). In conclusion, despite outcomes inferior to craniotomy, WBRT and gamma knife radiosurgery can provide palliation of neurological symptoms, even for patients not suitable for craniotomy.

Liver

Experience in the management of RCC lesions metastasized to the liver is limited when compared to other cancers that invade the liver, such as breast and colorectal carcinoma. In one series of 607 patients with reported hepatic metastases, renal metastases were found in 19% of patients (Motzer et al., 1999). The prognosis of hepatic metastasis is poor, with most patients having multiple concomitant sites of involvement by RCC. Most series reporting on RCC lesions in the liver are underpowered, preventing definitive conclusions in regard to prognostic factors for survival. In one of the largest series of hepatic metastasis in RCC patients, 10 patients were retrospectively reviewed (Alves et al., 2003). Eight of these patients had curative metastatic resections performed. Of the remaining two, one had positive margins on final pathological analysis and the other had a pulmonary metastasis that was resected the following month. Most lesions were detected metachronously (8/10) and all were asymptomatic with the lesions found on cancer surveillance imaging. Two-year survival rates were 56% with a median survival of 26 months. Unfortunately, the majority of the patients developed additional metastasis after the hepatic resection either in the liver or at other sites. As with brain, bone, and adrenal lesions, a longer disease-free interval from primary RNx (> 24 months) was associated with better outcomes; however, size < 50 mm was also significantly correlated with survival. In this series there was no mortality at 60 days postoperatively, yet another series reported a 31% (4/13 patients) perioperative mortality rate emphasizing the potential gravity of the operation (Stief et al., 1997). In spite of this, resection of hepatic metastases should be considered since long-term survival is a possibility. Indeed, 4 of the 10 patients in the former study were alive at 6, 18, 26, and 96 months after hepatic resection.

Other Sites

Renal cell carcinoma can metastasize to other areas of the body; however, this occurs at lower incidence than the sites described above. Pancreatic, esophageal, splenic, thyroid, and other sites have been detailed in the literature primarily as isolated case reports (Andoh et al., 2004; de los Monteros-Sanchez et al., 2004; Piardi et al., 1999; Sahin et al., 1998). Despite the small number of cases for each involved site, basic tenants of surgical management of RCC apply. These reports all stress that surgery for isolated metastasis consistently allows better survival over surgery in the face of multiple metastases. However, it is the responsibility of the surgeon to incorporate performance status, surgical morbidity, metastatic location, and the individual patient's history into the decision for surgery.

Cytoreductive Nephrectomy

Providing a detailed account of the current status and history of immunotherapy is not the aim of this chapter and will be covered elsewhere in this book; however, a brief overview will be provided to stress the importance of today's approach toward tumor immunobiology. Unlike conventional chemotherapy, immunotherapy is more specific for targeting malignant cells over normal dividing cells thus allowing more efficient tumor cell death.

The immune system is composed of the innate and adoptive immune system. Innate immunity includes macrophages, granulocytes, mast cells, and natural killer cells. These cells function to initiate inflammatory responses in order to initiate and sustain the adaptive immune system. The adaptive immune system is composed of B lymphocytes (humoral immunity) and T lymphocytes (cell mediated immunity). Upon stimulation, B lymphocytes become plasma cells and release antibodies. These antibodies function either to make antigens more readily able to be phagocytosed (also known as opsonization) or stimulate natural killer (NK) cells for antibody-dependent cell cytotoxicity. T helper CD4 cells and cytotoxic CD8 cells comprise the T lymphocytes. T lymphocytes are unlike B lymphocytes in that they are not able to be activated by direct contact with the antigen; instead the antigen must be presented to T cells in the form of a major histocompatibility complex (MHC). The MHC consists of class I [located on all nucleated cells except the testis and select central nervous system (CNS) neurons] and class II (processed antigens presented by antigen-presenting cells) antigens. An example of antigen presenting cells (APCs) is the dendritic cell (DC), which presents class II antigens to T cells. DCs are present throughout the body and stimulate primary antigen-dependent T cell responses by presenting the class II antigens to T cells. They derive their potency from the expression of co-stimulatory and adhesion molecules necessary for activation of naive T cells (Avigan, 2004).

Tumor cells possess specific antigens on their cell surface that can be recognized by the body's immune system. Cytotoxic T cells attack cancerous cells that possess class I antigens not recognized as "self" by the immune system. In addition, T helper cells recognize class II antigens from antigen-presenting cells (macrophages, dendritic cells, etc.) in order to augment cytotoxic T cells (via stimulatory cytokines) and the humoral immune system (stimulate production of additional antibodies directed against the particular antigen). Proinflammatory cytokines (tumor necrosis factor, interleukin, etc.) are released at the site of initial inflammation that ensues from cell killing of cancerous (foreign) cells, and these cytokines drive the APCs to further stimulate antibody production by the humoral system and can present the antigen via the MHC to T cells. For the T cells to become activated, stimulatory cytokines [IL, IFN, tumor necrosis factor (TNF), etc.] and the MHC complex must be present. From this knowledge of the numerous steps involved in the immune system, scientists have been able to target multiple pathways to kill cancer cells.

The introduction of IFN therapy was a medical breakthrough in immunotherapy, and it was the first immunobiological to be tested with cytoreductive nephrectomy in a prospective, randomized fashion Flanigan et al., 2001;

Mickisch et al., 2001). IFN functions to initiate a sequence of intracellular events after cell binding, which can lead to inhibition of replication in cancerous cells, suppression of cellular proliferation, and other immunomodulatory effects. The latter effects may encompass enhancement of NK cell activity, antibody-dependent cell cytotoxicity, or upregulation of MHC presentation to T lymphocytes. All of these efforts contribute to the antineoplastic effects of IFN-α. Monotherapy trials of IFN-α, using a variety of dosing schedules, have yielded response rates from 10% to 20% with a small number of patients attaining long-term survival (Minasian et al., 1993; Medical Research Council Renal Cell Collaborators, 1999).

IL-2 is a glycoprotein that is produced by a class of mature CD4 T helper cells. IL-2 binds to its receptor on T helper cells to promote clonal expansion and potentiate the activity of cytotoxic T cells. FDA approval for treatment of patients with metastatic RCC was based upon early trials using high-dose IL-2 (Fyfe et al., 1995). In this study, 254 patients with metastatic RCC were evaluated with high-dose IL-2. An overall objective response rate of 14% (5% CR; 9% PR) was achieved with an impressive median response duration of 19 months. Due to the morbidity and supportive care associated with the high-dose IL-2 regimen, lower doses of IL-2 have also been evaluated.

The National Cancer Institute completed a three-arm randomized study in 2003 to compare response rates and overall survival in metastatic RCC patients receiving high-dose intravenous (IV) IL-2, low-dose IV IL-2, and low-dose subcutaneous IL-2 (Yang et al., 2003). A median follow-up of 7.4 years was achieved in 400 patients. The treatment cohort was healthy with 85% performance status zero, and 98% had received prior nephrectomy. In regard to toxicity, across all three arms there were no IL-2-related deaths. A higher response rate was noted with high-dose IL-2 (21%) over low-dose IV IL-2 (13%, $p = 0.048$), but there was no detectable survival difference. Despite this, response durability and survival in CR patients receiving high-dose IL-2 were better

than low-dose IV IL-2 ($p = 0.04$). The response rate of subcutaneous IL-2 was similar to low-dose IV IL-2.

Recently the Cytokine Working Group in 2005 reported a prospective, randomized phase III trial comparing outpatient IL-2 and IFN-α2b relative to high-dose IL-2 in patients with metastatic RCC (McDermott et al., 2005). A significant difference in overall response rate was found for high-dose IL-2 delivery ($p = 0.018$), with a 23.2% overall response rate for high-dose IL-2 (22/95 patients) versus 9.9% for IL-2/IFN-α2b (9/91 patients). This is the first study to have shown a benefit of IL-2 with the primary tumor still in place; however, the benefit was found only in the high-dose IV IL-2 regimen. Outpatient IL-2/ IFN-α2b was essentially inactive in patients with metastatic RCC. Although no specific etiology has been found, it is likely that higher serum levels of IL-2 are needed to overcome the immune suppression associated with the primary tumor burden, and the implications seem to insinuate that the primary tumor can act to block the effectiveness of certain immunotherapy options or doses.

Retrospective reports have detailed the experience with cytoreductive nephrectomy as summarized in Table 8j-3. The largest retrospective series from the NCI included 195 patients treated with cytoreductive nephrectomy in preparation for IL-2 monotherapy (Walther et al., 1997). Of the 195 patients undergoing surgery, 45 (23%) had significant additional tumor resection besides nephrectomy. The overall response rate was 18%, which included a 4% complete response and 14% partial response rate. Unfortunately, 38% of the patients were unable to receive systemic immunotherapy due to rapid tumor progression, postoperative complications, or debilitated state. Although performance status was not provided in this study, patients were screened for absence of cardiac and renal disease, minimal pulmonary and/or hepatic dysfunction, and brain metastasis. Other smaller series have reported varying response rates (Table 8j-3). Variability in patient selection, particularly the distribution of patients with good versus poor performance status, limited versus extensive metastasis, and long versus short metastasis-free intervals probably account

TABLE 8j-3. Cytoreductive nephrectomy in preparation for immunotherapy: retrospective studies.[a]

Reference	Number of patients	Surgical mortality (%)	Unable to receive postoperative BMR therapy (%)	Overall response (%)[b]	CR (%)	PR (%)
Rackley et al. (1994)	37	1 (2.7)	8 (21.6)	3 (8.1)	0 (0.0)	3 (8.1)
Wolf et al. (1994)	23	0 (0.0)	6 (26.1)	3 (13.0)	2 (8.7)	1 (4.3)
Bennett et al. (1995)	30	5 (17)	23 (76.6)	4 (13.3)	3 (10.0)	1 (3.3)
Fallick et al. (1997)	28	1 (3.6)	2 (7.1)	11 (39.3)	5 (17.9)	6 (21.4)
Walther et al. (1997)	195	2 (1.0)	74 (37.9)	19 (17.8)	4 (3.7)	15 (14.0)
Figlin et al. (1997)	62	0 (0.0)	7 (11.3)	19 (34.5)	5 (9.1)	14 (25.5)
Levy et al. (1998)	66	2 (3.0)	12 (18.1)	–	–	–
Total[b]	441	11/441 (2.5)	132/441 (29.9)	59/375 (15.7)	19/375 (5.1)	40/375 (10.7)

Source: Adapted from Hafez and Montie (2004).

[a]BMR, biologic response modifier; CR, complete response; PR, partial response.

[b]Values as reported in each study. The calculations, however, are not always based upon intent-to-treat analysis and may be overestimations of true response rates.

for these varied results. In addition, some of these series calculated their response rates based on only those patients who received adjuvant immunotherapy after nephrectomy, effectively overestimating response rates. An intent-to-treat analysis would have been a more accurate reflection of the true response rate to therapy in these series.

As discussed above, one of the major concerns about cytoreductive nephrectomy is the risk of postoperative morbidity that could delay or prevent systemic therapy. The incidence of this phenomenon has ranged from 7% to 77%, with most series at the lower end of this range (Table 8j-3). Overall, 70% of patients in these series were able to proceed to systemic therapy. An important consideration is patient selection, which contributes to the variable results reported in these studies. Poor patient selection is particularly evident in the Bennett series, in which almost one-third of the patients had brain metastases, 43% had osseous lesions, 37% had hepatic metastases, and performance status was suboptimal or poor in a high percentage of patients (Bennett et al., 1995). Perioperative mortality is another concern about cytoreductive nephrectomy. In the collective series from Table 8j-3, a perioperative mortality rate of 2.5% was reported.

In an effort to reduce the perioperative morbidity and mortality associated with cytoreductive nephrectomy, Finelli and Walther designed two separate studies to investigate the use of minimally invasive techniques for cytoreductive nephrectomy (Finelli et al., 2004; Walther et al., 1999). In the study by Walther and colleagues, three treatment groups were compared: open nephrectomy, laparoscopic-assisted nephrectomy (surgery performed laparoscopically with a small incision made to finish the dissection and deliver the specimen intact), and pure laparoscopic nephrectomy with tissue morcellation (Walther et al., 1999). For open surgery, a median of 67 days elapsed before IL-2 was administered (range 50–151 days), whereas laparoscopic-assisted patients took a median of 60 days (range 47–63). The group that appeared to benefit most were those who had undergone pure laparoscopic surgery with tissue morcellation, as this group proceeded to systemic therapy within a median of 37 days (range 34–57 days). Minimally invasive surgery was performed with morbidity that was comparable to the traditional open approach and tumor morcellation was feasible even for large tumors. The authors concluded that laparoscopy offered a number of distinct advantages for cytoreduction in preparation for systemic therapy. In the study from the Cleveland Clinic by Finelli, laparoscopic nephrectomy with removal of the specimen through a muscle-splitting low Gibson or Pfannenstiel incision was associated with a median time to systemic therapy of 35 days (range 13–136 days) (Finelli et al., 2004). The extraction site used by Walther was subcostal, which differed from the site used in the later study by Finelli. The difference in extraction site by Walther may have been associated with prolonged time to receiving immunotherapy; however, this is strictly speculative. The median tumor size was similar in the two studies (Finelli = 8 cm; Walther = 9 cm).

In a follow-up study, Paulter and Walther reported on 31 attempted laparoscopic cytoreductive procedures at their institution (Pautler et al., 2001). Eleven cases required conversion to open nephrectomy, and blood loss was relatively high (750–3000 ml), especially when compared to other minimally invasive procedures. In addition, only 18 patients (58%) were eligible to proceed to immunotherapy postoperatively. When compared to the two studies above, blood loss was similar to a compared cohort of open nephrectomy (285 ml laparoscopic vs. 308 ml open); however, a smaller number of patients (8/22, 38%) went on to receive immunotherapy. Local invasion, obliteration of tissue planes, and enhanced neovascularity increase the potential morbidity of this procedure. Many centers still prefer to counsel these patients toward open surgery. A hand-assisted approach to minimally invasive cytoreductive nephrectomy would appear to be a reasonable alternative; however, there is a paucity of data in regards to this option.

Given the inconclusive data about cytoreductive nephrectomy and concerns about selection bias, a carefully designed and properly randomized and prospective trial was needed to determine the validity of this approach to metastatic RCC. The Southwest Oncology Group (SWOG) and European Organization for the Research and Treatment of Cancer (EORTC) completed trials in 2001 in which patients with advanced RCC were randomized to cytoreductive nephrectomy followed by systemic Intron A (IFN-α2b) therapy versus Intron A therapy alone (Flanigan et al., 2001; Mickisch et al., 2001). In SWOG trial 8949, a total of 246 patients were enrolled and 21 were declared ineligible primarily due to incorrect interpretation of the pathology or inadequate documentation at presentation (Flanigan et al., 2001). Fourteen of the 120 patients randomized to the nephrectomy plus IFN arm did not undergo surgery, and one of 121 patients randomized to the interferon only arm refused treatment. Analysis was based upon intent to treat (Table 8j-4). Overall, the survival advantage for the nephrectomy plus interferon arm (median survival 11.1 months RNx + IFN vs. 8.1 months IFN alone) was approximately 50%, and this persisted across all of the prestudy stratification points including performance status (0 versus 1), site of metastasis (pulmonary only versus other), and measurable disease (present versus absent). The study also demonstrated minimal surgical morbidity (two cardiac events, two infections, and one patient with hypotension, while 79.2% had no perioperative complications), and the combined operative and perioperative mortality was only 1%. Nearly all patients (98%) were able to proceed from nephrectomy to interferon therapy with a mean time of 19.9 days. Patients with good performance status were most likely to benefit from cytoreductive nephrectomy with a median survival of 17.4 months compared to 12.8 months in the interferon alone group. In the nephrectomy arm there were only three partial responders, and in the interferon arm there were two partial responders and one complete responder. Despite these disappointing

TABLE 8j-4. Survival analysis of nephrectomy followed by IFN-α2b versus IFN-α2b alone.[a]

Category	Median survival (months)		1-year survival (%)		p-value[b]
	IFN alone	Nx + IFN	IFN alone	Nx + IFN	
Not stratified	8.1	11.1	36.8	49.7	0.012
Stratification factor					
Measurable disease					0.010
Yes	7.8	10.3	34.7	46.6	
No	11.2	16.4	43.1	63.6	
Performance status[c]					0.080
0	11.7	17.4	49.2	63.6	
1	4.8	6.9	28.2	32.5	
Type of metastases					0.008
Lung only	10.3	14.3	41.5	58.5	
Other	6.3	10.2	34.6	45.1	

Source: Adapted from Flanigan et al., (2001).
[a] Nx, nephrectomy; IFN, interferon.
[b] p-values for the comparison of median survival between groups were derived with the log-rank test.
[c] Performance was scored as 0 or 1 indicating decreased activity.

numbers, a clear-cut survival advantage has been demonstrated for cytoreductive nephrectomy within the context of interferon-based systemic immunotherapy.

The EORTC study (EORTC 30947), which was designed using an identical format, demonstrated similar findings, although a few findings were unique and interesting (Mickisch et al., 2001). A smaller number of patients was included with 42 in the cytoreduction arm and 43 in the interferon alone arm. Eighty-five percent of the patients undergoing nephrectomy experienced no perioperative complications, and 40 of 41 patients were able to proceed to systemic immunotherapy. There were five complete responders in the nephrectomy arm compared to only one in the interferon only arm, while partial responders and patients with stable disease were similarly distributed between treatment arms. The time to progression and duration of survival were both in favor of the cytoreductive nephrectomy group. The median survival shifted from 7 months in the interferon alone arm to 17 months in the cytoreductive nephrectomy arm. The results in favor of cytoreductive nephrectomy were more impressive than in the SWOG trial. The congruence of results between these two independent trials supports the basic conclusions of these studies and has provided valuable information about cytoreductive nephrectomy.

In 2003, a combined analysis of the pooled data from SWOG 8949 and EORTC 30947 was published (Flanigan et al., 2004). A total of 331 patients were included with a median survival of 13.6 months for nephrectomy plus INF-α2b vs. 7.8 months for INF-α2b alone ($p = 0.002$). A 31% decrease in the risk of death was noted, and similar to each individual study, no significant response rate was noted for INF-α2b with or without prior nephrectomy (6.9% nephrectomy plus INF-α2b vs. 5.7% INF-α2b alone). In the combined study, only 5.6% did not proceed to immunotherapy, and the median time to initiation of INF-

α2b therapy was 19 days. Despite the impressive findings of the above two studies, the results must be understood in their correct context. There were no differences in the response rates to INF-α2b in either study (EORTC: 12% for INF-α2b alone and 19% for surgery plus INF-α2b; SWOG: 3.6% for INF-α2b alone and 3.3% for surgery plus INF-α2b).

Criticisms of the SWOG and EORTC trials include the following. The SWOG 8949 trial also took 7 years to complete in a multicenter fashion (up to 80 centers) to accrue 246 patients. Although randomized, the slow recruitment of patients raises concern of possible selection bias and whether the results can compare to the generalized population with advanced RCC (Cooney et al., 2004). In addition, when comparing the performance status of patients in the SWOG 8949 trial, there was a higher proportion of patients with a PS 1 in the INF-α2b alone group vs. the nephrectomy plus INF-α2b group (58.1% in INF-α2b vs. 45% in the nephrectomy plus INF-α2b group, $p = 0.04$). This may have implications for the survival benefit demonstrated in the cytoreductive nephrectomy group. Finally, quality of life data were not recorded in either study, which would have been important given the primary aim of survival benefits of aggressive surgery prior to immunotherapy. Regardless of the criticisms, both studies were crucial in determining whether a survival benefit is achievable in select patients with advanced RCC when cytoreductive nephrectomy is performed prior to immunotherapy.

While a survival benefit was apparent in both the SWOG and EORTC trials, some have questioned whether the survival might have been better if a different immunotherapeutic drug was used. This argument stems from the poor overall response seen with IFN-α2b. Based upon this concern, Pantuck identified 89 patients (out of 450 patients with a history of cytoreductive nephrectomy) who met the SWOG 8949 entrance criteria in the University of California–

Los Angeles (UCLA) department kidney database (Pantuck et al., 2001). The major difference was that IL-2 was used as the immunotherapeutic agent as opposed to IFN-α2b. The median survival for the surgery plus IL-2 arm was 16.7 months compared to 11.1 months in the RNx plus IFN-α2b arm of the SWOG trial. Although the UCLA data are retrospective and comparison to the SWOG trial is historical, the UCLA results support the prospective data favoring cytoreductive nephrectomy. Clearly, more work needs to be done in an effort to widen the inclusion criteria for patients with advanced RCC who could benefit from multimodality therapy.

While the above trials support cytoreductive nephrectomy as a valid option for the management of advanced RCC, physicians should be reminded that selection criteria must be enforced. Slaton reported that patients with metastatic RCC involving multiple organs, particularly the liver, spine, or brain, are at high risk for dying in the first 6 months after cytoreductive nephrectomy and are less likely to achieve palliation after surgery (Slaton et al., 2000). Wood and colleagues found that high grade tumors, particularly sarcomatoid variants, have a poor prognosis after cytoreductive nephrectomy and have suggested tumor biopsy as an adjunct prior to surgery (Wood et al., 2001). They also reported that patients with an elevated white blood cell count, which may be reflective of a paraneoplastic phenomenon, or an abnormal partial prothrombin time (PTT), which may reflect hepatic involvement or dysfunction, are less likely to benefit from cytoreductive nephrectomy. Based upon their experience, Fallick proposed the following criteria for cytoreductive nephrectomy: (1) the ability to perform > 75% debulking, (2) no CNS, bone, or liver metastasis, 3) adequate pulmonary and cardiac reserve, (4) an ECOG performance status of 0 or 1, and (5) predominant clear cell histology (Fallick et al., 1997). These criteria should be interpreted as relative rather that absolute contraindications due to the controversial nature of each. However, these recommendations are in accord with the SWOG 8949 trial, which demonstrated that relatively healthy patients with good performance status, and preferably with pulmonary only metastases, are the most likely to benefit from cytoreductive nephrectomy (Flanigan et al., 2001). As always, patient selection is the key component to the management of this group of patients.

Nephrectomy or Metastasectomy to Consolidate Therapy after Systemic Immunotherapy

Another approach to tumor cytoreduction is to reserve surgery for those who have demonstrated a favorable response to systemic therapy at their metastatic foci (Bex et al., 2002;Rackley et al., 1994; Sella et al., 1993). Proponents of this theory assert that a proportion of patients will be eliminated from receiving immunotherapy due to rapid disease progression, perioperative morbidity, and surgical mortality after initial cytoreductive nephrectomy.

Delay in initiation of immunotherapy during the perioperative recovery period and impairment of immunity from surgical stress have also been discussed as drawbacks to initial nephrectomy (Ben-Eliyahu et al., 1999; Ben-Eliyahu 2003; Eggermont et al., 1987). On the other hand, with the primary tumor removed, cell-mediated immunity should have an improved ability to eliminate residual metastatic disease, and additional immune cells should be available to interact with metastatic tumor cells. However, despite this postnephrectomy advantage, surgical stress can temporarily hamper the immune system and render the patient vulnerable to further metastasis, thus delaying or reducing the benefit of surgery prior to immunotherapy.

The phenomenon of rapid tumor progression at metastatic sites following removal of the primary tumor has been reported in up to 33% of cases and is yet another argument for initial immunotherapy rather than surgery (Bennett et al., 1995; Walther et al., 1993). General anesthesia, blood transfusions, open surgery, hypothermia, tissue damage, pain, and perioperative stress have been implicated in promoting immunosuppression during the perioperative period (Ben-Eliyahu 2003). As discussed previously, cytokines are cell messenger proteins released by immune cells as a means to regulate cell communication among the various immune system cells. As such, they regulate the production of other cytokines that function to augment or attenuate the inflammatory response. With surgery, a surge in proinflammatory cytokines (TNF-a, IL-1, IL-6, IL-8) may impair cell-mediated immunity (Lin et al., 2000). Research in mice has shown this effect to be temporary, lasting up to 2 weeks following surgery and resolved by 1 month (Eggermont et al., 1987).

One of the early reports of systemic immunotherapy followed by consolidative surgery was by Fleischmann, who reported on a small group of patients managed in this manner (Fleischmann and Kim 1991). This study group consisted of 10 patients with advanced RCC treated with IL-2 immunotherapy, of whom three had complete regression of disease outside the abdomen. Two of the latter were rendered disease free after surgical excision of the renal primary or a retroperitoneal recurrence, and these patients remained disease free for 9 and 18 months after surgery, respectively. This small study, which was published in 1991, has since served as a prototype for this approach to the management of patients with metastatic RCC.

Other studies have not demonstrated such favorable responses in patients treated with immunotherapy first. In 51 patients with metastatic RCC treated at the National Cancer Institute (NCI)with various immunotherapy regimens, including IL-2 and IFN- α, a complete response was seen in one and partial responses were seen in two at extrarenal sites, yielding an overall response rate of only 6% (Wagner et al., 1999). No responses were observed in the primary tumor itself. The three patients who demonstrated an objective response in their metastatic lesions underwent nephrectomy. Two had a combined partial response for 4 and 11 months before progression, while one patient experienced a durable complete response for more than 88 months. The median survival for the entire cohort was 13 months. This study highlights the major concerns about administering systemic immunotherapy upfront, which include (1) a lack of response in the primary tumor is a common finding in this setting and (2) overall response rates that appear to be lower than those achieved after cytoreduction. However, patient selection may confound interpretation of this study, as patients were selected for this protocol primarily based upon a predominance of disease at extrarenal sites. This group, which represented only 8.4% (51/607) of patients with metastatic RCC evaluated at the NCI during the study interval, appears to have had relatively advanced disease, with a predominance of visceral and bone metastases that may have contributed to the poor response rates in this series.

While administration of systemic therapy initially appears to have limitations, the reality is that many patients with metastatic RCC will not be reasonable candidates for cytoreductive nephrectomy and will be treated upfront with immunotherapy as dictated by their clinical status. Several recent studies suggest that surgical consolidation following immunotherapy may provide a potential benefit for a subgroup of these patients. Kim and Louie (1992) reviewed 14 separate clinical trials comprising a total of 399 patients treated with IL-2-based therapy with or without lymphokine-activated killer (LAK) cells and identified 62 patients (15.5%) with an objective response. This included 18 (4.5%) with a complete response and 44 (11%) with a partial response, 11 of whom underwent resection of residual disease within the lung, kidney, retroperitoneum, or pelvis to render them disease free. All 11 patients remained alive and without evidence of disease with a median follow-up of 21 months. Similarly, Krishnamurthi and colleagues (1998) reported on 14 patients treated with adjuvant surgery following biological response modifier therapy, nine with a partial response and five with stable disease. All were then rendered disease free by surgical excision of residual metastatic lesions and nephrectomy. Cancer-specific survival at 3 years was 82%, with seven patients (50%) alive and disease free with a mean follow-up of 41 months and three alive with recurrent disease with a mean follow-up of 48.3 months. Sella and colleagues (1993) reported similar results for surgery after INF-based therapy. They reviewed 17 patients who underwent nephrectomy and/or metastasectomy to consolidate therapy after initial immunotherapy and found cancer remaining in 15 patients (two had fibrosis only). Eleven patients remained disease free with a median follow-up of 12 months. Such retrospective studies suggest that adjuvant surgery can extend the survival of selected patients with metastatic RCC who exhibit an objective response or stabilization of disease with initial systemic therapy.

A small prospective study by Bex et al., in 2002 sought to evaluate the role of initial immunotherapy as selection for nephrectomy in patients with metastatic RCC. Sixteen patients were treated with subcutaneous IL-2 and INF-α. After the second doses, those with partial disease or stable disease underwent nephrectomy followed by two additional courses of immunotherapy. Consistent with the above referenced studies, no response was noted in the primary tumor. Of the 16, nine experienced stable disease, two had a partial response, and five had progressive disease after the first two courses of immunotherapy. All patients with progressive disease died at a median of 3 months compared to the 11.5 months (range 4–22) achieved in the cohort undergoing nephrectomy. Although no complete responses were noted after the two initial courses of immunotherapy, one patient with stable disease achieved a complete response (maintained for > 10 months). As such, Bex and colleagues presented the absence of disease progression following immunotherapy as selection criteria for nephrectomy. If validated by a randomized trial, this information would provide urologists and oncologists with information in an effort to spare select patients from unnecessary surgery.

Nephrectomy as a Component of Adoptive Immunotherapy

Nephrectomy has also been used as a vital component of adoptive immunotherapy protocols for the management of metastatic RCC. Perhaps the most encouraging initial results with these approaches came from the UCLA experience with IL-2 therapy along with tumor-infiltrating lymphocytes (TILs). In these protocols, TIL cells were harvested from the nephrectomy specimen, expanded in vitro, and reinfused along with IL-2 in an attempt to treat the remaining metastases. Many patients also received preoperative cytokines to improve the yield of TILs and in some cases CD8 cytotoxic lymphocytes were enriched to enhance responses. In 1997, Figlin and colleagues reported on 55 patients treated in this manner with an overall response rate of 34.6% (9.1% complete response and 25.5% partial response) and with a median duration of response of 14 months. Response rates were 43.5% in the 23 patients receiving CD8-enriched TILs compared to 28.2% in the remaining 32 patients who received standard TILs. There were no perioperative deaths and 89% of the patients were able to proceed to immunotherapy without significant delay. Based on these promising results, a prospective Phase III multicenter trial was initiated for patients with metastatic RCC randomized to receive either low-dose IL-2 monotherapy or combination CD8 TILs with low-dose IL-2 after nephrectomy (Figlin et al., 1999). Neither objective response rates nor 1-year survival rates were significantly different between the two groups (9.9% vs. 11.4% and 55% vs. 47%, respectively), and this trial was closed early after an interim analysis failed to demonstrate a potential advantage to TIL therapy. Difficulty in reliably preparing the CD8 TILs was encountered during this study and may have been related to the need for transport of the nephrectomy-derived specimen. When combined with concomitant patient selection issues, this may contribute to the divergent results reported in these series.

Role of Lymphadenectomy During Radical Nephrectomy

As described by Robson et al., in1969, RNx includes early ligation of the renal artery and vein, removal of the kidney outside Gerota's fascia, removal of the ipsilateral adrenal gland, and performance of a complete regional lymphadenectomy (LND) from the crus of the diaphragm to the aortic bifurcation. Despite Robson's findings, the therapeutic value of regional LND in all clinical stages of RNx is still debatable (Minervini et al., 2001; Pantuck et al., 2003a,b; Schafhauser et al., 1999). More accurate staging to allow correct surveillance and a lower risk of involved margin rate from the more extensive dissection for the LND can be beneficial for the patient. Furthermore, lymph node metastasis (N+ disease) has been shown to have a negative impact on survival, and preoperative knowledge of nodal disease can be useful for surgical planning (deKernion et al., 1978; Vasselli et al., 2001). In the preimmunotherapy era, deKernion reported on the role of nephrectomy for metastatic RCC and found that survival was decreased with the concomitant finding of positive lymph nodes (deKernion et al., 1978). Positive lymph nodes were strongly correlated with local recurrence at the renal fossa with less than 20% alive at 6 months when regional disease was not excised.

The clinical detection of lymph node metastasis correlates with an increase in lymph node size as a result of tumor infiltration; however, there is no preoperative radiographic study that can conclusively diagnose lymph node disease from RCC (Zagoria et al., 1990). Radiographic imaging to detect clinical nodal involvement is typically noted when nodal size increases to 1 cm; however, not all lymph nodes greater than 1 cm are cancerous. As shown by Studer, when 163 patients with RCC were reviewed by preoperative CT imaging, 43 were noted to have enlarged lymph nodes > 1 cm; however, pathological analysis revealed that only 18/43 (42%) of these were involved in RCC metastasis (Studer et al., 1990). These false-positive cases were attributed to inflammatory changes (i.e., from tumor necrosis) and/or follicular hyperplasia.

In an effort to increase staging accuracy at the time of radical lymphadenectomy, Terrone retrospectively evaluated the number of lymph nodes to be assessed for optimal RCC staging (Terrone et al., 2003). The extent of LND has been shown to correlate with survival in bladder and prostate cancer, but the correlation in RCC was previously unknown prior to this study (Barth et al., 1999; Leissner et al., 2000).

LND at the time of RNx was performed in 608 patients, and 13.6% were found to have N+ disease. A statistically significant association between the number of lymph nodes removed (13+) and the percentage with nodal involvement was discovered ($p < 0.01$). For locally advanced tumors, when 12 or less lymph nodes were removed, the pN+ rate was 19.7% in comparison to 32.2% pN+ when 13 or more nodes were removed.

Nonetheless, the role of LND at the time of surgery in patients with nodal disease and associated metastatic disease remains debatable. In a retrospective study to evaluate the role of LND at the time of RNx, Pantuck and colleagues at UCLA evaluated 900 patients from 1989 to 2000 who presented for surgery with a unilateral renal mass (Pantuck et al., 2003a). A preoperative radiographic work-up revealed 129/900 patients (14%) with clinically positive nodes (> 1 cm on CT or MRI scans) and 236/900 patients (26%) with distant metastasis only (N0M1). Of note, not all patients with N+ (lymph node positive) disease had concomitant metastatic disease (43/121 N+M0 vs. 86/121 N+/M1). LND was not performed during RNx in all subjects, and no standard template was employed. Despite this lack of formality, there was a statistically significant survival advantage in 112 patients with clinically positive lymph nodes who underwent LND compared to the 17 remaining patients with clinically positive nodes who did not undergo additional LND at the time of surgery ($p = 0.0002$). In general, N+ cases with associated LND were performed safely, and there was also a trend toward improved response to immunotherapy in those receiving LND with N+ disease (N+ disease plus LND = disease progression of 44%; N+ disease minus LND = disease progression of 56%; $p = 0.057$).

Additional studies support the data from Pantuck in which LND for locally advanced RCC impacts survival. Herrlinger evaluated 511 patients and divided them into 320 who underwent systematic LND vs. 191 with limited/no LND (Herrlinger et al., 1991). The operative mortality was less than 1% for systematic LND, and there was a 5-year survival benefit for pathological stage T1–3 tumors that had LND with RNx (66% vs. 58%). In a smaller study by Phillips and Messing in which 37 patients underwent RNx and later progressed, local control was also improved by LND (Phillips and Messing 1991).

Currently, there is no accepted standard template for LND at the time of RNx. Unsuspected lymph node involvement at the time of RNx is a rare phenomenon when adequate preoperative imaging has been performed; however, it is a possibility. Given the high false-positive rate reported by Studer, LND should be considered to allow more accurate pathological staging. For patients with locally or regionally advanced RCC, retrospective studies have shown a survival benefit and possible improved response to immunotherapy when LND has been performed. However, until prospective studies in this advanced cohort of patients are undertaken, definitive recommendations cannot be made.

Future Directions

While enthusiasm for TIL therapy has diminished, there are still a number of novel and promising approaches to adoptive immunotherapy that should be elaborated upon in future trials. In an effort to eradicate residual metastatic disease after cytoreductive nephrectomy, cancer immunotherapy will hopefully play a more involved part in therapy in the future. Immune tolerance toward malignant RCC cells is theorized to be due to a lack of necessary costimulatory signals required for the activation of T cell responses (Avigan, 2004). As researchers evaluate how to reverse tumor-induced anergy via presentation of the antigen in a manner to effectively prime T cells against RCC cells, hopefully the armamentarium of oncological therapies for metastatic RCC will expand. In addition, as our knowledge of the genetic pathways behind hereditary RCC has grown, drugs that target defective genetic pathways or take advantage of alternate genetic pathways in order to retard tumor growth have become the primary aim for treatment of advanced or metastatic RCC.

Active immunotherapy via tumor cell vaccine, gene-modified tumor vaccine, or a dendritic cell vaccine is characterized by induction of T cells from the respective tumor-bearing patient. A tumor cell vaccine has the advantage of targeting multiple different antigens present on tumor cells in an effort to maximize their effectiveness. An often cited article by Chang and colleagues involved a Phase II study in which 39 patients with metastatic RCC were treated with autologous irradiated tumor cells admixed with BCG to stimulate tumor-specific cells *in vivo* (Chang et al., 2001). Following vaccination, vaccine-primed lymph nodes were excised and secondarily activated with anti-CD3 monoclonal antibody. The activated cells were then reinfused with IL-2 via adoptive transfer. An overall response rate of 27% (four complete responses and five partial responses) was achieved with a median response duration of 35 months among the complete and partial responders. Although concomitant use of IL-2 did confound the response rates observed, the results were impressive.

Because of the technical difficulties and high costs of preparing patient-specific autologous tumor cell vaccines *ex vivo*, gene-modified tumor cell vaccines have evolved as a way to increase the stimulatory effects of tumor cell vaccine lines. By transducing a tumor cell with a stimulatory cytokine, researchers hope to enhance secondarily elicited humoral and cell-mediated immunity. A Phase I trial in 1997 sought to evaluate whether gene-modified tumor cells retrovirally transduced with granulocyte–macrophage colony-stimulating factor (GM-CSF) would cause an induction of immune response in 16 patients with metastatic RCC (Simons et al., 1997). GM-CSF is thought to attract APCs (i.e., dendritic cells) to the tumor site, theoretically in an effort to increase the potential concentration of cells presenting antigens to cytotoxic and helper T cells. The study was performed in a randomized, double-blinded, dose-escalating

fashion with RCC vaccine cells with and without GM-CSF gene transfer. No dose-limiting toxicities were encountered, and delayed type hypersensitivity (DTH) responses to autologous tumor cells and immune cell infiltration at vaccine sites were noted in the GM-CSF arm indicative of T cell immunity. A follow-up paper in 2005 from this group detailed the CD8 T cell response in two patients who showed a postvaccination DTH reaction associated with a partial clinical response (> 90% reduction in metastatic tumor volume) (Zhou et al., 2005). The results were encouraging in that GM-CSF vaccines were found to be able to induce *in vivo* CD8 T cell lines with diverse specificity that in theory could help recruit cell immunity against RCC tumors. Despite the encouraging results, the authors expressed their disappointment in not being able to isolate genes encoding tumor rejection antigens that could ultimately be used in renal tumor antigen-based vaccines. Eight RCC expressed antigens have been reported in the literature thus far; however, as with the above study, they are rarely expressed in RCC and subsequentlyare not applicable for vaccine therapy.

Phase I trials of a different gene modified autologous tumor cell vaccine utilizing B7-1 (CD80) instead of GM-CSF have also been described in a promising manner (Antonia et al., 2002; Frankenberger et al., 2005; Schendel et al., 2000). B7-1 is a costimulatory cytokine that is one of many cytokines that is responsible for activating T cells through binding CD28 ligands located on T cells. Expression of costimulatory molecules is restricted to APCs; however, by inducing tumor cells to express B7-1, an improved proliferation of primed T cells for RCC should theoretically ensue. Phase I trials have been encouraging with no major toxicities when combined with IL-2. Phase II trials are pending and will hopefully show enhanced tumor activity *in vivo*.

Vaccination with antigen-loaded DCs is a novel means of preserving the antigen-presenting and T cell-activating qualities of DCs while incorporating the antigenic nature of native tumor cells. These "DC tumor hybrids" have been studied and promising results have been published in a preliminary Phase I study in which 24 patients underwent vaccination with DC tumor hybrids. A partial response was noted in two patients, and eight experienced stable disease (Avigan, 2004). Transfection of DCs with nucleic acids, such as RNA, is another way to utilize DCs for activation of T cells against metastatic RCC cells. In this manner, RNA is translated into proteins and through intracellular processing is eventually presented on the surface of DCs. Theoretically, DCs could then be used to present RCC tumor antigen to naive and memory T cells to stimulate an immune response, even in cancers where no rejection antigens have been identified. An advantage of this concept is that minute amounts of RNA can be extracted from tumor cells and subsequently expanded to provide an unlimited supply of antigen. An extrapolation of this concept is that renal biopsy would be able to provide tissue with subsequent molecular expansion. A Phase I study of 12 patients with metastatic RCC displayed

RNA loaded DC hybrids were able to stimulate T cell responses *in vivo* (Dahm and Vieweg 2004). Based upon future directions of multimodality therapy to treat metastatic RCC, nephrectomy is a valuable step to allow elimination of the primary tumor volume and provide tumor antigens for further processing and inclusion in biological modifier therapy.

Conclusions

The paucity of effective therapy for metastatic RCC is a hurdle facing both urologists and patients. The key is to identify the subset of patients who will benefit from cytoreductive surgery and immunological therapy so that effective treatment can be delivered efficiently. As the mechanisms by which RCC alters immune responses are discovered, various pathways of treatment will hopefully become available to improve patient survival. Until then urologists should continue to proceed according to the outcomes derived from properly conducted prospectively randomized trials.

References

Althausen P, Althausen A, Jennings LC, et al. Prognostic factors and surgical treatment of osseous metastases secondary to renal cell carcinoma. *Cancer* 1997; 80: 1103–1109.

Alves A, Adam R, Majno P, et al. Hepatic resection for metastatic renal tumors: is it worthwhile? *Annals of Surgical Oncology* 2003; 10: 705–710.

Andoh H, Kurokawa T, Yasui O, et al. Resection of a solitary pancreatic metastasis from renal cell carcinoma with a gallbladder carcinoma: report of a case. *Surgery Today* 2004; 34: 272–275.

Antonia SJ, Seigne J, Diaz J, et al. Phase I trial of a B7-1 (CD80) gene modified autologous tumor cell vaccine in combination with systemic interleukin-2 in patients with metastatic renal cell carcinoma. *Journal of Urology* 2002; 167: 1995–2000.

Atkins MB, Regan M, McDermott D. Update on the role of interleukin 2 and other cytokines in the treatment of patients with stage IV renal carcinoma. *Clinical Cancer Research* 2004; 10: 6342S–6346S.

Avigan D. Dendritic cell-tumor fusion vaccines for renal cell carcinoma. *Clinical Cancer Research* 2004; 10: 6347S–6352S.

Barth PJ, Gerharz EW, Ramaswamy A, et al. The influence of lymph node counts on the detection of pelvic lymph node metastasis in prostate cancer. *Pathology, Research & Practice* 1999; 195: 633–636.

Ben-Eliyahu S, Page GG, Yirmiya R, et al. Evidence that stress and surgical interventions promote tumor development by suppressing natural killer cell activity. *International Journal of Cancer* 1999; 80: 880–888.

Ben-Eliyahu S. The promotion of tumor metastasis by surgery and stress: immunological basis and implications for psychoneuroimmunology. *Brain, Behavior, and Immunity* 2003; 17: S27–S36.

Bennett RT, Lerner SE, Taub HC, et al. Cytoreductive surgery for stage IV renal cell carcinoma.[see comment]. *Journal of Urology* 1995; 154: 32–34.

Bex A, Horenblas S, Meinhardt W, et al. The role of initial immunotherapy as selection for nephrectomy in patients with metastatic renal cell carcinoma and the primary tumor in situ. *European Urology* 2002; 42: 570–574.

Bui MH, Seligson D, Han KR, et al. Carbonic anhydrase IX is an independent predictor of survival in advanced renal clear cell carcinoma: implications for prognosis and therapy. *Clinical Cancer Research* 2003; 9: 802–811.

Bui MH, Visapaa H, Seligson D, et al. Prognostic value of carbonic anhydrase IX and KI67 as predictors of survival for renal clear cell carcinoma. *Journal of Urology* 2004; 171: 2461–2466.

Casamassima A, Picciariello M, Quaranta M, et al. C-reactive protein: a biomarker of survival in patients with metastatic renal cell carcinoma treated with subcutaneous interleukin-2 based immunotherapy. *Journal of Urology* 2005; 173: 52–55.

Chang AE, Li Q, Jiang G, et al. Phase II trial of autologous tumor vaccination, anti-CD3-activated vaccine-primed lymphocytes, and interleukin-2 in stage IV renal cell cancer. *Journal of Clinical Oncology* 2001; 21: 884–890.

Chow WH, Devesa SS, Warren JL, et al. Rising incidence of renal cell cancer in the United States [see comment]. *JAMA* 1999; 281: 1628–1631.

Cooney MM, Remick SC, Vogelzang NJ. A medical oncologist's approach to immunotherapy for advanced renal tumors: is nephrectomy indicated? [see comment]. *Current Urology Reports* 2004; 5: 19–24.

Dahm P, Vieweg J. Evolving immunotherapeutic strategies for the treatment of prostate and renal carcinomas. *AUA Update Series* 2004; 23: 25–32.

deKernion JB, Ramming KP, Smith RB. The natural history of metastatic renal cell carcinoma: a computer analysis. *Journal of Urology* 1978; 120: 148–152.

de los Monteros-Sanchez AE, Medina-Franco H, Arista-Nasr J, et al. Resection of an esophageal metastasis from a renal cell carcinoma. *Hepato-Gastroenterology* 2004; 51: 163–164.

Dernevik L, Berggren H, Larsson S, Roberts D. Surgical removal of pulmonary metastases from renal cell carcinoma. *Scandinavian Journal of Urology and Nephrology* 1985; 19(2):133–137.

Eggermont AM, Steller EP, Sugarbaker PH. Laparotomy enhances intraperitoneal tumor growth and abrogates the antitumor effects of interleukin-2 and lymphokine-activated killer cells. *Surgery* 1987; 102: 71–78.

Fallick ML, McDermott DF, LaRock D, et al. Nephrectomy before interleukin-2 therapy for patients with metastatic renal cell carcinoma. *Journal of Urology* 1997; 158: 1691–1695.

Ficarra V, Righetti R, D'Amico A, et al. Renal vein and vena cava involvement does not affect prognosis in patients with renal cell carcinoma. *Oncology* 2001; 61: 10–15.

Figlin RA, Pierce WC, Kaboo R, et al. Treatment of metastatic renal cell carcinoma with nephrectomy, interleukin-2 and cytokine-primed or CD8(+) selected tumor infiltrating lymphocytes from primary tumor. *Journal of Urology* 1997; 158: 740–745.

Figlin RA, Thompson JA, Bukowski RM, et al. Multicenter, randomized, phase III trial of CD8(+) tumor-infiltrating lymphocytes in combination with recombinant interleukin-2 in metastatic renal cell carcinoma. *Journal of Clinical Oncology* 1999; 17:2521–2529.

Finelli A, Kaouk JH, Fergany AF, et al. Laparoscopic cytoreductive nephrectomy for metastatic renal cell carcinoma. *BJU International* 2004; 94: 29129–29124.

Flanigan RC, Salmon SE, Blumenstein BA, et al. Nephrectomy followed by interferon alfa-2b compared with interferon alfa-2b alone for metastatic renal-cell cancer [see comment]. *New England Journal of Medicine* 2001; 345: 1655–1659.

Flanigan RC, Campbell SC, Clark JI, et al. Metastatic renal cell carcinoma. *Current Treatment Options in Oncology* 2003; 4: 385–390.

Flanigan RC, Mickisch G, Sylvester R, et al. Cytoreductive nephrectomy in patients with metastatic renal cancer: a combined analysis. *Journal of Urology* 2004; 171: 1071–1076.

Fleischmann JD, Kim B. Interleukin-2 immunotherapy followed by resection of residual renal cell carcinoma. *Journal of Urology* 1991; 145: 938–941.

Frankenberger B, Pohla H, Noessner E, et al. Influence of CD80, interleukin-2, and interleukin-7 expression in human renal cell carcinoma on the expansion, function, and survival of tumor-specific CTLs. *Clinical Cancer Research* 2005; 11: 1733–1742.

Franklin JR, Figlin R, Rauch J, et al. Cytoreductive surgery in the management of metastatic renal cell carcinoma: the UCLA experience. *Seminars in Urologic Oncology* 1996; 14: 230–236.

Fujikawa K, Matsui Y, Miura K, et al. Serum immunosuppressive acidic protein and natural killer cell activity in patients with metastatic renal cell carcinoma before and after nephrectomy. *Journal of Urology* 2000; 164: 673–675.

Fyfe G, Fisher RI, Rosenberg SA, et al. Results of treatment of 255 patients with metastatic renal cell carcinoma who received high-dose recombinant interleukin-2 therapy. *Journal of Clinical Oncology* 1995; 13: 688–696.

Gatenby RA, Gawlinski ET, Tangen CM, et al. The possible role of postoperative azotemia in enhanced survival of patients with metastatic renal cancer after cytoreductive nephrectomy. *Cancer Research* 2002; 62: 5218–5222.

Goetzl MA, Goluboff ET, Murphy AM, et al. A contemporary evaluation of cytoreductive nephrectomy with tumor thrombus: morbidity and long-term survival. *Urologic Oncology* 2004; 22: 182–197.

Goldfarb DA, Novick AC, Lorig R, et al. Magnetic resonance imaging for assessment of vena caval tumor thrombi: a comparative study with venacavography and computerized tomography scanning. *Journal of Urology* 1990; 144: 1100–1104.

Hafez KS, Montie JE. Indications and limitations of cytoreductive nephrectomy for metastatic renal cell carcinoma. *AUA Update Series* 2004; 23: 250–256.

Hatcher PA, Anderson EE, Paulson DF, et al. Surgical management and prognosis of renal cell carcinoma invading the vena cava. *Journal of Urology* 1991; 145: 20–24.

Herrlinger A, Schrott KM, Schott G, et al. What are the benefits of extended dissection of the regional renal lymph nodes in the therapy of renal cell carcinoma. *Journal of Urology* 1991; 146: 1224–1227.

Hinman F Jr. Kidney: excision. In: Hinman F Jr, Ed. Atlas of Urologic Surgery, 2nd ed. Philadelphia: W.B. Saunders Company, 1998.

Hock LM, Lynch J, Balaji KC. Increasing incidence of all stages of kidney cancer in the last 2 decades in the United States: an analysis of surveillance, epidemiology and end results program data. *Journal of Urology* 2002; 167: 57–60.

Jayson M, Sanders H. Increased incidence of serendipitously discovered renal cell carcinoma. *Urology* 1998; 51: 203–205.

Jemal A, Murray T, Ward E, et al. Cancer statistics. *Cancer Journal for Clinicians* 2005; 55: 10–30.

Jett JR, Hollinger CG, Zinsmeister AR, Pairolero PC. Pulmonary resection of metastatic renal cell carcinoma. *Chest* 1983; 84(4):442–445.

Kavolius JP, Mastorakos DP, Pavlovich C, et al. Resection of metastatic renal cell carcinoma. *Journal of Clinical Oncology* 1998; 16: 2261–2266.

Kierney PC, van Heerden JA, Segura JW, Weaver AL. Surgeon's role in the management of solitary renal cell carcinoma metastases occurring subsequent to initial curative nephrectomy: an institutional review. *Annals Surgery of Oncology* 1994; 1(4):345–352.

Kim B, Louie AC. Surgical resection following interleukin 2 therapy for metastatic renal cell carcinoma prolongs remission. *Archives of Surgery* 1992; 127: 1343–1349.

Klugo RC, Detmers M, Stiles RE, Talley RW, Cerny JC. Aggressive versus conservative management of stage IV renal cell carcinoma. *Journal of Urolology* 1977; 118(2):244–246.

Kollender Y, Bickels J, Price WM, et al. Metastatic renal cell carcinoma of bone: indications and technique of surgical intervention. *Journal of Urology* 2000; 164: 1505–1508.

Krishnamurthi V, Novick AC, Bukowski RM. Efficacy of multi-modality therapy in advanced renal cell carcinoma. *Urology* 1998; 51: 933–937.

Lammer J, Justich E, Schreyer H, et al. Complications of renal tumor embolization. *Cardiovascular & Interventional Radiology* 1985; 8: 31–35.

Lanigan D, Jurriaans E, Hammonds JC, et al. The current status of embolization in renal cell carcinoma—-a survey of local and national practice. *Clinical Radiology* 1992; 46: 176–178.

Lau WK, Zincke H, Lohse CM, et al. Contralateral adrenal metastasis of renal cell carcinoma: treatment, outcome and a review [see comment]. *BJU International* 2003; 91: 775–779.

Leissner J, Hohenfellner R, Thuroff JW, et al. Lymphadenectomy in patients with transitional cell carcinoma of the urinary bladder; significance for staging and prognosis. *BJU International* 2000; 85: 817–823.

Levy DA, Swanson DA, Slaton JW, Ellerhorst J, Dinney CP. Timely delivery of biological therapy after cytoreductive nephrectomy in carefully selected patients with metastatic renal cell carcinoma.

Lin E, Calvano SE, Lowry SF. Inflammatory cytokines and cell response in surgery. *Surgery* 2000; 127: 117–126.

Ljungberg B, Landberg G, Alamdari FI. Factors of importance for prediction of survival in patients with metastatic renal cell carcinoma, treated with or without nephrectomy. *Scandinavian Journal of Urology & Nephrology* 2000; 34: 246–251.

Marshall FF, Reitz BA. Technique for removal of renal cell carcinoma with suprahepatic vena caval tumor thrombus. *Urologic Clinics of North America* 1986; 13: 551–557.

Marshall FF, Reitz BA, Diamond DA. A new technique for management of renal cell carcinoma involving the right atrium: hypothermia and cardiac arrest. *Journal of Urology* 1984; 131: 103–107.

Masuda H, Kurita Y, Suzuki A, et al. Prognostic factors for renal cell carcinoma: a multivariate analysis of 320 cases. *International Journal of Urology* 1997; 4: 247–253.

McDermott DF, Regan MM, Clark JI, et al. Randomized phase III trial of high-dose interleukin-2 versus subcutaneous interleukin-2 and interferon in patients with metastatic renal cell carcinoma. *Journal of Clinical Oncology* 2005; 23: 133–141.

McNichols DW, Segura JW, DeWeerd JH. Renal cell carcinoma: long-term survival and late recurrence. *Journal of Urolology* 1981; 126(1):17–23.

Medical Research Council Renal Cell Collaborators. Interferon-alpha and survival in metastatic renal carcinoma: early results of a randomised controlled trial. *Lancet* 1999; 353: 14–17.

Mickisch GH, Garin A, van Poppel H, et al. Radical nephrectomy plus interferon-alfa-based immunotherapy compared with interferon alfa alone in metastatic renal-cell carcinoma: a randomised trial [see comment]. *Lancet* 2001; 358: 966–970.

Middleton RG. Surgery for metastatic renal cell carcinoma. *Journal of Urology* 1967; 97: 973–977.

Minasian LM, Motzer RJ, Gluck L, et al. Interferon alfa-2a in advanced renal cell carcinoma: treatment results and survival in 159 patients with long-term follow-up. *Journal of Clinical Oncology* 1993; 11: 1368–1375.

Minervini A, Lilas L, Morelli G, et al. Regional lymph node dissection in the treatment of renal cell carcinoma: is it useful in patients with no suspected adenopathy before or during surgery? *BJU International* 2001; 88: 169–172.

Montie JE, Stewart BH, Straffon RA, et al. The role of adjunctive nephrectomy in patients with metastatic renal cell carcinoma. *Journal of Urology* 1977; 117: 272–275.

Motzer RJ, Mazumdar M, Bacik J, et al. Survival and prognostic stratification of 670 patients with advanced renal cell carcinoma. *Journal of Clinical Oncology* 1999; 17: 2530–2540.

Motzer RJ, Russo P. Systemic therapy for renal cell carcinoma. *Journal of Urology* 2000; 163: 408–417.

Moudouni SM, Ennia I, Manunta A, et al. Factors influencing adrenal metastasis in renal cell carcinoma. *International Urology & Nephrology* 2003; 35: 141–147.

Naitoh J, Kaplan A, Dorey F, et al. Metastatic renal cell carcinoma with concurrent inferior vena caval invasion: long-term survival after combination therapy with radical nephrectomy, vena caval thrombectomy and postoperative immunotherapy. *Journal of Urology* 1999; 162: 46–50.

Neves RJ, Zincke H. Surgical treatment of renal cancer with vena cava extension. *British Journal of Urology* 1987; 59: 390–395.

Novick AC. Surgery of the kidney. In: Walsh PC, Retik AB, Vaughan ED Jr, et al. Eds. Campbells Urology, 8th ed. Philadelphia: W.B. Saunders, 2002.

Novick AC, Kaye MC, Cosgrove DM, et al. Experience with cardiopulmonary bypass and deep hypothermic circulatory arrest in the management of retroperitoneal tumors with large vena caval thrombi. *Annals of Surgery* 1990; 212: 472–477.

Novick AC, Campbell SC. Renal tumors. In: Walsh PC, Retik AB, Vaughan ED Jr, et al., Eds. Campbells Urology, 8th ed. Philadelphia: W.B. Saunders, 2002.

O'Dea MJ, Zincke H, Utz DC, et al. The treatment of renal cell carcinoma with solitary metastasis. *Journal of Urology* 1978; 120: 540–542.

Onufrey V, Mohiuddin M. Radiation therapy in the treatment of metastatic renal cell carcinoma. *International Journal of Radiation Oncology, Biology, Physics* 1985; 11: 2007–2009.

Pantuck AJ, Belldegrun AS, Figlin RA. Nephrectomy and interleukin-2 for metastatic renal-cell carcinoma [see comment]. *New England Journal of Medicine* 2001; 169: 1711–1712.

Pantuck AJ, Zisman A, Dorey F, et al. Renal cell carcinoma with retroperitoneal lymph nodes. Impact on survival and benefits of immunotherapy. *Cancer* 2003a; 97: 2995–3002.

Pantuck AJ, Zisman A, Dorey F et al. Renal cell carcinoma with retroperitoneal lymph nodes: role of lymph node dissection. *Journal of Urology* 2003b; 169: 2076–2083.

Paul R, Mordhorst J, Busch R, et al. Adrenal sparing surgery during radical nephrectomy in patients with renal cell cancer: a new algorithm. *Journal of Urology* 2001; 166: 59–62.

Pautler SE CP, Phillips JL, Pavlovich CP, Leach F, Linehan WM, Walther MM. Laparoscopic cytoreductive radical nephrectomy for metastatic renal cell carcinoma: a feasibility study. *Journal of Urology* 2001; 165: 185.

Phillips E, Messing EM. Role of lymphadenectomy in the treatment of renal cell carcinoma. *Urology* 1991; 41: 9–15.

Piardi T, D'Adda F, Giampaoli F, et al. Solitary metachronous splenic metastases: an evaluation of surgical treatment. *Journal of Experimental & Clinical Cancer Research* 1999; 18: 575–578.

Rackley R, Novick A, Klein E, et al. The impact of adjuvant nephrectomy on multimodality treatment of metastatic renal cell carcinoma. *Journal of Urology* 1994; 152: 1399–1403.

Robson CJ, Churchill BM, Anderson W. The results of radical nephrectomy for renal cell carcinoma. *Journal of Urology* 1969; 101: 297–301.

Sahin M, Foulis AA, Poon FW, et al. Late focal pancreatic metastasis of renal cell carcinoma. *Digestive Surgery* 1998; 15: 72–74.

Saitoh H, Nakayama M, Nakamura K, et al. Distant metastasis of renal adenocarcinoma in nephrectomized cases. *Journal of Urology* 1982; 127: 1092–1095.

Schafhauser W, Ebert A, Brod J, et al. Lymph node involvement in renal cell carcinoma and survival chance by systematic lymphadenectomy. *Anticancer Research* 1999; 19: 1573–1578.

Schendel DJ, Frankenberger B, Jantzer P, et al. Expression of B7.1 (CD80) in a renal cell carcinoma line allows expansion of tumor-associated cytotoxic T lymphocytes in the presence of an alloresponse. *Gene Therapy* 2000; 7: 2007–2014.

Sella A, Swanson DA, Ro JY, et al. Surgery following response to interferon-alpha-based therapy for residual renal cell carcinoma. *Journal of Urology* 1993; 149: 21–22.

Sheehan JP, Sun MH, Kondziolka D, et al. Radiosurgery in patients with renal cell carcinoma metastasis to the brain: long-term outcomes and prognostic factors influencing survival and local tumor control [see comment]. *Journal of Neurosurgery* 2003; 98: 342–349.

Siemer S, Lehmann J, Kamradt J, et al. Adrenal metastases in 1635 patients with renal cell carcinoma: outcome and indication for adrenalectomy. *Journal of Urology* 2004; 171: 2155–2159.

Simons JW, Jaffee EM, Weber CE, et al. Bioactivity of autologous irradiated renal cell carcinoma vaccines generated by *ex vivo* granulocyte-macrophage colony-stimulating factor gene transfer. *Cancer Research* 1997; 57: 1537–1546.

Skinner DG, Colvin RB, Vermillion CD, et al. Diagnosis and management of renal cell carcinoma. A clinical and pathologic study of 309 cases. *Cancer* 1971; 28: 1165–1177.

Skinner DG, Pritchett TR, Lieskovsky G, et al. Vena caval involvement by renal cell carcinoma. Surgical resection provides meaningful long-term survival. *Annals of Surgery* 1989; 210: 387–392.

Slaton JW, Balbay MD, Levy DA, et al. Nephrectomy and vena caval thrombectomy in patients with metastatic renal cell carcinoma. *Urology* 1997; 50: 673–677.

Slaton JW, Perrotte P, Balbay MD, et al. Reassessment of the selection criteria for cytoreductive nephrectomy in patients with metastatic renal cell carcinoma. *Journal of Urology* 2000; 163: 179.

Stief CG, Jahne J, Hagemann JH, et al. Surgery for metachronous solitary liver metastases of renal cell carcinoma. *Journal of Urology* 1997; 158: 375–377.

Studer UE, Scherz S, Scheidegger J, et al. Enlargement of regional lymph nodes in renal cell carcinoma is often not due to metastases. *Journal of Urology* 1990; 144: 243–245.

Swanson DA. Surgery for metastases of renal cell carcinoma. *Scandinavian Journal of Surgery* 2004; 93: 150–155.

Swierzewski DJ, Swierzewski MJ, Libertino JA. Radical nephrectomy in patients with renal cell carcinoma with venous, vena caval and atrial extension. *American Journal of Surgery* 1994; 168: 205–209.

Terrone C, Guercio S, De Luca S, et al. The number of lymph nodes examined and staging accuracy in renal cell carcinoma. *BJU International* 2003; 91: 37–40.

Tolia BM, Whitmore WF Jr. Solitary metastasis from renal cell carcinoma. *Journal of Urology* 1975; 114: 836–838.

Tsui K-H, Shvarts O, Barbaric Z, et al. Is adrenalectomy a necessary component of radical nephrectomy? UCLA experience with 511 radical nephrectomies. *Journal of Urology* 2000; 163: 437–441.

van der Poel HG, Roukema JA, Horenblas S, et al. Metastasectomy in renal cell carcinoma: a multicenter retrospective analysis. *European Urology* 1999; 35: 197–203.

Vasselli JR, Yang JC, Linehan WM, et al. Lack of retroperitoneal lymphadenopathy predicts survival of patients with metastatic renal cell carcinoma. *Journal of Urology* 2001; 166: 68–72.

Vis N, van der Gaast A, van Rhijn G, et al. A phase II trial of methotrexate-human serum albumin (MTX-HSA) in patients with metastatic renal cell carcinoma who progressed under immunotherapy. *Cancer Chemotherapy & Pharmacology* 2002; 49: 342–345.

Wagner JR, Walther MM, Linehan WM, et al. Interleukin-2 based immunotherapy for metastatic renal cell carcinoma with the kidney in place. *Journal of Urology* 1999; 162: 43–45.

Walther MM, Alexander RB, Weiss GH, et al. Cytoreductive surgery prior to interleukin-2-based therapy in patients with metastatic renal cell carcinoma. *Urology* 1993; 42: 250–258.

Walther MM, Yang JC, Pass HI, et al. Cytoreductive surgery before high dose interleukin-2 based therapy in patients with metastatic renal cell carcinoma. *Journal of Urology* 1997; 158: 1675–1678.

Walther MM, Lyne JC, Libutti SK, et al. Laparoscopic cytoreductive nephrectomy as preparation for administration of systemic interleukin-2 in the treatment of metastatic renal cell carcinoma: a pilot study. *Urology* 1999; 53: 496–501.

Wells IP, Hammonds JC, Franklin K. Embolisation of hypernephromas: a simple technique using ethanol. *Clinical Radiology* 1983; 34: 689–692.

Wolf JS Jr, Aronson FR, Small EJ, Carroll PR. Nephrectomy for metastatic renal cell carcinoma: a component of systemic treatment regimens. *Journal of Surgical Oncology* 1994; 55(1):7–13.

Wood CG, Huber N, Madsen L, et al. Clinical variables that predict survival following cytoreductive nephrectomy for metastatic renal cell carcinoma. *Journal of Urology* 2001; 165: 184.

Wronski M, Arbit E, Russo P, et al. Surgical resection of brain metastases from renal cell carcinoma in 50 patients. *Urology* 1996; 47: 187–193.

Wronski M, Maor MH, Davis BJ, et al. External radiation of brain metastases from renal carcinoma: a retrospective study of 119 patients from the M. D. Anderson Cancer Center. *International Journal of Radiation Oncology, Biology and Physics* 1997; 37: 753–759.

Yagoda A. Phase II cytotoxic chemotherapy trials in renal cell carcinoma: 1983–1988. *Progress in Clinical & Biological Research* 1990; 350: 227–241.

Yang JC, Sherry RM, Steinberg SM, et al. Randomized study of high-dose and low-dose interleukin-2 in patients with metastatic renal cancer. *Journal of Clinical Oncology* 2003; 21: 3127–3132.

Zagoria RJ, Dyer RB, Wolfman NT, et al. Radiology in the diagnosis and staging of renal cell carcinoma. *Critical Reviews in Diagnostic Imaging* 1990; 31: 81–115.

Zhou X, Jun do Y, Thomas AM, et al. Diverse CD8+ T-cell responses to renal cell carcinoma antigens in patients treated with an autologous granulocyte-macrophage colony-stimulating factor gene-transduced renal tumor cell vaccine. *Cancer Research* 2005; 65: 1079–1088.

Zisman A, Pantuck AJ, Chao DH, et al. Renal cell carcinoma with tumor thrombus: is cytoreductive nephrectomy for advanced disease associated with an increased complication rate? *Journal of Urology* 2002; 168: 962–967.

8k
Local Recurrence After Radical Nephrectomy for Renal Cell Carcinoma

M. Pilar Laguna

Introduction

Local recurrence after radical nephrectomy for renal cell carcinoma (RCC) is defined as the presence of recurrent cancer in the renal fossa or renal bed (after radical nephrectomy with curative intentions) (1).

Isolated renal fossa recurrence should not be mistaken for abdominal recurrence in other viscera or abdominal sites different from the surgical bed considered as distant metastases.

Classically recurrent disease at the renal bed or surgical site has been attributed to synchronic or asynchronic metastatic adrenal glands left *in situ* during radical nephrectomy, to residual disease in the regional lymph nodes, or to recurrent or residual disease in de Gerota's fat or in the psoas muscle.[2] However, incomplete tumoral resection, violation of the tumor, and spillage during primary surgery may also be the cause of the recurrence of ipsilateral fossa in spite of the presumed radicality.[3–5]

Local recurrence is a rare event and is frequently associated with disseminated disease.[6] Local fossa recurrence in association with distant metastatic disease is a poor prognostic factor with a 1-year survival rate of 14% vs. 40% among those without local recurrence.[7]

In the past two decades isolated local recurrence has been diagnosed with increased frequency owing to the routine use of a computed tomography (CT) scan in the follow-up after radical nephrectomy.[8] However, the liberal use of ultrasonography has led to a shift in the stage of the renal cancers at diagnosis and consequently less advanced stages are treated. As isolated local recurrence seems to be associated with advanced stages,[1,9–11] the incidence of such events should decrease, compensating for the effects of more strict imaging during follow-up.

In general little attention has been devoted to the subject of isolated local recurrence, with only case series reported. Most of these series include a small number of selected patients treated in a very long time frame. Isolated cases including recurrence in the vena cava have been described.[12–16]

Surgery, when possible, is accepted as the standard treatment, although other systemic treatments including immunotherapy, chemotherapy, and radiotherapy have been used in general with poor results.

Due to the nature of the above-mentioned case series evidence concerning local recurrence after nephrectomy and its treatment is low.[17]

Incidence

The overall incidence of local recurrence after radical nephrectomy in different series is variable. The presence of local recurrence has been classically described in 10–37% of the cases with metastatic disease.[11,18–21]

With the use of a CT scan even higher rates of local recurrence were reported. The incidence of local recurrence was found to be 41% in one autopsy series of patients dying of metastatic disease[22] up to 66% of patients with metastatic disease can also have a recurrence in the renal fossa when extensively evaluated by CT scan imaging.[23]

In spite of the widespread use of ultrasound and CT scan in the follow-up period after radical nephrectomy, the current incidence of isolated renal fossa recurrence after radical surgery is very low (between 0.8% and 4%).[11,18,24,25] A recent review of the literature comparing the outcomes of nephron-sparing surgery and radical nephrectomy indicates that the rate of local recurrence after radical nephrectomy is 0.4%.[26]

In the series of Stephenson including 435 cases after nephrectomy and excluding T4 tumors, 12 patients (2.7%) had local recurrence associated or not associated with distant metastases, with only four patients presenting isolated local recurrence (0.9%).[1]

Probably this incidence will steadily increase with increasing time from nephrectomy. In one of the best documented series the calculated incidence of isolated renal fossa recurrence among unilateral renal cell carcinoma (T1–3

TABLE 8k-1. Description of primary stages at nephrectomy according to 1997 TNM.

Reference	Number of patients	PT1	PT2	PT3a	PT3b	PT3c	PT4	NPA[a]
Schrödter[25,b]	13	1	4	5	1	–	2	–
Gogus[27]	10	1	5	–	3	1	–	–
Master[3]	14	2	2			10 pT3		
Itano[24]	30	13 pT1/2		4	12	1	–	–
Sandhu[4]	16	1	8	3	2	–	–	2
Tanguy[5,c]	16	0	7	5	2	–	–	2

[a]NPA, no pathology available of primary specimen.
[b]TNM not specified.
[c]1987 TNM.

No, Mo) without evidence of metastatic disease was 1.8% ± 0.4% at the 5-year follow-up, which increased to 2.3% ± 0.5% at the 10-year follow-up.[24]

Regarding the sex of the patient, the proportion of male to female oscillates between 2/1 and 4/3 in the present series.[3–5,9,24,25,27]

Risk Factors for Local (Fossa) Recurrence

Presumably recurrent carcinoma in the renal fossa may result from incomplete resection or persisting tumor in the regional contiguous lymph nodes[7] and represents a unique variant of advanced stage disease.[9]

Possible sources of local recurrence are incomplete tumoral resection, including thrombus in the vena renalis, the presence of tumoral node metastases, grossly or microscopic, and the presence of metastatic disease in the remaining adrenal gland.[4,6,9,11] Local recurrence is probably an expression of a remnant of microscopic disease or a form of metastatic disease.[24]

Spillage during primary surgery may be a potential source of contamination and may result in local recurrence.[4,5]

The risk and pattern of relapse of RCC after nephrectomy are associated with the pathological stage, with most recurrences occurring in patients with tumors extending beyond the capsule, T3–T4.[9,10] Abdominal relapse, including relapse in the retroperitoneum or in the renal bed, is significantly higher in the case of pT3a–b primary lesions.[1]

Local recurrence, however, can occur after any stage, although it happens more rarely after low primary stages.[9,10,28,29] In the series of Stephenson the incidence of local relapse was 14% after pT3 and only 1.8% when the primary lesion was pT1–2. Also in the case of pT3 lesions, local relapse seems to occur earlier, at a median follow-up of 12 months after primary surgery.[1]

Indeed, among patients presenting with isolated local recurrence the incidence of primary pT3 tumors seems to be higher than with other stages but is not exclusive.[3–5,24,25,27]

Table 8k-1 shows the pathological stage of the primary tumor in the most recent series.

The increasing incidence of local relapse related to the more advanced primary tumor has also been confirmed in the Integrated Stage Systems of the University of California–Los Angeles (UISS).[30] Local recurrence in the renal fossa bed was found during follow-up in 14.5% of the patients in the low-risk groups. For patients in the high-risk group this figure reached 25.8%.[30]

Patients with advanced T stage and lymph node involvement seem to be at higher risk of fossa recurrence.[8,23,28,31] It has been advocated that an extended lymphadenectomy at the time of the primary surgery may reduce the risk of local recurrence; however, this has never been definitively proven.[28,32] An analysis of the modern series on isolated local recurrence does not show that lymph node involvement at the moment of primary surgery is a risk factor.[3–5,9,24,25,27]

The impact of other known prognostic factors for recurrence of RCC such as histological subtype, cellular grade, or vascular invasion has not been assessed for isolated local recurrence. All histological subtypes can be the origin of a local recurrence, although there is a predominance or clear cell carcinoma.[3,24] This reflects the primary incidence and presentation of the different histological subgroups of RCC. It is, however, reasonable to think that some aggressive cellular forms such as sarcomatoid differentiation or the rare PEComas could recur more frequently in the renal bed.[33,34]

Fuhrman grade distribution in the radical nephrectomy specimen varied from 2 to 4,[4,25] although in some series grades 3 and 4 seem to be more frequent.[3] Fuhrman grade 1 is seldom found in the primary specimen.

Currently no biological or molecular marker has been identified as having a prognostic value in predicting the development of local recurrence.[35] Markers of tissue penetration may play a roll in the future in stratifying patients at risk for different patterns of metastasis.[36]

At present there are no data showing any difference in local recurrence after open or laparoscopic radical nephrectomy.

TABLE 8k-2. Series and outcomes of isolated renal/bed recurrence.

Reference	Number of patients[a]	Mean age (at recurrence)	Interval to recurrence[b] (months)	Symptoms present	Type of treatment	DFS[c]	Mean time DFS (months)
Schrödter[27]	13	62.3 (49–69)	45.5 (7–224)	15%	Surgery	5 (38%)	53
Gogus[27]	10	51.7 (26–74)	33.6 (3–68)	30%	Surgery± immunotherapy	7 (70%)	16.6
Master[3]	14	–	40 (5–180)	7%	Surgery± immunotherapy± IORT[d]	5 (36%)	66 (14–86)
Itano[24,e]	30	67 (35–85)	2.8 years (0.11–13.13)	60%	Surgery (10) Observation (9) Medical therapy (11)	51% 13% 18%	(5 years[e])
Sandhu[4]	14	57.4 (28.9–71.7)	2.2 years (0.27–14.46)	–	Surgery	5 (36%)	4–66
Esrig[9]	11	59 (41–73)	31 (2–84)	82%	Surgery	4 (36%)	85 (35–211)
Tanguay[5,f]	16	53 (23–74)	16.5 (5–71)	37%	Surgery± immunotherapy (7)	6 (37.5%)	37.5 (3–136)

[a]Number of patients: patients with pathological documented recurrence of RCC.
[b]Interval to recurrence: time from primary nephrectomy to diagnosis of local recurrence (mean or median).
[c]DFS, disease-free survival.
[d]IORT, intraoperative radiation therapy.
[e]Some patients in the surgical group also received additional treatment (four radiation and two immunotherapy).
[f]Three patients had previously treated metastases.

Detection of Local Recurrence

There is limited information in the literature regarding presentation. Local recurrence may be detected by imaging during routine follow-up or due to the presence of clinical symptoms.

The mean age at detection of the local recurrence varies from 52 to 67 years including some very young patients (Table 8k-2. The mean interval between the primary nephrectomy and the detection of the local recurrences varies from 16.5 to 45.5 months in the different series with some of the recurrences appearing very early after the primary nephrectomy and others after 15 years (Table 8k-2).

Routine Imaging

There is a paucity of data regarding the best schedule of imaging during follow-up after radical nephrectomy. In most of the modern protocols routine imaging of the retroperitoneum, by ultrasound or CT scan, is performed, although not frequently.[10,11,30]

In contrast with older series, local recurrence is now mostly detected by routine imaging during follow-up.[3,4,25,27] Most of the local recurrences are initially diagnosed by ultrasound and or confirmed later by CT scan[25,27] (Figs. 8k-1 and 8k-2). Abdominal relapse including relapse in the retroperitoneum was detected in the absence of symptoms, abnormal biochemical profile, or thoracic metastases detectable by chest X-ray in 1.4% of the patients in the series of Stephenson.[1]

Angiography was performed early in some of the series,[9,24] but is no longer recommended. Currently cross-sectional imaging, CT scan, and magnetic resonance imaging have

a higher sensitivity for the detection of local recurrence (Figs. 8k-3 and 8k-4).

Positron emission tomography scan is of limited usefulness, with a sensitivity of only 64%.[37]

In case of documented local renal fossa, distant metastasis in other organs should be ruled out by a CT scan of the thorax and a bone scan before a decision concerning therapy is made[4,25,27] (Fig. 8k-5).

Symptoms

The percentage of symptomatic patients at the diagnosis of local recurrence varies widely in the series from 7% to 82%[3–5,9,11,24,25,27] (Table 8k-2). While currently an early

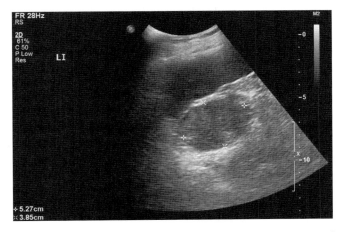

FIGURE 8k-1. Asymptomatic local recurrence (5.3 × 3.8 cm) diagnosed during follow-up ultrasound 10 years after left nephrectomy for clear cell carcinoma pT2 Nx M0 (without adrenalectomy).

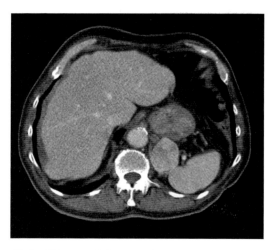

FIGURE 8k-2. CT scan of the same local recurrence of Fig. 8k–1. Diameters in cross-sectional imaging: 6 × 6 × 4.3 cm.

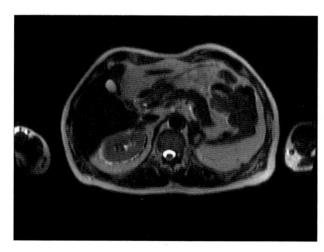

FIGURE 8k-4. Magnetic resonance imaging of the same case described in Fig. 8k–3. Solid nodular imaging of 1.4 cm diameter in the renal fossa.

diagnosis could be expected, before symptomatic disease, the series includes a significant number of patients diagnosed a long time ago before cross-sectional imaging and ultrasound were routinely performed.

The most frequently symptoms associated with a local recurrence are lassitude and fatigue, loss of appetite and weight, flank or abdominal pain, gross hematuria, abdominal bulging, and dyspnea.[3–5,9,24,25,27] Fever and anemia have also been described.[5]

In general, symptoms may be present in one-third of the patients, but they are unspecific and can also be found in cases of systemic recurrence.

Biopsy

Biopsy of the renal bed (or fossa) mass was regularly performed in the series at the Mayo Clinic for pathological tissue diagnosis, although it is not clear if this was in an open

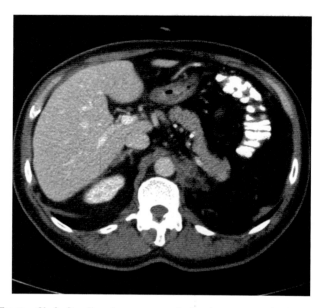

FIGURE 8k-3. Small and asymptomatic local recurrence in CT scan (2.2 × 1 cm) of the abdomen 17 months after radical nephrectomy because of RCC (pT3b NO MO).

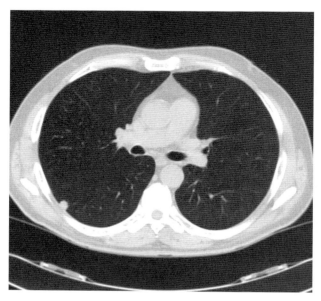

FIGURE 8k-5. CT scan of the thorax corresponding to the same case described in Figs. 8k–3 and 8k–4. Pulmonary metastasis of 1 cm diameter in the right lung.

or percutaneous way.[24] However, no references to a previous biopsy have been found in the other series.

Percutaneous biopsy may be indicated if no surgical treatment is expected and because some false-positive results have been described when the diagnosis is sustained only by CT.[25]

The choice between fine needle aspiration (FNA) and Tru-cut biopsy is dependent on the clinician's and the pathologist's expertise and is probably subjected to the same diagnostic limitations as in primary RCC.[38,39]

Postsurgery pathology of the local recurrence does not differ significantly from the primary RCC. Cell type and Fuhrman grade are similar to the primitive tumor, although a higher grade can be found in some cases.[4,25,27]

Treatment of Local Recurrence after Radical Nephrectomy

The first report, more than 35 years ago, proving that extended surgery for metastatic lesions of RCC prolonged survival is attributed to Skinner.[40]

Isolated local recurrence after radical nephrectomy results in a difficult therapeutic decision, mainly because it represents in itself a high risk of developing overt metastatic disease. However, isolated fossa recurrence may, at least potentially, behave in a manner similar to other isolated distant soft tissue metastases; thus, as in the latter, surgery may be indicated with the possibility of cure.[41,42]

Unfortunately, the increased sensitivity of a CT scan in the diagnosis of local recurrence has not translated into either an improved diagnosis of or an impairment in the development of distant metastasis.[8]

Local recurrence has an unfavorable prognostic, particularly if untreated, but treatment still remains controversial. At least two facts support the practice of an aggressive surgical treatment: the long time to disease progression in some cases of RCC[12,43] and the good results (long-term survival) obtained after excision of a solitary metastasis.[41,42,44]

It is generally accepted that when possible aggressive surgical treatment must be offered.[8] Surgical treatment provides the potential for cure when the disease is limited and can be completely excised. In some author's opinion surgery is the only potentially curative option.[9]

However, the effect of aggressive local surgery remains uncertain. The extreme rarity of isolated local recurrence after radical nephrectomy and the nature of the studies preclude definitive conclusions regarding the beneficial effects of surgery in prolonging survival, delaying metastases, or improving the quality of life. In spite of these limitations our nonstructured review of the literature supports the practice of total surgical excision when possible.

Surgical Excision

Resection of a local recurrence is a challenging, carrying a significant morbidity and mortality related to the extensive nature of the radical resection.[9,27]

Surgery is often difficult because of the ill-defined characteristics of the mass and the infiltration or growth within neighbor organs.[9] Although no recommendations have been made, it seems reasonable to perform this kind of surgery in centers of reference and as a matter of fact all the reports on surgical treatment of isolated fossa recurrence reflect the experience of reference centers.[3–5,9,24,25,27] This or the use of adjuvant therapies can in some cases result in a delay between the time of diagnosis and the time of surgical treatment. In some series, a median interval of 1.4 years has been found between the diagnosis of the recurrence and the surgical treatment.[4]

Various types of incisions have been described to approach the mass: lumbar between ribs 11 and 12, subcostal, transperitoneal, extension of the primitive incision to a Chevron-type,[3] midline, and thoracoabdominal transperitoneal or extraperitoneal.[3–5,9,24,25,27,45] The surgeon must be prepared to resect adjacent organs because of frequent invasion of the spleen, colon, or pancreas (Fig. 8k-6). Partial hepatectomy and the resection of psoas or quadratus lumorum muscles and diaphragm have also been described. In some cases complete macroscopic resection is impossible, particularly when infiltration of the vascular planes (great vessels) or the liver is present.[4,24,27]

Complete resection of the mass is not always possible in 10–25% of cases[4,24,27,45] and enucleation then represents the only valid option.

In spite of the macroscopically en bloc removal of the mass, in approximately one-third to one-half of the cases the histological examination may reveal positive resection

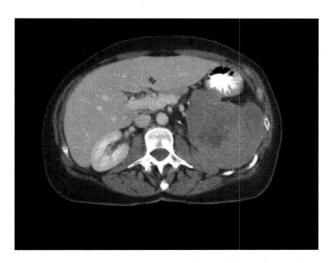

FIGURE 8k-6. Massive local recurrence (23 cm) 3 months after left nephroureterectomy because of PEComa. Surgical resection of the pancreatic tail was required as well as a partial left colectomy.

TABLE 8k-3. Operative data.[a]

Reference	Blood loss (median in ml)	Transfusion	Operative time (min)	Size of recurrence(cm)	Complications
Schrödter[25]	1.933 (300–3.500)	–	–	5.92 (2–10)	One wound seroma
Gogus[27]	–	–	–	8.45 (3–12)	One death colon leak
Master[3]	1.700[b]	Median 1 unit	450	6.35 (2–15)	42% (6 patients) pancreas leak in 29%
Itano[24]	2.800 (200–9.700)	67%	–	–	33% prolonged ileus, pneumonia, hydropneumothorax
Sandhu[4]	–	Median 2.5 units (0–12)	75 (60–135)	–	One wound infection, one chest infection, two incisional hernias
Tanguay[5]	950 (200–3.600)	–	–	–	31% subphrenic abscess, empyema, pneumonia, supraventricular tachycardia, pulmonary edema, and pyelonephritis

[a]Ranges are provided when available.
[b]Not recorded in three cases.

margins.[4,5] To ensure complete surgical resection a frozen section can be used at the surgeon's discretion.[5,25]

Complications are known to be high, varying from almost 0% to 43% (Table 8k-3). Intensive care requirements are not uncommon after this type of surgery, with up to 40% of the patients spending more than 1 day in the Intensive Care Unit.[3] Operative mortality is not negligible, accounting for 10–15% of the cases.[9,27]

The most frequent complication is the presence of a pancreatic leak following partial resection of the pancreas tail; this complication occurred in 29% of the patients in one series.[3] Management should be as conservative as possible, involving placement of percutaneous drains and the use of broad spectrum antibiotics. Other common complications are diarrhea, ileus, and pneumonia.

The mean hospital stay is approximately 10 days in most of the series.[3,5,25]

Other Treatment Strategies

No study has properly examined the role of systemic therapy in isolated fossa recurrence. In general, more than 50% of the patients included in the series have received some form of neoadjuvant treatment and are treated in an adjuvant setting with a combination of radiotherapy and immunotherapy. Systemic immunotherapy treatment seems to be of limited value in the treatment of local recurrence after radical nephrectomy. Early and more recent data indicate that patients with disease in the retroperitoneum and local recurrence of RCC generally do not respond well to immunotherapy and have a poor prognosis when treated only systemically.[46,47] Limited information concerning other types of treatment is available.

In the retrospective series of the Mayo Clinic[24] three different types of treatment were compared: observation (9 patients), medical therapy including chemotherapy or immunotherapy and radiation (11 patients), and complete surgical resection alone or in conjunction with additional therapy in 10 patients (4 receiving additional radiation and 2 postoperative immunotherapy). The reasons for the different choices are not clear, although comparison of basal characteristics among the three groups shows identical results. The mean follow-up in this series was 3.3 years with a median of 1.6 years. The 5-year cause-specific survival rates were 51% (SE 18), 18% (SE 12), and 13% (SE 12) for the surgical intervention, medical therapy, and observation groups, respectively.

Some authors suggest that an aggressive approach with a combination of systemic therapy and surgical resection is the best way to treat isolated fossa recurrence. In his series Tanguy shows a difference in the rates of disease-free patients depending on whether they were treated with a combination of biological therapy and surgery or they were treated with surgery alone (50% vs. 25%).[5] However, the small number of patients does not allow for conclusive statements.

Prophylactic radiotherapy of the surgical field has neither improved the disease-free survival nor diminished the rate of local recurrence in randomized studies,[20,50,51] thus suggesting its role in a curative setting after the diagnosis of local recurrence is minimal.

In fact, three randomized studies postoperatively delivered between 45 and 55 Gy to the tumor bed, suggesting only a positive local regional effect in case of nodal involvement but no effect at all on survival.[20,50,51] It is, however, worth mentioning that the data of the Sarcoma Study Group (National Cancer Institute) showed a better local control in the group treated by intraoperative radiation and external beam radiation than in the group treated only by intraoperative radiation.[52]

Intraoperative radiation therapy (IORT) has been used by some[3] in a mean dose of 1500 Gy (1200–2000) as a standard adjuvant treatment for RCC local recurrence. This adjuvant maneuver, however, failed to prevent reoccurrence in the renal fossa in 2 of the 10 patients treated and a difference in survival between those who received and those who did not receive intraoperative radiation was not apparent.[3]

Based on experimental studies showing enhancement of the effect of interleukin (IL)-2 by local tumor irradiation, a prospective study was launched in patients with progressive metastatic RCC combining immunochemotherapy [IL, interferon (IFN)-2a, and fluorouracil] with radiotherapy on the metastatic site.[53] Seven patients presented with local recurrence, of whom only three had no evidence of other sites. Of the four patients in whom the only target of radiation was the local fossa recurrence, three were able to discontinue all pain medication after the treatment and one reported remarkable pain relief. This study supports the fact that radiation therapy may be a useful palliative for symptomatic local recurrences not amenable to radical surgery. Together with selective embolization this has been used in anecdotal reports.[54] Guidelines on indications for the use of radiotherapy in RCC concluded that in case of local recurrence radiotherapy can be used as a palliative measure following a multidisciplinary team decision and after considering the prognostic factors. No standard dose is recommended.[49]

Other forms of ablation such as radiofrequency and thermal ablation have been used in the setting of local recurrence with the potential of reduced morbidity, but no consistent reports have been found in the literature and its durability and efficacy remain to be determined.[55,56]

Prognosis of Isolated Local Recurrence

It remains controversial whether an aggressive surgical approach can prolong survival. Although a long term survival can be attained by surgical resection interventions,[5,9] overall the occurrence of a local recurrence is an ominous sign with more than half of the patients developing distant metastasis and only one third surviving at long term. Survival after surgical resection can be equally attributed to the indolent course of the disease.

Development of Metastatic Disease

The heterogeneity of the series in regard to the type of patients included (with or without neoadjuvant treatment) and the variety of adjuvant treatments makes it difficult to assess the results. In fact two-thirds of the operated patients

developed distant metastasis and one-third also developed local recurrence.

Between 61% and 64% of the patients will develop distant metastasis both associated and not associated with recurrence in the renal fossa between 2 and 72 months after surgery.[3–5,9,24,25,27] The average time for the development of metastatic disease is around 17 months[5,25] (Table 8k-4).

Recurrence in the renal fossa may develop in 25–50% of the patients in spite of aggressive surgery and a totally macroscopic resected mass[3,4,24] usually in the course of the first year. Isolated recurrence in the fossa in the absence of distant metastasis is extremely rare.

The median time to local relapse was slightly longer for the development of recurrent tumor in the already treated fossa than for the development of distant metastases (2.4 vs. 4.3 years), although this was not significant in one series.[4]

Survival

Disease-free survival is described in Table 8k–2. The series are consistent that in the absence of metastatic disease or recurrence in the fossa, a long-term disease-free survival can be achieved in one-third of the patients. One- and 5-year overall crude and cause-specific survival was 66% and 28%, respectively, in the Mayo Clinic series.[24]

Specific cancer mortality increases with longer follow-up[3,5,25,27] and it is related to the development of distant metastasis (Table 8k-4). Depending on the mean-median follow-up of the series mortality varies from 22% at a mean time of 8.5 months[27] to 65% at a mean time of 17 months.[3] A slightly lower specific cancer mortality, 55% at a mean time of 23 months, has recently been described.[25] Non-cancer-related death seldom occurs.[9]

Prognostic Significance of Isolated Local Recurrence

In spite of the limited number of patients included in the series an effort to determine the local recurrence factors that may play a role in the course of the disease after surgery or other types of treatment has been made by some authors (Table 8k-5).

The presence of *tumor at the resection margin while microscopic or macroscopic* seems to be a significant factor in

TABLE 8k-4. Mortality and development of metastasis after treatment of isolated fossa recurrence.

Reference	Number of patients	Perioperative mortality	Follow-up	Metastasis	Cancer mortality	Mean time mortality
Schrödter[25]	13	0	36 months	8 (61.5%)	7 (54%)	23 (4–68) months
Gogus[27]	10	1 (10%)	16.6 months	2 (22%)	2 (22%)	3–14 months
Master[3]	14	0	34 months	–	9 (64%)	Mean 17 (±16) Median 14 (1–57)
Itano*[24]	30	0	3.3 years; median 1.6	25 (83%)	–	–
Sandhu[4]	14	0	1.65 years	9 (64%)	–	–
Esrig[9]	11	2 (18%)	1.0 years (0.25–6.5)	–	3 (33%)	–
Tanguay[5]	16	0	–	10 (62.5%)	4 (25%)	14.5 (9– 26)

TABLE 8k-5. Prognostic factors from the local recurrence for disease-free survival.

Prognostic factor	Significance/(reference)
Presence of tumor at resection margins	Adverse ($p < 0.05$)/(4)
Time to recurrence after nephrectomy	Shorter adverse time ($p < 0.05$)/(25)
Size of recurrence	Larger adverse time ($p < 0.06$)/(25)

predicting local and distant metastasis disease-free survival.[4] While this fact may be attributed to an inadequate surgical technique, it most likely indicates the aggressive nature of the disease.[4] In general, the presence of positive margins (macroscopic or microscopic) suggests a very bad prognosis with all the patients either dying shortly thereafter or presenting with metastases.[5]

In a recent series *time to recurrence after nephrectomy* was significantly longer (79.3 vs. 16.5 months) and the size of the recurrent tumor significantly smaller (4.3 vs. 7.2 cm) in the survivors.[25] The time to recurrence approached significance in the series of Master.[3] However, these two prognostic factors have not been confirmed by others.[27]

A cut-off of a 3-year interval between radical nephrectomy and the diagnosis of isolated local recurrence revealed a markedly although not significantly different postrecurrence survival time.[25] Patients with a longer disease-free interval after nephrectomy tend to demonstrate improved survival (RR 0.74), but the figure did not reach statistical significance.[24] Although most of the modern studies did not show statistical significance, considering the strong link between the disease-free interval from nephrectomy and survival in case of distant metastases,[57] there is a definitive trend to improved survival in those cases with a long disease-free interval between primary nephrectomy and the occurrence of local recurrence.

There was no survival advantage for patients who were symptomatic versus those who were asymptomatic ($p = 0.94$) in the Mayo Clinic series.[24] Other factors without statistical significance were the original T stage and size of the tumor. Primary histological type and Fuhrman grade do not bear any significance in the development of a local recurrence. The Fuhrman grade of patients who died was 3.22 versus grade 2 for survivors, which did not reach statistical significance ($p = 0.07$).[3]

One series suggests a better prognosis when local recurrence originates from the soft tissue in the renal fossa and does not involve the ipsilateral adrenal gland.[5]

Adjuvant treatment (radiotherapy, immunotherapy, and resection of isolated lung lesions) prior to the diagnosis of local recurrence does not have any impact on isolated fossa recurrence. There were no differences in postrecurrence survival or the interval between nephrectomy and recurrence in those groups that received adjuvant treatment and those that did not.[24,25] The mean time to recurrence and the mean

survival time in the adjuvant group therapy were 53 and 34.5 months, respectively, and were 38.7 and 39.4 months for the group that did not receive any adjuvant treatment.[25] IORT has no impact on survival; death in the group of patients receiving it was 60% vs. 75% in the group of patients who did not receive IORT.[3]

A detailed analysis of the different treatment groups in the series of Itano was carried out looking for factors accounting for the apparent survival benefit in the surgical group.[24] There were no statistical differences in original T stage grade or tumor size between those treated with surgery and those treated medically. However, patients who had undergone surgery were younger and had a longer median disease-free interval between nephrectomy and ipsilateral fossa recurrence (reflecting medical practice and possible bias in the study), although neither alone accounted for the apparent survival benefit in the regression analysis.[24] The mean comorbidity index was also similar in surgery and medically treated patients.[24] As expected, a higher comorbidity index was associated with a higher likelihood of death from comorbid disease.[24]

Surveillance After Radical Nephrectomy for the Diagnosis of Local Recurrence

If the goal is to diagnose local recurrence, two questions arises: how long do we have to follow the patients after radical nephrectomy and which patients have to be more intensively followed?

Local recurrence may appear either early in the course of the disease or very late, with local recurrences described as late as 15 years after nephrectomy. However, the incidence of isolated fossa recurrence is scarce and consequently it should be desirable to select patients at high risk of developing such an event to spare costs and social anguish.

While historically patients with pT3-4 tumors have a high risk of recurrence in the renal bed, those patients are also more prone to develop distant metastasis, with a poor prognosis, and are less suitable for a radical excision of the local recurrence.

On the other hand, at least theoretically, early detection should made local recurrence more amenable to surgery with a supposedly diminished morbidity. Probably the widespread use of ultrasound, easy to perform and cheaper than cross-sectional imaging, would obviate the matter of cost. However, ultrasound of an operated renal fossa may be difficult to evaluate and result in false-positive or false-negative results. Furthermore, there is no body of literature supporting the sensitivity and specificity of ultrasound in the rare event of local fossa recurrence.

A CT scan is currently the gold standard imaging technique in the diagnosis of local recurrence in the renal bed. In the presence of a basal postoperative CT scan, subsequent changes should be interpreted as a local recurrence. In the case of renal insufficiency or documented allergy to iodine contrast, an MRI should replace the CT scan.

Patients with advanced local staging at the time of nephrectomy (T3 or T4) should be followed every 6 months for the first 3 years with clinical assessment and chest X-ray, with an annual follow-up thereafter. The greater risk of abdominal relapse indicates they should receive surveillance with an abdominal ultrasound or CT scan at 6, 12, 24, and 36 months postoperatively if treatment is to be advised.[1] Based on the mean and median time of the appearance of the local recurrence (Table 8k-2), retroperitoneum scanning should be prolonged to at least 5 years if the goal is the diagnosis of a local recurrence.

References

1. Stephenson A.J., Chetner M.P., Rourke K., Gleave M.E., Signaevsky M., Palmer B., Kuan J., Brock G.B., Tanguay S. Guidelines for the surveillance of localized renal cell carcinoma based on the patterns of relapse after nephrectomy. J Urol, 2004, 172: 58–62.

2. Lorh M., Rohde D. Recidivtumor beim nierenkarzinom. Urologe A, 2005, 44: 358–368.

3. Master V.A., Gottschalk A.R., Kane C., Carroll P.R. Management of isolated renal fossa recurrence following radical nephrectomy. J Urol, 2005, 174: 473–477.

4. Sandhu S.S., Symes A., A'Hern R., Sohaib S.A., Eisen T., Gore M., Christmas T.J. Surgical excision of isolated renal-bed recurrence after radical nephrectomy for renal cell carcinoma. BJU Int, 2005, 95: 522–525.

5. Tanguay S., Pisters L.L, Lawrence D.D, Dinney C.P.N. Therapy of locally recurrent renal cell carcinoma after nephrectomy. J Urol, 1996, 155: 26–29.

6. De Kernion J.B., Belldegrun A. Renal tumours. In: Walsh PC, Retik AB, Stamey TA, et al (eds): Campbell's Urology, 5 ed. Philadelphia, W.B. Saunders, 1992, p. 1053

7. De Kernion J.B., Ramming K.P., Smith R.B. The natural history of metastatic renal cell carcinoma: a computer analysis. J Urol, 1978, 120: 148–152.

8. Campbell S.C., Novick A.C. Management of local recurrence following radical nephrectomy or partial nephrectomy. Urol Clin North Am, 1994, 21: 593–599.

9. Esrig D., Ahlering T.E., Lieskovsky G., Skinner D.G. Experience with fossa recurrence of renal cell carcinoma. J Urol, 1992, 147: 1491–1494.

10. Levy D.A., Slaton J.W., Swanson D.A., Dinney C.P. Stage specific guidelines for surveillance after radical nephrectomy for local renal cell carcinoma. J Urol, 1998, 159: 1163–1167.

11. Beisland C., Medby P.C., Beisland H.O. Presumed radically treated renal cell carcinoma. Recurrence of the disease and prognostic factors for subsequent survival. Scand J Urol Nephrol, 2004, 38: 299–305.

12. Froehner M., Manseck A., Lossnitzer A., Wirth M.P. Late local and pulmonary recurrence of renal cell carcinoma. Urol Int, 1998, 60: 248–250.

13. Bloom D.A., Kaufmann J.J., Smith R.B. Late recurrence of renal tubular carcinoma. J Urol, 1981, 126: 546–548.

14. Nakano E., Fujioka H., Matsuda M., Osafune M., Takaha M., Sonoda T. Late recurrence of renal cell carcinoma after nephrectomy. Eur Urol, 1984, 10: 347–349.

15. Takashi M., Hibi H., Ohmura M., Sato K., Sakata T., Ando M. Renal fossa recurrence of a renal carcinoma 13 years after nephrectomy: a case report. Int J Urol, 1997, 4: 508–511.

16. Minervini A., Salinitri G., Lera J., Caldarelli C., Caramella D., Minervini R. Solitary floating vena caval thrombus as a late recurrence of renal cell carcinoma. Int J Urol, 2004, 11: 239–242.

17. Oxford Centre for Evidence Based Medicine. Level of Evidence. May 2001. Available at http://www.cebmnet/levels-of-evidence.asp.

18. Alter A.J., Uehling D.T., Zwiebel W.J. Computed tomography of the retroperitoneum following nephrectomy. Radiology, 1979, 133: 663–668.

19. Rafla S. Renal cell carcinoma: natural history and results of treatment. Cancer, 1970: 25: 26–40.

20. Finney R. An evaluation of postoperative radiotherapy in Hypernephroma treatment: a clinical trial. Br J Urol, 1973, 45: 258–269.

21. Sease W.C., Belis J.A. Computerized tomography in the early postoperative management of renal cell carcinoma. J Urol, 1986, 136: 792–794.

22. Parienty R.A., Pradel J., Richard F., Khoury S. Recurrence after nephrectomy for renal cancer: CT recognition. Prog Clin Biol Res, 1982, 100: 409–415.

23. Phillips E., Messing E.M. Role of lymphadenectomy in the treatment of renal carcinoma. Urology, 1993, 41: 9–15.

24. Itano N.B., Blute M.L., Spotts B., Zincke H. Outcome of isolated renal cell carcinoma fossa recurrence after nephrectomy. J Urol, 2000, 164: 322–325.

25. Schrödter S., Hakenberg O.W., Manseck A., Leike S., Wirth M.P. Outcome of surgical treatment of isolated local recurrence after radical nephrectomy for renal cell carcinoma. J Urol, 2002, 167: 1630–1633.

26. Manikanadan R., Srinivasan V., Rane A. Which is the real gold standard for small-volume renal tumors? Radical nephrectomy versus nephron-sparing surgery. J Endourol, 2004, 18: 39–44.

27. Gogus C., Baltaci S., Beduk Y., Sahinli S., Kupeli S., Gogus O. Isolated local recurrence of renal cell carcinoma after radical nephrectomy: experience with 10 cases. Urology, 2003, 61: 926–929.

28. Giuliani L., Giberti C., Martorana G., Rovida S. Extensive surgery for renal cell carcinoma: Long-term results and prognostic factors. J Urol, 1990, 143: 468–473.

29. Stein M., Kuten A., Halpern J., Coachman N.M., Cohen Y., Robinson E. The value of postoperative irradiation in renal cancer. Radiother Oncol, 1992, 24: 41–44.

30. Lam J.S., Shvarts O., Leppert J.T., Pantuck A. J., Figlin R.A., Belldegrun A.S. Postoperative surveillance protocol for patients with localized and locally advanced renal cell carcinoma based on a validated prognostic nomogram and risk group stratification system. J Urol, 2005, 174: 466–472.

31. Uson A.C. Tumor recurrence in the renal fossa and or abdominal wall after radical nephrectomy for renal cell carcinoma. Prog Clin Biol Res, 1982, 100: 594–560.

32. Canfield S.E., Kamat A.M., Sanchez-Ortiz R.F., Detry M., Swanson D.A., Wood C.G. Renal cell carcinoma with nodal

metastases in the absence of distant metastatic disease (clinical stage TxN1–2Mo): the impact of aggressive surgical resection on patients outcome. J Urol, 2006, 175: 864–869.

33. Cangiano T., Liao J., Naitoh J., Dorey F., Figlin R. Sarcomatoid renal cell carcinoma: biologic behaviour, prognosis, and response to combined surgical resection and immunotherapy. J Clin Oncol, 1999, 17: 523–528.

34. Hornick J.L., Fletcher C.D. PEComa: what do we know so far? Histopathology, 2006, 48: 75–82.

35. Lam J.S., Leppert J.T., Figlin R.A., Belldegrun A.S. Role of molecular markers in the diagnosis and therapy of renal cell carcinoma. Urology, 2005, 66: 1–9.

36. Davidson B., Konstantinovsky S., Nielsen S., Dong H.P., Berner A., Vyberg M., Reich R. Altered expression of metastasis-associated and regulatory molecules in effusions from breast cancer patients: a novel model for tumor progression. Clin Cancer Res, 2004, 10: 7335–7346.

37. Majhail N.S., Urbain J.L., Albani J.M., Kanvinde M.H., Rice T.W., Novick A.C., Mekhail T.M., Olencki T.E., Elson P., Bukowski R.M. F-18 fluorodeoxyglucose positron emission tomography in the evaluation of distant metastases from renal cell carcinoma. J Clin Oncol, 2003, 21: 3995–4000.

38. Dechet C.B., Zincke H., Sebo T.J., King B.F., LeRoy A.J., Farrow G.M., Blute M.L. Prospective analysis of computerized tomography and needle biopsy with permanent sectioning to determine the nature of solid renal masses in adults. J Urol, 2003, 169: 71–74.

39. Eshed I., Elias S., Sidi A.A. Diagnostic value of CT-guided biopsy of indeterminate renal masses. Clin Radiol, 2004, 59: 262–267.

40. Skinner D.G., Vermillon C.D., Colvin R.B. The surgical management of renal cell carcinoma. J Urol, 1972, 107: 705–710.

41. Vogl U.M., Zehetgruber H., Dominkus M., Hejna M., Zielinski C.C., Haitel A., Schmidinger M. Prognostic factors in metastatic renal cell carcinoma: metastasectomy as independent prognostic variable. Br J Cancer, 2006, 95: 691–698.

42. Skinner D.G., Colvin R.B., Vermillion C.D., Pfister R.C., Leadbetter W.F. Diagnosis and management of renal cell carcinoma. A clinical and pathological study of 309 cases. Cancer, 1971, 28: 1165–1177.

43. Newmark J.R., Newmark G.M., Epstein J.I. et al. Solitary late recurrence of renal cell carcinoma. Urology, 1994, 43: 725–728.

44. McNichols D.W., Segura J.W., de Weerd J.H. Renal cell carcinoma: long term survival and late recurrence. J Urol, 1981, 126: 17–23.

45. Panchev P., Ianev K., Georgiev M., Kirilov S., Kumanov K.H. Fossa carcinoma–a relapse or rest carcinoma of the kidney. Khirurgiia, 2000, 56: 33–34.

46. Mani S., Todd M.B., Katz K., Poo W.J. Prognostic factors for survival in patients with metastatic renal cancer treated with biological response modifiers. J Urol, 1995, 154: 35–40.

47. Krigel R.L., Padavic-Shaller K.A., Rudolph A.R., Konrad M., Bradley E.C., Comis R.L. Renal cell carcinoma: treatment with recombinant interleukin 2 plus beta interferon. J Clin Oncol, 1990, 8: 460–467.

48. Kjaer M., Frederiksen P.L., Engelholm S.A. Postoperative radiotherapy in stage II and III renal adenocarcinoma: a randomized trial by the Copenhagen Renal Cancer Study group. Int J Radiat Oncol Biol Phys, 1987, 13: 665–672.

49. Beckendorf V., Bladou F., Farsi F., Kaemmerlen P., Negrier S., Philip T., Terrier-Lacombe M.J. Standards, options et recommendations pour la radiotherapie du cancer du rein. Cancer/Radiother, 2000, 4: 223–233.

50. Frydenberg M., Gunderson L., Hahn G., Fieck J., Zincke H. Preoperative external beam radiotherapy followed by cytoreductive surgery and intraoperative radiotherapy for local advanced primary or recurrent renal malignancies. J Urol, 1994, 152: 15–21.

51. Bussuti L., Jacopino B., Ferri C., Benati A. Adjuvant radiotherapy after simple nephrectomy for kidney carcinoma with extracapsular diffusion. 6th Annual ESTRO meeting, Lisbon, 25 May, 1987.

52. Sindelar W.F., Kinsella T.J., Chen P.W., DeLaney T.F., Tepper J.E., Rosenberg S.A. et al. Intraoperative radiotherapy in retroperitoneal sarcomas. Final results of a prospective randomized clinical trial. Arch Surg, 1993, 128: 402–410.

53. Brinkmann O.A., Bruns F., Gosheger G., Micke O., Hertle L. Treatment of bone metastases and local recurrence from renal cell carcinoma with immunochemotherapy and radiation. World J Urol, 2005, 23: 185–190.

54. Nickolissen R., Fallon B. Locally recurrent hypernephroma treated by radiation therapy and embolization. Cancer, 1985, 56: 1049–1051.

55. Rohde D., Albers C., Mahnken A., Tacke J. Regional thermoablation of local or metastatic renal cell carcinoma. Oncol Rep, 2003, 10: 753–757.

56. MacLaughlin C.A., Chen M.Y., Torti F.M., Hall M.C., Zagoria R.J. Radiofrequency ablation of isolated local recurrence of renal cell carcinoma after radical nephrectomy. AJR Am J Roentgenol, 2003, 181: 93–94.

57. Kavolius P., Mastorakos D.P., Pavlovich C., Russo P., Burt M.E., Brady M.S. Resection of metastatic renal cell carcinoma. J Clin Oncol, 1998, 16: 2261–2266.

9
Minimal Invasive Therapies

9a
Cryosurgery

Gyan Pareek, Brunolf W. Lagerveld, and Stephen Y. Nakada

Introduction

During the past decade there has been a resurgence of cryotherapy in the field of urology, particularly in the treatment of malignant lesions of the kidney. Much of the interest has been promoted by the advancement of radiographic technology and surgical instrumentation, along with the movement toward providing minimally invasive therapeutic options for patients. Currently, select kidney lesions are treated using cryotherapy. Although limited long-term survival data utilizing cryotherapy are available, recent series have provided compelling results, promoting interest in renal cryoablation. This chapter assesses the current status of cryotherapy, specifically the indications, techniques, and clinical results in treating kidney tumors.

Background

Cryotherapy destroys cells by consecutive rapid freeze and thaw cycles, leading to cellular necrosis at temperatures of −19.4°C or less.[1] Complete cell death of normal renal parenchyma is obtained with temperatures as low as −40°C in the targeted area. It has been suggested that for renal malignancies a temperature below −50°C is needed to create absolute cell death.[2] In addition to the depth of the temperature reached, the amount of treatment time at the low temperatures, thawing after a freeze cycle, and repetitive freeze cycles seem to enhance the lethal effect. Cell death is caused by direct cell destruction during the freeze cycles, by ischemia due to vascular injury, and indirectly by a molecular-based cellular response to freezing manifested by apoptosis.[3] The therapeutic use of cryoablation dates back to mid-nineteenth century England with the use of crushed ice and salt solutions capable of attaining temperatures of −20°C.[4] In 1961, Cooper and Lee introduced the first apparatus for cryotherapy, which paved the way for modern cryoablation.[5] Since then, tumors in various organs have been treated with cryoablation and probes of various shapes and sizes have been designed to improve tumor accessibility and ablation.

Noninvasive imaging modalities have led to an increase in the number of incidentally detected kidney masses. The result has been a stage migration to smaller lesions at initial diagnosis and the emergence of nephron-sparing surgery as a more prevalent treatment option for kidney tumors less than 4 cm. Nephron-sparing surgery is also appealing since approximately 15% of small solid contrast-enhanced lesions will be benign.[6] Currently, minimally invasive treatments in carefully selected patients includes laparoscopic partial nephrectomy and ablative procedures such as cryoablation, radiofrequency ablation, high-intensity focused ultrasound (HIFU), interstitial laser, microwave thermotherapy, and photon irradiation. The benefits of these minimally invasive therapies include nephron-sparing, decreased morbidity, decreased hospital stay, and shorter recovery. The current role of cryotherapy has continued to evolve since its initial introduction by Uchida and associates who performed the first kidney percutaneous cryosurgery in 1995.[7]

Indications

The optimal circumstances for renal cryotherapy is a peripheral, enhancing, well- circumscribed lesion less than 4 cm. In general, all patients with a small renal tumor are fit for cryotherapy. In particular, along with tumor characteristics, certain patient populations may benefit from kidney cryotherapy. They include elderly patients with comorbidities, particularly hypertension, diabetes, kidney stones, renal insufficiency, cerebrovascular accidents, and congestive heart failure. Other considerations include unique situations such as lesions less than 4 cm in a solitary or transplant kidney, along with certain hereditary conditions such as von Hippel–Lindau disease, tuberous sclerosis, and hereditary papillary renal cell carcinoma (HPRCC).[7,8] Contraindications to kidney cryoablation include locally advanced and/or metastatic disease and uncontrolled bleeding disorders. Other relative contraindications include lesions contiguous with bowel, great vessels, and/or tumor size of at least 5 cm.[8]

Preoperative Considerations

Routine preoperative preparation for renal cryoablation involves a thorough history and physical examination, along with a complete blood count, basic metabolic panel, urine analysis, and culture. Radiographic evaluation, to rule out metastatic disease, includes a chest radiograph and abdominal computed tomography (CT scan) with contrast in an early and delayed phase. A bone scan is reserved for patients with abnormal calcium and/or alkaline phosphatase levels. Magnetic resonance imaging (MRI) is indicated in patients with contrast allergy or renal insufficiency. The majority of patients require preoperative clearance from an internist or a specialist for the comorbidities. All patients should be notified of all possible treatment options, which include a detailed discussion about the limitations, expectations, and possible complications. An informed consent should be signed if indicated. Patients should be informed about the potential for performing a radical nephrectomy, laparoscopic or open, if the situation demands. A bowel preparation with 300 ml of magnesium citrate with a clear liquid diet a day prior to surgery can be performed. We usually admit patients on the day of surgery. Patients are usually typed but not cross-matched for blood. The procedure is coordinated with an experienced radiologist as intraoperative laparoscopic ultrasound is paramount for the success of the procedure.

Techniques

Overview

Operating Room and Team

The patient is placed in a flank position with the affected side up. The surgical team is positioned depending on the planned surgical approach. The primary surgeon, the first assistant, and the scrub nurse stand facing the abdomen (transperitoneal approach) and facing the spine (retroperitoneal approach). The laparoscopic monitors are stationed at the patient's shoulders and angled slightly toward the feet at a comfortable eye level to the operating personnel. The tower containing the laparoscopic insufflator, the light source, and the camera are positioned across the primary surgeon to facilitate monitoring of the pressure recordings. Next to the tower are the ultrasound machine and the computer that drives the freezing probes. The bottles of argon and helium gas are placed near the computer but should be secured from falling but be easy to change whenever they turn out to be empty during the procedure. The harmonic and electrocautery generator units are at the patient's feet across the primary surgeon. The suction irrigator/aspirator system is hung on the anesthetic pole on the side of the primary surgeon at the head end of the table. The scrub nurse's mayo stand is placed directly above the patient legs and the remaining laparoscopic instruments are placed on another table in an L-shaped configuration for easy access.

Patient Positioning

We routinely pad the operating table with two layers of foam to minimize the risk of neuromuscular injury. A Foley catheter and orogastric tube are inserted after induction of anesthesia. The patient is positioned in a semiflank position (15–20° from vertical) for a transperitoneal approach and full flank position for a retroperitoneal approach. The kidney rest is slightly elevated and the table flexed at the level of the twelfth rib. The down leg is flexed and the upper leg is placed straight with pillows oriented at right angles to the legs. Sequential compression devices and stockings are routinely used to prevent deep venous thrombosis. Two arm boards are placed side by side at the level of shoulder with foam padding. A foam roll is positioned two fingerbreadths below the axilla to prevent injury to the brachial plexus. Multiple pillows are placed between the upper extremities to support the upper arm. The patient is secured to the table with a safety strap over the lower extremities at the level of the calves. A cautery pad is strapped on the upper thigh and a 3-inch-wide cloth tape is used to strap the patient from the edge of the table to the other edge of the table. The upper torso is stabilized by using 3-inch-wide cloth tape from the edge of the table at the level of the shoulders and is split into two strips past the elbows and is attached to either side of the arm boards. All monitoring wires and intravenous lines are placed so that they are not under the patient at any point. A pneumatic warming device may be used on the upper torso to prevent hypothermia (Fig. 9a-1).

Surgical Mapping/Trocar Placement

Anatomic landmarks are marked on the patient's abdomen. We routinely delineate the midline, xyphoid process, costal margin, and the rib 12. The procedural steps vary by the type of surgical approach.

Transperitoneal Approach

The procedure is done by insufflating the peritoneal cavity through a Veress needle, midway between the umbilicus and the superior iliac crest just lateral to the rectus muscle.

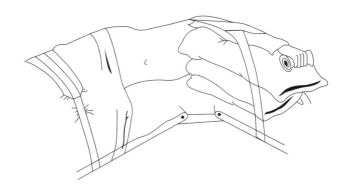

FIGURE 9a-1. Patient's positioning for laparoscopic transperitoneal cryoablation.

The drop-test confirms safe intraperitoneal needle placement. Furthermore, the first port placement and insufflating the peritoneal cavity can also be done via an open access procedure. The abdomen is insufflated up to 15 mm Hg pressure. A 10-mm or 5-mm nonbladed trocar is passed into the abdomen using an optiview system for the camera, depending on the surgeon's choice of using a 5- or 10-mm telescope. A second 10-mm port is placed at the lateral margin of the umbilicus and the third port is placed in a subcostal position, just lateral to midline, half way between the xyphoid and the umbilicus. The second and third ports could be 5 mm or 10 mm depending on the side of the lesion and the dominant hand of the surgeon. An additional 5-mm port may be necessary on the right side to retract the inferior margin of the liver about two fingerbreadths below the costal margin in the mid-axillary line. A Hasson cannula is utilized at the surgeon's discretion, most commonly in cases with previous abdominal surgery (Fig. 9a-2). Of course the configuration of the ports can be different according to the surgeon's preferences. It is important to make sure that there is enough space to come from the right angle with the probe(s) placement. Furthermore, it can be useful for all 10- to 12-mm ports, except for the one in the flank position, to be able to come from different directions with the ultrasound and the camera. In this way the needle placement and the ice development can be optimally monitored.

Retroperitoneal Approach

A Hasson cannula is inserted through a horizontal 2-cm incision and is placed 1 cm below and lateral to the tip of rib 12. The latissimus dorsi muscle fibers are bluntly separated and the retroperitoneum is entered by opening the anterior lamella of the thoracolumbar fascia. Blunt finger dissection is performed to develop space by pushing the peritoneum away from the psoas major muscle. Balloon

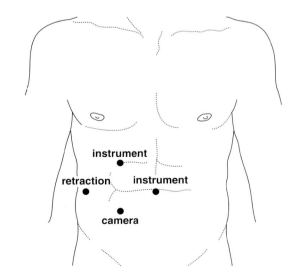

FIGURE 9a-2. Trocar placement for a transperitoneal approach.

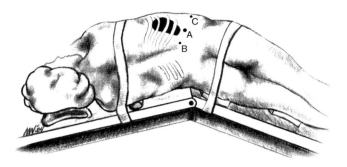

FIGURE 9a-3. Trocar placement for a retroperitoneal approach illustrating port sites for Hassan trocar (**A**) and 2.5-mm ports (**B** and **C**).

dilation of the retroperitoneal space is not routinely necessitated. If conservative measures to gain access to the retroperitoneal space fail, a trocar-mounted balloon could be used to develop adequate working space by instilling 800–1000 ml as described by Gill and his associates. A 10-mm blunt tip trocar is placed after removing the balloon dissection device and it is secured by inflating the internal retention balloon and cinching the external foam cuff. A Hassan cannula could also be used and it is tightly fixed by using fascial sutures around the trocar. Two more secondary ports are placed under vision, one 10/12-mm trocar is placed three fingerbreadths above the iliac crest in the anterior axillary line and the other 10/12-mm trocar is placed lateral to the erector spinae muscle just below rib 12 (Fig. 9a-3).

Exposure of the Lesion

The camera is inserted via the lower quadrant port and the surgeon operates with the subcostal and periumbilical ports in the transperitoneal approach. To obtain a comfortable position with "the eyes in the middle of the hands," some surgeons prefer to insert the camera in the middle port. The Harmonic scalpel is typically used to incise the line of Toldt and for subsequent exposure of the renal mass through the Gerota's fascia. In exophytic lesions it is usually straightforward, but mesophytic and endophytic lesions need intraoperative ultrasound to locate the lesions and exclude multicentric lesions. Ultrasound can also assess for other lesions in the remainder of the kidney. Extensive mobilization of colon, spleen, and hilum is not necessary. In medial located tumors of the lower pole it is sometimes necessary to identify the ureter and to mobilize it away from the intended ice ball. In the retroperitoneal approach, the camera is inserted via the middle port with the surgeon operating through the medial and lateral ports. Maintaining the orientation and identifying the psoas major muscle are very important in this approach. We routinely use laparoscopic ultrasound to help localize the renal mass and Gerota's fascia is incised and the renal mass is dissected by opening the perinephric fat. Once the renal lesion is identified and well exposed, the cryoablation technique is similar in both approaches. After finishing the procedure, hemostasis should be checked by lowering the pneumoperitoneum to 5 mm Hg and the larger abdominal ports are closed using a port closure device. We perform a simple closure of retroperitoneal ports.

Cryoablation

Cryotherapy of kidney tumors may be delivered by open, laparoscopic, or percutaneous approaches.[7, 10–21] Depending on the location of the lesion, the appropriate approach may be chosen. For example, posterior–lateral lesions may be approached percutaneously with imaging guidance (CT scan, MRI, or ultrasound), while more anterior lesions may be treated laparoscopically. However, posterior located upper pole tumors can be impossible to reach with the percutaneously image-guided technique because the kidney is not mobilized and the ribcage prevents a clear route toward the tumor with the probe(s). At our institutions the majority of lesions are treated laparoscopically. Furthermore, depending on surgeon preference and/or familiarity with anatomy, lesions may also be approached retroperitoneally.

After the approach is chosen, a stepwise protocol is used. The steps include mobilization of the kidney (open or laparoscopic), visualization of the lesion by ultrasound, minimal hilar and ureter dissection, and percutaneous or direct visualization of the probe placement. Before the probe placement a needle biopsy of the tumor can be taken for histology. In advance of the operation the exact size and configuration of the lesion are measured. A calculation of the number of probes needed is made. The placement of the probes should be checked with the aid of the intraoperative ultrasound, with the imaging technique chosen for the percutaneous approach. Thermometers can be placed in the lesion and outside of it in the normal parenchyma. The cryoablation starts with a freeze cycle with target tissues of −20°C. The cryolesion is readily visible as an ice ball on the ultrasound. The current thought is to await the disappearance of the cryolesion on ultrasound and refreeze according to the protocol described above. If the ultrasound image is not clear thawing is recommended until the temperature has reached 0°C in all thermometers. At the conclusion of the freeze and thaw cycles patience, on the part of the surgeon, is required at the time of probe removal. The probe disengages itself with time and manipulation of the probe prior to adequate thawing may result in bleeding from the probe track. Various hemostatic agents such as Surgicell, Gel Foam, and fibrin glue can be placed into the probe track after removal to ensure hemostasis.

Technological advances have led to the development of cryoprobes of various diameters and lengths to produce the desired cryolesion based on pretreatment planning. Most cryoprobes produce very low temperatures by allowing compressed gasses to boil at atmospheric pressures at the tip. Cryoablation is performed using an argon gas-based system that is operated on the Joule–Thompson principle. Based on the same principle helium gas can be used for active thawing. Cryoprobes are available in various diameters (1.47 mm, 2.4 mm, 3.0 mm, and 5.0 mm). Manufacturers now create

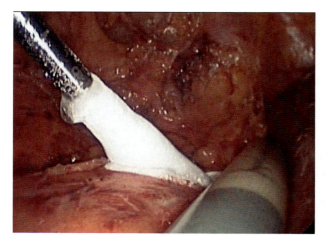

FIGURE 9a-4. Renal cryoablation with a single probe in progress with real-time ultrasound monitoring.

probes with different shapes of the ice ball at the end of the probe. The number and size of probes used in a case vary depending on the size and site of the tumor. Percutaneously approached lesions warrant the use of smaller probes; larger probes can be placed during laparoscopic procedures.

The procedure is begun with sonographic delineation of the lesion done under direct laparoscopic visualization or percutaneous ultrasound guidance. Figure 9a-4 illustrates typical cryolesions of a single probe and multineedle technique observed during a laparoscopic approach. The tumor is punctured with an appropriate sized probe(s) and cryoablation is initiated using two 10-minute freeze cycles followed by passive thaws. The freeze cycle is continued to 1 cm beyond the tumor margin. The cryolesion is monitored with real time ultrasonography performed by a radiologist experienced in laparoscopic ultrasound. Typically, an ice ball is generated during treatment. When probes are placed percutaneously, red rubber catheter tubing is placed around the probe to protect the skin and abdominal wall from cryoinjury. The skin can be rinsed with warm sterile saline to prevent frostbite. Before removal, passive thawing is allowed until the probe is loosened spontaneously. In renal cryotherapy, a piece of tightly rolled Surgicell (Ethicon, Somerville, NJ) is placed into the cryoprobe defect with injection of Tisseel (Baxter USA, Deerfield, IL) and held with direct pressure for 10 minutes. When thin probes are used the chance of bleeding is low. Compression of the bleeding probe site with surgicell is mostly sufficient. Postoperatively, a hematocrit is obtained.

Technical Considerations

Preoperative

The specific choices of probe design, number and size is determined based on the anatomical characteristics of the renal mass. Lesions near the renal hilum, lesions close to the collecting system and cystic lesions are generally not treated with cryotherapy at our institution.

Intraoperative

Intraoperative ultrasound, performed by an experienced radiologist, should be routinely used to delineate renal architecture as well as to rule out the possibility of multicentric disease and to guide proper probe placement. After defining the anatomy, we routinely perform double freeze and thaw cycles of 10 minutes duration each to achieve our goal of complete destruction of malignant cells. If indicated, multiple probes should be utilized to achieve adequate tumor kill. The importance of placing more than one cryoprobe to achieve adequate coverage of the whole tumor should not be overemphasized. We believe most of the recurrent tumors are persistent tumors that were missed in the earlier freezing. It is generally advised that a margin of 10-mm ice ball overlapping the tumor when performing intraoperative imaging is necessary to achieve adequate and dependable cell death. During and following treatment, venous bleeding is usually encountered, which could be controlled by pressure, packing with surgicell, and fibrin sealants as described earlier. Argon beam coagulation or laparoscopic suturing may be necessary on occasion. Patience on the part of the surgical team is required at the end of the procedure when assessing hemostasis. Intraabdominal pressures of 5 mm Hg should be utilized to assess hemostasis before concluding the procedure.

Patients should be advised to avoid strenuous activity for the next 2 weeks to prevent postoperative hemorrhage.

Follow-up

Radiographic imaging following cryotherapy establishes the effect of therapy. Many investigators have demonstrated that gadolinium-enhanced magnetic resonance imaging (MRI) is an effective means for posttreatment follow-up.[14,15] Other groups perform a contrast CT scan in the follow-up. Enhancement of a lesion at 30 days following treatment may be an ominous sign. Important criteria for assessing tumor recurrence with CT scan or MRI are lesion size and nodular enhancement. Rim enhancement with an increase in size is of more concern than rim enhancement alone.[12,13] In general, cryolesions demonstrate an increase in signal intensity on both T1- and T2-weighted images, but no enhancement (Fig. 9a-5). Serial MRIs, every 3 months after initial treatment, reveal a consecutive decrease in the size of the cryolesion by 40%.[15,16] The phenomena of no enhancement and decrease in size of the cryolesion are also seen with the CT scan during follow-up (Fig. 9a-6). Imaging of the lesion is performed every 3 months in the first year, every 6 months in the second year, and yearly thereafter. The role of renal biopsy in the follow-up remains questionable as long as the sensitivity is low, and thus leads to a definitive diagnosis.[17]

Pre-Gadolinium   Post-Gadolinium

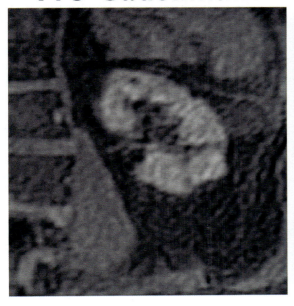
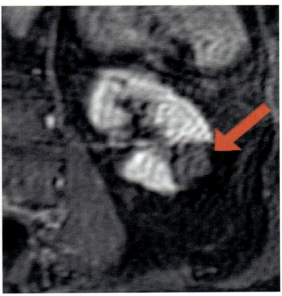

FIGURE 9a-5. Preoperative and postoperative MRI scan showing an exophytic enhancing renal mass (left) and nonenhancing cryoablated lesion.

(a)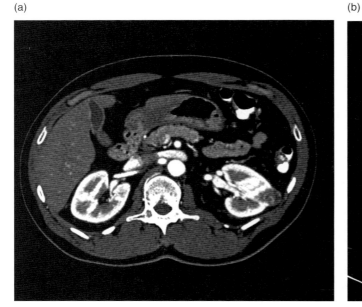

(b)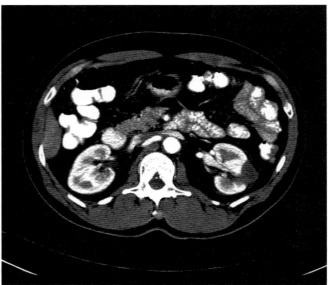

FIGURE 9a-6. (**A**) Preoperative CT scan with contrast showing an exophytic enhancing renal mass in the left kidney. (**B**) Postoperative CT scan with contrast showing the nonenhancing cryoablated lesion of (**A**) 3 months after surgery.

Results

To date, 10 laparoscopic series with a follow-up of 18 months provide the most abundant data for cryoablated kidney lesions. Only 3 of these, along with unpublished data from our institution, includes 20 or greater patients and are shown in Table 9a-1.[14–17] Gill et al.[20] reported their 3-year follow-up of laparoscopic kidney cryoablation in 56 patients with a total of 60 tumors. In 36 patients biopsies showed that the tumor was a renal cell cancer. All patients were treated with a double freeze–thaw cycle, under laparoscopic and ultrasonographic guidance. Follow-up consisted of MRI on postoperative day 1 and at months 3, 6, and 12 and semiannually thereafter until the cryolesion was no longer visible. In addition, CT-guided biopsies of all patients were performed at 6 months postoperatively. The mean patient age was 65 years. The mean preoperative tumor size was 2.3 cm (1.5–3.7 cm). Follow-up biopsies postcryoablation showed residual renal cancer in two patients (5.6%). New kidney lesions developed at a different site in three patients. At 3 years the overall patient survival and cryoablation-specific survival were 89% and 100%, respectively.

Recently, Cestari et al.[21] reported on 37 patients with a mean age of 64 years (range 29–89 years). The mean lesion diameter was 2.57 cm (range 10–60 cm). According to tumor position, 22 cases were approached transperitoneally and 15 retroperitoneoscopically. Postoperative follow-up included MRI on postoperative day 1 and 1, 3, 6, 12, 18, and 24 months after surgery, and annually thereafter. Six months following the surgical procedure biopsy of the site of the treated neoplasm was performed. The laparoscopic procedure was successfully completed in all cases. The mean operative time was 194 minutes (range 120–300 minutes) and mean blood loss was 165.3 ml (range 20–900 ml). The final histological evaluation revealed renal cell carcinoma in 29 cases and oncocytoma in 6, while 2 were reported as indefinite. All patients were discharged home after a mean of 3.8 days (range 3–7 days) and returned to normal social life after a mean of 7.3 days (range 5–9 days). Early and postoperative complications were evaluated. The mean diameter of the cryolesion on postoperative day 1 on MRI was 48.2 mm and it progressively decreased during follow-up. Of the 35 patients with at least 6 months of follow-up CT-guided biopsy was performed in 25, who were negative for neoplasm. One patient underwent

TABLE 9a-1. Laparoscopic cryoablation series (*n* <greater than> 20).

Year	Reference		Tumor size (cm)	OR time(minutes)	Blood loss(ml)	Mean follow-up(months)	Comp.
2003	Lee[19]	20	2.6	305	92.5	14.2	1
2004	Gill[20]	56	2.3	180	—	36	4
2004	Cestari[21]	37	2.5	194	163	20.5	4
2005	Wisconsin(unpublished)	35	2.5	136	57	14.3	1
2005	AMC Amsterdam(unpublished)	22	2.3	206	—	9	3
Total	5	170	2.4	204.2	104.2	18.8	13

a radical nephrectomy because of renal cell cancer near the cryoablated region that was negative at biopsy.

The University of Wisconsin laparoscopic series (unpublished data) includes 34 patients with a mean follow-up of 17.2 (1–50) months. There were 23 men and 11 women with 17 tumors on the right and 17 on the left side. Eighteen patients were treated retroperitoneoscopically and 16 transperitoneally. The mean tumor size was 2.7 cm. A double freeze, active thaw technique was utilized with two 10-minute freeze cycles. The mean operating time was 182 minutes and the mean blood loss was 40 ml. Usually, patients were discharged on the first postoperative day. Two lesions showed peripheral enhancement at the previously cryoablated site. One had peripheral rim enhancement with an increase in size of the cryoablated site with nodular enhancement in the subsequent follow-up scans and biopsy was consistent with active disease. This patient underwent partial nephrectomy. The other patient had no further nodular enhancement with a decrease in size of the cryoablated site. One patient developed nodular enhancement 9 months postoperatively with no previous rim enhancement.

The Academic Medical Center of Amsterdam laparoscopic series (unpublished data) includes 22 patients with a mean follow-up of 9 months (1–24 months). The mean age at treatment was 65.7 years (51–80 years). In total, 7 tumors were located on the right and 15 on the left in 12 men and 10 women. A laparoscopic approach was transperitoneal and retroperitoneal in 13 and in 9, respectively. In the last group one conversion to open cryoablation was needed due to hypercapnia. The mean tumor size was 2.3 cm (range 1.3–3.6 cm). All patients except for one had a functional contralateral kidney. In 16 patients a preoperative biopsy was taken. In six of these patients a renal cell cancer was proven. For the cryoablation 1.47-mm cryoneedles (Oncura) are used. A multineedle configuration is always needed. Depending on the size of the tumor the number of cryoneedles used varied from 3 to 10 needles. For monitoring the ice developing process both thermocouples as ultrasound are used. A double freeze cycle with passive thaw is always achieved. The mean operating time was 206 minutes (106–397 minutes). The mean number of days of postoperative stay in the hospital was 5 (range 1–32). All patients are followed up with contrast CT scan. So far no persistence or recurrence has occurred. During the entire follow-up no biopsies are performed.

Complications

Cryoablation for renal cell carcinoma aims to decrease morbidity by treating renal tumors *in situ*, eliminating the need for extirpation. The procedure may involve potential complications previously unassociated with renal tumor treatment. Recently, groups at medical centers with reported experience with cryoablation of renal tumors participated in a study in which each group submitted retrospective data regarding overall ablative treatment experience and associated complications. For each incident the nature of the complication, its associated morbidity, the necessity and nature of any subsequent interventions, and the final patient outcome were evaluated. Complications were divided into minor and major categories. Data were collected from groups at four institutions with a combined experience of 139 cases. The major and minor complication rates attributable to cryosurgery were 1.8% and 9.2%, respectively.[22] The five major complications reported included ileus, hemorrhage, conversion to open, scarring with ureteropelvic junction obstruction, and urinary leakage. Overall, the most common complication, as well as the most common minor complication, was pain or paresthesia at the probe insertion site.

Conclusions

Renal cryotherapy has been a well-investigated procedure and short-term results demonstrate it to be safe and efficacious. The predominant application in the kidney is for peripheral lesions less than 4 cm in patients who would benefit from nephron-sparing surgery. Long-term survival data will assess the true effectiveness of the treatment. The cytocidal effect and durability of cryoablation appear promising. Recently, Jang et al. demonstrated the long-term tumoricidal effect of cryotherapy in three patients who underwent radical nephrectomy an average of 275 days after laparoscopic cryoablation of renal tumors. Indications for surgery were positive postcryosurgery biopsies in two patients and a newly discovered metachronous lesion in one patient. Histopathology revealed no viable tumor in the nephrectomy specimens.[23] Although cryotherapy appears durable, the ideal treatment delivery system has yet to be defined. Real-time monitoring of cryolesions is still evolving and its accuracy is dependent on the skill and experience of the operator. There are not enough data regarding the treatment of tumor margins in the larger lesions and the safety of cryoablation for the lesions near the collecting system and kidney hilum. The next major challenge is the evaluation of clinical results. Limited postcryoablation imaging and biopsy results were reported. A decrease in size of the tumor, absence of growth, and lack of enhancement on CT/MRI may be viewed as oncological success. Rukstalis et al.[11] recommend routine follow-up biopsy, although to date only 6 months of biopsy data are available. Serial biopsies at regular intervals are ideal, but an optimal biopsy schedule is yet to be determined and biopsies are not without sampling errors and patient morbidity.

Future directions for renal cryotherapy include the administration of various adjunctive cryoenhancers in order to maximize cell death. These include the use of chemotherapeutic agents such as cyclophosphamide, 5-fluorouracil, and bleomycin.[24,25] These agents can be administered systemically or may be injected directly into the tumor. Additionally, technologies such as electrical impedance tomography are under investigation to improve real-time monitoring of the cryolesion at surgery.[26] The immune-mediated response following cryotherapy has also become an interesting area of research. At our institution, Hedican et al. recently reported survival advantages in a murine renal cancer model of cryotherapy over nephrectomy. The significance of these findings has become an intense area of research and immune system enhancers delivered at the time of cryotherapy are currently under investigation.[27]

References

1. Chosy SG, Nakada SY, and Lee FT, et al.: Monitoring kidney cryosurgery: predictors of tissue necrosis in swine. J Urol 159:1370–1374, 1998.
2. Gage AA, Baust J.: Mechanisms of tissue injury in cryosurgery. Cryobiology 37:171–186, 1998.
3. Hoffman NE, Bischof JC. The cryobiology of cryosurgical injury. Urology 60 (suppl 2a):40–49, 2002.
4. Arnott J: Practical illustrations of the remedial efficacy of a very low or anesthetic temperature I: In cancer. Lancet 2:257–259, 1850.
5. Cooper IS, Lee A: Cryostatic congelation: a system for producing a limited controlled region of cooling or freezing of biologic tissues. J Nerve Mental Dis 133:259–263, 1961.
6. Jacqmin D, van Poppel H, Kirkali Z, Mickisch G: Renal cancer. Eur Urol 39:361–369, 2001.
7. Uchida M, Imaide Y, Sugimoto, K, et al.: Percutaneous cryosurgery for kidney tumors. Br J Urol 45:132–137, 1995.
8. Fergany AF, Hafez KS, Novick AC: Long term results of nephron sparing surgery for localized kidney cell carcinoma: 10 year follow-up. J Urol 163:442–445, 2001.
9. Uzzo RG, Novick AC: Nephron sparing surgery for kidney tumors: indications, techniques and outcomes. J Urol 166:6–18, 2001.
10. Delworth MG, Pisters LL, Fornage BD, von Eisenbach AC: Cryotherapy for kidney cell carcinoma and angiomyolipoma. J Urol 155:252–254, 1996.
11. Rukstalis DB, Khorsandi M, Garcia FU: Clinical experience with open kidney cryoablation. Urology 57:34–39, 2001.
12. Gill IS, Novick AC, Soble JJ: Laparoscopic kidney cryoablation: initial clinical series. Urology 52:543–551, 1998.
13. Lowry PS, Nakada SY: Kidney cryotherapy: 2003 clinical status. Curr Opin Urol 13:193–197, 2003.
14. Shingleton WB, Sewell PE: Percutaneous kidney tumor cryoablation with MRI guidance. J Urol 165:773–776, 2001.
15. Ankem MK, Moon TD, Hedican SP, et al.: Is peripheral rim enhancement a sign of a recurrence of kidney cell carcinoma post cryoablation (abstract). J Urol 171(suppl), 2004.
16. Soble JJ, Gill IS, Novick AC, et al.: Ultrasound and MRI characteristics of laparoscopic kidney cryolesions (abstract). J Urol 161(suppl):368, 1999.
17. Richter F, Kasabian NG, Irwin RJ Jr, Watson RA, Lang EK: Accuracy of diagnosis by guided biopsy of renal mass lesions classified indeterminate by imaging studies. Urology 55(3):348–352, 2000.
18. Gill IS, Novick AC, Meraney AM, et al.: Laparoscopic kidney cryoablation in 32 patients. Urology 56(5):748–753, 2000.
19. Lee DI, McGinnis DE, Feld R, Strup SE: Retroperitoneal laparoscopic cryoablation of small kidney tumors: intermediate results. Urology 61(1):83–88, 2003.
20. Gill IS, Remer EM, Hasan WA, et al.: Renal cryoablation: outcome at 3 years. J Urol 173(6):1903–1907, 2005.
21. Cestari A, Guazzoni G, dell'Acqua V, et al.: Laparoscopic cryoablation of solid kidney masses: intermediate term follow-up. J Urol 172:1267–1270, 2004.
22. Johnson DB, Solomon SB, Su LM: Defining the complications of cryoablation and radiofrequency ablation of small renal tumors: a multi-institutional review. J Urol 172:874–877, 2004.
23. Jang TL, Wang, R, Kim, SC: Histopathology of human renal tumors after laparoscopic renal cryosurgery. J Urol 173(3):720–724, 2005.
24. Clarke DM, Baust JM, Van Buskirk RG, Baust JG: Chemo-cryo combination therapy: an adjunctive model for the treatment of prostate cancer. Cryobiology 43:274–285, 2001.
25. Mir LM, Rubinsky B: Treatment of cancer with cryochemotherapy. Br J Cancer 86:1658–1660, 2002.
26. Baust JG, Gage AA: Progress toward optimization of cryosurgery. Tech Cancer Res Treat 3:95–101, 2004.
27. Hedican SP, Wilkinson ER, Lee FT, Warner TF, Nakada SY: Cryoablation of advanced renal cancer has survival advantages in a murine model compared to nephrectomy. J Urol 171(4):Suppl., 2004 (abstract 778).

9b
Radiofrequency Ablation of Renal Masses

Michael C. Ost and Benjamin R. Lee

Introduction

Radiofrequency ablation (RFA) continues to emerge as an alternative treatment for renal tumors of an exophytic nature that are less than 4 cm in size. It is a beneficial minimally invasive treatment option that may be delivered laparosopically or percutaneously without general anesthesia. Significant advancements in energy-based treatments coupled with an increasing rate of incidentally detected small renal masses with sophisticated cross-sectional imaging[1] have given impetus to the refinement of alternative options in the treatment of these smaller renal masses. Trends in ablative techniques are following the trends of treatment efficacy demonstrated with nephron-sparing surgery for the definitive treatment of renal cell carcinoma (RCC).[2,3] Since the initial description to treat *in vivo* renal tumors by Zlotta and colleagues in 1997,[4] there have been refinements in RFA technology applied to a substantial cohort of patients over a relatively brief period of time. Short-term data have demonstrated radiographic and oncological efficacy, substantiating RFA as an additional minimally invasive treatment modality in the treatment of small renal tumors.

Indications, Safety, Physiological Effects, and Possible Postprocedure Complications

RFA has been approved in the United States by the Food and Drug Administration (FDA) for the treatment of soft tissue tumors. Much of the initial clinical experience with RFA has come from treatment of metastatic liver tumors.[5,6] Its use for ablation of renal tumors is still considered investigational. Within this investigational arena, RFA is indicated as a treatment for exophytic renal masses less than 4 cm in greatest dimension. It has been used to effectively treat both symptomatic metastatic RCC lesions for palliative purposes and isolated local RCC recurrences following radical nephrectomy.[8] Most importantly, RFA is primarily useful and indicated for treating renal lesions in patients with comorbidities that preclude a major surgical procedure such as partial nephrectomy or laparoscopic partial nephrectomy.

RFA may also be considered as an adjunct to hemostasis in patients undergoing laparoscopic partial nephrectomy[9,10] as RFA treatments have demonstrated the ability to coagulate and induce thrombosis and necrosis in renal tissue.[11,12] Gettman and associates, for example, used RFA as an adjunct to hemostasis during laparoscopic partial nephrectomy (LPN).[9] Ten patients underwent so-called radiofrequency (RF) coagulation-assisted LPN in which the RF probe was inserted under laparoscopic guidance and the tumor was ablated along with a margin of normal parenchyma. The tumor was then excised with laparoscopic scissors and the surgical bed was biopsied to confirm negative margins on frozen section. The mean tumor size was 2.1 cm and the median blood loss was 125 ml. All surgical margins were negative.

RFA prior to partial nephrectomy may aid in bypassing the time constraints and adverse effects associated with hilar control and clamping while maintaining excellent hemostasis.[13] The use of RFA is somewhat contraindicated in patients who have intraparenchymal tumors, as injury to the collecting system may result. Because of potential thermal injury to adjacent organs, laterally or posteriorly situated tumors are more amenable to treatment via image-guided percutaneous therapy, while medial or anterior lesions are better treated laparoscopically.

Typical minor morbidities associated with RFA include hematuria, perirenal hematoma formation, and discomfort at points of cutaneous probe insertion. Major morbidities associated with RFA have not been consistently reported although documented. Johnson et al. described a patient who developed a symptomatic uteropelvic junction (UPJ) obstruction following laparoscopic RFA treatment of a 2.3-cm exophytic biopsy proven renal cell carcinoma located on the medial-mid pole.[14] The patient ultimately underwent nephrectomy at 11 months posttreatment for a persistently obstructed collecting system with 8% overall function. Interestingly, no residual renal cell carcinoma was observed on pathological analysis. The experience with this patient, however, suggests that medial tumors near the collecting system should perhaps not be treated with RFA in order to minimize the potential complication of collecting system fibrosis and obstruction.

Thermal injury to collateral structures is therefore a potential complication during renal tumor RFA. A laparoscopic approach may have a slight advantage in this regard as critical structures may more readily be dissected away from tumors prior to treatment. In a percutaneous approach, thermocouples may monitor adjacent organ temperatures to avoid thermal injury. Experimental techniques to insure bowel protection during RFA sessions have been described. Farrell et al., for example, described two patients in whom a hydrodissection technique with sterile water was used under sonographic guidance to displace bowel in too close proximity to renal tumors prior to RFA treatments.[15] In addition, Kam et al. described the use of carbon dioxide dissection with balloon distraction to protect bowel segments during both percutaneous RFA and cryotherapy treatment of renal cell carcinomas.[16]

The impact of ablated tissue on the remaining kidney parenchyma was investigated by Johnson and colleagues.[17] In a cohort of 25 patients with 26 tumors treated with either laparoscopic RFA or percutaneous RFA, blood pressure measurements and serum creatinine levels were obtained preoperatively and at postoperative office visits. Using these objective endpoints with a minimum of 6 months follow-up, no patient experienced new onset hypertension or worsening of existing hypertension. In addition, no significant changes in mean serum creatinine or estimated creatinine clearance were observed. These findings indicate that RFA does not adversely affect surrounding renal parenchyma when small renal tumors are treated. Conversely, a case report from the same institution described a transiently induced acute renal failure following multiple site RFA combined with standard partial nephrectomy in a solitary kidney.[18] It was hypothesized that the cold ischemia time with hilar clamping (56 minutes) compounded the effect of the multiple RFA insults.

In a unique animal study, Ng and colleagues compared the systemic immune responses of RFA, cryotherapy, and surgical resection in a porcine liver model.[19] Better preservation of the systemic immune response has been demonstrated following minimally invasive procedures such as laparoscopic cholecystectomy when compared to open controls. In Ng's study, the systemic responses after RFA treatments, as measured by tumor necrosis-a and interleukin-1, were significantly less severe than those of cryotherapy. However, the increase in serum inflammatory markers and pneumonitis after RFA was substantial when compared to the hepatectomy group.

Su et al. demonstrated the short-term efficacy of percutaneous computed tomography (CT)-guided RFA of renal masses in 26 high-risk surgical patients.[20] After using a dry RFA technique in a cohort of patients with advanced age (>70 years), high ASA scores, or comorbidities, 13 treated renal lesions were followed for more than 1 year with 85% (11/13) demonstrating no residual enhancement or growth after treatment. Complications in this cohort of patients include the development of small hematomas, a liver burn, and a mortality secondary to aspiration pneumonia 2 days after an RFA treatment. Similarly, an 88% success rate was reported in a prospective study by Roy-Choudhury et al. in which percutaneous RFA was performed in 8 patients with 11 solid lesions. This cohort of patients was selected based on coexistent morbidity.[21]

There is merit to studies that investigate the efficacy of RFA in the treatment of small incidentally found renal masses (<4.0 cm) in patients older than 70 years of age. The greatest incidence of such tumors is found in those patients aged 70–90 years,[22] and it is not uncommon for the comorbidities present in this patient cohort to influence management decisions. Although it had been shown that conservative management of incidental contrast-enhancing renal masses may be a short-term safe alternative to more invasive therapies,[23] RFA is a minimally invasive option for those who wish to be treated.

The objective of a study by Zagoria and colleagues was to determine not only the success rate of percutaneus RFA in treating renal tumors, but also the risk of serious complications.[24] All ablations were accomplished with the impedance-based Radionics system. No serious complications occurred in their cohort of patients who had a 91% (20/22) radiographic success rate at an average of 7 months follow-up. Unlike other studies, a large percentage of patients (77%) had biopsy-proven renal cell carcinoma. In specific, complications reported within the first 24 hours of treatment included mild pain (15%), mild perinephric hematoma (33%), and mild pain and pneumothorax 4% (1/27). None of these complications required an intervention or prolonged hospital stay and no additional complications were found on follow-up clinical and radiographic evaluation.

Radiofrequency Ablation Mechanics, Delivery, and Equipment Specifications

Mechanism

The goal of RFA is the destruction of tissue using RF energy delivered through a probe inserted into the target tissue. RF energy is delivered in the form of alternating electrical current at very high frequency (over 400,000 Hz), causing agitation of tissue ions, which results in local production of heat through friction.[25,26] As tissue temperature rises, the tissue begins to desiccate and impedes the delivery of current to areas beyond the zone of desiccation, limiting the size of the ablation zone. It has been shown that heating tissue to 55–60°C for about 5 minutes results in irreversible cellular damage, and heating to over 60°C causes cell death and tissue coagulation.

Delivery

There are two basic types of RF delivery systems, impedance based and temperature based. Both types use probes with single or multiple tines, which are inserted into the target tissue to deliver alternating electrical current. Impedance-based systems are capable of sensing the rise in tissue impedance (essentially the resistance to flow of electrical current) as the tissue around the probe begins to desiccate, and they feed back to the generator to alter the delivery of current accordingly. Temperature-based RF systems use a similar mechanism to sense the change in tissue temperature around the probe, also feeding this information back to the generator, which again alters the delivery of current as appropriate to heat tissue to the desired target temperature. RF energy can be delivered either by an image-guided percutaneous route or laparoscopically under intraoperative ultrasound guidance.

Generators

Currently available RF generators include those from RITA Medical Systems, Radionics, and Medi-tech (formerly Radiotherapeutics, recently acquired by Boston Scientific) (Fig. 9b-1). The Model 1500 is the most recently introduced generator from RITA and is temperature based. It can deliver up to 150 W of power at 460 kHz. The Radionics and Medi-tech RF-3000 generators are impedance based and can deliver up to 200 W of power at 480 kHz. All generators require placement of disposable grounding pads on the patient, and these are provided with each kit.

Probes

Probes are configured as a needle that can be inserted into tissue and from which tines are deployed to create a target lesion. The RITA system uses the StarBurst XL probe, which is a 10-, 15-, or 25-cm-long, 14-gauge needle that houses nine tines that are deployed in front of the probe in a starburst configuration after the probe is inserted into the tissue (Fig. 9b-2a). This probe can be adjusted to create target lesions of 3–5 cm. Five of its nine tines have thermocouples to monitor local tissue temperature. The generator computes the average temperature of the five thermocouples to adjust energy delivery.

The Medi-tech system uses the LeVeen probe, which deploys multiple tines in an umbrella configuration (Fig. 9b-2b). The probe is placed by inserting a nonconducting cannula (available in various lengths) with a trocar

(a)

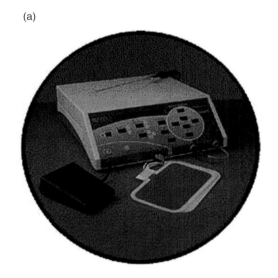

(b)

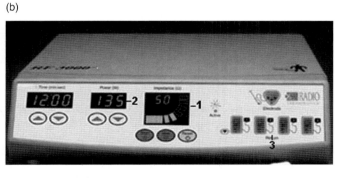

FIGURE 9b-1. (**A**) Temperature-based RITA Model 1500 Generator. (**B**) Impedance-based Medi-Tech RF 3000 Generator.

(a)

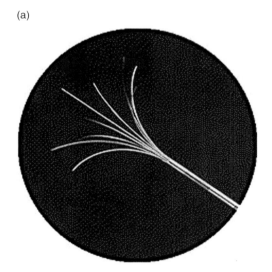

(b)

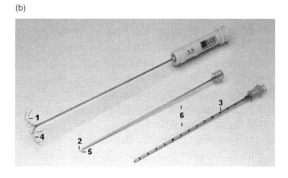

FIGURE 9b-2. (**A**) RITA StarBurst XL. (**B**) LeVeen Probe.

needle into the tissue. The tip of the trocar needle is echogenic, allowing positioning under ultrasound guidance. The needle is removed and the LeVeen probe is passed through the cannula, after which the tine array is deployed.

The Radionics system uses the Cool-tip probe, which circulates water internally in order to cool the tissue adjacent to the electrode, with the intent of delaying tissue desiccation so that energy can be delivered further from the electrode. Although used with an impedance-based generator, the Cool-tip probe also has a thermocouple to monitor local tissue temperature. It is designed as a single, straight, needle electrode, or cluster of three electrodes. The probe is 17 gauge and comes in lengths of 10, 15, 20, and 25 cm. It can create lesions 1–3 cm in diameter.

Imaging and Assessment of Ablated Margins

RFA probes are most often positioned under ultrasound or CT guidance, but may also be delivered laparoscopically with ultrasound assistance. A recent Phase II clinical trial using interactive magnetic resonance imaging (MRI) for guided RF interstitial thermal ablation of primary renal tumors[27] shows promise as an additional imaging modality during RFA treatments. Present day technology, however, does not allow for accurate real-time imaging of RF lesions as they are created; this is unlike cryolesions or lesions induced by high-intensity focused ultrasound (HIFU).[28] This is one of the main drawbacks of RF therapy and is an active area of ongoing research. Therefore, to confirm efficacy, initial follow-up imaging should be performed at 1, 3, and 6 months. Adequate imaging includes either a CT scan with and without intravenous contrast or, in patients with renal compromise, gadolinium-enhanced MRI. A treated lesion should show less than 10 Hounsfield units (HU) of enhancement on CT after contrast administration. MRI should show no evidence of qualitative enhancement after gadolinium infusion.

The natural posttreatment architectural and radiographic changes seen with RF ablated renal tissue differ from that of cryoablated tissue. Renal tumors successfully treated by cryoablation, for example, consistently demonstrate loss of enhancement and tissue retraction.[29] It has been a consistent observation that renal tumors successfully treated with RFA may not necessarily regress or decrease in size.

Matsumoto et al. described the *unique evolution* of RFA-treated lesions on contrast-enhanced CT (CE-CT) scan.[30] Sixty-four consecutive renal tumors were imaged with CE-CT at 6 weeks, 3 months, 6 months, and every 6 months after RFA treatments for a median follow up of 13.7 months. Biopsies of these tumors were taken before and after RFA and sent for permanent section, the majority of which were confirmed to be a renal carcinoma (41/64). Renal tumors were treated percutaneously ($n = 34$), laparoscopically ($n = 28$), or at open surgery ($n = 2$). The majority (62/64) of renal tumors

demonstrated an absence of contrast enhancement on CE-CT. Endophytically treated tumors developed a low density, nonenhancing, wedge-shaped defect with fat infiltration seen between the ablated tissue and normal parenchyma. Interestingly, treated exophytic tumors retained a configuration similar to that of the original lesion with a lack of contrast enhancement and minimal shrinkage. In particular, tumors treated percutaneously developed a peritumor scar or halo that demarcated ablated and nonablated tissue such as perirenal fat. In the rare instance of tumor persistence and recurrence ($n = 2$), enhancement (> 10 HU) was noted within the borders of treatment. In summary, the authors concluded that tumors successfully treated by RFA did not necessarily regress in size, showed no contrast enhancement, and occasionally retracted from normal parenchyma with fat infiltration.

The efficacy of a pure percutaneous ultrasound-guided RFA approach was investigated in a small series by Veltri et al.[31] Using the RITA Model 1500 generator with a Starburst Electrode needle under "real-time" ultrasound guidance (Technos, ESAOTE, Genoa, Italy), 13 patients with 18 tumors were treated. A retroperitoneal approach was utilized in all but two patients where a transperitoneal transhepatic approach was chosen in order to access tumors in the right upper pole. Patients were followed by ultrasound every 3 months and by CT and MRI every 6 months. At a mean follow-up of 14 months, the success rate after a single treatment in tumors less than 35 mm was 88.2%, which rose to 94.1% after a second treatment was needed in the largest lesion treated (75 mm).

Lewin and Colleagues sought to evaluate the efficacy and safety of interactive MRI in RFA ablation of renal tumors.[27] Ten patients with contraindications to surgical resection underwent a Phase II clinical trial using a 200-W RFA system with custom-fabricated MRI-compatible cool-tip electrodes guided by a 0.2-T MRI unit. All tumors were exophytic with a mean size of 2.3 cm; renal cell carcinoma was confirmed by biopsy in 50% (5/10) of the patients. Tumor recurrences were defined as hyperintense soft tissue signals within the RFA zone or margin on T2-weighted or STIR MR images or areas of abnormal contrast enhancement within the treated region on postcontrast images. At a mean follow-up of 25 months, there were no complications or evidence of tumor recurrence on MRI. It is important to note from this study that in 70% of the patients proactive MRI during the course of treatment ("MR fluoroscopic guidance") led to electrode repositioning and repeat RFA cycles to carry treatment to an endpoint of successful delivery. Although the total procedure time was calculated to be approximately 3 hours, this original report suggests that MRI may be a future "real-time" imaging choice in RFA renal tumor ablation. The overwhelming 100% success rate in this study was also demonstrated by Farrell et al.[32] and De Baere et al.[33] in earlier studies.

A common criticism of RFA therefore is the inability to monitor the proactive treatment of tumors with complete and clear real-time intraoperative imaging. To further address this limitation, experimental infrared thermography and thermocouple mapping have been used to assess RFA treatment margin adequacy in a porcine model.[34] Ogan et al. produced laparoscopic RFA lesions in pigs using the RITA generator and probe at target temperatures of 105°C. To assess the margins during the treatment, multiple thermocouples and a laparoscopic infrared camera were used to measure and map surface parenchymal temperatures. The results of histological analysis of the ablated lesions with NADH staining were correlated with mapped temperatures. The average diameter of gross lesions on the surface of the kidney measured 17.1 mm and 22.4 mm for 1-cm and 2-cm ablations, respectively. On gross histological examination the average depth of the lesions measured 19 mm for 1-cm ablations and 25 mm for 2-cm ablations. When using the laparoscopic infrared camera, the aforementioned surface measurements correlated with an average diameter of 16.1 mm and 15.9 mm for 1-cm and 2-cm ablations, respectively. At a threshold temperature of greater than 70°C for visual temperature change, the infrared camera identified the region of pathological necrosis during the RFA treatment. Most importantly perhaps was the finding that all cells within the intended ablation zones were nonviable by NADH analysis.

Radiofrequency Ablation Basic Research

With regard to renal tumors, experience with the technique in humans preceded experimental studies in animals. Zlotta and associates were the first to test RF energy for human kidney tumor ablation in 1997.[4] They ablated tumors ex vivo in four kidneys removed for localized RCC and treated three patients in vivo prior to nephrectomy. This study demonstrated the safety of RF application, as there were no adjacent organ injuries in the in vivo group, and target lesion size was comparable to the size of the observed lesions. Subsequent experimental studies have been performed in rabbits and pigs and have been directed at evaluating the correlation between the target and observed lesion size, the histological effects of RF on renal parenchyma, the physiological effects on renal function, and the efficacy of ablating implanted tumors.

Polascik and associates performed RF ablation of VX-2 tumors implanted under the renal capsule of rabbits.[35] They used a saline-augmented system in which saline is infused into the tumor during ablation. Saline infusion prevents tissue desiccation from occurring in proximity to the probe and may enhance ablation. Conclusions regarding the viability of tumor cells after treatment could not be made because this was not a survival study. In a later study, animals were sacrificed at 5, 10, and 15 days posttumor ablation, but the efficacy of therapy was difficult to assess because of the rapid development of occult metastases with the VX-2 model.[36] An additional study using VX-2 tumors in a rabbit model has further confirmed a high metastatic rate when using this experimental cell

line.[37] Most recently, Nakada and colleagues compared the efficacy of RFA, cryoablation, and radical nephrectomy in the treatment of implanted VX-2 carcinomas.[38] Interestingly, at animal sacrifice posttreatment RFA, cryoablation, and radical nephrectomy were all efficacious in the treatment of implanted VX-2 renal tumors compared with untreated controls and no significant difference was found between any of the three treatments.

Gill and co-workers subsequently performed a survival study in which normal renal parenchyma was ablated in pigs, using the LeVeen umbrella-type probe to create a 3.5-cm target lesion.[39] They showed no adverse effect on serum creatinine or hematocrit levels acutely or chronically. The renal lesions resorbed and autoamputated over time. Retrograde pyelography showed no evidence of urinary extravasation at any time point. In a related study, the same group described the histological changes over time following RF. They demonstrated the presence of coagulative necrosis in animals sacrificed on postoperative day 3 but not in animals sacrificed immediately after treatment. This raises the question of how to best assess the efficacy of RFA in tissue that is removed immediately after treatment, before coagulative necrosis has time to develop.

A porcine study similar to that of Gill was performed later by Crowley and colleagues.[40] In this study, both laparoscopic and CT-guided percutaneous RFA of normal renal parenchyma was accomplished with the LeVeen electrode. One of the ablations in the laparoscopic group resulted in a urinoma. One animal in the CT-guided percutaneous group suffered a major psoas injury from unrecognized extension of the electrode tines out of the kidney. This study highlights the potential for adjacent organ and urinary collecting system injuries with both laparoscopic and image-guided percutaneous approaches.

The question of whether hilar occlusion prior to RFA significantly alters the lesion size was answered by Corwin and associates, who found no statistical difference in the sizes of lesions created with or without hilar occlusion.[13] Conversely, a recent study on RFA with or without renal artery balloon occlusion in a porcine model demonstrated that RFA with arterial occlusion consistently provides larger thermal lesions than RFA without arterial occlusion.[41] Of concern in this study, however, were the induced renal infarctions peripheral to the thermal lesions when an occlusion balloon was deployed. In a similar porcine study, Chang and colleagues induced RFA lesions with normal blood flow or with interrupted renal blood flow using vascular clamping or renal artery embolization.[42] Obstruction of renal blood flow before and during RFA resulted in larger thermal lesions with potentially less variation in size compared with the lesions created with normal nonobstructed blood flow. It was concluded in this study that selective arterial embolization of the kidney vessels may be a useful adjunct to RFA of kidney tumors.

Gettman and associates compared RFA using an impedance-based system (Medi-tech) to ablation with a temperature-based system (RITA Medical) and found that both types of generators created lesions of similar shape.[43] Overall, there were no significant differences in ablation characteristics between the two types of generators. In a different porcine experiment, Nakada and colleagues compared bipolar and monopolar RFA of the kidney.[44] *In vivo* studies showed two distinct gross lesions with RFA, blanched or hemorrhagic. Using bipolar RFA, larger and more predominant blanched lesions were achievable than with monopolar RFA. Studies comparing monopolar and bipolar RFA in humans have not been performed to date.

Histological Assessment

RFA produces coagulative necrosis on standard hematoxylin and eosin (H&E) staining. However, at least 24–48 hours is required for coagulative necrosis to develop. Therefore, histological assessment of a lesion before 24 hours will not reveal signs of irreversible cell death. Several investigators have noted the remarkable degree of preservation of tissue architecture in acutely ablated lesions assessed by H&E (Fig. 9b-3). An alternative to histological analysis in these situations is assessment of cellular viability, which can be performed using the NADH stain (Fig. 9b-4). NADH is a ubiquitous coenzyme present in both cytoplasm and mitochondria. It is integral to oxidation–reduction reactions in glycolysis, the Krebs cycle, and in the production of adenosine triphosphate. NADH-diaphorase is an enzyme present in cellular constituents that catalyzes the reduction of substrates by transfer of free electrons from NADH, yielding reduced substrate and NAD. One such substrate is *p*-nitroblue tetrazolium, a compound that when reduced produces an insoluble, dark blue pigment deposited at the site of NADH-diaphorase activity. Diaphorase has been shown to be active only in

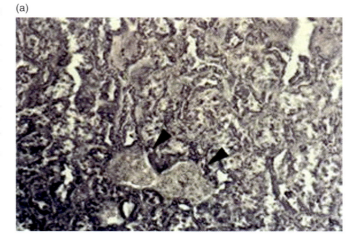

(a)

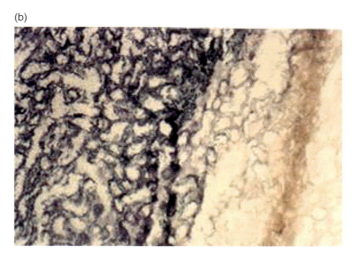

(b)

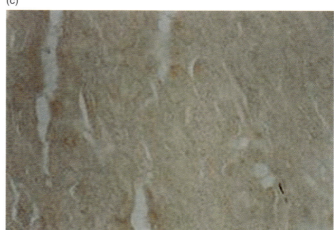

(c)

FIGURE 9b-4. (**A**) NADH stain of normal renal parenchyma. Arrowheads denote glomeruli. (**B**) Transition zone between unablated (left) and ablated (right) tissue on NADH stain. (**C**) Tissue section from the central zone of ablation showing lack of staining for NADH.

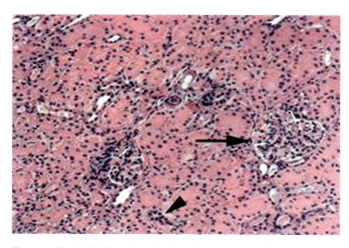

FIGURE 9b-3. H&E stain of ablated renal parenchyma showing extremely well-preserved architecture, glomerulus (arrow), and nuclear pyknosis (arrowhead).

viable cells, and its activity ceases immediately after cellular death. This staining method permits evaluation of tissue ablation based on a functional alteration, rather than on histological or morphological characteristics, which may be variably altered only after the intervention. With this stain, viable tissue appears blue, while nonviable tissue remains unstained and appears a tan color.

Marcovich et al. assessed RFA lesions with both H&E and NADH staining in a porcine model.[45] Ten kidneys underwent laparoscopic RFA of the upper and lower poles to a target temperature of 105°C. It was found that H&E staining of ablated tissue revealed a number of alterations in renal tubular histology at focal areas of treatment. Corresponding areas with NADH staining, however, showed the complete absence of staining, indicating the lack of cellular viability. In addition, there were no skip areas noted on NADH processed sections. The experimental findings of this study suggest that NADH staining should always be used to verify cellular death in RFA-treated lesions. In a follow-up study from the Long Island Jewish Medical Center, Tan et al. used the same porcine model to compare gross and microscopic pathological changes caused by saline-infused RFA vs. dry RFA.[46] No histopathological differences were seen between the two different RFA treatment modalities or if one vs. two wet RFA cycles were used. As in previous studies, NADH staining confirmed the lack of cellular viability; however, in these series of experiments it was noted that glomeruli were the last structures to lose viability in RFA-treated areas. It was concluded that RFA treatment of renal tissue is therefore *phasic* in nature and cell necrosis was ultimately *permanent*. An initial direct thermal phase causes acute cell death and a later subacute phase causes infarction of the distal arterial vascular supply to the ablated region, resulting in additional cell death and coagulative necrosis.

Most recently, Marguiles and colleagues reported on the acute histological effects of temperature-based RFA on pathological interpretation.[47] RFA was performed on 119 solid kidney tumors by percutaneous CT guidance, laparoscopically, or at the time of open surgery. Tumor specimens were obtained during percutaneous RFA using an 18-gauge TruCut needle, with a 5-mm cold-cup biopsy forceps during laparoscopy (or by partial nephrectomy if this was ultimately performed), and by incisional biopsy in the open cases. Overall, only 2.6% of specimens obtained before RFA and 5.7% obtained after RFA were nondiagnostic secondary to the paucity of tissue obtained. It was concluded that RFA of renal tumors causes predictable histological changes yet preserved tissue architecture. These *predictable* changes described in this cohort and previous studies included increased cytoplasmic eosinophilia, blood vessel dilation and blurring, nuclear elongation, and cytoplasmic dissolution. It is important to note that only H&E staining and not NADH analysis was used in this study and therefore tissue viability post-RFA, perhaps the most important pathological and oncological endpoint, was not assessed.

Clinical Studies and Oncological Outcomes: Laparoscopic versus Percutaneous Radiofrequency Ablation and Evaluation of Margin Status

To date approximately 16 clinical series of RF ablation have been reported in the literature. The majority of experience has come from reports on percutaneous delivery, although the laparoscopic approach and use during open nephrectomy has been described. Studies not mentioned in detail below have been cited elsewhere in the preceding text where relevant. Summaries of all studies may be found in Table 9b-1.

Laparoscopic Radiofrequency Ablation

Yohannes et al. were the first to describe laparoscopic radiofrequency ablation (L-RFA) of a solid renal mass.[48] Interestingly, this initial description was a retroperitoneal approach due to a prior history of transperitoneal open surgery in an elderly male (age 83) with significant comorbidities including renal insufficiency. Although the laparoscopic approach is gaining popularity among the minimally invasive community for the treatment of anterior renal tumors, there are presently few published studies that include cohorts of RFA cases performed only by this modality.

Jacomides et al.[49] presented the first sizable series of patients (n = 13 with 17 tumors) who underwent *in situ* laparoscopic RFA using a RITA Medical System. Ten of the treated patients proved to have focuses of renal carcinoma. In short-term follow-up (at least 6 weeks, mean of 9.8 months), 80% (8/10) of these patients did not have evidence of disease progression or radiographic recurrence by CT scan.

Figure 9b-5a demonstrates a CT scan of an enhancing exophytic lower pole renal mass that is positioned anteriorly. The patient with this mass was treated by laparoscopic wet RFA rather than a laparoscopic partial nephrectomy; a significant history of valvular heart disease requiring chronic oral anticoagulation therapy precluded an extirpative therapy. A follow-up CT scan (Fig. 9b-5b) demonstrated a successful treatment as evidenced by the lack of enhancement (<10 HU) after contrast administration (white arrow). Laparoscopic biopsy following RFA treatment revealed clear cell RCC with negative NADH staining.

Studies Investigating Both Laparoscopic and Percutaneous Radiofrequency Ablation

Hwang et al. recently reported on their intermediate outcomes on RFA-treated tumors in a cohort of 17 patients with 24 hereditary renal tumors.[50] A higher power 200-W cool-tip RF System (Radionics, Burlington, Massachusetts) was used under laparoscopic (n = 9) or percutaneous (n = 8) guidance

TABLE 9b-1. Radiofrequency ablation in the treatment of renal tumors.[a]

Study	Year	Average age	Number of patients treated	Number of tumors treated	Average tumor size (cm)	Overall average procedure time	Average blood loss	Success rates (radiographic)	Success rates (histological)	Follow-up
Hwang et al.[50]	2004	38	Lap (N = 9)	15	2.26	243 minutes ±29	67 ml ±9	92%		Median = 385 days
Lewin et al.[27]	2004	70	Perc (N = 8) Perc (N = 10)	9 10	2.26 2.3	3 hours ±27 minutes	NR	100%		25 months
Zagoria et al.[24]	2004	70	Perc (N = 22)	24	3.5	NR	NR	91%		7 months
Veltri et al.[31]	2004		Perc (N = 13)	18	Range 3.5–5.5			88.2%, 94.1% after salvage RFA		14 months
Jacomides et al.[49]	2003	59	Lap (N = 7) RFA assisted Lap partial (N = 5) Lap RFA + RFA assisted Lap partial (N = 1)	17	1.96	140 minutes 203 minutes	NR NA	80%		9.8 months
Su et al.[20]	2003	69	Perc (N = 29)	35	2.2 ± 0.7	NR	NA	85%		> 12 months for 13 selected patients
Gervais et al.[55]	2003	69	Perc (N = 34)	42	3.2	NR	NA	86%, 97% (after salvage RFA)		13.2 months
Mayo-Smith et al.[56]	2003	76	Perc (N = 32)	32	2.4	NR	NA	81%		9 months
Roy-Choudhury et al.[21]	2003		Perc (N = 8)	11	3	NR	NA	88%		17 months
Farrell et al.[32]	2003		Perc (N = 20)	27	1.7	NR	NA	100%		9 months
Ogan et al.[18]	2002	NR	Perc (N = 12)	13	2.3 ± 0.6	95 minutes	NA	93%		4.9 months
Pavlovich et al.[57]	2002	39	Perc (N = 21)	24	2.4 ± 0.4	NR	NA	79%		2 months
De Baere et al.[33]	2002	NR	Perc (N = 5)	5	3.3	NR	NR	100%		Median = 9 months
Rendon et al.[58]	2002	NR	Open (N = 4) then immediate nephrectomy Perc (N = 6) then delayed nephrectomy	5 4	2.4 (rad), 2.2 (gross)	NR	NR		20% 40%	NA NA
Matalga et al.[61]	2002	59.4	Open (N = 10) then immediate nephrectomy	10	3.2	NR	NR		80%	NA
Michaels et al.[61]	2002		Open (N = 15) then immediate nephrectomy	20	2.4				20%	NA
Total tumors treated				**321**						

[a] Lap, laparoscopic; Perc, percutaneous; NR, not recorded; NA, not applicable; RFA, radiofrequency ablation; rad, radical.

(a)

(b)

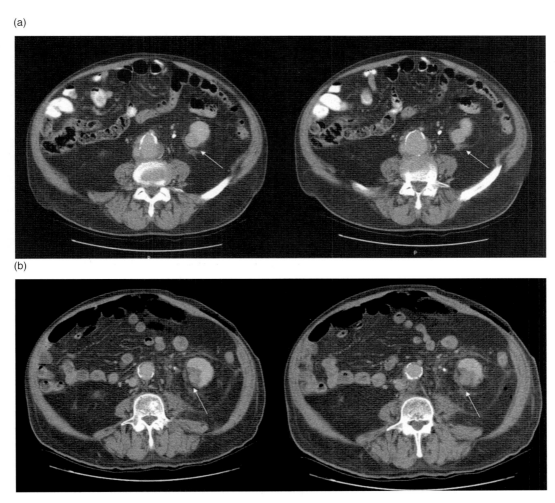

FIGURE 9b-5. (A) An enhancing, exophytic, lower pole renal mass (white arrow) treated by laparoscopic RFA. (B) Six-week follow-up CT scan of the mass treated in (A). Lack of enhancement on contrast CT (<10 HFU) indicating radiographic success (white arrow).

and all patients were followed for a minimum of 1 year. Of the 24 tumors treated, only 1 (4%) met radiographic criteria for recurrence on follow-up imaging (>10 HU enhancement). The recurrence was notable as it occurred in a central endophytic lesion that required intraoperative ultrasound for visualization and treatment. Similar to an induced fibrotic UPJ obstruction described by Johnson et al.,[17] one patient in this series whose tumor was adherent to the UPJ at the time of laparoscopic treatment developed a UPJ obstruction requiring an open repair. In this series a higher wattage-based system achieved a radiographic success rate of 92% at a minimum of 1 year follow-up.

Percutaneous Radiofrequency Ablation

The greatest clinical experience with RFA treatments of renal tumors has been with percutaneous delivery (Fig. 9b-6). In 1998, McGovern et al. were the first to report on the treatment of a 3.5-cm renal cell carcinoma via percutaneous placement of a needle electrode under ultrasound guidance.[51] Follow-up with CT at 3 months showed no evidence of radiographic recurrence. Since that time numerous case reports and small series combining RFA treatment with adjuvant modalities have been described. Hall et al., for example, successfully treated a 2.5 × 3.0-cm solid enhancing mass in a solitary kidney by combing percutaneous RFA with selective angioablation.[52] In the past 3 years, however, studies with sizable cohorts of patients have described percutaneous RFA treatments under CT, MRI, and ultrasound guidance with consistent success rates.

Ogan et al. reported on their experience with CT-guided percutaneous RFA in 12 patients with 13 tumors.[53] The RITA StarBurst probe was used to treat tumors with a mean size of 2.3 cm. A mean short-term follow-up at 4.9 months demonstrated radiographic success in 93% (12/13) of treated tumors without evidence of any major complications. Although all specimens in this study obtained before ablation were adequate for pathological diagnosis, it is important to note

(a)   (b)

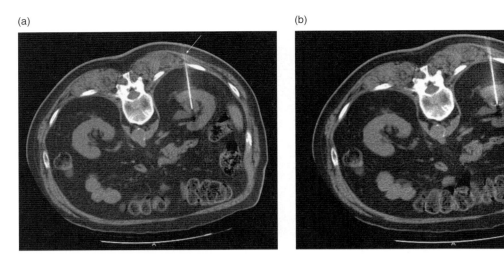

FIGURE 9b-6. Percutaneous RFA of a centrally located renal mass in a patient with multiple comorbidities. Prior to the procedure, a dual lumen catheter was placed retrograde into the collecting system for saline infusion to protect the collecting system. (**A**) RFA probe placed under CT guidance (white arrow). (**B**) Probe tines deployed (white arrow).

that only two RCCs were identified. Statistics such as the aforementioned should make one weary of the difference between *successful renal tumor ablation* and documented *successful RCC ablation*. Of course this is contingent on the adequacy of pre- or post-RFA tissue biopsies.

In an early small series, Gervais and associates percutaneously ablated nine tumors in eight patients under CT or ultrasound guidance using intravenous sedation.[54] Seven of the tumors were biopsied and found to be RCC prior to treatment. The mean tumor size was 3.3 cm (1.2–5.0 cm). The Radionics Cool-tip system was used. Four patient required additional treatments for complete tumor ablation. A large perinephric hematoma that obstructed the ureter and required placement of a stent occurred in one patient. Six-month follow-up demonstrated lack of enhancement in the exophytic tumors and in tumors less than 3 cm, while the larger, central tumors (>4.4 cm) required retreatment.

In a follow-up study, Gervais *et al.* evaluated 34 patients who underwent RFA of 42 RCCs during a 3.5-year period to assess factors that might influence technical success.[55] As in their initial study, the majority or tumors ($n = 38$) were ablated with the Radionics impedance-controlled 200-W generator under CT or ultrasound guidance. At an average follow-up of 13.2 months, there was an overall 86% technical success rate. When outcomes were stratified by size and location, 100% (29/29) of exophytic tumors (range 1.1–5.0 cm) were treated successfully, whereas only 45% (5/11) of central or mixed tumors were treated with success. Critical to this study therefore was the finding that for large tumors (>3 cm), location *is a significant predictor* of the technical success of the treatment. Among larger tumors, for example, those with a central component near large vessels or renal sinus were less likely to be treated successfully than those without such a component. Tumors such as these may therefore require repeat treatments at short intervals or are just not amenable to RFA treatments. In this

large series four complications occurred in a total of 54 ablation sessions: one minor hemorrhage, two major hemorrhages, and one ureteral stricture.

In a retrospective study from the Rhode Island Hospital, Mayo-Smith *el al.* reported on the results of 38 consecutive percutaneous RFA treatments in 32 patients using CT guidance with a 200-W generator in the majority.[56] Renal masses averaged 2.6 cm and the average treatment per mass was 2.4. Of the masses 44% (14/32) were documented to be RCCs, although all masses were solid on either CT or ultrasound. At an average of 9 months follow-up 81% (26/32) of patients had a successful radiographic treatment. Interestingly, the 19% (6/32) of patients who did not have an initial success returned for a second RFA session. Ultimately, 83% (5/6) of the masses requiring a salvage RFA treatment had a successful radiographic outcome for an overall success rate of 97%. Of concern in this report was one patient who had a single 5-mm metastasis in the skin at an electrode insertion site. This focal recurrence was resected without evidence of recurrence at 16 months follow-up. Similar to other studies, there was one collecting system injury manifested as a heat-induced caliceal stricture. Essential to this study was the finding that masses requiring a second treatment session were considerably larger than masses treated in a single session (3.5 cm vs. 2.4 cm, $p = 0.0013$), a significant finding confirmed in a recent study by Zagoria *et al.*[24]

Pavlovich and colleagues treated 24 tumors in 21 patients with hereditary forms of RCC including von Hippel–Lindau disease ($n = 19$) and papillary renal cancer ($n = 2$). CT- or ultrasound-guided percutaneous RF with the RITA system was the mode of treatment under general anesthesia or sedation.[57] The mean tumor size was 2.4 cm (1.5–3.0 cm), and at 2 months following ablation, 79% of the tumors demonstrated no contrast enhancement. The authors reported that in four of the five persistently enhancing tumors, four did not reach the target temperature during treatment. Only some minor complications occurred in this series including ipsilateral pain with hip flexion ($n = 2$) and cutaneous flank numbness ($n = 2$).

Clinical Studies Evaluating Margin Status

Radiographic success has been demonstrated to be a reliable surrogate endpoint in the short term. Ultimately, however, oncological efficacy is best demonstrated histologically with negative treatment margins. Hereditary renal tumors are likely to recur as a result of genetic predisposition; however, little debate exists regarding tumor recurrence in the face of negative pathological margins. To this end, studies have examined patients who have undergone treatment with RFA followed by immediate or delayed nephrectomy with the intent to examine margin status.

Rendon et al. treated 11 renal masses in 10 patients with RFA immediately before planned nephrectomy (Acute Group: four patients with five renal cell carcinomas) or 7 days before planned nephrectomy (Delayed Group: six patients with five renal cell carcinomas).[58] Rendon et al. had previously developed and tested a percutaneous RFA treatment technique in an in vivo porcine kidney model with efficacious radiographic results.[59] In their human study, a median of two RFA cycles was applied and the mean total heating time was just over 17 minutes when using a LeVeen Electrode with a RadioTherapeutics Corp. RF Generator. Final pathological examination without NADH staining demonstrated residual viable tumor in approximately 5% of the tumor volume in the acute group and in approximately 5–10% of the tumor volume in the delayed group. Areas of viable tumor were invariably present at the margins of treated tumors but not within the boundaries of properly heated areas. Findings of this study suggest that the absence of contrast enhancement on follow-up CT scan may not be an accurate predictor of tumor viability. Conversely, inadequate RFA heat delivery may have led to microscopic tumor persistence peripheral to zones of treatment. In this study use of an impedance-based system may have led to inadequate margin temperature delivery. Perhaps the development of sophisticated real-time imaging coupled with temperature monitoring at targeted margins will help to address this problem in the near future.

In a similarly designed prospective study, Matlaga and co-workers performed RFA using the Radionics device in 10 histologically proven RCCs immediately prior to open radical or partial nephrectomy.[60] The mean tumor size was 3.2 cm (1.4–8.0 cm). As assessed by NADH staining, tumor ablation was complete in 80% (8/10) of tumors with a mean treatment margin of 6.75 mm. Of the two tumors that were not completely ablated, neither reached a temperature greater than 70°C, and one of the tumors was 8 cm in diameter, far larger than would be recommended for treatment with RF. The higher histological success rate in

this study may be attributed to the use of a higher powered generator (200 W) with a saline-cooled tip probe as opposed to the 100-W non-saline-cooled probe used by Rendon et al.[58] The minimal charring observed with the saline-cooled Radionics device may allow for more accurate and evenly distributed temperature delivery and hence a more efficacious treatment.

Finally, using the RITA system Michaels and colleagues reported results of tumor ablation in 20 tumors just prior to partial nephrectomy.[61] They performed NADH staining on only the last five tumors in the series, but found incomplete ablation in four of these five. These tumors were well within the size range appropriate for treatment with RF. One possible reason for incomplete ablation might be that these tumors were treated for only 6 minutes. The manufacturer recommends two cycles of ablation of 5.5 minutes each (total of 11 minutes, with a cool-down period in between the cycles). Complications in this series of 20 tumors included a single thermal injury to the renal pelvis resulting in UPJ obstruction and two delayed calyceal leaks that resolved with stent placement.

Conclusions

RFA is an alternative minimally invasive treatment modality to address smaller (<4 cm) solid renal masses. It is an ideal treatment for renal tumors of this size in those patients with contraindications to laparoscopic partial nephrectomy or in those patents with recurrent hereditary renal tumors. As a general rule, posterior tumors are best served by a percutaneous approach and anterior, medial, or hilar-based tumors are better served via laparoscopic delivery. Morbidities are rare, but it is necessary to be wary of the risk factors for collecting system injures and the rarity of metastasis at electrode insertion sites. Risk factors for RFA failure or the need for salvage RFA treatment include larger tumors (>4 cm) and lack of an exophytic component. Clinical studies have demonstrated short-term success, defined radiographically. There are data proving oncological efficacy when NADH staining is used on nephrectomy specimens immediately following RFA treatments. Radiographic success, as defined by lack of enhancement on a follow-up CT scan, however, has served as a surrogate endpoint in the majority of these studies. Shortly, long-term follow-up data will provide definitive evidence regarding the oncological efficacy of RFA in the treatment of RCC.

References

1. Volpe A, Panzarella T, Rendon RA et al. The natural history of incidentally detected small renal masses. Cancer 2004;100(4):738–745.
2. Hafez KS, Fergany AF, Novick AC. Nephron sparing surgery for localized renal cell carcinoma: impact of tumor size on

patient survival, tumor recurrence and TNM staging. *J Urol* 1999;162:1930–1933.

3. Fergany AF, Hafez KS, Novick AC. Long-term results of nephron sparing surgery for localized renal cell carcinoma: 10-year follow-up. *J Urol* 2000;163:442–445.

4. Zlotta AR, Wildschutz T, Raviv G et al. Radiofrequency interstitial tumor ablation (RITA) is a possible new modality for treatment of renal cancer: ex vivo and in vivo experience. *J Endourol* 1997;11(4):251–258.

5. Wood TF, Rose DM, Chung M et al. Radiofrequency ablation of 231 unresectable hepatic tumors: indications, limitations, and complications. *Ann Surg Oncol* 2000;7(8):593–660.

6. Rossi S, Garbagnati F, Rosa L et al. Radiofrequency thermal ablation for treatment of hepatocellular carcinoma. *Int J Clin Oncol* 2002;7:225–235.

7. Rhode D, Albers C, Mahnken A et al. Regional thermoablation of local or metastatic renal cell carcinoma. *Oncl Rep* 2003;10(3):753–757.

8. McGlaughlin CA, Chen MY, Torti FM et al. Radiofrequency ablation of isolated local recurrence of renal cell carcinoma after radical nephrectomy. *Am J Roentgenol* 2003;181:93–94.

9. Gettman MT, Bishoff JT, Su LM et al. Hemostatic laparoscopic partial nephrectomy: initial experience with the radiofrequency coagulation-assisted technique. *Urology* 2001;58:8–11.

10. Corwin TP, Cadeddu JA. Radio frequency coagulation to facilitate laparoscopic partial nephrectomy. *J Urol* 2001;165:175–176.

11. Hsu THS, Fidler M, Gill IS. Radiofrequency of the kidney: acute and chronic histology in porcine model. *Urology* 2000;56(5):872–875.

12. Pritchard WF, Wray-Cahen D, Karanian JW et al. Radiofrequency cauterization with biopsy introducer needle. *J Vasc Interv Radiol* 2004;15;183–187.

13. Corwin TS, Lindberg G, Traxer O et al. Laparoscopic radiofrequency thermal ablation of renal tissue with and without hilar occlusion. *J Urol* 2001;166:281–284.

14. Johnson DB, Saboorian MH, Duchene DA et al. Nephrectomy after radiofrequency ablation-induced ureteropelvic junction obstruction: potential complication and long-term assessment of ablation adequacy. *Urology* 2003;62(2): xiv–xvi.

15. Farrell MA, Charboneau JW, Callstrom MR et al. Paranephric water instillation: a technique to prevent bowel injury during radiofrequency ablation. *Am J Roentgenol* 2003;181:1315–1317.

16. Kam AW, Littrup PJ, Walther MW et al. Thermal protection during percutaneous thermal ablation of renal cell carcinoma. *J Vasc Interv Radiol* 2004;15:753–758.

17. Johnson DB, Taylor GD, Lotan Y et al. The effects of radio frequency ablation on renal function and blood pressure. *J Urol* 2003;170:2234–2236.

18. Ogan K, Cadeddu JA, Sagalowsky AI. Radio frequency ablation induced acute renal failure. *J Urol* 2002;168:186.

19. Ng KK, Lam CM, Poon RT et al. Comparison of systemic responses of radiofrequency ablation, cryotherapy, and surgical resection in a porcine liver model. *Ann Surg Oncol* 2004;11(7):650–657.

20. Su L, Jarrett TW, Chan DY et al. Percutaneous computer tomography-guided radiofrequency ablation of renal masses in high surgical risk patients: preliminary results. *Urology* 2003;61(Suppl. A):26–33.

21. Roy-Choudhury SH, Cast JEI, Cooksey G, I et al. Early experience with percutaneous radiofrequency ablation of small solid renal masses. *Am J Roentgenol* 2003;180(6):1055–1061.

22. Chow WH, Devesa SS, Warren JL et al. Rising incidence of renal cell cancer in the United States. *JAMA* 1999;28:1628–1631.

23. Wehle MJ, Thiel DD, Petrou SP et al. Conservative management of incidental contrast-enhancing renal masses as safe alternative to invasive therapy. *Urology* 2004;64(1):49–52.

24. Zagoria RJ, Hawkins AD, Clark PE et al. Percutaneous CT-guided radiofrequency ablation of renal neoplasms: factors influencing success. *Am J Roentgenol* 2004;183:201–207.

25. Patterson EJ, Scudamore C, Owen DA et al. Radiofrequency ablation of porcine liver in vivo: effects of blood flow and treatment time on lesion size. *Ann Surg* 1998;227:559–565.

26. Scudamore CH, Lee SI, Patterson EJ et al. Radiofrequency ablation followed by resection of malignant liver tumors. *Am J Surg* 1999;177(5):411–417.

27. Lewin JS, Nour AG, Connell CF et al. Phase II clinical trial of interactive MR imaging-guided interstitial radiofrequency thermal ablation of primary kidney tumors: initial experience. *Radiology* 2004;232:835–845.

28. Hacker A, Michel MS, Koehrmann KU. Extracorporeal organotripsy for renal tumors. *Curr Opin Urol* 2003;13:221–225.

29. Rodriguez R, Chan DY, Bishoff JT et al. Renal ablative cryosurgery in selective patients with peripheral masses. *Urology* 2000;55(1):25–30.

30. Matsumoto ED, Watumull L, Johnson DB et al. The radiographic evolution of radio frequency ablated renal tumors. *J Urol* 2004;172:45–48.

31. Veltri A, De Fazio G, Malfitana V et al. Percutaneous US-guided RF thermal ablation for malignant renal tumors: preliminary results in 13 patients. *Eur Radiol* 2004;14:2303–2310.

32. Farrell MA, Charboneau WJ, DiMarco DS et al. Imaging-guided radiofrequency ablation of solid renal tumors. *Am J Roentgenol* 2003;180:1509–1513.

33. De Baere T, Kuoch V, Smayra T et al. Radio frequency ablation of renal cell carcinoma: preliminary clinical experience. *J Urol* 2002;167:1961–1964.

34. Ogan K, Roberts WW, Wilhelm DM et al. Infared thermography and thermocouple mapping of radiofrequency renal ablation to assess treatment adequacy and ablation margins. *Urology* 2003;62(1):146–151.

35. Polascik TJ, Hamper U, Lee BR et al. Ablation of renal tumors in a rabbit model with interstitial saline-augmented radiofrequency energy: preliminary report of a new technology. *Urology* 1999;53(3):465–471.

36. Munver R, Threatt CB, Delvecchio FC et al. Hypertonic saline-augmented radiofrequency ablation of the VX-2 tumor implanted in the rabbit kidney: a short-term survival pilot study. *Urology* 2002;60(1):170–175.

37. Lee J, Kim S, Chung G et al. Open radio-frequency thermal ablation of renal VX2 tumors in a rabbit model using a cooled-tip electrode: feasibility, safety, and effectiveness. *Eur Rad* 2003;13(6):1324–1332.

38. Nakada SY, Jerde TJ, Warner TF et al. Comparison of radiofrequency ablation, cryoablation, and nephrectomy in treating

implanted VX-2 carcinoma in rabbit kidneys. *J Endourol* 2004;18(5):501–506.

39. Gill IS, Hsu TH, Fox RL *et al*. Laparoscopic and percutaneous radiofrequency ablation of the kidney: acute and chronic porcine study. *Urology* 2000;56(2):197–200.

40. Crowley JD, Shelton J, Iverson AJ *et al*. Laparoscopic and computer tomography-guided percutaneous radiofrequency ablation of renal tissue: acute and chronic effects in an animal model. *Urology* 2001;57(5):976–980.

41. Kariya Z, Yamakado K, Nakatuka A *et al*. Radiofrequency ablation with and without balloon occlusion of the renal artery: an experimental study in porcine kidneys. *J Vasc Interv Radiol* 2003;14:241–245.

42. Chang I, Mikityansky I, Wray-Cahen D *et al*. Effects of perfusion on radiofrequency ablation in swine kidneys. *Radiology* 2004;231:500–505.

43. Gettman MT, Lotan Y, Corwin, TS *et al*. Radiofrequency coagulation of renal parenchyma: comparison of effects of energy generators on treatment efficacy. *J Endourol* 2002;16(2):83–88.

44. Nakada SY, Jerde TJ, Warner TF *et al*. Bipolar radiofrequency ablation of the kidney: comparison with monopolar radiofrequency ablation. *J Endourol* 2003;17(10):927–933.

45. Marcovich R, Aldana J, Morgenstern A *et al*. Optimal lesion assessment following acute radio frequency ablation of porcine kidney: cellular viability or histopathology? *J Urol* 2003;170(4 Pt 1):1370–1374.

46. Tan BJ, El-Hakim A, Morgenstern N *et al*. Comparison of laparoscopic saline infused to dry radio frequency ablation of renal tissue: evolution of histological infarct in the porcine model. *J Urol* 2004;172:2007–2012,

47. Margulis V, Matsumoto ED, Lindberg G *et al*. Acute histologic effects of temperature-based radiofrequency ablation on renal tumor pathologic interpretation. *Urology* 2004;64(4): 660–662.

48. Yohannes P, Pinto P, Rotariu P *et al*. Retroperitoneoscopic radiofrequency ablation of a solid renal mass. *J Endourol* 2001;15(8):845–849.

49. Jacomides L, Ogan K, Watumull L *et al*. Laparoscopic application of radio frequency energy enables in situ renal tumor ablation and partial nephrectomy. *J Urol* 2003;169: 49–53.

50. Hwang, JJ, Walther MM, Pautler, SE *et al*. Radio frequency ablation of small renal tumors: intermediate results. *J Urol* 2004;171:1814–1818.

51. McGovern FJ, Wood BJ, Goldberg SN *et al*. Radio frequency ablation of renal cell carcinoma via image guided needle electrodes. *J Urol* 1998;161:599–600.

52. Hall WH, McGahan JP, Link, DP *et al*. Combined embolization and percutaneous radiofrequency ablation of a solid renal tumor. *Am J Roentgenol* 2000;174:1592–1594.

53. Ogan K, Jacomides L, Dolmatch BL *et al*. Percutaneous radiofrequency ablation of renal tumors: technique, limitations, and morbidity. *Urology* 2002;60(6):954–958.

54. Gervais DA, McGovern FJ, Wood BY *et al*. Radio-frequency ablation of renal cell carcinoma: early clinical experience. *Radiology* 2000;217:665–772.

55. Gervais DA, McGovern FJ, Arelango RS *et al*. Renal cell carcinoma: clinical experience and technical success with radio-frequency ablation of 42 tumors. *Radiology* 2003;226: 417–424.

56. Mayo-Smith WW, Dupuy DE, Parikh PM *et al*. Imaging-guided percutaneous radiofrequency ablation of solid renal masses: techniques and outcomes of 38 treatment sessions in 32 consecutive patients. *Am J Roentgenol* 2003;180(6):1503–1508.

57. Pavlovich CP, Walther MM, Choyke PL *et al*. Percutaneous radio frequency ablation of small renal tumors: initial results. *Urology* 2002;167:10–12.

58. Rendon RA, Kachura JR, Sweet JM *et al*. The uncertainty of radio frequency treatment of renal cell carcinoma: findings at immediate and delayed nephrectomy. *J Urol* 2002;167: 1587–1592.

59. Rendon RA, Gertner MR, Sherar MD *et al*. Development of a radiofrequency based thermal therapy technique in an in vivo porcine model for the treatment of small renal masses. *J Urol* 2001;166:292–298.

60. Matlaga BR, Zagoria RJ, Woodruff RD *et al*. Phase II trial of radio frequency ablation of renal cancer: evaluation of the kill zone. *J Urol* 2002;168:2401–2405.

61. Michaels MJ, Rhee HK, Mourtzinos AP et al. Incomplete renal tumor destruction using radio frequency interstitial ablation. *J Urol* 2002;168;2406–2410.

9c
High-Intensity Focused Ultrasound

Michael Marberger

Introduction

Small, renal tumors detected incidentally in asymptomatic patients represent a rapidly growing segment of renal tumors coming to treatment today. About 20% of tumors 4 cm or less in diameter prove to be benign at histological examination and there is an inverse correlation between tumor size and the odds of having clear cell versus papillary and high-grade versus low-grade renal cell cancer (RCC) (Frank et al., 2003; Duchene et al., 2003). Although up to 26% of RCCs that are 3–4 inches in diameter are Fuhrman grade ≥ 3, and 36% $>$ pT3a and 8.4% have already spread systemically at the time of diagnosis (Remzi et al., 2006), many of these lesions tend to grow slowly (Volpe et al., 2004). Standard therapy, i.e., partial nephrectomy, has a substantial morbidity, even when performed laparoscopically in expert hands (Janetschek et al., 2000; (Gill et al., 2003). Given the low tendency to progress for the majority of small tumors and the fact that the largest increase in their incidence in past years occurred in the seventh to ninth decade age groups (Chow et al., 1999) with inherently high comorbidity, less invasive treatment options appear very attractive.

This can be achieved by targeted destruction of the tumor with energy-based ablation techniques. Small renal tumors are good targets, as they often have a spherical shape, are unifocal, and are surrounded by homogeneous renal parenchyma and perirenal fat. They are usually very accessible percutaneously or laparoscopically and real-time monitoring of tissue destruction can be attempted by intraoperative thermometry, ultrasonography, computed tomography (CT), or magnetic resonance imaging (MRI). Conversely, respiratory movement of the kidney and high renal perfusion pose real challenges for this approach. Needle puncture of the renal capsule immediately results in bleeding along the tract, with the risk of losing ablative energy and of tumor seeding. This is pronounced in proximity to large intrarenal vessels, which may drain ablative energy by conduction in a difficult to control manner and a significant factor that basically limits the approach to small, peripheral, and ideally exophytic tumors. Even then only a technique that destroys renal tissue so rapidly and with an adequate safety margin that

these energy losses are overcome can produce homogeneous lesions adequate for effective destruction of renal tumors. Preferably mechanical disruption of overlying structures and the tumor is avoided in the process of energy delivery, and ideally, this is performed by an extracorporeal no-touch approach.

At least theoretically, this is ideally achieved by high-intensity focused ultrasound (HIFU).

High-Intensity Focused Ultrasound

Mode of Action and Experimental Data

As an ultrasound wave propagates through biological tissues, it is progressively absorbed and energy is converted to heat. If the ultrasound beam is brought to a tight focus at a selected depth within the body, the high-energy density produced in this region results in temperatures exceeding the threshold level of protein denaturation. As a consequence, coagulative necrosis occurs. The energy drops sharply outside the focal zone, so that surrounding tissues remain unchanged. Utilization of these physical principles open a new prospective in minimally invasive therapy—targeted tissue ablation from an extracorporeal approach. The size and location of the ablated region depend on the shape of the piezoceramic element and its focusing system, ultrasound frequency, exposure duration, the absorption coefficient of the incident tissues, and the *in situ* intensity achieved (Madersbacher et al., 1995; Kennedy et al., 2003). With higher site intensities (>3500 W/cm³) cavitation phenomena occur, which are more difficult to control. In a multitude of experimental studies HIFU of malignant tumors has not been shown to cause tumor cell dissemination or an increased rate of metastases (Gelet et al., 1995).

Some of the first attempts at extracorporeal HIFU of renal tissue used a system of multiple piezoceramic elements arranged on a concave disk that targeted a common focal area. Derived from piezoelectric lithotriptors they generated site intensities in excess of 10,000 W/cm³ and hence predominantly cavitation induced lesions. Although studies on porcine

(a)

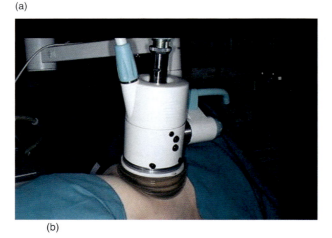

(b)

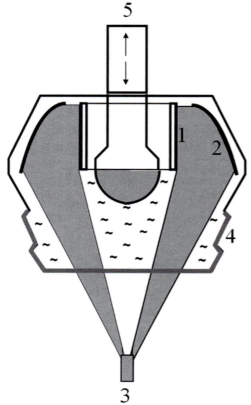

(a)

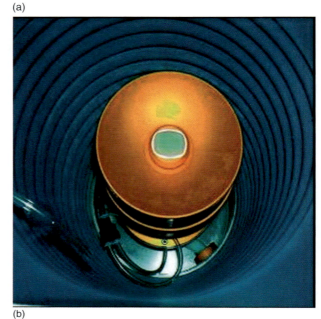

(b)

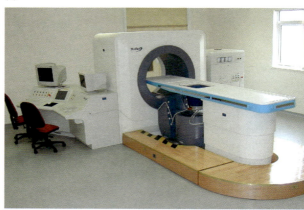

FIGURE 9c-2. The "Chongqin Haifu" System (Chongqin, China). Exchangeable transducers with US frequency varying from 0.8 to 3.2 MHz and focal lengths of 90–160 (**A**) are positioned in a degassed water bath below the treatment table (**B**). The patient lies above the transducer and the treatment zone is targeted with an integrated imaging B-mode transducer. (Courtesy of J. Kennedy, Oxford, UK.)

FIGURE 9c-1. Prototype for extracorporeal HIFU of renal tumors (Storz Medical, Switzerland). (**A**) Treatment module positioned with a mechanical arm to the patient's flank. (**B**) Ultrasound from a 1-MHz piezocylinder (1) is focused with a parabolic reflector (2) into a focal region of 3 × 12 mm (3). Energy is coupled to the skin with a flexible cushion (4) filled with degassed water. By changing the filling of the cushion, the focal depth can be varied from 3.5 to 8 cm. Targeting is controlled by ultrasonography with an integrated central B-mode transducer (5).

kidneys and limited clinical trials demonstrated renal lesions (Vallancien et al., 1991, 1992), focusing proved to be too unreliable for clinical use.

All systems presently employed for therapeutic HIFU have single transducers, which are focused either by having a concave shape or with acoustical lenses or multiple-element phased-array systems. The former are smaller and clinically have been mainly employed for intracavitary use, such as transrectal HIFU of the prostate (Madersbacher et al., 1995). As the focal lengths are smaller, frequencies in the 3–4 MHz range can be used. They produce smaller, but better defined lesions. A modified system of this type was recently developed for laparoscopic use, which in porcine kidneys permitted reproducible partial kidney ablation with no damage to surrounding structures (Paterson et al., 2003). For extracorporeal HIFU ablation penetration at

TABLE 9c-1. Clinical experience with HIFU of renal tumors.

Reference	System	Patients	Outcome	
			Radiological regression	Histological proof of necrosis
Vallancien et al., 1992	Extracorp. Pyrothec™ EDAP, France	4	—	Inconsistent tissue effects
Susani et al., 1992	Contact Sonablate 100™ Focus Surgery, U.S.	2	—	Sharply delineated coagulation necrosis within target
Köhrmann et al., 2002	Extracorp. Storz Medical, Switzerland	1	Partial in 2/3 tumors	—
Wu et al., 2003	Extracorp. Chongqing HAIFU™, China	13	3 complete 10 partial	—
Marberger et al., 2005	Extracorp. Storz Medical Chongqing HAIFU™, China	16	1/2 partial	14/14 very variable, always incomplete
		2	—	2/2 incomplete
Illing et al., 2005	Extracorp. Chongqing HAIFU™, China	8	4/6 partial	1/4 incomplete
Häcker et al., 2006	Extracorp. Storz Medical, Switzerland	19	—	15/19 variable thermal injury, no consistent necrosis

this frequency is too short, even in small laboratory animals (Adams et al., 1996). In the 1–1.5 MHz range penetration increases and in animal studies significant renal lesions were obtained at this frequency with an extracorporeal approach (Chapelon et al., 1992; Watkin et al., 1997).

Extracorporeal High-Intensity Focused Ultrasound: Clinical Experience

Using a prototype system based on a 1-MHz piezoelement focused at a depth of 10 cm with a parabolic reflector and with an integrated 3.5-MHz ultrasonic transducer for real time imaging Köhrmann et al. (2002) were able to achieve radiological regression of two of three tumors treated in a solitary kidney (Fig. 9c-1). Another system with exchangeable transducers of 0.8, 1.2, and 1.6 MHz and focal lengths of 100–160 mm has been tested extensively in China (Wu et al., 2002) (Fig. 9c-2). Site intensities of 5000–20,000 W/cm are targeted and the bubble formation in the tissue from cavitation effects is used for real-time ultrasound monitoring. To ablate larger volumes, the focal spot is moved continuously over the target zone, i.e., "painting" it rather than spacing one individual lesion next to another. In 13 patients with advanced renal cancer 3 renal tumors treated in this manner were ablated completely and 10 partially without significant complications (Wu et al., 2003). In contrast, a recent report on the use of these two systems for the treatment of 18 kidney tumors that were subsequently removed and examined histologically stated incomplete ablation of the tumors in all patients

(Marberger et al., 2005). Other authors reported a similar experience (Table 9c-1).

The disappointing results mainly stem from difficult targeting because of the respiratory movements of the kidney, the complexity of acoustical interphases from intervening structures of the abdominal wall and ribs, and the acoustic inhomogeneities within the tumor. These problems could be overcome by individualizing treatment parameters, if a reliable method were available for on-line assessment of the treatment effect. As standard thermosensors cannot be used with HIFU because of acoustical interference, at present this is mainly attempted by complex MRI thermometry (Damianou et al., 2004). The magnetic resonance signal from tissue is inherently sensitive to temperature. The most common strategies in use to date for monitoring temperature during clinical applications of thermal therapy have been phase mapping with rapid gradient echo sequences and/or magnitude imaging with T1-weighted sequences. In addition to the intrinsic MR tissue signal approaches using exogenous chemical agents with highly sensitive temperature-dependent MR signals or contrast-containing liposomes with temperature-dependent permeabilities are being studied (Mulkern, 2005, Jacobs et al., 2005). Movement of the target can at least in in vivo experiments be partly corrected for by using multichannel focused ultrasonic systems that track motion of tissues in real-time 3D. The approaches mainly utilized for this either use iterative reversal mirror technology with a beacon signal from the target or tracking 3D ultrasonic speckle noise backscatter changes with phased-array transducers electronically, thus basically combining motion tracking and feedback electronic steering of the HIFU beam (Fink et al., 2005). Multiprobe systems of small aperture confocal HIFU transducers (Chauhan et al., 2005) or phased array HIFU transducers (Rivers et al., 2005) also theoretically permit more flexible targeting and circumventing of interposed structures such as ribs. These approaches are presently being studied extensively and may ultimately help overcome the barriers extracorporeal HIFU of the kidney encounter today. The other approach presently being pursued to avoid disturbing interphases is bringing the HIFU transducer directly to the tumor by using laparoscopic HIFU transducers (Orvieto et al., 2006).

Until these problems are overcome, and in contrast to the use of HIFU in other organs, such as the treatment of breast cancer, uterine fibroids, or prostate cancer, HIFU ablation of kidney tumors must therefore still be categorized as strictly experimental at this time.

References

Adams JB, Moore RG, Anderson JA et al. High intensity focused ultrasound ablation of rabbit kidney tumors. J Endourol 1996;10:71–75.

Chapelon JY, Margonari J, Theillere Y et al. Effect of high energy focused ultrasound on kidney tissue in the rat and the dog. Eur Urol 1992;22:147–152.

Chauhan S, Hryanto A, Haecker A, Stephan M, Koehrmann KV. A multiprobe multi-route system for automated control of HIFU beam. Proceedings of the 5th International Symposium Ther. Ultrasound, Boston, 2005.

Chow WH, Devesa SS, Warren JL et al. Rising incidence of renal cell cancer in the United States. JAMA 1999;281:1628–1631.

Damianou C, Pavlou M, Velev O et al. High intensity focused ultrasound ablation of kidney guided by MRI. Ultrasound Med Biol 2004;30:397–404.

Duchene DA, Lotan Y, Caddedu JA et al. Histopathology of surgically managed renal tumors: analysis of a contemporary series. Urology 2003;62:827–830.

Fink M, Pernot M, Tanter M. 3D real-time motion tracking for ultrasound therapy. Proceedings of the 5th International Symposium Ther. Ultrasound, Boston, 2005.

Frank I, Blute ML, Cheville JC et al. Solid renal tumors: an analysis of pathological features related to tumor size. J Urol 2003;170:2217–2220.

Gelet A, Chapelon JY. Effect of high-intensity focused ultrasound on malignant cells and tissues. In: Marberger M, Ed. Application of Newer Forms of Therapeutic Energy in Urology. London: Oxford, 1995:107–114.

Gill IS, Martin SF, Desai MM et al. Comparative analysis of laparoscopic versus partial nephrectomy for renal tumors in 200 patients. J Urol 2003;170:64–68.

Hacker A, Dinter D, Michel MS, Alken P: Extracorporeally induced ablation of renal tissue by high intensity focused ultrasound. BJU Int 2006;97:779.

Illing RO, Kennedy JE, WU F, Ter Haar GR, Protheroe AS, Friend PJ, Gleeson FV, Cranston DW, Philips RR, Middleton MR. The safety and feasibility of extracorporeal high-intensity focused ultrasound (HIFU) for the treatment of liver and kidney tumours in a Western population. Br J Cancer 2005;93:890–895.

Jacobs M, Herskovits E, Hyun K. Uterine fibroids: Diffusion-weighted MR imaging for monitoring therapy with focused ultrasound surgery——preliminary study. Radiology 2005; 236:196.

Janetschek G, Jeschke K, Peschel R. Laparoscopic surgery for stage 1 renal cell carcinoma: radical nephrectomy and wedge resection. Eur Urol 2000;38:131–138.

Kennedy J et al. High-intensity focused ultrasound in the treatment of solid tumors. Net Rev Cancer 2005;5:321–327.

Köhrmann KU, Michael MS, Gaa H et al. High intensity focused ultrasound as non invasive therapy for multifocal renal cell carcinoma: case study and review of the literature. J Urol 2002;167:2397–2403.

Madersbacher S, Vingers L, Marberger M et al. Effect of high-intensity focused ultrasound on human prostate cancer in vivo. Cancer Res 1995;55:3346–3351.

Marberger M, Schatzl G, Cranston D et al. Extracorporeal ablation of renal tumors with high intensity focused ultrasound. BJU Int 2005;95:52–55.

Mulkern RV. Basic strategies for temperature monitoring with MR. Proceedings of the 5th International Symposium Ther. Ultrasound, Boston, 2006.

Orvieto M, Lyon M, Mikhail A, Rapp D, Fedew R, Seip R, Sanghvi N. Laparoscopic renal tissue ablation with high intensity focused ultrasound: The video. J Urol 2006;175, Suppl.

Paterson RF, Barret E, Siqueria TM et al. Laparoscopic partial kidney ablation with high intensity focused ultrasound. J Urol 2003;169:347–351.

Remzi M, Özsoy M, Klingler HC, Susani M, Waldert M, Seitz C, Schmidbauer J, Marberger M. Are small renal tumors harmless? Analysis of histopathological features according to tumor size in tumors 4cm or less in diameter. J Urol 2006;176:896–899.

Rivens I, Civale J, Ter Haar G. A phased striparray HIFU transducer. Proceedings of the 5th International Symposium Ther. Ultrasound, Boston, 2005.

Susani M, Madersbacher S, Kratzik C, Marberger M. Morphology of tissue destruction induced by focused ultrasound. Eur Urol 1993;23:24.

Ter Haar G, Kennedy J, Wu F et al. Dosimetric considerations. In: Andrew MA, Crum LA, Vaezy S, Eds. Proceedings of the 2nd International Symposium Ther., Ultrasound. Seattle: University of Washington, 2003:307–313.

Vallancien G, Chartier Kastle E, Chopin D et al. Focused extracorporeal pyrotherapy: experimental results. Eur Urol 1991;20: 211–219.

Vallancien G, Haroun M, Veillon B et al. Extracorporeal pyrotherapy feasibility study in man. J Endourol 1992;6:171–181.

Volpe A, Panzarella T, Rendon RA et al. The natural history of incidentally detected small renal masses. Cancer 2004;15: 738–745.

Watkin NA, Morris SB, Rivens H et al. High intensity focused ultrasound ablation of the kidney in a large animal model. J Endourol 1997;11:191–196.

Wu F, Chen WZ, Bai J et al: Tumor vessel destruction resulting in high intensity focused ultrasound in patients with solid malignancies. Ultrasound Med Biol 2002;28:535–542.

Wu F, Wang ZB, Chen WZ et al. Preliminary experience using high intensity focused ultrasound for the treatment of patients with advanced stage renal malignancy. J Urol 2003;170:2237–2240.

9d
Current Status of Photodynamic Therapy for Renal Tumors

Surena F. Matin and Avigdor Scherz

Introduction

Photodynamic therapy (PDT) is a highly unique form of therapy. It is important to differentiate this from heat-based laser treatments such as interstitial laser coagulation, laser thermal ablation, or laser interstitial thermal therapy. In all these cases, thermal energy is used primarily for tissue ablation. In contrast, PDT relies on a photochemical and photobiological reaction that generates free radicals, causing tissue injury and tumor ablation. The clinical experience with these technologies in the field of urology is limited, and the clinical experience with renal tumors is lacking. The state of the art at present exists on the laboratory bench, in animal preclinical laboratories, and in our imaginations. Currently, internationally approved indications for PDT include age-related macular degeneration, skin disorders, lung cancer, esophageal cancer, gastric cancer, cervical dysplasia, and cervical cancer. It has also been used for treatment of brain, head and neck, bladder, and prostate cancers.[1] Intravascular applications for treatment of vascular disease are being investigated.[2] In the field of urology, PDT has primarily been investigated for the diagnosis and treatment of bladder cancer[3,4] and has just entered Phase II/III clinical trials with patients who failed radiation therapy of localized prostate cancer.[5] Thus, given the sparse laboratory and clinical experience that is available for treatment of renal tumors, the majority of this chapter will focus on the science of PDT, some of the photosensitizers available, promising technologies on the horizon, and some preclinical data on treatment of renal tissue.

PDT relies on three interacting components: drug, light, and molecular oxygen. The drug is a photosensitizer, usually delivered intravenously. However, oral application of PDT agent's precursor is possible, and topical creams are used for dermatological applications. Light of a specific wavelength that activates the photosensitizer is delivered (from lasers or white lamps) at a specific time interval after drug administration. This generates reactive oxygen species (ROS). Primarily, but not exclusively, this involves singlet oxygen, which causes organelle (largely mitochondria), cellular, and microvascular damage. New sensitizers such as Tookad (palladium-bacteriopheophorbide, WST-09, Steba-Biotech, Paris, France), used in the treatment of localized prostate cancer,[6] generate a relatively large concentration of hydroxyl and superoxide radicals responsible for the observed thrombogenic effect of the small tumor blood vessels. The generation of oxygen free radicals also depletes oxygen levels with resulting local hypoxia. These multiple mechanisms result in direct or indirect (via nutrients and oxygen deprivation) cytotoxicity. It was suggested that both anoxic and programmed processes (via mitochondrial damage initiating the apoptotic cascade) play a role in the observed tumor cell death.[7]

PDT has unique properties that have made it an attractive form of treatment for neoplastic disease. Targeting is one of these unique properties. In addition to direct targeting by the laser fiber into the tissue of interest, some photosensitizers were reported to have higher affinity for tumor cells, tumor cell organelles, and tumor microvasculature. This "double-targeting" is expected to confine the treatment to the abnormal area in question and reduce the collateral damage. Vascular damage and collapse are important mechanisms of tissue ablation in addition to direct cytotoxicity and induction of apoptosis during PDT.[8,9]

As stated at the beginning, PDT does not rely on heat generation for efficacy. It is thus important to note that thermal damage typically will start occurring above 200 mW/cm^2 of light fluence.[10] For this reason, most applications for PDT will use light fluence at less than or up to this point. However, when photoexcitation is performed on circulating sensitizers such as in vascular-targeted PDT (VTP) the thermal effect is less pronounced, allowing for higher light regimens.[11]

Following traditional application of PDT, light is usually applied at a lag period following sensitizer's administration. This period (several hours to a few days) was meant to allow for a selective accumulation of the sensitizer in the tumor cells.[12] However, with the new generation of vascular-targeted sensitizers light is applied during (e.g., Tookad) or shortly after (e.g., Visudine) drug administration.[13–15]

The history of PDT began with initial studies at the Mayo Clinic in the 1960s using derivatives of hematoporphyrin to assist with visualization of tumors.[16] Researchers at Roswell Park Cancer Institute are credited with most of the subsequent clinical development and experience with porphyrin-based PDT. A purified form of hematoporphyrin eventually became commercially available as Photofrin® (Porfimer sodium, Axcan Scandipharm Inc., Birmingham, AL).[17] This first-generation photosensitizer has significant light absorption at no more than 640 nm. Light at this wavelength range does not penetrate tissues as well as longer wavelengths (partly because of absorption by endogenous porphyrins) and is one of the limiting aspects of the first-generation photosensitizers. Other limitations include a long half-life (probably because of high affinity to serum albumin) and significant, prolonged skin phototoxicity.[18, 19] Since this initial development, a variety of other porphyrin and nonporphyrin photosensitizers have become available. Many of these novel photosensitizers have been developed for a variety of specific indications, have specific pharmacokinetic properties, and require specific light activation parameters (Table 9d-1).

Besides porphyrin-based compounds, aminolevulinic acid (ALA) is another popular compound used for PDT. ALA is an intermediary in the heme pathway, forming the primary backbone of porphyrin synthesis.[20] It was discovered that following exogenous administration of this compound, increased levels of protoporphyrin IX (PPIX) were detected in tumor tissues,[21] this latter compound being photochemically active. Exogenously administered ALA thus acts as a prodrug, leading to increased PPIX synthesis allowing for photodynamic therapy. ALA may be given orally and has a shorter half-life than hematoporphyrin derivatives, qualities that are felt to make this a superior agent for PDT of certain conditions.[21] ALA-induced PPIX synthesis appears to have selectivity for tumor tissues. This may be because of increased tissue permeability and cell uptake, as well as less breakdown of PPIX by tumor cells.[4] In the end, tumor cells accumulate higher concentrations of this photosensitizer. One of the first medical uses of ALA administration was for visualization of tumors, and this continues to play a role in the diagnosis of a variety of neoplasms.[20, 21] Efforts at improving the pharmacokinetics and lowering the dose of the ALA are underway in an attempt to improve cancer therapy and lower toxicity.[22]

PDT using ALA has also been found to rapidly alternate responses to growth factors and cytokines via receptor-mediated events,[23] including reduction of endothelial growth factor receptor (EGFR) levels, which is overexpressed in many cancers, including RCC. PDT-treated cells experienced a greater than 99% reduction in EGFR, with surviving cells regaining 80% of pretreatment expression 72 hours posttreatment.[23] EGFR overexpression in neoplastic tissue is associated with any malignant actions, such as invasiveness, proliferation, and angiogenesis. A novel approach to this problem has been to conjugate the photosensitizer to monoclonal antibodies in order to improve targeting as well as cytotoxicity. Using an EGFR antibody conjugated to a porphyrin derivative, it has been demonstrated that such photosensitizer immunoconjugates were highly selective for EGFR overexpressing cells.[24]

Photochemistry and Photobiology of Photodynamic Therapy

The spearhead of PDT is oxygen molecules that become excited (type II), negatively charged, or turn into hydroxyl radicals (type I) by *in situ* interaction with the photoexcited sensitizer.[6] Nonexcited oxygen molecules are naturally found in their ground, triplet state. The symmetry of this state makes the chemical interaction of molecular oxygen with other molecules (e.g., oxidation) unfavorable. Upon excitation, oxygen molecules can temporally reside in the excited singlet state and the symmetry of this state allows for oxidation of many biomolecules including nonsaturating lipids, lipoproteins, and some peptides.[25] Injury of cellular membranes

TABLE 9d-1. Photosensitizers in clinical or preclinical use.

Drug	Alternate name	Maximum activation wavelength (nm)	Time to Phototherapy
Porfimer sodium	Photofrin®	630	40–50 hours
Aminolevulinic acid (ALA)	Levulan®	630	6–8 hours
ALA methyl ester (topical)	Metvix®	570–670	3 hours
Tin etiopurpurin	Purlytin®	665	24 hours
Lutetium texaphyrin	Antrin®	732	18–24 hours
Benzoporphyrin derivative-Monoacid Ring A (BPD-MA)	Visudyne®	690	15 minutes
mTHPC	Foscan®	652	4 days
N-Aspartyl chlorin e6	Npe6	664	4–8 hours
Indium chloride methyl pyropheophorbide MV6401	Photopoint®	664	60–90 minutes
WST09	Tookad®	760	During administration

because of these interactions at high singlet oxygen concentrations can initiate necrosis or apoptosis of the target cells depending on the impaired membrane compartment. Thus, impairment of the mitochondrial membrane is expected to initiate apoptosis by means of protease release while the impairment of proton pumps in the cell membrane results in a rapid cell lysis.[8,26] Other forms of biological interactions include impairment of the tubulin structure or direct interaction with nuclear factors.[27,28] Electron transfer to molecular oxygen from the triplet state of the excited sensitizer initially results in the formation of superoxide radicals.[6] Housekeeping enzymes such as superoxide dismutase maintain low superoxide radical concentration. However, at sufficiently high concentrations these radicals generate extensive peroxidation, resulting in lethal protein denaturation and impairment of cell membranes as described above. Additionally, interactions of superoxide radicals with traces of reducing metals leads to hydroxyl radical formation.[25] Hydroxyl radicals may also form in the absence of metal traces as recently demonstrated for the new sensitizer Tookad.[6] Importantly, superoxide dismutation to hydrogen peroxide is an important step in hydroxyl radical formation. The high reactivity of hydroxyl radicals makes them very potent toxic reagents. The ROS life times are short and, therefore, their direct toxicity is spatially limited. Thus, with most photosensitizers in use today the direct PDT damage is limited to the field of illumination.

Although from its early days PDT was shown to affect both the cellular and vascular compartments of the treated tissue,[29] efforts are currently mostly aimed at sensitizers that present preferential accumulation in tumor cells. Following recent studies, the advantage of creating a burst of oxygen radicals in the tumor vasculature has been widely recognized as having major advantages and some developmental efforts are now focusing on the tumor blood vessels as a major therapeutic target.[18,19,30] The drawbacks of currently used drugs have been realized for quite some time and have inspired an extensive search for second-generation sensitizers that present more ideal factors for clinical use, such as chemical purity; strong absorption at long wavelengths (to allow for deeper tissue penetration); high yield of ROS generation; no undesired phototoxicity in skin, eyes, or mucous epithelia; rapid clearance, stability, and ease of packaging; and finally, specificity and localization of damage.

Preclinical Experience with Renal Photodynamic Therapy for Renal Tumors

Currently, PDT typically consists of five steps:

1. Administration of a photosensitizer, usually intravenously (IV). It should be noted that nearly all photosensitizers are handled in low-light conditions, as exposure to ambient light may bleach the drug. Drug vials, syringes, and IV lines are usually covered, such as with aluminum foil, to prevent this phenomenon.
2. Allowing a specific time period for retention or accumulation of photosensitizers in the target tissue.
3. Illumination of the target tissue (transcutaneously for superficial lesions or interstitially via optical fibers for internal organs) with consequent local generation of cytotoxic ROS.
4. Development of tumor necrosis and tumor eradication.
5. Tissue remodeling and healing.

A number of preclinical studies in animal models are currently underway using novel vascular-targeted PDT (VTP). These studies indicate that treatment can be applied laparoscopically, with localized damage to the area of treatment and no evidence of damage to the remaining kidney, either from laser or drug exposure (Fig. 9d-1). Histological evaluation indicates interesting findings (Fig. 9d-2. These

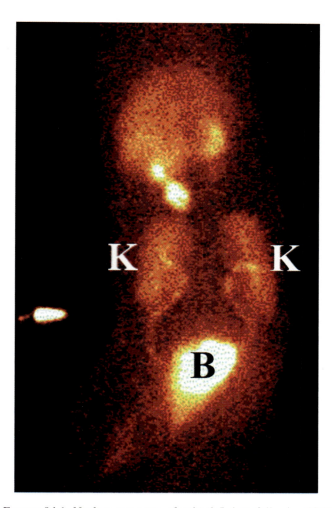

FIGURE 9d-1. Nuclear renogram of animal 5 days following PDT using a novel-vascular targeted agent (WST-09) showing normal and bilaterally symmetric renal function. The right kidney (on the left side of the image) was treated. The kidneys are labeled as "K" and the bladder as "B."

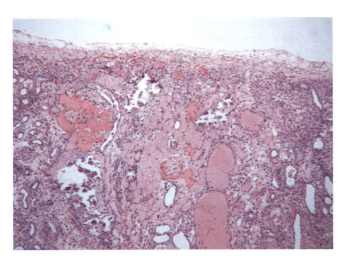

FIGURE 9d-2. Hematoxylin and eosin stain of treated kidney showing areas of necrosis, variable loss of tubules, and intense infiltration by lymphocytes in the interstitium. Vascular damage is indicated by thrombosis of interstitial and glomerular capillaries, hypertrophy of the tunica medialis, and endothelial hypertrophy of the interstitial blood vessels. Original magnification 100×.

studies at present have been limited to low doses of drug–light combinations, with resulting small areas of treatment effect (S.F. Matin et al., unpublished work). An even newer generation of VTP, which is water soluble (WST-11), will be part of the next series of preclinical investigations using larger doses of drug and higher light fluence.

Indications and Contraindications

There is very little evidence-based data on which to establish indications and contraindications for this emerging technology. Partly, this will depend on the determination of individual and interrelated kinetics of light fluence delivery and drug pharmacokinetics, which have still not been determined. Preclinical research for renal cell carcinoma (RCC) has been hampered by the lack of a large animal tumor model. However, important data can be extrapolated from other ablative technologies for which more extensive clinical experience has become available. Specifically, cryoablation and radiofrequency ablation (RFA) have accumulated considerable laboratory and clinical experience. Based on this experience, we can establish certain parameters for the initial application of this unique technology to the clinical treatment of renal tumors. We are thus dependent, initially, on in vitro and small animal models, such as with use of a mouse RCC (Renca), rabbit VX2 tumor, or Ecker rat model. Large animal models are then usually used to evaluate treatment safety with respect to the normal kidney. In vitro research can be used to initially establish oncocidal selectivity and activity. Small animal models are then used to determine cancer lethality and selectivity, as well as initial doses and safety parameters

to a limited degree. Subsequently, large animal models help establish the safety and feasibility of renal treatment delivery systems in a setting more closely similar to the human, but the oncological efficacy is extrapolated from prior in vitro and small animal data and the response of the normal tissue. Thus, the initial clinical application of PDT will likely be limited to one of two protocol-based settings: (1) intent-to-treat therapy of small renal tumors with close radiographic follow-up, as has been done with cryoablation and RFA, or (2) as part of an "ablate and resect" strategy, as has been done with liver and some renal RFA trials.[31] In the latter situation, trials are performed to establish the treatment kinetics and efficacy of cancer kill, and are not employed as primary curative therapy. This latter strategy has the advantage of immediate pathological evaluation, while for the intent-to-treat strategy, only radiographic and clinical correlates (e.g., survival and recurrence) are utilized, which require a longer time for the determination of efficacy. The caveat of treat-and-resect trials is that sufficient time for physiological necrosis responses needs to be anticipated, and the type of histological assessment (such as type of viability stain) carefully considered.

As experience with cryoablation and RFA has shown, accurate targeting is a critical factor in successful treatment. Whether employed percutaneously or during laparoscopy, the ability to perform real-time, image-guided surveillance will be a critically important aspect of treatment. This may require the use of radioopaque laser fibers with computed tomography (such as during percutaneous therapy), or hyperechoic optical fibers for use with ultrasound during laparoscopic surgery. Regarding contraindications, in general, patients with porphyria or uncontrolled coagulopathy are not candidates for PDT. As more information becomes available with greater experience, refinements in proper patient selection are anticipated.

Morbidity

One of the most common and troubling side effects of PDT is skin phototoxicity. Patients frequently have to limit sun exposure for days or weeks after drug administration. Newer compounds such as Tookad display extremely fast clearance rates from the entire circulation body. One hour after application of Tookad, no skin toxicity was seen in either animal models or human trials.[15] The favorable characteristics of these newer generation compounds hold the key in delivering the long-awaited promise of PDT.

Future Horizons

Since PDT is already a somewhat challenging procedure requiring synchronization of drug and light delivery, it is unlikely that making the process additionally complex will aid in pushing this science to a medically feasible setting. Continued development of novel photosensitizers that can perform molecular targeting is one area of promising work in oncology.[24] New forms of light distribution will also help in expanding the range of treatment by PDT as well as its ease of application.[32]

One very new and interesting alternative to traditional porphyrin-based derivatives is the use of bacteriochlorophyll. Tookad (WST-09) is a promising agent from this novel family in which the central magnesium ion has been replaced by a palladium ion. *In vitro* and *in vivo* studies have shown that Tookad is a vascular agent with dramatically different effects on tumor and nontumor tissues in preclinical studies.[33] In addition, the drug remains sequestered in the vascular compartment.[34,35] This has led to significant improvements in toxicity and selectivity. In a Phase I/II trial of WS-T09 in patients with recurrent prostate cancer after radiation therapy, no skin phototoxicity was seen, even when patients were challenged with skin light application.[15] Furthermore, drug clearance is rapid. One of the most unique properties of this compound, however, is the vascular selectivity, or "vascular-targeted" application, whereby the most significant damage occurs to the tumor microvasculature, owing largely to the fact that the compound is restricted to the vascular space. On a practical level, since illumination is performed within minutes of injection, no separate clinic visit or prolonged waiting time is necessary as is the case with nearly all other compounds presently available. Another mechanistic advantage of this compound is that maximal light absorption occurs at the visible near-infrared range of 760 nm. This is significant in that this higher wavelength penetrates deeper into tissues than the lower wavelengths used for other forms of PDT. This process also depends to some degree on the pigmentation of tissue.[10]

In summary, PDT has at present limited current applications in urology, and its role in the treatment of RCC is in the initial preclinical stage. The availability of vascular-targeted PDT, which is more selective and less toxic than treatment with older generation drugs, holds limitless promise for the minimally invasive and cancer-specific treatment of RCC.

References

1. Dougherty TJ. An update on photodynamic therapy applications. Journal of Clinical Laser Medicine & Surgery 2002;20(1):3–7.
2. Kereiakes DJ, Szyniszewski AM, Wahr D, et al. Phase 1 drug and light dose-escalation trial of motexafin lutetium and far red light activation (phototherapy) in subjects with coronary artery disease undergoing percutaneous coronary intervention and stent deployment. Circulation 2003;108:1310.
3. Shackley DC, Briggs C, Whitehurst C, et al. Photodynamic therapy for superficial bladder cancer. Expert Review of Anticancer Therapy 2001;1(4):523–530.
4. Frimberger D, Zaak D, Hofstetter A. Endoscopic fluorescence diagnosis and laser treatment of transitional cell carcinoma of the bladder. Seminars in Urologic Oncology 2000;18(4):264–272.
5. Weersink RA, Bogaards A, Gertner M, et al. Techniques for delivery and monitoring of TOOKAD (WST09)-mediated photodynamic therapy of the prostate: clinical experience and practicalities. Journal of Photochemistry and Photobiology 2005;79:211–222.
6. Vakrat-Haglili Y, Weiner L, Brumfeld V, et al. The microenvironment effect on the generation of reactive oxygen species by Pd-bacteriopheophorbide. Journal of the American Chemical Society 2005;127:6487–6497.
7. Agarwal ML, Clay ME, Harvey EJ, et al. Photodynamic therapy induces rapid cell death by apoptosis in L5178Y mouse lymphoma cells. Cancer Research 1991;51:5993–5996.
8. Nieminen AL. Apoptosis and necrosis in health and disease: role of mitochondria. International Review of Cytology—-a Survey of Cell Biology 2003;224:29–55.
9. Agostinis P, Buytaert E, Breyssens H, Hendrickx N. Regulatory pathways in photodynamic therapy induced apoptosis. Photochemical & Photobiological Sciences 2004;3:721–729.
10. Svaasand LO. Photodynamic and photohyperthermic response of malignant tumors. Medical Physics 1985;12(4):455–461.
11. Abels C. Targeting of the vascular system of solid tumours by photodynamic therapy (PDT). Photochemical & Photobiological Sciences 2004;3(8):765–771.
12. Castano AP, Demidova TN, Hamblin MR. Mechanisms in photodynamic therapy: part three—-photosensitizer pharmacokinetics, biodistribution, tumor localization and modes of tumor destruction. Photodiagnosis and Photodynamic Therapy 2005;2:91–106.
13. Keam SJ, Scott LJ, Curran MP. Verteporfin—-a review of its use in the management of subfoveal choroidal neovascularisation. Drugs 2003;63:2521–2554.
14. Schreiber S, Gross S, Brandis A, et al. Local photodynamic therapy (PDT) of rat C6 glioma xenografts with Pd-bacteriopheophorbide leads to decreased metastases and increase of animal cure compared with surgery. International Journal of Cancer 2002;99(2):279–285.
15. Weersink RA, Forbes J, Bisland S, et al. Assessment of cutaneous photosensitivity of TOOKAD (WST09) in preclinical animal models and in patients. Photochemistry and Photobiology 2005;81:106–113.
16. Moan J, Peng Q. An outline of the hundred-year history of PDT. Anticancer Research 2003;23:3591–3600.
17. Dougherty TJ, Gomer CJ, Henderson BW, et al. Photodynamic therapy. Journal of the National Cancer Institute 1998;90(12):889–905.
18. Mazor O, Brandis A, Plaks V, et al. WST11, A Novel Water-soluble bacteriochlorophyll derivative; cellular uptake, pharmacokinetics, biodistribution and vascular-targeted photodynamic activity using melanoma tumors as a model. Photochemistry and Photobiology 2005;81:342–351.
19. Brandis A, Mazor O, Neumark E, et al. Novel water-soluble bacteriochlorophyll derivatives for vascular-targeted photodynamic therapy: synthesis, solubility, phototoxicity and the effect of serum proteins. Photochemistry and Photobiology 2005;81:983–993.
20. Fukuda H, Casas A, Batlle A. Aminolevulinic acid: from its unique biological function to its star role in photodynamic therapy. International Journal of Biochemistry & Cell Biology 2005;37(2):272–276.
21. Ackroyd R, Kelty C, Brown N, Reed M. The history of photodetection and photodynamic therapy. Photochemistry and Photobiology 2001;74(5):656–669.

22. Casas A, Batlle A. Rational design of 5-aminolevulinic acid derivatives aimed at improving photodynamic therapy. Current Medicinal Chemistry Anti Cancer Agents 2002;2(4): 465–475.

23. Wong TW, Tracy E, Oseroff AR, Baumann H. Photodynamic therapy mediates immediate loss of cellular responsiveness to cytokines and growth factors. Cancer Research 2003;63(13):3812–3818.

24. Savellano MD, Hasan T. Photochemical targeting of epidermal growth factor receptor: a mechanistic study. Clinical Cancer Research 2005;11:1658–1668.

25. Halliwell B, Gutteridge JMC. Free Radicals in Biology and Medicine, 3 ed. New York: Oxford University Press, 1999.

26. Castano AP, Demidova TN, Hamblin MR. Mechanisms in photodynamic therapy: part two—cellular signaling, cell metabolism and modes of cell death. Photodiagnosis and Photodynamic Therapy 2005;2:1–23.

27. Rosenkranz AA, Jans DA, Sobolev AS. Targeted intracellular delivery of photosensitizers to enhance photodynamic efficiency. Immunology and Cell Biology 2000;78(4): 452–464.

28. Matroule J-Y, Piette J. Nuclear factor-kB activation by singlet oxygen produced during photosensitization. Methods in Enzymology 2000;319:119–129.

29. Dougherty TJ. Photosensitization of malignant tumors. Seminars in Surgical Oncology 1986;2(1):24–37.

30. Kramer B. Vascular effects of photodynamic therapy. Anticancer Research 2001;21(6B):4271–4277.

31. Michaels MJ, Rhee HK, Mourtzinos AP, et al. Incomplete renal tumor destruction using radio frequency interstitial ablation. Journal of Urology 2002;168:2406–2410.

32. Chen J, Keltner L, Christophersen J, et al. New technology for deep light distribution in tissue for phototherapy. Cancer Journal 2002;8(2):154–163.

33. Vardi IY, Koudinova NV, Leibovitch I, et al. Photodynamic therapy of renal cell carcinoma (RCC) xenografts in mice, using a second generation photosensitizer— Tookad (WST09). Journal of Urology 2004;171(4):261.

34. Huang Z, Chen Q, Luck D, et al. Studies of a vascular-acting photosensitizer, Pd-bacteriopheophorbide (Tookad), in normal canine prostate and spontaneous canine prostate cancer. Lasers in Surgery and Medicine 2005;36(5): 390–397.

35. Borle F, Radu A, Monnier P, van den Bergh H, Wagnieres G. Evaluation of the photosensitizer Tookad for photodynamic therapy on the Syrian golden hamster cheek pouch model: Light dose, drug dose and drug-light interval effects. Photochemistry and Photobiology 2003;78(4):377–383.

10a
Complicated Cysts and Cystic Carcinomas

Morton A. Bosniak and Gary M. Israel

Introduction

Complicated cysts remain one of the more difficult lesions of the kidney to diagnose correctly and manage properly. While some cystic lesions can be classified as benign and left alone, others are obviously malignant and need to be surgically removed. However, there remain a sizable number of cases that are difficult to diagnose with imaging studies. Some of these cystic masses need to be removed while others can be watched and followed expectantly with imaging studies to ensure benignity. This chapter will describe the techniques and imaging findings to help evaluate these complicated cysts so that the proper management of these lesions is achieved.

Techniques of Examination

While it is not appropriate to go into great detail on technical aspects of the performance of imaging studies in this chapter, it must be stressed that high-quality imaging studies are essential for accurate diagnosis and the use of exploratory surgery (including laparoscopic surgery) or ablative techniques in a complicated cystic lesion in lieu of an adequate imaging study is felt to be inappropriate. While the technical details of the imaging studies are of less concern, the urologist needs to be able to evaluate an examination and know when it is adequate and hopefully to be knowledgeable enough to join in with the imager in the interpretation. The most important diagnostic modality in the characterization of renal masses, in general, is the computed tomography (CT) scan, but sonography and magnetic resonance imaging (MRI) also have important roles.

Sonography is of value in characterizing simple renal cysts and minimally complex cysts that contain a few hairline thin septa. It is therefore useful in the triaging of renal masses detected on urography or incidentally discovered on sonography or when found on a CT scan that was performed without intravenous contrast medium. If a mass meets the sonographic criteria of a cyst (well-marginated and anechoic with a sharp posterior wall and increased through transmission) this diagnosis can be accepted with total confidence. Lesions that do not fulfill these criteria cannot be diagnosed as a benign cyst and require further study.[32] Recent advances in ultrasound technology have increased the reliability and usefulness of sonography, but as yet these advances have not had a significant impact on the diagnosis and imaging workup of complicated cystic renal masses.[53]

MRI can also play an important role in imaging masses in the kidney, and this will be demonstrated and discussed further later in this chapter. It is of particular value in patients with allergy to iodinated contrast agents. MRI has contrast resolution superior to CT and therefore can be helpful in some cases of questionable enhancement on CT.[31] MRI is also increasingly being used to avoid ionizing radiation.

CT is the most important imaging study to evaluate renal masses. Whether or not a lesion enhances with intravenous contrast is the most important criteria in separating benign and malignant masses. This is why a CT scan is not complete if the examination does not include acquisitions performed before as well as after contrast injection. Lesions that do not enhance (therefore are avascular) can be considered benign. Masses that enhance with contrast are likely to be malignant; however, some will be benign such as some hemorrhagic or chronically infected cysts or multilocular cystic nephromas.[4,6]

Characterization of Cystic Renal Masses

Renal cysts and cystic renal masses are so common and varied in appearance and complex pathologically that it is best to classify them by their imaging appearance. In 1986, Bosniak proposed a classification of renal cystic lesions based on their imaging appearance and suggested an appropriate management approach.[3] The classification system, which has become known as the Bosniak cyst classification system, has been modified over the years to adjust for further experience with these lesions and the improvement in imaging equipment.[4–7,29,30] The classification is used worldwide because it is a framework for communication about cystic lesions among physicians.[1,16,39,43]

The Bosniak cyst classification system is based on imaging characteristics including the number and thickness of septa, wall thickness, calcification, attenuation of fluid within the cyst, and, most important, enhancement of tissues in the lesion. The details of the system are listed in Table 10a-1. In general, the classification divides cystic lesions into five categories. Category I and II are benign and need no further evaluation. Categories III and IV need surgical intervention since Category IV lesions are malignant and Category III cysts are lesions in which malignancy cannot be excluded. Category IIF lesions are believed to be benign but in these cysts, benignity must be proven by follow-up studies.[30]

Category I

Simple benign cysts are the most common of all cystic lesions in the kidney and are said to be present in more than 50% of the population over the age of 50 years.[36] These cysts should never cause a problem in diagnosis (although they can become infected or can become enlarged and cause renal obstruction). Category I cysts contain clear fluid, are sharply marginated with a thin smooth wall, and do not enhance with intravenous contrast. They are equally easy to diagnose on sonography (as noted above) and on MRI where they are clearly seen on T2-weighted images as sharply defined hyperintense lesions.[31]

TABLE 10a-1. The Bosniak renal cyst classification system.

Category I
These are benign simple cysts. They have hairline-thin walls and do not contain septa or calcifications. They measure water density and do not enhance with contrast material.

Category II
These cysts are minimally complicated and may contain a few hairline thin septa. Fine calcification or a short segment of slightly thickened calcification may be present in the wall or septa but no measurable enhancement is present. Uniformly high-attenuation lesions (high-density cysts) less than 3.0 cm that are sharply marginated and do not enhance are also included in this group. These are benign lesions and need no further study.

Category IIF (F for follow-up)
These cysts may contain multiple hairline thin septa. Minimal "perceived" but not measurable enhancement of these septa or its wall can be seen and there may be minimal smooth thickening of the septa or wall. The cyst may contain calcification that may be thick and nodular, but no measurable contrast enhancement is present. There are no enhancing soft tissue components. Totally intrarenal nonenhancing high-attenuation lesions that are greater than 3.0 cm are also included in this category. These lesions require follow-up examinations to prove their benignity.

Category III
These cysts are indeterminant masses that include both benign and malignant lesions. They have grossly thickened irregular or smooth walls or septa in which measurable enhancement is present. These lesions generally require surgical intervention.

Category IV
These are clearly malignant cystic masses that have all the characteristics of Category III lesions but also contain enhancing soft-tissue areas adjacent but independent of the wall or septa. These lesions need surgical removal.

Category II

These cysts are also benign. They have many of the criteria of Category I cysts but may contain a few hairline thin smooth septa. Calcification can occur in the wall or septa but is thin and smooth and most important is not associated with any soft tissue that enhances. In fact, no measurable enhancement is present in the lesion (Figs. 10a-1 and 10a-2).

Perceived Enhancement

With the newer CT scanners in which very thin sections are obtained and with the use of higher doses of contrast medium injected rapidly, "perceived" enhancement in the wall or septa of these benign lesions can be seen, which is believed to be secondary to contrast medium filling of capillaries in these structures. We call this "perceived enhancement" because it cannot be measured, but it can be subjectively seen by comparing precontrast and postcontrast CT images side by side. This must not be confused with measurable enhancement, which can be measured and quantified and is seen in surgical lesions (Category III and Category IV).[32]

High Attenuation Cysts

Also in Category II are some high attenuation cysts (high-density cysts). These cysts contain fluid that has a higher attenuation than water density fluid in simple cysts. They measure greater than 20 Hounsfield units (HU) and as high as approximately 100 HU depending on their contents. If the increased attenuation is due to high protein content, the attenuation will be in the lower range and can be shown to be clear fluid on sonography. High attenuation cysts of approximately 50 HU or above generally contain

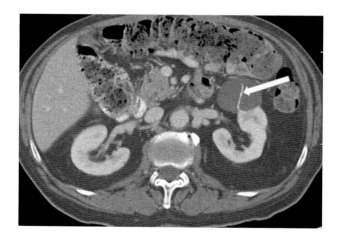

FIGURE 10a-1. An 84-year-old man with a Category II renal cyst. Axial contrast-enhanced CT image demonstrates a cystic renal mass in the left kidney. The cystic mass does not enhance with intravenous contrast, has a hairline thin wall, and contains a septation that has slightly thickened but smooth calcification (arrow) consistent with a Bosniak Category II cyst.

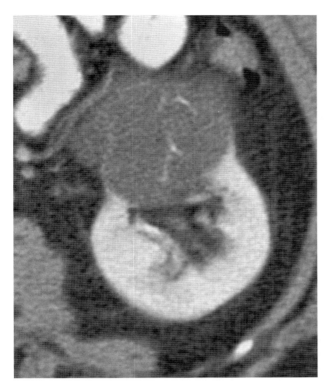

FIGURE 10a-2. A 52-year-old female with a Category II cyst in the left kidney. Axial contrast-enhanced CT image demonstrates a minimally complicated cyst in the left kidney that contains fine calcification in thin septa. (Reprinted from Israel GM, Bosniak MA. Renal imaging for diagnosis and staging of renal cell carcinoma. Urol Clin N Am 2003;30:499–514.).

blood products and cannot be diagnosed by sonography since they will demonstrate internal echoes due to the debris within them. However, they can be diagnosed definitively by CT if they are less than 3.0 cm in size, a portion of the wall extends outside the contour of the kidney (so that at least a portion of its margination can be appreciated), and, most importantly, it does not enhance with contrast. It is generally accepted that if these criteria are met, these lesions can be considered Category II benign cysts and do not need follow-up studies, cyst puncture, or biopsy[3,6,30] (Fig. 10a-3). High-density cysts are difficult lesions to evaluate since the thickness of the wall and the internal composition of the lesion cannot be assessed because of the high attenuation fluid inside the lesion, which masks these structures. Therefore the major diagnostic criterion used in evaluating these cysts is the presence or absence of enhancement. Therefore the highest quality examination needs to be performed to correctly diagnose these lesions. MRI because of its superior contrast resolution can sometimes be helpful in evaluating possible enhancement in questionable cases. These are relatively common lesions, and are often seen in patients with autosomal dominant polycystic kidney disease (ADPKD). However, if the high-density cyst is totally

intrarenal (so that its margination is difficult to evaluate) and/or is greater than 3.0 cm in size, the lesion should be placed in Category IIF and followed (as noted in the next section).[6,7,30,33]

Category IIF (F for Follow-up)

This category (which was added to the classification subsequent to its initial description) includes cases that are somewhat more complex than Category II but not complicated enough to be put into Category III, which would require surgical intervention (in most cases). Category IIF lesions are believed to be benign, but since they have more complex features when compared to Category II cysts, their benignity must be proven by follow-up examinations to demonstrate no change in the lesion. In a reported series of 42 Category IIF lesions, 40 proved to be benign on follow-up of 2 years or more. Two cases showed progression on follow-up (within 1 and 1.5 years) and proved to represent malignancies.[30] Both patients are alive and well 3 and 5 years after surgical removal. Compared to Category II lesions, Category IIF lesions may contain multiple hairline thin septa. The septa and cyst wall may be minimally thicker but *smooth*, and again with perceived enhancement but without measurable enhancement. Calcification can be thicker and nodular and even extensive as long as there is no measurable enhancement in the associated tissues[6,7,30,32,33] (Figs. 10a-4 to 10a-7).

Calcification

Calcification per se is not a sign of malignancy in a cystic lesion. Calcification in a solid lesion, of course, is usually indicative of malignancy. When calcification is seen in the wall or septa of a cystic lesion and there is no associated measurable tissue enhancement, a diagnosis of benignity can be made[29](Figs. 10a-6 and 10a-7). As noted above, the calcification in Category II lesions is smooth and thin. When the calcification is thicker and more extensive (without associated tissue enhancement) the lesion is considered Category IIF and follow-up studies are obtained. Calcification associated with a grossly thickened (often irregular) wall or septa that has measurable enhancement is a surgical lesion (Category III or IV). The lesion is considered surgical not because of the calcification, but because of the measurable enhancement within the wall/septa of the cystic mass.[29,32,33]

Follow-up Studies

Generally, the first follow-up examination for a Category IIF lesion should be obtained 6 months after the initial study. If the lesion is unchanged, additional follow-up examinations should be performed at yearly intervals for a minimum of 5 years. The length of time that follow-up studies need to be performed has yet to be determined since the growth rate of these cystic lesions has not been established, but apparently they have a slow rate of growth.[10] The length of follow-up

(a)   (b)

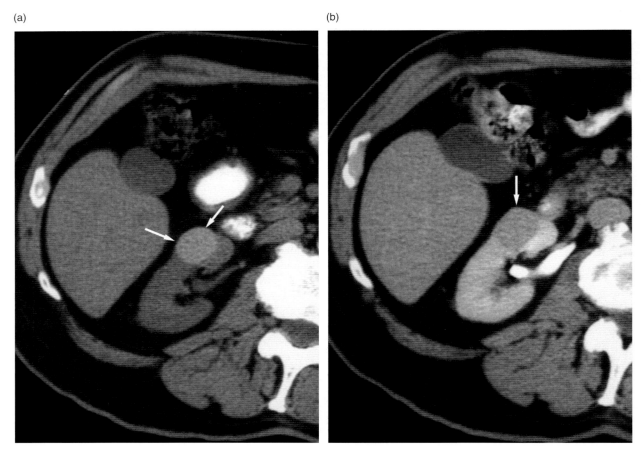

FIGURE 10a-3. High attenuation cyst. Category II cyst. (**A**) CT scan performed without intravenous contrast reveals a 3.0-cm high-density mass on the anterior surface of the right kidney (arrows). The mass is homogeneous and measures 80 HU. (**B**) Contrast-enhanced scan reveals the mass (arrow) to be well marginated and homogeneous. It measures 81 HUN, indicating that it is avascular and represents a high attenuation cyst. If the examination was performed only with contrast, the lesion might have been thought to represent a solid renal tumor. High attenuation renal cysts that are totally intrarenal and over 3 cm in size are classified as Category IIF and should have follow-up studies to prove benignity.

also depends on a number of factors including the patient's age as well as the size and complexity of the lesion. A minimum of a 5-year follow-up period is considered adequate for most Category IIF lesions to show that a moderately complex cystic lesion is stable. However, in younger patients a longer follow-up may be necessary. After 5 years, examinations could be performed at 2–3 year intervals. Many patients and physicians do not want to continue follow-up studies after 3 years, which is probably adequate in less complex Category IIF lesions and in older patients. Obviously, further experience is necessary to determine the proper interval and length of follow-up necessary in these cases.[30]

In general, CT studies should be performed initially as the follow-up examination. This will allow for a precise and direct comparison of the thickness of the septa and wall of the lesion when compared to the initial CT scan. MRI can be performed for follow-up, particularly in young patients, to reduce radiation exposure. Although CT and MRI examinations are often compatible in terms of assessing cystic renal lesions, at times they are not equivalent. Septa are more prominent and obvious on MRI studies, so comparing a CT scan with a subsequent MRI study can, at times, be difficult on the initial changeover to MR from CT.[34] Subsequent examinations will be easier to compare. If a lesion grows slightly, this change should not be considered troublesome because even benign simple cysts grow. If the septa and wall of the lesion are unchanged, this finding supports benignity and continued follow-up is recommended. However, if an increase in the thickness or in the irregularity of the wall or septa is seen, surgical exploration is necessary because either finding indicates malignancy. If this follow-up strategy is used, it is essential that these studies are performed on a timely basis and both the patient and physician should take on the responsibility that follow-up studies are performed.

It is possible to argue that all Category IIF lesions should be surgically removed. That assertion may be true in some young patients or in those uncomfortable with the follow-up

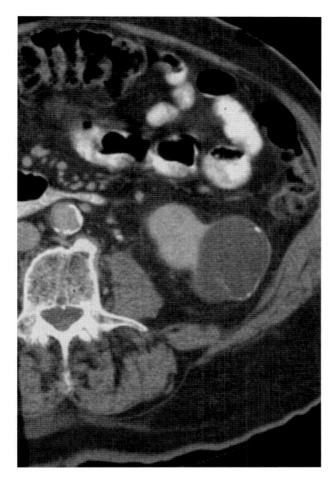

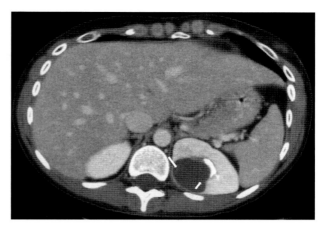

FIGURE 10a-5. Contrast-enhanced image from a CT scan demonstrates a mild to moderately complex cystic left renal mass that contains barely perceptible septa (arrow) and "perceived" enhancement of a slightly thickened wall. This lesion is believed to be benign but falls between Bosniak Categories II and IIF. There may be interobserver variability in characterizing the lesion, and some may be more comfortable placing it in Category IIF. In such cases, follow-up examinations to proven benignity rather than surgery or biopsy is appropriate. (Reprinted from Israel GM, Bosniak MA. An update of the Bosniak renal cyst classification system. Urology 2005;66:484–488.).

FIGURE 10a-4. A 43-year-old male with a Category IIF left renal cyst. An axial contrast-enhanced CT image demonstrates a 4-cm cystic lesion that has a smooth, but slightly thickened and calcified wall and septation. Follow-up examinations performed up to 4 years later (not shown) demonstrated no change in the lesion, consistent with a benign cyst. (Reprinted from Israel GM, Bosniak MA. Renal imaging for diagnosis and staging of renal cell carcinoma. Urol Clin N Am 2003;30:499–514.).

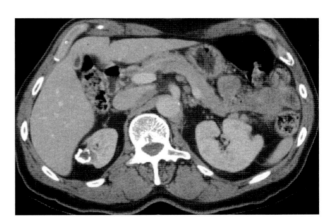

FIGURE 10a-6. A 68-year-old man with a calcified cystic mass (Category IIF). An axial image from a contrast-enhanced CT examination shows a 1.5-cm complex cystic mass that has a thick and nodular calcified wall, but no evidence of soft tissue enhancement. Follow-up examinations through 5 years showed no change in mass or amount of calcification. [Reprinted from Israel GM, Bosniak MA. Follow-up CT studies for moderately complex cystic renal masses (Bosniak Category IIF). AJR 2003;181:627–633.].

approach, but an interventional approach does not seem appropriate for the general population. In a reported series,[30] only 5% of Category IIF lesions were found to be malignant on follow-up studies and then they were surgically removed. As discussed later in the pathological aspects section of this chapter, these malignant cystic lesions may represent a low-grade variant of renal cell carcinoma.[20,37,47] They are associated with a better prognosis than other renal malignancies,[10,14] have less tendency to metastasize,[10,14,38,47] and are of "low malignant potential".[20] Therefore, in those few cases in which a diagnosis of malignancy is delayed until follow-up examinations reveal the true nature of the lesion, the welfare of the patient does not appear to be compromised and surgical removal of all Category IIF cysts cannot be justified. The possible use of cyst biopsy in these cases is discussed later in this chapter.

Category III Cysts

Category III cysts are truly "indeterminate" lesions because it is uncertain on the basis of imaging studies whether they are benign or malignant and therefore they require surgical intervention. This category contains both benign and malignant lesions. The benign lesions include acute and

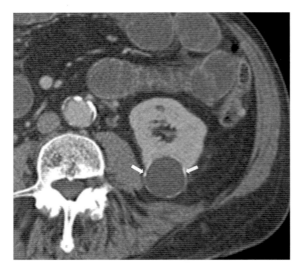

FIGURE 10a-7. A 61-year-old male with a Category IIF cyst. A contrast-enhanced CT image demonstrates a mild to moderately complex cystic left renal mass that contains slightly thickened but smooth calcification (arrows) in its wall. The noncalcified portions of the wall are minimally thickened but do not measurably enhance. This lesion was believed to be benign, but follow-up studies were obtained for up to 3 years without change to indicate benignity. (Reprinted from Israel GM, Bosniak MA. An update of the Bosniak renal cyst classification system. Urology 2005;66:484–488.).

chronically infected cysts, hemorrhagic cysts (often secondary to trauma), and benign cystic tumors such as some multilocular cysts, multiseptated cysts, and multilocular cystic nephroma (Figs. 10a-8 to 10a-11).

The malignant lesions in this category include multilocular cystic renal cell carcinoma and cystic malignancies that have undergone total central necrosis and liquefaction (Figs. 10a-12 to 10a-15). Imaging criteria include a grossly thickened, enhancing wall or septa; calcification may be present and complex fluid within the lesion is often present. These findings are more extensive and pronounced when compared to Category IIF lesions since in Category III lesions the wall or septa are thicker and often are irregular with measurable enhancement. It was initially thought that approximately 50% of Category III lesions were benign and 50% malignant. However, these figures vary in the literature depending mainly on whether cases that are on the borderline between Category IIF and III are placed in either one of these categories. Obviously if more Category IIF cases are put into Category III, more benign lesions will be found in Category III. Category III lesions at times can be so complex that often at surgical inspection or at gross pathology a firm diagnosis cannot be established and operative biopsy is not definitive in some cases.[10] Finally, even following removal of the tumor, pathological diagnosis might be difficult in some cases requiring multiple histological sections and a diagnosis

(a)   (b)

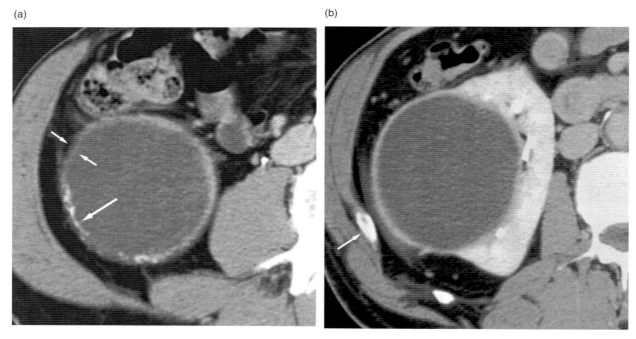

FIGURE 10a-8. A Category III lesion in a 55-year-old male with a history of automobile trauma and multiple inferior right rib fractures. (A) A contrast-enhanced axial CT examination demonstrates a cystic lesion with a thick enhancing wall (short arrows) and mural calcification (long arrow) extending off the lower pole of the right kidney. (B) An image approximately 5 cm cephalad to (A) demonstrates that the lesion is immediately adjacent to a previously fractured rib (arrow). Because of the likelihood that this lesion was posttraumatic, the surgical approach was modified to exploratory. Resection of the lesion was performed, confirming a hemorrhagic cyst. (Reprinted from Israel GM, Bosniak MA. Calcification in cystic renal masses: is it important in diagnosis? Radiology 2003;226:47–52.).

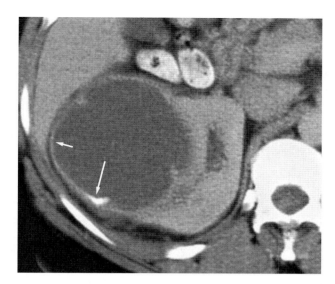

FIGURE 10a-9. A Category III lesion in a 42-year-old female with fever, leukocytosis, right flank pain, and a prior history of urinary tract infection. A contrast-enhanced axial CT examination demonstrates an irregular cystic mass with a thick enhancing wall (short arrows) and mural calcification (long arrow). Because of the probability of infection, the lesion was aspirated and pus was recovered. Catheter drainage was then instituted in treatment. The diminished nephrogram seen in this case was due to a poor contrast injection. (Reprinted from Israel GM, Bosniak MA. Calcification in cystic renal masses: is it important in diagnosis? Radiology 2003 226:47–52.).

of benignity is made only after multiple sections fail to reveal malignant cells

Category IV Cysts

Category IV cysts are malignant lesions and need surgical removal. Their imaging appearance may include all the findings described in Category III as well as the existence of solid enhancing areas within the lesion or adjacent to the wall of the lesion. This diagnosis should be made with close to 100% accuracy. Category IV lesions include multilocular cystic renal cell carcinomas, unilocular papillary cystadenocarcinomas, necrotic carcinomas that have undergone cystic necrosis, and tumor in the wall of a cyst. These lesions contain more solid enhancing (vascularized) tissue and therefore may be more aggressive than malignant Category III cysts (Figs. 10a-16 to 10a-21).

Interpretation of Imaging Studies

Because these cystic lesions can be complex, interobserver variation in interpretation of imaging studies of these cases can occur.[54] There also are reports in the literature that incorrectly describe or apply the Bosniak cyst classification or omit the important IIF category.[13,22,41,44,51] Category I and Category IV lesions should be easy to diagnose but Category

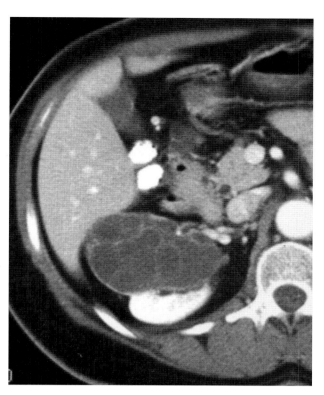

FIGURE 10a-10. A 56-year-old woman with a Bosniak Category III renal cyst. A contrast-enhanced image from a CT scan demonstrates a complex cystic right renal mass that has a thickened wall and septa in which measurable enhancement could be demonstrated. The mass is centrally located extending into the renal sinus and on other images (not shown) to the renal pelvis. Its imaging appearance, which when combined with the patient's gender and age, suggests a multilocular cystic nephroma. However, since a cystic renal cell carcinoma cannot be excluded, nephrectomy was performed. A multilocular cystic nephroma was confirmed at pathology.

II, IIF, and II lesions, at times, can be more difficult. The ability to confidently diagnose these lesions will improve as more experience is gained. However, if there is uncertainty as to which category a lesion should be placed, in general, it should be placed in the higher category and treated appropriately. If there is uncertainty in the diagnosis of a Category II lesion it should be placed in Category IIF and followed. If there is a problem differentiating between Category IIF and III it should be placed in Category III and treated surgically. Differentiating Category III and IV lesions is less of a problem since they are both surgical lesions. If a surgeon is operating on too many benign lesions, then an adjustment in the criteria for categorization would be in order.

Pseudoenhancement

It has been shown that renal cysts on occasion may show artificial apparent enhancement of 10 HU or more on contrast-enhanced CT. This phenomenon is called "pseudoenhancement" and potentially can lead to the

(a)   (b)

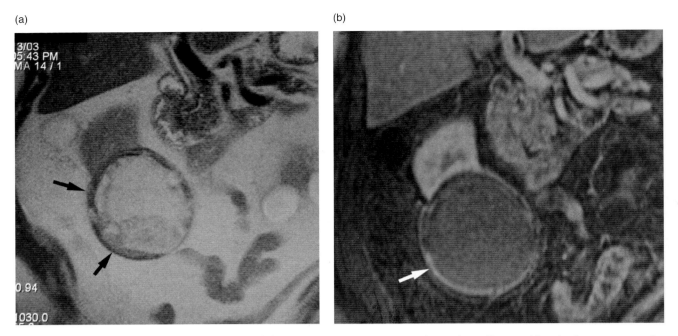

FIGURE 10a-11. A Category III hemorrhagic cyst. (A) A coronal T2-weighted MR image in a 69-year-old male demonstrates a 9-cm complex mass in the right kidney that has a thickened wall (arrows) and shows heterogeneous internal components. (B) A coronal gadolinium-enhanced fat-suppressed T1-weighted MR image shows enhancement within the thickened wall of the mass (arrow), but no enhancement of the internal components, consistent with a Category III mass. A renal neoplasm could not be excluded and surgery was recommended. The patient has refused surgical intervention, and this mass is unchanged for 10 years, and likely represents a benign complex hemorrhagic cyst. (Reprinted from Israel GM, Bosniak MA. Cystic renal masses. Magn Reson Imaging Clin N Am 2004;12:403–412.)

(a)   (b)

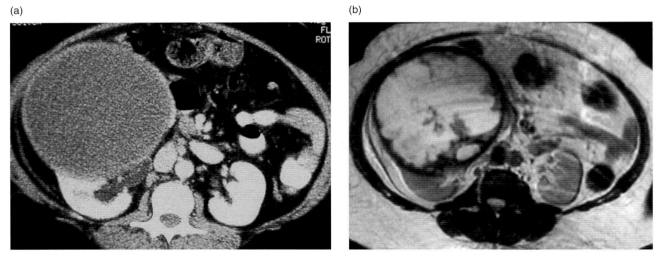

FIGURE 10a-12. A Category III cystic carcinoma. (A) An axial contrast-enhanced CT scan in a 57-year-old female shows a 15-cm mass in the right kidney that has a thickened, irregular, and enhancing wall (arrows), consistent with a Category III mass. (B) An axial T2-weighted MR image, obtained 4 days after the CT scan, shows further thickness and irregularity of the wall (arrows), which is not appreciated on the CT scan. Also notice that the central aspect of the mass appears to be very homogeneous on the CT scan; the MR image shows that the mass is heterogeneous and complex and there was no enhancement of its internal components. At surgical pathology, this mass represented a renal cell carcinoma that had undergone cystic necrosis and was filled with hemorrhagic debris. (Reprinted from Israel GM, Bosniak MA. Cystic renal masses. Magn Reson Imaging Clin N Am 2004;12:403–412.)

(a)   (b)

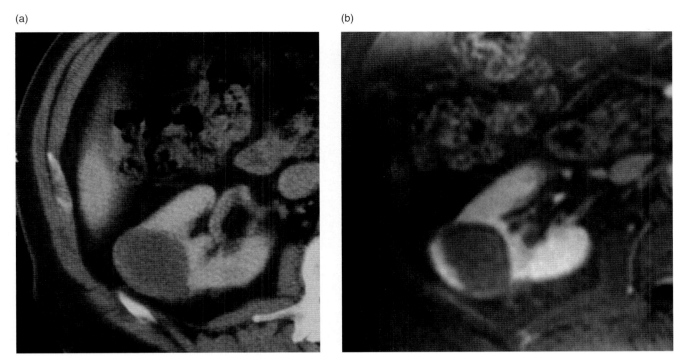

FIGURE 10a-13. A 65-year-old male with a pathologically proven renal cell carcinoma. (A) An axial contrast-enhanced CT image shows a cystic mass in the right kidney that has an enhancing thickened and irregular wall typical of a Category III lesion. (B) Gadolinium-enhanced fat-suppressed T1-weighted (3.6/1.6/12°) image shows enhancing soft tissue associated with the wall of the cyst, upgrading the lesion to Category IV on MR imaging. (Reprinted from Israel GM, Hindman N, Bosniak MA. Comparison of CT and MRI in the evaluation of cystic renal masses. Radiology 2004;231:365–371.).

mischaracterization of a renal cyst as a renal neoplasm.[2,9,12,15] Pseudoenhancement on CT is thought to be secondary to the image reconstruction algorithm used in helical scanners, to adjust for beam-hardening effects.[2,46] Pseudoenhancement is relatively easy to suspect when a mass appears as a simple cyst and measures 10 HU or less on the unenhanced CT examination. However, when a mass measures greater than 10 HU on an unenhanced CT examination, and "enhances" approximately 10–15 HU after contrast, it is difficult to know if this represents pseudoenhancement of a benign cyst or true enhancement within a renal neoplasm. In such cases, sonography or MR can be used as a problem-solving modality to prove the existence of a cyst.[32]

The Role of Magnetic Resonance Imaging

Although the Bosniak cyst classification system was developed and based only on CT findings it is commonly applied to other imaging modalities including ultrasound and MRI.

As noted earlier, the use of ultrasound is limited to diagnosing Category I and some minimally complicated

Category II lesions. More complex cystic masses on sonography require CT for further evaluation and categorization. On the other hand, MRI does have a role in evaluating cystic renal masses and as mentioned before is often used when iodinated contrast is contraindicated.[31] In addition, many cystic renal masses are incidentally discovered when performing MRI for another reason.

Therefore it is necessary to be able to accurately characterize these cystic masses with this modality. It has been shown that MRI can be used reliably to evaluate most cystic renal masses using the Bosniak cyst classification.[34] MRI may demonstrate some septa that are not depicted at CT, and may also show additional thickness of the septa and wall of some lesions. particularly on T2-weighted images (Figs. 10a-12 to 10a-14). Also, the superior contrast resolution of gadolinium-enhanced T1-weighted MR images compared to CT may demonstrate definitive enhancement in renal lesions that show only equivocal enhancement at CT (Fig. 10a-21). Therefore, it is possible that a cystic renal mass will be placed in a higher cyst category with MRI when compared to CT in some cases. This is not a problem in most cases; however, it can create uncertainty in patient management in masses that appear as Category IIF on CT but Category III on MRI. Further experience is needed to determine the proper management of these cases in which CT and MRI differ.

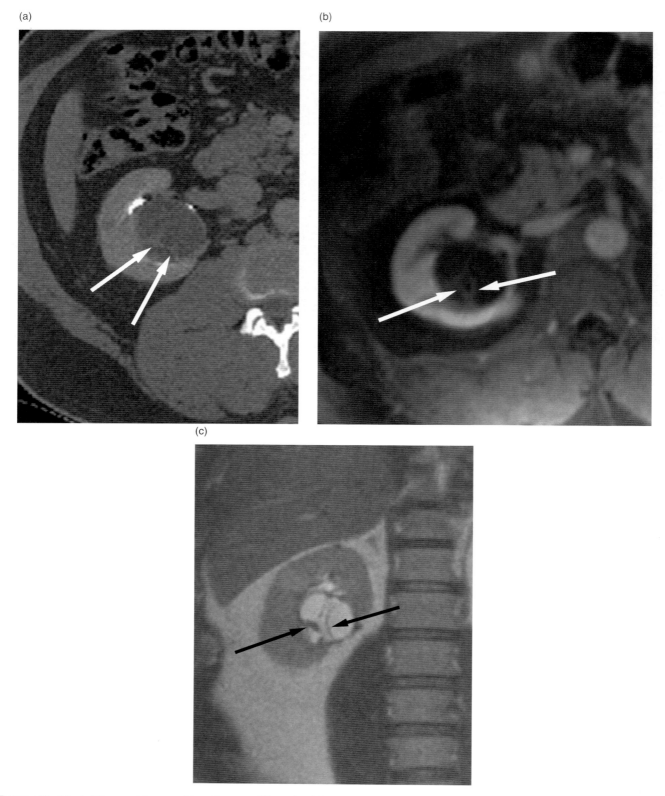

FIGURE 10a-14. A 56-year-old man with a Category III cystic right renal mass. (A) An axial contrast-enhanced CT image demonstrates a cystic right renal mass that contains enhancing thickened and irregular septa (arrows) consistent with a Category III mass. (B) An axial gadolinium-enhanced fat-suppressed T1-weighted MR image (3.6/1.6/12°) also demonstrates enhancing thickened and irregular septa (arrows) within the mass, similar to those depicted on the CT image. (C) A coronal T2-weighted MR image (8/65/180°) better delineates the septa (arrows) within the mass. A multiloculated cystic renal cell carcinoma was diagnosed at surgical pathology. (Reprinted from Israel GM, Bosniak MA. How I do it: evaluating renal masses. Radiology, 2005;236:441–450.)

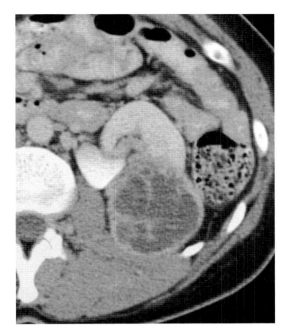

FIGURE 10a-15. A 32-year-old female with a multiseptated Category III left renal mass. A contrast-enhanced axial CT examination reveals a multiseptated, thick-walled mass extending from the posterior surface of the left kidney. The mass has enhancing somewhat irregular septa and wall and is clearly a surgical lesion. Nephrectomy revealed a multiloculated renal cell carcinoma.

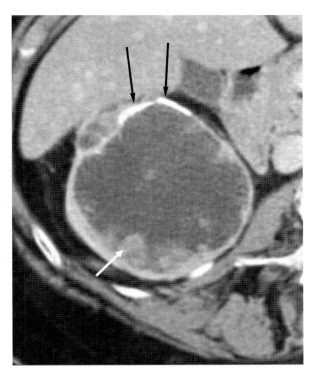

FIGURE 10a-17. A Category IV lesion in an 86-year-old female. A contrast-enhanced axial CT examination demonstrates a complex cystic lesion containing mural calcification (long arrow), wall enhancement, and obvious enhancing soft tissue components (short arrow). Surgical removal revealed a renal cell carcinoma with cystic necrosis. (Reprinted from Israel GM, Bosniak MA. Calcification in cystic renal masses: is it important in diagnosis? Radiology 2003;226:47–52.)

Percutaneous Biopsy

The role of cyst puncture and percutaneous biopsy in cystic lesions of the kidney is controversial and open to differences of opinion. There are those who believe that these procedures are valuable tools in the evaluation of many of these "indeterminate" cystic lesions;[22,40,51] however, others (including the authors of this chapter) believe that the technique is an unnecessary invasive procedure of limited value, particularly in cystic masses.[8,18,26,28,49,52]

Cyst puncture clearly has a role in diagnosing a cystic appearing mass that might represent a chronic abscess or infected cyst. If there is some clinical history suggesting that a complicated cystic mass might be due to infection, cyst puncture is indicated.

If pus is obtained, drainage can be performed. If hemorrhagic fluid is obtained, surgery is indicated. Percutaneous biopsy has a limited role in cystic lesions because many of the so called "indeterminate masses" that are biopsied are Category IIF, which need only follow-up studies to prove their benignity (as previously discussed). The truly "indeterminate" cystic masses (Category III) require surgery, whether the biopsy is positive or negative for malignant cells. A

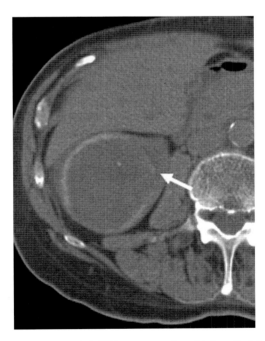

FIGURE 10a-16. An axial CT image reveals a thick-walled lesion in the right kidney which enhanced following contrast administration. There is a small focus of tissue (arrow) which enhanced with contrast that is not in the wall or septum that makes it a Category IV lesion. At pathology, a papillary cystadenocarcinoma (unilocular cystic carcinoma) was diagnosed.

(a)   (b)

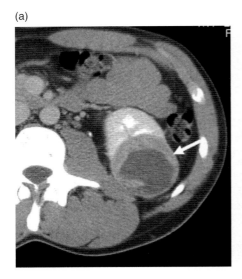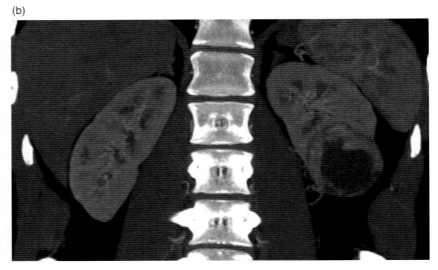

FIGURE 10a-18. A 24-year-old man with Category IV cystic carcinoma. Axial (**A**) and coronal multiplanar reformatted (**B**) CT images demonstrate a cystic mass at the lower pole of the left kidney that has a grossly thickened enhancing wall (arrow) and nodular regions of soft tissue enhancement. At surgical pathology, a renal cell carcinoma was diagnosed.

positive biopsy merely confirms the need for surgery and a biopsy result that is negative for malignancy does not alter patient management because there will be uncertainty as to whether a sampling error is present. The patient may still have a malignancy and therefore surgical exploration of the lesion is still necessary (unless clinically contraindicated). In some cystic renal carcinomas, the cystic architecture dominates the morphological appearance of the tumor and there is less solid tissue to sample. In addition, the total population of malignant cells is small in these lesions.

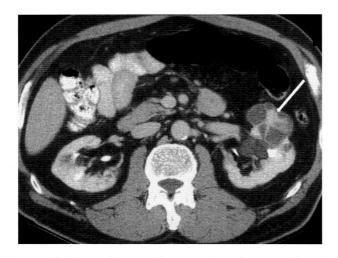

FIGURE 10a-19. A 48-year-old man with a Category IV cystic carcinoma. An axial contrast-enhanced CT image demonstrates a 4.5-cm complex cystic left renal mass that has a moderately thickened wall, grossly thickened septa, and enhancing soft tissue (arrow) centrally. At surgical pathology, a multiloculated cystic renal cell carcinoma was diagnosed.

Characterizing these masses as a renal malignancy at times may be difficult for the pathologist, even when the entire specimen is examined. In addition, once a cystic renal mass is biopsied, the natural history could be changed. If it is decided to perform follow-up examinations on the basis of a negative biopsy, it might be difficult to know if the change in the mass is secondary to a change in its nature or a response to the instrumentation. Lastly, although reportedly rare, biopsy of a neoplastic lesion can cause needle tumor tracking and in cystic masses, potential spillage and implantation of malignant cells.[8,19,21] Complications such as hemorrhage and infection have also been reported.[8,21] Therefore, a meticulous evaluation of high-quality imaging studies combined with follow-up studies (when necessary) will characterize the overwhelming majority of lesions Percutaneous biopsy, therefore, is an unnecessary procedure in most complicated cyst cases.

Clinical Considerations

The clinical aspects of each case such as the patient's age and comorbidities as well as the size and location of the mass in the kidney also affect the treatment options.[33] Decisions as to management are dependent on the combination of imaging findings, clinical factors, and available treatment options. For example, a Category IIF mass (which requires follow-up examinations) may now be treated with laparoscopic partial nephrectomy. This surgical approach might be appropriate in a young patient with a small exophytic Category IIF cyst to alleviate the need for long-term follow-up examinations, and in some cases to alleviate patient anxiety while ruling out the possibility (albeit very small) of malignancy. This

(a)   (b)

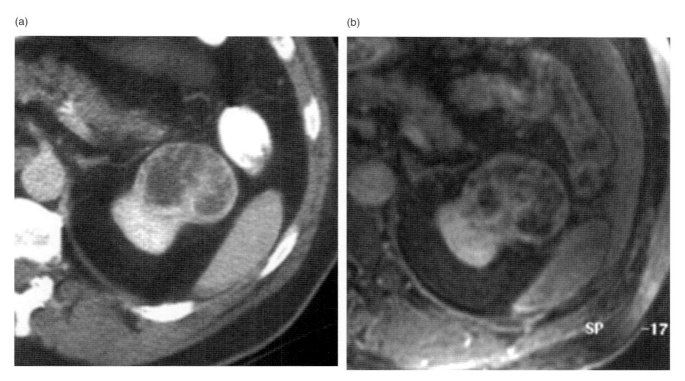

FIGURE 10a-20. A 56-year-old female with a Bosniak Category IV cystic lesion in the left kidney. (A) An axial image from a contrast-enhanced CT scan shows a complex cystic mass that contains a grossly thickened and enhancing wall and enhancing soft tissuecomponents. (B) Axial gadolinium-enhanced fat-suppressed T1-weighted (3.4/1.4/12°)MR image demonstrates similar findings when compared to the CT examination. This lesion was surgically removed and a cystic renal cell carcinoma was found. (Reprinted from Israel GM, Hindman N, Bosniak MA. Comparison of CT and MRI in the evaluation of cystic renal masses. Radiology 2004;231:365–371.)

(a)   (b)

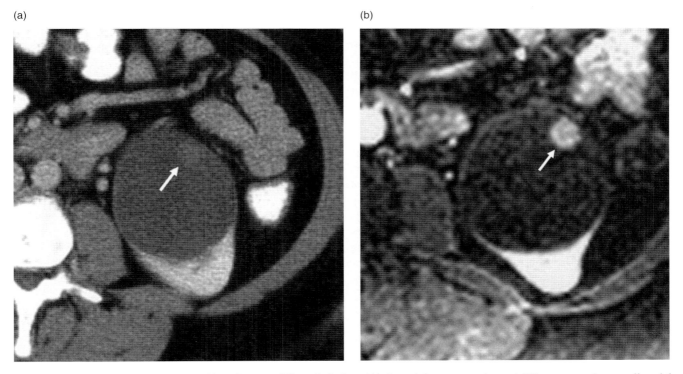

FIGURE 10a-21. A 48-year-old female with a Category IV cystic lesion. (A) An axial contrast-enhanced CT scan reveals a small nodule (arrow) in the lateral wall of a large cyst in the left kidney. (B) Gadolinium-enhanced fat-suppressed T1-weighted MR image (4.2/1.2/12°) shows the enhancing nodule to better advantage. Pathology revealed a renal cell carcinoma in the wall of a cyst.

same lesion in an elderly patient would be managed with follow-up studies. Obviously the age and clinical condition of the patient dictate patient management. While Category III lesions are surgical lesions, in an elderly patient who is a poor surgical risk, a watchful waiting approach can be a prudent management choice in some instances. Also, the size and location of the lesion might affect the management decision. If the lesion is amenable to laparoscopic removal (or tumor ablation techniques) this might affect the decision on management in a questionable case. In the end, each case must be individualized to the various clinical factors, imaging findings, and the experience and skills of the urologist. Certainly, there can be more than one way to manage these cases.

Pathological Considerations

Cystic renal neoplasms include the malignant lesions multi-locular cystic renal cell carcinoma (Figs. 10a-14, 10a-15, and 10a-19, unilocular papillary cystadenocarcinoma (Fig. 10a-16), renal carcinomas that have undergone cystic necrosis (Figs. 10a-12, 10a-17, and 10a-18), carcinoma in a cyst wall (Fig. 10a-21), and the benign lesion multilocular cystic nephroma (Fig. 10a-10).[23,25]

Multilocular Cystic Renal Cell Carcinoma

Multilocular cystic renal cell carcinoma (MCRCC) represents a variant of clear cell renal carcinoma. It is reported to make up 3.5–6% of conventional renal cell carcinomas.[50] A cystic RCC is considered to be an MCRCC if not more than 25% of the cystic lesion is composed of solid areas;[14] however, others use 10% solid tissue as the cutoff.[47] However, some pathologists consider lesions with little or no significant soft tissue mass but only microscopic findings in the septa or walls containing aggregates of epithelial cells with clear neoplasm as MCRCC.[20] It is these extensively cystic renal neoplasms with minimal soft tissue that are Category III lesions in imaging, while lesions with gross soft tissue elements are Category IV. In any event, MCRCC appears to be a less aggressive neoplasm with a low malignant potential.[10,14,20,37,38,47,48] Published reports indicate that they are usually Fuhrman nuclear grade 1. Their prognosis is excellent and there are almost no reports of metastases in these cases. These finding justify the watchful waiting approach suggested for some of these mildly complex lesions (Category IIF). Likewise there is few data on growth rate since these lesions are taken out usually when incidentally discovered. Our own observations and the observations of others[10,20] along with the pathological findings would indicate a slow growth rate for these tumors. In fact, some pathologists[20,37] believe that those lesions without solid elements but only septa lined with cells with clear cytoplasm are lesions with a "cystic growth pattern, and no, or at most little, malignant potential."[20]

Unilocular Papillary Cystadenocarcinoma

Unilocular cystic renal cell carcinomas are less common than MCRCC. These lesions have a unilocular cystic growth pattern (cystadenocarcinoma).[23] Microscopically, these lesions show papillary fronds lining the cyst cavity. Occasionally, mural tumor nodules occur. At times, they can be difficult to differentiate with imaging studies from a previously solid RCC that has undergone extensive cystic necrosis. When presenting with a mural nodule, unilocular papillary cystadenocarcinoma can look very much like a tumor in the wall of a simple cyst.

Renal Carcinoma with Cystic Necrosis

Renal carcinoma can undergo cystic degeneration. It can be from rapid tumor growth or from tumor regression.[48] These lesions can be differentiated from MCRCC pathologically and usually by imaging studies. Lesions with cystic degeneration tend to have thicker irregular walls and do not contain septa. They will appear as Category III or IV lesions depending on whether some solid elements remain. They contain considerable bloody debris particularly well seen on T2-weighted MR studies.

Tumor in the Wall of a Cyst

Occasionally a mass of tumor tissue (enhancing tissue) is seen in the wall of what appears to be a simple cyst[23] (Fig. 10a-21). This is thought to represent the origination of a tumor in the epithelial wall of the cyst, but some of these represent unilocular cystic renal cell carcinoma and the whole lesion is cancerous. In either case these lesions are easy to diagnose on imaging studies and can be classified as Category IV because of the enhancing solid element of the lesion.

Cystic Nephroma (Multilocular Cystic Nephroma)

Multilocular cystic nephroma (MCN) is an uncommon benign neoplasm of uncertain origin. Unfortunately it cannot be differentiated by imaging from multilocular cystic renal cell carcinoma as it contains multiple cystic locules separated by septa, similar to MCRCC[17,24,35,45] (Fig. 10a–10). The septa in MCN contain spindle-shaped fibroblasts and cells resembling smooth muscle cells.[27] No solid elements are seen and they appear as Category III lesions at imaging. MCN is often found in males below 2 years of age and in females age 40–60 years (some authors believe they are different tumors).[20] These lesions tend to be large, usually located in the central portion of the kidney, and often portions of them actually herniate into the renal pelvis.[56] They are benign, but sarcomatoid degeneration has been reported as a rare event.[45] Even though the lesion can be suspected in many cases based on the imaging appearance and the age and sex of the patient, removal is necessary (except in poor operative risk patients) because it cannot be safely differentiated from a cystic malignancy.

Localized Cystic Disease of the Kidney

This benign entity is also called "segmental cystic disease" because it represents a collection of simple cysts clustered together in a segment or localized portion of the kidney[55] (Fig. 10a-22). It is essential to differentiate this collection of cysts from a multilocular cystic renal cell carcinoma or multiloculur cystic nephroma. This can be done by realizing that these is no capsule or pseudocapsule around the cysts, that there is intervening normal renal tissue between the cysts, and that there usually are one or more cysts in the kidney at some distance from the main aggregate of cysts. With good imaging studies and an awareness of this entity this condition should be recognized for what it is to avoid unnecessary surgical intervention. Most of these cases can be easily recognized. However, if there is uncertainty in the diagnosis, a follow-up approach can be used to ensure benignity. Occasionally, the entire kidney is involved and the condition has been described incorrectly as unilateral ADPKD. However, localized cystic disease is not familial and has no manifestations of adult polycystic kidney disease.

Miscellaneous Cystic Diseases

Other cystic diseases include ADPKD and the cystic disease associated with tuberous sclerosis. Cystic neoplasms are associated with von Hippel–Lindau disease[11] and an increased incidence of renal cancer is seen in patients with acquired

cystic disease.[42] Echinococcus cystic disease of the kidney can mimic a Category III lesion and a relevant history is needed for diagnosis.[57] A cyst that has been traumatized may become a chronic hemorrhagic cyst with reactive changes in the wall that may become thickened and in which calcium may be deposited. These cysts contain bloody fluid and debris and can mimic a cystic degenerating neoplasm from which they cannot be differentiated by imaging studies (Category III lesions) (Figs. 10a-8 and 10a-11) and require pathological evaluation of the wall of the lesion for diagnosis. The same is true of a chronically infected cyst. These lesions can develop a thickened wall, sometimes with calcium deposition within it (Fig. 10a-9). Debris is often present within the cyst. They cannot be differentiated from cystic degenerating neoplasms by imaging studies and are included with Category III lesions. Diagnosis is possible if a history of prior infection is ascertained, which should lead to needle puncture to obtain pus or infected fluid for diagnosis and drainage.

Conclusions

Imaging findings in the various complicated cystic lesions of the kidney are presented along with a management approach based on these findings. Certainly other approaches may be equally effective. Clearly, it is important to accurately separate surgical from nonsurgical lesions and to limit the number of benign lesions that undergo surgical exploration and removal. New surgical techniques have provided safe nephron-sparing surgery, but the use of a follow-up noninterventional approach also seems reasonable in many of these cases. Hopefully we will continue to advance our imaging and surgical techniques so that patients will receive the best possible management.

(a)   (b)

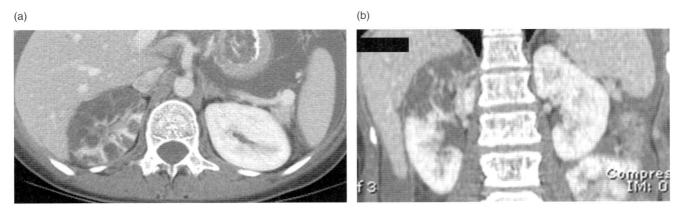

FIGURE 10a-22. A 42-year-old man with localized cystic disease in one portion of the kidney. (**A**) An axial CT scan reveals an unusual collection of cysts clustered together at the upper pole of the right kidney. The cysts are bunched together suggesting the possibility that they represent a single cystic mass. However, there is no capsule or pseudocapsule around them. The apparent septa represent attenuated renal tissue between the cysts. Note the more obvious simple cysts medially. Unassociated abdominal ascites is present. (**B**) A coronal multiplanar formatted image from the CT scan demonstrates the segmental distribution of the clumps of cysts.

Acknowledgment

The authors would like to acknowledge the contribution of Tony Jalandoni for his work in digital photography.

References

1. Aronson S, Frazier HA, Balwah JD et al. Cystic renal masses: usefulness of the Bosniak classification. Urol Radiol 1991;13:83–90.
2. Birnbaum BA, Maki DD, Chakraborty DP et al. Renal cyst pseudoenhancement: evaluation with an anthropomorphic body CT phantom. Radiology 2002;225:83–90.
3. Bosniak MA. The current radiological approach to renal cysts. Radiology 1986;158:1–10.
4. Bosniak MA. Difficulties in classifying cystic lesions of the kidney. Urol Radiol 1991;13:91–93.
5. Bosniak MA. Problems in the radiologic diagnosis of renal parenchymal tumors. Urol Clin North Am 1993;20:217–230.
6. Bosniak MA. Diagnosis and management of patients with complicated cystic lesions of the kidney. AJR 1997;169:819–821.
7. Bosniak MA. The use of the Bosniak classification system for renal cysts and cystic tumors. J Urol 1997;157:1852–1853.
8. Bosniak MA. Should we biopsy complex cystic renal masses (Bosniak category III)? (letter) AJR Am J Roentgenol 2003;181:1425–1426.
9. Bosniak MA, Rofsky NM. Problems in the detection and characterization of small renal masses. Radiology 1996;198:638–641.
10. Bielsa O, Lloreta J, Gelabert-Mas A. Cystic renal cell carcinoma: pathological features, survival and implications for treatment. Br J Urol 1998;82:16–20.
11. Choyke PL, Glenn GM, McClennan M. Hereditary renal cancers. Radiology 2002;26:33–46.
12. Chung EP, Herts BR, Linnel G et al. Analysis in changes in attenuation of proven renal cysts on different scanning phases of triphasic MDCT. AJR 2004;182:405–410.
13. Cloix P, Martin X, Pangaud C et al. Surgical management of complex renal cysts: a series of 32 cases. J Urol 1996;156:28–30.
14. Corica FA, Iczkowski KA, Cheng L et al. Cystic renal cell carcinoma is cured by resection: a study of 24 cases with long term follow-up. J Urol 1999;161:408–411.
15. Coulam CH, Sheafor DH, Leder RA et al. Evaluation of pseudoenhancement of renal cyst during contrast-enhanced CT. AJR 2000;174:493–498.
16. Curry NS, Cochran ST, Bissada NK. Cystic renal masses: accurate Bosniak classification requires adequate renal CT. AJR 2000;175:339–342.
17. Dalla-Palma, LPozi-Mucelli F, di Donna A et al. Cystic renal tumors: US and CT findings. Urol Radiol 1990;12:67–73.
18. Dechet CB, Zincke H, Sebo TJ et al. Prospective analysis of computerized tomography and needle biopsy with permanent sectioning to determine the nature of solid masses in adults. J Urol 2003;169:71–74.
19. Denton KJ, Cotton DW, Nakielny RA et al. Secondary tumour deposits in needle biopsy tracts: an underestimated risk. (letter) J Clin Pathol 1990;43:83.
20. Eble JN, Bonsib SM. Extensively cystic renal neoplasms: cystic nephroma, cystic partially differentiated nephroblastoma, multilocular cystic renal cell carcinoma, and cystic hamartoma of the renal pelvis. Semin Diagn Pathol 1998;15:2–20.
21. Herts BR, Baker ME. The current role of percutaneous biopsy in the evaluation of renal masses. Semin Urol Oncol 1995;13:254–261.
22. Harisinghani MG, Maher MM, Gervais DA et al. Incidence of malignancy in complex cystic renal masses (Bosniak category III): should imaging-guided biopsy precede surgery? AJR 2003;180:755–758.
23. Hartman DS, Davis CJ, Johns T et al. Cystic renal cell carcinoma. Urology 1986;28:145–153.
24. Hartman DS, Davis CJ, Sanders RC et al. The multiloculated renal mass: considerations and differential features. RadioGraphics 1987;7:29–52.
25. Hartman DS, Choyke PL, Hartman MS. A practical approach to the cystic renal mass. RadioGraphics 2004;24:S101–S104.
26. Hayakawa M, Hatano T, Tsuji A et al. Patients with renal cysts associated with renal cell carcinoma and the clinical implications of cyst puncture: a study of 223 cases. Urology 1996;47:643–646.
27. Hopkins JK, Giles HW Jr, Wyatt-Ashmead J et al. Cystic nephroma. RadioGraphics 2004;24:589–583.
28. Horwitz CA, Manivel JC, Inampudi S et al. Diagnostic difficulties in the interpretation of needle aspiration material from large renal cysts. Diag Cytopathol 1994;11:380–383.
29. Israel GM, Bosniak MA. Calcification in cystic renal masses: is it important in diagnosis? Radiology 2003;226:47–52.
30. Israel GM, Bosniak MA. Follow-up CT studies for moderately complex cystic renal masses (Bosniak category IIF). AJR 2003;181:627–633.
31. Israel GM, Bosniak MA. MR imaging of cystic renal masses. Magn Reson Imaging Clin N Am 2004;12:403–412.
32. Israel GM, Bosniak MA. How I do it: evaluating renal masses. Radiology 2005;236:441–450.
33. Israel GM, Bosniak MA. An update of the Bosniak renal cyst classification system. Urology 2005;66:484–488.
34. Israel GM, Hindman N, Bosniak MA. Comparison of CT and MRI in the evaluation of cystic renal masses using the Bosniak classification system. Radiology 2004;231:365–371.
35. Kettritz U, Semelka RC, Siegelman ES et al. Multilocular cystic nephroma: MR imaging appearance with current techniques, including gadolinium enhancement. J Magn Reson Imaging 1996;6:145–148.
36. Kissane JM. Congenital malformations. In: Hepinstall RH, ed. Pathology of the Kidney. Boston: Little Brown, 1974, 69–119.
37. Kirsh EJ, Strauss FS II, Goldfisher ER et al. Benign adenomatous multicystic kidney tumor (Perlmann's tumor) and renal cortical carcinoma with adenomatous multicystic features. 12 cases. Urology 1999;53:65–70.
38. Koga S, Nishikido M, Hayashi T et al. Outcome of surgery in cystic renal cell carcinoma. Urology 2000;56:67–70.
39. Koga S, Nishikido M, Inuzuka S et al. An evaluation of Bosniak's radiological classification of cystic renal masses. BJU Int 2000;86:607–609.
40. Lang EK, Macchia RJ, Gayle B et al. CT-guided imaging of indeterminate renal cystic masses (Bosniak 3 and 2F): accuracy and clinical management. Eur Radiol 2002;12:2518–2524.
41. Laven BA, Orvieto MA, Rapp DE et al. Malignant B-cell lymphoma in renal cyst wall. Urology 2004;64:590.

42. Levine E. Renal cell carcinoma in uremic acquired renal cystic disease: incidence, detection and management. Urol Radiol 1992;13:203–210.

43. Levy P, Helenon O, Merran S et al. Cystic tumors of the kidney in adults: radio-histopathologic correlations. J Radiol 1991;80:121–133.

44. Limb J, Santiago L, Kaswick J et al. Laparoscopic evaluation of indeterminate renal cysts: long-term follow-up. J Endourol 2002;16:79–82.

45. Madewell JE, Goldman SM, Davis CJ et al. Multilocular cystic nephroma: a radiologic-pathologic correlation of 58 patients. Radiology 1983;146:309–321.

46. Maki DD, Birnbaum BA, Chakraborty DP et al. Renal cyst pseudoenhancement: beam hardening effects on CT numbers. Radiology 1999;213:468–472.

47. Murad T, Komaiko W, Oyasu R. Multilocular cystic renal cell carcinoma. Am J Clin Pathol 1991;95:633–637.

48. Nassir A, Jollimore J, Gupta R et al. Multilocular cystic renal cell carcinoma: a series of 12 cases and review of the literature. Urology 2002;60:421–427.

49. Renshaw AA, Granter SR, Cibas ES. Fine needle aspiration of the adult kidney. Cancer 1997;81:71–88.

50. Reuter VE, Presti JC Jr. Contemporary approach to the classification of renal epithelial tumors. Semin Oncol 2000;27:124–137.

51. Richter F, Kasabian NG, IrwinJr RJ et al. Accuracy of diagnosis by guided biopsy of renal mass lesions classified indeterminate by imaging studies. Urology 2000;55:348–352.

52. Rybicki FJ, Shu KM, Cibas EM et al. Percutaneous biopsy of renal masses: sensitivity and negative predictive value stratified by clinical setting and size of masses. AJR 2003;180: 1281–1287.

53. Schmidt T, Hohl C, Haage P et al. Diagnostic accuracy of phase-inversion tissue harmonic imaging versus fundamental B-mode sonography in the evaluation of focal lesions of the kidney. AJR Am J Roentgenol 2003;180:1639–1647.

54. Siegel CL, McFarland EG, Brink JA et al. CT of cystic renal masses: analysis of diagnostic performance and interobserver variation. AJR 1997;169:813–818.

55. Slywotzky CM, Bosniak MA. Localized cystic disease of the kidney. AJR Am J Roentgenol 2001;176:843–849.

56. Uson AC, Melikow M. Multilocular cysts of kidney with intrapelvic herniation of "daughter" cyst: report of 4 cases. J Urol 1963;89:341–348.

57. von Sinner WN, Hellstrom M, Kagevi I et al. Hydatid disease of the urinary tract. J Urol 1993;149:577–580.

10b
Nephron-Sparing Surgery for Central Renal Tumors

Sascha Pahernik and Joachim W. Thüroff

Introduction

Surgery is the gold standard for treatment of renal cell carcinoma (RCC). Nephron-sparing surgery (NSS) has become a standard strategy for treating selected renal tumors.[1-3] NSS for RCC is indicated for treatment of bilateral renal tumors, for tumors in a solitary kidney, and when total renal function is impaired or at risk, e.g., in diabetic nephropathy when radical nephrectomy would result in renal failure and hemodialysis. NSS for RCC with an elective indication, such as in the presence of a normal contralateral kidney, has become accepted for small incidental tumors. The outcome of patients with RCC treated with cone resection, wedge resection, or partial nephrectomy in the elective setting is excellent and is comparable to results obtained by radical nephrectomy.[4,5]

In patients with centrally localized tumors, preservation of renal parenchyma must be weighed against the risk of compromising oncological efficacy. Thus, NSS for centrally localized tumors is general limited to imperative indications. As a consequence, surgery for centrally localized tumors poses unique challenges for surgical and clinical management. Under elective indication, NSS for centrally localized tumors may be justified if the tumor is of uncertain type,[6] thus avoiding nephrectomy for a possible benign tumor. A renal tumor is defined as central (1) when a small tumor is surrounded by normal parenchyma and may not even be detectable on intraoperative inspection or palpation and (2) when a larger tumor develops into the renal hilum and contacts or invades the renal collecting system or major renal veins. Intraoperative ultrasound may be necessary to localize the tumor with certainty.

Materials and Methods

Patients

Since 1969 NSS for centrally located renal tumors has been performed for 74 cases at our institution. Nine patients with a palliative indication for NSS had metastases prior to surgery. NSS preceded planned resection of metastasis in these patients. Tumors completely surrounded by normal parenchyma were defined as centrally localized. Preoperative imaging included renal ultrasound, intravenous pyelography (IVP), as well as computed tomography (CT) or magnetic resonance imaging (MRI) of the kidneys. Arteriography was not routinely performed. The average patient age at surgery was 57.3 years (range: 25.5–78.6 years). The mean follow-up is 5.8 years (range: 0.4–23.4 years).

The indication for NSS was imperative in 56 cases and elective in 18. Among the 56 patients with an imperative indication, 18 patients had bilateral synchronous renal tumors, 32 patients had a solitary kidney, and 4 patients had chronic renal failure. Of the 32 patients with a solitary kidney, 14 patients had had previous nephrectomy because of RCC. The time interval for patients with metachronous bilateral RCC between radical nephrectomy and NSS for treatment of the centrally localized tumor in the remaining contralateral kidney was a mean of 9.1 years (range: 1.2–26.9).

Surgical Technique

NSS for tumors in a central location is a nonstandardizable surgical technique. Surgical access is generally gained by an extraperitoneal flank incision. The kidney is freed from the surrounding fatty tissue except for fat adhering to the tumor and is carefully inspected for any possible satellite lesions. Intraoperative ultrasound is routinely performed to determine tumor extension and check for previously undetected tumors. At least 30 minutes prior to ischemia 1.25 mg of the angiotensin-converting enzyme (ACE) inhibitor enalaprilate is administered intravenously. In addition, 20% mannitol (1 ml/kg body weight) is given and good intraoperative hydration is ensured.[7] After clamping the artery with a bulldog or Edwards clamp, renal hypothermia is induced by external cooling with slush ice. It is usually not necessary to clamp the renal vein because we expect no temperature dissipation when the renal artery is clamped. The tumor is resected—-if possible—-with a surgical margin of a few millimeters of renal parenchyma.

The choice of surgical strategy depends on the size and location of the tumor and the number of tumors per kidney. Small central tumors adjacent to the hilum are resected using an intrasinusal dissection technique. Larger central tumors are resected by a transparenchymal approach. For transparenchymal incision, the segmental renal arteries are localized by Doppler ultrasound and marked on the renal surface with ink before clamping the renal artery.[8] The parenchymal incision is made between the vessels to avoid ischemic injury. For blunt and sharp dissection, neurosurgical brain spatulas are used. Multiple biopsies are obtained from the renal margins of resection and are sent separately from the resected complete tumor obtain frozen sections to determine the surgical margins. However, recent data provide evidence that a smaller margin may be adequate.[9,10] Although local recurrence is more likely in the presence of RCC at the surgical margin, it is not inevitable.[9] A positive frozen section may be addressed by a more extended resection, tissue ablation, nephrectomy, in particular in an elective setting, or closure. The latter strategy acknowledges the inherent uncertainty of frozen section findings. Small vessels are coagulated and large vessels are oversewn with 4/0 polyglycolic acid, which does not melt during the following coagulation. An argon beam laser and infrared coagulator are used for coagulation. Both instruments provide the required hemostasis from parenchymal bleeding. The noncontact argon laser does so by superficial tissue carbonization, while the infrared contact coagulator produces heat necrosis of tissue of 1–3 mm depth depending on the exposure time (1–5 seconds), with little carbonization and tissue adherence. Hence, in addition to providing hemostasis, infrared coagulation may be used for nonsurgical extension of the safety margin of resection. In addition, alternatively, hemostatic or hemostyptic agents such as Tachosil, Tachocomb, or Floseal can be used. With both techniques, most monofilament sutures tend to melt, so that braided sutures should be used preferably for ligation or oversewing. Suspected leakage from the renal collecting system by an undetected injury can be evaluated by puncture of the renal pelvis and injection of methylene blue. When partial resection of the collecting system is also required, a nephrostomy catheter is placed before reconstruction of the collecting system. A 6-8 F polyurethane ureteric stent is used as a nephrostomy and fixed by a 5/0 polyglytone pursestring suture. The opened calyces and renal pelvis are reconstructed with 6/0 polyglycolic acid. Suspected intrahilar injury of the renal pelvis or caliceal opening is evaluated by aspirating the renal pelvis, which serves the additional purpose of removing clots, and injecting methylene blue. Defects of the renal fibrous capsule are covered with a free peritoneal patch or an absorbable polyglactin mesh. Alternatively, hemostatic or hemostyptic agents such as Tachosil or Tachocomb might be used. The kidney can usually be closed by suturing the renal fibrous capsule without using parenchymal sutures, which damage preserved renal parenchyma and tend to tear through the

tissue. However, if the defect is too large, parenchymal sutures become necessary. The renal fibrous capsule is closed with a running monofilament mattress suture of 4/0 or 5/0 poly-p-dioxanone; this is a very important step for hemostasis. When the perirenal fat is lost, the mobilized kidney is embedded in greater omentum to prevent adhesions between the kidney and the surrounding tissue and to avoid ureteral kinking. In this series, no *ex vivo* tumor excisions are included.

Results

The intraoperative course was unremarkable in all cases. All tumor resections were performed *in situ* and bench surgery techniques were not required. Two patients (2.7%) died within the first 30 postoperative days because of heart failure from myocardial infarction in one patient and pulmonary edema in the other patient. The collecting system was opened in 25 patients (33.9%), in seven of whom (9.5%) a urinary extravasation developed. Urinary extravasation was treated in all cases with retrograde insertion of a ureteric catheter and in three patients additionally with percutaneous drain insertion. In one of these patients, secondary nephrectomy had to be performed because of sepsis. Postoperative hemorrhage occurred in three patients requiring open surgical reintervention in two and superselective arterial embolization in one patient. Acute renal failure requiring consecutive temporary hemodialysis occurred in four patients (5.4%). Renal function recovered after a mean of 8 weeks in three of these four patients. Chronic renal failure requiring hemodialysis developed in three patients (4.3%) after a mean of 3.8 years including the one patient with postoperative acute renal failure, in whom kidney function did not recover. Serum creatinine in the remainder (no dialysis) was 1.21 mg/dl (range: 0.51–2.8 mg/dl) at the latest follow-up.

The pathological features of NSS for centrally located tumors can be summarized as follows. Histological examination revealed benign tumors in 10 patients (13.5%), which were oncocytoma in 7 patients, angiomyolipoma in two patients, and an atypical cyst in one patient. The remaining 64 patients had RCC. Of the 64 patients with RCC, 51 patients (79.6%) had clear cell RCC, 9 (14.0%) had papillary RCC, and 4 (5.4%) had chromophobe RCC. The mean tumor size was 3.5 cm (range: 1.2–8.0 cm). Thirty-six patients (56.2%) had stage pT1a, 21 patients (32.8%) pT1b, three patients (4.7%) pT2, and four patients (6.3%) pT3. Fourteen patients (21.9%) had grade 1 RCC, 40 (62.5%) had grade 2, and 10 (15.6%) had grade 3 tumors.

At the time of surgery, nine patients (12.2%) had metastatic disease. They are excluded from further analysis with respect to tumor progression. Among the 55 patients without systemic disease, a total of 20 died, nine from tumor progression of RCC. The estimated overall survival rates at 1, 5, and 10 years were 94.4%, 76.1%, and 62.5%, respectively. The cancer-specific survival rates at 1, 5, and 10 years were 96.1%,

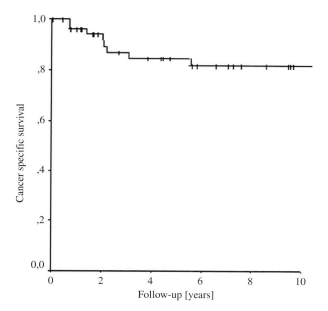

FIGURE 10b-1. Cancer-specific survival rates of NSS for centrally localized RCC (*n* = 55). Cancer-specific survival rates at 1, 5, and 10 years are 96.1%, 84.6%, and 81.7%, respectively.

84.6%, and 81.7%, respectively (Fig. 10b-1). Local tumor recurrence occurred in nine patients. The mean interval from nephron-sparing surgery to local tumor recurrence was 3.1 years (range: 0.2–12.3 years). The estimated local recurrence-free rates at 1, 5, and 10 years were 98.1%, 88.6%, and 85.5%, respectively (Fig. 10b-2).

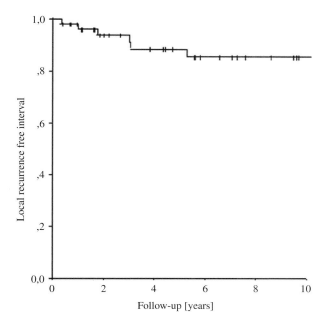

FIGURE 10b-2. Local recurrence-free interval of NSS for centrally localized RCC (*n* = 55). The local recurrence-free rates at 1, 5, and 10 years are 98.1%, 88.6%, and 85.5%, respectively.

Discussion

NSS for small, peripherally localized renal tumors is now generally accepted since it results in excellent local tumor control with disease-free survival rates comparable to those of radical nephrectomy. In elective NSS, selection for organ preservation is biased by oncological safety of resection from tumor size, location, and safe resectability. Thus, NSS for centrally localized tumors is mostly performed for imperative indications, since these locations mostly do not favor organ-sparing resection, but are justified to avoid subsequent hemodialysis and transplantation. Improvements in surgical technique and increased surgical experience have made it possible to approach even centrally located tumors previously considered inaccessible by NSS.[11,12] The Cleveland clinic compared the technical and oncological aspects of NSS between central and peripheral small RCCs;[11] NSS for central tumors proved to be technically more demanding, as evidenced by increased ischemia time and an increased incidence of opening of the collecting system. However, complication rates, renal function, and oncological outcome were comparable to NSS for peripheral lesions. These data were supported by our earlier series analyzing 33 patients undergoing NSS for centrally localized tumors.[12] In the present series, 18 patients underwent NSS for elective indications mostly because of the uncertain nature of the tumor. However, 14/18 (77.8%) were found to have RCC. After ensuring negative frozen margins and complete tumor resection, the decision was made to leave the kidney *in situ*. Elective NSS of centrally located tumors should be reserved for these selected patients. Diligent patient compliance is a prerequisite to ensure adequate follow-up studies. The current series also includes nine patients in whom metastatic disease was diagnosed preoperatively. The justification for performing surgery of any kind in such patients was curative in intent by combining renal surgery with resection of metastases.

NSS for centrally located renal tumors poses unique surgical challenges. Intraoperative ultrasound is a technical advance that facilitates NSS, in particular in a central location[8] to identify the tumor and to assess the tumor margins and the depth of the tumor extension. Extracorporeal surgery can be useful for excision of a central tumor, but all tumors of our series were amenable to *in situ* resection with arterial clamping and surface cooling. Such surgery is done under time constraints, since this type of cold ischemia time is limited to about 60 minutes. Postoperative complications requiring intervention in our series included urinary extravasation (9.5%), acute renal failure (5.4%), hemorrhage (4%), and sepsis (1.2%). In case of relevant postoperative bleeding from the kidney, angiography with the option of superselective embolization[13] of an arterial bleeding is an option. If there is no arterial bleeding detectable by angiography, conservative management is preferable to surgical revision as the latter carries the risk of nephrectomy. A urinary fistula or a urinoma is verified by the determination of creatinine concentration from the drainage fluid. Imaging usually includes ultrasonography and IVP or CT. Drainage of the collecting system by retrograde placement of a ureteric catheter usually solves the problem of extravasation. When a JJ stent is placed, continuous bladder drainage is required to prevent continued extravasation by reflux. Large urinomas must be drained, which can usually be done percutaneously by ultrasound-guided placement of a drain. In all cases of urinary extravasation (fistula, urinoma), antibiotic treatment is mandatory. Acute renal failure secondary to ischemic tubular necrosis is mostly temporary and requires temporary hemodialysis in cases of a solitary kidney or preexistent chronic renal failure. Dilation of the upper urinary tract as a sign of impaired urinary drainage may be caused by blood clots. If patients are symptomatic (fever, pain), drainage by means of a ureteric catheter or stent and antibiotics are required.

The major concern for justifying NSS for the treatment of RCC is the oncological safety of the strategy. In our series, the disease-specific survival rates at 5 and 10 years were 84.6% and 81.7%, respectively, which is comparable to other studies analyzing NSS for treatment of RCC under imperative indications.[14-16] In 14 patients with elective NSS for centrally localized RCC, we did not observe any case of tumor progression.

Our data indicate that resection of centrally localized kidney tumors is technically feasible with an acceptable complication rate. Most importantly, local tumor control is ensured. In addition, benign tumors may be diagnosed and excised without removing the kidney. Avoiding hemodialysis in imperative indications of NSS is the major gain for quality of life of these patients.

References

1. Novick, A. C., Stewart, B.H., Straffon, R.A., Banowsky, L.H.: Partial nephrectomy in the treatment of renal adenocarcinoma. J Urol, 118:932, 1977.
2. Marberger, M., Pugh, R.C., Auvert, J., Bertermann, H., Costantini, A., Gammelgaard, P.A. et al.: Conservation surgery of renal carcinoma: the EIRSS experience. Br J Urol, 53:528, 1981.
3. Bazeed, M.A., Scharfe, T., Becht, E., Jurincic, C., Alken, P., Thuroff, J.W.: Conservative surgery of renal cell carcinoma. Eur Urol, 12:238, 1986.
4. Butler, B.P., Novick, A.C., Miller, D.P., Campbell, S.A., Licht, M.R.: Management of small unilateral renal cell carcinomas: radical versus nephron-sparing surgery. Urology, 45:34, 1995.
5. Lerner, S.E., Hawkins, C.A., Blute, M.L., Grabner, A., Wollan, P.C., Eickholt, J.T. et al.: Disease outcome in patients with low stage renal cell carcinoma treated with nephron sparing or radical surgery. J Urol, 155:1868, 1996.
6. Marshall, F.F.: Is nephron-sparing surgery appropriate for a small renal-cell carcinoma? Lancet, 348:72, 1996.
7. Humke, U., Uder, M.: Renovascular hypertension: the diagnosis and management of renal ischaemia. BJU Int, 84:555, 1999.
8. Thuroff, J.W., Frohneberg, D., Riedmiller, R., Alken, P., Hutschenreiter, G., Thuroff, S. et al.: Localization of segmental arteries in renal surgery by Doppler sonography. J Urol, 127:863, 1982.
9. Sutherland, S.E., Resnick, M.I., Maclennan, G.T., Goldman, H.B.: Does the size of the surgical margin in partial nephrectomy for renal cell cancer really matter? J Urol, 167:61, 2002.
10. Castilla, E.A., Liou, L.S., Abrahams, N.A., Fergany, A., Rybicki, L.A., Myles, J. et al.: Prognostic importance of resection margin width after nephron-sparing surgery for renal cell carcinoma. Urology, 60:993, 2002.
11. Hafez, K.S., Novick, A.C., Butler, B.P.: Management of small solitary unilateral renal cell carcinomas: impact of central versus peripheral tumor location. J Urol, 159:1156, 1998.
12. Black, P., Filipas, D., Fichtner, J., Hohenfellner, R., Thuroff, J.W.: Nephron sparing surgery for central renal tumors: experience with 33 cases. J Urol, 163:737, 2000.
13. Poulakis, V., Ferakis, N., Becht, E., Deliveliotis, C., Duex, M.: Treatment of renal-vascular injury by transcatheter embolization: immediate and long-term effects on renal function. J Endourol, 20:405, 2006.
14. Ghavamian, R., Cheville, J.C., Lohse, C.M., Weaver, A.L., Zincke, H., Blute, M.L.: Renal cell carcinoma in the solitary kidney: an analysis of complications and outcome after nephron sparing surgery. J Urol, 168:454, 2002.
15. Saranchuk, J.W., Touijer, A.K., Hakimian, P., Snyder, M.E., Russo, P.: Partial nephrectomy for patients with a solitary kidney: the Memorial Sloan-Kettering experience. BJU Int, 94:1323, 2004.
16. Blute, M.L., Itano, N.B., Cheville, J.C., Weaver, A.L., Lohse, C.M., Zincke, H.: The effect of bilaterality, pathological features and surgical outcome in nonhereditary renal cell carcinoma. J Urol, 169:1276, 2003.

10c
Bilateral Renal Masses

Bradley C. Leibovich and Michael L. Blute

Introduction

Radical nephrectomy remains the accepted "gold standard" of care for clinically localized renal cell carcinoma (RCC) with a normal contralateral kidney due to proven long-term efficacy and continued lack of systemic therapeutic options. Clinicians will occasionally encounter patients with bilateral renal masses or masses in solitary kidneys who require special consideration to surgical approach. Hereditary and familial forms of RCC include tuberous sclerosis, von Hippel–Lindau (VHL) syndrome, Birt–Hogg–Dube syndrome, and familial papillary clear cell RCC. RCC occurring in the setting of these syndromes generally occurs at a younger age and is often bilateral and multifocal.[1] Hereditary factors are covered elsewhere in this text; we review the literature and our clinical approach to patients with bilateral renal masses or masses in solitary kidneys.

Incidence

Bilateral RCC is generally considered to be uncommon; in 1967 Villegas et al. reviewed the available literature consisting of only 39 cases.[2] The published incidence of bilateral RCC is approximately 1–4%.[2–8] Vermillion et al. reported the Massachusetts General Hospital experience with 12 bilateral renal mass patients and reported an incidence of 1.8% based on six bilateral cases of 329 total cases between 1935 and 1965.[7] Patel et al.[5] reported on 46 patients with sporadic bilateral renal tumors in a tertiary referral center that represented 4.25% of all patients with nonmetastatic renal tumors at their institution. Of the 5100 patients in the Mayo Clinic nephrectomy registry, there are 197 patients (3.8%) with synchronous bilateral renal masses and 230 cases (4.5%) of renal masses in solitary kidneys. The incidence of contralateral recurrence of RCC after prior nephrectomy in a large retrospective review from our registry was determined to be 1.2%.[9] The true incidence of solitary kidneys with masses and bilaterality is, however, difficult to ascertain as the majority of published data emanates from tertiary referral

centers and likely reflects a biased data set with overrepresentation of such difficult cases.

Histology

The behavior of solid renal tumors is related to histology, and in the case of bilateral masses, the clinician must always consider the possibility of benign renal masses,[10,11] metastatic lesions,[12,13] and other non-RCC histology such as lymphoma.[14–18] Dechet et al.[10] reported the benign nature of oncocytoma and noted that 5% of cases were bilateral and 6% of cases were multifocal. In general, renal biopsy and imaging findings are not considered to be good predictors of RCC histology compared with pathological examination of a surgical specimen after radical nephrectomy (RN) or nephron-sparing surgery (NSS).[19] However, in the case of bilateral renal masses, especially those with infiltrative growth patterns or other imaging features suggestive of metastatic lesions or lymphoma, percutaneous biopsy should be considered prior to intervention (see Fig. 10c-1).

Patients with bilateral RCC may also be more likely to have histological subtypes, which will behave in an indolent fashion. Siemer et al. have previously shown that non-clear cell histology, specifically papillary RCC, is more prevalent in bilateral RCC than in unilateral RCC.[20] Bani-Hani et al. noted the overrepresentation of papillary RCC also appears to apply to asynchronous bilateral RCC in a large series from our institution.[9] Cheville et al. reviewed 2385 patients with RCC and found that multifocality was present in 11% of patients with papillary RCC versus 2% each for patients with clear cell or chromophobe RCC.[21] Furthermore, they report a cancer-specific survival rate of 87% for papillary and chromophobe RCC versus 69% for clear cell RCC.

Several investigators have attempted to ascertain if bilateral renal tumors represent simultaneously occurring primary tumors or metastases from one kidney to the contralateral kidney. A large series from our institution suggested that bilateral RCC represents multiple *de novo* primary tumors rather than metastatic events.[22] Kume et al. examined 10 nonpapillary bilateral RCC tumors and found five patients

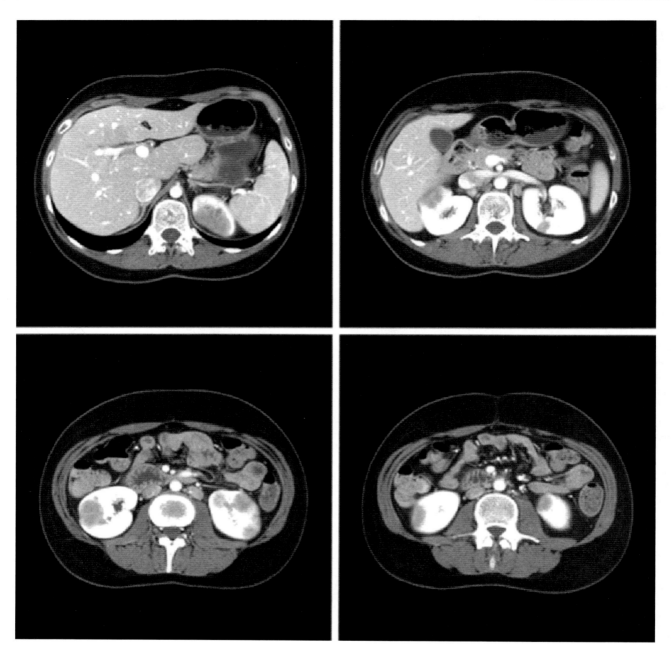

FIGURE 10c-1. This patient presented with bilateral renal masses. However, the appearance was atypical for RCC. Renal biopsy revealed histiocytosis.

with VHL mutation.[23] Three of the five had concordant mutations and two had discordant mutations suggesting that a slight majority of cases in this small series was metastatic in origin. In contrast, another study of VHL mutation in 43 bilateral synchronous non-VHL clear cell RCC cases revealed a 56% rate of VHL gene mutation.[24] However, only one patient had identical mutations in the right and left kidneys suggesting that the majority of bilateral cases were independent events. Kito et al. found via DNA microsatellite analysis that asynchronous bilateral RCCs were of clonal origin and the subsequent lesions were likely to be a

metastatic events while synchronous bilateral RCC was more likely to be due to multiple primary tumors that were genetically distinct.[25] A recent study by Itano et al. examined the pathological features, DNA ploidy, proliferation, and image mophometry of right and left RCC specimens in patients with bilateral synchronous tumors.[26] They noted that despite a high concordance of histological subtype, significant heterogeneity of morphology, DNA ploidy, and proliferation were suggestive of separate *de novo* renal tumors rather than clonal origin. Ultimately, more sophisticated analysis of genetic aberrations in bilateral RCC will not only clarify this issue,

TABLE 10c-1. Results of imperative nephron-sparing surgery.

Reference	Number of patients	Cause specific survival(%)	Local recurrence(%)	Mean follow-up (months)
Novick (1977)[33]	17	83	NR[a]	NR
Smith	36	72	8	3–117
Novick (1986)[35]	33	85	6	45
Bazeed	29	93	7	36
Provet	33	91	3	36
Moll (1993)[32]	47	94	4	35

[a]NR, not reported.

but may also identify the factors that predispose for bilateral RCC in the absence of heritable RCC syndromes.

Surgical Therapy

Potentially curative options for patients with solid renal masses that are bilateral or in solitary kidneys include RN and NSS. Ablative techniques are useful as adjuncts to surgery, especially in the setting of small local recurrences in a kidney after NSS (discussed elsewhere in this chapter). Historically, bilateral renal masses have been treated with bilateral nephrectomy rendering the patient anephric,[27] or with subsequent transplantation.[28] Alternatively, when experience with NSS was still limited, bilateral masses were occasionally treated with bench surgery and autotransplantation.[29,30] With increased experience and excellent outcomes with NSS,[31–35]

most patients with a solid mass in a solitary kidney or bilateral masses are treated with *in situ* NSS (Table 10c-1).

Currently, the surgical approach to the patient with bilateral solid masses is based on presentation, patient comorbidities, tumor size and location, surgeon experience and comfort with complex NSS, and the clinical status of the retroperitoneal lymph nodes. Most often, patients with bilateral masses have an obvious discrepancy in the complexity of the renal masses as illustrated in Fig. 10c-2. Surgeon preference varies; however, we advocate approaching the kidney with the larger more complex mass first via a transabdominal exposure. The advantage to treating the larger mass first is that if it is necessary to abandon treatment for the contralateral kidney and perform staged operations, the more threatening mass is already treated. When the first kidney is treated by a radical nephrectomy and the patient is doing well intraoperatively, contralateral NSS can be undertaken in the same operative procedure. If bilateral NSS is planned and the

(a)

(b)

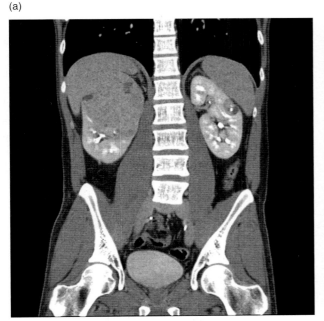
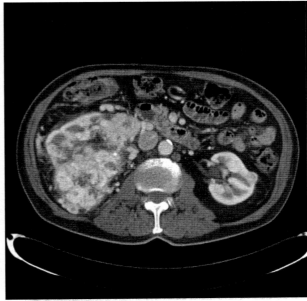

FIGURE 10c-2. (A) This patient had an incidental finding of bilateral renal masses. A transabdominal approach was utilized and bilateral NSS was performed in the same setting. The larger right-sided mass was removed first. (B) This patient had the larger right-sided mass removed first via a transabdominal approach and radical nephrectomy. However, since a tumor thrombus necessitated occlusion of the left renal vein, the small left renal mass was left for a second, staged operation.

kidney remains well perfused with adequate urine output throughout the more complex procedure, the less complex NSS on the contralateral kidney can be undertaken in the same operation. Staged operations are preferred by some surgeons and are also recommended if there is any doubt as to thr viability of a kidney, or if the patient is unstable intraoperatively. It is critical for the surgeon to recognize that bilateral renal masses are associated with multifocality.[22] Therefore, we routinely expose the entire surface of the kidney in the course of NSS leaving fat adherent to the renal mass only, allowing careful inspection for additional lesions.

Details of surgical technique are covered elsewhere in this text. However, we have noted that when assessing a tumor for NSS, urologists often take into consideration the perceived need for a rim of at least 1 cm of normal uninvolved parenchyma. There are few data to support this practice. Novick et al.[33] reported a series of enucleations performed for RCC at the Mayo Clinic and Cleveland Clinic between 1970 and 1983.[35] Their 3-year actuarial survival was 90% and local tumor recurrence occurred in only two patients (6%). Lerner et al. compared the outcomes of NSS in 185 patients with RN in 209 matched patients in 1996.[36] NSS consisted of partial nephrectomy in 82 patients and enucleation in 87 patients. They found no difference in the rate of cancer death or progression to metastases between patients treated by partial nephrectomy versus enucleation. Recently, Sutherland et al. directly examined the issue of surgical margins for NSS by quantifying the thickness of uninvolved tissue surrounding the tumor in 44 partial nephrectomy specimens.[37] The mean and median size of negative margins was 0.25 and 0.2 cm, respectively (range 0.05–0.7) and three patients had positive surgical margins. One patient with positive surgical margins had multiple local and systemic recurrences. None of the other patients had tumor recurrence with a mean follow-up for this series of 49 months. The authors conclude that only a minimal margin of less than 5 mm is required when performing NSS. We have found that with modern techniques of *in situ* NSS, including enucleation where appropriate, it is rare to have a situation in which a patient must be rendered anephric due to synchronous bilateral renal masses.

Outcome

Outcome from several modern series of bilateral RCC with emphasis on preservation of renal parenchyma is summarized in Table 10c-2; 5-year cancer-specific survival ranges from 70% to 93%. Figure 10c-3 illustrates cancer-specific survival for the current total experience at our institution with 197 cases of bilateral renal masses.

Two studies have addressed survival after bilateral RN and dialysis. Black et al. reported a 44% survival at 5 years in six patients after bilateral RN and dialysis.[27] They also reviewed the published literature at the time, which consisted of 14 reported cases. Of the 14 patients three died of tumor-related causes and six died of tumor-unrelated causes at a median of 1.1 years. Charmes et al. reported a 5-year survival of 16% in a series of 31 patients rendered anephric after bilateral RN and dialysis.[27,38] Although comparison of these series to series of patients largely managed with renal conservation is inappropriate due to likely differences in extent of disease at the time of presentation, preservation of renal function may offer a survival advantage.

Preservation of renal function is also advantageous with regard to quality of life. Clark et al. reported results of administering validated questionnaires on quality of life and impact and stress of cancer to 97 patients two had undergone either RN or NSS for localized renal cell carcinoma.[39] The RN and NSS groups were similar in overall quality of life, and both groups were similar to age-matched controls who had not undergone surgery for renal cell carcinoma. However, they found that a greater quantity of remaining renal parenchyma was associated with better self-reported physical health, less daily anxiety regarding cancer, less concern regarding cancer recurrence, and less impact of cancer on overall health. Quality of life after therapy for localized RCC was assessed in 15 RN and 51 NSS cases by Shinohara et al.[40] Patients treated with NSS had a significantly higher score on physical function in a standardized quality of life questionnaire than patients treated with radical nephrectomy ($p < 0.05$). NSS patients were also found to have less postoperative fatigue, sleep disturbance, pain, and constipation than patients who had RN.

TABLE 10c-2. Survival with bilateral renal cell carcinoma.[a]

Reference	Number of patients	5-year CSS	Local recurrence	Median follow-up (months)
Grimaldi, 1998[3]	29	93%	NR	52
Gacci, 2001[41]	46	92%	9%	92
Blute, 2000[44]	94[b]	81%	5%	50
Lundstam, 2003[42]	43	70%	NR	61
Patel, 2003[5]	46	83%	4%	74
Blute, 2003,[22c]	32 clear cell	80%	9%	
	12 papillary	83%	8%	91

[a]NR, not reported; CSS, cancer-specific survival.
[b]All patients had bilateral synchronous tumors.
[c]Series limited to bilateral synchronous subtype concordant renal cell carcinoma.

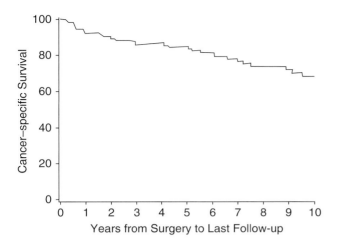

FIGURE 10c-3. Kaplan–Meier estimate of cancer-specific survival for 197 patients treated surgically at the Mayo Clinic for bilateral renal masses.

Gacci et al. reported on imperative NSS in 62 patients with RCC 46 of whom had either bilateral tumors (synchronous and asynchronous) or a solitary kidney.[41] The median follow-up in this retrospective review was 92 months. RCC recurrence was observed in 28% of patients overall with four patients having recurrence in a renal remnant alone, three patients having local recurrence and concurrent metastatic RCC, and five patients having distant metastases alone. The probability of survival was 100%, 92%, and 82% at 2, 5, and 10 years, respectively.

Lundstam et al. reported long-term results of NSS for RCC in 87 patients, 43 of whom had bilateral disease (28 synchronous).[42] They noted that cancer-specific survival at 5 years was 80% for all patients and 70% for patients with bilateral RCC. No difference was seen between those patients with synchronous and asynchronous presentation.

Patel et al. conducted a retrospective review of the Memorial Sloan-Kettering Cancer Center experience with bilateral sporadic renal tumors.[5] Of the 92 renal tumors in 46 patients 42% were managed with RN and 57% were managed with NSS. Seven patients were managed with bilateral NSS. Histology was clear cell in 66% and papillary in 14% with 76% concordant histology between subtypes of tumors in each patient. Survival was noted to be similar to a group of 1029 patients with unilateral RCC. With a median follow-up of 74 months, 5-year cancer-specific survival was 83% and 82% for bilateral and unilateral RCC, respectively. Patel et al. noted no difference in survival for patients with synchronous versus asynchronous presentation in their study,[5] although this is controversial.[8,34,43] Both Marberger et al.[43] and Zincke et al.[8] have reported superior survival for synchronous tumors versus asynchronous tumors.

Blute et al. analyzed a series of 94 patients with sporadic synchronous bilateral renal masses from the Mayo Clinic.[44] Of 94 patients, 85 (90%) had cancer in at least one kidney;

71 (76%) had bilateral synchronous RCC and 14 had unilateral cancer with a contralateral benign synchronous mass. Bilateral benign tumors were found in nine patients (10%). Cancer-specific survival among the 85 patients with at least one RCC was 81%, 59%, and 59% at 5, 10, and 15 years, respectively. Multivariate analysis revealed that metastasis-free survival was associated with nuclear grade and cancer-specific survival was associated with tumor size. The surgical approach was assessed with regard to outcome. Unilateral RN with contralateral NSS was performed in 61 patients, bilateral NSS in 20 patients, and bilateral RN in 4 patients. Multivariate analysis revealed that the surgical approach was not associated with outcome. Likewise, the type of NSS (extended partial nephrectomy versus enucleation) did not impact outcome.

A subsequent study by Blute et al. compared a select cohort of 44 patients with bilateral nonhereditary RCC to 1714 cases of unilateral clear cell RCC and 322 cases of unilateral papillary RCC.[22] Of the 44 patients, 32 had bilateral synchronous clear cell RCC and 12 had bilateral synchronous papillary RCC. Clinical and pathological features were similar among patients with unilateral RCC and patients with bilateral RCC with the exception of a higher rate of multifocal RCC. Multifocality was observed in 28% and 33% of bilateral synchronous clear cell and papillary RCC compared with 2% and 7% of unilateral clear cell and papillary RCC. When controlled for stage, histology, tumor size, nuclear grade, and the presence of histological tumor necrosis, there was no statistical difference in cancer-specific survival or metastasis-free survival between patients with bilateral and unilateral RCC. However, patients with bilateral RCC were at higher risk of local recurrence than patients with unilateral RCC despite controlling for the same covariates.

Complications

Complications in several large series of NSS are summarized in Table 10c-3. The rates of complications in the Mayo Clinic Nephrectomy registry for patients with bilateral renal masses or masses in a solitary kidney are summarized in Tables 10c-4 and 10c-5, respectively. Blute et al. specifically addressed the likelihood of complications in bilateral synchronous tumors based on whether the operations were staged (7 patients) or done in one operative setting (37 patients).[22] Among the staged patients, 43% had some complication while only 11% had complications among those that were not staged, although this did not reach statistical significance (Table 10c-6). Considering the complexity of surgery, including the frequent requirement for clamping of the renal hilar vessels, the number of overall complications for this patient population appears acceptably low.

TABLE 10c-3. Complications of nephron-sparing surgery.

	Lerner[45] (n = 169)[a]	Morgan[46] (n = 104)	Belldegrun[47] (n = 146)	Lau[48] (n = 164)	Duque[49] (n = 64)	Ghavamian†[50] (n = 76)
Postoperative bleeding	0	1 (0.9%)	3 (2.0%)	2 (1.2%)	3 (4.5%)	1 (1.6%)
Urine leak	3 (1.8%)	1 (0.9%)	2 (1.4%)	3 (1.8%)	6 (9.1%)	2 (3.2%)
Acute renal failure	0	NR[b]	NR	0	10 (15.1%)[c]	8 (12.7%)
Repeat open surgery	NR	NR	3 (2.0%)	1 (0.6%)	2 (3.0%)	7 (11.1%)
Myocardial infarction	1 (0.5%)	1 (0.9%)	2 (1.4%)	1 (0.6%)	0	NR
Death	1 (0.5%)	2 (1.9%)	3 (2.0%)	0	0	0

[a]For patients who underwent *in situ* partial nephrectomy.
[b]NR, not reported.
[c]Nephron-sparing surgery in patients with solitary kidneys.

TABLE 10c-4. Surgical complications for 197 patients with bilateral synchronous disease.

Surgical complication	N (%)
Intraoperative death	0 (0.0)
Perioperative death	0 (0.0)
Hemorrhage	5 (2.5)
Deep vein thrombosis	0 (0.0)
Pulmonary embolism	1 (0.5)
Myocardial infarction	0 (0.0)
Wound infection	6 (3.1)
Abscess	1 (0.5)
Urine leak	7 (3.6)
Sepsis	0 (0.0)
Acute renal failure	11 (5.6)
Dialysis	5 (2.5)
Kidney loss	3 (1.5)
Additional surgery	21 (10.7)
Ileus	15 (7.6)
Pneumothorax	2 (1.0)
Any surgical complication	46 (23.4)

TABLE 10c-6. Early complications after surgical management of bilateral synchronous clear cell or papillary renal cell carcinoma.[a]

	Staged	Not staged	
Number of patients	7	37	
Number (%) early complications			
Hemorrhage	0	1 (2.7)	
Urine leakage or extravasation	1 (14.3)	1 (2.7)	
Acute renal failure	2 (28.6)	1 (2.7)	
Kidney loss	1 (14.3)	1 (2.7)	
Additional surgical procedure	3 (42.9)	3 (8.1)	
Any complication[b]	3 (42.9)	4 (10.8)	p = 0.068

Source: Adapted from Blute et al. (2003).[22]
[a]No patients had deep vein thrombosis, pulmonary embolism, myocardial infarction, wound infection, sepsis, abscess, ileus, or pneumothorax.
[b]Some patients had more than one complication.

Conclusions

Bilateral renal tumors and tumors in solitary kidneys are relatively rare and present a difficult surgical problem. Clinicians must be aware of the increased incidence of multifocality and the potential for unique histology. In some clinical scenarios, biopsy may be indicated if there is concern for non-RCC histology. The surgeon should attempt to remove all disease with negative surgical margins while preserving as much bulk of normal renal parenchyma as possible. This can often be accomplished in a single transabdominal operation, which does not increase complication rates. Despite earlier reports to the contrary, current data indicate that patients may have long-term cure rates equivalent to cases of unilateral RCC.

TABLE 10c-5. Surgical complications for 254 procedures in a solitary kidney.

Surgical complication	N (%)
Intraoperative death	1 (0.4)
Perioperative death	3 (1.2)
Hemorrhage	6 (2.4)
Deep vein thrombosis	1 (0.4)
Pulmonary embolism	2 (0.8)
Myocardial infarction	2 (0.8)
Wound infection	3 (1.2)
Abscess	4 (1.6)
Urine leak	11 (4.3)
Sepsis	3 (1.2)
Acute renal failure	30 (11.8)
Dialysis	15 (5.9)
Kidney loss	3 (1.2)
Additional surgery	28 (11.0)
Ileus	14 (5.5)
Pneumothorax	0 (0.0)
Any surgical complication	65 (25.6)

References

1. Linehan, W.M., M.M. Walther, and B. Zbar, The genetic basis of cancer of the kidney. Journal of Urology, 2003. **170**(6 Pt 1):2163–2172.
2. Villegas, A.C., Bilateral primary malignant renal tumors of dissimilar histogenesis: report of 2 cases and review of the literature. Journal of Urology, 1967. **98**(4):450–455.

3. Grimaldi, G., V. Reuter, and P. Russo, Bilateral non-familial renal cell carcinoma. Annals of Surgical Oncology, 1998. **5**(6):548–552.

4. Hubmer, G. and P.H. Petritsch, Organ-preserving surgery for renal cell carcinoma in patients with a solitary kidney or bilateral tumors. Seminars in Surgical Oncology, 1988. **4**(2):133–136.

5. Patel, M.I., et al., Long-term follow-up of bilateral sporadic renal tumors. Urology, 2003. **61**(5):921–925.

6. Sethney, T., et al., Bilateral asynchronous renal tumors. Journal of Urology, 1983. **129**(1):123–125.

7. Vermillion, C.D., D.G. Skinner, and R.C. Pfister, Bilateral renal cell carcinoma. Journal of Urology, 1972. **108**(2):219–222.

8. Zincke, H. and S.K. Swanson, Bilateral renal cell carcinoma: influence of synchronous and asynchronous occurrence on patient survival. Journal of Urology, 1982. **128**(5):913–915.

9. Bani-Hani, A.H., et al., Associations with contralateral recurrence following nephrectomy for renal cell carcinoma using a cohort of 2,352 patients. Journal of Urology, 2005. **173**(2): 391–394.

10. Dechet, C.B., et al., Renal oncocytoma: multifocality, bilateralism, metachronous tumor development and coexistent renal cell carcinoma. Journal of Urology, 1999. **162**(1):40–42.

11. Fairchild, T.N., D.H. Dail, and G.E. Brannen, Renal oncocytoma—-bilateral, multifocal. Urology, 1983. **22**(4): 355–359.

12. Becker, W.E. and P.F. Schellhammer, Renal metastases from carcinoma of the lung. British Journal of Urology, 1986. **58**(5):494–498.

13. Mitnick, J.S., et al., Metastatic neoplasm to the kidney studied by computed tomography and sonography. Journal of Computer Assisted Tomography, 1985. **9**(1):43–49.

14. Cupisti, A., et al., Bilateral primary renal lymphoma treated by surgery and chemotherapy. Nephrology Dialysis Transplantation, 2004. **19**(6):1629–1633.

15. Tornroth, T., et al., Lymphomas diagnosed by percutaneous kidney biopsy. American Journal of Kidney Diseases, 2003. **42**(5):960–971.

16. O'Sullivan, A.W., et al., Bilateral primary renal lymphoma. Irish Journal of Medical Science, 2003. **172**(1):44–45.

17. O'Riordan, E., et al., Primary bilateral T-cell renal lymphoma presenting with sudden loss of renal function. Nephrology Dialysis Transplantation, 2001. **16**(7):1487–1489.

18. Bhatia, S., et al., Primary bilateral renal lymphoma. American Journal of Surgical Pathology, 1996. **20**(2):257.

19. Dechet, C.B., et al., Prospective analysis of computerized tomography and needle biopsy with permanent sectioning to determine the nature of solid renal masses in adults. Journal of Urology, 2003. **169**(1):71–74.

20. Siemer, S., et al., Bilateral kidney tumor. Therapy management and histopathological results with long-term follow-up of 66 patients. Urologe A, 2001. **40**(2):114–120.

21. Cheville, J.C., et al., Comparisons of outcome and prognostic features among histologic subtypes of renal cell carcinoma. American Journal of Surgical Pathology, 2003. **27**(5): 612–624.

22. Blute, M.L., et al., The effect of bilaterality, pathological features and surgical outcome in nonhereditary renal cell carcinoma. Journal of Urology, 2003. **169**(4):1276–1281.

23. Kume, H., et al., Genetic identification of bilateral primary or metastatic nonpapillary renal cell carcinoma. BJU International, 2000. **86**(3):208–212.

24. Boelter, C., et al., Von Hippel-Lindau mutations in bilateral synchronous clear cell renal cell carcinoma. Presented at the American Urological Association. Abstract 104515, 2003.

25. Kito, H., et al., Distinct patterns of chromosomal losses in clinically synchronous and asynchronous bilateral renal cell carcinoma. Journal of Urology, 2002. **168**(6):2637–2640.

26. Itano, N.B., et al., Is there pathologic concordance among non-von Hippel Lindau patients with synchronous bilateral renal cell carcinoma? Presented at the North Central Section of American Urological Association, Scottsdale, Arizona, November 4, 2000.

27. Black, J., et al., Bilateral nephrectomy and dialysis as an option for patients with bilateral renal cancer. Nephron, 1988. **49**(2):150–153.

28. Jochimsen, P.R., P.M. Braunstein, and J.S. Najarian, Renal allotransplantation for bilateral renal tumors. JAMA, 1969. **210**(9):1721–1724.

29. Zincke, H., et al., Treatment of renal cell carcinoma by in situ partial nephrectomy and extracorporeal operation with autotransplantation. Mayo Clinic Proceedings, 1985. **60**(10):651–662.

30. Zincke, H., et al., Treatment of renal cell carcinoma by in situ partial nephrectomy and extracorporeal operation with autotransplantation. Mayo Clinic Proceedings, 1985. **60**(10):651–662.

31. Marshall, F.F., et al., The feasibility of surgical enucleation for renal cell carcinoma. Journal of Urology, 1986. **135**(2):231–234.

32. Moll, V., E. Becht, and M. Ziegler, Kidney preserving surgery in renal cell tumors: indications, techniques and results in 152 patients. Journal of Urology, 1993. **150**(2 Pt 1):319–323.

33. Novick, A.C., et al., Partial nephrectomy in the treatment of renal adenocarcinoma. Journal of Urology, 1977. **118**(6):932–936.

34. Novick, A.C., et al., Conservative surgery for renal cell carcinoma: a single-center experience with 100 patients. Journal of Urology, 1989. **141**(4):835–839.

35. Novick, A.C., et al., Surgical enucleation for renal cell carcinoma. Journal of Urology, 1986. **135**(2):235–238.

36. Lerner, S., et al., Disease outcome in patients with low stage renal cell carcinoma treated with nephron sparing or radical surgery. Journal of Urology, 1996. **155**:1868–1873.

37. Sutherland, S.E., et al., Does the size of the surgical margin in partial nephrectomy for renal cell cancer really matter? Journal of Urology, 2002. **167**(1):61–64.

38. Charmes, J.P., et al., Prognosis on dialysis of 31 patients after bilateral nephrectomy for bilateral renal cancer. Nephron, 1989. **52**(4):365–366.

39. Clark, P.E., et al., Quality of life and psychological adaptation after surgical treatment for localized renal cell carcinoma: impact of the amount of remaining renal tissue. Urology, 2001. **57**(2):252–256.

40. Shinohara, N., et al., Impact of nephron-sparing surgery on quality of life in patients with localized renal cell carcinoma. European Urology, 2001. **39**(1):114–119.

41. Gacci, M., et al., Imperative indications for conservative surgery for renal cell carcinoma: 20 years' experience. Urologia Internationalis, 2001. **67**(3):203–208.

42. Lundstam, S., et al., Nephron-sparing surgery for renal cell carcinoma—-long-term results. Scandinavian Journal of Urology & Nephrology, 2003. **37**(4):299–304.

43. Marberger, M., et al., Conservation surgery of renal carcinoma: the EIRSS experience. British Journal of Urology, 1981. **53**(6):528–532.

44. Blute, M.L., et al., Management and extended outcome of patients with synchronous bilateral solid renal neoplasms in the absence of von Hippel-Lindau disease. Mayo Clinic Proceedings, 2000. **75**(10):1020–1026.

45. Lerner S.E., et al., Disease outcome in patients with low stage renal cell carcinoma treated with nephron sparing or radical surgery. Journal of Urology, 1996. **155**(6):1868–1873.

46. Morgan W.R. and H. Zincke, Progression and survival after renal-conserving surgery for renal cell carcinoma: experience in 104 patients and extended followup. Journal of Urology, 1990. **144**(4):852–857; discussion 857–858.

47. Belldegrun, A., K.H. Tsui, J.B. deKernion, and R.B. Smith, Efficacy of nephron-sparing surgery for renal cell carcinoma: analysis based on the new 1997 tumor-node-metastasis staging system. Journal of Clinical Oncology, 1999. **17**(9):2868–2875.

48. Lau W.K., M.L. Blute, A.L. Weaver, V.E. Torres, and H. Zincke. Matched comparison of radical nephrectomy vs nephron-sparing surgery in patients with unilateral renal cell carcinoma and a normal contralateral kidney. Mayo Clinic Proceedings, 2000. **75**(12):1236–1242.

49. Duque J.L., K.R. Loughlin, M.P. O'Leary, S. Kumar, and J.P. Richie, Partial nephrectomy: alternative treatment for selected patients with renal cell carcinoma. Urology, 1998. **52**(4):584–590. Review.

50. Ghavamian R., J.C. Cheville, C.M. Lohse, A.L. Weaver, H. Zincke, and M.L. Blute, Renal cell carcinoma in the solitary kidney: an analysis of complications and outcome after nephron sparing surgery. Journal of Urology, 2002. **168**(2): 454-459.

10d
Old and Fragile Patients

Dmitry Y. Pushkar and Alexander V. Govorov

Introduction

In most countries the increasing longevity of the general population is a current demographic evolution. In 1998 there were 60 million individuals older than 65 years in the European Union accounting for 16% of the population.[129] As the median age of the world's population continues to increase so will the number of elderly patients requiring surgery. In the same way the number of cases of renal cell carcinoma (RCC) is steadily increasing,[56] particularly in patients 65 years or older. Renal cancer accounts for approximately 3% of all diagnosed malignancies and up to 95,000 deaths per year worldwide[98] and is primarily a disease of the elderly.[56] The mean age at the time of diagnosis is from 66[98] to 70 years.[79]

Physiological changes accompanying aging are numerous and they affect almost every organ system. These changes are accompanied by a high incidence of multiple adverse events, especially for hospitalized elderly patients. Hospitalization and surgery in the elderly population are associated with a delirium (defined as an acute decline in attention and cognition) occurring in 15–53% of older patients postoperatively and in 70–87% of those in intensive care,[43,44] a higher rate of falls (4–11/1000 patient-days),[70] a 32% incidence of functional decline,[101] and a 10–15% rate of adverse drug events (typical for elder patients),[39] among other risks.[61] Because of these observations it is becoming increasingly necessary to understand the impact of aging on both the diagnosis and treatment of RCC in elderly and fragile people.

Evaluation of Performance Status and Comorbidities

Outcome studies of the elderly are confounded primarily by coexisting medical conditions that are more prevalent with increasing age[31] and that may affect therapeutic decision making and survival. The study of Patard[92] confirmed the prognostic value of an important clinical variable in RCC: an altered health condition at diagnosis.

In oncological surgery outcome depends not only on the biological aggressiveness of the particular tumor, but also on the overall health of the individual patient.[82] This statement is particularly relevant for many patients undergoing nephrectomy given the advanced age and comorbidity frequently encountered in this population. Of particular importance is the identification of treatable comorbidities to optimize the patient's functional status preoperatively.

The evaluation of functional status plays a unique role in the assessment of older cancer patients. While performance status has been the traditional method for oncologists to assess the impact of a cancer patient's disease, older cancer patients may require a more thorough evaluation of their functional status. The evaluation of functional status provides information that can predict outcomes and may provide information that can be utilized to improve function. There are many different methods available to assess functional status and individual assessment of functional status in the context of a geriatric assessment may be important components of the care older cancer patients receive.[33]

Anesthesiologists assign the American Society of Anesthesiologists (ASA) score as a method of classifying preoperative surgical risk. Whereas the ASA score has a general definition and it has been associated with mortality rates,[126] the classification is somewhat subjective and may be prone to variation.[74]

The Charlson comorbidity index (a validated comorbidity index developed to classify comorbid conditions prospectively, which may impact mortality for patients with various medical diagnoses) identifies specific medical conditions and assigns a number representing a weighted risk for each condition.[15] Thus the index represents the additive risk from all comorbid conditions; it has been associated with 1-year mortality rates. Although it is a more objective risk stratification model, the Charlson index has been criticized as being poorly generalizable because it is based on a limited index population.[15] Nevertheless, because of its simplicity and predictive ability, multiple important and recent studies have relied on the Charlson index or administrative modifications thereof for postoperative outcomes analysis.[5,80,88]

Gettman et al.[34] analyzed the Charlson comorbidity index as a predictor of outcome after surgery for RCC and concluded that the Charlson index did not predict cause-specific survival in a cohort of surgically treated patients, and that prospective assessment of comorbidity in patients treated with surgery versus conservative therapy is warranted. A prospective study of comorbidity in patients treated with surgery versus conservative therapy may further address the effect of comorbid disease on clinical outcome.[34] Although the Charlson index was reported to be a better measure of comorbidity in retrospective studies,[27] assessment of comorbidity with other validated measures may also have strengthened the observations in the study. In addition, developing a comorbidity index specific to RCC may be warranted to assess the effect of preexisting medical conditions on outcome after surgery.[34]

General health status is often measured by the Eastern Cooperative Oncology Group performance status (ECOG-PS). This is a four-grade scoring system: 0, normal activity; 1, restricted in physically strenuous activity but ambulatory; 2, bedridden less than 50% of the time; and 3, completely bedridden. In other words, ECOG-PS defines performance as the ability to perform the daily activities of life, such as housework and self-care. ECOG performance status is a recognized prognostic factor for either localized or metastatic tumors.[114] The ECOG-PS score has been demonstrated to be one of the most important independent predictors of survival in patients with localized and advanced RCC and it has been incorporated into validated integrated staging systems.[127,128] On this basis other authors also integrated symptoms and performance status in mathematical algorithms predicting survival in RCC.[54,124]

However, ECOG-PS does not include measures of presenting signs and symptoms and it is not surprising that other parameters that predict survival can be identified. To better predict prognosis the findings of Kim et al.[55] suggest that ECOG-PC should be expanded to include indices of cachexia, which can be important in patients with RCC and significant comorbidities. ECOG performance status is an important predictor of bone metastasis in patients with presumed RCC lesions. A bone scan should be performed in patients with an ECOG score greater than 0 regardless of T stage, but is unnecessary in those presenting with an ECOG score of 0.[106]

At present there is no universally accepted tool for the measurement of medical comorbidity among patients treated with radical, partial or laparoscopic nephrectomy and comparisons of nephrectomy outcomes among individual surgeons and institutions are limited by the absence of rigorous risk adjustment instruments.

Prognostic and Hereditary Factors

The precise determination of prognostic factors is an essential step in the evaluation of patients with RCC not only to initiate new adjuvant treatments but also to predict disease evolution. Because conventional chemotherapy or immunotherapy provides only limited efficacy, a better understanding of prognostic factors would enable a better selection of patients to avoid ineffective treatment and to identify those who might benefit from earlier initiation of conventional therapy and finally those who should be directly enrolled in new therapeutic trials.[77] In our opinion, this is particularly important in the elderly and in patients with significant comorbidities.

Type of presentation, performance status, and comorbidity are the most important clinical prognostic factors (patient-related factors). Despite all the studies done to detect prognostic factors, the only significant parameters are the traditional ones: performance status, stage, grade, and histological type.[60] Age has no independent prognostic value.[49]

The number of elderly end stage renal disease patients has increased markedly[41] and hemodialysis treatment is the most widely used form of renal replacement therapy in the elderly.[28] A higher rate of detection of RCC (with RCC arising in 1–2% in these patients)[47,63,75] has been observed among patients with chronic renal failure undergoing hemodialysis, particularly among those with acquired renal cystic disease (ARCD), which[12,16,102] develops in up to 80% of patients with end-stage renal failure. The overall relative risk of RCC is 5- to 100-fold higher in patients with end-stage renal failure.[47,63,75] RCC arises in 1–2% in patients with ARCD.

All patients on dialysis suffer from an increased risk of cancer of the genitourinary tract. In particular, the native kidneys represent a considerable risk factor as underlying kidney disease predisposes to malignancy such as analgesic nephropathy or cystic kidney disease.[94] The risk of developing RCC is 30–40 times greater compared with the general population. The standardized incidence rate has been reported to be 7. For these reasons regular urological examinations are mandatory, with particular emphasis on the native kidneys.[67] It has been recommended that screening should be carried out with ultrasonography or computed tomography (CT) beginning during the third year on dialysis in younger and healthier patients.[18,87]

Recently Ishikawa[46] summarized 489 RCCs occurring in Japan in patients receiving dialysis. In Japan more than 50% of the dialysis patients with RCC had spent more than 10 years on dialysis compared to only 2.5% of such patients in the United States.[72] Of the patients in this study 17% have actually received more than 20 years of dialysis. The incidence of RCC was more than 10 times that in the normal population. The incidence in the Japanese study was almost four times higher in patients who had been receiving dialysis more than 10 years than in a previously reported series from the United States.[72]

Malignant tumors have a major impact on morbidity and mortality in patients after transplantation. The risk of cancer in patients on renal replacement therapy is even higher after transplantation than with dialysis.[8] Malignancy in kidney graft recipients can develop in three different ways: malignancies can occur *de novo*, be recurrent after transplantation, or derive from the donor organ.

The data of Murphy suggest that posttransplant patients, usually considered to have weakened status, have nearly double (1.85 times) the risk of developing RCC when compared to a historical, nontransplant cohort in the general population. The increased risk for development of RCC in posttransplant patients does not appear to be significantly affected by age, gender, ethnicity, or time from renal transplant.[84]

The probability of developing RCC by the seventh decade of life in von Hippel–Lindau (VHL) disease patients is 70%[69] and is a major cause of their mortality. Up to 95% of patients with VHL disease who survive to between ages 60 and 70 years have a solid or cystic renal lesion. The solid tumors are recurrent low-grade clear cell carcinomas.[99] Generally, screening for RCC is limited to target populations. Patients with VHL and patients with end-stage renal failure (preferably male, on hemodialysis, with a long life expectancy) are target populations for screening for RCC.[56] Patients treated by hemodialysis for chronic renal insufficiency who retain their native kidneys often develop cystic disease in their kidneys and later a kidney tumor. As noted above, they should be checked regularly as they are known to be at risk.[60]

Artificial neural networks (ANN) are more often used in prostate cancer patients, but there are some ANNs for prediction of 5-year survival status in patients with RCC.[38] We believe that developing an ANN to predict individual survival in old and fragile patients might be helpful for selection of the candidates for surgery or nonsurgical treatment.

Recently different novel systems for staging and predicting survival for RCC have been proposed. In particular, Zisman combined 1997 TNM, Fuhrman grading system, and ECOG performance status and identified five groups with significantly different survival patterns.[127] However, the relevance of performance status could be potentially correlated with the high number of advanced RCC patients analyzed in these series.[29,113,127]

Another well-known postoperative prognostic nomogram to predict disease recurrence for RCC, developed by Kattan et al.[54] did not take into account the Eastern Cooperative Oncology Group performance status and needs further validation in old and fragile patients. The combination of already known prognostic factors or the postoperative prognostic nomogram is highly attractive and easy to use but remains to be validated by large multicenter studies including elderly and low performance status patients.

Diagnostic Tests and Surgery

Diagnostic tests in old patients are not essentially different from those in young patients. In our opinion special preoperative preparation may be necessary only in limited categories of patients with significant comorbidities, and particularly in cases of continuous anticoagulation therapy or in patients with end-stage renal failure.

The indications and application of percutaneous biopsy for renal masses are rather limited in all patients. Biopsies can be performed in cases of suspected metastatic disease, or in the elderly to obtain a diagnosis and to avoid radical nephrectomy.[56]

CT is the gold standard in detecting and characterizing renal masses and staging RCCs. Ultrasound also plays a key role in the early diagnosis of RCCs.[100] Both technologies are widely used in examining all patients including the elderly and patients with a weakened state. Magnetic resonance imaging (MRI) may be useful in patients with renal insufficiency[100] since there is no nephrotoxic effect at the doses used with the MR contrast media (gadolinium chelates).

An interesting observation is that higher proportions of women and the elderly are noted within the incidentally detected cohorts.[10,17,62] This can be explained, at least in part, by more frequent physician visits by females and the elderly.[62]

Significant advances in the diagnosis, staging, and treatment of patients with RCC (including old and fragile patients) in the past 2 decades have resulted in improved survival of a select group of patients and an overall change in the natural history of the disease.

Radical nephrectomy is the "gold standard" curative treatment for patients with localized RCC.[116] Despite the risk of such major surgery in the elderly, radical nephrectomy remains a treatment option in healthy elderly patients. Constant advances in surgical procedures, anesthesia, and postoperative care provide this opportunity to elderly patients. However, patient benefit must be associated with an acceptable postoperative outcome and sufficient life expectancy.

In elderly patients with small tumors the morbidity and mortality of nephrectomy need to be balanced against the risks posed by the tumor. There are few published data about symptom control in those who forego radical surgery for advanced age and/or comorbidity. For patients with a short life expectancy the morbidity of a large procedure may offset the modest survival benefit.[83]

Usually patients older than 75 years have a lower preoperative hemoglobin and higher complication and transfusion rates after nephrectomy as described by Fornara et al.[30] Anemia with a hemoglobin concentration less than 10 mg/dl was also found to be a prognostic factor associated with the poor outcome by some investigators, but this remains controversial.[35,123] Han et al.[40] performed a retrospective analysis to determine the operative morbidity in patients with substantial comorbidities requiring renal surgery (n = 551). They found little difference in perioperative morbidity in patients undergoing radical nephrectomy regardless of their preoperative ASA status. Intermediate-risk patients (ASA classification 3, n = 297) did have a greater estimated blood loss, leading to greater transfusion rates. However, no increase occurred in intraoperative or postoperative morbidity. High-risk patients (ASA classification 4, $n = 17$) also had greater transfusion rates as well as a greater rate of complications occurring more than 24 hours after surgery. It was concluded that partial or radical nephrectomy can be offered to patients with comorbid conditions.

The ideal indication for nephron-sparing surgery (NSS) in the presence of a normal contralateral kidney is the presence of an easily resectable, small (4 cm diameter or less), solitary, exophytic renal tumor in a patient who is not a candidate for surveillance and whose medical condition is good enough to undergo surgery and to benefit from it. Relative indications include those patients in whom the contralateral kidney has preexisting renal disease or its future function is threatened (patients with stone disease, chronic pyelonephritis, renal artery stenosis, vesicoureteral reflux, chronic renal obstruction from congenital or acquired causes, or systemic diseases such as diabetes, hypertension, and nephrosclerosis). The risk and benefits of NSS must be considered individually in such patients, because the age of the patient at the time of presentation, comorbidities, and risk of disease progression might influence their remaining renal function:[51] e.g., in older patients with baseline renal insufficiency or increased surgical risk, partial nephrectomy may confer a warm ischemic insult and a somewhat higher complication rate.[24]

According to Shirasaki et al.,[105] NSS should be considered in patients with one or more risk factors (preoperative hypertension, diabetes, proteinuria, and a patient age >65 years), positively correlating with postoperative deterioration of renal function.

It is known that although patients undergoing open NSS experience more procedure-related complications, these are generally minor and include perirenal or intrarenal hemorrhage and urinary fistula that can, almost always, be managed by minimally invasive techniques.[109] The laparoscopic NSS had a longer renal warm-ischemia time compared with the open approach and was associated with more frequent and more severe intraoperative complications and more postoperative urological complications.[37]

Generally, in contemporary series, the complication rate for open partial nephrectomy ranges from 4% to 30%,[95] while the complication rate for laparoscopic partial nephrectomy ranges from 10% to 33%.[37,64,95] Although several complications were minor in these series, major complications occurred as well. Patients were not stratified by their ASA score and comorbidities, so complications could not be categorized by patient health.

Clearly, for patients for whom the risk associated with treatment is greater than that of observation (patients with high ASA scores, multiple medical comorbidities, age of ≥75 years, and a limited expected life span), watchful waiting is a reasonable option.[7] Besides, a critical consideration when contemplating major cancer surgery in the elderly patient

often is the length of time it would take for the patient to resume usual physical activities.[89] Valid concerns about the possible untoward sequelae of a prolonged period of convalescence and physical inactivity on the suboptimal cardiovascular and musculoskeletal status of the elderly often mitigate against major open cancer surgery in this patient population.[42]

Undoubtedly, age alone should not exclude elderly patients from definitive treatment at the outset. But morbidities of open and laparoscopic NSS in elder patients make watchful waiting a viable option, which could be a possible explanation for the lack of published data concerning partial nephrectomy in elderly patient group.

The follow-up frequency after NSS can be tailored according to the prognostic risk factors of each individual patient.[57] Improved perioperative care and changes in patient care strategies have given us the opportunity to reexamine certain practices. For many procedures limited postoperative hospitalization has become normal and it has been shown to have no adverse effect on patient morbidity or outcome.[14] On the other hand, patients who require radical nephrectomy are a diverse population who may often have more significant comorbidities that result in prolonged hospital stay.

The surgical approach for radical nephrectomy is determined by the size and location of the tumor and by patient-related factors. The open procedure is usually done through a transperitoneal (midline or chevron) incision to allow early access to the vessels. Some still prefer an extended subcostal extraperitoneal or transperitoneal incision.[58] The disadvantages of a transperitoneal approach are longer postoperative ileus and possible late intraabdominal adhesions. A thoracoabdominal approach is seldom required but can be used in patients with large upper pole tumors.[115]

Most patients undergoing radical nephrectomy because of RCC are middle aged or elderly and they seem to have risk factors for renal insufficiency. Thus, the remaining kidney after unilateral nephrectomy possibly shows more damage in these middle aged and elderly patients than in younger populations. However, few studies have evaluated renal function after unilateral nephrectomy in older populations[66,120] and few studies have addressed clinical guidelines of elderly patient care after radical or partial nephrectomy. Indeed, the relationship between postoperative renal function and preoperative risk factors is not well understood and it is necessary to determine preoperative factors predicting postoperative renal function[48] that may influence the decision on whether to perform a radical nephrectomy or a nephron-sparing procedure.

Taking into consideration that older patients are liable to have many more complications that can affect renal function that the younger population, Ito et al.[48] evaluated preoperative risk factors for predicting postoperative renal function in middle aged and elderly patients treated with radical nephrectomy. They concluded that in their study older age, male sex, hypertension, diabetes mellitus, proteinuria, preoperative serum creatinine, blood urea nitrogen, and serum potassium were significantly associated with postoperative renal function on univariate analysis, while preoperative serum creatinine, hypertension, and proteinuria were significant independent predictors on multivariate analysis.[48]

Stephenson et al.[109] reviewed the early complications of radical nephrectomy and partial nephrectomy in a large contemporary cohort using a standardized grading scale and concluded that patient age, operative time, and pathological stage were significant predictors of postoperative complications in a multivariate analysis.

The laparoscopic approach in the elderly population has significant favorable advantages. Smaller and strategically placed incisions are associated with decreased pain, decreased narcotic use, and earlier mobility,[13,36,111] all of which have a positive impact on postoperative respiratory drive and pulmonary function.[25] Investigators have observed that patients undergoing laparoscopic procedures experience decreased pulmonary complications, particularly compared with operations previously requiring an upper abdominal incision.[32] Decreased narcotic use and shorter hospitalization may not only lower the incidence of delirium and confusion in hospitalized elderly patients, but also may decrease hospital-associated complications and help lower the high cost of care generally associated with older patients.[74] The question that remains is whether the indications for urological laparoscopy can be extended to older people, despite the higher risk of and lower tolerance to complications in these patients, so that they can also benefit from the advantages of laparoscopy.

Laparoscopy has some features carrying a higher risk, particularly for elderly patients with compromised cardiovascular and pulmonary function.[117] Creating a pneumoperitoneum can cause cardiovascular changes similar to those of heart failure.[110] The increase in both systemic and pulmonary vascular resistance raises the cardiac afterload, which results in a decrease in cardiac output. The preload is also increased, as indicated by measurements of the central venous and right atrial pressures. The situation can be complicated if laparoscopically induced oliguria is not taken into consideration since inadvertent overhydration can lead to hemodilution and congestive heart failure.[117]

All the above mentioned pathophysiological changes are more pronounced when laparoscopic surgery is prolonged. Most of these concerns were raised in the early development of laparoscopic surgery when experience was being gained and operative times were long.[81,121] Currently, with faster procedures, a better understanding of the effects of pneumoperitoneum, and increased surgical experience, laparoscopic procedures are being used in patients with greater comorbidity.[117] Moreover, greater age has not been shown to be a predictor of a higher complication rate or a worse postoperative course in laparoscopic general surgical procedures.[4,45,96] Data on elderly patients undergoing laparoscopy for urological diseases are sparse, either because these patients are included in larger series of patients of all ages[13] or because there are only a few such patients in the infrequent existing publications.

Three prior reports of minimally invasive urological surgery in elderly patients have been published.[42,76,117] In the report by McDougall et al.,[76] five patients aged >80 years had laparoscopic radical nephrectomy (LRN) or nephroureterectomy. The postoperative course was excellent, with only one medical complication (atrial fibrillation), despite all patients being relatively ill (mean ASA physical status of 3) and the series being early in the experience, as is indicated by the long operative duration (range 6.75–10.6 hours).

Shorter LRNs were reported by Hsu et al.,[42] in which the outcomes of 11 laparoscopic and six open radical nephrectomies in patients aged ≥80 years were compared. The advantages of laparoscopic surgery were confirmed by reduced analgesic requirements, earlier oral intake, shorter hospital stay, and faster convalescence in the laparoscopy group. Complications, operative times, and average blood loss were similar in the open and laparoscopy groups, which indicated that once experience has been gained laparoscopy provides an excellent alternative to open surgery for tumor nephrectomy even in patients aged >80 years.[117]

Varkarakis et al. evaluated the efficacy and outcome of LRN in patients aged >75 years and compared the results with those obtained from patients younger than this undergoing laparoscopic surgery for the same indication.[117] With 28 patients aged >75 years and 14 aged >80, it is the largest series of elderly patients undergoing LRN yet reported. There was no difference between the older and younger groups in complications rates and postoperative variables; furthermore, the operative duration, estimated mean blood loss, and tumor size were comparable, indicating that the tumors treated were of similar surgical difficulty. The only statistically significant difference was the higher ASA score in the older group, but this did not affect the final outcome of surgery. This is in line with the results reported by Massie et al.,[73] where elderly patients had higher ASA scores but the laparoscopic procedure was associated with lower morbidity than open surgery. A laparoscopic approach appears to offer advantages in these older patients. However, it has been reported that in several open procedures (e.g., cholecystectomy, total hip replacement), increasing age and higher ASA scores are associated with a prolonged hospital stay, higher complication rates, and more office visits after discharge.[19]

So Varkarakis et al.[117] concluded that elderly patients (>75 years old) should not be excluded from LRN, even though they usually have more comorbidities than younger patients, and that careful preoperative preparation, intraoperative monitoring, and attentive postoperative care make laparoscopy in these patients as promising as in their younger counterparts. These findings are consistent with those in multiple prior studies documenting decreased pain, improved bowel function, and more rapid recovery in patients undergoing laparoscopic renal and adrenal surgery compared with open surgery.[13,36] Hand-assisted laparoscopic surgery is especially useful when patient comorbidities require a rapid procedure.[86]

To determine whether age and comorbidity are predictors of outcome in patients undergoing laparoscopic renal and adrenal surgery, Matin et al.[74] performed a single center, retrospective study. They concluded that the findings in their study are consistent with data from other surgical disciplines suggesting that age 65 years or older is not a significant independent predictor of adverse outcomes after laparoscopic surgery. On the other hand, as measured by the Charlson index, comorbidity is associated with a higher risk of postoperative complications when comparing those with an index of less than versus greater than 3. They found no statistically significant associations between higher ASA score and perioperative complications overall. Patients with a higher ASA score were more likely to receive blood transfusions. Age 65 years or older did not appear to increase the incidence of intraoperative, postoperative, or late operative complications on univariate or multivariate analyses. However, age 65 years or older was predictive of increased hospitalization (approximately 1 day) after major renal and adrenal laparoscopic surgery.

Older patients with a history of abdominal surgery and with multiple comorbidities should be advised that if laparoscopic simple or radical nephrectomy is planned, there is a higher probability of blood transfusion.[91]

Many patients who need radical nephrectomy are in the sixth and seventh decades of life, corresponding to the age at which these diseases typically present. Many older patients have previously undergone an abdominal operation. The data of Seifman et al.[103] indicate that operative and major complication rates are higher in patients who have undergone a previous open abdominal operation if the transperitoneal laparoscopic route is elected. In their series these patients were approximately 8 years older and had more medical comorbidities, as reflected in the higher ASA score, which may place the patient at a higher risk for complications.

Desai et al.[23] showed that operative morbidity and complications after LRN were similar with transperitoneal or retroperitoneal approaches, but in their opinion the retroperitoneal approach may be preferred in patients with multiple prior transperitoneal surgeries in the area of interest as well as in morbidly obese patients.

Treatment of Metastatic Renal Cell Carcinoma

General condition, which combines symptoms and comorbidity, is a prognostic factor that has been identified based on most series. Thus, an ECOG performance status of 2 or greater not only is an independent prognostic factor associated with shorter survival[26,35] but also predicts a poorer response to immunotherapy.[65] Nevertheless, it is difficult to discern whether the treatment is less effective because the performance status is low or whether the performance status is low because the tumor is more aggressive.[77]

Discussing treatment options for advanced metastatic RCC (mRCC) according to performance status, Vogelzang concluded that a nephrectomy should be strongly considered before immunotherapy only in PS 0 patients, should be considered in PS 1 patients, and should not be done in PS 2 patients.[118] In the same paper Bui and Belldegrun noted that the most favorable responses to immunotherapy are seen in patients with high performance status (ECOG 0-1), no concomitant underlying diseases, and good cardiac, respiratory, and renal function.[118] Therefore, patient selection is of paramount importance, especially because interleukin-2 (IL-2) can produce significant side effects, such as azotemia, hypotension, pulmonary edema, and renal failure.

For these reasons patients with metastatic RCC who have a good ECOG-PS are more likely to respond to immunotherapy[127] and, therefore, at most centers IL-2-based immunotherapy is administered only to patients with good PS.

Concerning nephrectomy followed by immunotherapy in patients with significant comorbidities, it is obvious that careful patient selection is critical and patients with inadequate cardiac or pulmonary function or concurrent illnesses should not be considered.[49] Indeed Mickisch also suggested that patients with inadequate cardiac or pulmonary function or concurrent illness are ineligible for immunotherapy a priori.[78] Generally only patients with an ECOG performance status of 0 or 1 are selected for high-dose IL-2 therapy.[90] Bad performance status (WHO $\geq$ 1) is a risk factor for a short survival in patients with mRCC.[9]

Analyzing survival in a cohort of patients with mRCC treated with gemcitabine plus 5-fluorouracil-based regimens Stadler et al. concluded that poor performance status was one of the independent risk factors for poor survival.[108]

In all studies that have been reported using either chemotherapy or immunotherapy in metastatic RCC, several prognostic factors consistently predict for a better outcome regardless of the therapy that has been used.[119] So patients with a bad performance status have a poor prognosis independent of any other factors.

Minimally Invasive Therapies

Surgery continues to be the standard treatment for RCC but with increased understanding of the natural history of RCC, and because of patient demand, alternative minimally invasive therapies have begun to play a role in the treatment of this disease. Increasingly small renal lesions are being diagnosed in the elderly, who present a high operative risk. Furthermore, as RCC is a slow growing tumor, a less invasive procedure may be preferable in patients with kidney failure and those who have a limited life expectancy due to another disease.[68] Energy-based ablation techniques have been developed for the subset of patients in whom surgery is contraindicated.[20]

Less invasive therapies that have the potential of avoiding open surgery and better preserving renal function are being investigated. Examples of these minimally invasive techniques are cryotherapy, microwave thermal therapy, interstitial laser fiberoptic heating, radiofrequency heating, high-intensity focused ultrasound, and high-energy shock waves. Depending on the modality, these therapies can be delivered during open surgery, laparoscopically, percutaneously, or even extracorporeally.[97] Because critical long-term data are currently lacking, all these energy-based techniques remain developmental in nature.

These techniques [particularly cryotherapy and radiofrequency ablation (RFA)] are justifiably applied in patients of advanced age or with medical comorbidities who may not be suitable for extirpative surgery.[1] RFA could be considered an alternative treatment for elderly patients with multiple comorbidities at high risk for surgery and in patients with an impaired contralateral renal function.[11] The appropriate indications for renal RFA continue to be refined, but generally RFA is indicated in case of small (<4 cm) peripheral tumors in patients who are not surgical candidates.[125] Treatment with RFA does not appear to have an effect on renal function or blood pressure. Even in patients with limited renal reserve these indicators of broad renal damage remain stable.[50] Although the long-term oncological effects remain to be confirmed, RFA appears to be a medically safe therapy for patients with small renal tumors and for patients with significant comorbid conditions.

Cryoablation of renal lesions is indicated in peripheral tumors 3.5 cm or less in size and those at least 0.5 cm away from the collecting system. The procedure can be performed during open surgery, laparoscopic surgery, and hand-assisted laparoscopic surgery or percutaneously with CT guidance. The latter technique requires a high-speed helical CT scanner to monitor the growth of the ice ball and minimize the risk of injury to the collecting system and subsequent uriniferous pseudocyst formation or fistula. The direct vision approaches require intraoperative real time ultrasound monitoring during the freeze–thaw cycles for the same reason.

Minimally invasive therapy for renal tumors can potentially offer curative outcome while conferring several intraoperative and postoperative surgical advantages over open surgery: mainly faster recovery and improved renal preservation. Intermediate-term results of renal cryoablation have been promising. On the other hand, the clinical outcomes from RFA of renal tumors have been controversial, and more treatment data are needed before its true clinical efficacy and renal applicability can be determined.

Newer thermal energy-based strategies, such as high-intensity focused ultrasound (HIFU), laser-induced and microwave thermotherapy, and strategies such as intracavitary photon radiation await additional investigations in animal and Phase I clinical trials before they can be widely employed in the management of renal tumors.[59]

Until the long-term efficacy of cryotherapy and RFA is better defined, ablative therapies should be reserved for patients who may be poor candidates for laparoscopic or open surgery.[6] If long-term results are favorable RFA should prove

to be an attractive treatment option for small renal masses in patients at risk for multiple renal tumors or with other relative contraindications to surgery.[93]

When performed at selected centers, renal cryoablation may be a reasonable treatment option in the older patient with comorbid disease who desires minimally invasive treatment for a small, exophytic, peripherally located tumor.[22]

Laparoscopic renal cryosurgery is especially well suited for older patients or patients with multiple comorbidities.[85] It is a viable and safe therapeutic option, especially for small incidental lesions and patients with many comorbidities. Laparoscopic renal cryosurgery has some advantages compared to partial nephrectomy in that there is less blood loss, it does not involve renal hilar clamping and warm ischemia, does not involve technically difficult suturing, does not result in urine leaks, decreases the need for ureteral stenting and is effective in patients on anticoagulation.[85]

Another minimally invasive technique for the treatment of patients with renal malignancy is HIFU. The preliminary experience of Wu et al. suggests that HIFU is a safe and feasible modality in the treatment of patients with renal malignancy, but the long treatment (median hours therapy–5.4) and anesthesia time can raise potential risks, particularly to patients in a weakened state.[122]

Recent developments in minimal-access surgery are radically changing RCC treatment options and this must be acknowledged in evaluating the contemporary role of transarterial embolization (TAE) in the treatment of RCC. Renal tumors may be treated with percutaneous cryosurgery, percutaneous ultrasound ablation, or TAE in those unable (i.e., old and fragile patients) to undergo open surgery for Stage I–III RCC. Munro et al. described the results of TAE in the cohort of 25 patients divided into two groups for analysis.[83] The first group was composed of 11 patients (median age 73 years) with Stage IV RCC and the second group was composed of 14 patients with localized disease (Stages I–III) who were unable or unwilling to undergo radical nephrectomy; they were generally elderly (median age 80 years). The embolizing agent was ethanol, usually combined with stainless-steel coils (85% of cases). After analyzing the procedural pain, fever, hospital stay, survival, and symptom control it was concluded that contemporary renal embolization has a role in palliating symptoms derived from the primary tumor in patients with advanced (Stage IV) disease and for those with less advanced disease who refuse radical surgery. Because embolization is associated with minimal morbidity and complications, it can be a treatment option for elderly and patients with a weakened state. Its efficacy remains to be proven, however.

Observation

Although surgery remains the treatment of choice for most solid renal masses some patients, especially those with significant comorbid conditions, may benefit from nonoperative management if the tumor histological type and grade could be determined. Dechet et al.[21] hoped to provide evidence that certain patients, such as those with significant comorbid conditions, may benefit from percutaneous needle biopsy and permanent section to distinguish those who should undergo surgical intervention and those in whom observation would be preferable. After analyzing the radical or partial nephrectomy results in 100 patients, it was concluded that the nondiagnostic rate for CT and needle biopsy was 20% and 31%, respectively, and specificity was low, so routine preoperative CT and subsequent needle biopsy to guide treatment decision making are not recommended. Rather, cases must be decided individually, especially in some patients with significant comorbid conditions.

For elderly patients, patients with multiple comorbid conditions, and patients with poor contralateral renal function, patients and/or physicians may elect to observe the evolution of small renal masses out of fear of possible complications. As more benign small incidental tumors are being discovered, in addition to the aging of the population, treatment of these patients may raise questions. In a selected group of patients, particularly the elderly and patients with poor medical condition, observation may represent a valid option. In a study of Kassouf et al.[52] only five of the 24 patients demonstrated growth of the renal mass after a mean follow-up of 31.6 months. Of the five patients with tumor growth four underwent surgery and the pathology revealed localized RCC. Metastasis did not develop in any patient. We agree with Seigne who wrote in an editorial comment that "clearly one can be relatively comfortable observing small renal masses in ill patients with a limited life expectancy."[104]

Baird et al. documented long-term survival in patients with RCC in whom the primary tumor was left *in situ* and treatment was limited to palliative and symptomatic measures. They concluded that such patients with or without metastatic disease can survive for a considerable period with no aggressive surgical or systemic measures, and such intervention may offer no significant advantage in outcome and survival over supportive treatment alone.[3]

This conclusion should be kept in mind when choosing a treatment strategy for elderly patients and for patients in a weakened state.

Although the growth rates of small RCCs vary widely, growth is slow for most tumors. Therefore, Kato et al.[53] advocate that for elderly patients or those at risk for surgery, nonsurgical watchful waiting is an acceptable alternative if the initial follow-up indicates that the lesion has a slow growth rate.

Conclusions

In the second half of the twentieth century the average life expectancy has increased, which in part reflects the success of public health interventions.[2]

The number of individuals 65 years or older is estimated to at least double in the next 50 years,[130] with a disproportionately higher number requiring medical and surgical care.[31] The increased popularity of minimally invasive urological surgery has important implications for the growing number of aging people. Few reports in the urological literature have focused on this segment of the population.

In fact, in a MEDLINE search of the urological literature we found only a few contemporary studies that specifically assessed this population.[42,76,117] The goal of any cancer surgery is definitive therapy for the primary tumor and preservation of the quality of life.[107] In all patients, but particularly in the elderly, the treatment must not be worse than the disease. When treating elderly patients, doctors are often reluctant to propose surgical treatment because of the risk of perioperative morbidity and mortality.[71] Concomitant medical problems such as cardiovascular and pulmonary disease make elderly patients less tolerant of surgical blood loss or anesthetic complications. In addition, postoperative pain and limited ambulation predispose these patients to deep venous thrombosis, pulmonary embolism, and atelectasis or pneumonia. However, modern intraoperative and postoperative management has made open surgery in this population possible and reasonably safe.[117] It is our conclusion that radical nephrectomy can be performed in well-selected older patients and should not be withheld based on age alone.

This surgery requires a multidisciplinary approach and careful preoperative assessment, especially for cardiopulmonary and neurological status. An adapted surgical technique and increased vigilance in the perioperative period result in acceptable morbidity and hospital stay. Patients with impaired renal function, nephropathy, significant calculus disease, or comorbid conditions such as diabetes, nephritis, or hypertension are considered candidates for NSS.[59] Alternative models of preoperative risk stratification and the development of standardized, well-defined criteria for classifying perioperative adverse events should be explored to improve future surgical outcome analyses.[74]

One of the frequent motivations of patients to observe small renal masses is the fear of pain and possible complications associated with surgery. It is possible that this perception and fear of morbidity will change in the next few years with the rapidly increasing use of laparoscopy, which is associated with less pain and faster recovery. Laparoscopic surgery has been widely adopted at many centers, mainly because it allows for a faster recovery; it is largely the older patient who benefits from the advantages of laparoscopy, e.g., reduced requirements for postoperative analgesia and early oral intake. The absence of a large muscle-splitting incision minimizes postoperative pain and therefore decreases the need for sedating analgesics; confusion, agitation, and ileus are therefore kept to a minimum.[112] This also helps early postoperative pulmonary function, as deep breathing is not inhibited by pain or narcotics. In addition, early resumption of oral intake helps minimize nutritional problems, which are more frequent in elderly patients.[117]

As the worldwide incidence of elderly patients suffering from end-stage renal disease has increased almost 3-fold in the past 20 years, new strategies for the treatment of such patients have been developed.[28] Patients who are poor surgical candidates and those with hereditary-based renal tumors who are at risk of multiple renal operations would benefit from less invasive treatment modalities by avoiding surgical morbidity and potentially better preserving renal function.[59]

New minimally invasive technologies are being applied to decrease operating time, pain, morbidity, and hospital stay. Tumor ablative treatment modalities include cryosurgery, RFA, HIFU, and laser and microwave coagulation. Although some reports suggested that complete tumor eradication is not always achieved with these novel approaches, they may nevertheless delay local tumor progression in elderly patients.[97] Furthermore, the percutaneous approach with the patient under local anesthesia may allow ablation of renal tumors in patients judged poor surgical candidates because of multiple comorbid conditions.[52]

As is always the case, general guidelines are merely constructs to help the clinician and the patient (particularly old and fragile) choose the most appropriate therapy given the intricacies of the individual situation; they should not be construed as absolute laws but should help to place therapy on a more rational basis.

References

1. Anderson CJ, Havranek EG. Minimally invasive ablative techniques in renal cancer. BJU Int 2004;93:707–709.
2. Anonymous. Trends in aging, United States and worldwide. MMWR Morb Mortal Wkly Rep 2003;52:101.
3. Baird AD, Woolfenden KA, Desmond AD et al. Outcome and survival with nonsurgical management of renal cell carcinoma. BJU Int 2003;91(7):600–602.
4. Bammer T, Hinder RA, Klaus A et al. Safety and long-term outcome of laparoscopic antireflux surgery in patients in their eighties and older. Surg Endosc 2002;16:40–42.
5. Begg CB, Riedel ER, Bach PB et al. Variations in morbidity after radical prostatectomy. N Engl J Med 2002;346:1138–1144.
6. Belldegrun AS, Schulam PG, Kim HI. Minimally invasive options for treatment of renal cell carcinoma. Kidney Cancer J 2004;1(2):14–17.
7. Bhayani SB. Small renal cell carcinoma. Cont Urol 2005;Dec:40–45.
8. Birkeland S, Lokkegaard H, Storm H. Cancer risk in patients on dialysis and after renal transplantation. Lancet 2000;355:1886–1887.
9. Bleumer I, Oosterwijk E, De Mulder P et al. Immunotherapy for renal cell carcinoma. Eur Urol 2003;44:65–75.
10. Bos SD, Mellema CT, Mensink HJ. Increase in renal cell carcinoma in the northern part of the Netherlands. Eur Urol 2000;37:267–270.
11. Brausi M, Castagnetti G, Gavioli M et al. Radio frequency ablation of renal tumours does not produce complete tumour destruction: results of a phase II study. Eur Urol 2004;suppl. 3:14–17.
12. Buccianti G, Maisonnevue P, Ravasi B et al. Cancer among patients on renal replacement therapy: a population based survey in Lombardy, Italy. Int J Cancer 1996;66:591–593.
13. Cadeddu JA, Ono Y, Clayman RV et al. Laparoscopic nephrectomy for renal cell cancer: evaluation of efficacy and safety: a multicenter experience. Urology 1998;52:773–777.
14. Chang SS, Cookson MS, Hassan JM et al. Routine postoperative intensive care monitoring is not necessary after radical cystectomy. J Urol 2002;167(3):1321–1324.
15. Charlson ME, Pompei P, Ales KL et al. A new method of classifying prognostic comorbidity in longitudinal studies: development and validation. J Chronic Dis 1987;40:373.
16. Chen KS, Lai MK, Huang CC et al. Urologic cancers in uremic patients. Am J Kidney Dis 1995;25:694–700.
17. Chow WH, Devesa SS, Warren JL et al. Rising incidence of renal cell cancer in the United States. JAMA 1999;281:1628–1631.
18. Cohn EB, Campbell SC. Screening for renal cell carcinoma. In: Brukowski RM, Novick AC, Eds. Renal Cell Carcinoma. Totowa, NJ: Humana Press, 2000, pp. 93–109.
19. Cullen DJ, Apolone G, Greenfield S et al. ASA-PS and age predict morbidity after three surgical procedures. Ann Surg 1994;220:3–9.
20. De Baere T, Kuoch V, Smayra T et al. Radio frequency ablation of renal cell carcinoma: preliminary clinical experience. J Urol 2002;167(5):1961–1964.
21. Dechet CB, Zincke H, Sebo TJ et al. Prospective analysis of computerized tomography and needle biopsy with permanent sectioning to determine the nature of solid renal masses in adults. J Urol 2003;169(1):71–74.
22. Desai MM, Gill IS. Renal tumors: clarifying the role of cryoablation. Cont Urol 2002;14(9):35–51.
23. Desai MM, Strzempkowski B, Matin SF et al. Prospective randomized comparison of transperitoneal versus retroperitoneal laparoscopic radical nephrectomy. J Urol 2005;173(1):38–41.
24. Desai MM, Aron M, Gill IS. Laparoscopic partial nephrectomy versus laparoscopic cryoablation for the small renal tumor. Urology 2005;66(Suppl 5A):23–28.
25. Eden CG, Haigh AC, Carter PG et al. Laparoscopic nephrectomy results in better postoperative pulmonary function. J Endourol 1994;8:419.
26. Elson PJ, Witte RS, Trump DL. Prognostic factors for survival in patients with recurrent or metastatic renal cell carcinoma. Cancer Res 1988;48:7310.
27. Extermann M. Measuring comorbidity in older cancer patients. Eur J Cancer 2000;36:453–471.
28. Fabrizii V, Horl W. Renal transplantation in the elderly. Curr Opin Urol 2001;11:159–163.
29. Ficarra V, Prayer-Galetti T, Novella G et al. Incidental detection beyond pathological factors as prognostic predictor of renal cell carcinoma. Eur Urol 2003;43:663–669.
30. Fornara P, Doehn C, Friedrich HJ et al. Nonrandomized comparison of open flank versus laparoscopic nephrectomy in 249 patients with benign renal disease. Eur Urol 2001;40:24–31.
31. Francis J.: Perioperative management of the older patient. In: Hazzard WR, Andres R, Bierman EL et al., Eds. Principles of Geriatric Medicine and Gerontology, 4th ed. New York: McGraw-Hill, 1999.

32. Fried GM, Clas D, Meakins JL. Minimally invasive surgery in the elderly patient. Surg Clin North Am 1994;74: 375.

33. Garman KS, Cohen HJ. Functional status and the elderly cancer patient. Crit Rev Oncol 2002;43(3):209–217.

34. Gettman MT, Boelter CW, Cheville JC et al. Charlson comorbidity index as a predictor of outcome after surgery for renal cell carcinoma with renal vein, vena cava or right atrium extension. J Urol 2003;169(4):1282–1286.

35. Giberti C, Oneto F, Martorana G et al. Radical nephrectomy for renal cell carcinoma: long-term results and prognostic factors on a series of 328 cases. Eur Urol 1997;31:40.

36. Gill IS, Kavoussi LR, Clayman RV et al. Complications of laparoscopic nephrectomy in 185 patients: a multi-institutional review. J Urol 1995;154:479–483.

37. Gill IS, Matin SF, Desai MM et al. Comparative analysis of laparoscopic versus open partial nephrectomy for renal tumors in 200 patients. J Urol 2003;170:64–68.

38. Gomha M, Mosbah A, Showky S et al. A neural network for prediction of 5-year survival status in patients with renal cell carcinoma treated by radical nephrectomy. BJU Int 2002;90(suppl. 2):104.

39. Gray SL, Sanger M, Lestico MR et al. Adverse drug events in hospitalized elderly. J Gerontol A Biol Sci Med Sci 1998;53:M59.

40. Han K-R, Kim HL, Pantuck AJ et al. Use of American Society of Anesthesiologists physical status classification to assess perioperative risk in patients undergoing radical nephrectomy for renal cell carcinoma. Urology 2004;63:841–847.

41. Horl WH. Renal medicine and renal transplantation (editorial comment). Curr Opin Urol 2001;11:131–132.

42. Hsu TH, Gill IS, Fazeli-Matin S et al. Radical nephrectomy and nephroureterectomy in the octogenarian and nonogenarian: comparison of laparoscopic and open approaches. Urology 1999;53:1121–1125.

43. Inouye SK. Delirium in hospitalized elderly patients: recognition, evaluation and management. Conn Med 1993;57:309.

44. Inouye SK. Delirium in older persons. N Engl J Med 2006;354:1157–1165.

45. Iroatulam AJ, Chen HH, Potenti FM et al. Laparoscopic colectomy yields similar morbidity and disability regardless of patient age. Int J Colorectal Dis 1999;14:155–157.

46. Ishikawa I. Present status of renal cell carcinoma in dialysis patients in Japan: questionnaire study in 2002. Nephron Clin Pract 2004;97:11–16.

47. Ishikawa I, Saito Y, Shikura N et al. A ten year prospective study on the development of renal cell carcinoma in dialysis patients. Am J Kidney Dis 1990;16:452–458.

48. Ito K, Nakashima J, Hanawa Y et al. The prediction of renal function 6 years after unilateral nephrectomy using preoperative risk factors. J Urol 2004;171(1):120–125.

49. Jacqmin D, Van Poppel H, Kirkali Z et al. Renal cancer. Eur Urol 2001;39(3):1–9.

50. Johnson DB, Taylor GD, Lotan Y et al. The effects of radio frequency ablation on renal function and blood pressure. J Urol 2003;170(6):2234–2236.

51. Joniau S, Vander Eeckt K, Van Poppel H. The indications for partial nephrectomy in the treatment of renal cell carcinoma. NCP Urology 2006;3(4):198–205.

52. Kassouf W, Aprikian AG, Laplante M et al. Natural history of renal masses followed expectantly. J Urol 2004;171(1): 111–113.

53. Kato M, Suzuki T, Suzuki Y et al. Natural history of small renal cell carcinoma: evaluation of growth rate, histological grade, cell proliferation and apoptosis. J Urol 2004;172(3):863–866.

54. Kattan MW, Reuter V, Motzer RJ et al. A postoperative prognostic nomogram for renal cell carcinoma. J Urol 2001;166:63–67.

55. Kim HL, Belldegrun AS, Freitas DG et al. Paraneoplastic signs and symptoms of renal cell carcinoma: implications for prognosis. J Urol 2003;170(5):1742–1746.

56. Kirkali Z, Obek C. Clinical aspects of renal cell carcinoma. EAU Update Series 2003;1:189–196.

57. Kirkali Z, Van Poppel H. Developments in organ preserving treatments for renal cell cancer: open surgery. Eur Urol 2004;suppl. 3:9–13.

58. Kirkali Z, Van Poppel H, Tuzel E et al. A prospective survey of surgical approaches in clinically localized renal cell carcinoma. Urol Oncol 2002;2:169–174.

59. Lam JS, Shvarts O, Pantuck AJ. Changing concepts in the surgical management of renal cell carcinoma. Eur Urol 2004;45:692–705.

60. Lang H, Jacqmin D. Prognostic factors in renal cell carcinoma. EAU Update Series 2003;1:215–219.

61. Leape LL, Brennan TA, Laird N et al. The nature of adverse events in hospitalized patients. Results of the Harvard Medical Practice Study II. N Engl J Med 1991;324:377–384.

62. Lee CT, Katz J, Fearn PA et al. Mode of presentation of renal cell carcinoma provides prognostic information. Urol Oncol 2002;7(4):135–140.

63. Levine E. Renal cell carcinoma in uremic acquired renal cystic disease: incidence, detection and management. Urol Radiol 1992;13:203–210.

64. Link RE, Bhayani SB, Allaf ME et al. Exploring the learning curve, pathological outcomes and perioperative morbidity of laparoscopic partial nephrectomy performed for renal mass. J Urol 2005;173:1690–1694.

65. Lissoni P, Barni S, Ardizzoia A et al. Prognostic factors of the clinical response to subcutaneous immunotherapy with interleukin-2 alone in patients with metastatic renal cell carcinoma. Oncology 1994;51:59.

66. Ljungberg B, Alamdari FI, Holmberg G et al. Radical nephrectomy is still preferable in the treatment of localized renal cell carcinoma. A long-term follow-up study. Eur Urol 1998;33:79–85.

67. Lutz J, Heemann U. Tumours after kidney transplantation. Curr Opin Urol 2003;13(2):105–109.

68. Mabjeesh NJ, Avidor Y, Matzkin H. Emerging nephron sparing treatments for kidney tumours: a continuum of modalities from energy ablation to laparoscopic partial nephrectomy. J Urol 2004;171(2):553–560.

69. Maher ER, Kaelin WG Jr. von Hippel-Lindau disease. Medicine (Baltimore) 1997;76:381–391.

70. Mahoney JE. Immobility and falls. Clin Geriatr Med 1998;14:699.

71. Margiotta SJ, Horvitz JR, Willis IH et al. Cholecystectomy in the elderly. Am J Surg 1994;156:509–512.

72. Marshall FF. Urological survey: Editorial comment. J Urol 2005;173(2):410.

73. Massie MT, Massie LB, Marrangoni AG et al. Advantages of laparoscopic cholecystectomy in the elderly and in patients with high ASA classifications. J Laparoendosc Surg 1993;3:467–476.

74. Matin SF, Abreu S, Ramani A et al. Evaluation of age and comorbidity as risk factors after laparoscopic urological surgery. J Urol 2003;170(4):1115–1120.

75. Matson MA, Cohen EP. Acquired cystic kidney disease: occurrence, prevalence and renal cancers. Medicine 1990;69: 217–226.

76. McDougall EM, Clayman RV. Laparoscopic nephrectomy and nephroureterectomy in the octogenarian with a renal tumour. J Laparoendosc Surg 1994;4:233.

77. Mejean A, Oudard S, Thiounn N. Prognostic factors of renal cell carcinoma. J Urol 2003;169(3):821–827.

78. Mickisch GH. Surgical treatment of advanced disease for renal cell cancer. Eur Urol 2003; EAU Update Series 1:230–236.

79. Mickisch GH, Carballido J, Hellsten S et al. Guidelines on renal cell cancer. Eur Urol 2001;40:252–255.

80. Miller DC, Taub DA, Dunn RL et al. The impact of comorbid disease on cancer control and survival following radical cystectomy. J Urol 2003;169(1):105–109.

81. Monk TG, Weldon BC, Lemon D. Alterations in pulmonary function during laparoscopic surgery. Anesth Analg 1993;76:5274.

82. Montie JE, Wood DP. The risk of radical cystectomy. Br J Urol 1989;63:483.

83. Munro NP, Woodhams S, Nawrock JD et al. The role of transarterial embolization in the treatment of renal cell carcinoma. BJU Int 2003;92:240–244.

84. Murphy MJ, Waukesha WI, Langenstroer P. Renal cell carcinoma in the transplant patient. J Urol 2004;171(4)suppl: 491.

85. Nadler RB, Kim SC, Rubenstein JN et al. Laparoscopic renal cryosurgery: the Northwestern experience. J Urol 2003;170(4):1121–1125.

86. Nelson CP, Wolf JS. Comparison of hand assisted versus standard laparoscopic radical nephrectomy for suspected renal cell carcinoma. J Urol 2002;167(5):1989–1994.

87. Novick AC, Campbell SC. Renal tumors. In: Walsh PC, Retik AB, Vaughan ED, Eds. Campbell's Urology. Philadelphia: Saunders, 2002, pp. 2672–2731.

88. O'Connell RL, Lim LL. Utility of the Charlson comorbidity index computed from routinely collected hospital discharge diagnosis codes. Methods Inf Med 2000;39:7.

89. Orihuela E, Cubelli V. Management and results in elderly patients with urologic cancer. Semin Urol 1987;5: 134–140.

90. Pantuck AJ, Zisman A, Dorey F et al. Renal cell carcinoma with retroperitoneal lymph nodes: role of lymph node dissection. J Urol 2003;169(6):2076–2083.

91. Parsons JK, Jarrett TJ, Chow GK et al. The effect of previous abdominal surgery on urological laparoscopy. J Urol 2002;168(6):2387–2390.

92. Patard JJ, Leray E, Rodriguez A et al. Correlation between symptom graduation, tumour characteristics and survival in renal cell carcinoma. Eur Urol 2003;44:226–232.

93. Pavlovich CP, Walther MM, Choyke PL et al. Percutaneous radio frequency ablation of small renal tumours: initial results. J Urol 2002;167(1):10–15.

94. Penn I. Occurrence of cancers in immunosuppressed organ transplant recipients. Clin Transplant 1998;28:171–194.

95. Ramani AP, Desai MM, Steinberg C et al. Complications of laparoscopic partial nephrectomy in 200 cases. J Urol 2005;173:42–47.

96. Reissman P, Agachan F, Wexner SD. Outcome of laparoscopic colorectal surgery in older patients. Am Surg 1996;62: 1060–1063.

97. Rendon RA, Kachura JR, Sweet JM et al. The uncertainty of radio frequency treatment of renal cell carcinoma: findings at immediate and delayed nephrectomy. J Urol 2002;167(4):1587–1592.

98. Ries A, Eisner M, Kosary C et al. SEER Cancer Statistics Review 1973–1999. National Cancer Institute, Bethesda, 2002: http://seer.cancer.gov/csr/1973–1999/,2002.

99. Roupret M, Hopirtean V, Mejean A et al. Nephron sparing surgery for renal cell carcinoma and von Hippel-Lindau disease: a single center experience. J Urol 2003;170(5):1752–1755.

100. Roy C, Buy X, Ghali S. Imaging in renal cell cancer. EAU Update Series 2003;1:209–214.

101. Sager MA, Franke T, Inouye SK et al. Functional outcomes of acute medical illness and hospitalization in older persons. Arch Intern Med 1996;156:645.

102. Sasagawa I, Terasawa Y, Imai K et al. Acquired cystic disease of the kidney and renal carcinoma in hemodialysis patients: ultrasonographic evaluation. Br J Urol 1992;70:236–239.

103. Seifman BD, Dunn RL, Wolf JS. Transperitoneal laparoscopy into the previously operated abdomen: effect on operative time, length of stay and complications. J Urol 2003;169(1): 36–40.

104. Seigne J. Editorial comment. J Urol 2004;171(1):113.

105. Shirasaki Y, Tsushima T, Saika T et al. Kidney function after nephrectomy for renal cell carcinoma. Urology 2004;64:43–47.

106. Shvarts O, Lam JS, Kim HL et al. Eastern Cooperative Oncology Group performance status predicts bone metastasis in patients presenting with renal cell carcinoma: implication for preoperative bone scans. J Urol 2004;172(3):867–870.

107. Soulié M, Straub M, Gamé X et al. A multicenter study of the morbidity of radical cystectomy in select elderly patients with bladder cancer. J Urol 2002;167(3):1325–1328.

108. Stadler WM, Huo D, George C et al. Prognostic factors for survival with gemcitabine plus 5-fluorouracil based regimens for metastatic renal cancer. J Urol 2003;170(4):1141–1145.

109. Stephenson AJ, Hakimi AA, Snyder ME et al. Complications of radical and partial nephrectomy in a large contemporary cohort. J Urol 2004;171(1):130–134.

110. Struthers AD, Cuschieri A. Cardiovascular consequences of laparoscopic surgery. Lancet 1998;352:568–570.

111. Swanson DA, Borges PM. Complications of transabdominal radical nephrectomy for renal cell carcinoma. J Urol 1983;129:704.

112. Tichener JL, Levine M. Surgery as a Human Experience. The Psychodynamics of Surgical Practice. New York: Oxford University Press, 1960, pp. 242–246.

113. Tsui K-H, Shvarts O, Smith RB et al. Renal cell carcinoma: prognostic significance of incidentally detected tumors. J Urol 2000;163:426–430.

114. Tsui K-H, Shvarts O, Smith RB et al. Prognostic indicators for renal cell carcinoma: a multivariate analysis of 643 patients using the revised 1997 TNM staging criteria. J Urol 2000;163:1090–1095.

115. Van Poppel H. Conservative vs radical surgery for renal cell carcinoma. BJU Int 2004;94:766–768.

116. Van Poppel H, Deroo F, Joniau S. Open surgical treatment of localized renal cell cancer. Eur Urol 2003; EAU Update Series 1:220–225.

117. Varkarakis I, Neururer R, Harabayashi T et al. Laparoscopic radical nephrectomy in the elderly. BJU Int 2004;94: 517–520.

118. Vogelzang NJ, Bui MH, Belldegrun AS. Radical nephrectomy: is it necessary for metastatic RCC? Cont Urol 2002;14(12): 16–33.

119. Whelan P. The medical treatment of metastatic renal cell cancer. Eur Urol 2003; EAU Update Series 1:237–246.

120. Wishnow KI, Johnson DE, Preston D et al. Long-term serum creatinine values after radical nephrectomy. Urology 1990;35:114–116.

121. Wittgen CM, Andrus CH, Fitzgerald SD et al. Analysis of the hemodynamic and ventilatory effects of laparoscopic cholecystectomy. Arch Surg 1991;126:997–1000.

122. Wu F, Wang ZB, Chen WZ et al. Preliminary experience using high intensity focused ultrasound for the treatment of patients with advanced stage renal malignancy. J Urol 2003;170(6):2237–2240.

123. Yasunaga Y, Shin M, Miki T et al. Prognostic factors of renal cell carcinoma: a multivariate analysis. J Surg Oncol 1998; 68:11.

124. Yaycioglu O, Roberts WW, Chan T et al. Prognostic assessment of nonmetastatic renal cell carcinoma: a clinically based model. Urology 2001;58:141–145.

125. Zelkovic PF, Resnick MI. The promise of radiofrequency ablation. Cont Urol 2004;16(4):39–45.

126. Zenilman ME. Surgery in the elderly. Curr Probl Surg 1998;35:99.

127. Zisman A, Pantuck A, Dorey F et al. Improved prognostication of renal cell carcinoma using an integrated staging system. J Clin Oncol 2001;19:1649–1657.

128. Zisman A, Pantuck AJ, Wieder J et al. Risk group assessment and clinical outcome algorithm to predict the natural history of patients with surgically resected renal cell carcinoma. J Clin Oncol 2002;20:4559–4566.

129. Les hommes et les femmes: condensé de l'Annuaire Eurostat. In: Communautés européennes. Luxembourg City in Luxembourg State, Luxembourg: Office des publications officielles des communautés européennes, 1998, p. 2.

130. U.S. Bureau of the Census, Statistical Abstracts of the United States: 1998. Washington D.C.: U.S. Government Printing Office, 1998.

Obesity and Coumadin in Kidney Cancer

10e.i
Obesity and Kidney Cancer

Louis S. Liou, Emil Kheterpal, and Richard K. Babayan

Introduction

The diagnosis of renal carcinoma has evolved in recent years with earlier detection via advanced imaging, such as computed tomography (CT) scans and magnetic resonance imaging (MRI). This has led to a variety of nephron-sparing approaches to this disease. This chapter will deal with the special complicating factor of obesity (Chapter 10e.ii will deal with anticoagulation therapy), which can significantly alter the surgeon's approach to treatment, and review the ways in which it affects the disease process as well as treatment approaches. A review of the current literature regarding this condition will be included, but no specific recommendations can be given, as this factor must be individualized when dealing with different tumor sizes, locations, and other mitigating circumstances in the decision-making process.

Obesity

The word obesity is derived from the Latin word *obesitas* and is defined in *Webster's Third New International Dictionary* as "a bodily condition marked by excessive generalized deposition and storage of fat" (*Webster's Third New International Dictionary, Unabridged.* (Merriam-Webster, 2002), http://unabridged.merriam-webster.com) (Fig. 10e.i-1). However, the clinical definition of obesity is usually dependent on measuring the body mass index (BMI), which is the weight in kilograms divided by the square of the height in meters. A normal BMI is between 18.5 and 24.9 while overweight is between 25 and 29.9, obese is 30–39.9, and 40 or over is morbidly obese. Although it takes into account the proportion of the person, it does not distinguish between the bodily distribution of this weight and what tissue (fat or muscle) is making up the bulk of the weight. Therefore, this measurement alone cannot be entirely accurate as body morphology also plays a role in determining the overall health and risk factor of a patient. Hence, the concept of visceral obesity or abdominal girth

has been used in place of BMI. In addition, people identified with a higher risk obesity profile will also manifest systemic pathology with insulin resistance, which is described as the "metabolic syndrome." The clinical definition is the presence of three or more of the following criteria: (1) abdominal obesity (waist circumference >102 cm in men and >88 cm in women), (2) hypertriglyceridemia (>150 mg/dl), (3) low high-density lipoprotein (HDL) (<40 in men and <50 in women), and (4) high blood pressure (>130/85) and high fasting glucose (>110 mg/dl) (Cossrow and Falkner 2004). Insulin resistance syndrome and obesity have become a major problem in the United States and affects over 30% of the population and may contribute to over 300,000 deaths per year. The incidence of severe obesity has also increased, but the trend of increasing childhood obesity is most disturbing with a current prevalence rate of 15% in children aged 6–19 years. Obesity is known to cause many medical conditions such as adult-onset diabetes, hypertension, cardiac disease, sleep apnea, osteoarthritis, and stroke. Other medical conditions that may be affected by obesity are benign prostatic hypertrophy, dyslipidemia, asthma, cataracts, and depression (Stein and Colditz 2004). The two largest prospective studies of BMI and overall mortality were the Cancer Prevention Studies. Part I and II enrolled over 300,000 and 1,000,000 participants but both found an overall increase of 40–100% mortality in people with BMI >30 (Stevens et al., 1998); (Calle et al., 2002). The association with cancer has been documented in many retrospective and prospective studies. A recent large prospective trial, following more than 900,000 adults over a 16-year period, found that when the BMI was >40, both men and women had a cancer death rate that was 52% and 62% higher, respectively. The study found a significant association between obesity and cancer of the esophagus, colon, rectum, liver, gallbladder, pancreas, and kidney. Significant trends were found in stomach and prostate cancer in men and breast, uterus, cervix, and ovarian cancer in women. It has been estimated that the obesity pattern in this country could account for 14% and 20% of all cancer deaths in men and women, respectively (Calle et al., 2003).

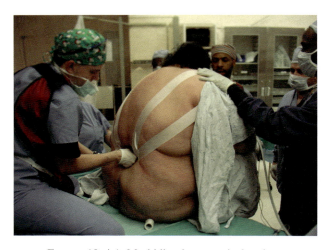

FIGURE 10e.i-1. Morbidly obese surgical patient.

Epidemiological Evidence of Obesity and Kidney Cancer

The link between kidney cancer and obesity has been shown both retrospectively and prospectively. A quantitative review of the literature between 1966 and 1998 for BMI and kidney cancer found 24 unique studies and based their quantitative summary analysis on 14 studies that evaluated each sex separately. Most of these studies were population-based case-controlled studies and all except for one study had a positive association of kidney cancer with obesity while all but four were statistically significant. The authors found a 1.07 relative risk for each unit increase of BMI and estimated that 27% and 29% of kidney cancer in men and women, respectively, were the result of obesity (Bergstrom et al., 2001). Another case-controlled study showed a 5.9 times higher risk of renal cell carcinoma (RCC) in people with the highest BMI. In addition, the onset of obesity at a young age (20 years old), which was maintained throughout adulthood, was also a risk factor. This suggests that obesity may play a role in both the initiation and development of RCC. In general, many case-controlled studies have found that obesity increases the risk for RCC and that women are at a higher risk than men (Amling 2004). In a 20-year period in the Yorkshire region of England, obesity rates tripled, with 21% of women and 17% of men being clinically obese. In parallel, the incidence of RCC has also increased overall by 86% (2.8–5.2 cases per 100,000), with a 80% increase in men and a 90% increase in women. This increased incidence occurred in all age groups as well as all socioeconomic groups (Tate et al., 2003). The African-American population has had the most rapid rate of kidney cancer increase in the United States with a diminished prognosis when compared to white patients (Chow et al., 1999). This may be explained by the fact that this ethnic group is more susceptible to insulin resistance and has a higher incidence of obesity-related hypertension and diabetes (Cossrow and Falkner 2004).

Prospective studies have also implicated obesity in kidney cancer. In one Swedish study, 363,992 men who had at least one physical examination during the time period of 1971–1992 were followed until their death or the year 1995. The men in the highest 2/8 BMI and the middle 3/8 BMI were twice as likely and had a 30–60% greater risk of developing RCC than the bottom 3/8 BMI subjects ($p <0.001$). There was also an independent association of elevated blood pressure with kidney cancer ($p <0.001$ for diastolic and $p <0.007$ for systolic). This risk could be altered if the high blood pressure was treated. Finally, this study found that cigarette smoking was also a risk factor as well (Chow et al., 2000). Another Swedish cohort study included over 28,000 men and women hospitalized with a diagnosis of obesity and found that there was a 33% higher cancer risk, with RCC having the second highest increased risk (Wolk et al., 2001). Dietary factors, such as a diet high in protein and animal fat and low in vegetables and fruits, have also contributed to the increased risk of developing RCC (Amling 2004).

Prognosis of Renal Cell Cancer in Obese Patients

Since the epidemiological evidence of the relationship between obesity and kidney cancer is convincing, many studies have looked at whether obesity impacts survival of kidney cancer. In a retrospective study at a single institution, 683 patients were surgically treated for kidney cancer over a 7-year period. BMI did not correlate with stage (Schips et al., 2003) and was not predictive of patient survival in a multivariate analysis (Schips et al., 2004). However, patients with a BMI of greater than 25 did have a better outcome in a univariate analysis. The M.D. Anderson Cancer Center reported their findings in a 14-year series of 400 patients undergoing nephrectomy for kidney cancer. BMI, time to metastasis, and pathological stage were found to be the best predictors of cancer-specific death in a multivariate analysis. A BMI over 25, a longer time to metastasis, and a lower stage were all good prognostic factors, while normal BMI with pT3 or higher and metastasis within 19 months of surgery conferred the worst prognosis (Kamat et al., 2004). Therefore, the data that obesity is a risk factor for kidney cancer but can be protective once the patient undergoes a nephrectomy are puzzling. All these studies were retrospective with the Schips articles using self-reported height and weight on admission preoperatively while the M.D. Anderson series were based on the measured height and weight at initial office evaluation. The majority of both series had no presenting complaints, but it is conceivable that each patient may have been at various tumor biology states and the BMI reflected the stable growth state prior to cancer cachexia. In addition, none of these studies reported the RCC subtype (conventional clear, papillary chromophobe, collecting duct, medullary) (Reuter and Presti 2000) when evaluating BMI. Since it is known that some subtypes have a better prognosis than others but it is not known if obesity increases the risk of all subtypes, there could be subgroups of patients that BMI affects more profoundly. This question was addressed by a study from Memorial Sloan-Kettering Cancer Center. The study retrospectively reviewed 1159 partial or radical nephrectomy cases with 98% having BMI data. It found that clear cell type was associated with the obese BMI ($p = 0.002$ for BMI $\geq$ 30) but that there was no adverse impact on survival with increasing BMI but rather a trend to better prognosis. In addition, operative time and blood loss were significantly increased with BMI ($p = 0.05$) while pathological stage and metastasis were not significantly associated (Donat et al., 2006). Certainly, multiinstitutional prospective studies will be needed to investigate this issue. In conclusion, BMI may be protective in patients with localized kidney cancer but it does not appear to be predictive of the stage of disease, although it is correlated with the clear cell subtype.

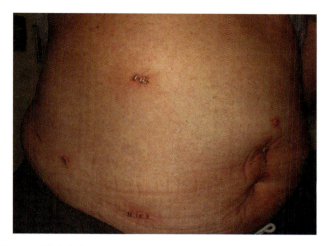

FIGURE 10e.i-2. Laparoscopic port sites in the obese surgical patient.

Surgical Treatment of Renal Cell Cancer in the Obese Patient

The predominant treatment modality of kidney cancer is still surgery and with an increasing BMI associated with RCC, surgery in the obese can be challenging. The transabdominal approach necessitates entry through the pannus or the thick anterior abdominal wall. However, in a flank approach, even obese patients are less obese over the rib cage and the pannus is falling away from the surgical incision. With the advent of laparoscopy, multiple studies have been published demonstrating the efficacy and advantage of this technique over the open approach. In a Cleveland Clinic retrospective study, 21 obese patients (BMI >30) who underwent laparoscopic renal and adrenal surgery were compared to a historical control group that underwent open surgery. The laparoscopic group had statistically a significant lower blood loss, a faster resumption of oral intake and ambulation, a lower narcotic requirement, and shorter hospital stays. Both operating time and complications were not significantly different (Fazeli-Matin et al., 1999). The same group has also published a case report of a retroperitoneoscopic radical nephrectomy in a superobese (BMI = 77) patient (Abreu et al., 2004). The advantages of the laparoscopic retroperitoneal versus transperitoneal approach to the kidney lie in the early control of the hilum to limit blood loss and the avoidance of peritoneal contents, which in obese people may represent a much greater benefit to technical feasibility than in the normal patient. However, the port placement and the laparoscopic instruments may need to be adjusted for this patient population (Fig. 10e.i-2). One other study has shown that in a series of 50 laparoscopic retroperitoneal radical nephrectomies, three open conversions were performed, one for bleeding and two for interference of the technique by obesity (Cicco et al., 2001). Another study compared laparoscopic radical nephrectomies in 69 patients with normal BMI with 32 patients with BMI >30. It was concluded that there were no significant differences in mean operative time, hospital stay, time to ambulation, open conversion rate, and complication rate and that obesity should not be considered a contraindication to laparoscopic surgery (Fugita et al., 2004). Finally, hand-assisted laparoscopic (HAL) nephrectomy was shown to be feasible in the obese patient when compared to patients with normal BMIs, but there was a longer operative time and convalescence (Stifelman et al., 2003). This may be due to the limitations of the length of the surgeon's arm when utilized in the obese habitus and to the fact that the intraabdominal approach is more difficult with increased fat. In conclusion, minimally invasive laparoscopic surgery for the obese patient with kidney cancer can be beneficial, but alterations in technique and instruments with increased surgical skill sets will be needed.

Molecular Mechanism of Obesity in Renal Cell Cancer

Syndrome X, metabolic syndrome, or insulin resistance syndrome was described by Gerald Reaven and has been closely linked to the development of diabetes and cardiovascular disease (Reaven et al., 2004). In addition, insulin resistance increases the risk of cancer. Metabolic syndrome and obesity are probably influenced by both genetics and the environment. There are genetic animal models of obesity such as the *ob* and *db* strains of mice that have defects in the leptin receptor and are markedly heavier than their genetically normal wild-type counterparts (Fig. 10e.i-3). There are human patients who also have these defects and some of these people can have their obesity reversed with leptin administration. However, none of these hereditary models has shown

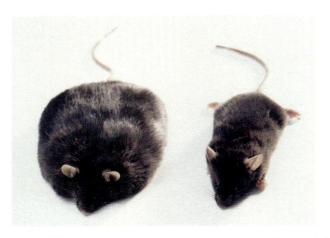

FIGURE 10e.i-3. Wild-type and ob mice. http://www.blc.arizona.edu/
INTERACTIVE/NUTRITION5.95/ob_gene.html
http://www.hhmi.org/genesweshare/d130.html.

an increased incidence of kidney tumors, although the number of patients is small.

A familial history of kidney cancer in either a first- or second-degree relative can increase the risk (OR = 2.5) of kidney cancer (Gago-Dominguez et al., 2001). There are many types of hereditary kidney cancers, each with a specific subtype of RCC. The most prevalent genetic defect is in the VHL gene locus 3p25–26. The familial version has different phenotypes that result from different genotypes. The syndrome can result in clear cell carcinoma of the kidney as well as pheochromocytomas, retinal angiomas, central nervous system hemangioblastomas, pancreatic cysts or adenocarcinomas, epididymal cystadenomas, and endolymphatic sac tumors. In addition, there are hereditary papillary RCC (HPRCC) that are associated with the MET protooncogene on 7q (Novick and Campbell 2002), Birt–Hogg–Dube (17p12-q11.2), which is associated with benign skin lesions and renal tumors (Khoo et al., 2001), and tuberous sclerosis, which is associated with an increased incidence of angiomyolipomas. However, none of these adult kidney tumor syndromes has obesity specifically associated with them (Cohen and Zhou 2005).

One specific hereditary syndrome that has both a predilection for RCC and obesity is a variant of the WAGR (Wilm's tumor, aniridia, genitourinary abnormalities, and mental retardation) syndrome. The usual genetic defect is a deletion in 11p13, which contains the aniridia gene (PAX6) and the Wilm's tumor suppressor gene (WT1). However, in the variant where the deletion is at 11p12p14 there is also severe obesity. One subject at age 13 and 16 had BMIs of 65/144 and 130/160, respectively. It has been postulated that obesity is a phenotypical manifestation of the 11p deletion and that therefore an obesity gene might be in that region (Gul et al., 2002).

Obesity results from the excess supply of energy. This energy is converted to increased storage within adipocytes and, therefore, more fat. There are many factors that can contribute to the metabolic imbalance, and one of the primary components is insulin. It plays a central role in glucose homeostasis and the anabolic process in cell growth. Hyperinsulinemia is a result of obesity and many neoplastic processes also result in hyperglycemia and insulin resistance. The increased rate of insulin resistance in both the developed and developing world is secondary to both dietary factors and the diminished rate of exercise. Dietary factors such as increased saturated high-fat foods, omega-6 fats, and the concentrated and refined carbohydrates can contribute to insulin resistance while plant diets, omega-3 fats, and dairy products may increase insulin sensitivity. Also, exercise will increase insulin sensitivity while a sedentary life-style will increase resistance (Boyd 2003).

Insulin works via the insulin receptors that are found in all cells, normal or neoplastic, and has both metabolic and growth-promoting effects. It also acts in a manner similar to insulin-like growth factor-I (IGF-I) or somatomedin C and both bind to their respective tyrosine kinase receptors, insulin receptor (IR) and IGF-IR. The metabolic effects increase the substrates needed for cellular expansion and include stimulation of glucose transport, glucose utilization, amino acid transport, and protein synthesis. The growth-promoting effects included stimulation of RNA/DNA synthesis, cell proliferation, cell differentiation, and cell survival (O'Dell and Day 1998; Boyd 2003). Serum IGF-I levels have been shown to be an independent predictor of prognosis in patients with RCC and the receptor is also markedly increased in the cancer. In addition, both leptin and prealbumin were shown to be inversely related to RCC prognosis, although this finding was not found in a multivariate analysis (Rasmuson et al., 2004). These receptors and growth factors may activate many pathways such as mitogen-activated protein (MAP) and the phosphoinositol-3-kinase/AKT cascade, both of which are increased in kidney cancer but are not prognostic factors (Manning, 2004). Finally, in the insulin-resistant state, there is also a chronic state of inflammation. Serum cytokines such as interleukin-6 (IL-6) and C-reactive protein (CRP) are elevated while cyclooxygenase-2 is increased in the tissue. These have also been shown to be prognostic in the outcome of patients with kidney cancer (Boyd 2003).

Insulin growth factor II is somatomedin A and also works through IGF-IR and IR. It is found in 11p15, spans 30 kp, and consists of four promoters and nine exons. IGF-II knockout mice have significant fetal growth retardation and in humans continue to be expressed postnatally. This gene is imprinted, but with relaxation or loss of imprinting, IGF-II levels increase and the resultant genetic disease is Beckwith–Wiedemann syndrome. This is characterized by increased unilateral growth and a risk of Wilm's tumor. However, the loss of IGF-II imprinting has also been seen in other cancers and is implicated in obesity. The rare ApaI polymorphism in the 3′ UTR region of IGF-II mRNA results in lower body mass while increased serum IGF-II levels are correlated with larger BMIs (O'Dell and Day O'Dell).

All three members of the insulin growth factors (insulin, IGF-I, and IGF-II) interact with insulin-like growth factor binding proteins (IGFBP) and the most predominant in the serum is IGFBP-3. Of the IGFs 90% are complexed to this protein. The membranous forms may enhance the action of IGFs by bringing the IGFs to the cell while the soluble forms may inhibit activity by sequestering the IGFs and preventing binding to the cellular targets (Pollak 2000). We have found that the number one gene that consistently emerged from different microarray papers as significantly different between normal kidney and clear cell kidney cancer was IGFBP-3 (Lenburg et al., 2003; Liou et al., 2004). In addition, the protein appears to be increased in only the clear cell subtype of kidney cancer while it is rare in papillary and not found in chromophobe variants (Takahashi et al., 2005). This is consistent with the finding that BMI is positively correlated with the clear cell subtype and may play a role in both BMI and kidney cancer (Donat et al., 2006). Further work to elucidate the etiology of IGFBP-3 elevation as well as its clinical relevance still needs to be done. There are many new technologies that have contributed a large amount of knowledge to the study of tumor biology. The challenge will be to integrate this knowledge into the application of kidney cancer treatment.

Kidney cancer is composed of many subtypes. However, all of the epidemiological data support an association with obesity. The newly described metabolic syndrome and insulin resistance may play a role in the etiology and the tumor biology. There is increasing evidence that the insulin pathway genes play a role in kidney cancer, and more work into integrating this information into clinical practice is needed. Finally, obesity presents a challenge to the current treatment for kidney cancer, which is surgical extirpation. Variations of this approach and use of newer technologies, such as laparoscopy, retroperitoneoscopy, and minimally invasive ablation techniques, help to provide the urological surgeon with addition tools to circumvent the anatomic obstacles presented by the obese patient.

References

Abreu, S. C., J. H. Kaouk, et al. (2004). Retroperitoneoscopic radical nephrectomy in a super-obese patient (body mass index 77 kg/m^2). *Urology* **63**(1): 175–176.

Amling, C. L. (2004). The association between obesity and the progression of prostate and renal cell carcinoma. *Urol Oncol* **22**(6): 478–484.

Bergstrom, A., C. C. Hsieh, et al. (2001). Obesity and renal cell cancer—a quantitative review. *Br J Cancer* **85**(7): 984–990.

Boyd, D. B. (2003). Insulin and cancer. *Integr Cancer Ther* **2**(4): 315–329.

Calle, E. E., C. Rodriguez, et al. (2002). The American Cancer Society Cancer Prevention Study II Nutrition Cohort: rationale, study design, and baseline characteristics. *Cancer* **94**(2): 500–511.

Calle, E. E., C. Rodriguez, et al. (2003). Overweight, obesity, and mortality from cancer in a prospectively studied cohort of U.S. adults. *N Engl J Med* **348**(17): 1625–1638.

Chow, W. H., S. S. Devesa, et al. (1999). Rising incidence of renal cell cancer in the United States. *JAMA* **281**(17): 1628–1631.

Chow, W. H., G. Gridley, et al. (2000). Obesity, hypertension, and the risk of kidney cancer in men. *N Engl J Med* **343**(18): 1305–1311.

Cicco, A., L. Salomon, et al. (2001). Results of retroperitoneal laparoscopic radical nephrectomy. *J Endourol* **15**(4): 355–359; discussion 375–376.

Cohen, D. and M. Zhou. (2005). Molecular genetics of familial renal cell carcinoma syndromes. *Clin Lab Med* **25**(2): 259–277.

Cossrow, N. and B. Falkner. (2004). Race/ethnic issues in obesity and obesity-related comorbidities. *J Clin Endocrinol Metab* **89**(6): 2590–2594.

Donat, S. M., E. W. Salzhauer, et al. (2006). Impact of body mass index on survival of patients with surgically treated renal cell carcinoma. *J Urol* **175**(1): 46–52.

Fazeli-Matin, S., I. S. Gill, et al. (1999). Laparoscopic renal and adrenal surgery in obese patients: comparison to open surgery. *J Urol* **162**(3 Pt 1): 665–669.

Fugita, O. E., D. Y. Chan, et al. (2004). Laparoscopic radical nephrectomy in obese patients: outcomes and technical considerations. *Urology* **63**(2): 247–252; discussion 252.

Gago-Dominguez, M., J. M. Yuan, et al. (2001). Family history and risk of renal cell carcinoma. *Cancer Epidemiol Biomarkers Prev* **10**(9): 1001–1004.

Gul, D., G. Ogur, et al. (2002). Third case of WAGR syndrome with severe obesity and constitutional deletion of chromosome (11)(p12p14). *Am J Med Genet* **107**(1): 70–71.

Kamat, A. M., R. P. Shock, et al. (2004). Prognostic value of body mass index in patients undergoing nephrectomy for localized renal tumors. *Urology* **63**(1): 46–50.

Khoo, S. K., M. Bradley, et al. (2001). Birt-Hogg-Dube syndrome: mapping of a novel hereditary neoplasia gene to chromosome 17p12-q11.2. *Oncogene* **20**(37): 5239–5242.

Lenburg, M. E., L. S. Liou, et al. (2003). Previously unidentified changes in renal cell carcinoma gene expression identified by parametric analysis of microarray data. *BMC Cancer* **3**: 31.

Liou, L. S., T. Shi, et al. (2004). Microarray gene expression profiling and analysis in renal cell carcinoma. *BMC Urol* **4**: 9.

Manning, B. D. (2004). Balancing Akt with S6K: implications for both metabolic diseases and tumorigenesis. *J Cell Biol* **167**(3): 399–403.

Novick, A. C. and S. C. Campbell. (2002). Renal tumors. In: *Campbell's Urology*. P.C. Walsh, A.B. Retik, E.D. Vaughan, and A.J. Wein, Eds. Philadelphia: Saunders, pp. 2673–2731.

O'Dell, S. D. and I. N. Day. (1998). Insulin-like growth factor II (IGF-II). *Int J Biochem Cell Biol* **30**(7): 767–771.

Pollak, M. (2000). Insulin-like growth factor physiology and cancer risk. *Eur J Cancer* **36**(10): 1224–1228.

Rasmuson, T., K. Grankvist, et al. (2004). Serum insulin-like growth factor-1 is an independent predictor of prognosis in patients with renal cell carcinoma. *Acta Oncol* **43**(8): 744–748.

Reaven, G., F. Abbasi, et al. (2004). Obesity, insulin resistance, and cardiovascular disease. *Recent Prog Horm Res* **59**: 207–223.

Reuter, V. E. and J. C. Presti, Jr. (2000). Contemporary approach to the classification of renal epithelial tumors. *Semin Oncol* **27**(2): 124–137.

Schips, L., R. Zigeuner, et al. (2003). Do patients with a higher body mass index have a greater risk of advanced-stage renal cell carcinoma? *Urology* **62**(3): 437–441.

Schips, L., K. Lipsky, et al. (2004). Does overweight impact on the prognosis of patients with renal cell carcinoma? A single center experience of 683 patients. *J Surg Oncol* **88**(2): 57–61; discussion 61–62.

Stein, C. J. and G. A. Colditz. (2004). The epidemic of obesity. *J Clin Endocrinol Metab* **89**(6): 2522–2525.

Stevens, J., J. Cai, et al. (1998). The effect of age on the association between body-mass index and mortality. *N Engl J Med* **338**(1): 1–7.

Stifelman, M. D., T. Handler, et al. (2003). Hand-assisted laparoscopy for large renal specimens: a multi-institutional study. *Urology* **61**(1): 78–82.

Takahashi, M., V. Papavero, et al. (2005). Altered expression of members of the IGF-axis in clear cell renal cell carcinoma. *Int J Oncol* **26**(4): 923–931.

Tate, R., R. Iddenden, et al. (2003). Increased incidence of renal parenchymal carcinoma in the Northern and Yorkshire region of England, 1978-1997. *Eur J Cancer* **39**(7): 961–967.

Wolk, A., G. Gridley, et al. (2001). A prospective study of obesity and cancer risk (Sweden). *Cancer Causes Control* **12**(1): 13–21.

10e.ii
Coumadin and Kidney Cancer

Louis S. Liou, Emil Kheterpal, and Richard K. Babayan

Introduction

The diagnosis of renal carcinoma has evolved in recent years with earlier detection via advanced imaging, such as computed tomography (CT) scans and magnetic resonance imaging (MRI). This has led to a variety of nephron-sparing approaches to this disease. This chapter will deal with anticoagulation therapy (Chapter 10e.i dealt with obesity), which can significantly alter the surgeon's approach to treatment, and review the ways in which it affects the disease process as well as treatment approaches. A review of the current literature regarding this therapy will be included, but no specific recommendations can be given, as this factor must be individualized when dealing with different tumor sizes, locations, and other mitigating circumstances in the decision-making process.

Cancer and Thrombosis: Pathogenesis

The main therapeutic modality for kidney cancer is surgery and surgical consideration in an anticoagulated patient is of principal concern. Currently, over 2 million patients are on oral anticoagulation (OAC) therapy mainly for venous thromboembolism (VTE), atrial fibrillation, and artificial heart valves. However, OAC is utilized in cancer patients because of their increased risk of VTE, although this is controversial. Kidney cancer has a unique link to thromboembolism within the venous system and surgery to remove both the primary cancer as well as the tumor thrombus can be curative (Fig. 10e.ii-1). Therefore, this chapter will first explore the known etiology of cancer and thromboembolism and the methodology/risk of anticoagulation with bridging therapy for discontinuation or resumption of perioperative anticoagulation. Finally, the discussion will focus on how this may impact on surgical treatment of kidney cancer.

The association between cancer and thrombosis was first noted by Trousseau in 1865. Since his initial observation, thromboembolic disease is recognized as both an early clinical sign of underlying malignancy (Caine et al., 2002) and as the second most frequent cause of death in cancer patients (Donati, 1995). After accounting for subclinical thromboembolic events, the incidence of venous thromboembolism in all cancer patients likely exceeds 15%, which represents the clinically detectable VTE (Rickles and Levine 1998; Johnson et al., 1999). Likewise, the impact of a hypercoagulable-induced state in cancer patients is demonstrated by the 2-fold increased risk of recurrent thromboembolism (TE) (Levitan et al., 1999; Caine et al., 2002) and postoperative deep vein thrombosis (DVT) compared with noncancer patients (De Cicco, 2004). The magnitude of the problem of VTE in cancer patients is further illustrated by the rate of VTE detection in as much as 50% of autopsy series (Deitcher, 2003). The pathogenic mechanisms resulting in a prothrombotic state are multiple and interdependent.

The best-characterized prothrombotic substances released by tumor cells are tissue factor (TF) and cancer procoagulant (CP). Tissue factor is a transmembrane glycoprotein that can be expressed on normal resting cells in response to proinflammatory stimuli; however, tumor cells constitutively express TF and also induce macrophage expression of TF via direct receptor binding and activation of factor VII (Caine et al., 2002; De Cicco, 2004). Increased levels of TF complex with factor VII to initiate catalysis of factor X to factor Xa and subsequent thrombin formation. Recent studies have demonstrated that TF expression alters a tumor cell phenotype, not only enhancing procoagulant activity but also increasing *in vitro* tumor cell invasion and growth (Sampson and Kakkar, 2002). Cancer procoagulant, similarly, is a vitamin K-dependent cysteine protease that directly activates factor X, independent of factor VII and TF, and activates platelets in a dose-dependent manner (Lee, 2002). It has been found to be elevated exclusively on malignant cells (De Cicco, 2004), including renal cancer (Gordon et al., 1979; Mandala et al., 2003). Another factor recently identified as being overexpressed on several tumor cell lines is hepsin, a transmembrane serine protease. It has demonstrated the ability to activate factor VII independent of TF and catalyze the generation of low levels of factor X in the absence of factor VII (Sampson and Kakkar, 2002). Coagulation is also promoted by the inhibition of fibrinolysis, the suppression of anticoagulant factors, and the inflammatory response to tumor-specific

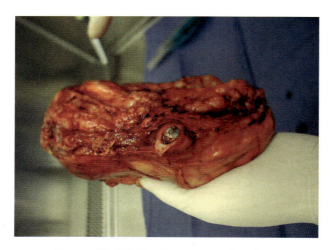

FIGURE 10e.ii-1. Renal vein tumor thrombus.

antigens. Fibrin is lysed through the action of plasmin, which is derived from plasminogen through the action of plasminogen activator (Walsh-McMonagle and Green, 1997). Plasminogen activator inhibitor type-1 (PAI-1), a direct inhibitor of this pathway that is typically released by platelets and endothelial cells, has been elaborated by a variety of cancer cells (Nachman and Hajjar, 1991). Furthermore, the typical physiological response to cancer cells is characterized by the release of inflammatory mediators, i.e., tumor necrosis factor (TNF) and interleukin-1 (IL-1). These cytokines may induce TF expression by endothelial cells and tumor-associated macrophages, activate platelets, downregulate the protein C pathway via suppression of the surface receptor thrombomodulin, and induce PAI-1 expression by endothelial cells (Caine et al.,, 2002; De Cicco 2004).

Renal Cell Carcinoma–Coagulapathy Relationship

Renal cell carcinoma (RCC) is a relatively uncommon tumor that is considered to arise from the proximal convoluted tubule and is associated with thromboembolic disease. A study by Zacharski and colleagues concluded that activation of the host coagulation mechanism may be factor VII dependent; however, they noted that factors VII and X were present in the pericellular spaces of tumor cells and absent in normal and perivascular tissue. Furthermore, they performed a literature review of coagulation-related studies of RCC that observed elevated fibrinogen levels in RCC, which declined following nephrectomy, local inhibition of fibrinolysis around the tumor, and coagulant activity independent of factor VII (Zacharski et al., 1986). A more recent study by Forster and colleagues compared TF expression in tumor tissue and tumor-free parenchyma of patients with RCC. Although they observed a greater concentration of TF in nonmalignant tissue compared with tumor tissue, they detected *de novo* expression within tumor tissue. This was significant because all the

RCC specimens were of a clear cell type, which is a histological subtype that originates from the proximal tubules and that is normally TF negative (Forster et al., 2003). Zacharski et al., (1998) detected hepsin that localized by specific staining exclusively to tumor cell membranes in all seven cases and was absent in tumor-free tissue; hence, they suggested that hepsin served as an activator of thrombin generation.

Thromboembolism

Although prophylactic anticoagulation of patients with malignancy alone is controversial (Thodiyil et al., 2001), patients with a history of VTE, mechanical heart valves, and atrial fibrillation with associated comorbidities are orally anticoagulated. The management of these patients with concurrent cancer may be complicated by an elevated risk of both VTE and bleeding (Thodiyil et al., 2001; Mandala et al., 2003). The risk of recurrent VTE and major bleeding in cancer patients is 3- to 6-fold higher than in noncancer patients during warfarin treatment (Mandala et al., 2003).

Mechanical Heart Valve

Warfarin therapy is clinically important in the management of patients with mechanical heart valves and its absence results in 15% mortality in patients who develop valve-associated thrombosis (Douketis, 2002; Garcia et al., 2004), an annual risk of stroke of approximately 4% (Dunn and Turpie, 2003), and an estimated incidence of thromboembolic event between 9% and 22% (Douketis, 2002). The risk of embolism is reduced by 75% in anticoagulated patients (Kearon and Hirsh, 1997; Dunn and Turpie, 2003). Multiple factors influence the risk of thrombosis such as type of heart valve replacement, valve site, and prior history of thrombosis (Douketis, 2002; Jafri and Metha, 2004). Newer generation heart valves are associated with a lower incidence of arterial embolism. Table 10e.ii-1 summarizes risk according to previously mentioned factors. The absolute risk of thromboembolism was estimated as 0.17–0.42% during a 6- to 8-day perioperative period after interruption of warfarin therapy (Douketis, 2002).

Atrial Fibrillation

Patients with atrial fibrillation can be categorized as high risk or intermediate risk depending on their age and other comorbidities. Patient at high risk for TE include those who are older than 75 years and have a history of hypertension, LV dysfunction, and diabetes. (Douketis, 2002; Jafri and Metha, 2004). The average risk of systemic embolization in patients with nonvalvular atrial fibrillation without OAC is 4–5% per year; however, risks rose to 12% per year in patients with previous cerebral embolism (Kearon and Hirsh, 1997; Douketis, 2002). Table 10e.ii-2 illustrates the relative risk of stroke when chronic atrial fibrillation is associated with

TABLE 10e.ii-1. Risk factors for thromboembolism.

Thromboembolism risk category	Valve location and type
High risk	Any mitral valve
	Aortic valve
	Caged-ball (Starr-Edwards) Single-leaflet tilting disc (Bjork-Shiley, Medtroin-Hall, or Omnicarbon)
Moderate risk	Aortic valve
	Bileaflet tilting disc (St. Jude or Carbomedics) with two or more risk factors
Low risk	Aortic valve
	Bileaflet tilting disc (St. Jude or Carbomedics) with less than two risk factors

Source: Douketis (2002).

TABLE 10e.ii-2. Risk factors for stroke in patients with chronic atrial fibrillation.

Risk factor[a]	Relative risk of stroke
Previous stroke, TIA, or systemic embolism	2.0–2.9
Age	1.6–1.8
Hypertension	1.6–2.0
Diabetes	1.6–1.7
LV dysfunction	2.5

Source: Douketis (2002).
[a]TIA, transient ischemic attack; LV left ventricular.

specific risk factors. Anticoagulant therapy reduces the overall risk by two-thirds (Kearon and Hirsh, 1997).

History of Venous Thromboembolism

Patients with recent VTE are generally treated with warfarin since chronic anticoagulation reduces the risk by approximately 80% (Kearon and Hirsh, 1997; Jafri and Metha, 2004). During the first month after VTE, patients are at high risk (40%) of recurrence; however, the risk of an acute episode declines significantly over the following months, with a subsequent risk of 10% during the second and third months and 5% at the end of 3 months of anticoagulation (Kearon and Hirsh, 1997; Douketis, 2002; Jafri and Metha, 2004; Spyropoulos, 2005). However, patients with comorbidities such as cancer, chronic disease, or antiphospholipid antibodies are at an overall greater inherent risk (Douketis, 2002).

An important note should be added for patients with a recent (<3 month) history of VTE who undergo surgery because of an associated 100-fold increased risk of recurrent VTE (Kearon and Hirsh, 1997; Douketis, 2002; Dunn and Turpie, 2003; Spyropoulos, 2005). This is especially important when considering perioperative management following a recent episode of VTE. During the first month after an acute episode, patients have a 1.0% absolute increased risk of recurrence. Although postoperative heparin doubles the risk of bleeding, administration of intravenous heparin results in a net reduction of morbidity in these patients because of the high risk of VTE. Similarly, postoperative anticoagulation is associated with decreased morbidity during the second and third months. After 3 months, the administration of postoperative anticoagulation is controversial because of the greater risk of bleeding than an acute episode of a VTE. As a result, it has been suggested that after 3 months the benefits of intravenous heparin after surgery were outweighed by the risk of major bleeding, but low-molecular-weight heparin (LMWH) may be used because of the lower risk of associated bleeding (Kearon and Hirsh, 1997).

Current Bridging Recommendations

Multiple factors must be considered during perioperative management of patients on long-term OAC therapy. A patient's previous history of bleeding, especially with invasive procedures, is an important determinant in assessing surgical bleeding risk, as is the use of antiplatelet and nonsteroidal antiinflammatory medications. Furthermore, the clinical consequence of a thrombotic or bleeding event should be identified: main hepatic vein (MHV) thrombosis is fatal in 15% of patients, arterial thromboembolism results in death or major disability in 70% of patients, venous thromboembolism has an estimated death or disability rate of approximately 5%, and postoperative major bleeding has a fatality rate of approximately 3% (Spyropoulos, 2005).

Clinical studies have demonstrated the equal safety and efficacy of the use of LMWH and unfractionated heparin (UFH) in bridging therapy (Douketis, 2002; Jafri and Metha, 2004; Spyropoulos, 2005). Table 10e.ii-3 presents a summarized risk stratification of thromboembolism and anticoagulation recommendations of the Seventh American College of Chest Physician Consensus Conference.

In patients with renal insufficiency, UFH is the anticoagulant of choice because, unlike LMWH, it is not cleared primarily by the kidney. The Food and Drug Administration does not recommend the use of LMWHs in patients with a creatinine clearance less than 30 ml/min (Jafri and Metha, 2004). Physicians must be aware of the fact that if LMWH is used in such patients, bioaccumulation may go undetected since the activated partial thromboplastin time (aPTT) will not be increased; as a result, these patients will be at an elevated risk of intraoperative and postoperative bleeding. If LMWH is used, antifactor Xa should be measured 4 hours after administration of an LMWH dose to evaluate the anticoagulant effect, with a targeted level of 0.5–1.5 U/ml. In addition, in patients with a history of previous heparin-induced thrombocytopenia, both UFH and LMWH should be avoided. Instead lepirudin or argatroban, direct thrombin inhibitors, may be safely administered in patients with heparin-induced thrombocytopenia (HIT) (Douketis, 2002).

The management of patients on long-term OAC is not an exact science; however, it is important to be aware of the increased risk of thrombotic events associated with abrupt

TABLE 10e.ii-3. Patient risk stratification and perioperative management recommendations.[a]

	High risk	Moderate risk	Low risk

Mechanical prosthetic heart valve	Recent (<1 month) stroke or TIA
	Any mitral valve
	Caged ball or single leaflet-tilting disc
	Aortic valve
		Bileaflet-tilting disc
		Aortic valve and ≥ 2
		  stroke risk factors
			Bileaflet tilting disc
			Aortic valve and <2
			  stroke risk factors

Chronic AF	Recent (<1 month) stroke or TIA Rheumatic mitral valvular heart disease	Chronic AF and ≥ 2 stroke risk factors	Chronic AF and >2 stroke risk factors

Previous episode of VT	Recent (<3 months) episode of VT
	Active cancer
	Major comorbid disease
	Antiphospholipid antibody
		VT within the past 6 months
		VT occurring in association with
		  previous interruption of warfarin
		  therapy
			None of the previously
			  stated

Anticoagulation	Full dose of UFH or LMWH	Prophylactic or higher dose UFH or LMWH	Optional

Source: Guidelines from the Seventh American College of Chest Physician Consensus Conference.
[a]TIA, transient ischemic attack; AF, atrial fibrillation; VT, ventricular tachycardia; UFH, unfractionated heparin; LMWH, low-molecular-weight heparin.

TABLE 10e.ii-4. Perioperative bridging protocol for patients on OAC.[a]

Instructions regarding warfarin use	1. Stop at least 4 days prior to surgery
	2. Check INR 1 day prior to surgery
	  If <1.5, proceed with surgery
	  If 1.5–1.8, consider low-level reversal with vitamin K
	  If >1.8, recommend reversal with vitamin K (either 1 mg SC or 2.5 mg PO)
	3. Recheck INR the day of surgery
	4. Restart maintenance dose of warfarin the evening of surgery
	5. Daily INR until in therapeutic range (>1.9)

Instructions regarding IV UFH use	1. Should start at least 2 days prior to surgery at therapeutic dose using a validated, aPTT-adjusted, weight-based nomogram (i.e., 80 U/kg bolus dose IV followed by maintenance dose of 18 U/kg/h IV) 2. Discontinue 6 hours prior to surgery 3. Restart no less than 12 hours postoperatively at the previous maintenance dose once hemostasis is achieved 4. Discontinue IV UFH when INR is in the therapeutic range (>1.9)

Instructions regarding LMWH use	1. Should start at least prior to surgery at BID therapeutic dose (i.e., enoxaparin 1 mg/kg SC BID or
	  dalteparin 100 IU/kg SQ BID)
	2. Discontinue at least 12 hours prior to surgery (if surgery is in the early morning consider holding previous
	  evening dose)
	3. Restart the usual therapeutic dose within 12–24 hours after surgery once hemostasis is achieved
	4. Discontinue LMWH when INR is in the therapeutic range (>1.9)
	5. LMWH should be used in patients undergoing spinal or epidural anesthesia using ASRA guidelines

Source: Spyropoulos (2005).
[a]OAC, oral anticoagulation; INR, international normalized ratio; aPTT, activated partial thromboplastin time; UFH, unfractionated heparin; LMWH, low-molecular-weight heparin; ASRA, American Society of Regional Anesthesia.

discontinuation of warfarin compared with a gradual, or stepwise, reduction (Spyropoulos, 2005). Generally, it takes approximately 4 days after stopping warfarin to reduce the international normalized ratio (INR) from a steady-state value of 2.0 or 3.0 to a value of 1.5, at which point surgery may be performed safely, and approximately 3–5 days to reach therapeutic INR after OAC resumption. The temporary discontinuation of warfarin exposes the patient to the risk of thromboembolism equivalent to 1 day without anticoagulation before surgery and 1 day after surgery (Jafri and Metha, 2004).

In a recent literature review, Spyropoulos offers an explicit bridging algorithm that accounts for the preoperative transition based on TE risk and postoperative anticoagulation regimen after accounting for procedural bleeding risk. This protocol is presented in Table 10e.ii-4. Of note, patients with a high risk of TE and a high risk of bleeding should restart LMWH or UFH at therapeutic doses. However, in patients with a moderate risk of TE and high risk of bleeding, LMWH or UFH may either be restarted or held until hemostasis is achieved (Spyropoulos, 2005). Patients who are also on antiplatelet medications, such as aspirin, ticlopidine, or clopidogrel, should stop these medications at least 7 days prior to surgery, since they cause irreversible inhibition of platelet function for the duration of the 7- to 10-day platelet life span (Jafri and Metha, 2004).

Complications of Nephrectomy

Radical Nephrectomy

Radical nephrectomy is the gold standard curative operation for patients with localized RCC. Currently, open radical nephrectomy remains the preferred technique for patients with RCC and any of the following characteristics: (1) major venous or vena caval involvement, (2) local tumor invasion, (3) massive tumor size, and (4) gross lymphadenopathy. In these settings, the ability of laparoscopic radical nephrectomy to achieve complete tumor excision is not established (Novick, 2004). However, laparoscopic and hand-assisted radical nephrectomies have proven to be an effective alternative with similar complication rates and improved postoperative recovery compared to open surgery (Shuford et al., 2004).

Cookson and colleagues retrospectively compared the early complications among 74 consecutive patients who were treated with open, hand-assisted, or laparoscopic radical nephrectomies. Patients in the three groups had similar preoperative characteristics, including preoperative hematocrit. The estimated intraoperative blood loss declined from open to hand-assisted to pure laparoscopic nephrectomies; however, this trend was accompanied by a statistically significant increased rate of transfusion, with the pure laparoscopic procedure associated with the highest transfusion rate. The greater blood loss intraoperatively in open radical nephrectomies is consistent with studies by Andrews et al. and Clayman et al. (Dunn et al., 2000; Simon et al., 2004).

According to most studies intraoperative bleeding and postoperative bleeding are not significant morbidities associated with radical nephrectomies. Therefore, radical and laparoscopic techniques have similar surgical outcomes and complications, of which bleeding is not a significant morbidity.

Partial Nephrectomy

Open nephron-sparing surgery for renal tumors less than or equal to 4 cm has a cancer control equivalent to that of open radical nephrectomy. The emergence of laparoscopic partial nephrectomy has demonstrated similar oncological results; however, the complication rates, primarily postoperative bleeding, and urine leak may be higher than for open nephron-sparing surgery (Kim et al., 2003).

In a study by Ramani and colleagues, 18 of 200 consecutive patients (9%) who underwent laparoscopic partial nephrectomy had hemorrhagic complications, which were defined as bleeding requiring transfusion or therapeutic intervention. Hemorrhage was stratified according to intraoperative (3.5%), postoperative (2%), and delayed hemorrhage (4%). Intraoperative bleeding could be attributed to systemic coagulopathy in only one of seven patients; otherwise bleeding was a result of clamping malfunction or multiple renal arteries. Furthermore, they noted that use of a bioadhesive, FloSeal, reduced the intraoperative hemorrhage rate from 9.5% to 3%. More importantly, postoperative bleeding (prior to discharge) occurred in four patients (2%) all on postoperative day 2; in all these patients, complete hemostasis was reported intraoperatively after hilar unclamping. All four patients responded to conservative treatment with either bed rest or transfusion. Delayed hemorrhage occurred at a mean of 16 days postoperatively in eight patients, only three of whom had no identifiable precipitating event. When comparing the conclusions of another study by Van Poppel et al. that suggested that larger tumor size and central location increased the risk of postoperative hemorrhage, Ramani and colleagues stated that 67% of patients who developed hemorrhage had a central tumor infiltrating to a depth of 2.2 cm and abutting the renal sinus (Ramani et al., 2005).

Another retrospective study by Kavoussi and colleagues that reviewed 217 laparoscopic partial nephrectomy cases recorded a 1.8% (4 of 217) rate of postoperative bleeding that required transfusion. They concluded that major postoperative complications including delayed renal hemorrhage were slightly lower than the rate published in a series of open partial nephrectomies; however, they noted higher intraoperative blood loss (385 ml vs. 150 ml). They also documented a perioperative blood transfusion rate of 6.9% and a rate of delayed renal hemorrhage of 1.8% compared with the previously documented 3.0% (Link et al., 2005). In a retrospective study by Gill and colleagues that compared laparoscopic partial nephrectomies with laparoscopic cryoablation, they noted a postoperative hemorrhage rate of 6% (10/153). However, with the inclusion of intraoperative renal hemorrhage, the risk of hemorrhage approached 10% (Gill et al., 2005).

With an overall disease-specific survival rate of 97% and local recurrence rate of 0.9%, laparoscopic nephron-sparing surgeries offer a favorable alternative to open partial nephrectomies (Link et al., 2005). The increased use of improved hemostatic adjuvants, such as tissue sealants and glues, the harmonic scalpel, and other new instrumentation, has allowed laparoscopic surgery to be performed with less blood loss. Nonetheless, it is important to lower pressures at the conclusion of surgery to assess bleeding at sites obscured by pneumoperitoneum that may subsequently cause late postoperative bleeding (Varkarakis et al., 2005).

Nephrectomy in Patients on Long-Term Oral Anticoagulation Therapy

In a recent study Kavoussi and colleagues investigated the hemorrhagic and thromboembolic complications of chronically anticoagulated patients after laparoscopic renal/adrenal surgery. In this retrospective study, they reviewed the records of 787 patients of whom 25 had laparoscopic renal/adrenal surgery and were chronically anticoagulated with warfarin. The perioperative management of these patients included cessation of warfarin 3–4 days before surgery, reduction of INR preoperatively to 1.5, bridging with either UFH (17 of 25) or LMWH (8 of 25), discontinuation of UFH 6 hours before surgery and restarted 12 hours after surgery, and resumption of warfarin 24–36 hours postoperatively. Of the 25 patients, six patients (24%) required transfusions compared with 5.2% of the control group (those not on OAC).

Two of six patients (8%) had definitive evidence of postoperative bleeding compared with 0.9% in the control group. In an addendum, they stated that in the other four transfused patients there was neither an increase in intraoperative blood loss nor evidence of postoperative bleeding demonstrated by CT; rather these patients had a lower transfusion threshold secondary to their coexisting cardiac comorbidities. Although intraoperative blood loss and thromboembolic events were not statistically different between the two groups, they concluded that the incidence of postoperative bleeding and the possibility of transfusion were statistically higher in chronically anticoagulated patients (Varkarakis et al., 2005).

Bridging Recommendations in Urological Patients with Renal Cell Carcinoma

There has been no definitive literature on the perioperative approach to patients on OAC who have kidney cancer surgery. However, urological procedures are associated with an increased risk of postoperative bleeding, partly due to the presence of urokinase that is produced by the genitourinary epithelium (Douketis, 2002). Urokinase is present in high concentration in the urine and plays a central role in extracellular matrix degradation, cell migration, and invasion. Moreover, it is a major activator of fibrinolysis in the extravascular compartment, and studies have shown greater expression of urokinase in malignant tissue, specifically human RCC, in comparison to normal tissue. In addition, the kidneys are a highly vascular organ system, receiving 25% of the total cardiac output.

To provide general bridging recommendations, it is important to examine the risks associated with bridging of patients undergoing urological procedures associated with

a high risk of bleeding. Although it is difficult to extrapolate, one such procedure that was documented as having a high risk of bleeding is a transurethral prostatectomy (TURP) (Douketis et al., 2004). Many of the studies that report outcomes of TURPs in patients on OAC are small case series. Several management strategies have been employed to investigate the possible complications. These strategies include complete discontinuation of warfarin preoperatively with resumption within 48 hours postoperatively (Mulcahy et al., 1975), continuation of warfarin during the procedure with the administration of fresh frozen plasma at the end of surgery (if needed) (Parr et al., 1989), bridging with intravenous UFH 2 days preoperatively and postoperatively (Tscholl et al., 1980), and finally bridging with LMWH (Dotan et al., 2002). It is important to note that only with continued warfarin treatment was there an associated increased rate of transfusion. In addition, none of the series had VTE complications, although the underlying risk was not always provided. However, bridging with LMWH resulted in a prolonged hospital stay, although without bleeding or VTE complications. The provided data can be used as a guide to laparoscopic partial nephrectomies that may be grouped with TURPs as having a high risk of bleeding.

Before providing recommendations, it is important to understand the management options and their rationales. The management options include (1) complete cessation of warfarin preoperatively with resumption postoperatively, (2) bridging with intravenous UFH or LMWH preoperatively with resumption of only warfarin postoperatively, and (3) bridging preoperatively and postoperatively with intravenous UFH or LMWH. When choosing a management plan, it is important to weigh the risks of VTE against the risks of bleeding from the procedure. For example, in a patient with a mitral mechanical heart valve undergoing radical nephrectomy, bridging with intravenous UFH or LMWH would be imperative; similarly, in a 65-year-old patient with VTE greater than

TABLE 10e.ii-5. Perioperative bridging recommendations.[a]

Risk of TE	Procedure	Type	Recommendations
High risk	Radical nephrectomy	Open, HAL, or laparoscopic	Bridging with full dose of UFH or LMWH as per the protocol in Table 10e.ii-4
	Partial nephrectomy	Open, HAL	Bridging with full dose of UFH as per Table 10e.ii-4
		Laparoscopic	Bridging preoperatively with prophylactic or higher dose of UFH or LMWH as per Table 10e.ii-4, with resumption of only warfarin postoperatively.
Moderate risk	Radical nephrectomy	Open, HAL, or laparoscopic	Bridging with prophylactic or higher dose of UFH or LMWH as per the protocol in Table 10e.ii-4
	Partial nephrectomy	Open, HAL	Bridging with prophylactic or higher dose of UFH or LMWH as per the protocol in Table 10e.ii-4
		Laparoscopic	Bridging preoperatively with prophylactic or higher dose of UFH or LMWH as per Table 10e.ii-4; with resumption of only warfarin postoperatively
Low risk	Radical nephrectomy	Open, HAL, or laparoscopic	Bridging optional
	Partial nephrectomy	Open, HAL	Bridging optional
		Laparoscopic	No bridging with UFH or LMWH

[a]TE, thromboembolism; HAL, hand-assisted laparoscopy; UFH, unfractionated heparin; LMWH, low-molecular-weight heparin.

6 months ago undergoing a partial nephrectomy, temporary warfarin cessation without bridging seems logical. However, a quandary arises in patients at high risk of both VTE and bleeding. Surgeons must then consider the absolute need for surgery (given the patient's expected life span) or possibility of minimally invasive alternatives, such as renal cryoablation or radiofrequency ablation, which do not have long-term (5-year) data available but are associated with decreased blood loss and numbers of postsurgical bleeding (Gill et al., 2005).

Conclusions

In summary, thrombosis is a common sign of underlying malignancy and is a subsequent cause of death in patients with cancer. Many urological-based surgical procedures are associated with considerable postoperative bleeding. Radical nephrectomy remains the curative standard for RCC, although this approach is associated with high intraoperative blood loss and low postoperative bleeding. In contrast, partial nephrectomy utilizing laparoscopy for the management of RCC is associated with low intraoperative blood loss and high postsurgical bleeding. The clinical and surgical challenge remains in the patient on long-term OAC requiring partial or radical nephrectomy. In this patient setting, the incidence of postoperative bleeding requiring transfusion must be balanced with the prevention of thrombosis through perioperative bridging of OAC. Close and careful management requires critically timed discontinuation of warfarin therapy prior to surgery with pharmacological bridging using UFH and LMWH therapy. While tumor prothrombotic substances have been characterized along with typical physiological responses to inflammatory mediators, more needs to be learned about the role of the tumor biology and thrombus process. Thus, in patients with RCC, a careful choice of surgical approach must be balanced with the clinical management of coagulation status to ensure optimal patient outcome (Table 10e.ii-5).

References

Caine, G. J., P. S. Stonelake, et al. (2002). The hypercoagulable state of malignancy: pathogenesis and current debate. *Neoplasia* **4**(6): 465–473.

De Cicco, M. (2004). The prothrombotic state in cancer: pathogenic mechanisms. *Crit Rev Oncol Hematol* **50**(3): 187–196.

Deitcher, S. R. (2003). Cancer-related deep venous thrombosis: clinical importance, treatment challenges, and management strategies. *Semin Thromb Hemost* **29**(3): 247–258.

Donati, M. B. (1995). Cancer and thrombosis: from Phlegmasia alba dolens to transgenic mice. *Thromb Haemost* **74**(1): 278–281.

Dotan, Z. A., Y. Mor, et al. (2002). The efficacy and safety of perioperative low molecular weight heparin substitution in patients on chronic oral anticoagulant therapy undergoing transurethral prostatectomy for bladder outlet obstruction. *J Urol* **168**(2): 610–613; discussion 614.

Douketis, J. D. (2002). Perioperative anticoagulation management in patients who are receiving oral anticoagulant therapy: a practical guide for clinicians. *Thromb Res* **108**(1): 3–13.

Douketis, J. D., J. A. Johnson, et al. (2004). Low-molecular-weight heparin as bridging anticoagulation during interruption of warfarin: assessment of a standardized periprocedural anticoagulation regimen. *Arch Intern Med* **164**(12): 1319–1326.

Dunn, A. S. and A. G. Turpie. (2003). Perioperative management of patients receiving oral anticoagulants: a systematic review. *Arch Intern Med* **163**(8): 901–908.

Dunn, M. D., A. J. Portis, et al. (2000). Laparoscopic versus open radical nephrectomy: a 9-year experience. *J Urol* **164**(4): 1153–1159.

Forster, Y., A. Meye, et al. (2003). Tissue specific expression and serum levels of human tissue factor in patients with urological cancer. *Cancer Lett* **193**(1): 65–73.

Garcia, D. A., W. Ageno, et al. (2004). Perioperative anticoagulation for patients with mechanical heart valves: a survey of current practice. *J Thromb Thrombolysis* **18**(3): 199–203.

Gill, I. S., E. M. Remer, et al. (2005). Renal cryoablation: outcome at 3 years. *J Urol* **173**(6): 1903–1907.

Gordon, S. G., J. J. Franks, et al. (1979). Comparison of procoagulant activities in extracts of normal and malignant human tissue. *J Natl Cancer Inst* **62**(4): 773–776.

Jafri, S. M. and T. P. Metha. (2004). Periprocedural management of anticoagulation in patients on extended warfarin therapy. *Semin Thromb Hemost* **30**(6): 657–664.

Johnson, M. J., M. W. Sproule, et al. (1999). The prevalence and associated variables of deep venous thrombosis in patients with advanced cancer. *Clin Oncol (R Coll Radiol)* **11**(2): 105–110.

Kearon, C. and J. Hirsh. (1997). Management of anticoagulation before and after elective surgery. *N Engl J Med* **336**(21): 1506–1511.

Kim, F. J., K. H. Rha, et al. (2003). Laparoscopic radical versus partial nephrectomy: assessment of complications. *J Urol* **170**(2 Pt 1): 408–411.

Lee, A. Y. (2002). Cancer and thromboembolic disease: pathogenic mechanisms. *Cancer Treat Rev* **28**(3): 137–140.

Levitan, N., A. Dowlati, et al. (1999). Rates of initial and recurrent thromboembolic disease among patients with malignancy versus those without malignancy. Risk analysis using Medicare claims data. *Medicine (Baltimore)* **78**(5): 285–291.

Link, R. E., S. B. Bhayani, et al. (2005). Exploring the learning curve, pathological outcomes and perioperative morbidity of laparoscopic partial nephrectomy performed for renal mass. *J Urol* **173**(5): 1690–1694.

Mandala, M., G. Ferretti, et al. (2003). Venous thromboembolism and cancer: new issues for an old topic. *Crit Rev Oncol Hematol* **48**(1): 65–80.

Mulcahy, J. J., R. O. Bradenburg, et al. (1975). Transurethral prostatic resection in patients with prosthetic cardiac valves. *J Urol* **113**(5): 642–643.

Nachman, R. L. and K. A. Hajjar. (1991). Endothelial cell fibrinolytic assembly. *Ann NY Acad Sci* **614**: 240–249.

Novick, A. C. (2004). Laparoscopic and partial nephrectomy. *Clin Cancer Res* **10**(18 Pt 2): 6322S–6327S.

Parr, N. J., C. S. Loh, et al. (1989). Transurethral resection of the prostate and bladder tumour without withdrawal of warfarin therapy. *Br J Urol* **64**(6): 623–625.

Ramani, A. P., M. M. Desai, et al. (2005). Complications of laparo-scopic partial nephrectomy in 200 cases. *J Urol* **173**(1): 42–47.

Rickles, F. R. and M. N. Levine. (1998). Venous thromboem-bolism in malignancy and malignancy in venous thromboem-bolism. *Haemostasis* **28 Suppl 3**: 43–49.

Sampson, M. T. and A. K. Kakkar. (2002). Coagulation proteases and human cancer. *Biochem Soc Trans* **30**(2): 201–207.

Shuford, M. D., E. M. McDougall, et al. (2004). Complications of contemporary radical nephrectomy: comparison of open vs. laparoscopic approach. *Urol Oncol* **22**(2): 121–126.

Simon, S. D., E. P. Castle, et al. (2004). Complications of laparoscopic nephrectomy: the Mayo Clinic experience. *J Urol* **171**(4): 1447–1450.

Spyropoulos, A. C. (2005). Perioperative bridging therapy for the at-risk patient on chronic anticoagulation. *Dis Mon* **51**(2-3): 183–193.

Thodiyil, P. A., D. C. Walsh, et al. (2001). Thromboprophylaxis in the cancer patient. *Acta Haematol* **106**(1-2): 73–80.

Trousseau, A. (1865). Phlegmasia alba dolens. *Clinique Medicale de l'Hotel-Dieu de Paris. London: The New Syndeham Society* **3**: 94–99.

Tscholl, R., W. Straub, et al. (1980). Electroresection of the prostate in patients treated with heparin. *J Urol* **124**(2): 221–222.

Varkarakis, I. M., S. Rais-Bahrami, et al. (2005). Laparoscopic renal-adrenal surgery in patients on oral anticoagulant therapy. *J Urol* **174**(3): 1020–1023; discussion 1023.

Walsh-McMonagle, D. and D. Green. (1997). Low-molecular-weight heparin in the management of Trousseau's syndrome. *Cancer* **80**(4): 649–655.

Zacharski, L. R., V. A. Memoli, et al. (1986). Coagulation-cancer interaction in situ in renal cell carcinoma. *Blood* **68**(2): 394–399.

Zacharski, L. R., D. L. Ornstein, et al. (1998). Expression of the factor VII activating protease, hepsin, in situ in renal cell carcinoma. *Thromb Haemost* **79**(4): 876–877.

10f
Embolization

Theo M. de Reijke and Otto M. van Delden

Introduction

Transarterial embolization for renal cancer was first described in 1973.[1] At that time it was applied to patients with metastatic disease with symptoms from the affected kidney and as a preoperative tool to facilitate radical nephrectomy.

Following this first description, a number of centers published their results using different techniques.[4,6,7,18,29–31,38–42,45,46] These publications all originate from the 1970s and 1980s, when approximately one-third of patients presented with metastatic disease at initial presentation. Today most patients present with early disease, where even organ-preserving modalities are the first choice of treatment. The indications for embolization in case of a renal cancer have also been modified as a result of improved imaging and surgical techniques and the introduction of effective adjuvant treatment leading to more aggressive surgery in case of metastatic disease.[14,15,32] While preoperative embolization has been almost completely abandoned, palliative vascular occlusion may still have a role.

Technique

Before the embolization procedure a urine culture should be obtained if a urinary tract infection is suspected in order to perform the procedure under antibiotic coverage. If no infection is present generally no antibiotics are prescribed.

As severe loin pain and/or nausea may develop during the embolization procedure the patient should have an intravenous line put in before starting the procedure to enable immediate administration of pain medication. Alternatively, pain medication can be started prior to beginning the procedure.

Renal angiography is usually performed from a common femoral approach using a 5 French sheath. Alternatively, a brachial approach may be used in some situations (e.g., access through the groin is not possible or there is difficulty in catheterizing the renal artery from a femoral approach). A flush aortogram with a pigtail catheter should be performed initially to assess the localization and the number of renal arteries as well as the potential collateral arterial tumor supply from lumbar arteries (Figs. 10f-1 and 10f-2). The renal artery is selected using a cobra-type or Simm-type catheter. Selective angiography is then performed to determine the exact localization of the tumor and the branches supplying the tumor. The tumor is usually markedly hypervascular and is rapidly recognized by its pathological vasculature. Parasitic capsular tumor vessels are often observed. Arteriovenous shunting may also be seen in the tumor, which may be important since it influences the choice of the embolization material to be used. Subsequently, the catheter can be left in the main stem of the renal artery to embolize the whole kidney or the tumor feeders can be selectively catheterized in an attempt to embolize only the tumor and spare as much normal renal parenchyma as possible. Care should be taken to obtain a stable catheter position to prevent dislocation and possible inadvertent embolization of nontarget organs or tissue.

Embolization can be performed with many different materials (Table 10f-1, but the most commonly used categories are fluids/sclerosants (e.g., alcohol), particles (e.g., polyvinyl alcohol), or steel coils. When using fluids, the main renal artery can be temporarily occluded using an occlusion balloon to prevent backflow of the sclerosant into the aorta. Similarly, when using particles, these should be slowly injected using constant fluoroscopic monitoring and this should be terminated when there is still some slow antegrade flow in the renal artery. Gelfoam pledgets may also be used for embolization and these are safe and effective. However, gelfoam produces a nonpermanent type of embolization, because it is quickly resorbed by the body and recanalization of the embolized vessels may develop in a matter of days.

The choice between these materials depends on the specific anatomical circumstances and the operator's preference. In general, embolization with small particles (e.g., polyvinyl 350–500 μm) or sclerosants (e.g., alcohol) is desirable, because it creates occlusion of the distal arterial supply to the tumor. This prevents early recanalization or collateral arterial vascularization of the tumor. Significant arteriovenous

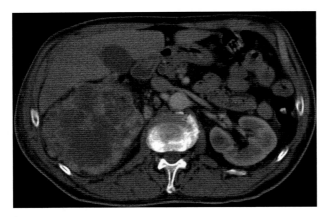

FIGURE 10f-1. Contrast-enhanced CT scan of large unresectable renal cell carcinoma in the right kidney, giving rise to massive hematuria.

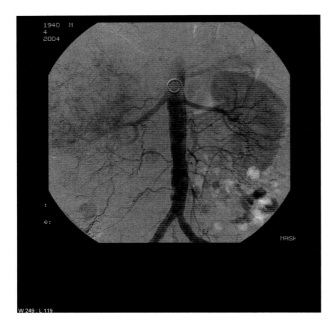

FIGURE 10f-2. The same patient as in Fig. 10f–1. Angiography and subsequent embolization were performed to control the hematuria. A flush aortogram shows the large hypervascular tumor mass with numerous pathological vessels in the right kidney.

shunting precludes the use of fluids or small particles as embolic agents, because these may enter the systemic circulation and induce necrosis of nontarget organs.

Many operators prefer to further occlude the main renal artery with coils after initial peripheral embolization with particles. No significant differences in procedural results have been reported between the use of particles combined with coils versus sclerosants. However, the use of alcohol requires significant skill from the operator and is associated with more pain.

TABLE 10f-1. Agents used for embolization of renal cell carcinoma.

Absolute alcohol
Autologous muscle particles
Avitene® (microfibrillar collagen hemostat)
Coils (metal/steel/mini/Gianturco/GAW)
Collagen
Detachable balloons
Dura particles
Ethibloc® (oily contrast-labeled amino acid)
Fibrospum
Gelatine foam/Gelfoam®
Gelatine sponge/Gelaspon®
Gelfoam prepared with BCG
Histoacryl®
Ivalon® (polyvinyl alcohol)
ICBA (isobutyl-2-cyanoacrylate)
Lyodura
MMC (microencapsulated or nonencapsulated mitomycin C)
Palacos® (methylmethacrylate)
Spongostan®
Tachotyp flocculi®
Thrombin
Vilan®

The embolization procedure is usually finished when a control angiogram shows complete occlusion of the main renal artery and all collateral branches feeding the tumor (Fig. 10f-3). In experienced hands a complete embolization procedure should generally not take longer then 45 minutes.

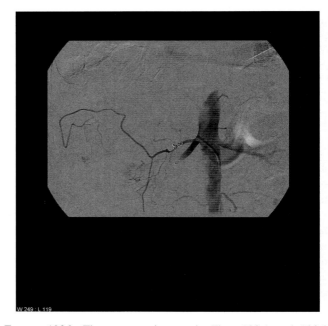

FIGURE 10f-3. The same patient as in Figs. 10f–1 and 10f–2. Selective series of the right renal artery after embolization with polyvinyl alcohol particles and coils. Some filling of a pathological branch is still seen. This was further embolized with particles and coils until all flow to the tumor had ceased.

The patient is usually admitted to the hospital after the procedure in order to observe if complications develop.

Outcome of Renal Embolization for Different Indications

Following the first descriptions of renal artery occlusion the main indications were palliative treatment for symptoms of an inoperable renal tumor, e.g., pain and hematuria, and paraneoplastic symptoms, e.g., hypercalcemia, erythrocytemia, hypertension, and preoperative embolization, to facilitate subsequent surgery; today these indications for preoperative embolization have almost been abandoned.[2] It was originally suggested that it would facilitate subsequent surgery by reducing the size and vascularity of the tumor. Following initial encouraging reports, other investigators found no benefits for preoperative embolization, and a survey among urologists from the UK demonstrated a decline in its use if results of 1983 were compared with those of 1992, 60% and <0.2%, respectively.[9,27,44,47]

However, if a patient presents with metastatic disease and intractable pain due to a local tumor mass and/or recurrent hematuria, palliative nephrectomy and embolization are two possible approaches. However, the collateral or parasitic blood supply of the affected kidney will result in revascularization and the reappearance of symptoms if the affected kidney is embolized. Palliative embolization should thus be offered in situations in which life expectancy is considered to be short. The results from palliative embolization are reasonable, although the reported series described only a small number of patients. Nurmi et al. described 20 patients who were embolized for pain control and hematuria.[37] A good result was obtained for pain in three out of six patients and hematuria was controlled in 11 out of 14 patients. No prolongation of survival time was evident, and all the patients died of renal adenocarcinoma within 38 months. Marx et al. obtained control of the hematuria in 13 out of the 13 patients embolized, although three of them relapsed.[30] Jacobs et al. reported one patient with malignant hypercalcemia related to a renal cell cancer who became normocalcemic following renal embolization, despite metastatic bone lesions.[21] Finally, in a series of 25 patients Munro et al. demonstrated that 17 out of 25 (68%) reported no further problems from their primary tumor (pain or hematuria) following embolization.[35] Kalman and Varenhorst reviewed the available literature on the role of palliative arterial embolization, but they could not assess the role of renal embolization due to the considerable variation in presentation and selection criteria.[22]

Palliative embolization could be offered to the patient either for treatment of the involved kidney or treatment of symptomatic metastases. In particular, the presence of bone metastases can induce complaints of uncontrollable pain and surgery is usually not indicated if multiple lesions are present.

Immunotherapy is also not likely to control the pain, although local radiation of the painful metastases is usually the first choice. Embolization of the bone metastases has been shown to be advantageous as a palliative measure for pain relief and also in case a local surgical resection is contemplated by reducing blood loss during the surgery.[8,28]

Spontaneous regression of renal cell cancer metastases following nephrectomy is a rare event. The incidence is estimated to be in the range of 0.8%.[12] Spontaneous regression is mostly reported in lung lesions, but regression of other soft tissue and bone lesions has been reported.[10–12,16] The hypothesis is that renal cell cancer is an immunogenic tumor, which is why embolization has also been evaluated in the frame of combination therapy. The concept of preoperative renal embolization was based on the hypothesis that the host immune response was stimulated; therefore the tumor necrosis in the delay between embolization and nephrectomy would create an autovaccine that would upregulate the natural antitumor activity of the immune system in patients.[3,36] In 1980 Swanson et al. presented the results of a series of 50 patients with primary metastatic renal cell cancer who underwent a nephrectomy following prior renal embolization some days before.[43] A response was seen in 18 patients, a complete response in seven patients (median range of 18 months), a partial response in five patients (median range of 12 months), and stable disease in six patients (median range of 18 months). Because of these surprising data the European Organization for Research and Treatment of Cancer Genito-Urinary (EORTC-GU) group initiated a pilot study using the same concept.[25] Nephrectomy was performed 2–6 days following embolization of the renal artery of a biopsy-confirmed renal cell cancer with metastases. Twenty-five patients with an average age of 60 years were included in this study. One patient died following nephrectomy, one patient had a complete response (at 36 months there was no evidence of disease), six patients had stable disease (at 14, 17, 18, 19, 24, and 31 months), and 18 patients had no response (death within 1–11 months). The South West Oncology Group reported a similar study in 30 patients.[19] No complete remissions were found and a 28% 1-year survival and a 7-month median survival were realized, which is similar to other series in which no therapy or palliative nephrectomy was performed.

Based on the outcome of these series preoperative embolization in patients with metastatic disease does not result in better survival.

However, Zielinski et al. reported a series of 474 patients with renal cell cancer who underwent radical nephrectomy over a period of 15 years.[48] Of this group of patients 118 had a preoperative renal embolization. For this group, they matched 116 patients who underwent a radical nephrectomy without prior embolization. Preoperative embolization was shown to be an important prognostic factor influencing survival. The overall 5- and 10-year survival for 118 patients embolized before nephrectomy was 62%

and 47%, respectively, and it was 35% and 23%, respectively, for the matched group of 116 patients treated with surgery alone. Of course, these data have to be interpreted with caution because it was not a prospective randomized study.

Another possible indication could be renal occlusion in combination with intravascular drug targeting. Kato *et al.* examined chemoembolization using ethylcellulose microencapsulation of mitomycin C.[23] There was a high-sustained drug activity in the target sites with a low-sustained drug level in the systemic circulation. In all, 173 patients were treated with this chemoembolization technique using a single dose in 137 patients and repeated doses (two to five) in the rest of the patients.[24] In 18/124 evaluable tumors a reduction of >50% was observed in tumor size, 22/124 tumors showed a size reduction between 25% and 49%, and in 25/124 tumors a <24% size reduction was demonstrated. One tumor increased in size. Side effects included fever (28%), pain (25%), gastrointestinal discomfort (10%), myelosuppression (5%), renal dysfunction (3%), hepatic dysfunction (2%), distant embolization (1%), and skin ulcer (1%). When the results of the chemoembolization were compared with a contemporary group of patients undergoing nephrectomy an improved survival was found only in patients with Stage II and III disease, but not in patients with Stage I and IV disease. The concept has not been reproduced by other groups and this approach has been abandoned.

Since patients now present more frequently with localized tumors due to the increased use of imaging techniques

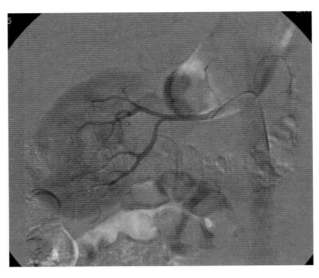

FIGURE 10f-5. Selective angiogram of the right kidney showing a small arterial branch filling the false aneurysm (arrow).

for other indications where renal sparing surgery might be indicated, this type of surgery could induce postoperative vascular complications, e.g., postoperative hemorrhage (0–5.6%) and pseudoaneurysms.[20] Angiography enables very precise visualization of extravasation of contrast material in the renal fossa. Percutaneous superselective embolization of the feeding vessels is then indicated to treat the bleeding, because open surgery usually results in nephrectomy. The superselective embolization is successful in most of the cases (80%) and has not been shown to impair renal function (Figs. 10f-4–10f-7).

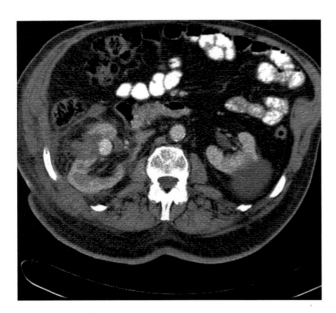

FIGURE 10f-4. CT scan with intravenous contrast showing a false aneurysm in the right kidney after partial right nephrectomy. There is also some hemorrhage around the right kidney with some infiltration of the perinephric fat.

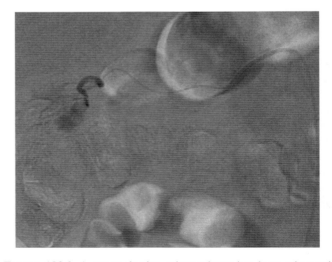

FIGURE 10f-6. A superselective microcatheter has been advanced into the small arterial branch, which supplies the false aneurysm.

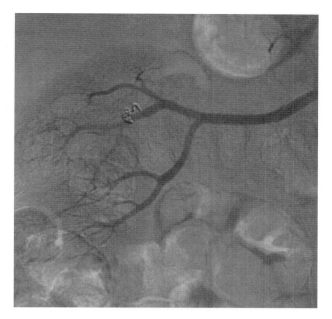

FIGURE 10f-7. Completion angiogram after embolization of the small supplying branch of the false aneurysm with multiple small micro-coils. No more filling of the false aneurysm is seen.

Complications and How to Prevent Them

Before considering renal embolization the diagnosis of a renal cell cancer should be substantiated. The complications can be divided in those induced by the specific embolization procedure and those due to angiography in general. Complications related to the angiographic procedure include systemic sequelae such as contrast-induced renal failure and allergic or anaphylactic reactions to the contrast media. Contrast-induced renal failure can be prevented by reducing the contrast load as much as possible and by taking preventive periprocedural measures such as hyperhydration. Adverse contrast reactions are now very rare due to the use of newer generation contrast media. Local complications of the angiographic procedure include puncture site hematoma or dissection/thrombosis of the access vessel. In experienced hands the combined angiography-related complication rate should be less than 5%.

The specific embolization-related complications are the result of the necrosis created by the procedure. If a major vessel is occluded, subsequent necrosis will be induced. This will result in a postinfarction syndrome, usually seen 1–3 days following the renal artery occlusion, with systemic effects such as loin pain, fever, nausea, and vomiting. On a computed tomography (CT) scan or ultrasound images following renal embolization gas formation can be seen from the infarcted tissue due to the necrosis, which is not necessarily a sign of infection.[13] Patients can also develop transient or persistent hypertension. These effects cannot be predicted. Since necrosis is induced due to the embolization, it is mandatory to rule out infection in the affected kidney

before the embolization procedure. A positive urine culture mandates antibiotic coverage during the procedure. It is not known if this antibiotic coverage should be given to everyone. Because of the possibility of the induction of severe pain, the patient should have a well-running intravenous drip in order to administer morphine in case severe pain is developing. An epidural catheter may be placed before the procedure. Due to the local reaction around the kidney, patients can also develop a paralytic ileus. If renal embolization is indicated preoperatively, the optimal interval between embolization and surgery is probably less than 48 hours in order to reduce the distress caused by the postinfarction syndrome.

Major complications following renal embolization can be the reflux of embolic material into the systemic circulation leading to occlusion of nontarget vessels and to ischemia of the intestines, spinal cord, or renal failure (intoxication of the contralateral kidney by contrast medium or arteria testicularis).[17, 26, 34] In 121 renal tumor embolizations a mean complication rate of 9.9% was reported with a mortality of 3.3%.[26] The complication rate of renal embolization as a palliative measure was approximately four times as high compared to preoperative embolization due to the performance status of these patients and the size of the tumor mass.

There are insufficient data to compare the complication rates of different embolization materials. One study reported increased complications if Ivalon® was used compared to gelfoam; however, definite conclusions cannot be drawn and the published studies are outdated.[26]

Future Applications

Since more small renal lesions are now being identified, which leads to more renal-sparing techniques such as partial nephrectomy, cryosurgery, high-frequency tumor ablation, and high-intensity focused ultrasound, there may be a possible renewed role for embolization. In particular, if cryosurgery or radiofrequency techniques are applied, high blood flow compromises the effect of the ablative techniques. If the tumor is very selectively occluded the effect could possibly be improved and following the procedure the effect could be evaluated immediately.

As previously described, a combination of embolization and systemic therapy did not improve the results; however, we may now have more active drugs for patients with metastatic disease. It is generally accepted that before systemic therapy the affected kidney should be removed, but this will lead to "overtreatment" of a number of patients who will not react to subsequent systemic therapy.[14, 15, 32] Recently, a series was published in which patients were first treated with systemic therapy and if there was an effect they then underwent radical nephrectomy.[5]

Presystemic therapy embolization could possibly improve the results, but again this has to be proven in randomized studies.

References

1. Almgard LE, Fernstrom I, Haverling *et al.* Treatment of renal adenocarcinoma by embolic occlusion of the renal circulation. *Br J Urol* 1973;45:474–479.

2. Altaffer LF 3rd, Chenault OW Jr. Paraneoplastic endocrinopathies associated with renal tumors. *J Urol* 1979;122:573–577.

3. Bakke A, Gothlin JH, Haukaas SA *et al.* Augmentation of natural killer cell activity after arterial embolization of renal carcinomas. *Cancer Res* 1982;42:3880–3883.

4. Belis JA, Horton JA. Renal artery embolization with polyvinyl alcohol foam particles. *Urology* 1982;19:224–227.

5. Bex A, Kerst M, Mallo H *et al.* Interferon alpha 2b as medical selection for nephrectomy in patients with synchronous metastatic renal cell carcinoma: a consecutive study. *Eur Urol* 2006;49:76–81.

6. Bucheler E, Hupe W, Hertel EU *et al.* Katheterembolisation von Nierentumoren. *Rofo* 1976;124:134–138.

7. Buzelin JM, Bourdon J, Mitard D *et al.* L'Embolisation de l'artère rénale. *J Urol Nephrol* 1974;80:541–553.

8. Chatziioannou AN, Johnson ME, Pneumaticos SG *et al.* Preoperative embolization of bone metastases from renal cell carcinoma. *Eur Radiol* 2000;10:593–596.

9. Christensen K, Dyreborg U, Andersen JF *et al.* The value of transvascular embolization in the treatment of renal carcinoma. *J Urol* 1985;133:191–193.

10. DeWeerd JH, Hawthorne NJ, Adson MA. Regression of renal cell hepatic metastasis following removal of primary lesions. *J Urol* 1977;117:790–792.

11. Doolittle KH. Spontaneous remission of solitary bony metastasis after removal of the primary kidney carcinoma. *J Urol* 1976;116:803–804.

12. Fairlamb DJ. Spontaneous regression of metastases of renal cancer: a report of 2 cases including the first recorded regression following irradiation of a dominant metastasis and review of the world literature. *Cancer* 1981;47:2102–2106.

13. Fischedik AR, Peters PE. CT-Untersuchungen nach Äthanolembolisation maligner Nierentumoren. *Fortschr Rontgenstr* 1986;144:76–79.

14. Flanigan RC, Salmon SE, Blumenstein BA *et al.* Nephrectomy followed by interferon alfa-2b compared with interferon alfa-2b alone for metastatic renal-cell cancer. *N Engl J Med* 2001;345:1655–1659.

15. Flanigan RC, Mickisch G, Sylvester R *et al.* Cytoreductive nephrectomy in patients with metastatic renal cancer: a combined analysis. *J Urol* 2004;171:1071–1076.

16. Freed SZ, Halperin JP, Gordon M. Idiopathic regression of metastases from renal cell carcinoma. *J Urol* 1977;118:538–542.

17. Gang DL, Dole KB, Adelman LS. Spinal cord infarction following renal artery embolization. *JAMA* 1977;237:2841–2842.

18. Georgi M, Marberger M, Kaufmann A. Embolisation eines inoperablen Nierentumors durch intraarterielle Applikation von Thrombin bei Ballonverschluss der Nierenarterie. *Dtsch Med Wochenschr* 1975;100:2428–2429.

19. Gottesman JE, Crawford ED, Grossman HB *et al.* Infarction-nephrectomy for metastatic renal carcinoma. Southwest oncology group study. *Urology* 1985;25:248–250.

20. Heye S, Maleux G, Van Poppel H *et al.* Hemorrhagic complications after nephron-sparing surgery: angiographic diagnosis and management by transcatheter embolization. *AJR* 2005;184:1661–1664.

21. Jacobs JA, Ring EJ, Wein AJ. New indications for renal infarction. *J Urol* 1981;125:243–245.

22. Kalman D, Varenhorst E. The role of arterial embolization in renal cell carcinoma. *Scand J Urol Nephrol* 1999;33:162–170.

23. Kato T, Nemoto R, Mori H *et al.* Sustained/release properties of microencapsulated mitomycin C with ethylcellulose infused into the renal artery of the dog. *Cancer* 1980;46:14–21.

24. Kato T, Nemoto R, Mori H *et al.* Arterial chemoembolization with microencapsulated anticancer drug. An approach to selective cancer chemotherapy with sustained effects. *JAMA* 1981;245:1123–1127.

25. Kurth KH, Cinqualbre J, Oliver RTD *et al.* Embolization and subsequent nephrectomy in metastatic renal cell carcinoma. *Prog Clin Biol Res* 1984;153:423–436.

26. Lammer J, Justich E, Schreyer H *et al.* Complications of renal tumor embolization. *Cardiovasc Intervent Radiol* 1985;8:31–35.

27. Lanigan D, Jurriaans E, Hammonds JC *et al.* The current status of embolization in renal cell carcinoma——a survey of local and national practice. *Clin Radiol* 1992;46:176–178.

28. Layalle I, Flandroy P, Trotteur G *et al.* Arterial embolization of bone metastases: is it worthwhile? *J Belge Radiol* 1998;81:223–225.

29. Marberger M, Georgi M. Balloon occlusion of the renal artery in tumor nephrectomy. *J Urol* 1975;114:360–363.

30. Marx FJ, Chaussy Ch, Moser E. Grenzen und Gefahren der palliativen Embolisation inoperabler Nierentumoren. *Urologe A* 1982;21:206–210.

31. Menachem YB, Crigler CM, Corriere JN. Elective transcatheter renal artery occlusion prior to nephrectomy. *J Urol* 1975;114:355–259.

32. Mickisch GH, Garin A, van Poppel H *et al.* Radical nephrectomy plus interferon-alfa-based immunotherapy compared with interferon alfa alone in metastatic renal-cell carcinoma: a randomised trial. *Lancet* 2001;358:966–970.

33. Montie JE, Stewart BH, Straffon RA *et al.* The role of adjunctive nephrectomy in patients with metastatic renal cell carcinoma. *J Urol* 1977;117:272–275.

34. Mukamel E, Hadar H, Nissenkorn I *et al.* Widespread dissemination of gelfoam particles complicating occlusion of renal circulation. *Urology* 1979;14:194–197.

35. Munro NP, Woodhams S, Nawrock JD *et al.* The role of transarterial embolization in the treatment of renal cell carcinoma. *BJU Int* 2003;92:240–244.

36. Nakano H, Nihira H, Toge T. Treatment of renal cancer patients by transcatheter embolization and its effects on lymphocyte proliferative responses. *J Urol* 1983;130:24–27.

37. Nurmi M, Satokari K, Puntala P. Renal artery embolization in the palliative treatment of renal adenocarcinoma. *Scand J Urol Nephrol* 1987;21:93–96.

38. Pontonnier F, Plante P, Mourlan D *et al.* Embolisation rénale dans le traitement des tumeurs du rein. *Sem Hop* 1981;57:929–933.

39. Rosenkrantz H, Sands JP, Buchta KS *et al.* Renal devitalization using 95 per cent ethyl alcohol. *J Urol* 1982;127:873–875.

40. Schulman CC, Struyven J, Giannakopoulos X *et al.* Preoperative embolization of renal tumors—comparison of different methods. *Eur Urol* 1980;6:154–157.
41. Steckenmesser R, Bayindir S, Rothauge CF *et al.* Embolisation maligner Nierentumoren. *Rofo* 1976;125:251–257.
42. Stösslein F, Schöpke W, Porstmann W *et al.* Die prä-operative Nierenembolisierung maligner Tumoren bei externen Patienten. *Z Urol Nephrol* 1981;74:721–728.
43. Swanson DA, Wallace S, Johnson DE. The role of embolization and nephrectomy in the treatment of metastatic renal carcinoma. *Urol Clin North Am* 1980;7:719–730.
44. Teasdale C, Kirk D, Jeans WD *et al.* Arterial embolisation in renal carcinoma: a useful procedure? *Br J Urol* 1982;54:616–619.
45. Tehlen M, Bruhl P, Gerlach F *et al.* Katheterembolisation von metastasierten Nierenkarzinomen mit Butyl-2-Cyanoacrylate. *Rofo* 1976;124:232–235.
46. Turner RD, Rand RW, Bentson JR *et al.* Ferromagnetic silicone necrosis of hypernephromas by selective vascular occlusion to the tumor: a new technique. *J Urol* 1975;113:455–459.
47. Wallace S, Chuang VP, Swanson D *et al.* Embolization of renal carcinoma. *Radiology* 1981;138:563–570.
48. Zielinski H, Szmigielski S, Petrovich Z. Comparison of preoperative embolization followed by radical nephrectomy with radical nephrectomy alone for renal cell carcinoma. *Am J Clin Oncol* 2000;23:6–12.

10g
Benign Tumors of the Kidney

Doddametikurke R. Basavaraj and Adrian Joyce

Introduction

Renal lesions can be congenital or acquired. Currently, many renal lesions come to light incidentally during a radiological investigation for nonspecific upper abdominal symptoms. Often an ultrasound scan is the initial imaging modality that detects a renal lesion. Space-occupying lesions of the kidney can be cystic, solid, or indeterminate and sonographic criteria for diagnosing a simple renal cyst are well established and further investigation or treatment is seldom necessary in the majority of cases. Bosniak's classification helps the clinician to define the nature of cystic and indeterminate renal masses and the probability of their malignant potential (Bosniak, 1986). By general convention, most solid space-occupying lesions of the kidney are presumed to be malignant until proved otherwise and are managed accordingly. Benign tumours of the kidney, per se, are very rare and distinguishing a benign from a malignant renal lesion on clinical or radiological grounds can be very difficult.

This chapter aims to review the common benign tumors of the kidney, with the emphasis on their diagnosis, pathology, and treatment.

Classification

Benign neoplasms can arise from almost any of the constituents of renal tissue. Common benign tumors include (Table 10g-1):

- Adenoma
- Angiomyolipoma
- Cystic nephroma

There are three types of renal adenomas—-papillary adenoma, metanephric adenoma, and renal oncocytoma (Liu et al. 2002), differentiated by their immunostaining features (Table 10g-2). In the early literature the term renal adenoma was used to describe papillary adenoma.

Papillary Adenoma

Papillary adenoma (PA), defined as minute cortical foci of proliferating epithelium, is a frequently occurring lesion in adult human kidneys (Holm-Nielsen and Olsen 1988). PA constitutes the commonest renal neoplasm affecting over 40% of the general population (Grignon and Eble 1998). They are small well-differentiated tumors of the renal cortex usually seen at autopsy or in nephrectomy specimens removed for renal cell carcinoma (RCC). The majority are solitary lesions; however, 25% are multicentric, with a male-to-female ratio of 3:1. They are more common in patients with von Hippel–Lindau (VHL) disease and acquired renal cystic disease associated with end-stage renal failure. The prevalence in end-stage renal failure patients pretransplant is 14% (Denton et al., 2002).

Pathology

Although grouped under the term benign renal neoplasia, no clinical, histological, or immunohistochemical criteria differentiate PA from renal carcinoma. Histologically, a well-circumscribed lesion showing tubulopapillary architecture has a uniform basophilic or eosinophilic cell appearance with monotonous nuclear and cellular characteristics and features suggesting malignant potential, e.g., nuclear pleomorphism, significant mitotic activity, and lymphovascular invasion are absent. Cytogenetically, however, they are similar to that of renal papillary cell carcinoma and it has been speculated that this may represent an adenoma–carcinoma progression sequence (Kiyoshima et al., 2004). Well-differentiated cells with a diploid DNA histogram and a nuclear surface area less than 32 mm^2 are thought to favor a diagnosis of adenoma (Ganzen et al., 1991). No hemorrhage or necrosis was noted in a series of 59 renal adenomas (Hashine and Sumiyoshi 1996. Traditionally tumors < 3 cm were regarded as benign, but tumors >5 ml have been shown to metastasize; thus current thinking suggests that all lesions >5 mm have malignant potential. Faria et al. (1994) identified two distinct groups of adenomas according to size, histological type, and extent of

TABLE 10g-1. Classification of benign renal tumors.

Renal adenoma
Papillary adenoma
Metanephric adenoma
Oncocytoma
Angiomyolipoma
Cystic nephroma
Miscellaneous
Fibroma
Leiomyoma
Hemangioma
Lymphangioma
Neurogenic tumor

sclerosis, and suggested that small adenomas of the mixed tubulopapillary type with basophilic cells have little or no malignant potential, whereas, adenomas with a solid or papillary pattern with clear cells are potentially malignant. PA shows the histochemical features of the distal tubule, suggesting differentiation to a distal tubule-like histology (Suzuki et al., 1989).

Diagnosis

In clinical practice, standard cross-sectional renal imaging protocols are most likely to miss lesions measuring less than 5 mm and thus these are the lesions that most likely can be considered truly benign.

Management

Lesions larger than 5 mm, which are detected incidentally on imaging, should be deemed to be malignant and managed accordingly. Renal exploration with wedge resection or alternatively other minimally invasive ablative therapies can be strongly considered for all such clinically evident lesions, after appropriate consideration of patient age, comorbidity, and other relevant factors (Novick and Campbell, 2002).

Another problematic area can be found when these lesions are discovered during organ retrieval for transplantation. A case of renal cortical adenoma in a kidney harvested from a live donor has been reported (Jones et al., 2003). In this case the kidney was not transplanted as the risk of malignant transformation with immunosuppression could not be adequately determined and the donor elected not to have the kidney reimplanted. When faced with a similar situation during a live

TABLE 10g-2. Immunostaining features of renal adenomas.

	Epithelial membrane antigen	Cytokeratin 7
Papillary adenoma	Positive	Positive
Metanephric adenoma	Negative	Negative/focally positive
Oncocytoma	Positive	Negative

Source: Liu et al. (2002).

or cadaveric transplant, a full and frank discussion should take place between the recipient, pathologist, transplant surgeon, and nephrologist. The theoretical risk of potential malignancy should be weighed against the status of access for renal support available to the patient, the life expectancy of the recipient, the quality of life posttransplant, and the scarcity of supply of organs for transplantation.

Metanephric Adenoma

Metanephric adenoma (MA) is a recently recognized rare tumor of the kidney with a propensity for a benign clinical outcome. Over 80 well-documented cases have been reported (Pins et al., 1999). An MA originates from the distal tubules, is generally less than 1 cm in dimension, and is located in the renal cortex (Longoni et al., 2004). It is commonly encountered in middle-aged women and has a female-to-male ratio of 2:1. The etiology is unknown, but associations with smoking, tubular nephrosclerosis, and dialysis have been postulated. Although commonly an incidental finding, this lesion may present as a palpable mass or with hematuria or loin pain. An interesting association is seen with polycythemia, which resolves after surgical excision of the lesion.

Pathology

The cut surface of the tumor displays a tan to gray or yellow color, and tumors generally form well-circumscribed masses. Calcification, cysts, hemorrhage, and necrosis have been described. Microscopically, these tumors are composed of small epithelial cells that form small acini, and within the tumor these acini are tightly packed with scant intervening stroma. The cells have very scanty pale pink cytoplasm with regular nuclei and may occasionally show indentation and overlapping glomeruloid bodies, which are composed of lobulated papillary projections (Davis et al., 1995). The category of metanephric tumors has recently become broadened to include metanephric adenomas, adenofibromas, and stromal tumors, and it appears to comprise a continuous histological spectrum (Kuroda et al., 2003b).

Previously these tumors have been incorrectly designated as Wilms' tumor, nephroblastomatosis, or an unusual tubular carcinoma of the kidney. However, immunohistochemistry using immunostains such as keratin AE1, cytokeratin (CK) 7, CD56, CD57, and WT1 can help to differentiate RCC from Wilms' tumor and MA. Muir et al. (2001) demonstrated that MA was strongly and diffusely positive for CD57 and WT1 and was focally positive for CK7 and keratin AE1, whereas papillary RCC was negative for CD57 and WT1 but showed strong staining for CK7 and keratin AE1. These immunohistochemical features indicate that MA and RCC are not closely related entities. The staining patterns of both MA and Wilms' tumor reflect developing nephrons, with positive expression of CD56, CD57, and WT1, supporting the belief that they are closely related.

Diagnosis

Distinctive imaging characteristics to confidently diagnose this entity do not exist. MA shows up as a hyperechoic lesion on an ultrasound scan and calcification has been seen in such lesions. On computerized tomography (CT) the lesion has higher attenuation than the adjacent normal renal parenchyma and enhances with contrast injection. The CT and ultrasound findings correlate with the pathological features of a high nuclear-to-cytoplasmic ratio and psammomatous calcifications (Chaudhary et al., 2004; Fielding et al., 1999).

The ability to make a preoperative diagnosis of this condition by biopsy or aspiration cytology is appealing. The aspirates are cellular and are composed of many small-to-large tightly packed clusters of cells and short papillae. Occasional tubules, rosettes, and glomeruloid-like structures are seen. Cells show scanty cytoplasm; small, oval-to-round nuclei, and minute or absent nucleoli. Atypia, pleomorphism, necrosis, and mitosis are absent (Granter et al., 1997).

Management

Apart from isolated case reports in children (Drut et al., 2001; Renshaw et al., 2000), a uniformly benign clinical course has been associated with metanephric adenoma. However, given its relatively recent identification, rarity, and the lack of clinical, radiographic, or cytological means to establish a definite diagnosis, metanephric adenoma must remain primarily a pathological diagnosis. Treatment should be consistent with managing a similar malignant renal neoplasm.

Oncocytoma

Renal oncocytoma (RO) is a benign tumor affecting the kidney. It can also occur in other endocrine organs, e.g., adrenal, thyroid, parathyroid, and salivary glands. An estimated 3–7% of renal tumors are oncocytomas, which are thought to arise from the intercalated cells of the collecting duct (Storkel, 1993). The age at presentation and male preponderance are similar to that of RCC, with a mean age at presentation of 65 years and male-to-female ratio of 2–2.5:1. The majority of the tumors, ranging from 58% to 83%, are asymptomatic and the remainder present with loin pain or bleeding. Most tumors are unifocal, but 2–12% are multifocal and 4–12% are bilateral (Tickoo et al., 1999). It may be inherited in some families (Weirich et al., 1998).

Pathology

Grossly, the tumors are well circumscribed but not truly encapsulated. The cut surface of the tumor is characteristically mahogany brown or dark red in color, and larger tumors tend to have the characteristic central stellate scar that is seen in 33–80% of the cases. Necrosis, a feature commonly

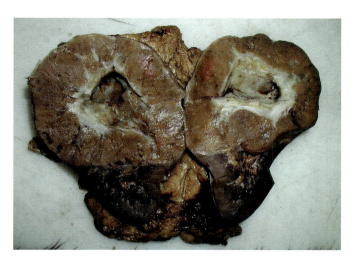

FIGURE 10g-1. Cut section of renal oncocytoma showing a stellate-shaped scar.

noticed in RCC, is not seen, but hemorrhage can occasionally be found (Fig. 10g-1).

Histologically, these tumors contain a finely granular cytoplasm with an edematous, myxomatous, or hyalinized stroma within a nested, tubulocystic, solid, or trabecular pattern (Kuroda et al., 2003a). Uniformity in cellular size and color, a round to polygonal shape, and abundant fine granular cytoplasm are consistent characteristic findings (Figs. 10g-2 and 10g-3). Ultrastructurally, these tumor cells are packed with abundant mitochondria, which account for an intensely eosinophilic cytoplasm on light microscopy. Most oncocytomas are cytologically low grade; however, prominent nucleoli are not uncommon, and conspicuous pleomorphism or cellular atypia has been reported in 12–30% of cases and is generally accepted within the diagnosis of renal oncocytoma if all other diagnostic criteria are met (Amin et al., 1997).

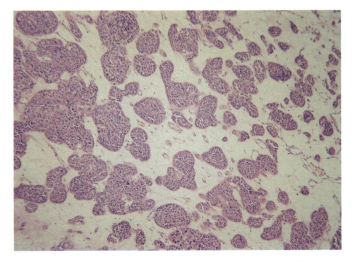

FIGURE 10g-2. Renal oncocytoma ×200: cluster of cells in an edematous stroma.

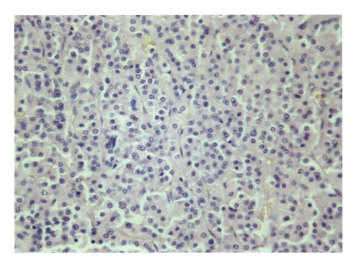

FIGURE 10g-3. Renal oncocytoma ×400: cells with abundant eosinophilic cytoplasm forming occasional tubules.

presence of numerous microvesicles in the cytoplasm is typical for a chromophobe RCC. Several findings suggest the existence of a close relationship between chromophobe RCC and RO. Both tumors share a phenotype of intercalated cells of the collecting duct system and mitochondrial DNA alterations. A few cases of coexistent oncocytoma and chromophobe RCC have been described, designated as renal oncocytosis. In addition, oncocytic variants of chromophobe RCCs with ultrastructural features similar to those of RO have been reported. The existence of a chromophobe adenoma, which is the benign counterpart of chromophobe RCC and which shows loss of chromosomes Y and 1, has recently been suggested. Although almost all ROs behave in a benign fashion, some cases that caused metastasis or resulted in death have also been described and, therefore, further studies are needed to resolve these problems and also to elucidate the genetic mechanisms responsible for the occurrence of RO (Kuroda et al., 2003a).

A small cell variant of oncocytoma has been described that can be confused with a malignant tumor (Hes et al., 2001). The malignant characteristics of lymphovascular invasion, perinephric extension, and necrosis are rarely seen and their impact on patient prognosis is inconclusive. Such tumors are best considered "atypical oncocytomas" (Chao et al., 2002).

Oncocytoma versus Chromophobe Renal Cell Carcinoma

The histological separation of RO from chromophobe RCC is of great importance prognostically (Table 10g-3). On electron microscopy, the most striking feature in RO is the diffuse distribution of round and uniform mitochondria, with a scarcity of all other cytoplasmic organelles, whereas the

Diagnosis

There are no unique clinical or radiological features that can confidently differentiate an RO from an RCC. The following radiological findings favor a diagnosis of RO:

- A homogeneous tumor with or without a central stellate scar on CT (Levine and Huntrakoon, 1983).
- A "spoke-wheel" appearance of tumor arterioles, the "lucent rim sign" of the capsule, and a homogeneous capillary nephrogram phase on angiography (Weiner and Bernstein, 1977).
- Increased uptake on technetium-99m sestamibi images (Gormley et al., 1996).
- A well-defined capsule, central stellate scar, and distinctive intensities on T1 and T2 images of magnetic resonance imaging (MRI) (Harmon et al., 1996).

TABLE 10g-3. Differentiating features of oncocytoma and chromophobe renal cell carcinoma (RCC).

	Oncocytoma	Chromophobe RCC
Necrosis/hemorrhage	Rare	Common
Stellate scar	Common	Rare
Architecture	Tubulocystic, organoid or mixed	Sheets of cells aligned along fibrovascular septae
Cell type	Single cell type showing abundant granular, eosinophilic cytoplasm	Two cell types showing clear reticular cytoplasm and granular, eosinophilic cytoplasm
Multiple nuclei	Rare	Common
Nuclei	Round and uniform	Wrinkled "raisinoid" nuclei
Mitochondria	Abundant	Variable
Microvesicles	Focal collections	Abundant
Hale's colloidal iron stain	Focal positivity	Diffuse positivity
Kidney specific cadherin	Negative	Positive
Cytokeratin 7	Negative or weak focal staining	Strong cytoplasmic staining
Cathepsin H	Strong cytoplasmic staining	Negative or weak focal staining

Sources: Chao et al. (2002), Cochand-Priollet et al. (1997), Mazal et al. (2005), Tickoo and Amin (1988), Skinnider and Jones (1999), and Tickoo et al. (2000).

Davidson et al. (1993) used the CT criteria of homogeneity alone or with the presence of a centrally located stellate area of low attenuation to distinguish RO from RCC. Overall, 67% of ROs were given readings that were consistent with the correct diagnosis. More importantly, however, 42% of adenocarcinomas less than 3 cm and 16% of tumors larger than 3 cm were also read as ROs. Their study concluded that the CT findings alone lacked sufficient predictive value to distinguish benign from malignant tumors. A "spoke-wheel" pattern has been described on dual-phase helical CT (Bandhu et al., 2003) and in patients with poor renal function magnetic resonance imaging (MRI) is a useful imaging modality. A low-intensity homogeneous mass on the T1-weighted images, which appears as increased intensity on T2 images, the presence of a capsule, central scar, or stellate pattern, and the absence of either hemorrhage or necrosis are features to suggest an oncocytoma. The optimal MRI to evaluate renal masses should include T1-weighted spin echo images and without gadolinium, T2-weighted images, and gradient recalled echo images (Harmon et al., 1996).

The role of fine needle aspiration cytology in the preoperative diagnosis of renal oncocytoma is still debated. Although most tumors demonstrate the classic cytological features, a specific diagnosis using conventional smears or even core biopsies can be difficult. Cytological morphology combined with ancillary studies, including immunostaining with cytokeratin and vimentin antibodies, and Hale's colloidal iron stain may be necessary to differentiate renal oncocytoma from renal cell carcinoma. In difficult cases electron microscopy can provide additional information for diagnostic confirmation (Liu and Fanning, 2001).

Management

Given the uncertainty of a definitive preoperative clinical or radiological diagnosis, the management of an individual case should be aggressive and follow the general oncological principles of managing an RCC. The coexistence of RCC and RO is not uncommon and is seen in 10–32% of patients with RO (Licht et al., 1993). If RO is suspected then nephron-sparing surgery is desirable if the tumor size and location are amenable.

Angiomyolipoma

Angiomyolipoma (AML) is a relatively common polymorphic neoplasm affecting the kidney; it was first identified by Fisher in 1911 and was designated AML by Morgan in 1951. These lesions have also been described in other viscera. They consist of mature adipose tissue, smooth muscle, and thick-walled vessels in varying proportions. Often commonly described as a hamartoma, meaning the abnormal proliferation of tissues that are normally present in the organ, it has been argued that AML is actually a choristoma since fat and smooth muscle are not normal kidney components (Dickinson et al., 1998). In a renal ultrasound series carried out on 17,941 healthy adults without any signs of urinary tract malignancy, the prevalence of angiomyolipoma was 0.13%, which was similar to that of renal cell carcinoma (Fujii et al., 1995). Approximately 20% of AMLs are found in patients with tuberous sclerosis syndrome (TS), an autosomal-dominant disorder characterized by mental retardation, epilepsy, and adenoma sebaceum, a distinctive skin lesion. Penetrance for each of these traits is far from complete, and only approximately 50% of patients with TS develop AMLs (Eble, 1998). The differentiating features of TS associated and sporadic AML are listed in Table 10g-4. In patients with TS, AML is often accompanied by cysts and occasionally by RCC.

In non-TS patients, a study of 48 cases of AML revealed an average age at diagnosis of 50 years with 94% of cases seen in women (Steiner et al., 1993). They are rarely diagnosed before puberty in patients without tuberous sclerosis. Larger lesions are more common in women than in men and they occasionally grow rapidly during pregnancy. These features suggest that hormones may play a role in stimulating the growth of AML (Eble, 1998), and the presence of estrogen and progesterone receptors or both in more than 25% of the tumors has been found (L'Hostis et al., 1999).

Pathology

Renal AML is a benign tumor histologically characterized by the proliferation of spindle, epithelioid, and adipose cells in concert with many thick-walled blood vessels (Figs. 10g-4

TABLE 10g-4. Features of TS-associated and sporadic AML.[a]

	TS-associated AML	Sporadic AML
Distribution	20%	80%
Mean age at presentation	30 years	Fifth or sixth decade
Female to male predominance	2 to 1	More pronounced
Multiple tumors	97%	13%
Accelerated growth	Common	Uncommon
Acute hemorrhage	44%	14%
Mean growth rate/year	20%	5%

Sources: Novick and Campbell (2002) and Nelson and Sanda (2002).
[a]TS, tuberous sclerosis; AML, angiomyolipoma.

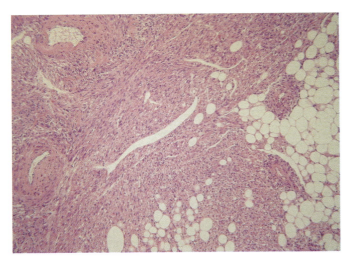

FIGURE 10g-4. Cut section of renal angiomyolipoma with hemorrhage.

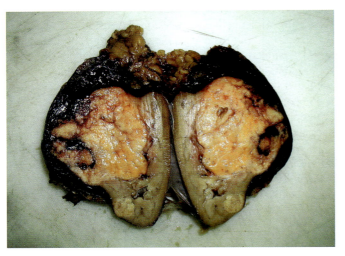

FIGURE 10g-5. Angiomyolipoma ×400: smooth muscle, thick-walled blood vessels, and fat are intermingled.

and 10g-5). HMB-45 immunoreactivity, a marker of ultrastructural striated organelles that closely resemble premelanosomes, aids the diagnosis of AML. The immunophenotypic and ultrastructural profiles of renal AML based on the phenotypic cell type (epithelioid, spindle, and adipocytic cell) support a common cell line (Stone et al., 2001). Perivascular epithelioid cells have been proposed as the commonest progenitor cells in renal AML. The triphasic distribution of tissue elements is altered in the epithelioid variant of AML, which is predominantly composed of myogenic elements (Cho et al., 2004). Rarely AML may mimic a liposarcoma, leiomyoma, or lymphangiomyoma. Though AMLs are benign lesions, rarely extension of the tumor along the vein and lymph node involvement are indicative of more aggressive behavior (Cittadini et al., 1996). This is more commonly documented with large central tumors. Many cases of

inferior vena caval involvement have been described (Islam et al., 2004), but few cases of malignant transformation with metastases have been reported (Takahashi et al., 2003). Fifteen cases of AML associated with RO have been reported with or without associated tuberous sclerosis complex (Blute et al., 1988; Pillay et al., 2003).

Diagnosis

AML is commonly an incidental finding on ultrasound. Rarely the classic triad of clinical presentation of flank pain, palpable tender mass, and gross hematuria is seen, but other features include nausea, vomiting, fever, hypertension, anemia, renal failure, and hemorrhage-induced hypotension (Nelson and Sanda, 2002). After RCC, AML is the second commonest renal cause of retroperitoneal hemorrhage. If AML is detected incidentally on imaging the possibility of an undiagnosed or subclinical TS complex should also be considered and the necessary investigations and appropriate referral initiated.

AML is the most hyperechoic renal neoplasm on ultrasound (US), due to a combination of factors including high fat content, multiple tissue interfaces, and extensive vascular tissue (Lemaitre et al., 1997). Since 8–47% of small RCCs can also be hyperechoic, a CT scan is essential in the initial diagnosis of AML (Fig. 10g-6). Detecting the existence of fat in a renal lesion on CT is diagnostic of AML and is the only radiological feature that can help differentiate AML from RCC (Bosniak et al., 1988). Measuring single voxel values in the hypoattenuating areas on nonenhanced thin sections (3 or 1.5 mm) is essential for the CT diagnosis of small (<1.0 cm) renal AML (Kurosaki et al., 1993). Tissue attenuation of less than −10 HU before contrast administration is consistent with fat. The presence of discrete contrast-enhancing lesions

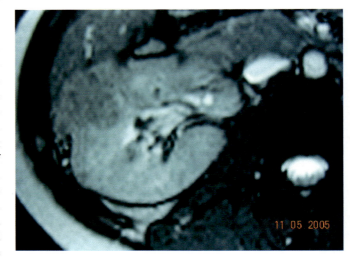

FIGURE 10g-6. CT scan showing enhancing hypoechoic lesion— AML.

within an enlarging AML may mimic malignancy (Vander-Brink et al., 2004). A few cases of RCC containing fat density have also shown calcification, which has never been reported within an AML (Lemaitre et al., 1997).

On MRI, the fat component of an angiomyolipoma shows a high signal intensity on unenhanced T1-weighted images and lower intensity on T2-weighted images, while it is generally isointense relative to retroperitoneal fat. Fat suppression techniques can sometimes be particularly helpful to differentiate RCC since RCC usually has a low signal intensity on T1 and high intensity on T2. Similarly, MRI can differentiate angiomyolipoma from RCC (Uhlenbrock et al., 1988); it is particularly useful when the CT results are inconclusive or for evaluation during pregnancy.

Angiography has no role in the primary diagnosis of AML. The role of fine needle aspiration cytology in the diagnosis of AML is limited; based on radiological and cytological criteria, AML can be mistaken for RCC or liposarcoma (Crapanzano, 2005). Immunocytochemical analysis of the aspirate with HMB-45, a marker of perivascular epithelioid cells, may increase the accuracy of diagnosis of AML (Bonzanini et al., 1994).

Complications

Complications of AML are rare but often severe depending on the size and content of the lesion. Some of the following complications can be diagnosed on CT scan:

- Compression of the pyelocalyceal system
- Intralesional bleeding
- Extralesional bleeding resulting in significant subcapsular, perirenal, pararenal, intrarenal, or parapelvic hematoma
- Cystic degeneration (Antonopoulos et al., 1996)

Some patients, especially those with tubercus sclerosis complex and multiple AML, can present with renal insufficiency or failure. Renal insufficiency can be a result of compression and/or replacement of normal parenchyma by the tumor.

Treatment

The natural history of renal AML is not well described. The basis for management is renal preservation (Khaitan et al., 2001). Current management options include careful surveillance, selective embolization of the tumor, nephron-sparing surgery, and total nephrectomy. Tumors less than 4 cm tend to be asymptomatic and generally do not require intervention, whereas tumors over 8 cm are responsible for significant morbidity and generally require treatment. Tumors of intermediate size are less predictable (Dickinson et al., 1998).

Patients with small, asymptomatic renal AML can be kept under close surveillance (Kennelly et al., 1994), and individuals who choose such conservative management

should probably avoid contact sporting activities where flank or abdominal impact is a possibility (Bardot and Montie, 1992). In a prospective study of 26 patients with renal AML, verified by CT, follow-up by sonographic monitoring was sufficient as long as the sonostructure remained unchanged (Hobarth et al., 1993).

Selective embolization of AML is an accepted intervention in patients presenting acutely with bleeding or considered to have features of increased risk of hemorrhage (Figs. 10g-7 and 10g-8). The principal advantages of selective embolization for angiomyolipoma include the preservation of functional renal parenchyma, the ability to embolize bleeding vessels selectively, and circumvention of the need for a surgical incision or anesthesia. Various materials have been used for embolization, including absorbable gelatin sponge, absolute alcohol, iodized oil, polyvinyl alcohol particles,

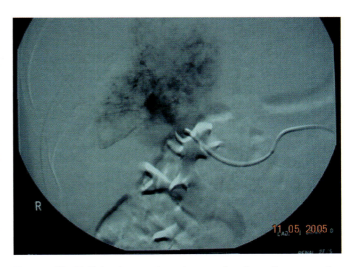

FIGURE 10g-7. Selective renal angiogram showing a hypervascular lesion with microaneurysms consistent with angiomyolipoma.

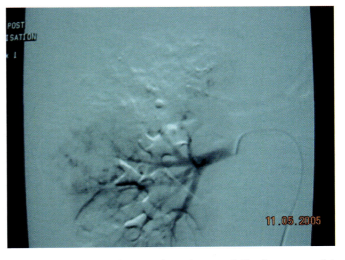

FIGURE 10g-8. Selective renal angiogram following successful embolization.

and metal coils (Lee et al., 1998). Of patients undergoing selective renal embolization 85% may develop postembolization syndrome characterized by fever and flank pain (Nelson and Sanda, 2002). This inflammatory response can be debilitating. Treatment with a short-term (2 weeks) tapering dose of prednisolone has been successful in reducing the effects of postembolization syndrome (Bissler et al., 2002). In a retrospective review, embolization was technically successful in all 30 lesions found in 19 patients. During a mean follow-up of over 4 years, recurrence was noted in 30% of lesions, all associated with TS complex, and the median time from embolization to recurrence was over 6 years (Kothary et al., 2005).

If surgical intervention is warranted, nephron-sparing surgery can be performed with a high success rate in renal AML. Long-term follow-up studies reveal no local tumor recurrences and stable renal function even in patients with solitary kidneys (Heidenreich et al., 2002). Open or laparoscopic nephrectomy can be considered for those cases in which there has been extensive renal replacement by the AML, or when nephron-sparing surgery is not feasible either due to the location or the size of the AML lesion, or if malignancy is suspected in a large lesion, or when there is failure to control hemorrhage by embolization techniques (Nelson and Sanda, 2002).

Follow-up

Evidence-based data from prospective studies to guide follow-up are lacking and there is a need to develop a clear surveillance strategy to aid early detection of lesions with the potential for complications. This includes the appropriate frequency of surveillance for patients in different age groups and at different stages of AML development, based on the growing knowledge of the natural history of this condition. A CT or MRI may be required for early detection of a large aneurysm within the tumor, which may be missed on ultrasound (Simmons et al., 2003). Lesions below 4 cm can be followed up with ultrasound annually and larger lesions may need CT or MRI every 6–12 months depending on the rate of growth.

Multilocular Cystic Nephroma

Multilocular cystic nephroma (MCN) is a rare benign tumor of the kidney grouped among the cystic nongenetic disorders (Morga Egea et al., 2004). Metastasis or local recurrence has not been reported in such cases (Gonzalez-Crussi et al., 1982) and the age distribution is bimodal, with presentation occurring usually in the first 2 to 3 years of life and again in the fourth and fifth decade (Upadhyay and Neely, 1989). Male children are more commonly affected, whereas in adults there is female predominance. Children tend to present with an asymptomatic abdominal mass detected

on routine physical examination, whereas adults tend to be symptomatic with abdominal pain, hematuria, urinary tract infection, or hypertension (Madewell et al., 1983). Most cases of MCN are nonfamilial, unilateral, and unifocal. Tumor growth is unpredictable, varying from months to years.

Pathology

MCN is a segmental purely cystic mass characterized by multiple septations composed entirely of differentiated tissues without blastemal elements (Agrons et al., 1995). Grossly these lesions are well circumscribed, encapsulated, and most often centrally located (Fig. 10g-9). Microscopically, the cysts are lined with cuboidal epithelial cells arranged in a hobnail pattern, and the intervening stroma is characteristic for its pronounced cellularity (Figs. 10g-10 and 10g-11) (Novick and Campbell, 2002).

Diagnosis

MCN usually presents with clinical and radiological features indistinguishable from a malignant renal neoplasia. Certain distinctive radiological features have been described that may help in determining a possible diagnosis of MCN, e.g., a mass on plain radiography may show a curvilinear calcification in 10–20% of cases. Intravenous urography and retrograde pyelography are helpful when renal pelvic herniation of the tumor is recognized and CT scanning shows a multilocular, septated centrally situated mass (Madewell et al., 1983). All MCN by definition will fall into Bosniak's class III classification (Bosniak, 1986). Avascular or hypovascular lesions are commonly seen on angiography, but hypervascular lesions have also been described. Enhancement within the septa on CT or MRI is not uncommon.

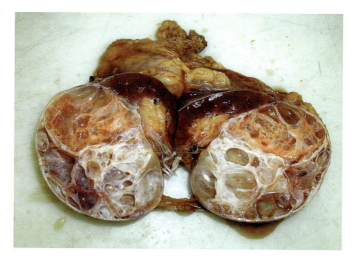

FIGURE 10g-9. Multilocular cystic nephroma: cysts have a smooth inner surface and contain clear yellow fluid.

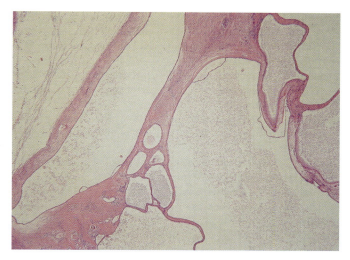

FIGURE 10g-10. Multilocular cystic nephroma: cysts are separated by fibrous septae.

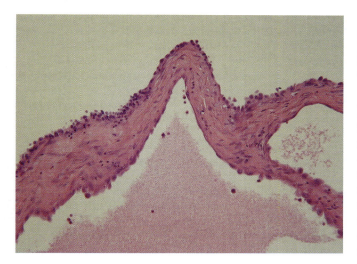

FIGURE 10g-11. Multilocular cystic nephroma: the septae are lined with flat/cuboidal pithelium arranged in a hobnail pattern.

There is insufficient information concerning the accuracy of percutaneous biopsy to make a definitive decision for management of most of these lesions (Hartman et al., 1987).

In children the differential diagnosis includes other pediatric cystic renal masses that may require different treatment stratagems:

- Wilms' tumor with cyst formation
- Cystic clear cell sarcoma
- Cystic mesoblastic nephroma
- Cystic RCC
- Multicystic dysplastic kidney
- Segmental multicystic dysplasia in a duplicated renal collecting system (Agrons et al., 1995)

Management

MCN may radiologically mimic a cystic Wilms' tumor or cystic RCC mandating a nephrectomy or a nephron-sparing surgery (Gonzalez-Crussi et al., 1982; Castillo et al., 1991). If the preoperative clinical suspicion is strong, an intraoperative frozen section diagnosis may help avoid radical surgery (Morga Egea et al., 2004).

Miscellaneous Benign Tumors

Many other rare benign tumors arising from various mesenchymal derivatives within the kidney and its environs have been described, mainly as case reports. These tumors include leiomyoma (Di Palma and Giardini, 1988), solitary fibrous tumor (Gelb et al., 1996; Magro et al., 2002), benign fibrous histiocytoma, hemangiopericytoma, and benign peripheral nerve sheath tumors (Magro et al., 2002), lipoma etc.

Role of Radiological Studies in the Diagnosis of Benign Renal Tumors

RO and AML have certain radiological characteristics favoring their diagnosis. A tumor that contains fat, as determined with CT or MRI, can be confidently diagnosed as AML without further diagnostic intervention (Davidson et al., 1997). A diagnosis of RO only by radiological means is less certain; in a retrospective review of MRI in a case series, specific criteria for the different types of benign and small malignant tumors were identified (Dombrovskii, 2001). Spiral CT can show many of the key imaging features of small renal masses used to distinguish between benign and malignant lesions. However, despite the theoretical benefits of volumetric CT, some lesions remain indeterminate and require surgical removal for a definitive diagnosis (Silverman et al., 1994).

Role of Biopsy in the Diagnosis of Benign Renal Tumors

Recent easy access and improvements in renal imaging techniques have resulted in an increase in the diagnosis of incidental small renal lesions. A preoperative diagnosis in such cases mandates fine needle aspiration cytology or needle biopsy. However, about 15% of the samples are deemed unsatisfactory for diagnostic purposes (Truong et al., 1999), although in a recent report of 54 percutaneous core biopsies, sufficient material for analysis was available in all samples (Jaff et al., 2004). Core biopsies using 18-gauge needles would be more reliably diagnostic than 20-gauge needles (Johnson et al., 2001). Concurrence of needle biopsy with final histopathology is about 85% (Hara et al., 2001), although 100% accuracy has been claimed (Caoili et al., 2002). Renal fine needle aspiration can provide an accurate diagnosis in most instances but has limitations and pitfalls. Low-grade RCC has to be differentiated from oncocytoma, angiomyolipoma, renal infarct, and reactive conditions. A sensitivity, specificity, positive predictive value, and negative predictive value of 92.5%, 91.9%, 89.9%, and 94.0%, respectively, have been shown (Zardawi, 1999). A high negative predictive value is useful in reassuring patients with a radiological and cytological benign lesion. However, a negative fine needle aspiration does not exclude malignancy in the presence of radiological suspicion.

Needle biopsy is not widely undertaken for diagnosing renal masses for three primary reasons:

- Tumor spread due to needle tract seeding has been reported after percutaneous 18-gauge needle biopsy of the renal lesion (Gibbons et al., 1977; Slywotzky and Maya, 1994).
- Concern has been raised regarding complications such as hemorrhage after needle biopsy.
- Most importantly, biopsy results often do not affect the subsequent management of renal masses, including angiomyolipoma, since a negative biopsy does not exclude the possibility of malignancy.

References

Agrons, G. A., B. J. Wagner,et al. (1995). Multilocular cystic renal tumor in children: radiologic-pathologic correlation. *Radiographics* **15**(3): 653–669.

Amin, M. B., T. B. Crotty, et al. (1997). Renal oncocytoma: a reappraisal of morphologic features with clinicopathologic findings in 80 cases. *Am J Surg Pathol* **21**(1): 1–12.

Antonopoulos, P., C. Drossos, et al. (1996). Complications of renal angiomyolipomas: CT evaluation. *Abdom Imaging* **21**(4): 357–360.

Bandhu, S., S. Mukhopadhyaya, et al. (2003). Spoke-wheel pattern in renal oncocytoma seen on double-phase helical CT. *Australas Radiol* **47**(3): 298–301.

Bardot, S. E. and J. Montie. (1992). Renal angiomyolipoma: current concepts of diagnosis and management. *AUA Update Series* **11**(39): 306–311.

Bissler, J. J., J. Racadio, et al. (2002). Reduction of postembolization syndrome after ablation of renal angiomyolipoma. *Am J Kidney Dis* **39**(5): 966–971.

Blute, M. L., R. S. Malek, et al. (1988). Angiomyolipoma: clinical metamorphosis and concepts for management. *J Urol* **139**(1): 20–24.

Bonzanini, M., M. Pea, et al. (1994). Preoperative diagnosis of renal angiomyolipoma: fine needle aspiration cytology and immunocytochemical characterization. *Pathology* **26**(2): 170–175.

Bosniak, M. A. (1986). The current radiological approach to renal cysts. *Radiology* **158**(1): 1–10.

Bosniak, M. A., A. J. Megibow, et al. (1988). CT diagnosis of renal angiomyolipoma: the importance of detecting small amounts of fat. *AJR Am J Roentgenol* **151**(3):497–501.

Brunelli, M., J. N. Eble, et al. (2003). Metanephric adenoma lacks the gains of chromosomes 7 and 17 and loss of Y that are typical of papillary renal cell carcinoma and papillary adenoma. *Mod Pathol* **16**(10): 1060–1083.

Caoili, E. M., R. O. Bude, et al. (2002). Evaluation of sonographically guided percutaneous core biopsy of renal masses. *AJR Am J Roentgenol* **179**(2): 373–378.

Castillo, O. A., E. T. Boyle, Jr., et al. (1991). Multilocular cysts of kidney. A study of 29 patients and review of literature. *Urology* **37**(2): 156–162.

Chao, D. H., A. Zisman, et al. (2002). Changing concepts in the management of renal oncocytoma. *Urology* **59**(5): 635–642.

Chaudhary, H., M. Raghvendran, et al. (2004). Correlation of radiological and clinical features of metanephric neoplasms in adults. *Indian J Cancer* **41**(1): 37–40.

Cho, N. H., H. S. Shim, et al. (2004). Estrogen receptor is significantly associated with the epithelioid variants of renal angiomyolipoma: a clinicopathological and immunohistochemical study of 67 cases. *Pathol Int* **54**(7): 510–515.

Cittadini, G., Jr., F. Pozzi Mucelli, et al. (1996). Aggressive renal angiomyolipoma. *Acta Radiol* **37**(6): 927–932.

Cochand-Priollet, B., V. Molinie, et al. (1997). Renal chromophobe cell carcinoma and oncocytoma. A comparative morphologic, histochemical, and immunohistochemical study of 124 cases. *Arch Pathol Lab Med* **121**(10): 1081–1086.

Crapanzano, J. P. (2005). Fine-needle aspiration of renal angiomyolipoma: cytological findings and diagnostic pitfalls in a series of five cases. *Diagn Cytopathol* **32**(1): 53–57.

Davidson, A. J., W. S. Hayes, et al. (1993). Renal oncocytoma and carcinoma: failure of differentiation with CT. *Radiology* **186**(3): 693–696.

Davidson, A. J., D. S. Hartman, et al. (1997). Radiologic assessment of renal masses: implications for patient care. *Radiology* **202**(2): 297–305.

Davis, C. J., Jr., J. H. Barton, et al. (1995). Metanephric adenoma. Clinicopathological study of fifty patients. *Am J Surg Pathol* **19**(10): 1101–1114.

Denton, M. D., C. C. Magee, et al. (2002). Prevalence of renal cell carcinoma in patients with ESRD pre-transplantation: a pathologic analysis. *Kidney Int* **61**(6): 2201–2209.

Dickinson, M., H. Ruckle, et al. (1998). Renal angiomyolipoma: optimal treatment based on size and symptoms. *Clin Nephrol* **49**(5): 281–286.

Di Palma, S. and R. Giardini. (1988). Leiomyoma of the kidney. *Tumori* **74**(4): 489–493.

Dombrovskii, V. I. (2001). [Magnetic resonance imaging in the diagnosis of benign renal parenchymal epithelial tumors: MRI–-pathomorphological comparison]. *Vestn Rentgenol Radiol* (3): 42–50.

Drut, R., R. M. Drut, et al. (2001). Metastatic metanephric adenoma with foci of papillary carcinoma in a child: a combined histologic, immunohistochemical, and FISH study. *Int J Surg Pathol* **9**(3): 241–247.

Eble, J. N. (1998). Angiomyolipoma of kidney. *Semin Diagn Pathol* **15**(1): 21–40.

Faria, V., M. Reis, et al. (1994). Renal adenoma: identification of two histologic types. *Eur Urol* **26**(2): 170–175.

Fielding, J. R., A. Visweswaran, et al. (1999). CT and ultrasound features of metanephric adenoma in adults with pathologic correlation. *J Comput Assist Tomogr* **23**(3): 441–444.

Fujii, Y., J. Ajima, et al. (1995). Benign renal tumors detected among healthy adults by abdominal ultrasonography. *Eur Urol* **27**(2): 124–127.

Ganzen, T. N., S. M. Sekamova, et al. (1991). [Kidney adenoma]. *Arkh Patol* **53**(7): 48–55.

Gelb, A. B., M. L. Simmons, et al. (1996). Solitary fibrous tumor involving the renal capsule. *Am J Surg Pathol* **20**(10): 1288–1295.

Gibbons, R. P., W. H. Bush, Jr., et al. (1977). Needle tract seeding following aspiration of renal cell carcinoma. *J Urol* **118**(5): 865–867.

Gonzalez-Crussi, F., J. M. Kidd, et al. (1982). Cystic nephroma: morphologic spectrum and implications. *Urology* **20**(1): 88–93.

Gormley, T. S., M. J. Van Every, et al. (1996). Renal oncocytoma: preoperative diagnosis using technetium 99m sestamibi imaging. *Urology* **48**(1): 33–39.

Granter, S. R., J. A. Fletcher, et al. (1997). Cytologic and cytogenetic analysis of metanephric adenoma of the kidney: a report of two cases. *Am J Clin Pathol* **108**(5): 544–549.

Grignon, D. J. and J. N. Eble. (1998). Papillary and metanephric adenomas of the kidney. *Semin Diagn Pathol* **15**(1): 41–53.

Hara, I., H. Miyake, et al. (2001). Role of percutaneous image-guided biopsy in the evaluation of renal masses. *Urol Int* **67**(3): 199–202.

Harmon, W. J., B. F. King, et al. (1996). Renal oncocytoma: magnetic resonance imaging characteristics. *J Urol* **155**(3): 863–867.

Hartman, D. S., C. J. Davis, et al. (1987). The multiloculated renal mass: considerations and differential features. *Radiographics* **7**(1): 29–52.

Hashine, K., Y. Sumiyoshi, et al. (1996). [A morphological study of renal adenoma and latent renal cell carcinoma in autopsy cases]. *Nippon Hinyokika Gakkai Zasshi* **87**(3): 667–675.

Heidenreich, A., A. Hegele, et al. (2002). Nephron-sparing surgery for renal angiomyolipoma. *Eur Urol* **41**(3): 267–273.

Hes, O., M. Michal, et al. (2001). Small cell variant of renal oncocytoma—a rare and misleading type of benign renal tumor. *Int J Surg Pathol* **9**(3): 215–222.

Hobarth, K., H. C. Klingler, et al. (1993). Value of routine sonography in the diagnosis and conservative management of renal angiomyolipoma. *Eur Urol* **24**(2): 239–243.

Holm-Nielsen, P. and T. S. Olsen. (1988). Ultrastructure of renal adenoma. *Ultrastruct Pathol* **12**(1): 27–39.

Islam, A. H., T. Ehara, et al. (2004). Angiomyolipoma of kidney involving the inferior vena cava. *Int J Urol* **11**(10): 897–902.

Jaff, A., V. Molinie, et al. (2004). Evaluation of imaging-guided fine-needle percutaneous biopsy of renal masses. *Eur Radiol* 12(3) : 53–56.

Johnson, P. T., L. N. Nazarian, et al. (2001). Sonographically guided renal mass biopsy: indications and efficacy. *J Ultrasound Med* **20**(7): 749–753.

Jones, J. R., K. J. Woodside, et al. (2003). Renal cortical adenoma incidentally found during living donor nephrectomy. *Prog Transplant* **13**(2): 94–96.

Kennelly, M. J., H. B. Grossman, et al. (1994). Outcome analysis of 42 cases of renal angiomyolipoma. *J Urol* **152**(6 Pt 1): 1988–1991.

Khaitan, A., A. K. Hemal, et al. (2001). Management of renal angiomyolipoma in complex clinical situations. *Urol Int* **67**(1): 28–33.

Kiyoshima, K., Y. Oda, et al. (2004). Multicentric papillary renal cell carcinoma associated with renal adenomatosis. *Pathol Int* **54**(4): 266–272.

Kothary, N., M. C. Soulen, et al. (2005). Renal angiomyolipoma: long-term results after arterial embolization. *J Vasc Interv Radiol* **16**(1): 45–50.

Kuroda, N., M. Toi, et al. (2003a). Review of renal oncocytoma with focus on clinical and pathobiological aspects. *Histol Histopathol* **18**(3): 935–942.

Kuroda, N., M. Tol, et al. (2003b). Review of metanephric adenoma of the kidney with focus on clinical and pathobiological aspects. *Histol Histopathol* **18**(1): 253–257.

Kurosaki, Y., Y. Tanaka, et al. (1993). Improved CT fat detection in small kidney angiomyolipomas using thin sections and single voxel measurements. *J Comput Assist Tomogr* **17**(5): 745–748.

L'Hostis, H., C. Deminiere, et al. (1999). Renal angiomyolipoma: a clinicopathologic, immunohistochemical, and follow-up study of 46 cases. *Am J Surg Pathol* **23**(9): 1011–1020.

Lee, W., T. S. Kim, et al. (1998). Renal angiomyolipoma: embolotherapy with a mixture of alcohol and iodized oil. *J Vasc Interv Radiol* **9**(2): 255–261.

Lemaitre, L., M. Claudon, et al. (1997). Imaging of angiomyolipomas. *Semin Ultrasound CT MR* **18**(2): 100–114.

Levine, E. and M. Huntrakoon. (1983). Computed tomography of renal oncocytoma. *AJR Am J Roentgenol* **141**(4): 741–746.

Licht, M. R., A. C. Novick, et al. (1993). Renal oncocytoma: clinical and biological correlates. *J Urol* **150**(5 Pt 1): 1380–1383.

Liu, J. and C. V. Fanning. (2001). Can renal oncocytomas be distinguished from renal cell carcinoma on fine-needle aspiration specimens? A study of conventional smears in conjunction with ancillary studies. *Cancer* **93**(6): 390–397.

Liu, L., C. Zhang, et al. (2002). Clinicopathological observation of renal adenomas. *Zhonghua Bing Li Xue Za Zhi* **31**(3): 204–207.

Longoni, E., G. L. Berti, et al. (2004). Metanephric adenoma: case report and review of the literature. *Arch Ital Urol Androl* **76**(3): 121–123.

Madewell, J. E., S. M. Goldman, et al. (1983). Multilocular cystic nephroma: a radiographic-pathologic correlation of 58 patients. *Radiology* **146**(2): 309–321.

Magro, G., V. Cavallaro, et al. (2002). Intrarenal solitary fibrous tumor of the kidney report of a case with emphasis on the differential diagnosis in the wide spectrum of monomorphous spindle cell tumors of the kidney. *Pathol Res Pract* **198**(1): 37–43.

Mazal, P. R., M. Exner, et al. (2005). Expression of kidney-specific cadherin distinguishes chromophobe renal cell carcinoma from renal oncocytoma. *Hum Pathol* **36**(1): 22–28.

Morga Egea, J. P., L. O. Fontana Compiano, et al. (2004). [Multilocular cystic nephroma. A diagnostic and therapeutic challenge. Report of two cases]. *Arch Esp Urol* **57**(4): 431–434.

Morgan, G. S., J. V. Straumfjord, and E. J. Hall. (1951). Angiomyolipoma of the kidney. *J Urol* **65**: 525.

Muir, T. E., J. C. Cheville, et al. (2001). Metanephric adenoma, nephrogenic rests, and Wilms' tumor: a histologic and immunophenotypic comparison. *Am J Surg Pathol* **25**(10): 1290–1296.

Nelson, C. P. and M. G. Sanda. (2002). Contemporary diagnosis and management of renal angiomyolipoma. *J Urol* **168**(4 Pt 1): 1315–1325.

Novick, A. C. and S. C. Campbell. (2002). *Renal Tumours*. Philadelphia: W. B. Saunders Company.

Pillay, K., J. Lazarus, et al. (2003). Association of angiomyolipoma and oncocytoma of the kidney: a case report and review of the literature. *J Clin Pathol* **56**(7): 544–547.

Pins, M. R., E. C. Jones, et al. (1999). Metanephric adenoma-like tumors of the kidney: report of 3 malignancies with emphasis on discriminating features. *Arch Pathol Lab Med* **123**(5): 415–420.

Renshaw, A. A., D. R. Freyer, et al. (2000). Metastatic metanephric adenoma in a child. *Am J Surg Pathol* **24**(4): 570–574.

Silverman, S. G., B. Y. Lee, et al. (1994). Small (< or = 3 cm) renal masses: correlation of spiral CT features and pathologic findings. *AJR Am J Roentgenol* **163**(3): 597–605.

Simmons, J. L., S. A. Hussain, et al. (2003). Management of renal angiomyolipoma in patients with tuberous sclerosis complex. *Oncol Rep* **10**(1): 237–241.

Skinnider, B. F. and E. C. Jones. (1999). Renal oncocytoma and chromophobe renal cell carcinoma. A comparison of colloidal iron staining and electron microscopy. *Am J Clin Pathol* **111**(6): 796–803.

Slywotzky, C. and M. Maya. (1994). Needle tract seeding of transitional cell carcinoma following fine-needle aspiration of a renal mass. *Abdom Imaging* **19**(2): 174–176.

Steiner, M. S., S. M. Goldman, et al. (1993). The natural history of renal angiomyolipoma. *J Urol* **150**(6): 1782–1786.

Stone, C. H., M. W. Lee, et al. (2001). Renal angiomyolipoma: further immunophenotypic characterization of an expanding morphologic spectrum. *Arch Pathol Lab Med* **125**(6): 751–758.

Storkel, S. (1993). [Carcinoma and oncocytoma of the kidney. Phenotypic characteristics and prognostic features]. *Veroff Pathol* **140**: 1–165.

Suzuki, M., T. Nikaido, et al. (1989). Renal adenoma. Clinico-pathological and histochemical studies. *Acta Pathol Jpn* **39**(11): 731–736.

Takahashi, N., R. Kitahara, et al. (2003). Malignant transformation of renal angiomyolipoma. *Int J Urol* **10**(5): 271–273.

Tickoo, S. K. and M. B. Amin. (1998). Discriminant nuclear features of renal oncocytoma and chromophobe renal cell carcinoma. Analysis of their potential utility in the differential diagnosis. *Am J Clin Pathol* **110**(6): 782–787.

Tickoo, S. K., V. E. Reuter, et al. (1999). Renal oncocytosis: a morphologic study of fourteen cases. *Am J Surg Pathol* **23**(9): 1094–1101.

Tickoo, S. K., M. W. Lee, et al. (2000). Ultrastructural observations on mitochondria and microvesicles in renal oncocytoma, chromophobe renal cell carcinoma, and eosinophilic variant of conventional (clear cell) renal cell carcinoma. *Am J Surg Pathol* **24**(9): 1247–1256.

Truong, L. D., T. D. Todd, et al. (1999). Fine-needle aspiration of renal masses in adults: analysis of results and diagnostic problems in 108 cases. *Diagn Cytopathol* **20**(6): 339–349.

Uhlenbrock, D., C. Fischer, et al. (1988). Angiomyolipoma of the kidney. Comparison between magnetic resonance imaging, computed tomography, and ultrasonography for diagnosis. *Acta Radiol* **29**(5): 523–526.

Upadhyay, A. K. and J. A. Neely. (1989). Cystic nephroma: an emerging entity. *Ann R Coll Surg Engl* **71**(6): 381–383.

VanderBrink, B. A., R. Munver, et al. (2004). Renal angiomyolipoma with contrast-enhancing elements mimicking renal malignancy: radiographic and pathologic evaluation. *Urology* **63**(3): 584–586.

Weiner, S. N. and R. G. Bernstein. (1977). Renal oncocytoma: angiographic features of two cases. *Radiology* **125**(3): 633–635.

Weirich, G., G. Glenn, et al., (1998). Familial renal oncocytoma: clinicopathological study of 5 families. *J Urol* **160**(2): 335–340.

Zardawi, I. M. (1999). Renal fine needle aspiration cytology. *Acta Cytol* **43**(2): 184–190.

10h
Bone Metastases

10h.i
Radiotherapy

Padraig R. Warde and Mary K. Gospodarowicz

Introduction

Approximately one-third of patients with renal cell carcinoma (RCC) have metastatic disease at the time of diagnosis and approximately 50% of patients undergoing potentially curative surgery for clinically localized disease will develop distant metastases during the course of their illness.[1,2] Symptomatic bone metastases are a major clinical problem in many of these patients and have been reported to develop in 30% of patients after treatment for presentations with localized disease.[3] The median survival of patients with bone metastases has been reported to be approximately 12 months.[3] However, approximately 5–10% of patients with metastatic RCC survive for more than 5 years, which emphasizes the need for an aggressive approach to achieve durable symptom control in patients with symptomatic skeletal disease.[4]

Bone metastases in RCC are typically lytic and predominantly affect the axial skeleton.[3] While most patients have extensive bony involvement, a proportion of patients present with solitary lesions; a frequency as high as 45% was reported in one series.[3] Fractures, spinal cord compression, and hypercalcemia are common complications of bone metastasis in RCC and have a significant detrimental effect on quality of life. RCC has historically been considered less responsive to radiotherapy (RT) than other tumors and this was confirmed by *in vitro* experiments.[5,6] In a series of 76 human cell types studied by Deschavanne and Fertil, RCC cell lines were demonstrated to be the least radiosensitive.[6] However, multiple clinical studies of palliative RT in this setting have demonstrated symptomatic relief with or without demonstrable tumor regression.[2,7–12]

In this chapter, we attempt to address the role of localized and wide-field radiation therapy for bone metastases from RCC and also discuss the possible applications of newer RT approaches such as extracranial stereotactic RT and radioimmunotherapy.

Evaluation of Patients with Bone Metastases

Symptoms from bony metastatic disease include intermittent or constant bone pain, bone marrow suppression, hypercalcemia, pathological fractures, and spinal cord or nerve roots compression. Clinical evaluation typically includes a thorough history, physical examination, bone scan, plain radiographs, and serum alkaline phosphatase. However, benign processes such as healing fractures, arthritis, Paget's disease, other bone infections, and inflammatory diseases may lead to false-positive bone scan imaging. For this reason, suspicious areas on a bone scan should be confirmed by plain radiographs and/or cross-sectional imaging as necessary. If spinal cord compression is suspected clinically, computed tomography (CT), myelography, or magnetic resonance imaging (MRI) should be performed. In a study by Bayley et al., prostate cancer patients with bone metastases without neurological signs were screened for occult spinal cord compression using MRI. Thirty-two percent of patients have subarachnoid or spinal cord compression and the extent of disease on the bone scan was predictive for an increased risk of occult spinal disease.[13]

Localized External Beam Radiation Therapy

External beam radiation therapy remains one of the most effective and cost-efficient methods of relieving pain of bone metastases from all primary tumor sites. Despite numerous studies, there is still no consensus on the optimal dose fractionation scheme. Retrospective studies have documented improvement in pain in 80–90% of cases without inducing serious hematological or gastrointestinal toxicity.[14–17] However, RCC patients contributed only a small proportion of the patients in those trials. Four prospective studies of RT for metastatic RCC have been reported.[18–20]

Two studies included treatment with combined RT and chemoimmunotherapy in a small number of patients, making the interpretation of the impact of RT difficult.[18,20] Huegenin et al. examined the palliative benefit of RT in patients with metastatic RCC and melanoma.[19] Significant pain response was observed in 56% of patients with bone metastases from RCC, with a median duration of 2.4 months. Although the study focused on palliative endpoints, there were problems with missing data and the exclusive use of physician-assessed outcomes. Lee et al. recently reported the results of a prospective Phase II study to assess the impact of RT on symptoms and quality of life in patients with metastatic RCC.[7] Of 31 patients entered on this trial, 24 had symptomatic bony metastases. All patients were treated with a dose of 30 Gy in 10 fractions over 2 weeks. Of 23 evaluable patients, 83% ($n = 19$) experienced site-specific pain relief following RT and 48% ($n = 11$) have not required associated increase in analgesic medication. The median duration of site-specific pain response was 3 months. Global quality of life was improved in 33% ($n = 8$) of evaluable patients.

Dose/Fractionation

Several prospective randomized trials evaluating different dose-fractionation schemes in patients with bone metastases from different primary sites have been reported. Price et al. reported results in 288 patients randomized to 8 Gy given in a single fraction and to 30 Gy given in 10 daily fractions.[21] Pain was monitored using a self-assessed diary along with a record of analgesic intakes. The median survival for all patients was 5 months, and there was no difference between 8 Gy and 30 Gy in overall response or duration of response at 1 year. However, a large proportion of patients was lost to follow-up. The same group later conducted another study of 270 patients randomized to a single 4 Gy or a single 8 Gy treatment.[22] The median survival for all patients was 8 months, but treatment with a single 4 Gy produced a lower overall response rate (53%) than the 8 Gy (76%).[37]

A number of other large-scale multicenter trials compared the efficacy of 8 Gy single treatment against multiple treatments[23–28] (Table 10h.i-1). The Bone Pain Working Party in the UK studied 765 patients and found no difference in the extent and duration of pain relief between single treatment and five fractions.[27] The Dutch Bone Metastases study of 1171 patients found no difference in pain relief or quality of life following treatment with 8 Gy or 24 Gy.[23] However, in the Bone Pain Trial Working Party trial, retreatment was more frequent in the single-dose (8 Gy) group (29.1%) than in the multifraction (24 Gy) group (9.8%); in the study by Steenland et al.[23] 25% of patients required retreatment in the single fraction group and only 7% in the multifraction group.

Recent surveys in North America suggest that radiation oncologists prefer protracted treatment schemes despite evidence showing similar efficacy between a single treatment of 8 Gy and multiple fractionations.[29–31] On the other hand,

European oncologists have now adopted a single treatment of 8 Gy as standard practice for patients with uncomplicated metastatic bone pain.[32]

In patients with bone metastases from RCC, the relationship between radiation dose and clinical response has been studied in several retrospective studies with conflicting results.[9–11] Onufrey[7] noted significantly higher response rates in patients treated with a time dose fractionation (TDF) value greater than 70 when compared with a TDF value of less than 70 (65% vs. 25%). Using the same TDF model, Halperin et al.[9] have not identified any correlation between equivalent dose and palliative response, with the overall response rate of 77% for painful bony metastasis. Dibiase et al.,[10] using the linear quadratic model with an α/β ratio of 10, reported an overall symptomatic response rate of 86% and concluded that a biologic effective dose (BED) greater than 50 was associated with significantly higher complete response rates. In the study by Lee et al.[7] from Princess Margaret Hospital in Toronto, a dose of 3000 cGy in 10 fractions was used since it represented the most commonly employed schedule in prior studies. It represented a reasonable tradeoff between delivering a potentially effective dose and providing a treatment schedule for these patients that is not unduly protracted. The chosen dose of 3000 cGy in 10 fractions is equivalent to a TDF of 62 or BED_{10} of 39. Although this did not meet the thresholds of TDF greater than 70 or BED_{10} greater than 50 determined to be significant by Onufrey and Dibiase, respectively, a high pain response rate was achieved.

Wide-Field/ Half-Body External Beam Radiation

Half-body irradiation (HBI) is a useful treatment approach in patients with multiple painful bone metastases. Single fraction HBI has been shown in retrospective and prospective Phase I and II studies to provide pain relief in 70–80% of patients.[33–36] Pain relief is usually apparent within 24–48 hours. Toxicities include bone marrow suppression and gastrointestinal side effects such as nausea and vomiting in upper abdominal radiation and may be controlled with ondansetron or dexamethasone.[37] Pulmonary toxicity is minimal provided the lung dose is limited to 6 Gy (corrected dose).[38] Fractionated HBI has also been investigated and some studies have suggested better results with this approach as compared to single fraction TBI.[39,40]

Radionuclides

Patients with metastatic RCC often present with multiple bone metastases requiring external beam radiation to several parts of the skeleton, frequently requiring more than one course of palliative RT. Radiopharmaceuticals are radioactive

TABLE 10h.i-1. Results of randomized trials in palliative radiation therapy.[a]

Author/institution treatment arms	Total number of patients	Percentage with prostate cancer	CR or PR		Frequency of reirradiation	
			Low dose	High dose	Low dose	High dose
UK Bone Pain Working Party[27] 8 Gy vs. 20 Gy/5#	765	34%	57% CR 78% PR	58% CR 78% PR	23%	10%
Dutch Bone Group[23] 8 Gy vs. 24 Gy/6#	1171	23%	37% CR 72% PR	33% CR 69% PR	25%	7%
Nielsen et al.[25] 8 Gy vs. 20 Gy/5#	241	33%	12% CCR 15% CR 62% PR	12% CCR 17% CR 74% PR	20%	12%
Jeremic et al.[26] 4 Gy (vs. 6 Gy) vs. 8 Gy	327	16%	21% CR 59% Min	32% CR 78% Min	42%	38%
Gaze et al.[28] 10 Gy vs. 22.5 Gy/5#	280	20%	15% CCR 39% CR 84% Min	14% CCR 42% CR 89% Min	N/A	N/A
Niewald et al.[24] 20 Gy/5# vs. 30 Gy/15#	100	10%	33% CR 77% Min	31% CR 86% Min	N/A	N/A
Hoskin et al.[22] 4 Gy vs. 8 Gy	270	13%	36% CR 44% PR	39% CR 69% PR	20%	9%
Price et al.[21] 8 Gy vs. 30 Gy/10#	288	8%	35% CR 84% Min	27% CR 84% Min	n = 15	n = 4

[a]Cr, complete response; PR, partial response; CCR, complete cytogenetic remission; N/A, not applicable.

agents administered intravenously that localize specifically to reactive bone sites and deliver radiation to metastatic areas in a highly localized manner.[41] Strontium-89 and samarium-153 have an affinity for bone and concentrate in areas of bone turnover. The exact mechanism of action of radiopharmaceuticals in relieving pain of bone metastases is not known, but is assumed to be the result of destruction of tumor cells in the bone.

There is little information available on the efficacy of these agents in metastatic RCC. Most studies have been done in patients with metastatic breast cancer, prostate cancer, and lung cancer.[41] Indeed, both strontium-89 and samarium-153 accumulate preferentially in osteoblastic lesions and as the skeletal changes in RCC are predominantly lytic this strategy may not be very effective. Two systematic reviews of the role of radiopharmaceuticals in the palliation of painful bone metastases has recently been published.[41,42] In both reviews it was concluded that these agents should be considered as a possible option for the palliation of multiple sites of bone pain from metastatic cancer where pain control with conventional means is not achieved and there is increased activity on a bone scan.

Stereotactic Radiotherapy

In numerous clinical studies brain metastases treated with gamma-knife radiation therapy have given local control rates in excess of 85%. The application of a similar radiation technique has become possible in extracranial sites in the past decade due to the development of stereotactic body-frame and high-precision radiation techniques. Wersall et al. have reported results of extracranial stereotactic RT in 50

patients with metastatic disease in various sites including bone.[43] The most common dose fractionation schemes used were 8 Gy × 4, 10 Gy × 4, and 15 Gy × 3 over approximately a week. With a median follow-up of 37 months, a complete response based on radiological criteria was seen in 30% of cases and 60% of patients had either a partial response or no evidence of disease progression. No data were provided on symptom control and side effects were generally mild. The results of this study suggested that local control of disease (and control of local symptoms) can be achieved with high dose/fraction stereotactic RT in approximately 90% of cases.

The survival time after surgery for patients with solitary metastases of RCC, especially if localized to lung or bone, is relatively long (35–50%).[44,45] In these cases, aggressive local therapy using surgery or RT is indicated.

Radioimmunotherapy

Radioimmunotherapy (RIT) involves a form of biologically targeted radiopharmaceutical treatment in which a radioactive isotope (typically a short-range, high-energy β emitter) is chemically bound to a target-specific monoclonal antibody or fragment.[46] Thus, these radioimmunoconjugates combine the targeting specificity of the humoral immune system with the known cell-killing power of high-energy RT. Two RIT agents have been approved for clinical use, yttrium-90 ibritumomab tiuxetan and iodine-131 tositumomab. Both of these agents target the CD20 molecule found on the surface of normal and malignant B cells and are indicated for the management of indolent B cell lymphoma and other related conditions. Another agent,[131] IcG250, has been investigated in patients with metastatic RCC though results to date have been disappointing. Future work in this area will likely focus on patients with solitary small lesions, perhaps after surgical resection.

Conclusions

The most common approach to the management of bone metastasis in cancer is to reduce symptoms and to prevent complications such as fracture or spinal cord compression. In patients in the final phases of disseminated cancer, palliation of symptoms and improving the quality of life are the overarching concerns. Most studies reflect these concerns. However, not all patients with bone metastasis are in the terminal phase of their illness. Some survive for prolonged periods of time. In such patients, local control of metastasis is the optimal outcome. This may be accomplished with surgery or combination of surgery and RT. In cases where surgery is not feasible or optimal, aggressive treatment with RT may produce local control. Local control has been obtained with a high single RT dose using stereotactic RT in the brain. The introduction of image-guided precision RT techniques has facilitated research in applying extracranial stereotactic RT to clinical practice. This is one of the exciting areas of research in the radical treatment of oligometastatic disease. Recent studies suggested that the use of image-guided radiotherapy (IGRT) and intensity-modulated radiotherapy (IMRT) may not only result in an improved local control and reduced toxicity in conventional fractionation prescriptions, but should facilitate the use of novel high-dose per fraction treatments. Furthermore, there is preliminary laboratory evidence that the endothelial apoptosis and microvascular dysfunction contribute significantly to tumor lethality following single high-dose RT and such approaches may result in enhanced local tumor control.[47,48]

Recent advances in systemic therapy of renal cell cancer may pave the way toward a more aggressive treatment of metastasis, especially solitary or oligometastasis. Further research is needed both to identify patients who are most likely to benefit from aggressive treatment of metastasis and to identify optimal treatment protocols to improve local control and decrease treatment toxicity.

References

1. Motzer RJ, Bander NH, Nanus DM: Renal-cell carcinoma [see comment]. N Engl J Med 335:865–875, 1996.
2. Figlin RA: Renal cell carcinoma: management of advanced disease. J Urol 161:381–166, 1999; discussion 386–387.
3. Zekri J, Ahmed N, Coleman RE, et al.: The skeletal metastatic complications of renal cell carcinoma. Int J Oncol 19:379–382, 2001.
4. Motzer RJ, Mazumdar M, Bacik J, et al.: Survival and prognostic stratification of 670 patients with advanced renal cell carcinoma. J Clin Oncol 17:2530–2540, 1999.
5. Fertil B, Malaise EP: Intrinsic radiosensitivity of human cell lines is correlated with radioresponsiveness of human tumors: analysis of 101 published survival curves. Int J Radiat Oncol Biol Phys 11:1699–1707, 1985.
6. Deschavanne PJ, Fertil B: A review of human cell radiosensitivity in vitro. Int J Radiat Oncol Biol Phys 34:251–266, 1996.
7. Lee J, Hodgson D, Chow E, et al.: A phase II trial of palliative radiotherapy for metastatic renal cell carcinoma. Cancer 104:1894–1900, 2005.
8. Fossa SD, Kjolseth I, Lund G: Radiotherapy of metastases from renal cancer. Eur Urol 8:340–342, 1982.
9. Halperin EC, Harisiadis L: The role of radiation therapy in the management of metastatic renal cell carcinoma. Cancer 51:614–617, 1983.
10. DiBiase SJ, Valicenti RK, Schultz D, et al.: Palliative irradiation for focally symptomatic metastatic renal cell carcinoma: support for dose escalation based on a biological model. J Urol 158:746–749, 1997.
11. Onufrey V, Mohiuddin M: Radiation therapy in the treatment of metastatic renal cell carcinoma. Int J Radiat Oncol Biol Phys 11:2007–2009, 1985.
12. Seitz W, Karcher KH, Binder W: Radiotherapy of metastatic renal cell carcinoma. Sem Surg Oncol 4:100–102, 1988.
13. Bayley A, Milosevic M, Blend R, et al.: A prospective study of factors predicting clinically occult spinal cord compression in patients with metastatic prostate carcinoma. Cancer 92:303–310, 2001.
14. Arcangeli G, Micheli A, Giannarelli D, et al.: The responsiveness of bone metastases to radiotherapy: the effect of site, histology and radiation dose on pain relief. Radiother Oncol 14:95–101, 1989.
15. Jensen NH, Roesdahl K: Single-dose irradiation of bone metastases. Acta Radiol Ther Phys Biol 15:337–339, 1976.
16. Schocker JD, Brady LW: Radiation therapy for bone metastasis. Clin Orthopaed Related Res 169:38–43, 1982.
17. Vargha ZO, Glicksman AS, Boland J: Single-dose radiation therapy in the palliation of metastatic disease. Radiology 93:1181–1184, 1969.
18. Brinkmann OA, Bruns F, Prott FJ, et al.: Possible synergy of radiotherapy and chemo-immunotherapy in metastatic renal cell carcinoma (RCC). Anticancer Res 19:1583–1587, 1999.
19. Huguenin PU, Kieser S, Glanzmann C, et al.: Radiotherapy for metastatic carcinomas of the kidney or melanomas: an analysis using palliative end points. Int J Radiat Oncol Biol Phys 41:401–405, 1998.
20. Redman BG, Hillman GG, Flaherty L, et al.: Phase II trial of sequential radiation and interleukin 2 in the treatment of patients with metastatic renal cell carcinoma. Clin Cancer Res 4:283–286, 1998.
21. Price P, Hoskin PJ, Easton D, et al.: Prospective randomised trial of single and multifraction radiotherapy schedules in the treatment of painful bony metastases. Radiother Oncol 6:247–255, 1986.
22. Hoskin PJ, Price P, Easton D, et al.: A prospective randomised trial of 4 Gy or 8 Gy single doses in the treatment of metastatic bone pain. Radiother Oncol 23:74–78, 1992.
23. Steenland E, Leer JW, van Houwelingen H, et al.: The effect of a single fraction compared to multiple fractions on painful bone metastases: a global analysis of the Dutch Bone Metastasis

Study. [see comment] [Erratum appears in Radiother Oncol 1999 Nov;53(2):167.] Radiother Oncol 52:101–109, 1999.

24. Niewald M, Tkocz HJ, Abel U, et al.: Rapid course radiation therapy vs. more standard treatment: a randomized trial for bone metastases. Int J Radiat Oncol Biol Phys 36:1085–1089, 1996.

25. Nielsen OS, Bentzen SM, Sandberg E, et al.: Randomized trial of single dose versus fractionated palliative radiotherapy of bone metastases. Radiother Oncol 47:233–240, 1998.

26. Jeremic B, Shibamoto Y, Acimovic L, et al.: A randomized trial of three single-dose radiation therapy regimens in the treatment of metastatic bone pain. Int J Radiat Oncol Biol Phys 42: 161–167, 1998.

27. 8 Gy single fraction radiotherapy for the treatment of metastatic skeletal pain: randomised comparison with a multifraction schedule over 12 months of patient follow-up. Bone Pain Trial Working Party. Radiother Oncol 52:111–121, 1999.

28. Gaze MN, Kelly CG, Kerr GR, et al.: Pain relief and quality of life following radiotherapy for bone metastases: a randomised trial of two fractionation schedules. Radiother Oncol 45: 109–116, 1997.

29. Duncan G, Duncan W, Maher EJ: Patterns of palliative radiotherapy in Canada. Clin Oncol (Royal College of Radiologists) 5:92–97, 1993.

30. Chow E, Danjoux C, Wong R, et al.: Palliation of bone metastases: a survey of patterns of practice among Canadian radiation oncologists. [see comment] Radiother Oncol 56:305–314, 2000.

31. Ben-Josef E, Shamsa F, Williams AO, et al.: Radiotherapeutic management of osseous metastases: a survey of current patterns of care. Int J Radiat Oncol Biol Phys 40:915–921, 1998.

32. Bentzen SM, Hoskin P, Roos D, et al.: Fractionated radiotherapy for metastatic bone pain: evidence-based medicine or...? [comment] Int J Radiat Oncol Biol Phys 46:681–683, 2000.

33. Salazar OM, Rubin P, Hendrickson FR, et al.: Single-dose half-body irradiation for palliation of multiple bone metastases from solid tumors. Final Radiation Therapy Oncology Group report. Cancer 58:29–36, 1986.

34. Kuban DA, Delbridge T, el-Mahdi AM, et al.: Half-body irradiation for treatment of widely metastatic adenocarcinoma of the prostate. J Urol 141:572–574, 1989.

35. Fitzpatrick PJ, Rider WD: Half body radiotherapy. Int J Radiat Oncol Biol Phys 1:197–207, 1976.

36. Hoskin PJ, Ford HT, Harmer CL: Hemibody irradiation (HBI) for metastatic bone pain in two histologically distinct groups of patients. Clin Oncol (Royal College of Radiologists) 1:67–69, 1989.

37. Quilty PM, Kirk D, Bolger JJ, et al.: A comparison of the palliative effects of strontium-89 and external beam radiotherapy in metastatic prostate cancer. Radiother Oncol 31: 33–40, 1994.

38. Van Dyk J, Keane TJ, Kan S, et al.: Radiation pneumonitis following large single dose irradiation: a re-evaluation based on absolute dose to lung. Int J Radiat Oncol Biol Phys 7:461–467, 1981.

39. Salazar OM, Sandhu T, da Motta NW, et al.: Fractionated half-body irradiation (HBI) for the rapid palliation of widespread, symptomatic, metastatic bone disease: a randomized Phase III trial of the International Atomic Energy Agency (IAEA). [see comment] Int J Radiat Oncol Biol Phys 50:765–775, 2001.

40. Zelefsky MJ, Scher HI, Forman JD, et al.: Palliative hemiskeletal irradiation for widespread metastatic prostate cancer: a comparison of single dose and fractionated regimens. Int J Radiat Oncol Biol Phys 17:1281–1285, 1989.

41. Bauman G, Charette M, Reid R, et al.: Radiopharmaceuticals for the palliation of painful bone metastasis—a systemic review. Radiother Oncol 75:258–270, 2005.

42. Finlay IG, Mason MD, Shelley M: Radioisotopes for the palliation of metastatic bone cancer: a systematic review. [see comment]. Lancet Oncol 6:392–400, 2005.

43. Wersall PJ, Blomgren H, Lax I, et al.: Extracranial stereotactic radiotherapy for primary and metastatic renal cell carcinoma. Radiother Oncol 77:88–95, 2005.

44. Loizzi M, Sollitto F, Sardelli P, et al.: Endothoracic nodules in patients who under-went nephrectomy for renal cell carcinoma. Results of surgical resection. Minerva Med 94:103–110, 2003.

45. Kavolius JP, Mastorakos DP, Pavlovich C, et al.: Resection of metastatic renal cell carcinoma. J Clin Oncol 16:2261–2266, 1998.

46. Pohlman B, Sweetenham J, Macklis RM: Review of clinical radioimmunotherapy. Expert Rev Anticancer Ther 6:445–461, 2006.

47. Ling CC, Yorke E, Fuks Z: From IMRT to IGRT: frontierland or neverland? Radiother Oncol 78:119–122, 2006.

48. Fuks Z, Kolesnick R: Engaging the vascular component of the tumor response. Cancer Cell 8:89–91, 2005.

10h.ii
Surgery

Ignace R. Samson and Friedl C. Sinnaeve

Introduction

Renal cell carcinoma (RCC) belongs, together with lung, prostate, breast, and thyroid carcinoma, to the group of bone-seeking tumors due to the fact that bone metastases are common in these tumors. But there are several publications, mainly in the orthopedic literature, dealing only with the surgical treatment of bone metastases from RCC.[1,2,9,10,17,18,20,23,29,35,39,45] These metastases are considered a special group because compared to the other four groups, the metastases of RCC show some peculiar features. Although most of the metastases are located in the common metastatic regions of the skeleton (ribs, vertebrae, pelvis, humerus, and femur), distant metastases—-below the elbow and the knee—-and even acrometastases[1,12,28,31] have been described. A second feature is the occasional late development of a solitary bone metastasis, sometimes 3, 5, and even more years after the diagnosis and treatment of the kidney tumor. The bone metastases of RCC are also known to be very vascular tumors, sometimes with an unexpected high blood loss during surgical treatment. Even a simple incisional biopsy can be a hazardous undertaking if the fact that the osteolytic bone lesion is a metastasis of RCC is not known. And last but maybe most important, the effect of medical treatment and radiotherapy on the bone metastases has often been disappointing and unpredictable. Hopefully the availability of new treatment modalities (bisphosphonates, tyrosine kinase inhibitors, vaccination immunotherapy, etc.)[7,16,24,25,27,30,33,36,37,41,46] will delay or diminish the genesis and development of bone metastases in RCC.

Although long-lasting disease-free survival after the treatment of solitary bone metastases of RCC has been reported, for most patients with skeletal metastases treatment is usually palliative. In planning the treatment, the focus should be on the preservation of a good quality of life by controlling pain, by trying to preserve or to restore early ambulatory function, and by reducing the need for and the time of hospitalization. The use of only one or a combination of the three modalities of local treatment—-radiotherapy, embolization, and surgery—-should be considered, taking into account the extent of the metastatic disease (solitary versus multiple bone lesions, only skeletal versus multiple system metastases), the time of appearance of the bone metastases (synchronous versus metachronous), and the general condition of the patient or, more correctly, the life expectancy. As a consequence, a multimodality approach implies a multidisciplinary approach and forethought.

Diagnosis and Staging

The time of development of bone metastases of RCC is unpredictable. However, bone metastases can often be detected synchronous with the renal tumor and the renal tumor may often be detected in the staging of a painful osteolytic bone lesion. The presence of the "flow-void" sign[6] on magnetic resonance imaging (MRI) of the bone lesion should prompt the clinician to further examine the kidneys with ultrasonography and/or computed tomography (CT) (Fig. 10h.ii-1). If one metastatic bone lesion is detected, a careful search for other metastases (bone, lungs, and brain) should be done, because the presence of more than one bone metastasis, particularly the presence of metastases to more than one system (e.g., bone and lung), worsens the prognosis and can influence the type of local treatment chosen.[13]

The role of bone scintigraphy in the staging of RCC is not clear.[15,19] It can be false positive (e.g., asymptomatic Paget or enchondromas), but it can also be false negative. The uptake of the tracer in bone metastases of RCC is often only modest (Fig. 10h.ii-2). The osteolytic lesion itself is usually "cold," but may be surrounded by a "warm" or even a "hot" rim. Although most lesions in the limbs can be detected this way, small (but sometimes large) lesions in the axial skeleton, especially in the vertebrae and the pelvis, are easily missed. Review of the staging (preferable helical) CT of the trunk in a bone window setting is more sensitive and more reliable in excluding or detecting bone metastases in these regions (Fig. 10h.ii-3). The probability of detecting bone metastases on bone scintigraphy in an asymptomatic patient is also low. For these reasons a bone scan is not routinely used in the staging of an RCC in a patient without orthopedic symptoms.

(a)

(b)

(c)

(d)

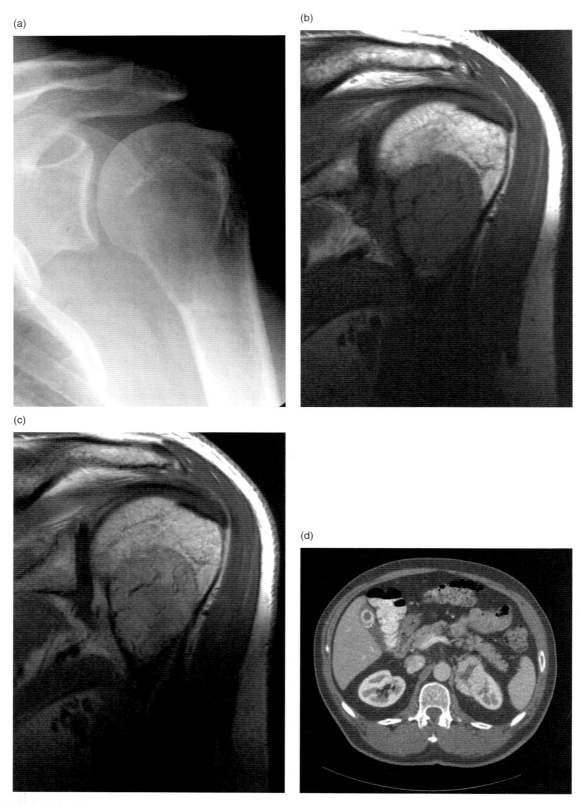

FIGURE 10h.ii-1. Male, 62 years old, presenting with increasing pain and limitation of motion in the left shoulder and upper arm over a period of 6 months. Radiographs of the left shoulder show a geographic osteolytic lesion in the proximal metaphysis of the humerus (**A**). An MRI with T1-weighted images clearly demonstrates the lesion, which is isointense to muscle, but contains multiple tubular structures with low signal intensity (**B**). After administration of gadolinium contrast, the tumor stains homogeneously while the tubular structures remain of low signal intensity (**C**). Because of the presence of this "flow-void" sign, a metastasis of RCC was suspected. A CT of the abdomen showed a tumor of 6 cm diameter in the anterior part of the upper pole of the right kidney (**D**).

(a)

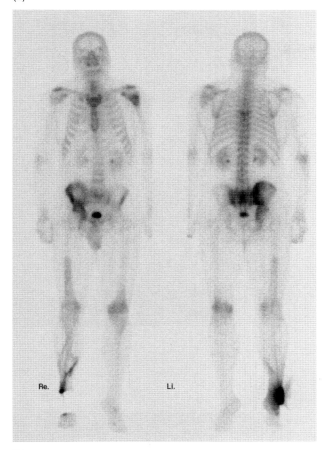

(a)

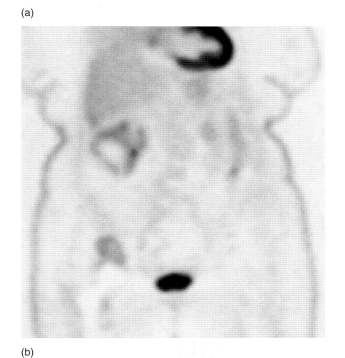

(b)

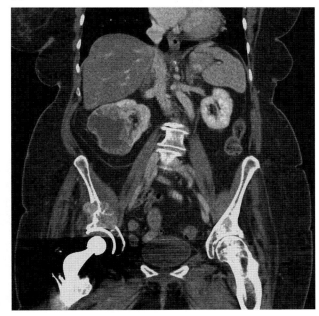

(b)

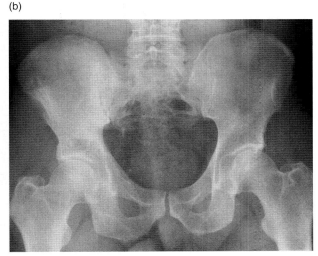

FIGURE 10h.ii-2. The same patient as in Fig. 10h.ii-1. The bone scintigraphy shows moderate uptake of the tracer in the left proximal humerus. Marked tracer uptake is noted in the sacrum and right hemipelvis. Moderate tracer uptake is also noted in the distal half of the right femur, in the left femoral condyles, and in the sixth thoracic vertebra. Due to a partial paravenous injection, there is an artifact in the right ankle region (**A**). Complementary radiographs of the asymptomatic regions showed Paget's disease in all of them, most clearly seen on the X-rays of the pelvis (**B**).

FIGURE 10h.ii-3. Female, 74 years old, with a right total hip arthroplasty performed 10 years previously. She also has seronegative rheumatoid arthritis, under treatment with low-dose methotrexate for 12 years. Radiographs of the pelvis revealed a slowly growing osteolytic bone lesion in the right acetabulum. Because a lymphoma was suspected, a fluorodeoxyglucose positron emission tomography (FDG-PET) scan was performed (**A**). There was a moderate FDG uptake in the osteolytic bone lesion in the right acetabulum, but the scan was also very suspicious for a large necrotic tumor in the right kidney. The CT with coronal reconstructions more clearly depicts the large right kidney tumor and the lobulated osteolytic metastatic bone lesion in the right acetabulum (**B**).

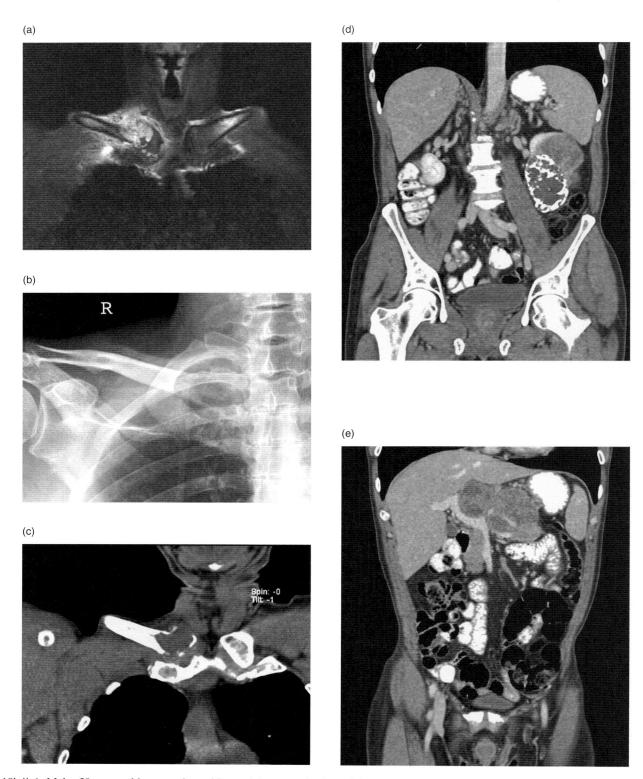

FIGURE 10h.ii-4. Male, 58 years old, presenting with a painless tumefaction of the sternal part of the right clavicle, much more easily assessed on MRI (**A**) and CT (**C**) than on plain radiographs (**B**). On CT of the abdomen a very large and partly calcified left kidney tumor was detected (**D**), with a paraaortic lymph node and large pancreatic metastases (**E**). An incisional biopsy of the lesion in the clavicle confirmed the diagnosis of a metastasis of a clear cell carcinoma.

The appearance of bone metastases can also be metachronous, occurring several months and even many years after the diagnosis of the RCC. In particular, if there is a long time interval between the treatment of the RCC and the development of an osteolytic bone lesion, the diagnosis is not always straightforward. Once again the detection of the "flow-void" sign on the MRI of the bone lesion suggests the diagnosis. Sometimes histological confirmation (fine needle aspiration, core biopsy, or incisional biopsy) is necessary. As mentioned previously, bone metastases of RCC are highly vascular tumors. A biopsy can therefore be complicated by massive bleeding during surgery or by the formation of a large hematoma afterward. This is important as it is in a subgroup of these patients (solitary metachronous bone metastasis with a long—more than 2 year—disease-free interval) that a wide resection of the metastasis with curative intent should be considered.[1,2,9,18,20,23] Contamination of the surrounding tissue by a bleeding biopsy site should therefore be avoided.

Most often patients complain of pain, especially with movement (upper limb, spine) or weight bearing (pelvis and lower limb). On radiographs, the lesions are mostly large and osteolytic, with thinning or destruction of the cortex and sometimes a periosteal reaction, pointing out the danger of a pathological fracture. Pathological fractures are usually preceded by increasing pain for several weeks. If located superficially (e.g., the clavicle or scapular spine) or distally in the appendicular skeleton (e.g., hand or finger or foot), a slowly enlarging mass can be the presenting symptom (Fig. 10h.ii-4). Lesions in the spine can present with neurological signs of radicular pain or paresis, due to the extension of the tumor into the spinal canal with compression of the myelum (above the L1–L2 level) or the radices (at or below L2). Radicular pain can also be caused by a metastasis located posterolaterally in the vertebral body or around the neural foramen (pedicle, superior and inferior articular processes, vertebral end of a rib) (Fig. 10h.ii-5).

If one or more of these symptoms are present at the time of diagnosis of the renal tumor or develops in the following years, appropriate imaging should be performed. Radiographs and bone scintigraphy are indicated for lesions in the limbs. CT is the most reliable and sensitive imaging modality for bone lesions in the axial skeleton (spine, ribs, pelvis, and scapula).

Over the past few years, several prognostic factors have been identified[3,5,8,26,38,40] and scoring systems have been developed.[21,22] They are primarily used for planning or for the evaluation of the effect of medical treatment (interferon, interleukin-2), but are also helpful in planning the treatment of skeletal metastases. Not surprisingly, some of these prognostic factors have also been noticed in retrospective studies regarding the outcome of the surgical treatment of bone metastases of RCC.[1,18,29]

Positive prognostic signs regarding the time of survival are a good general condition, a primary tumor less than 7 cm in maximal diameter, the possibility of or a history of nephrectomy for the primary tumor, the possibility that the primary tumor and all metastatic lesions can be removed, metastases in a single organ system (in casu bone), metastases in the appendicular skeleton, a solitary lesion, and, for metachronous metastases, a disease-free interval of more than 1, but preferable more than 2 years.

Unfavorable signs are constitutional symptoms, a high-grade histology, especially with the presence of tumor necrosis or sarcomatoid features, the presence of tumor thrombus, and changes in the blood examination (low hemoglobin, elevated white blood cell count, elevated alkaline phosphatases, hypercalcemia, and elevated lactate dehydrogenase). The presence of regional lymph node metastases is not consistently shown to be an important factor.

In conclusion, when bone metastases of RCC are detected (synchronous or metachronous), a thorough evaluation is mandatory before planning treatment. This evaluation should consist of a physical examination (including inspection, palpation, and evaluation of motion of the limbs, the shoulder and pelvic girdles, and the spine, as well as a neurovascular evaluation of the limbs), a blood examination, a bone scintigraphy, radiographic evaluation of all suspect regions detected by the physical examination or on the bone scan, a CT of the chest and abdomen, and a CT of the brain. If there is doubt regarding the nature of any of the detected bone lesions, magnetic resonance imaging (MRI) and sometimes CT can be helpful in distinguishing metastatic disease from incidentally found and often benign bone pathology.

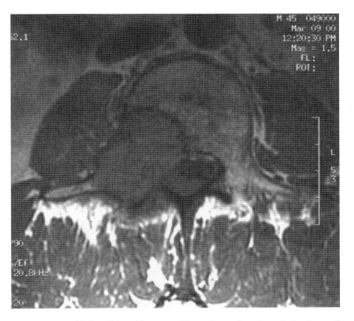

FIGURE 10h.ii-5. This 45-year-old patient developed back and right thigh pain 26 months after a left radical nephrectomy for RCC, which had been detected with ultrasonography performed for arterial hypertension. The MRI (T1-weighted images without contrast enhancement) shows a metastasis in the right posterolateral part of the vertebral body of L3, extending into and expanding the right pedicle and base of the transverse process.

In the case of synchronous bone metastases with a high risk for or presenting with a pathological fracture, the treatment of the metastases should be planned and performed synchronous with or even before the treatment of the primary tumor (if a nephrectomy is possible) to maintain or restore safe mobilization of the patient as soon as possible.

Surgical Treatment of Bone Metastases

The treatment of metastatic bone disease is usually palliative. The aim is to diminish pain and to maintain or to restore as soon as possible a normal and safe ambulatory function for the rest of the patient's life. For bone metastases of some other tumors, simple osteosynthesis (interlocking nails in long bones, pedicular screw fixation in the spine) in conjunction with radiation therapy and very effective medical treatment (chemotherapy, hormonal therapy, bisphosphonates, etc.) is usually sufficient.

Unfortunately the effect of radiotherapy and medical treatment on the bone metastases of RCC is usually disappointing, although promising results have been reported with the use of zoledronic acid[24,33,36] in prolonging the time to development as well as the incidence of skeletal events, the latter being defined as the occurrence of a pathological fracture or the need for radiotherapy or surgery to prevent or treat pathological fractures. Another factor that is important is the observation that in patients with bone metastases from RCC a survival of more than 2 years is not uncommon. The surgery for bone metastases of RCC should for this reason also focus on a lasting local control at the treated sites, with a durable strong fixation or reconstruction to prevent the need for further operations (Fig. 10h.ii-6). For this reason a more aggressive surgical treatment has to be considered, ranging from simple but thorough curettage to wide resection and reconstruction.[1,2,4,10,43] Amputations are also sometimes indicated, not only for distant metastases, but also for more proximally located lesions.[2,20]

There are two distinct ways of treating both metastatic as well as primary bone lesions. The first is called translesional. During surgery, the lesion is opened and removed from inside out. This way the bulk of the tumor is removed, but it can be expected that tumor cells remain at the periphery, unless the tumor is clearly demarcated with a fibrotic capsule or a sclerotic bone rim. To kill these remaining cells, additional measures are necessary. These can be mechanical (high-speed burr), chemical (phenol), or physical (cryosurgery, radiotherapy). If the remaining bone defect is large, with a high risk for fracture of the affected bone, it should be filled and bridged over. For metastatic disease the defect is usually filled with polymethylmethacrylate (PMMA) bone cement and bridged with an intramedullary nail or a plate and screws.[4,44] Bone metastases of RCC are notorious for being highly vascular lesions. For translesional resections at or below the elbow or the knee, a tourniquet can be used from the moment the surgeon is ready to open the lesion. In more proximally located metastases or for lesions in the pelvis or spine, preoperative embolization is advisable, with the surgery being planned within 24–48 hours[14,20,44] (Fig. 10h.ii-7).

Massive preoperative bleeding can also be prevented by extralesional surgical treatment in which the lesion is removed en bloc, without opening it. If the dissection around the lesion is close to or through the pseudocapsule, it is called a marginal resection. If a cuff of normal tissue remains around the lesion, the resection is called wide. This minimizes the risk for local recurrence of the disease. There are some bones that can be removed this way without causing mechanical instability or impairment of function, the so-called expendable bones (e.g., clavicle, iliac wing, a single rib, fibula), hence no bony or prosthetic reconstruction of the resulting skeletal defect is necessary. Usually, however, the remaining defect has to be reconstructed. In treating metastatic disease it is important to decrease as much as possible the postoperative morbidity and the time of revalidation, as these patients usually have only a limited life expectancy. The reconstruction should therefore be chosen in such a way as to allow early mobilization and full weight bearing. The two reconstruction materials most often used are massive allogenic bone segments and metal prosthetic implants, sometimes combined in so-called APCs (Allograft-Prosthetic Composite).[1,4,20,32,42] Allografts are most often used to reconstruct intercalary resections in long bones (Fig. 10h.ii-8). They should be combined with rigid internal fixation to allow early motion and loading. The time to consolidation of the osteotomy sites is negatively affected by the use of preoperative or postoperative radiotherapy, which can lead to nonunion and ultimate failure of the reconstruction. APCs are most often used if reinsertion of important muscle tendons (e.g., at the proximal humerus and the proximal tibia) is thought to be important to maintain muscle strength around the affected joint (Fig. 10h.ii-9). On the other hand, temporary protection, and sometimes immobilization of the reconstructed joint, is necessary to allow healing of the tendon sutures. In addition, in this type of reconstruction, bony healing of the osteotomy site is influenced by previous or postoperatively planned radiation therapy. Certainly after transarticular resections of a bone segment lacking major tendon insertions (e.g., distal humerus and distal femur), reconstruction with a cemented resection prosthesis is the first choice (Figs. 10h.ii-10 and 10h.ii-11).

Although it may look as if an extralesional resection with reconstruction is much more radical than a translesional curettage and stabilization, the opposite can be true. For example, a metastasis in the femoral head or neck can more easily and with less blood loss be treated with a simple wide resection and implantation of a standard total hip prosthesis than by attempting to retain the hip joint with a curettage and cementing.

Although seemingly very drastic, an amputation is sometimes the simplest and a well-tolerated treatment.

(a)   (b)   (c)

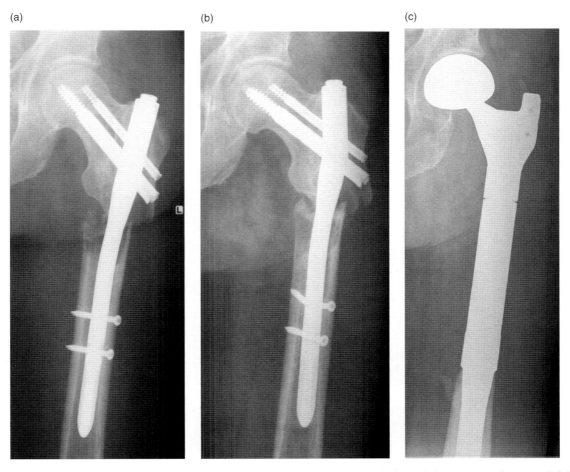

FIGURE 10h.ii-6. Male, 77 years old, who 6 years ago had a right radical nephrectomy for an RCC. Four years later a painful osteolytic metastasis in the left proximal femur developed. During radiation treatment he developed a pathological fracture treated with osteosynthesis (**A**). Due to a nonunion of the fracture, the metal implants finally broke (**B**). To allow quick mobilization of the patient with full weight bearing, surgery consisted of a proximal femoral resection and reconstruction with a biarticular proximal femoral resection prosthesis (**C**).

Especially for lesions in the phalanges of the hand or feet, and even for metastases in the metacarpal or metatarsal bones (with the exception of the bones of the thumb), a finger or toe amputation or a ray resection offers quick relief of pain while maintaining a good functional result.[11, 12, 28, 31] Also in patients suffering from pain, where other treatments (e.g., even high-dose radiotherapy) have failed, more "conservative" surgery will not produce a good functional result, and in whom the metastatic disease is not immediately life threatening, even a forequarter or a hindquarter amputation should be considered as an option for palliation of pain or for local control of the disease.[2, 20]

Metastases to the spine deserve special attention.[4, 14, 34, 39] Most of the metastases to the spine are located in the vertebral bodies, although invasion of the posterior elements (e.g., spinous process, lamina) is also possible. Destruction of the bone may cause progressive pain and pathological fractures due to loss of mechanical strength, but more importantly, extension of the tumor in the spinal canal endangers neurological function. The development of paresis is a medical

emergency and in these circumstances immediate evaluation of the location and the extent of the metastatic disease is necessary. Radiographs of the spine to evaluate the alignment of the spine and to identify osteolytic lesions or pathological fractures, combined with an MRI with contrast enhancement to detect small lesions and more importantly the location and the extent of the invasion of the spinal canal, are the most informative examinations. The feasibility of surgery should be evaluated by the spine surgeon, as this is the quickest way to decompress the dural sac and its contents. The same principles of treatment (translesional or extralesional resection) can be applied, although of course, due to the specific anatomy of the vertebral column, an extralesional resection is a much more extensive intervention[34] (Fig. 10h.ii-12). Once again, it is necessary to be aware of the highly vascular nature of this type of metastases, which is why preoperative angiography with embolization of the feeding segmental vessels is advisable. As a general rule, a metastasis located in the vertebral body with compression of the dura mater and its contents from the ventral side is usually

(a)

(b)

(c)

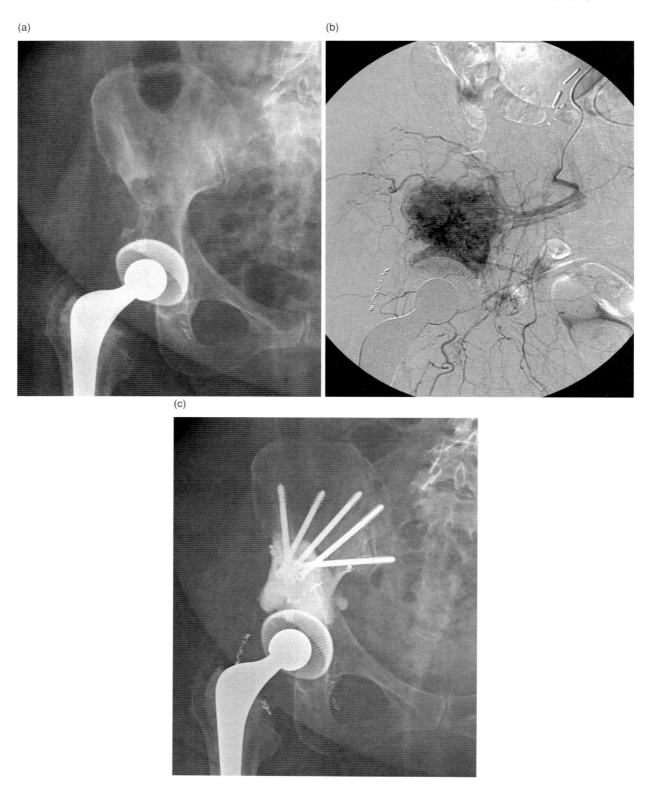

FIGURE 10h.ii-7. The same patient as in Fig. 10h.ii–3. Because of the slow growth of the metastasis in the pelvis, she first underwent a right radical nephrectomy. The radiographs show the geographic osteolytic metastasis in the roof of the acetabulum and the caudal part of the iliac bone with high risk for pathological fracture and protrusion of the hip arthroplasty (**A**). Preoperative angiography shows the extremely vascular nature of the RCC metastasis (**B**), for which a careful embolization of all feeding vessels was done at the same time. The following day a translesional resection was done with thorough curettage of the tumor and filling of the bone defect with bone cement, supplemented with screws (**C**). After healing of the wound, radiation therapy was started, with administration of a total dose of 39 Gy in fractions of 3 Gy.

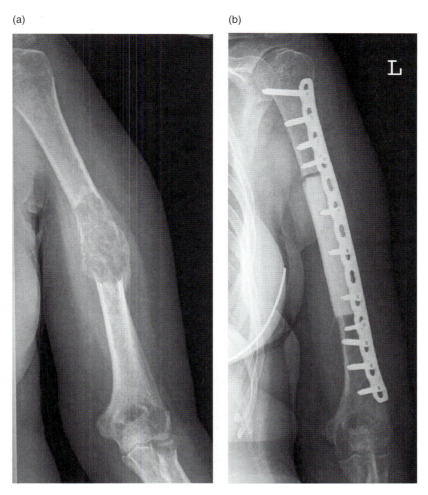

(a) (b)

FIGURE 10h.ii-8. Female, 67 years old, presenting with a pathological fracture of the diaphysis of the left humerus (**A**). Seven years before a radical left nephrectomy for RCC had been performed. Further staging showed no other lesions, except for two subpleural long nodules on the left side of only 5 mm. A punction biopsy confirmed the diagnosis of metastasis of RCC. A wide intercalary resection with preservation of the radial nerve was done. The skeletal defect was reconstructed with an intercalary allograft of the humerus, fixed with a long locking plate and screws. The medullary canal of the allograft was filled with bone cement to increase its strength (**B**).

treated by a so-called anterior approach (e.g., via lumbotomy or thoracotomy). Compression of the dura posteriorly by a metastasis located in the neural arch, is approached from the dorsal side. To be able to mobilize the patient safely shortly after surgery, internal fixation of the affected segment with vertebral body screws and rods anteriorly or pedicular screw fixation posteriorly is usually necessary.

If confronted with a patient suffering from skeletal metastases of RCC, two questions should be answered: when is there an indication for surgery and what type of intervention (intralesional or extralesional) should be performed (Fig. 10h.ii-13).

Pathological fractures of the long bones are an indication for surgery, even if the patient is in a poor general condition. If the latter is the case, and even if the patient is bedridden, internal fixation of the fractured limb(s) will palliate the pain and will facilitate nursing. If there is a life expectancy of several months, at least rigid internal fixation and radiotherapy are indicated, but an intralesional resection with reconstruction and adjuvant radiotherapy should be considered. For intraarticular pathological fractures prosthetic replacement of the involved articulation and the affected bone segment is indicated.

If the patient presents with pain and a fracture seems imminent, surgery is also indicated to relieve pain and to preserve or to restore function. If several negative prognostic factors are present, an intralesional resection with internal fixation and adjuvant radiotherapy probably will suffice to preserve local control for the rest of the patient's life. If, on the other hand, several good prognostic factors are identified, a wide resection and reconstruction should be considered, as this technique has been shown to minimize the risk for local recurrence. In these cases, adjuvant radiation therapy is probably superfluous.

(a)   (b)   (c)

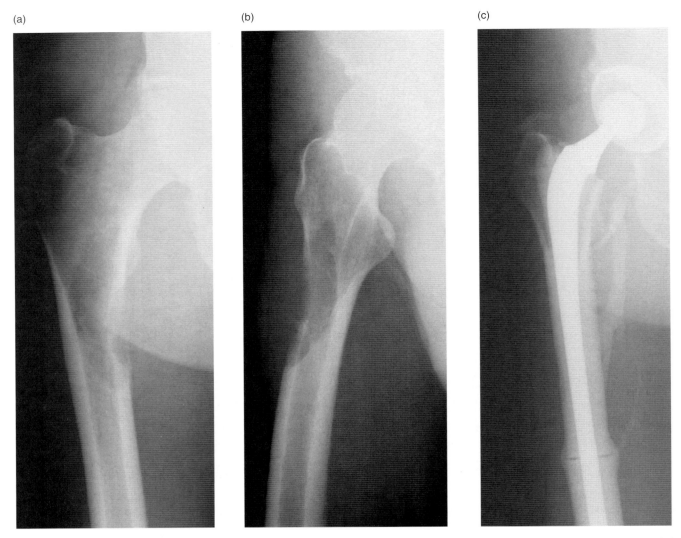

Figure 10h.ii-9. Male patient, 45 years old, referred for an increasing mechanical type of pain in the right leg. Radiographs of the right proximal femur show a geographic osteolytic bone lesion in the subtrochanteric region of the right proximal femur (**A**) with a large cortex defect anteriorly (**B**). A large left kidney tumor was easily demonstrated with ultrasonography. Further staging with CT and bone scintigraphy revealed no other metastatic lesions. Because the bone metastasis was considered as being a high risk for fracture, a wide resection of the right proximal femur was done, reconstructed with an allograft and a long-stem total hip arthroplasty (**C**). Two weeks later a radical left nephrectomy was done. Lung metastases were detected 6 months later. He died with widespread multisystem metastatic disease (bone, lungs, brain) 32 months after the diagnosis of the kidney cancer.

(a) (b)

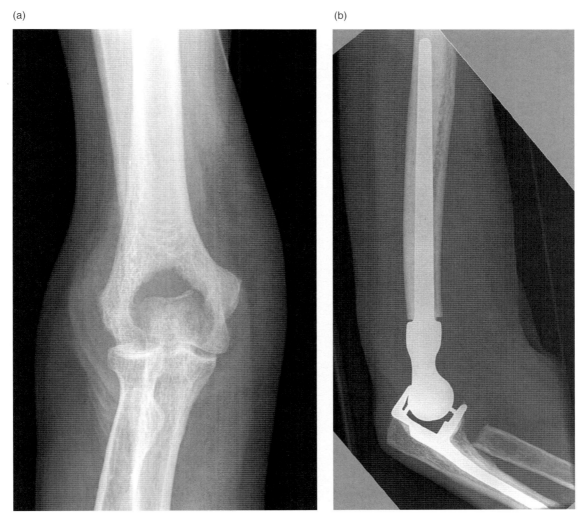

FIGURE 10h.ii-10. Female, 78 years old, developed pain in the right elbow, accompanied by unexplained loss of weight. Radiographs of the right elbow show a geographic pure osteolytic lesion of the distal epiphysis and metaphysis of the humerus (**A**). A large left kidney tumor was detected on ultrasonography and confirmed with CT. A wide transarticular distal humerus resection, reconstructed with a revision type total elbow prosthesis, was done first (**B**), followed by a radical left nephrectomy 2 weeks later. She regained full function in the right elbow, but died with widespread metastatic disease 22 months later.

(a)   (b)

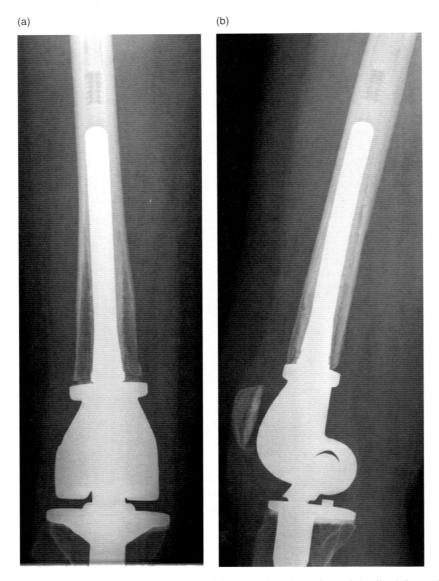

FIGURE 10h.ii-11. Female, 54 years old, in whom a solitary painful osteolytic lesion of the right distal femoral epiphysis was detected 30 months after treatment for breast carcinoma and after a radical left nephrectomy for RCC, which was coincidentally discovered in the staging of the breast tumor. A cemented distal femoral prosthesis was used after wide resection of the metastasis of her RCC, resulting in an almost normal function of the knee and allowing immediate full weight bearing. Radiographs in anteroposterior (**A**) and lateral (**B**) views 4 years after the surgery do not show any sign of loosening or local recurrence.

(a)   (b)

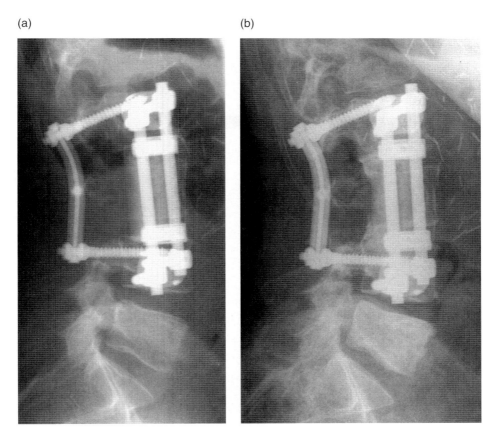

FIGURE 10h.ii-12. The same patient as in Fig. 10h.ii–5. Radiotherapy failed to improve his back and leg pain. Further evaluation did not show other metastasis. For these reasons an extralesional resection was performed through a combined dorsal and right lateral approach after preoperative angiography and embolization. Reconstruction was done with an intercalary cortical femur allograft, in combination with anterior and posterior fixation with screws, rods, and a plate (A). Although he has been treated for several other bone, lung, and even brain metastases in the meantime, this reconstruction remains solid and without the development of local recurrence 6 years later (B).

(a)   (b)   (c)

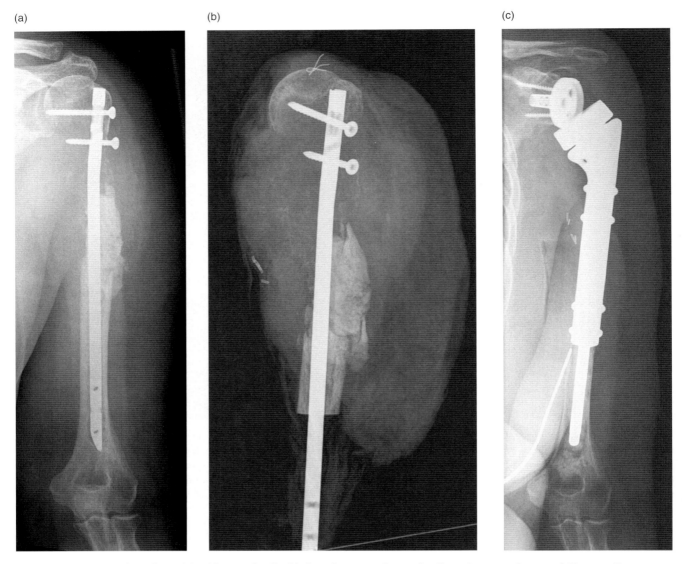

FIGURE 10h.ii-13. Female patient with a history of radical left nephrectomy for renal cell carcinoma at the age of 41 years. Twenty years later an osteolytic lesion in the diaphysis of the left humerus developed. Staging showed an RCC in the upper pole of the remaining right kidney and two lung metastases. Shortly after the diagnosis a pathological fracture of the left humerus arose, for which she was treated with curettage, cementing, and nailing, followed by radiotherapy. Unfortunately, there was progressive osteolytic destruction of the proximal humerus together with soft tissue extension (**A**), with which she presented in our department. The proximal half of the humerus together with the medullary nail was marginally resected [(**B**) shows a radiograph of the resected specimen] and the resulting defect was reconstructed with a large resection prosthesis of the humerus and shoulder (**C**). Eighteen months later she developed a soft tissue metastasis on the dorsal side of the scapula, but no signs of local recurrence in the left shoulder and upper arm.

For asymptomatic small lesions an attitude of waiting can be adopted, with clinical and radiographic follow-up.

There is evidence that zoledronic acid diminishes the risk for skeletal complications in patients with RCC, including local progression. Newer medical treatments that are becoming available or are under investigation may also diminish the risk for the development of or the progression of metastatic disease in these patients. If this goes hand in hand with a better quality of life and an increasing life expectancy, this will hopefully diminish the need for surgery, but at the same time may increase the need for wide (extralesional) resections and long-lasting reconstructions.

References

1. Althausen R, Althausen A, Jennings LC et al. Prognostic factors and surgical treatment of osseous metastases secondary to renal cell carcinoma. Cancer. 1997;15:1103–1109.

2. Baloch KG, Grimer RJ, Carter SR et al. Radical surgery for the solitary bony metastasis from renal-cell carcinoma. J Bone Joint Surg Br. 2000;82:62–67.

3. Beisland C, Medby PC, Beisland HO. Presumed radically treated renal cell carcinoma. Recurrence of the disease and prognostic factors for subsequent survival. Scand J Urol Nephrol. 2004;38:299–305.

4. Bohm P, Huber J. The surgical treatment of bony metastases of the spine and limbs. J Bone Joint Surg Br. 2002;84: 521–529.

5. Campbell SC, Flanigan RC, Clark JI. Nephrectomy in metastatic renal cell carcinoma. Curr Treat Options Oncol. 2003;4:363–372.

6. Choi JA, Lee KH, Jun WS et al. Osseous metastasis from renal cell carcinoma: "flow-void" sign at MR imaging. Radiology. 2003;228:629–634.

7. Doehn C, Jocham D. Vaccination immunotherapy: an update. Scand J Surg. 2004;93:163–169.

8. Donskov F, von der Maase H. Impact of immune parameters on long-term survival in metastatic renal cell carcinoma. J Clin Oncol. 2006;24:1997–2005.

9. Durr HR, Maier M, Pfahler M et al. Surgical treatment of osseous metastases in patients with renal cell carcinoma. Clin Orthop Relat Res. 1999;367:283–290.

10. Fuchs B, Trousdale RT, Rock MG. Solitary bone metastasis from renal cell carcinoma: significance of surgical treatment. Clin Orthop Rel Res. 2005;431:187–192.

11. Fusetti C, Kurzen P, Bonaccio M et al. Hand metastasis in renal cell carcinoma. Urology. 2003;62:141.

12. Ghert MA, Harrelson JM, Scully SP. Solitary renal cell carcinoma metastasis to the hand: the need for wide excision or amputation. J Hand Surg. 2001;26A:156–160.

13. Han KR, Pantuck AJ, Bui MH et al. Number of metastatic sites rather than location dictates overall survival of patients with node-negative metastatic renal cell carcinoma. Urology. 2003;61:314–319.

14. Heary RF, Bono CM. Metastatic spinal tumors. Neurosurg Focus. 2001;5:1–8.

15. Henriksson C, Haraldsson G, Aldenborg F et al. Skeletal metastases in 102 patients evaluated before surgery for renal cell carcinoma. Scand J Urol Nephrol. 1992;26:363–366.

16. Huland E, Heinzer H. Renal cell carcinoma: novel treatments for advanced disease. Curr Opin Urol. 2003;13:451–456.

17. Jackson RJ, Loh SC, Gokaslan ZL. Metastatic renal cell carcinoma of the spine: surgical treatment and results. J Neurosurg. 2001;94(1 Suppl):18–24.

18. Jung ST, Ghert MA, Harrelson JM et al. Treatment of osseous metastases in patients with renal cell carcinoma. Clin Orthop Relat Res. 2003;409:223–231.

19. Koga S, Tsuda S, Nishikido M et al. The diagnostic value of bone scan in patients with renal cell carcinoma. J Urol. 2001;166:2126–2128.

20. Kollender Y, Bickels J, Price WM et al. Metastatic renal cell carcinoma of bone: indications and technique of surgical intervention. J Urol. 2000;164:1505–1508.

21. Leibovich BC, Cheville JC, Lohse CM et al. A scoring algorithm to predict survival for patients with metastatic clear cell carcinoma: a stratification tool for prospective clinical trials. J Urol. 2005;174:1759–1763.

22. Leibovic BC, Han KR, Bui MH et al. Scoring algorithm to predict survival after nephrectomy and immunotherapy in patients with metastatic renal cell carcinoma: a stratification tool for prospective clinical trials. Cancer. 2003;98: 2566–2575.

23. Les KA, Nicholas RW, Rougraff B et al. Local progression after operative treatment of metastatic kidney cancer. Clin Orthop Relat Res. 2001;390:206–211.

24. Lipton A, Colombo-Berra A, Bukowski RM et al. Skeletal complications in patients with bone metastases from renal cell carcinoma and therapeutic benefits of zoledronic acid. Clin Cancer Res. 2004;10:6397s–6403s.

25. Mancuso A, Sternberg CN. New treatments for metastatic kidney cancer. Can J Urol. 2005;12(Suppl 1):66–70; discussion 105.

26. Mekhail TM, Abou-Jawde RM, Boumerhi G et al. Validation and extension of the Memorial Sloan-Kettering prognostic factors model for survival in patients with previously untreated metastatic renal cell carcinoma. J Clin Oncol. 2005;23: 832–841.

27. Morabito A, De Maio E, Di Maio M et al. Tyrosine kinase inhibitors of vascular endothelial growth factor receptor in clinical trials: current status and future directions. Oncologist. 2006;11:753–764.

28. Perdona S, Autorino R, Gallo L et al. Renal cell carcinoma with solitary toe metastasis. Int J Urol. 2005;12:401–404.

29. Pongracz N, Zimmerman R, Kotz R. Orthopaedic management of bony metastases of renal cancer. Semin Surg Oncol. 1988;4:139–142.

30. Pyrhonen SO. Systemic therapy in metastatic renal cell carcinoma. Scand J Surg. 2004;93:156–161.

31. Ritter HG, Ghobrial I. Renal cell carcinoma with acrometastasis and scalp metastasis. Mayo Clin Proc. 2004;79:76.

32. Rolf O, Gohlke F. Endoprosthetic elbow replacement in patients with solitary metastasis resulting from renal cell carcinoma. J Shoulder Elbow Surg. 2004;13:656–663.

33. Saad F, Lipton A. Zoledronic acid is effective in preventing and delaying skeletal events in patients with bone metastases secondary to genitourinary cancers. BJU Int. 2005;96: 964–969.

34. Sakaura H, Hosono N, Mukai Y et al. Outcome of total en bloc spondylectomy for solitary metastasis of the thoracolumbar spine. J Spinal Disord Tech. 2004;17:297–300.

35. Smith EM, Kursch ED, Makley J *et al*. Treatment of osseous metastases secondary to renal cell carcinoma. *J Urol*. 1992;148:784–787.

36. Smith MR. Zoledronic acid to prevent skeletal complications in cancer: corroborating the evidence. *Cancer Treat Rev*. 2005;31(Suppl 3):16–25.

37. Tannir N, Jonasch E, Pagliaro LC *et al*. Pilot trial of bone-targeted therapy with zoledronate, thalidomide, and interferon-gamma for metastatic renal cell carcinoma. *Cancer*. 2006;107:497–505.

38. Tongaonkar HB, Kulkarni JN, Kamat MR. Solitary metastases from renal cell carcinoma: a review. *J Surg Oncol*. 1992;49: 45–48.

39. Ulmar B, Catalkaya S, Naumann U *et al*. Surgical treatment and evaluation of prognostic factors in spinal metastases of renal cell carcinoma. *Z Orthop Ihre Grenzgeb*. 2006;144:58–67.

40. Uygur MC, Usubutun A, Ozen H *et al*. Prognostic factors and the role of nephrectomy in metastatic renal cell carcinoma. *Int Urol Nephrol*. 1998;30:681–687.

41. van Spronsen DJ, de Weijer KJ, Mulders PF *et al*. Novel treatment strategies in clear-cell metastatic renal cell carcinoma. *Anticancer Drugs*. 2005;16:709–717.

42. Weber KL, Lin PP, Yasko AW. Complex segmental elbow reconstruction after tumor resection. *Clin Orthop Relat Res*. 2003;415:31–44.

43. Wedin R, Bauer HC, Wersall P. Failures after operation for skeletal metastatic lesions of long bones. *Clin Orthop Relat Res*. 1999;358:128–139.

44. Wunder JS, Ferguson PC, Griffin AM *et al*. Acetabular metastases: planning for reconstruction and review of results. *Clin Orthop Relat Res*. 2003;415(Suppl):S187–S197.

45. Yadav R, Ansari MS, Dogra PN. Renal cell carcinoma presenting as solitary foot metastasis. *Int Urol Nephrol*. 2004;36:329–330.

46. Zekri J, Ahmed N, Coleman RE *et al*. The skeletal metastatic complications of renal cell carcinoma. *Int J Oncol*. 2001;19:379–382.

11
Medical Management

11a
Immunotherapy

Edith Huland, Hans Heinzer, and Hartwig Huland

Introduction

Improvement of Prognosis by Cytokines

Untreated metastatic renal cell carcinoma (mRCC) has a dismal prognosis, treatment options are limited, and cure is rare. Without cytokine therapy median survival in metastatic disease is some 7 months, with nearly no long-term survivors beyond 3 years (Table 11a-1). The use of interferon-α (IFN-α) and interleukin-2 (IL-2) has favorably changed the natural course of advanced RCC, leading to median survival times of 12–24 months and long-term survival of more than 5 years in up to about 20% of patients (Table 11a-2). Immunotherapy using IFN-αimproves survival significantly by 30 weeks as shown in 160 randomized patients. High-dose IL-2 in selected cases induces long-term complete responses. Tyrosine kinase inhibitors, recently approved in the United States, so far failed to show a significant survival benefit. Sorafenib was tested in the largest randomized double-blind placebo controlled multi-center study of advanced renal cell cancer today (903 patients) and survival interim analysis, based on 220 deaths, did not reach significance. Immunotherapy is still the only option for patients who aim at survival and complete responses. Systemic therapy, however, is limited to patients with good performance status. Both cytokines induce cancer remissions and prolong life in well-selected patients and are considered standard care for those fit to tolerate systemic treatment-related side effects. Optimum treatment effects seem to be dose dependent. In similar risk groups higher doses of IL-2 monotherapy show a tendency to increase the numbers of complete long-term responses (Yang, 2003a).

Spontaneous Regression of Metastatic Renal Cell Carcinoma

Spontaneous tumor regressions, possibly mediated by the body´s own immune mechanisms, are occasionally reported in mRCC, but cannot be expected to change the natural course of this fatal disease. The overall incidence reported in the literature is less than 1%. Nephrectomy does not induce spontaneous remission. It is rare, short-lived, and does hardly translate into survival. A most extraordinary high response rate of 6% was reported in 99 patients with mRCC in a placebo-controlled population; the duration of regressions though was very short, 2–13 months, with only one ongoing response of 9 months at the time of publication. In addition, more than 90% of these patients were dead within 20 months (Gleave, 1988). Spontaneous remission does not substitute for effective therapy.

Influence of Risk Factors and Comorbidity on Treatment Success

The success of systemic cytokine therapy is without doubt influenced significantly by the patient´s risk factors and comorbidity. Because of the toxicity, approved doses of systemic IL-2 and IFN-α have to be limited to well-selected patients in good general condition. Treating fewer or unselected patients will induce even more aggressive toxicities, and consequently will lead more frequently to reduced doses, to reduced treatment times, and to unfavorable treatment results. Common frequent toxicities of systemic cytokine administration include fever, fatigue, and malaise, and more seriously, high-dose systemic IL-2 treatment can cause vascular leak syndrome and severe life-threatening infections. In attempts to improve success and tolerability, treatment intensity and duration, doses and intervals, the type of application, and the use of cytokine combinations have been varied considerably in different studies. The design of study protocols is often significantly influenced by the toxicity of systemic cytokine therapy and selection for systemic immunotherapy is determined by the patient's ability to tolerate its side effects rather than their therapeutic need. Approved therapies today define exclusion criteria for patients with risk factors or comorbidities, which leaves a significant number of patients without treatment options. As we all need to speak the same language, a common standardized use of risk factors in RCC patients is a goal to aim at.

TABLE 11a-1. Median survival (months), progression free survival (months), and overall survival (percent of patients surviving at 1, 2, 3, 4, and 5 years) in publications reporting a total of 1980 mRCC patients without IL-2- and IFN-α-based therapies.[a]

Author, year	Patient No.	Therapy	Risk	PFS (months)	Median survival(months)	1 year survival (%)	2 year survival (%)	3 year survival (%)	4 year survival (%)	5 year survival (%)
Bacoyiannis, 2002	29	Vinblastine/INF-μ	Mixed	3.2	12.6					0
Bacoyiannis, 2002	40	Vinblastine/INF-μ/ 13 CRA	Mixed	3.9	9.5					0
Bennouna, 2003	59	Folfox-4	Mixed	3.0	10.6			0	0	
Brinkmann, 2004	37	Mistletoe	Mixed	<2	5	0				
Dutcher, 2003	39	INF-μ	Mixed	1.4	7		10	<10		
Drucker, 2003	18	Chemotherapy (ZD 1839)	Mixed	<4						
Elson, 1988	610	Chemotherapy or none	Mixed		7		<10			
Fizazi, 2003	16	Chemotherapy (irinotecan)	Mixed		8	19				
Fossa, 1994	159	Chemotherapy	Mixed				8			<5
Gleave, 1988 (part)	90	Placebo	Good	1.9	15.7		<10			
Gleave, 1988 (part)	91	INF-μ	Good	1.9	12.2		25			
Haas, 2003	21	Chemotherapy	Mixed	<2	10				0	
Minor, 2002	29	Thalidomide	Mixed	2.3	3.5					
MRCRCC, 1999	176	Medroxyprogesterone	Mixed	<3	6	31	12			
Pyrhönen, 1999	81	Vinblastine	Mixed		8.4	38.3		5.1	1.3	0
Patel, 1978	166	Chemotherapy and other	Mixed			24		4		<4
Royston, 2004	175	Medroxyprogesterone	Mixed		6	28	13	6	2	<1
Shamash, 2003	28	Chemotherapy	Mixed	3.9–4.8	6–10	0–40	0–20	0		
Yang, 2003a	76	Bevazizumab LD/HD	Good	3–4.8						<20

[a]PFS, progression free survival; IFN, interferon.

Danger of Life-Threatening Side Effects

Systemic immunotherapy has to be restricted to patients willing and able to tolerate side effects. Unselected patients hardly benefit from therapy but are in even greater danger of experiencing severe and possibly life-threatening toxicity. In well-selected patients today it is possible to manage toxicities and reduce treatment-related risks by measures of stringent therapy control and comedication, to ease therapy and improve compliance. Experienced staff and a well-informed patient are both important to achieve the best risk-to-benefit ratios.

Physiological Application: Local Cytokine Therapy

Cytokines are physiologically local hormones. Systemic toxicity is directly related to intravascular cytokine concentrations. Local application of cytokines is generally well tolerated, does not lead to systemic toxicity, and provides a tool to control local tumor growth without the toxicity associated with systemic application; therefore it is particularly suitable for patients unable to tolerate systemic side effects. It also may be used to enhance systemic therapy. Wide experience has been gained using inhalation of IL-2; more than 50 centers have published their own experience and some 800 patients have been reported worldwide (Nakamoto, 1997; Heinzer, 1999; Pizza, 2001; Huland, 2003; Merimsky, 2004; Barutca, 2004; Michelson, 2005; Melichar, 2005). Inhalation of IL-2 represents a local application in mRCC to eradicate or control metastatic lung disease, especially in patients unfit for or resistant to systemic cytokine therapy. In 2003 an orphan designation for the inhalation use of IL-2 was granted by the EMEA (European agency for the evaluation of medicinal products) (http://www.emea.eu.int/pdfs/human/comp/opinion/122803-en.pdf. access 18.8.2003).

Metastatic Renal Cell Carcinoma: "Orphan" Disease

mRCC is a rare disease and—in particular in subselected groups—it may hardly be cost efficient to develop therapies and/or will require a long time until sufficient numbers of patients are recruited for therapy studies. Rare diseases, also called "orphan diseases," may qualify for "orphan designations" of approval authorities enabling companies to receive special support to develop therapies in promising medical fields of life-threatening diseases without treatment alternatives. In mRCC orphan designations have been granted by approval authorities in various countries to facilitate the development of and meet an urgent need for effective therapies.

Immunotherapy

"Three decades of extensive clinical investigation have identified only two agents that have an effect on survival for patients with mRCC: treatment with high-dose bolus IL-2 achieved durable responses in a small proportion of highly selected patients. A modest survival benefit for interferon-alpha therapy in mRCC was observed in two phase III trials comparing interferons-alpha with vinblastine or medroxyprogesterone" (Motzer, 2003).

Without IL-2- or INF-α-based therapies nearly all patients are reported to die within 3 years (Table 11a-1). Using IL-2- or INF-α-based therapies a notable prolongation of survival leading to a 20–25% 5-year survival in patients with low-risk factors and good performance status may be achieved (Table 11a-2). High-risk patients do not benefit from systemic cytokine therapy, but may find treatment options in local (e.g., IL-2 inhalation) therapies.

Although the complete mechanism of action of IL-2 and IFN-α is poorly understood, the induction of antitumor immunity by these cytokines in murine models has been linked both to the direct killing of tumor cells by activated T cells and natural killer (NK) cells, as well as to antiangiogenic effects. IL-2 has no direct effect and IFN-α has only a minor growth inhibitory effect on cancer cells. Lymphocytes and monocytes are required to carry out antitumor mechanisms. Intratumoral immune cells ("tumor infiltrating lymphocytes") are prognostically favorable and can be found in huge amounts in primary and metastatic renal cancer. They have been reported to become 50–100 times more cytotoxic than peripheral mononuclear cells by incubation with IL-2. Increasing intratumoral lymphocyte subsets (CD 3, CD 4, CD8, CD 57) are positive prognostic factors for survival (Donskov, 2004). For optimum results in experimental animal therapy rather high doses were required as well as a long-term IL-2-triggered stimulation of mononuclear cells (e.g., incubation for at least 3 days) to improve outcome. Both induction of killer activity as well as proliferation seem to be important to mediate optimum anticancer activity. It is established that only three variables determine T cell G_1 progression to DNA replication: IL-2 concentration, IL-2 receptor density, and the duration of the IL-2 receptor interaction (Smith, 1998). All are variables of the local immune response and local T cell proliferation. T cell clonal proliferation after antigen challenge is obligatory for immune responsiveness and immune memory.

Many schedules, combinations, and variable doses using IL-2 and IFN-α have previously been published, sometimes together with chemotherapy, such as 5-fluorouracil (5-FU) or vinblastine, and treatment results as discussed are occasionally quite controversial. Appraisal of outcomes always has to take into consideration patient selection, comorbidity, risk stratification, as well as applied doses and treatment times.

TABLE 11a-2. Median survival (months), progression-free survival (months), and overall survival (percent of patients surviving at 1, 2, 3, 4, and 5 years) in publications reporting a total of 11,297 mRCC patients *with* IL-2- and IFN-a-based therapies.[a]

	Patient No.	IL-2 ± IFN-α-based therapy	Risk	PFS (months)	Median survival (months)	1 year survival (%)	2 year survival (%)	3 year survival (%)	4 year survival (%)	5 year survival (%)
Allen, 2000	55	IL-2/ IFN-α/5-FU	Mixed	4	11	45				
Atzpodien, 2004	341	IL-2- and INF-α-based therapy	Good							
Part A	132	IL-2- and INF-α-based therapy	Good	7	25			37		20
Part B	146	IL-2- and INF-α-based therapy	Good	6	27			41		20
Part C	63	INF-α-based therapy	Good	5	16			21		<20
Atzpodien, 2003a	425	IL-2- and INF-α-based therapy	Good		20					16
Part		IL-2- and INF-α-based therapy	Good		32					27
Part		IL-2- and INF-α-based therapy	Median		18					11
Part		IL-2- and INF-α-based therapy	Poor		8					5
Atzpodien, 2002		IL-2- and INF-α-based therapy	Good	6	13		45			16
Bex, 2002	22	Pegylated INF-α	Mixed	4,0	13			0		
Bordin, 2000	92	IL-2	Mixed			58		17		9
Bukowski, 2002	57	Pegylated INF-α	Good	<3	13.2	50	30	<20		
Bukowski, 2004	309	IL-2- and INF-α-based therapy								
Part	59	IL-2- and INF-α-based therapy	Good		28.6			30	20	
Part	215	IL-2- and INF-α-based therapy	Median		14.6			18	10	
Part	35	IL-2- and INF-α-based therapy	Poor		4.5			0		
Bukowski, 2004	1134	IL-2- and INF-α-based therapy	Mixed		12	50	30	20	15	10
Buzio, 2001	50	IL-2- and INF-α-based therapy	Good					47		
Clark et al., 1999	19	IL-2- and INF-α-based therapy	Poor		6	16				
Clark, 2002	47	IL-2 + INF-α	Mixed	2	13		20			
Coppin, 2000	3089	IL-2/INF-α	Mixed		11.6		22			
Dutcher, 2003	49	INF-α and INF-γ	Mixed	2,9	10.9		18	<10		
Figlin, 1997	203	HD IL-2	Good		18	61	40	31		
Fossa, 1992	178	INF-α based therapy	Mixed							9
Part		INF-α based therapy	Good							13
Part		INF-α based therapy	Median							6
Part		INF-α based therapy	Poor							0
Fossa, 1994	136	INF-α	Mixed							9
Fisher, 2000	255	HD IL-2 IV	Good		16.3			24		19
Flanigan, 2004	331	INF-α ± op	Mixed							
Part	161	INF-α with nephrectomy	Mixed		13.6	55	28	20	14	10
Part	163	INF-α without nephrectomy	Mixed		7.8	36	18	12	6	<5

Author, year	n	Therapy	Risk								
Gez, 2002	62	L-2/INF-α/5-FU	Good								
Gold, 2000	123	HD IL-2 z.Tl LAK	Good			19		30			20
Huland, 2003	197	IL-2-based therapies (+ INF-α)	Poor								
Part	94	Inhaled IL-2	Poor			47	28	23			21
Part	103	Systemic IL-2 (SC/IV)	Poor			26	10	1			0
Libra, 2003	56	HD IL-2 continuous IV	Good		20		41				21
Minasian, 1993	159	INF-α	Mixed		11, 4						3
Merimsky, 2004	40	Inhaled IL-2	Poor	8.7	13						<10
Motzer, 2002	463	INF-α	Mixed	4.7							
Part	80	INF-α	Good (no risk)	8.1	30	83	55	45			20
Part	269	INF-α	Median (1–2 risks)	5.1	14	58	31	17			<10
Part	88	INF-α	Poor (3–5 risks)	2.5	5	20	6	2			
Michelson, 2005	51	Inhaled IL-2	Mixed	8.6	23						
MRCRCC, 1999	167	INF-α	Mixed	4		43					
vNegrier, 2002	782	IL-2 or INF-α or both	Mixed	12.8	8.5	17.4		4			
O'Brien, 2004	59	IL-2/ INF-α/5-FU	Mixed		10	53	21	16			5
Part	17	IL-2/ INF-α/5-FU	Good		24		40				
Part	24	IL-2/ INF-α/5-FU	Median		22		38				
Part	16	IL-2/ INF-α/5-FU	Poor		10		6				
Olencki, 2001	20	IL-2/ INF-α/5-FU	Mixed		13.6	50		5	0		
Olencki, 2001	26	IL-2/ INF-α/5-FU	Mixed		22.3			20	<20		
Rogers, 2000	33	IL-2 SC and INF-α SC	Mixed		10	45	30	22	10		
Royston, 2004	172	INF-α	Mixed		45	22	12	5			3
Sleijfer, 1992	27	IL-2 SC	Mixed		12		20				
van Herpen, 2000	51	IL-2/ INF-α /5-FU	Mixed	5	16.5	65	35				
Yang, 2003b	400	IL-2, HD IV, LD IV and SC	Good	20	20	20—30	18–28	15—25			15—18

IL, interleukin; IFN, interferon; PFS, progression free survival; 5-FU, 5-fluorouracil; op, operation.

Clinical studies in mRCC have led to the approval of subcutaneous IL-2 (Europe), continuous intravenous IL-2 (Europe), as well as high-dose bolus intravenous IL-2 therapy (United States) and subcutaneous and intramuscular IFN-α (Europe). Approved systemic therapy is limited to well-selected patients.

Cytokine-based immunotherapy is considered standard in the treatment of mRCC today. Long-term survival and even cure seem possible in a small but substantial subgroup of patients.

Indications/Contraindications

A number of therapeutic schemes have been approved for mRCC or advanced RCC. Patient selection and safety measures for those therapies are well defined. In addition, therapeutic schemes using combinations have been established in routine clinical use and their value is supported by numerous studies.

Interferon-α-2a, Subcutaneous or Intramuscular Application (EU Approved)

IFN-α SC or IM, approved in Europe, is an outpatient therapy. Doses initially are increased from week 1 [3 × 3 million international units (MIU)] to week 2 (3 × 9 MIU) and to week 3 (3 × 18 MIU). This schedule has been based on the first randomized study to demonstrate prolonged survival by using IFN-α-2a for mRCC patients (Pyrhönen, 1999). The total dose to be used in the approved schedule is some 700 MIU in 3 months and the treatment duration is recommended to be 3–12 months, depending on the absence of progression. For patients unable to tolerate IFN-α-2a at 18 million units per injection, the dose may be reduced to 9 million units. Patients with heart disease (including anamnestic heart disease) are excluded from approved therapy as fever and tachycardia may place such patients in danger. In addition, patients with severe impairment of kidney, liver, bone marrow, or central nervous function do not qualify for the approved schedule as well as patients with seizure disorder. Pyrhönen, (1999)has reported a nearly twice as long median survival of 67.6 weeks for the 79 patients receiving IFN-α-2a plus vinblastine compared to 37.8 weeks for the 81 patients treated with vinblastine only (p = 0.0049). Overall response rates were 16.5% for patients treated with IFN-α-2a plus vinblastine and 2.5% for patients treated with vinblastine alone (p = 0025). Treatment with the combination was associated with constitutional symptoms and abnormalities in laboratory parameters, but no toxic deaths were reported.

A survival benefit for the interferon group was also suggested when comparing megestrol with IFN-α (MRCRCC, 1999). Patients with mRCC were randomly assigned to SC IFN-α (three doses—5 MU, 5 MU, 10 MU—for the first week, then 10 MU three times per week for

a further 11 weeks; n = 174) or oral medroxyprogesterone acetate (MPA; 300 mg once daily for 12 weeks; n = 176). Data are available for 335 patients (167 IFN-α, 168 MPA). There was a 28% reduction in the risk of death in the IFN-α group and IFN-α gave an improvement in 1-year survival (MPA 31% survival, IFN-α43%) and an improvement in median survival of 2.5 months (MPA 6 months, IFN-α8.5 months).

The efficacy of IFN-α in mRCC to improve response rates has been evaluated using a variety of preparations, doses, and schedules; an overall response rate of approximately 15% is reported.

Interferon-α Combination with Chemotherapy

Efforts to improve the antitumor efficacy of IFN-α have included combination with chemotherapy, especially vinblastine or 5-FU. However randomized trials comparing IFN-α plus vinblastine to IFN-α alone showed no survival difference between the two groups indicating no value of adding vinblastine to IFN-α (Fossa, 1992; Neidhart, 1991).

Interferon-α-2b, Pegylated

Pegylated IFN-α-2a produces a lower peak serum concentration and a longer exposure time but levels of 1.5–6.0 mg/kg/week did not result in higher efficacy or reduced toxicity in patients with mRCC as compared to standard IFN-α-2a treatment (Bex, 2004).

Interleukin-2, Subcutaneous Application (EU Approved)

This is the only IL-2-based outpatient scheme approved. Subcutaneous IL-2 mediates antitumor responses and reduces toxicities associated with IV IL-2 administration. SC IL-2 was evaluated in a Phase II setting. Eighty unselected, consecutive patients with mRCC or recurrent RCC received IL-2 on an outpatient basis, 5 days per week for 4 or 6 consecutive weeks. During the first 5-day cycle, a dose of 18 MIU IL-2 was administered once a day; during subsequent cycles the dose after the first 2 days was reduced to 9 MIU, which is the basis for the approved doses and time intervals in Europe (Table 11a-3). To circumvent flu-like symptoms, all patients received a maximum oral dose of 3 g acetaminophen daily. Three (4%) complete responses (CR) and 6 (8%) partial responses (PR) were observed, and 44 (57%) patients had stable disease (SD). Response durations were 64, 29, and 29+ months for the CR and 2, 6, 8, 11, 32, and 47 months for the PR. The median length of survival of all patients was 12 months, whereas the median survival of responders and nonresponders was 35+ and 10+ months, respectively (p <0.001). Side effects included fever, chills, nausea, vomiting, and transient inflammation and induration at the injection sites. Side effects completely disappeared after

TABLE 11a-3. Interleukin-2 subcutaneous (SC) scheme as approved in Europe.[a]

	Day 1	Day 2	Day 3	Day 4	Day 5
Week 1	18 M IU IL-2 SC	18 M IU IL-2 SC	18 M IU IL-2 SC	18 M IU IL-2 SC	18 M IU IL-2 SC
Week 2	18 M IU IL-2 SC	18 M IU IL-2 SC	9 M IU IL-2 SC	9 M IU IL-2 SC	9 M IU IL-2 SC
Week 3	18 M IU IL-2 SC	18 M IU IL-2 SC	9 M IU IL-2 SC	9 M IU IL-2 SC	9 M IU IL-2 SC
Week 4	18 M IU IL-2 SC	18 M IU IL-2 SC	9 M IU IL-2 SC	9 M IU IL-2 SC	9 M IU IL-2 SC
Week 5					
Week 6	18 M IU IL-2 SC	18 M IU IL-2 SC	18 M IU IL-2 SC	18 M IU IL-2 SC	18 M IU IL-2 SC
Week 7	18 M IU IL-2 SC	18 M IU IL-2 SC	9 M IU IL-2 SC	9 M IU IL-2 SC	9 M IU IL-2 SC
Week 8	18 M IU IL-2 SC	18 M IU IL-2 SC	9 M IU IL-2 SC	9 M IU IL-2 SC	9 M IU IL-2 SC
Week 9	18 M IU IL-2 SC	18 M IU IL-2 SC	9 M IU IL-2 SC	9 M IU IL-2 SC	9 M IU IL-2 SC

[a] In nonprogressive patients treatment cycles from week 1 to week 8 may be repeated. IL, interleukin.

cessation of IL-2 (Sleijfer, 1992; Nieken, 1996). However, in unselected patients treatment-related death has been reported (Sleijfer, 1992).

Patients with an Eastern Co-Operative Oncology Group (ECOG) scale of 2 or greater (Table 11a-4), significant heart disease, infectious disease requiring antibiotics, $pO_2 < 60$ mm Hg, severe organ diseases, brain metastases, seizure disorders, or all patients in whom all three of the following prognostic factors are present—performance status of ECOG 1 or greater, more than one organ with metastatic disease sites, and a period of less than 24 months between initial diagnosis of the primary tumor and date of evaluation of treatment—are excluded from approved SC or continuous intravenous (IV) (see below) IL-2 therapy in Europe. It is also recommended that patients with leukocytes <4000/mm³, thrombocytes <100,000/mm³, hematocrit <30%, elevated

creatinine or bilirubin in serum, autoimmune disease, foreign organ transplants (danger of rejection!), or who require steroid therapy be excluded.

Patients strictly selected according to the approved criteria achieve favorable median survival times of 24 months, which seems to mainly result from long-term stabilization of their (previously progressive) disease (H. Heinzer and H. Huland, unpublished) rather than from response by tumor reduction.

Interleukin-2, Constant Intravenous (EU Approved)

This has been the first therapeutic scheme ever approved for mRCC. Preclinical studies suggest a steep dose–response relationship for the anticancer effect of IL-2; however, trans-

TABLE 11a-4. Performance status: Karnofsky and Elson.

Karnofsky scale	Karnofsky definition	ECOG scale	ECOG definition
100%	Normal, no complaints, no evidence of disease	0	Fully active, able to carry on all predisease performance without restriction
90	Able to carry on normal activity: minor symptoms of disease	I	Restricted in physically strenuous activity but ambulatory and able to carry out work of a light or sedentary nature, e.g., light housework, office work
80	Normal activity with effort: some symptoms of disease	I	
70	Cares for self: unable to carry on normal activity or active work	II	Ambulatory and capable of all self care but unable to carry out any work activities; up and about more than 50% of waking hours
60	Requires occasional assistance but is able to care for needs	II	
50	Requires considerable assistance and frequent medical care	III	Capable of only limited self care, confined to bed or chair more than 50% of waking hours
40	Disabled: requires special care and assistance	III	
30	Severely disabled: hospitalization is indicated, death not imminent	IV	Completely disabled; cannot carry on any self care; totally confined to bed or chair
20	Very sick, hospitalization necessary: active treatment necessary	IV	
10	Month moribund, fatal processes progressing rapidly	IV	
0	Dead	V	Dead

Sources: Doyle D, Hanks G, MacDonald N. *Oxford Textbook of Palliative Medicine*. New York: Oxford University Press, 1993;109. Schag CC, Heinrich RL, Ganz PA. Karnofsky performance status revisited: reliability, validity, and guidelines. *J Clin Oncol* 1984;2:187–193. Oken MM, Creech RH, Tormey DC, et al. Toxicity and response criteria of the Eastern Cooperative Oncology Group. *Am J Clin Oncol* 1982;5:649–655.

lation of high-dose IL-2 to humans was known to be complicated by major toxicities, including hypotension, capillary leak phenomena, and fluid retention. Different from IV bolus or SC application, continuous intravenous application has the advantage of allowing a very close treatment control as infusion may be stopped at any time in case of unacceptable toxicity. In an attempt to develop a manageable approach to dose-intense IL-2, a continuous infusion schedule, 18×10^6 IU IL-2/m^2/day for 5 days, was reported by West, (1987). This treatment resulted in complete and partial remission as well as stabilization of mRCC. One cycle of the approved scheme consists of 2×5 days CIV therapy separated by 2–6 days and followed by 3 weeks of rest and may be repeated in those stable or responding to therapy. Patient selection and safety measures for the approved scheme are identical to those for SC IL-2.

Interleukin-2, High-Dose Bolus Application (US Approved)

IV high-dose bolus application is the most toxic scheme approved in mRCC, requiring stringent patient selection and the use of specialized intensive care unit facilities. Approval in the United States was granted on the basis of seven Phase II clinical trials including 255 patients in whom 600,000 or 720,000 IU/kg was administered by 15-minute IV infusion every 8 hours for up to 14 consecutive doses over 5 days as clinically tolerated with maximum support, including pressors (Fyfe, 1995). Within 1 week, using this intense regimen, an 80 kg patient may receive up to 800 MIU IL-2, compared to up to 150 MIU IL-2 using CIV or up to 90 MIU IL-2 using SC IL-2 as approved in Europe.

Using high-dose bolus IV IL-2, two identical cycles of treatment are scheduled with a 5- to 9-day period of rest, and courses may be repeated every 6–12 weeks in stable or responding patients. The overall objective response rate reported was 14%, with 5% complete responses and 9% partial responses, which occurred in all sites of disease, including bone, intact primary tumors, and visceral metastases, and in patients with large tumor burdens or bulky individual lesions. ECOG performance status was the only predictive prognostic factor for response to IL-2. While treatment was associated with severe acute toxicities, these generally reversed after therapy was completed. A total of 4% of patients died of adverse events judged to be possibly or probably treatment-related. Fyfe, (1995) concluded that high-dose IL-2 appears to benefit some patients with mRCC by producing durable CRs or PRs and recommend that despite severe acute treatment-associated toxicities, IL-2 should be considered for initial therapy of patients with appropriately selected mRCC.

Selection of patients for this therapy is a critical issue. The U.S. product information for high-dose bolus IL-2 (September, 2000) states that "Careful patient selection is mandatory prior to the administration of proleukin" and

"experience in patients with ECOG PS >1 is extremely limited." It adds that even "patients with normal cardiovascular, pulmonary, hepatic, and central nervous system (CNS) function may experience serious, life-threatening or fatal adverse events. Adverse events are frequent, often serious and sometimes fatal." It excludes patients with significant cardiac (abnormal thallium stress test), pulmonary, renal, hepatic, or CNS impairment, CNS metastases, or organ allografts and recommends extreme caution in patients with a normal thallium stress test and normal pulmonary function who have a history of cardiac or pulmonary disease. Administration in a hospital setting requires an intensive care facility and specialists skilled in cardiopulmonary or intensive care medicine must be available. A detailed description of "warnings," "precautions," and "contraindications" in the product information sheet gives further insight into an essential and stringent selection process of patients. An excellent survey about precautions and how to deal with treatment-related toxicities has been published by Schwartzentruber (2001). It is reported that treatment-related deaths have not occurred in recent years, which may be a result of a learning curve as well as the result of considerable dose reductions in clinical use from the approved 14 doses given per 5 days down to an average of 7 doses per 5 days (Kammula, 1998).

Local Interleukin-2-Based Immunotherapy

Therapies using local delivery of cytokines are intended to mimic their physiological mode of action. Their toxicity profile differs fundamentally from systemic cytokines. Systemic side effects occur in a dose-dependent manner whenever IL-2 is present in the vascular system where it physiologically cannot be found. Since no intravascular IL-2 concentrations arise, systemic side effects such as fever and flu-like symptoms are largely absent. In addition, large IL-2 losses via the kidneys—typical of IV administration—can be avoided. Therapeutic effects of local application are mainly limited to local tumor control. However, systemic immunomodulation, e.g., increase in eosinophils or IL-2 receptors, is present during exclusive local therapy.

Inhaled IL-2 is the most commonly used local application of IL-2 in mRCC. In patients fit for systemic therapy inhalation does not substitute for systemic application but rather can be used in addition to systemic treatment to intensify therapy. Most patients treated so far, however, are high-risk patients not suitable or unresponsive to systemic approved therapy and inhaled IL-2 was their only treatment option left to control lung metastases and prevent suffocation (Huland, 2003; Merimsky, 2004).

Aerosol Interleukin-2 as Only Therapy

Currently only well-selected patients with mRCC are treated with systemic IL-2. A significant number of patients with comorbidity, however, do not benefit from systemic immunotherapy and are excluded from approved immunotherapy because they cannot tolerate approved schedules and experience significant toxicity. These patients as well as those unresponsive to approved schedules constitute a group with unmet high medical need. Of these patients 60–70% present with lung metastases and therefore are candidates for either IL-2 inhalation alone or, depending on their comorbidities, inhalation in combination with systemic therapy, radiation, operation, etc. Inhalation use of IL-2 does not lead to absorption into the blood. It therefore induces local (generally minor) side effects such as cough but no systemic toxicity. Because of significant toxicity a considerable number of patients cannot tolerate systemic cytokine therapy using IL-2 and/or IFN-α. Their median progression-free survival (PFS) is about 2 months, their median survival is below 6 months, and their overall survival is well below 3 years. IL-2 aerosol in patients with pulmonary, pleura, or mediastinal metastases prevents suffocation and achieves long-term PFS, and long-term overall survival similar to high-dose systemic IL-2 but without the toxicity associated with it. It is the only outpatient cytokine therapy with good quality of life, allowing employment or family care during treatment. Inhalation consistently induces a dose-dependent immunomodulation in the lung. Total cells, activation markers, IL-5 production, and nitric oxide increase. Major side effects are cough and fatigue. Inhalation therapy is reported to be a mode of treatment that preserves the patient's quality of life, more than all other modes of IL-2 administration (Merimsky, 2004). In a multicenter study from Israel, 11 centers reported 40 patients with progressive pulmonary metastases of RCC and significant risk factors treated with inhalation of IL-2 who were not candidates for other treatment options (Merimsky, 2004) and did not tolerate any systemic IL-2 application. Twenty-five patients

had at least another extrapulmonary site involved and 22 reported pulmonary symptoms (dyspnea, cough, and hemoptysis) prior to the start of treatment. Outpatient treatment was well tolerated. While only one partial response was seen (2.5%), the long-term disease control rate was high (55%). Median PFS evaluated by an external radiologist was 8.7 months. This is more than the expected median survival for this group and represents the longest PFS reported in patients with high-risk criteria (Table 11a-2). For example, 40 placebo-treated patients (Yang, 2003b) had a PFS of 2.5 months only (Table 11a-1) and after 8 months 95% were in progress.

Aerosol Interleukin-2 Plus Low-Dose Systemic Interleukin-2

A multicenter study (Huland, 2003) compared the clinical response, survival, and safety of 94 "high-risk" patients treated clinically mainly with aerosol IL-2 (inhaled; INH) with 103 patients, comparable "high-risk" historical controls from approval studies, who received IL-2 systemically (SYST group) at the registered dose and schedule in Europe for SC administration. All patients fulfilled today's exclusion criteria to (EU) approved systemic IL-2 therapy. The median survival in the INH group was 12 months and 6.3 months in the SYST group (Fig. 11a-1). Survival in high-risk patients treated with systemic cytokine-based immunotherapy has consistently been reported to be 6 months or less, and no relevant 5-year survival has ever been reported in this group (Tables 11a-1 and 11a-2). The probability of survival at 5 years was 21% for the INH group and 0 for the SYST group. More patients responded (CR, PR, SD) in the INH group (45%) compared to the SYST group (33%). Responding patients of the INH group had a better long-term survival than responders from the SYST group (Fig. 11a-2). The quality

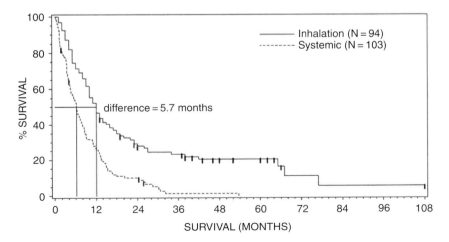

FIGURE 11a-1. Kaplan–Meier overall survival curve of high-risk patients* with mRCC treated with either inhaled IL-2 and very low dose SC IL-2 (INH group, solid line) or systemically administered IL-2 (rhIL-2 SYS group, dotted line). Only INH patients (*n* = 94) on (mainly) inhaled IL-2 had a long-time survival benefit. No SYS patient survived 5 years in the systemic treated group (*n* = 103). [*High risk = documented exclusion criteria for EU approved systemic (SC or IV) IL-2 therapy.]

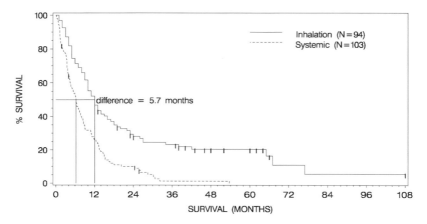

FIGURE 11a-2. Kaplan–Meier survival curve of high-risk patients* with mRCC responding (CR/PR/SD) to IL-2 based immunotherapy. More patients on inhaled IL-2 (45%, 42 of 94 patients, solid line) responded compared to systemic IL-2 (33%, 34 of 103 patients, dotted line) and more patients survived long term on inhaled IL-2 than on systemic IL-2. [*Documented exclusion criteria for approved (Europe) systemic (SC or IV) IL-2 therapy.]

of life during treatment is essentially unimpaired (Heinzer, 1999) and patients are able to fulfill their social role during therapy. Inhalation of IL-2 is efficacious and safe in high-risk mRCC patients with pulmonary metastases who have no other treatment option available.

Nebulizer Device

Modern nebulizer devices decrease the amount of IL-2 required for aerosol therapy down to 25–50% of that before, reducing treatment costs significantly. Approximately 6 × 9 MIU IL-2 per week is required for inhalation therapy, less than the amount required for any of the approved schedules. Not all nebulizers are suitable for cytokine aerosol generation. For example, they have to maintain temperature to preserve biological activity. For patient mobility small and easy to carry as well as battery-driven devices are optimal.

Interleukin-2 and Interferon-α Combination Therapy

IFN-α upregulates the expression of HLA class 1 and tumor-associated antigens, thereby possibly increasing the immunogenicity of tumor cells, and increasing their susceptibility to IL-2-mediated cell lysis. Combinations of IFN-α and IL-2 have been studied in patients with RCC, both with and without cytotoxic agents, by several groups (Allen, 2000; Atzpodien, 2003a; Gez, 2002; Negrier, 1998; Neri, 2002; van Herpen, 2000; Vogelzang, 1993). Most of the combined regimens were used outpatient and those using higher doses of cytokines are reported to be associated with prolonged survival. There are distinct and probably very important differences in the doses of IL-2 and IFN-α between the various protocols using the same substances. This needs to be taken into consideration as it cannot be expected that cytokine effects are independent of doses.

Atzpodien and Kirchner (1995) reported that SC IL-2, SC IFN-α and IV 5-FU achieve a 5-year survival up to 27% in a subgroup of patients with very good prognostic factors. Treatment was effective, safe, and well tolerated in patients selected for a good and intermediate risk profile (Atzpodien, 2004), but is associated with considerable flu-like systemic toxicity. Comedication (e.g., antiinflammatory and antiemetic) before and during therapy is mandatory to control flu-like symptoms. A rapid deterioration of quality of life within the first 3 weeks of this treatment was reported to be possibly associated with complete response (Atzpodien, 2003b). A multicenter Phase II trial of SC administration of IL-2 and IFN-α was tolerated well in an outpatient setting but required frequent dose adjustments. It confirmed response rates and median survival durations similar to those observed with high-dose IL-2 alone or high dose IL-2 and IFN (Dutcher, 1997). Using considerable lower cytokine doses (about 20–50% of the originally reported schedules) as well as shorter treatment times, similar combination regimens largely failed to produce identical results (Rathmell, 2004; mcdermott, 2005; Henriksson, 1998; Negrier, 1998, 2000). This may indicate that dose and treatment time are important parameters that need to be considered carefully (Huland,1998). Rathmell, (2004) investigated a treatment time of 4 weeks (Atzpodien 8 weeks) and a total dose of 108 MIU (Atzpodien 324 MIU) of IL-2 and a total dose of IFN-α of 60 MIU (Atzpodien 234 MIU). It was concluded that this regimen has no significant antitumor activity and report a median PFS of 2.8 months. Negrier (1998, 2000) reported results of an 8-week combination schedule with doses reduced to a total dose of 216 MIU (Atzpodien 324 MIU) of IL-2 and a total dose of IFN-α of 72 MIU (Atzpodien 234 MIU). McDermott in 2005 reported results of a 4-week therapy with 198 MIU of IL-2 (Atzpodien 324 MIU) and 108 MIU of IFN-α(Atzpodien 234 MIU) in a Phase III trial comparing a short-term and low-dose combination regimen with monotherapy of high-dose bolus IL-2. He found a higher response rate (23 versus 10%) for the high-dose bolus therapy with a trend toward better median survival (17.5 versus 13 months). Henriksson´s 6-week schedule consisted of a total of 180 MIU IL-2 (Atzpodien 324 MIU), and 140 MIU IFN-α (Atzpodien 234 MIU) also was reported to be of little efficacy (Henriksson, 1998), with survival similar to the group receiving tamoxifen. In addition, in this study most patients did receive much less than this planned dose. Only 40 of the 65 patients in the treatment arm received 75% or more of the intended dose; 25 of the patients received less than 75% of the intended dose and five of them less than 25% of the intended dose. It probably confirms the fact that adequate patient selection is critical and only those fit and willing to perform therapy should be included in systemic cytokine schemes. Adequate patient selection may be recognized by almost identical numbers of patients intended to be treated and patients treated. Large differences between those numbers may indicate inaccurate selection and require specific attention before designing further trials in order to learn how to optimize patient selection.

Cytokines Other Than Interleukin-2 or Interferon-α

Other single cytokines as well as combination schemes did not produce an outcome better or even similar to IFN-α or IL-2 in mRCC. Toxicity, however, often is equal or even worse. Single-agent IFN-γ therapy, for example, has had minimal or no activity in patients with RCC (Gleave, 1988). Furthermore, the combination of IFN-α and IFN-γ does not improve the results of IFN-α alone (De Mulder, 1995). In a randomized prospective trial in 95 patients with detailed risk stratification the IFN-γ-treated group A failed to demonstrate activity and the combination of IFN-γ- and IFN-α-treated group B achieved a response rate similar to IFN-α alone. The median survival of group A was 7 months compared to 10.9 months in group B and the PFS was 1.4 versus 2.9 months. Responses were seen in group B only and four of five responders were at "good risk." A better survival was found for "good risk" patients possibly because "good risk patients are able to continue treatment long enough to produce a therapeutic effect" (Drucker, 2003). No response is reported in 15 patients with RCC and a good risk profile with a combination therapy of IV IL-12 and low-dose SC IL-2 (Gollop, 2003).

Interleukin-2- and Interferon-α-Based Therapies and Nephrectomy

Data of two identically designed studies support the use of nephrectomy in addition to cytokine therapy to improve survival compared to cytokine therapy alone in patients who present with good performance status. The Southwest Oncology Group (SWOG) randomly assigned 246 patients presenting with mRCC to immediate IFN-α (5 mU/m^2 three times weekly) or to initial nephrectomy followed by IFN-α (Flanigan, 2001, 2004). Although few responses to INF therapy were observed, the median survival was significantly better for patients undergoing cytoreductive nephrectomy (11.1 versus 8.1 months). A similar benefit was noted in an identically designed trial of 83 patients with metastatic disease, sponsored by the EORTC (Mickisch, 2001). Both time to progression (5 versus 3 months) and median survival duration (17 versus 7 months) significantly favored nephrectomy prior to immunotherapy.

Adjuvant Interleukin-2- and/or Interferon-α-Based Cytokine Therapies

Adjuvant cytokine application does not improve the natural course of patients at risk to relapse in mRCC (Atzpodien, 2005; Clark, 2003). In a randomized study Atzpodien (2005) reported a decreased survival in the adjuvant-treated group; however, the number of node-positive patients was larger in that group as well.

Results and Outcome: Response, Survival, and Quality of Life

What Is the Most Important Outcome?

According to an ASCO guideline, "survival is the most important outcome of cancer treatment and toxicity, both short- and long-term, is vitally important. Patient outcomes (e.g., survival and quality of life) should receive higher priority than cancer outcomes (e.g., response rate)" (ASCO, 1996).

Prolonged survival has been reported with both IL-2 and IFN-α; however, systemic therapy using cytokines in approved doses decreases quality of life significantly and has raised the crucial question about a "netto" benefit, e.g., improved survival plus improved or maintained quality of life. In well-selected patients using approved therapy a 10–20% 5-year survival can be reached while those patients without cytokine therapy are nearly all dead within 3 years. Not all patients, however, will benefit from systemic treatment; some may experience toxicity only. As the individual outcome cannot be predicted accurately, patients need to be well informed to make their own choices to accept or deny systemic cytokine therapy under these premises.

The indication for local cytokine therapy may be easier as toxicity is not a key issue. Inhalation of IL-2 is particularly favorable considering cancer outcome according to ASCO´s guideline—increase survival and maintain quality of life. IL-2 inhalation therapy maintains quality of life for considerable periods of time (Heinzer, 1999) and increases survival, especially in patients at risk (Huland, 2003).

TABLE 11a-5. Total number and percent response rate in correlation with performance status ECOG 0 and ECOG 1 mRCC patients receiving high dose bolus intravenous (IV) IL-2.[a]

mRCC	All responding patients (number and %)	Patients with performance status ECOG 0 (number and %)	Patients with performance status ECOG 1 (number and %)
Complete response	17 of 255 (7%)	14 of 166 (8%)	3 of 89 (3%)
Partial response	20 of 255 (8%)	16 of 166 (9%)	4 of 89 (4%)
Total	37 of 255 (15%)	30 of 166 (17%)	7 of 89 (7%)

Source: Fyfe (1995); adapted from product information Proleukin, Chiron, USA.

[a]Experience in patients with ECOG >1 is extremely limited. mRCC, metastatic renal cell carcinoma; IL, interleukin.

Remission Rate

In contrast to the conclusion of a previous publication in 2000, in a recent update of a Cochrane review the difference in remission rate between immunotherapy arms was found to correlate poorly with the differences in median survival. The most recent conclusion is that remission rate is not a good surrogate or intermediate outcome for survival for advanced renal cancer (Coppin, 2005). Unfortunately the Cochrane review did not correlate response rate to performance status and this may explain the current confusion. It is well known that remission rate correlates directly with performance status and assessments of remission rate need to take this in consideration. For example, high-dose bolus IL-2 achieves a 17% objective response rate in ECOG 0 patients and only 7% in ECOG 1 patients (Table 11a-5). To assess treatment efficacy it is therefore mandatory to compare remission rates in subgroups of various performance status as well as various prognostic groups. In groups of identical risk profile, the survival of patients with a partial response or stable disease has repeatedly been significantly better than that of patients who exhibited progressive disease (Figlin, 1997; Huland, 2003). Because mRCC may progress rapidly any correct assessment of remission rate requires a measurement of parameters within a very narrow time window before treatment starts, e.g., usually a maximum of 4 weeks prior to treatment start is recommended. Taking this into consideration, the instrument response rate may still be a useful surrogate parameter.

Progression-Free Survival

PFS in mRCC *without* IL-2- or IFN-α-based immunotherapy is about 2 months and ranges between 1 and 5 months (Table 11a-1). Using approved cytokine therapy with IL-2 or IFN-α (Table 11a-2) an average of 5–6 months and a range of 2–8.7 months are reported. A PFS of 6 months or longer requires either a low-risk status with good prognostic factors plus systemic IL-2 and/or IFN-α

therapy (Atzpodien, 2002, 2004 ; Motzer, 2002) or may be achieved by well-tolerated local application of mainly or exclusively inhaled IL-2 therapy, even in poor risk patients (Merimsky, 2004; Michelsen, 2005).

Survival

Independent of therapeutic activities, survival in mRCC is significantly influenced by risk factors and performance status is among the most important ones. Distinct ranges in survival times in unselected groups are frequent and survival comparing cytokine-based immunotherapy may more reliably be assessed in comparable risk groups. Detailed stratification of study patients according to prognostic factors is obligatory.

Median survival in mRCC *without* IL-2- or IFN-α-based immunotherapy ranges between 3.5 and 15.7 months (Table 11a-1); *with* IL-2- or IFN-α-based immunotherapy (Table 11a-2) median survival shows a tendency to be increased to 6–28.6 months.

Overall survival at 3 years *without* IL-2- or IFN-α-based immunotherapy is well below 10% (Table 11a-1). *With* IL-2- or IFN-α-based immunotherapy a 3-year survival in good risk groups is reported to be about 30–40%, in median risk groups some 15–25%, and in poor risk groups 0–6% (Table 11a-2), again with the particular exemption of local inhaled immunotherapy resulting in a 23% survival in a poor risk group (Table 11a-2; Huland, 2003).

Quality of Life

Systemic therapy is linked to a decrease in quality of life during therapy. Antiinflammatory and antiemetic comedications are frequently required and a distinct measurable decrease of quality of life using the instrument of EORTC QLQC30 to measure quality of life before and at 3 weeks of therapy seems to be predictive for success of therapy (Atzpodien, 2004). Steroids may not be used to treat such toxicities as this abrogates treatment success.

Little impairment in quality of life has to be expected using local therapy such as inhaled IL-2. During therapy Heinzer (1999) reported an unimpaired and stable quality of life for patients for more than a year, with a small decrease at week 4 of therapy. For this analysis EORTC QLQC30 was used before at 1 month, 3 months, 6 months, 9 months, and 12 months of therapy. Patients on IL-2 inhalation therapy are able to perform their social role, e.g., job or family care, with nearly no limitations.

Prognostic Factors

Variants of important prognostic factors in metastatic disease have been published, including performance status, disease-free survival after nephrectomy, disease to treatment interval, nephrectomy status, number of metastatic sites, as well as hematological parameters such as serum lactate dehydrogenase level, hemoglobin level, and serum calcium level.

The better a patient's performance level, as measured by either the Karnofsky or ECOG scale (Table 11a-4), the greater likelihood for long-term survival as well as for response to immunotherapy. In addition, these patients are likely to have decreased morbidity with therapy. Patients who have a 2-year or longer disease-free interval after nephrectomy have a better prognosis, while those who have a recurrence within 1 year have a 2-year survival rate that approaches zero.

Prediction of Survival Based on Prognostic Factors

In 1988, Elson et al. published an analysis of 670 patients who had not been treated with IL-2 or IFN-α. This multivariate analysis resulted in five groups with different median survival and still probably gives very accurate estimates for mRCC patients who do not receive cytokine immunotherapy. Favorable predictors of survival in this model include a performance status of 0 (ECOG, Eastern Cooperative Oncology Group), diagnostic time interval from initial diagnosis (>1 year), absence of recent weight loss, absence of prior cytotoxic chemotherapy, and one metastatic site only. Patients with this favorable combination have a predicted median survival of 12.8 months. With an increasing number of risk factors survival decreases to a median of 7.7 months, 5.3 months, 3.4 months, and 2.1 months, respectively.

Palmer et al. in 1992 considered the following three risk factors——ECOG score (0 versus1), number of metastasis sites (1 versus 2 or more), and diagnostic time interval (DTI) (more than 24 months versus less than 24 months)——and created four groups of patients: "very low risk" with no risk factors (ECOG 0 and one metastatic site and DTI more than 24), "low risk" with one risk factor, "medium risk" with two risk factors, and "high risk" with three risk factors. Median survival for each subgroup is 28, 17, 10, and 5 months, respectively. The model was validated in an independent cohort of 125 patients with RCC treated with SC rIL-2 and predicted for survival accurately. By determining the risk group category in which patients may fall, treating physicians may be better equipped to decide on patient management. The model may also be of value to stratify patients in clinical trials.

In a retrospective review of 463 patients with advanced RCC treated in six prospective clinical trials and followed long term, Motzer (2002) identified prognostic factors for outcome with IFN-α treatment. The median overall survival and time to progression were 13 and 4.7 months, respectively. Five factors independently predicted for poorer survival: Karnofsky PS <80%, serum lactate dehydrogenase (LDH) >1.5 times the upper limit of normal, corrected serum calcium >10 mg/dl (2.5 mmol/liter), serum hemoglobin below the lower limit of normal, and less than 12 months from initial diagnosis to use of IFN-α. Prognosis differed significantly for those with none (good risk), one or two (intermediate risk), or three or more risk factors (poor risk). The good risk patients had higher rates of median survival (30 months versus 14 months and 5 months for intermediate and poor risk patients) and survival at 1 year (83% versus 58% and 20%), 2 years (55% versus 31% and 6%), and 3 years (45 versus 17% and 2%).

Negriers et al. (1998) identified clinical predictors of rapid disease progression (e.g., within 10 weeks of treatment initiation) in a randomized trial of IL-2 plus IFN-α or either agent as monotherapy and included the presence of more than one site of metastatic disease, a progression-free interval less than 1 year, and the presence of liver metastases or mediastinal node involvement. Patients with all of these characteristics had a >70% chance of rapid disease progression and a median survival of only 6 months.

Figlin et al. in 1997 identified the presence of prior nephrectomy and a time from nephrectomy to treatment of more than 6 months as favorable predictors of survival in patients receiving IL-2-based therapy. Patients who began immunotherapy at least 6 months after nephrectomy had the best median survival and a 46% 3-year survival rate.

McDermatt in 2005 published results of the Cytokine Working Group trial that suggested the greatest degree of benefit for high-dose IL-2 as compared to low-dose IL-2 with or without IFN in patients with the primary tumor intact and/or those with hepatic or bone metastases.

Taken together these analyses are in agreement with the main thesis that the presence of more risk factors correlates with lower patient life expectancy.

Morbidity

Toxicity and Management

In 1985 Rosenberg described the IV bolus application of IL-2 in "pharmacological" doses, which for the first time resulted in complete and long-term remissions in some patients with advanced RCC and melanoma, a remarkable treatment success. However, short-term infusion of 50–60 MIU IL-2 three times daily for 5 days caused life-threatening side effects including a 4% treatment-related death rate and excluded most patients from treatment (Rosenberg, 1985). The use of this U.S. approved therapy calls for very extensive patient monitoring, requiring intensive care units, intensive cotherapy, and significant expertise. Physiologically IL-2 cannot be found in the vascular system. It is produced by immune cells locally in the tissue and local vascular leakage by local IL-2 may promote transit of immune mediators from the vascular system to the inflammatory site. A "pharmacological" IV bolus application of IL-2 results in a general leakage ("vasculary oder capillary leakage") with potentially very dangerous toxicities (severe edema, loss of intravascular volume) (Lotze, 1986; Cotran, 1988).

SC application and continuous IV application of IL-2, both approved in Europe, result in less serious but still considerable toxicity. SC therapy of IL-2 can be given outpatient like SC therapy of IFN-α. In addition, and different from IFN-α, SC IL-2 generally leads to local nodal inflammation at the injection site and may cause considerable local discomfort. Systemic IL-2- or IFN-α-based therapies using the approved schedules still do require stringent patient selection and comedication to control systemic side effects is mandatory. Systemic therapies impair quality of life significantly (Atzpodien, 2003a). Systemic side effects of IL-2 and IFN-α are quite similar and their management is generally comparable. Usually they are not managed by reducing the amount of drug given. Instead, treatment is halted temporarily until the side effects subside; then therapy can be resumed.

Typical cytokine-related toxicities include dose-dependent flu-like symptoms (e.g., fever, chills, fatigue, myalgias, and arthralgias), weight loss, depression, anemia, leukopenia, and abnormal renal and liver function tests. Side effects are more prominent in older patients or comorbid patients. Side effects are not immediately present but usually develop during the first treatment days and careful monitoring of patients during this induction period is advisable. After treatment cessation toxicity in general resolves completely and there is no particular permanent damage to be expected. Guidelines for the management of cytokine therapy can be found in the product information as well as in the literature and must be followed closely in the management of the most toxic high-dose bolus IV schedules (Schwartzentruber, 2001). It is advisable to combine systemic cytokine therapy from the first treatment start with antiinflammatory medication to make therapy tolerable and improve the patient´s compliance.

Inhaled IL-2 does not require comedication but in about 50% of patients medication to control cough and usually moderate bronchospasm may be needed. Again steroids, even local (e.g., inhaled), should not be used as this abrogates local immunomodulation and treatment efficacy.

Interleukin-2 and Interferon-α Combinations

Despite the often overlapping toxicities some patients tolerate combination therapies better than intense monotherapies, suggesting that the toxicity profile of both substances cannot be regarded as identical.

Atypical Contrast Media Allergy

Atypical contrast media reactions in patients associated with systemic (Oldham, 1990; Zukiwski, 1990; Abi-Aad, 1991; Fishman, 1991) as well as local (Heinzer, 1992) IL-2 therapy have been reported and considerable acute toxicity has been observed. Use of diagnostic procedures with iodinated contrast media in patients with a history of IL-2 immunotherapy needs to be restrictive and requires special

attention. Patients need to know about this rare but important toxicity of cytokine immunotherapy and as a precaution receive written information to inform colleagues involved in diagnostic procedures.

Controversies

How Important Are Spontaneous Remissions?

Spontaneous remissions rarely occur, but there is still concern that they may mimic treatment success in studies. The number of spontaneous remissions, however, is well below responses using cytokine therapy (Oliver, 1989). Response rate is a surrogate parameter with several limitations. It is known that prognostic parameters influence remission rates of therapy significantly. It is unknown if this may be similar for spontaneous remission. In addition, some infections may increase immune responsiveness leading to "spontaneous" remissions. Hepatitis A infection, for example, preceded a spontaneous remission of liver metastases in one patient of the publication by Oliver (1989) (R.T. Oliver, personal communication). With very few exceptions (Vogelzang, 1992) spontaneous remission does not transfer into long-term survival (Gleave, 1988). In general, survival seems to be the preferred parameter to assess efficacy of treatment.

Is Efficacy of Immunotherapy Altogether Questionable?

"The results of the subcutaneous cytokine regimen seem disappointing" (Negrier, 2000).

"IL-2 and/or IFN-α are routinely used for treating patients with metastatic renal cell cancer. However, results have been disappointing with a majority of treatment failure" (Negrier, 2002). "This study does not support the use of SC IFN or IL-2 in mRCC patients with intermediate prognosis" (Negrier, 2005).

Apart from the already mentioned problem of different (reduced) doses, when comparing "the use of SC IFN or IL-2 in mRCC" disappointing results may also reflect inadequate patient selection. In approved schedules careful patient selection is obligatory by regulatory agencies. Measures to be taken are usually to be found in the summary of product characteristics and to follow them closely is advisable and probably important for treatment success. For many groups reporting disappointing results, it is either unclear how many of their patients do or do not qualify for approved SC cytokine therapy. In the French studies this may well be a significant number. According to the European approval for SC IL-2, for example, patients with a combination of ECOG 1 plus more than one metastatic site, plus a diagnostic treatment interval of less than 2 years, have to be excluded from therapy as no benefit by SC IL-2 can be expected. Negrier et al. in 2000 report the presence of several of these risk factors in their patient group in high numbers, 68% of patients have a metastases-free interval of less than a year, 20% have an ECOG of 1, and 76% have more than one metastatic site; in a different patient group (Negrier, 2005), again, the Karnofsky score was ≤80 in 39% of patients and the time from initial diagnosis to metastases was <1 year in 66% of patients. It may well be that a significant number of patients, unfit for SC cytokines as defined by approval authorities, were included in their studies. Those patients are known to benefit little from systemic cytokines and therefore should not be burdened with cytokine toxicity.

Systemic cytokine therapy is not indicated for every unselected patient. It has to be used in those fit for it. For example, high-dose IV bolus IL-2 therapy has produced very consistent results with a stringent and uncompromised patient selection required for this demanding therapy.

Significance of Survival Benefit

In a recent Cochrane review only a "modest" survival benefit was attributed to patients on cytokine immunotherapy. Using INF-α a doubling of survival from 37.8 to 67.6 weeks for well-selected patients has been reported (Pyrhönen, 1999). The number of patients who respond to systemic cytokine immunotherapy is not 100% but is limited to a subgroup. This survival benefit therefore results from patients in whom (long-term) disease control is achieved. Survival prolongation in individual patients may be quite long and really worthwhile. The use of the word "modest" therefore does not adequately reflect the possible benefit of a patient responding to immunotherapy and may mislead an individual when making a treatment decision.

What Is the "Real Value" of Immunotherapy?

"The value of IL-2 for patients with renal cancer lies in the small probability that this drug can be curative for some patients with metastatic disease" (Yang, 2003).

This rigid limitation of a treatment value to very few patients is disputable. Cure is extremely rare in patients with metastatic disease. Using high-dose IV IL-2 in 155 patients 8 patients experienced an ongoing complete remission at the time of publication (Yang, 2003b) and not all 8 patients will finally be cured. Do we unnecessarily treat the other 147 patients? The data of Tables 11a-1 and 11a-2 show that there is long-term survival in patients receiving cytokine therapy and this may well be due to patients experiencing a partial response or a long-term stabilization of their disease. Few patients without IL-2- or IFN-α-based therapy survive more than 3 years; however, with those cytokines for the first time a relevant 5-year survival in mRCC patients is achieved. It needs to be realized that disease arrest is beneficial in many areas such as diabetes, dialysis, and heart diseases and we may need to learn for oncological diseases as well that a significant delay of disease progression can be achieved;

however, the disease may not be finally eradicated by therapy.

How to Improve Interleukin-2-Induced Treatment Success?

Other than in Europe, in the United States a high-dose bolus IV application of IL-2 in well-selected patients is used and is often reported to be the "gold standard." IL-2 was more clinically active at higher doses using IV bolus therapy than at lower doses in a recently published randomized comparison (Yang, 2003b) echoing animal therapy results of the initial IL-2 development. A further dose increase in patients using systemic application, however, is not feasible. In reality high-dose bolus IV applications have rather been reduced. Since 1998 the maximum number of administered IL-2 doses during the first cycle of therapy decreased from an initial median of 13 doses to 7 doses per first treatment cycle (1998, 1998). Increasing doses at the tumor site will require other measures such as local applications as high-dose bolus IV therapy is already too toxic to be further escalated.

Systemic Interleukin-2 Application

A three-arm study published by Yang in 2003 compared SC IL-2, high-dose IV bolus IL-2 and low dose bolus IV IL-2. Six of 96 patients responded in the high-dose IV group and 2 of 93 in the SC group. No survival difference was found but there was a tendency in high-dose IV patients to experience more complete responses. This study cannot be used to provide evidence for the superiority of the application of IV versus SC, as the SC dose used was rather low and no high-dose SC schedule has been included. Unfortunately, no conclusion can be drawn comparing the approved SC schedule in Europe and the approved high-dose bolus IV application in the United States. The study design (Yang, 2003b) used only about 40% lower doses (310 MIU in 6 weeks) than those used in the approved SC IL-2 therapy in Europe (558 MIU in 8 weeks). In addition, nonprogressive patients in Europe may continue treatment according to SC IL-2 approval and receive on an average two 8-week-cycles. Furthermore, Yang et al. included patients with ECOG 2 (4 of 94) in the SC group only but not in the high-dose IV bolus group (0 of 96). Inclusion of unfavorable prognostic patients has a proven impact on overall treatment results. ECOG 2 is an exclusion criteria for SC IL-2 as approved in Europe and experience in patients with ECOG >1 is extremely limited using a high-dose IV bolus IL-2 as approved in the United States. ECOG 2 patients have not been reported to benefit from U.S. high-dose bolus IV or from SC EU approved IL-2 schemes.

Until today, there is no evidence that the type of systemic application is a key issue. However, the data indicate that the dose administered may be important. Increasing the dose beyond a high-dose IV bolus IL-2, however, will require local applications because of toxicity.

Local Interleukin-2 Application

"Delivery of high local concentrations of IL-2 may more closely mirror the normal physiological production of IL-2, which is normally produced at high concentration in a localized way" (Lotze, 2000).

This is how Lotze in 2000 described possible future roles for IL-2 therapy. IL-2 can be applied in many different ways. Systemic therapy is called "pharmacologic" as IL-2 is not naturally present in the vascular system and local application has been termed "physiologic" as it mimics cytokine action physiologically. Systemic side effects are usually absent using local delivery, since no intravascular IL-2 concentrations occur. Inhalation is the most frequent local use of IL-2 in mRCC. It controls pulmonary and mediastinal metastases in patients with mRCC, administered either alone in patients with no systemic treatment alternatives or additional to standard systemic therapy. It does not generally substitute for systemic therapy and the effect of inhalation is mainly local. Inhalation induces significant local responses in the lung (Figs 11a–3 to 11a–6), long-lasting median PFS time (8.7 months, Merimsky et al., 2004), and long-term survival (21% for 5 years; Huland, 2003). This cannot be explained by a better prognosis in "lung metastases only" disease. Once lung metastases are the only metastatic site, they may be cured by complete resection. Incomplete resection in those patients, however, has no better outcome than metastatic disease in general. In recent reports all incomplete resected patients were dead after 4 years (Hofmann, 2005) or 3 years (Pitz, 2003), respectively. Without effective cytokine therapy long-term survival cannot be expected. For inoperable patients unfit for systemic cytokines local inhaled IL-2 is the only method of effective tumor control.

How Important Is Progression-Free Survival and Stabilization of Disease?

Merimsky et al. (2004) found the longest PFS in high-risk patients (8.7 months) reported so far but only 1 of 40 patients responded. The majority of patients experienced an effective growth control of their tumors. Therefore Merimsky et al. reassessed and modified the definition of response criteria in biological therapy. Stable disease should be regarded as a favorable outcome, a paradigm shift, discussed by other authors as well. The rate of stabilization achieved with IL-2 inhalation was much higher than the spontaneous regression or stabilization of mRCC. The duration of stabilization was significant and probably led to improvement in survival. Therefore, "disease arrest may be regarded as a true response. Consequently, long-term stable disease or a longer time to progression might be a more appropriate treatment end point for biologicals and some of the cytotoxics, than the traditional definitions of response. It should be remembered that from the patient's point of view, stabilization, although traditionally defined as no response, is of course better than progression, especially when it is achieved by a treatment with acceptable side-effects" (Merimsky, 2004).

Are Prospective Randomized Controlled Trials the Only Way to Create Evidence?

Results from six studies ($n = 963$) (Coppin, 2000) indicate that IFN-α is superior to controls when comparing survival. There is a lack of placebo-controlled studies and of randomized controlled studies comparing IL-2 to controls resulting in a controversy about the conclusiveness of treatment effects.

(a)

(b)

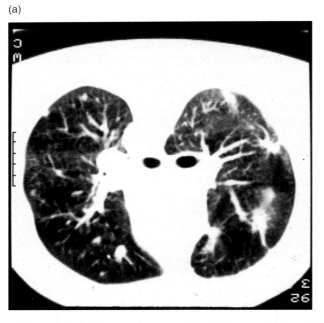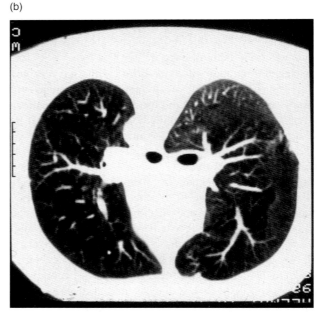

FIGURE 11a-3. Computed tomography (CT) scan of a lung before (**A**) and after 6 months (**B**) of mainly inhaled IL-2 therapy.

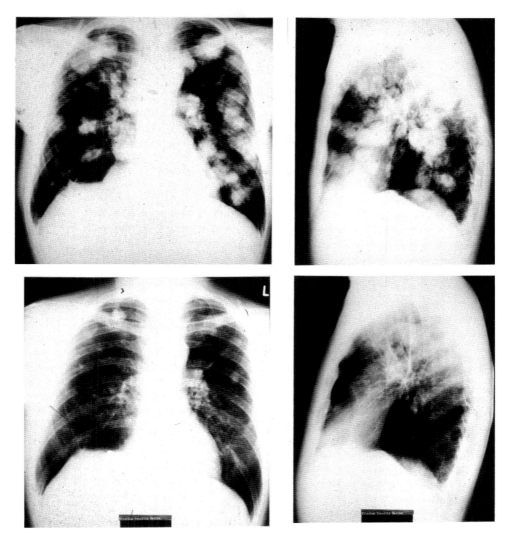

FIGURE 11a-4. X-Ray of patient before and after 9 months of mainly inhaled IL-2 therapy. This is the first patient who ever inhaled IL-2.

It is often stated that evidence should be created only by using randomized designs; however, numerous studies have failed to prove the superiority of a randomized design and observational studies have been shown to give similar information: "We found little evidence that estimates of treatment effects in observational studies reported after 1984 are either consistently larger than or qualitatively different from those obtained in randomized, controlled trials" (Benson, 2000). "It is shown that it has not been demonstrated up to now that well-designed and analyzed observational studies would have yielded results that are distinct or even qualitatively different from results of similar randomized clinical trials" (Koch, 1998). "The results of well-designed observational studies (with either a cohort or a case-control design) do not systematically overestimate the magnitude of the effects of treatment as compared with those in randomized, controlled trials on the same topic" (Concato 2000). "Overall, there is good concordance between randomized trials and nonran-

domized studies, in particular prospective ones, but discrepancies do occur sometimes" (Ioannidis, 2001). There is solid evidence that observational studies do give similar information, which is especially important in a rare and life-threatening disease, as randomized studies require twice as many patients and twice as much time and cost twice as much. A top highlight in this controversy is a systematic review of a British group evaluating randomized controlled trials for parachute use to prevent death and major trauma related to gravitational challenge (Smith, 2003).

Current Limitations of Management and Future Horizons

Today therapy is available for patients with good performance status willing and able to tolerate treatments with considerable toxicity, typically "flu-like" and significantly

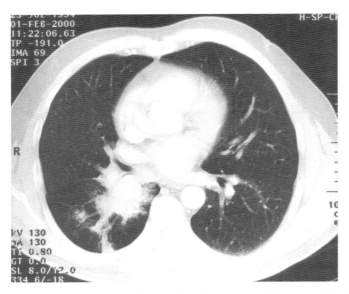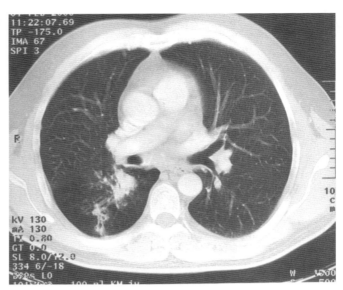

FIGURE 11a-5. CT scan of lung before (**A**) and after 12 months (**B**) of mainly inhaled IL-2 therapy. Treatment started in 3/2000; following partial response this patient was operated on for residual metastases in 3/2002 and 5/2005. He is free of disease 5 years after treatment started (5/2005).

impairing quality of life. Two cytokines, recombinant IL-2 (aldesleukin, Proleukin from Chiron) and recombinant IFN-2α (Roferon from Roche), are approved and used for systemic treatment of mRCC in various countries. To achieve a positive risk-to-benefit ratio strict patient selection is required, respecting contraindications defined by regulatory authorities. Despite the considerable pressure of a life-threatening disease, contraindications should not be ignored as this may put patients in significant, even acute, danger and may result not only in lack of effectivity but in significant toxicity during the final phase of a patient's life. Properly selected patients may experience response or disease arrest and long-term survival using cytokine immunotherapy. But even in selected patients treatment duration using systemic therapy is limited by toxicity and some may experience

toxicity without benefit, as not every patient responds. Systemic application does not use the full potential of cytokines. In patients who are not candidates for systemic cytokines, IL-2 given by inhalation is reported to achieve long-term PFS (Merimsky, 2004) and long-term overall survival (Huland, 2003) similar to high-dose systemic IL-2 (Yang, 2003b) but without the toxicity associated with it. Local therapy offers a wide field for development and cytokine therapy should not be limited to toxic systemic applications but should expand further to well-tolerated local applications with the potential to control local tumor progression. Nontoxic schedules are the key for better use of the high antitumor potential of cytokines.

We do not have a perfect answer to the question of how to treat mRCC today. However, our patients are better off

(a)   (b)

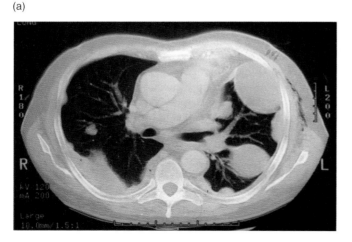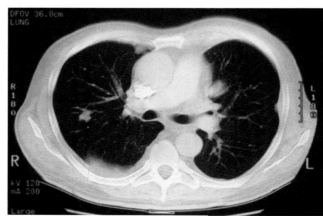

FIGURE 11a-6. CT scan of a lung before (**A**) and after 10 weeks (**B**) of mainly inhaled IL-2 therapy.

than patients several years ago. As we know today, cytokine-based immunotherapy induces "objective responses," which may lead to immediate symptomatic relief and may justify treatment for this reason only. We also now know that significant survival benefit and complete response, perhaps even cure, can be achieved in selected patients. A breakthrough in patient outcome is that a group of "high-risk" patients can now be treated and can achieve a long-term survival remarkably similar to that achieved in high-dose systemic therapy. Today we know that immunotherapy does not always have to be toxic and that variations of applications improve patient outcome significantly. Patients who can be treated with IL-2- or INF-α-based therapies are not candidates for experimental first-line therapies using new agents with unknown effectivity and toxicity. New agents need a good preclinical rationale, may be applied in patients for whom no treatment alternative with IL-2- or INF-α-based therapies exists, and preferably should be tested for survival prolongation in a randomized way. This is sometimes problematic due to the low number of patients in stratified subpopulations. Risk stratification may substitute for randomization. Well-designed observational studies are reported to provide results within the same magnitude of treatment effects as randomized trials today (Benson, 2000; Concato, 2000; Koch, 1998). Detailed information about therapeutic effects, risk stratification, and survival in advanced RCC is available today for standard immunotherapeutic schedules and allows optimum trial designs. In the interest of our patients, the primary goal of new studies should focus on improving patient outcome, defined as survival with a good quality of life.

References

Abi-Aad AS, Figlin RA, Belldegrun A et al. Metastatic renal cell cancer: IL-2 toxicity induced by contrast agent injection. *J Immunother* 1991;10(4):292–295.

Allen MJ, Vaughan M, Webb A et al. Protracted venous infusion 5-fluorouracil in combination with subcutaneous IL-2 and interferon-alpha in patients with metastatic renal cell cancer: a phase II study. *Br J Cancer* 2000;83(8):980–985.

ASCO. Guidelines outcomes of cancer treatment for technology assessment and cancer treatment guidelines. *ASCO* 1996;14: 671–679.

Atzpodien J, Lopez Hänninen EL, Kirchner H et al. Multiinstitutional home-therapy trial of recombinant human interleukin-2 and interferon-alpha-2 in progressive metastatic renal cell carcinoma. J Clin Oncol 1995;13: 497–501.

Atzpodien J, Hoffmann R, Franzke M et al. Thirteen-year, long-term efficacy of interferon-alpha-2 and interleukin-2-based home therapy in patients with advanced renal cell carcinoma. *Cancer* 2002;95:1045–1050.

Atzpodien J, Küchler T, Wandert T et al. Rapid deterioration in quality of life during interleukin-2- and interferon-alpha-based home therapy of renal cell carcinoma is associated with a good outcome. *Br J Cancer* 2003a;89:50–54.

Atzpodien J, Royston P, Wandert T et al. Metastatic renal carcinoma comprehensive prognostic system. *Br J Cancer* 2003b;88(3): 348–353.

Atzpodien J, Kirchner H, Jonas U et al. Interleukin-2 and interferon-alpha-2a-based immunochemotherapy in advanced renal cell carcinoma: a prospectively randomized trial of the German Cooperative Renal Carcinoma Chemoimmunotherapy Group (DGCIN). *J Clin Oncol* 2004;22(7):1188–1194.

Atzpodien J, Schmitt E, U Gertenbach U et al. Adjuvant treatment with interleukin-2- and interferon-alpha-2a based chemoimmunotherapy in renal cell carcinoma post tumour nephrectomy: results of a prospectively randomized trial of the German Cooperative Renal Carcinoma Chemoimmunotherapy Group (DGCIN). *Br J Cancer* 2005;92:843–846.

Bacoyiannis C, Dimopoulos MA, Kalofonos HP et al. Vinblastine and interferon-gamma combination with and without 13-cis retinoic acid for patients with advanced renal cell carcinoma. *Oncology* 2002;63:130–138.

Barutca S, Meydan N, Barlak A. Prevention of interleukin-2-induced severe bronchospasm with salbutamol. *J Aerosol Med* 2003;16(2):183–184.

Bennouna J, Delva R, Gomez F et al. A phase II study with 5-fluorouracil, folinic acid and oxaliplatin (folfox-4 regimen) in patients with metastatic renal cell carcinoma. *Oncology* 2003;64:25–27.

Benson K, Hartz AJ. A comparison of observational studies and randomized trials. *N Engl J Med* 2000;342(25):1878–1886.

Bex A, Kerst M, Mallo H et al. A phase 2 study of pegylated interferon-alpha-2b (Pegintron) for patients with metastatic renal cell carcinoma after removal of the primary tumour. EAU Poster Session 16 2004, 290.

Bordin V, Giani L, Meregalli S et al. Five-year survival results of subcutaneous low-dose immunotherapy with interleukin-2 alone in metastatic renal cell cancer patients. *Urol Int* 2000;64:3–8.

Brinkmann OA, Hertle L. Combined cytokine therapy vs mistletoe treatment in metastatic renal cell cancer: clinical comparison of therapy success with combined administration of interferon-alpha-2b, interleukin-2, and 5-fluorouracil compared to treatment with mistletoe lectin. *Onkologe* 2004;978–985.

Bukowski R, Ernstoff MS, Gore ME et al. Pegylated interferon-alpha-2b treatment for patients with solid tumors: a phase I/II study. *J Clin Oncol* 2002;20(18):3841–3849.

Bukowski RM, Negrier S, Elson P. Prognostic factors in patients with advanced renal cell carcinoma: development of an international kidney cancer working group. *Clin Cancer Res* 2004;10:6310–6314.

Buzio C, Andrulli S, Santi R et al. Long-term immunotherapy with low-dose interleukin-2 and interferon-alpha in the treatment of patients with advanced renal cell carcinoma. *Am Cancer Soc* 2001;92(9):2286–2296.

Clark JI, Gaynor ER, Martone B et al. Daily subcutaneous ultra-low-dose interleukin-2 with daily low-dose interferon-alpha in patients with advanced renal cell carcinoma. *Clin Cancer Res* 1999;5:2374–2380.

Clark JI, Kuzel TM, Lestingi TM et al. A multi-institutional phase II trial of a novel inpatient schedule of continuous interleukin-2 with interferon-alpha-2b in advanced renal cell carcinoma: major durable responses in a less highly selected patient population. *Ann Oncol* 2002;13:606–613.

Clark JI, Atkins MB, Urba WJ et al. Adjuvant high-dose bolus interleukin-2 for patients with high-risk renal cell carcinoma: a cytokine working group randomized trial. *J Clin Oncol*, 2003;21(16):3133–3140.

Concato J, Shah N, Horwitz RI. Randomized, controlled trials, observational studies, and the hierarchy of research designs. *N Engl J Med* 2000;342(25):1887–1892.

Coppin C, Porzsolt F, Kumpf J et al. Immunotherapy for advanced renal cell carcinoma (Cochrane Review). *Cochrane Database Syst Rev* 2000;3:CD001425.

Coppin C, Porzsolt F, Awa A et al. Immunotherapy for advanced renal cell cancer. *Cochrane Database Syst Rev* 2005;1:CD001425.

De Mulder PH, Oosterhof G, Bouffioux C et al. EORTC (30885) randomized phase III study with recombinant interferon-alpha and recombinant interferon-alpha and -gamma in patients with advanced renal cell carcinoma. The EORTC Genitourinary Group. *Br J Cancer* 1995;71(2):371–375.

Donskov F, Bennedsgaard KM, Hokland M et al. Leukocyte orchestration in blood and tumour tissue following interleukin-2 based immunotherapy in metastatic renal cell carcinoma. *Cancer Immunol Immunother*,2004;53:729–739.

Drucker B, Bacik J, Ginsberg M et al. Phase II trial of ZD1839 (IRESSA^TM) in patients with advanced renal cell carcinoma. *Invest New Drugs* 2003;21:341–345.

Dutcher JP, Fisher RI, Weiss G et al. Outpatient subcutaneous interleukin-2 and interferon-alpha for metastatic renal cell cancer: five-year follow-up of the Cytokine Working Group Study. *Cancer J Sci Am* 1997;3(3):157–162.

Dutcher JP, Fine JP, Krigel RL et al. Stratification by risk factors predicts survival on the active treatment arm in a randomized phase II study of interferon-gamma plus/minus interferon-alpha in advanced renal cell carcinoma (E6890). *Med Oncol* 2003;20(3):271–281.

Elhilali MM, Gleave M, Fradet Y et al. Placebo-associated remissions in a multicentre, randomized, double-blind trial of interferon-gamma-1b for the treatment of metastatic renal cell carcinoma. *BJU Int* 2000;86:613–618.

Elson PJ, Witte RS, Trump DL. Prognostic factors for survival in patients with recurrent or metastatic renal cell carcinoma. *Cancer Res* 1988;48:7310–7313.

Figlin R, Gitlitz B, Franklin J et al. Interleukin-2-based immunotherapy for the treatment of metastatic renal cell carcinoma: an analysis of 203 consecutively treated patients. *Cancer J Sci Am* 1997;3(1):92–97.

Fisher RI, Rosenberg SA, Fyfe G. Long-term survival update for high-dose recombinant interleukin-2 in patients with renal cell carcinoma. *Cancer J Sci Am* 2000;1:55–57.

Fishman JE, Aberle DR, Moldawer NP et al. Atypical contrast reactions associated with systemic interleukin-2 therapy. *Am J Roentgenol* 1991;156(4):833–834.

Fizazi K, Rolland F, Chevreau C et al. A phase II study of irinotecan in patients with advanced renal cell carcinoma. *Am Cancer Soc* 2003;98:61–65.

Flanigan RC, Salmon SE, Blumenstein BA et al. Crawford ED nephrectomy followed by interferon-alpha-2b compared with interferon-alpha-2b alone for metastatic renal-cell cancer. *N Engl J Med* 2001;345(23):1655–1659.

Flanigan RC, Mickisch G, Sylvester R et al. Cytoreductive nephrectomy in patients with metastatic renal cancer: a combined analysis. *J Urol* 2004;171:1071–1076.

Fossa SD, Martinelli G, Otto U et al. Recombinant interferon-alpha-2a with or without vinblastine in metastatic renal cell carcinoma: results of a European multi-center phase III study. *Ann Oncol* 1992;3(4):301–305.

Fossa SD, Kramar A, Droz JP. Prognostic factors and survival in patients with metastatic renal cell carcinoma treated with chemotherapy or interferon-alpha. *Eur J Cancer* 1994;30A: 1310–1314.

Fyfe G, Fisher RI, Rosenberg SA et al. Results of treatment of 255 patients with metastatic renal cell carcinoma who received high-dose recombinant interleukin-2 therapy. *J Clin Oncol* 1995;13:688–696.

Gez E, Rubinov R, Gaitini D et al. Interleukin-2, interferon-alpha, 5-fluorouracil, and vinblastine in the treatment of metastatic renal cell carcinoma: a prospective phase II study: the experience of Rambam and Lin Medical Centers 1996–2000. *Cancer* 2002;95(8):1644–1649.

Gleave ME, Elhilali M, Fradet Y et al. Interferon-gamma-1b compared with placebo in metastatic renal cell carcinoma. *Mass Med Soc* 1998;338:1265–1306.

Gold PJ, Thompson JA, Markowitz DR et al. Metastatic renal cell carcinoma: long-term survival after therapy with high-dose continuous-infusion interleukin-2. *Cancer J Sci Am* 1997;3: 85–91.

Gollop JA, Veenstra KG, Parker RA et al. Phase I trial of concurrent twice-weekly recombinant human interleukin-12 plus low-dose IL-2 in patients with melanoma or renal cell carcinoma. *J Clin Oncol* 2003;21(13):2564–2573.

Haas NB, Giantonio BJ, Litwin S et al. Vinblastine and estramustine phosphate in metastatic renal cell carcinoma: a phase II trial of the Fox Chase Network. *Cancer* 2003;98(9):1837–1841.

Heinzer H, Huland E, Huland H. Adverse reaction to contrast material in a patient treated with local interleukin-2. *Am J Roentgenol* 1992;158(6):1407.

Heinzer H, Mir TS, Huland E et al. Subjective and objective prospective, long-term analysis of quality of life during inhaled interleukin-2 immunotherapy. *J Clin Oncol* 1999;17:3612–3620.

Heinzer H, Toma M, Huland E et al. Survival analysis in patients with pulmonary metastatic renal cell carcinoma treated by inhaled interleukin-2 compared to prognostic stratification models. *Eur Urol* 2003;1(2):99A.

Heinzer H, Huland E, Huland H Long-time survival (> 4 yrs) in non resectable pulmonary metastatic renal cell carcinoma and aerosol interleukin-2 therapy. EAU, Poster Session 16: Treatment and prognosis in renal cell carcinoma 2004, 289.

Henriksson R, Nilsson S, Colleen S et al. Survival in renal cell carcinoma—-a randomized evaluation of tamoxifen vs interleukin-2, interferon-alpha (leucocyte) and tamoxifen. *Br J Cancer* 1998;77(8):1311–1317.

Hernberg M, Virkkunen P, Bono P et al. Interferon-alpha-2b three times daily and thalidomide in the treatment of metastatic renal cell carcinoma. *J Clin Oncol* 2003;21(20):3770–3776.

Hofmann HS, Neef, H, Krohe K et al. Prognostic factors and survival after pulmonary resection of metastatic renal cell carcinoma. *Eur Urol* 2005;48:77–82.

Huland E, Heinzer H. Survival in renal cell carcinoma. *Br J Cancer* 2000;82(1):246–247.

Huland E, Heinzer H. Renal cell carcinoma—-innovative medical treatments. *Curr Opinion Urol* 2004;14:239–244.

Huland E, Burger A, Fleischer J et al. Efficacy and safety of inhaled recombinant interleukin-2 in high-risk renal cell cancer patients compared with systemic interleukin-2: an outcome study. *Fol Biol* 2003;49:183–190.

Ioannidis JPA, Haidich AB, Pappa M et al. Comparisons between randomized and non-randomized evidence. BMC Meeting Abstracts: 9th International Cochrane Colloquium 2001, 1:4.

Kammula US, White DE, Rosenberg SA. Trends in the safety of high dose bolus interleukin-2 administration in patients with metastatic cancer. *Cancer* 1998;83(4):797–805.

Koch A, Abel U. Die Rolle der Randomisation in klinischen Studien. *Forsch Komplementarmed* 1998;5(1):121–124.

Libra M, Talamini R, Crivellari D et al. Long-term survival in patients with metastatic renal cell carcinoma treated with continuous intravenous infusion of recombinant interleukin-2: the experience of a single institution. *Tumori* 2003;89(4):400–404.

Lotze MT. The future role of interleukin-2 in cancer therapy. *Cancer J Sci Am* 2000;6(1):58–60.

McDermott DF, Regan MM, Clark JI et al. Randomized phase III trial of high-dose interleukin-2 versus subcutaneous interleukin-2 and interferon in patients with metastatic renal cell carcinoma. *J Clin Oncol* 2005;1;23(1):133–141.

Medical Research Council Renal Cancer Collaborators (MRCRCC). Interferon-alpha and survival in metastatic renal carcinoma: early results of a randomized controlled trial. *Lancet* 1999;353:14–17.

Melichar B, Solichova D, Svobodova I, Melicharova K. Neopterin in renal cell carcinoma: inhalational administration of interleukin-2 is not accompanied by a rise of urinary neopterin. *Luminescence* 2005;20:311–314

Merimsky O, Gez E, Weitzen R et al. Targeting pulmonary metastases of renal cell carcinoma by inhalation of interleukin-2. *Ann Oncol* 2004;15:610–612.

Merimsky O, Gez E, Weitzen R et al. Targeting pulmonary metastases of renal cell carcinoma by inhalation of interleukin-2. *Ann Oncol* 2004;15:610–612.

Michelson G, Esteban E, Garcia-Giron C et al. Review of inhaled recombinant interleukin-2 in patients with renal cell carcinoma with pulmonary metastases. *ASCO* 2005;4756:441.

Mickisch GH, Garin A, van Poppel H et al. Radical nephrectomy plus interferon-alpha-based immunotherapy compared with interferon-alpha alone in metastatic renal-cell carcinoma: a randomized trial. *Lancet* 2001;358(9286):966–970.

Minasian LM, Motzer RJ, Gluck L et al. Interferon-alpha-2a in advanced renal cell carcinoma: treatment results and survival in 159 patients with long-term follow-up. *J Clin Oncol* 1993;11(7):1368–1375.

Minor DR, Monroe D, Damico LA et al. A phase II study of thalidomide in advanced metastatic renal cell carcinoma. *Invest Drugs* 2002;20:389–393.

Motzer RJ. Renal cell carcinoma: a priority malignancy for development and study of novel therapies. *J Clin Oncol* 2003;21(7):1193–1194.

Motzer RJ, Bacik J, Murphy BA et al. Interferon-alpha as a comparative treatment for clinical trials of new therapies against advanced renal cell carcinoma. *J Clin Oncol* 2002;20(1):289–296.

Nakamoto T, Kasaoka Y, Mitani S, Usui T. Inhalation of interleukin-2 combined with subcutaneous administration of interferon for the treatment of pulmonary metastases from renal cell carcinoma. *Int J Urol* 1997;4:343–348.

Negrier S, Escudier B, Lasset C et al. Recombinant human interleukin-2, recombinant human interferon-alpha-2a, or both in metastatic renal-cell carcinoma. Groupe Francais d'Immunotherapie. *N Engl J Med* 1998;338(18):1272–1278.

Negrier S, Escudier B, Lasset C et al. Recombinant human interleukin-2, recombinant human interferon-alpha-2a, or both in metastatic renal-cell carcinoma. Groupe Francais d'Immunotherapie. *N Engl J Med* 1998;338(18):1272–1278.

Negrier S, Caty A, Lesimple T et al. Treatment of patients with metastatic renal carcinoma with a combination of subcutaneous interleukin-2 and interferon-alpha with or without fluorouracil. *J Clin Oncol* 2000;18(24):4009–4015.

Negrier S, Escudier B, Gomez F et al. Prognostic factors of survival and rapid progression in 782 patients with metastatic renal carcinomas treated by cytokines: a report from the Groupe Francais d'Immunotherapie. *Ann Oncol* 2002;13(9):1460–1468.

Negrier S, Perol D, Ravaud et al. Do cytokines improve survival in patients with metastatic renal cell carcinoma (MRCC) of intermediate prognosis: results of the prospective randomized PERCY Quattro trial. LBA4511. *ASCO* 2005.

Neidhart JA, Anderson SA, Harris JE et al. Vinblastine fails to improve response of renal cancer to interferon-alpha-n1: high response rate in patients with pulmonary metastases. *J Clin Oncol* 1991;9(5):832–836.

Neri B, Doni L, Gemelli MT et al. Phase II trial of weekly intravenous gemcitabine administration with interferon and interleukin-2 immunotherapy for metastatic renal cell cancer. *J Urol* 2002;168(3):956–958.

Nieken J, Sleijfer DT, Buter J et al. Outpatient-based subcutaneous interleukin-2 monotherapy in advanced renal cell carcinoma: an update. *Cancer Biother Radiopharm* 1996;11(5): 289–295.

O'Brien MF, Rea D, Rogers E et al. Interleukin-2, interferon-alpha and 5-fluorouracil immunotherapy for metastatic renal cell carcinoma: the all Ireland experience. *Eur Urol* 2004;45(5): 613–618.

Oldham RK, Brogley J, Braud E. Contrast medium "recalls" interleukin-2 toxicity. *J Clin Oncol* 1990;8(5):942–943.

Olencki T, Peereboom D, Wood L. Phase I and II trials of subcutaneously administered rIL-2, interferon-alpha-2a, and fluorouracil in patients with metastatic renal carcinoma. *J Cancer Res Clin Oncol* 2001;127(5):319–324.

Oliver RT, Nethersell AB, Bottomley JM. Unexplained spontaneous regression and interferon-alpha as treatment for metastatic renal carcinoma. *Br J Urol* 1989;63(2):128–131.

Palmer PA, Vinke J, Philip T et al. Prognostic factors for survival in patients with advanced renal cell carcinoma treated with recombinant interleukin-2. *Ann Oncol* 1992;3(6):475–480.

Patel NP, Lavengood RW. Renal cell carcinoma: natural history and results of treatment. *J Urol* 1978;119(6):722–726.

Pizza G, De Vinci C, Lo Conte G, et al. Immunotherapy of metastatic kidney cancer. *Int J Cancer* 2001;94(1):109–120.

Pulkkanen K, Kataja V, Johansson R. Systemic capillary leak syndrome resulting from gemcitabine treatment in renal cell carcinoma: a case report. *J Chemother* 2003;15(3):287–289.

Pyrhönen S, Salminen E, Ruutu M et al. Prospective randomized trial of interferon-alpha-2a plus vinblastine versus vinblastine alone in patients with advanced renal cell carcinoma. *J Clin Oncol* 1999;17:2859–2867.

Rathmell WK, Malkowicz SB, Holroyde C et al. Phase II trial of 5-fluorouracil and leucovorin in combination with interferon-alpha and interleukin-2 for advanced renal cell cancer. *Am J Clin Oncol* 2004;27(2):109–112.

Ravaud A, Trufflandier N, Ferrière JM et al. Subcutaneous interleukin-2, interferon-alpha-2b and 5-fluorouracil in metastatic renal cell carcinoma as second-line treatment after failure of previous immunotherapy: a phase II trial. *Br J Cancer* 2003;89:2213–2218.

Rogers E, Bredin H, Butler M et al. Combined subcutaneous recombinant interferon-alpha and interleukin-2 in metastatic renal cell cancer: results of the Multicentre All Ireland Immunotherapy Study Group. *Eur Urol* 2000;37(3):261–266.

Roigas J, Deger S, Taymoorian K et al. Effects of 13-cis-retinoic acid on chemoimmunotherapy of metastatic renal cell carcinoma—results of a retrospective analysis. *Cancer Biother Radiopharm* 2003;18(2):157–163.

Rosenberg SA, Lotze MT, Muul LM et al. Observations on the systemic administration of autologous lymphokine activated killer cells and recombinant interleukin-2 to patients with metastatic cancer. *N Engl J Med* 1985;313(23):1485–1492.

Royston P, Sauerbrei W, Ritchie A. Is treatment with interferon-alpha effective in all patients with metastatic renal carcinoma: a new approach to the investigation of interactions? *Br J Cancer* 2004;90:794–799.

Schwartzentruber DJ Guideline for the safe administration of high-dose interleukin-2. *J Immunother* 2001;24:284–293.

Shamash J, Steele JP, Wilson P et al. IPM chemotherapy in cytokine refractory renal cell cancer. *Br J Cancer* 2003;88:1516–1521.

Sleijfer DT, Janssen RAJ, Buter J et al. Phase II study of subcutaneous interleukin-2 in unselected patients with advanced renal cell cancer on an outpatient basis. *J Clin Oncol* 1992;10:1119–1123.

Smith KA. Interleukin-2: inception, impact, and implications. *Science* 1988;240:1169–1176.

Smith GCS, Pell JP. Parachute use to prevent death and major trauma related to gravitational challenge: systematic review of randomized controlled trials. *BMJ* 2003;327:1459–1461.

van Herpen CM, Jansen RL, Kruit WH et al. Immunochemotherapy with interleukin-2, interferon-alpha and 5-fluorouracil for progressive metastatic renal cell carcinoma: a multicenter phase II study. Dutch Immunotherapy Working Party. *Br J Cancer* 2000;82(4):772–776.

Vogelzang NJ, Priest ER, Borden L. Spontaneous regression of histologically proved pulmonary metastases from renal cell carcinoma: a case with 5-year followup. *J Urol* 1992;148(4):1247–1248.

Vogelzang NJ, Lipton A, Figlin RA. Subcutaneous interleukin-2 plus interferon-alpha-2a in metastatic renal cancer: an outpatient multicenter trial. *J Clin Oncol* 1993;11(9):1809–1816.

West WH, Tauer KW, Yannelli JR et al. Constant-infusion recombinant interleukin-2 in adoptive immunotherapy of advanced cancer. *N Engl J Med* 1987;316(15):898–905.

Yang JC, Haworth L, Sherry RM et al. A randomized trial of bevacizumab, an anti-vascular endothelial growth factor antibody, for metastatic renal cancer. *N Engl J Med* 2003a;349(5):427–434.

Yang JC, Sherry RM, Steinberg SM et al. Randomized study of high-dose and low-dose interleukin-2 in patients with metastatic renal cancer. *J Clin Oncol* 2003b;21(16):3127–3132.

Zukiwski AA, David CL, Coan J et al. Increased incidence of hypersensitivity to iodine-containing radiographic contrast media after interleukin-2 administration. *Cancer* 1990;65(7):1521–1524.

11b
Antiangiogenic Therapies in Renal Cell Carcinoma

Karen L. Reckamp, Robert M. Strieter, and Robert A. Figlin

Introduction

Renal cell carcinoma (RCC) growth and metastases have been associated with primary tumor-associated angiogenesis resulting from the mutation or hypermethylation of the von Hippel–Lindau (VHL) gene with subsequent hypoxia-inducible factor (HIF) activation accompanied by the downstream effects of vascular endothelial growth factor (VEGF) induction.[14,18]

Angiogenesis in the tumor environment is important for cancer growth, invasion, and metastasis. The balance between proangiogenic and antiangiogenic factors determines the overall angiogenesis in the tumor microenvironment. Angiogenesis stimulating factors and inhibiting factors are listed in Table 11b-1. VEGF has been studied extensively in RCC as an important component of net angiogenesis. Recently, a randomized Phase II study in cytokine refractory patients demonstrated that using the neutralizing humanized monoclonal antibody to VEGF, bevacizumab, resulted in a significant prolonged time to progression in patients with metastatic RCC.[48] Additional Phase II and III trials of bevacizumab alone and in combination are in progress. Inhibitors of VEGF receptor tyrosine kinases have also demonstrated promising activity in clear cell RCC.[9,35,41] However, other factors that regulate angiogenesis in both a positive and a negative manner are clearly involved in this process, and are under investigation.

Angiogenesis

Embryonic vascular development is a complex series of events during which endothelial cells differentiate, proliferate, migrate, and undergo maturation into an organized network of vessels. The first step in blood vessel development is vasculogenesis, the process through which mesodermal precursors differentiate into endothelial cells and assemble into primitive vascular networks.[42] Remodeling and expansion of these primary vessels into arteries, veins, and capillaries of different sizes constitute angiogenesis. Angiogenesis occurs via the sprouting of new blood vessels from existing vessels and by the splitting of large blood vessels into smaller blood vessels. It is highly regulated in normal adult tissues, but in cancer, tumor growth depends on angiogenesis. Angiogenesis facilitates tumor growth and metastasis and, therefore, antiangiogenic therapy may have broad therapeutic potential. A variety of proangiogenic and antiangiogenic molecules are produced by cancer cells, endothelial cells, stromal cells, blood cells, and the extravascular matrix. Delivery of the drug to the target site in the vasculature is efficient, as the endothelial cells are in direct contact with the blood supply. Furthermore, targeting the tumor vasculature, which is derived from the normal host blood vessels rather than the genetically unstable tumor cells directly, may also limit the development of drug resistance.[7]

Vascular Endothelial Growth Factor Family

Blood vessel and lymphatic development depends on members of the VEGF family of proteins and their receptors. VEGF-A, VEGF-B, VEGF-C, VEGF-D, VEGF-E, and placenta growth factor (PlGF) bind to receptor tyrosine kinases inducing receptor dimerization and activation and the transduction of signals that direct cellular functions.[7,10] All VEGFs belong to the cysteine knot growth factor family and are secreted as dimeric glycoproteins. They all contain an approximately 100-amino acid VEGF homology domain characterized by the precise spacing of eight cysteine residues, which are involved in intramolecular and intermolecular disulfide bonds.[10] These glycoproteins belong to a structural superfamily of growth factors that also includes platelet-derived growth factor (PDGF) and transforming growth factor-β.

Key signals regulating embryonic cell growth and differentiation, as well as the remodeling and regulation of adult tissues by VEGFs, are mediated by a family of tyrosine kinase receptors and by nontyrosine kinase receptors neuropilins 1 and 2 (NRP-1, NRP-2).[10] The VEGF receptor (VEGFR) family includes VEGFR-1 (Flt-1), VEGFR-2 (KDR/Flk-1),

TABLE 11b-1. Angiogenesis stimulatory and inhibitory factors.[a]

Proangiogenic	Antiangiogenic
Acidic and basic FGF	aaATIII
Angiopoietin-I	Angiopoietin-2
Hepatocyte growth factor	Angiostatin
Interleukin-8 (CXCL8)	Endostatin
Placenta growth factor	Histidine-rich glycoprotein
PDGF	Interferon-α, -β, -γ
TGF-α and -β	Platelet factor-4
TNF-α	Prolactin fragment
VEGF	Thrombospondin-1 and -2
	TIMPs 1, 2, and 3
	CXCL9, CXCL10, CXCL11

[a]FGF, fibroblast growth factor; PDGF, platelet-derived growth factor; TGF, transforming growth factor; TNF, tumor necrosis factor; VEGF, vascular endothelial growth factor; ATIII, anti-thrombin III; TIMPs, tissue inhibitors of metalloproteinases.

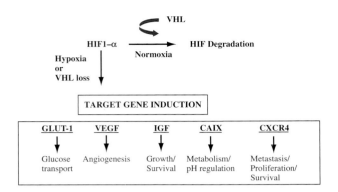

FIGURE 11b-1. VHL, hypoxia, and RCC tumorigenesis. In RCC, the hypoxia-induced pathway is linked to VHL loss. Accumulation of HIF results in upregulation of genes and proteins involved in RCC tumorigenesis, such as glucose transport, angiogenesis, cell growth and survival, metabolism and pH control, and metastasis.[37]

and VEGFR-3 (Flt-4), which belong to a superfamily of receptor tyrosine kinases characterized by extracellular immunoglobulin homology domains and a split tyrosine kinase intracellular domain.[10] The VEGF receptors have partly overlapping, but independent roles in vascular development and maintenance, and the expression levels of their genes modulate the different types of vessels in tissues.

von Hippel–Lindau/Hypoxia-Inducible Factor Pathway

The *VHL* gene was identified and named based on its functional role in the hereditary cancer syndrome von Hippel–Lindau disease. VHL syndrome is an autosomal dominant hereditary cancer syndrome, characterized by the development of highly vascular tumors such as hemangioblastomas of the central nervous system (classically in the cerebellum) and retina, often in association with clear cell RCC and pheochromocytomas.[23] VHL syndrome patients have germline mutations in one copy of the *VHL* gene, and the tumors that develop in these patients have a mutation or deletion of the remaining allele. Somatic, biallelic *VHL* inactivation also occurs extremely frequently in nonhereditary cases of RCC, accounting for up to 70% of these cases.[13,14,18] Thus, *VHL* may be the most important tumor suppressor in RCC.

VHL exerts its tumor suppressor function by negative regulation of the hypoxia-inducible factors HIF1α and HIF2α. A third HIF gene has been identified but has not been critically linked to the pathway described below. The VHL protein forms a multimeric complex with elongin B, elongin C, Cul2, and Rbx1, which target HIF for ubiquitin-mediated degradation under normoxic conditions.[19,24] HIF must undergo proline hydroxylation (a posttranslational modification mediated by the oxygen-dependent enzyme prolyl hydroxylase) in order to bind the VHL complex.

HIF accumulates under hypoxic conditions in normal cells because they are no longer proline hydroxylated and therefore are unable to bind VHL and undergo degradation.[8,20,21] In contrast, cells lacking VHL (due to gene mutation) contain constitutive, high levels of HIF, irrespective of changes in ambient oxygen.[32] HIF binds to hypoxia-response elements (HREs), which results in the activation of numerous hypoxia-response genes. These include genes involved in angiogenesis (e.g., VEGF, VEGF receptor-1, adrenomedullin, PDGF, SDF-1/CXCL12, CXCR4), anaerobic metabolism (e.g., GLUT1), pH regulation (e.g., carbonic anhydrase-IX), and apoptosis (e.g., NIP3, NIX), among others (Fig. 11b-1).[17] Recent data using genetic models have demonstrated that HIF1α is a critical effector of cellular transformation mediated by VHL loss, leading to enhanced interest in the concept that HIF and/or HIF-regulated genes may be appropriate therapeutic targets.[25,31,37] The signaling pathway linking VHL loss, HIF activation, and angiogenic growth factors provides a compelling molecular explanation for the well-known histological observation of intense angiogenesis in RCC.

Hypoxia-Inducible Factor in the PI3K/AKT/mTOR Pathway

Recent data suggest that mammalian target of rapamycin (mTOR) can play a critical role in angiogenesis, raising the interesting possibility that the clinical activity of rapamycin and other mTOR inhibitors in RCC might be explained through this mechanism. There are two distinct potential scenarios that must be considered—one involving the role of mTOR in regulating HIF (and angiogenesis) through the phosphatidylinositol-3-kinase (PI3K)/AKT pathway in tumor cells and the second implicating mTOR in the endothelial cell response to VEGF.

Recent data clearly place HIF in the PI3K/AKT pathway downstream of mTOR. For example, constitutively active alleles of PI3K or AKT are sufficient to induce VEGF mRNA and even angiogenesis.[22,50,51] These effects are blocked by rapamycin and other mTOR inhibitors. Similarly, the receptor tyrosine kinase Her-2/neu upregulates HIF protein expression in breast cancer cells through the PI3K/AKT/mTOR pathway, and this upregulation is blocked by the PI3K inhibitor LY294002 and by rapamycin. In these experiments, HIF is most likely upregulated by increased translation of HIF mRNA (which contains 5′-untranslated sequences sensitive to the mTOR effector S6K) rather than through HIF stabilization (as occurs with VHL loss).[27,43] Therefore, mTOR inhibitors can have antiangiogenic activity by downregulation of HIF in tumor cells, particularly in the setting of PI3K/AKT pathway dysregulation. In addition, recent data have shown that rapamycin is able to decrease HIF-1 levels in TSC2 null cells, indicating that TSC2 regulates HIF by inhibiting mTOR.[3]

Indirect Antiangiogenic Effects of mTOR Inhibition

In addition to direct effects on tumor cells, mTOR inhibitors can also have antiangiogenic activity through indirect effects on endothelial cells in the tumor microenvironment. Endothelial cells respond to VEGF stimulation by VEGFR receptor phosphorylation and subsequent activation of several signaling proteins, including PI3K.[12] Activation of PI3K is critical for VEGF-mediated endothelial cell proliferation, survival, and migration as well as AKT-mediated activation of endothelial nitric oxide synthase (eNOS), as demonstrated using pharmacological inhibitors.[5,11] Similarly, rapamycin is also able to inhibit VEGF-dependent human umbilical vein endothelial cell (HUVEC) proliferation as well as VEGF-induced HUVEC tubular formation.[4,49] In fact, rapamycin-coated coronary artery stents appear remarkably effective in preventing restenosis in patients with coronary artery disease who undergo angioplasty.[6,34] The importance of this mechanism in tumor models was recently demonstrated by showing antitumor activity of rapamycin in vivo against cells that were resistant to rapamycin in vitro. Therefore, the activity of mTOR inhibitors in RCC might be explained solely on the basis of an effect on the tumor vasculature (analogous to VEGF antibody) without invoking a direct antitumor mechanism.[15]

Identification of Molecular Markers of Angiogenesis

The VEGF family is involved in distinct signaling pathways controlling angiogenesis and/or lymphangiogenesis (Table 11b-2). Understanding the expression of these markers will individualize the selection of target-specific therapies based on the tumor biology and optimize the benefit of agents targeting these pathways in RCC. A tissue microarray was constructed from paraffin-embedded clear cell and papillary RCC nephrectomy specimens to evaluate the role of the VEGF family in RCC. Immunohistochemistry was performed with antibodies directed against VEGF-A, VEGF-C, VEGF-D, VEGFR-1, VEGFR-2, and VEGFR-3. In the VEGF angiogenesis pathway, papillary RCC demonstrated a higher mean expression of VEGF-A (57% vs. 37%, $p < 0.0001$) and VEGFR-2 (49% vs. 37%, $p < 0.0001$) than clear cell RCC, while there was no difference observed in the expression of VEGFR-1 ($p = 0.53$).[28] Within the lymphangiogenesis pathway, clear cell RCC demonstrated a higher mean expression of VEGF-D (51% vs. 41%, $p = 0.033$), while papillary RCC demonstrated a higher mean expression of VEGFR-3 (13% vs. 3%, $p = 0.0002$) within the tumor epithelium and no difference was seen in the mean expression of VEGF-C ($p = 0.33$).[28] These data suggests that patients with papillary RCC should also be considered for therapies

TABLE 11b-2. The vascular endothelial growth factor (VEGF) family of growth factors and receptors.

Growth factors	
VEGF-A	Most potent direct-acting angiogenic protein; expression leads to endothelial cell proliferation, angiogenesis, and increased vascular permeability
VEGF-B	Structurally closely related to VEGF-A; very stable and not upregulated by factors that induce expression of VEGF-A
VEGF-C	30% identical to VEGF-A and is synthesized as a precursor protein; VEGF-C gene expression is regulated by growth factors and inflammatory cytokines but not by hypoxia
VEGF-D	61% sequence identity with VEGF-C secreted as a precursor protein
VEGF-C and VEGF-D	Regulate the growth of lymphatic vessels
Receptors	
VEGF-1 (Flt-1)	High-affinity receptor for VEGF-A, VEGF-B, and PIGF
VEGF-2 (KDR/Flk-1)	High-affinity receptor for VEGF-C, VEGF-D, and VEGF-E; major mediator of physiological and pathological effects of VEGF-A on vascular endothelial cells
VEGF-3 (Flt-4)	High-affinity receptor for VEGF-C and VEGF-D; major signaling pathway for lymphangiogenesis

targeting the VEGF-A pathway, which so far have been limited to patients with clear cell RCC. Furthermore, significant expression of VEGFR-1, VEGFR-2, and VEGFR-3 was found within the tumor epithelium demonstrating that VEGFR expression does not appear to be limited to the endothelium of blood and lymphatic vessels.

Survival and metastatic patterns in clear cell RCC were also evaluated. When analyzed as continuous variables, univariate predictors of hematogenous spread to distant metastases included VEGFR-1 ($p = 0.006$) and VEGFR-2 ($p = 0.02$) expression on the tumor epithelium and VEGF-A ($p = 0.009$), VEGFR-1 ($p = 0.006$), and low endothelial expression of VEGFR-3 ($p = 0.0003$), all univariate predictors of lymph node involvement.[26] Low VEGFR-3 expression was retained as an independent predictor of lymph node involvement in multivariate analysis ($p = 0.01$) with a 4-fold increase in risk of lymphatic metastasis. When evaluating disease-specific survival, VEGF-A ($p = 0.0004$), VEGFR-1 ($p < 0.0001$), VEGFR-2 ($p = 0.01$), and VEGFR-3 ($p = 0.008$) in tumor-associated endothelium were significant in univariate models. Only low endothelial expression of VEGFR-3 was retained as an independent predictor of survival in multivariate analysis ($p = 0.02$).[26] These findings suggest that decreased expression of VEGFR-3 is an independent predictor of both nodal metastases and poor disease-free survival.

CXC Chemokines in Renal Cell Carcinoma Angiogenesis

CXC chemokines are important for enhancing immunity, regulating angiogenesis, and mediating tumor cell metastases. They are a cytokine family in which members display either angiogenic or angiostatic activity. CXC chemokines are heparin-binding proteins that display disparate roles in the regulation of angiogenesis. They have four highly conserved cysteine amino acid residues, with the first two cysteines separated by a nonconserved amino acid residue.[2,29,47] A second structural domain within the CXC chemokine family also dictates their functional activity. The NH_2-terminus of several CXC chemokines contains three amino acid residues (Glu-Leu-Arg; the "ELR" motif), which precedes the first cysteine amino acid residue of the primary structure of these cytokines.[2,29,47] Members that contain the "ELR" motif (ELR$^+$) are equipotent angiogenic factors with basic fibroblast growth factor (bFGF) and VEGF.[47] In contrast, members that lack the ELR motif (ELR$^-$) and are interferon (IFN) inducible, inhibit angiogenesis.[47] Therefore, on both structural and functional levels the CXC chemokine family plays an integral role in the promotion or inhibition of angiogenesis relevant to RCC.

The importance of the ELR$^+$ CXC chemokines and their receptor, CXCR2, in RCC tumor growth and angiogenesis has been shown in a murine model (R.M. Strieter, 2005, personal communication). Preclinical models have demonstrated the integral role of CXC chemokines in the regulation of angiogenesis in metastatic RCC. ELR$^+$ CXC chemokines promote angiogenesis through CXCR2. The angiostatic members of the CXC chemokine family include CXCL4, CXCL9, CXCL10, and CXCL11.[2,46,47] Interferon-inducible CXC chemokines (CXCL9, CXCL10, and CXCL11) act through their putative receptor, CXCR3, and promote cell-mediated immunity and inhibit angiogenesis (i.e., "immunoangiostasis"). Interleukin (IL)-2 is the major agonist for the expression of CXCR3 on Th1 cells, which promote antitumor immune responses. Furthermore, a recent study demonstrated a strong correlation between CXCR3 expression and survival in patients with advanced melanoma,[36] suggesting its importance in tumor growth and invasion. Another study demonstrated that systemic priming with IL-2 could lead to a kinetic expression of chemokine receptor, CXCR3, from peripheral blood mononuclear cells (PBMCs) of patients with metastatic RCC receiving standard therapy with high-dose IL-2.[40] CXCR3 expression on circulating mononuclear cells of patients with metastatic RCC also increased in response to high-dose IL-2 therapy. CXCR3 expression on CD4, CD8, and natural killer (NK) cells rose in response to high-dose IL-2 treatment. The induction of CXCR3 expression of PBMCs was most pronounced in a patient with a complete response to therapy. Chemokines have been found to display pleiotropic activity, such as recruitment of specific subsets of leukocytes and regulation of angiogenesis.[45] On the basis of the ability of IFN-inducible CXC chemokines (CXCL9, CXCL10, CXCL11) to promote Th1 immunity and inhibit angiogenesis, they have a potential biological role in promoting tumor regression.

Immunoangiostasis may be optimized by first priming the systemic pool of PBMCs to upregulate the expression of CXCR3 by using less than maximally tolerated systemic administration of IL-2. The second step includes increasing the chemotactic gradient in order to target these cells to the tumor using a stimulus of local tumor overexpression of CXCR3 ligands (IFN-inducible CXC chemokines). The effect of this temporal and spatial therapy would enhance selective and specific extravasation of Th1 cells into the tumor, enhance Th1-mediated immunity in situ to tumor-associated antigens, increase the expression of local IFNs, augment the local expression of CXCR3 ligands, amplify in situ Th1-mediated immunity, and at the same time promote CXCR3 ligand-related angiostasis—the concept of immunoangiostasis. While investigators have focused on CXCR3 and its ligands in tumor immunity, the missing link to ultimately improve this response was the mechanism to increase CXCR3 on PBMCs through the concept of systemic priming with IL-2. In other words, overexpression of a CXCR3 ligand alone at the local tumor level will not be sufficient to recruit PBMCs to the tumor unless they are primed and activated with upregulated expression of CXCR3. Therefore, both components of the CXCR3/CXCR3 ligand biological axis must be optimized for recruitment of mononuclear cells.

Bevacizumab

A revolutionary advance contributing to an improved understanding of pathways underlying RCC has been the recognition of VEGF-A, an important regulator of tumor-induced angiogenesis. This focus on the molecular genetics of RCC has paved the way for the development of new agents designed to block VEGF-A signaling and impede the cascade of events leading up to tumor formation. Such a blockade has been shown to inhibit tumor growth in a variety of models, including genetic models of cancer. Recently, bevacizumab, a neutralizing antibody to VEGF-A, has been shown to prolong the time to progression in patients with metastatic clear cell RCC. A recent randomized Phase II clinical trial to evaluate the activity of bevacizumab in 116 cytokine-refractory patients with metastatic RCC demonstrated significant prolongation of time to progression in patients receiving high-dose antibody.[48] The probabilities of being progression free for patients given high-dose antibody, low-dose antibody, or placebo were 64%, 39%, and 20% at 4 months, respectively, and 30%, 14%, and 5% at 8 months, respectively.

The most common toxicities seen with bevacizumab were hypertension (20%) and proteinuria (7%). Grade 3 toxicities were seen in 33% of the high-dose arm and in 5% of the low-dose arm (vs. 0% with placebo).[48] Recently, the combination of bevacizumab and erlotinib was studied as first- or second-line treatment for metastatic RCC with a response rate of 25% and a stable disease rate of 61%.[16,44] Currently, randomized, prospective Phase II and III trials are evaluating bevacizumab in combination in previously untreated patients either alone or in combination with erlotinib or IFN-α.

Sorafenib (BAY 43-9006)

BAY 43-9006 (Bayer Pharmaceuticals, West Haven, CT, http://www.bayerpharma-na.com and Onyx Pharmaceuticals, Richmond, CA, http://onyx-pharma.com) is an orally bioavailable biaryl urea Raf kinase inhibitor that has demonstrated inhibition in Ras-dependent human tumor xenograft models.[30] Activated Ras promotes cell proliferation through the Raf/MEK/ERK pathway by binding to and activating Raf kinase. BAY 43-9006 has also demonstrated direct inhibition of VEGFR-2, VEGFR-3, and PDGFR-β. Xenograft models treated with daily BAY 43-9006 also demonstrated significant inhibition of tumor angiogenesis, as measured by anti-CD31 immunostaining.

Following activity demonstrated in Phase I trials and the randomized discontinuation trial reported by Ratain et al.,[38,39] Phase III trials were pursued. The TARGETs (Treatment Approaches in Renal Cancer Global Evaluation Trial) group recently reported results from the randomized Phase III trial of sorafenib (BAY 43-9006).[9] Patients who had received one prior systemic therapy for advanced RCC were randomized to receive oral sorafenib, 400 mg twice a day (n = 384) or

placebo (n = 385). Seven patients (2%) demonstrated a partial response (PR) according to Response Evaluation Criteria In Solid Tumors (RECIST) criteria and 78% had stable disease over the course of the study. Tumor shrinkage was observed in the majority of patients (74%) treated with sorafenib. Preliminary data from this trial demonstrated a significant improvement in progression-free survival (PFS) for patients on sorafenib compared to placebo (24 weeks vs. 12 weeks, $p < 0.0001$).

Sorafenib was well tolerated with manageable side effects. Toxicities were most commonly Grade 1 or 2 and included rash/desquamation (31%), diarrhea (30%), hand–foot skin reaction (26%), alopecia (23%), fatigue (18%), pruritus (14%), anorexia (9%), hypertension (8%), and dry skin (7%). Grade 3/4 toxicities included hypophosphatemia (11%), elevated lipase (10%), and lymphopenia (9%). Current efforts include treatment of previously untreated patients with sorafenib, or its use in combination with other targeted agents.

Sunitinib (SU11248)

SU11248 (Pfizer, Inc., La Jolla, CA, http://www.pfizer.com) is an orally bioavailable oxindole small-molecule tyrosine kinase inhibitor of VEGFR-2 and PDGFR-β. Inhibition of VEGF-induced proliferation of endothelial cells and PDGF-induced proliferation of mouse fibroblast cells has been demonstrated in vitro.[33] Growth inhibition of various implanted solid tumors and eradication of larger, established tumors have been demonstrated in mouse xenograft models.

SU11248 was investigated in two sequentially conducted single-arm, multicenter phase II trials in advanced RCC patients failing initial cytokine therapy (Trial 1, n = 63 and Trial 2, n = 106).[35] Trial 1 included patients with any RCC histology and Trial 2 included only patients with clear cell histology. Patients were treated with oral SU11248, 50 mg daily on a 4-weeks-on/2-weeks-off cycle. Of 63 patients enrolled in Trial 1, 25 (40%) achieved a PR, 18 (28%) had stable disease, and 16 (25%) had progression as the best response. Of 25 patients who achieved a PR, the median duration of response was 12.5 months (range 2.2–19.4); eight remain progression free at 21+ to 24+ months from the start of therapy (six patients remain on SU11248 and two patients off SU11248 after being rendered no evidence of disease by surgery). The median time to PR was 2.3 months (range: 0.8–13.6). The median time to progression (TTP) was 8.7 months and the median survival was 16.4 months. Of 106 patients enrolled in Trial 2, preliminary data show that 40 (38%) achieved a PR, 1 (1%) had a complete response, 25 (23%) had stable disease, and 33 (31%) had progression as the best response.

Toxicities were most commonly Grade 1 or 2 in both trials and included fatigue (38% and 22%), diarrhea (26% and 16%), nausea (19% and 13%), and stomatitis (19 and 14%). Grade 3/4 toxicities included neutropenia (13% and 13%),

TABLE 11b-3. Metastatic renal cell carcinoma trials.[a]

Regimen	Sponsor	Status
Phase III sorafenib vs. placebo	Bayer/Onyx	Completed
Phase II sorafenib vs. IFN	Bayer/Onyx	Accruing
Phase III SU 11248 vs. IFN	Pfizer	Completed
Phase III bevacizumab +IFN vs. IFN	Genentech	Accruing
Phase III CCI-779 + IFN vs. IFN vs. CCI-779	Wyeth	Completed
Phase II bevacizumab ± erlotinib	Genentech	Completed
Bevacizumab + HD IL-2	Chiron/Genentech	Accruing
Bevacizumab + sorafenib	Genentech	Accruing
SU 11248 in bevacizumab refractory patients	Pfizer	Accruing
E2804-6 arm combination trial	ECOG	In development

[a]IFN, interferon; HD, high dose; IL, interleukin; ECOG, Eastern Cooperative Oncology Group.

anemia (10% and 6%), and elevated lipase (21% and 15%) and amylase (8% and 3%) without clinical signs of pancreatitis. A randomized Phase III trial versus IFN-α monotherapy in untreated metastatic RCC patients is ongoing.

A Phase II clinical trial of AG-013736, an oral small molecule inhibitor of VEGFR-1, VEGFR-2, and PDGFR-β, enrolled a total of 52 patients who had failed a cytokine-based therapy.[41] The best response as assessed by RECIST criteria was PR in 21 patients (40%). With a median follow-up of 1 year (235–387 days), 13 patients (25%) have progressed, 3 (6%) have discontinued for adverse events, and 36 (69%) remain on study with response or stable disease. The median TTP has not been reached, and only one patient with PR has relapsed (after 232 days of therapy). Drug-related hypertension was observed in 17 patients (33%), and one patient was discontinued for worsening hypertension. Other related toxicities were mostly Grade 1/2 events including fatigue (29%), nausea (29%), diarrhea (27%), hoarseness (19%), anorexia (17%), and weight loss (15%). Grade 3/4 toxicities related to AG-013736 in more than one patient include hypertension (12%), aggravated hypertension (6%), diarrhea (6%), fatigue (6%), blister (4%), and limb pain (4%). There were no cases of neutropenia or thrombocytopenia above Grade 1.

CCI-779

In 2004, Atkins et al.[1] evaluated the efficacy and safety of three different doses of CCI-779 in patients with advanced refractory RCC. All included patients had extensive disease and had been heavily pretreated without success. One hundred and eleven patients were randomized to receive CCI-779 (IV) 25 mg/week in a 30-minute continuous infusion ($n = 36$), or 75 mg/week ($n = 38$), or 250 mg/week ($n = 37$). Response rates were similar between groups with an objective response of 5.6% in the 25 mg group, 7.9% in the 75 mg group, and 8.1% in the 250 mg group. The median time to progression was 6.3, 6.7, and 5.2 months, respectively. Analysis showed a probability of 2-year survival of 24%, 26%, and 36% for each of the groups, with a median survival duration of 13.8, 11, and 17.5 months respectively.

Toxicities seen with CCI-779 included hyperglycemia (17%), hypophosphatemia (13%), anemia (9%), and hypertriglyceridemia (6%). Treatment was generally well tolerated, with no significant differences in the percentage of patients who presented Grade 1–4 toxic events in the three study arms. No treatment-related deaths were reported. A randomized, placebo-controlled trial of IFN-α versus IFN-α plus CCI-779 versus CCI-779 awaits completion and reporting of the results.

Conclusions

Angiogenesis has been implicated in regulating RCC growth and metastases. There is increasing evidence for the involvement of multiple angiogenic factors in this diverse process. The inhibition of angiogenesis, either directly through VEGF and its receptors or indirectly through signaling pathways, has shown efficacy in advanced RCC, primarily of the clear cell histology and in the cytokine refractory setting. The importance of these agents in the adjuvant setting and in combination with other targeted agents in metastatic disease is currently being evaluated. Clinical trials in these areas are ongoing and will help to determine mechanisms of angiogenesis in RCC (Table 11b-3). In addition, delineation of how angiogenic-dependent genes and proteins modulate the malignant phenotype will provide novel insights in kidney cancer pathogenesis.

References

1. Atkins MB, Hidalgo M, Stadler WM et al. Randomized phase II study of multiple dose levels of CCI-779, a novel mammalian target of rapamycin kinase inhibitor, in patients with advanced refractory renal cell carcinoma. *J Clin Oncol* 2004;22:909–918.
2. Belperio JA, Keane MP, Arenberg DA et al. CXC chemokines in angiogenesis. *J Leukoc Biol* 2000;68:1–8.
3. Brugarolas JB, Vazquez F, Reddy A et al. TSC2 regulates VEGF through mTOR-dependent and -independent pathways. *Cancer Cell* 2003;4:147–158.

4. Dayanir V, Meyer RD, Lashkari K *et al*. Identification of tyrosine residues in vascular endothelial growth factor receptor-2/FLK-1 involved in activation of phosphatidylinositol 3-kinase and cell proliferation. *J Biol Chem* 2001;276:17686–17692.

5. Dimmeler S, Fleming I, Fisslthaler B *et al*. Activation of nitric oxide synthase in endothelial cells by AKT-dependent phosphorylation. *Nature* 1999;399:601–605.

6. Duda SH, Pusich B, Richter G *et al*. Sirolimus-eluting stents for the treatment of obstructive superficial femoral artery disease: six-month results. *Circulation* 2002;106:1505–1509.

7. Dvorak HF. Vascular permeability factor/vascular endothelial growth factor: a critical cytokine in tumor angiogenesis and a potential target for diagnosis and therapy. *J Clin Oncol* 2002;20:4368–4380.

8. Epstein AC, Gleadle JM, McNeill LA *et al*. C. elegans EGL-9 and mammalian homologs define a family of dioxygenases that regulate HIF by prolyl hydroxylation. *Cell* 2001;107:43–54.

9. Escudier B, Szczylik C, Eisen T *et al*. Randomized phase III trial of the Raf kinase and VEGFR inhibitor sorafenib (BAY 43–9006) in patients with advanced renal cell carcinoma (RCC). *J Clin Oncol* 2005;23:S648 (abstract 4510).

10. Ferrara N, Gerber HP, LeCouter J. The biology of VEGF and its receptors. *Nat Med* 2003;9:669–676.

11. Fulton D, Gratton JP, McCabe TJ *et al*. Regulation of endothelium-derived nitric oxide production by the protein kinase AKT. *Nature* 1999;399:597–601.

12. Gerber HP, McMurtrey A, Kowalski J *et al*. Vascular endothelial growth factor regulates endothelial cell survival through the phosphatidylinositol 3′-kinase/AKT signal transduction pathway. Requirement for Flk-1/KDR activation. *J Biol Chem* 1998;273:30336–30343.

13. Gnarra JR, Glenn GM, Latif F *et al*. Molecular genetic studies of sporadic and familial renal cell carcinoma. *Urol Clin North Am* 1993;20:207–216.

14. Gnarra JR, Tory K, Weng Y *et al*. Mutations of the VHL tumour suppressor gene in renal carcinoma. *Nat Genet* 1994;7:85–90.

15. Guba M, von Breitenbuch P, Steinbauer M *et al*. Rapamycin inhibits primary and metastatic tumor growth by antiangiogenesis: involvement of vascular endothelial growth factor. *Nat Med* 2002;8:128–135.

16. Hainsworth JD, Sosman JA, Spigel DR *et al*. Phase II trial of bevacizumab and erlotinib in patients with metastatic renal carcinoma (RCC). *J Clin Oncol* 2004;22:14S (abstract 4502).

17. Harris AL. Hypoxia—a key regulatory factor in tumour growth. *Nat Rev Cancer* 2002;2:38–47.

18. Herman JG, Latif F, Weng Y *et al*. Silencing of the VHL tumor-suppressor gene by DNA methylation in renal carcinoma. *Proc Natl Acad Sci USA* 1994;91:9700–9704.

19. Ivan M, Kaelin WG Jr. The von Hippel-Lindau tumor suppressor protein. *Curr Opin Genet Dev* 2001;11:27–34.

20. Ivan M, Kondo K, Yang H *et al*. HIFalpha targeted for VHL-mediated destruction by proline hydroxylation: implications for O2 sensing. *Science* 2001;292:464–468.

21. Jaakkola P, Mole DR, Tian YM *et al*. Targeting of HIF-alpha to the von Hippel-Lindau ubiquitylation complex by O2-regulated prolyl hydroxylation. *Science* 2001;292:468–472.

22. Jiang BH, Jiang G, Zheng JZ *et al*. Phosphatidylinositol 3-kinase signaling controls levels of hypoxia-inducible factor 1. *Cell Growth Differ* 2001;12:363–369.

23. Kaelin WG. Molecular basis of the VHL hereditary cancer syndrome. *Nat Rev Cancer* 2002;2:673–682.

24. Kondo K, Kaelin WG Jr. The von Hippel-Lindau tumor suppressor gene. *Exp Cell Res* 2001;264:117–125.

25. Kondo K, Klco J, Nakamura E *et al*. Inhibition of HIF is necessary for tumor suppression by the von Hippel-Lindau protein. *Cancer Cell* 2002;1:237–246.

26. Lam JS, Leppert JT, Yu H *et al*. Expression of the vascular endothelial growth factor family in tumor dissemination and disease free survival in clear cell renal cell carcinoma. *J Clin Oncol* 2005;23:16S (abstract 4538).

27. Laughner E, Taghavi P, Chiles K *et al*. HER2 (neu) signaling increases the rate of hypoxia-inducible factor 1alpha (HIF-1alpha) synthesis: novel mechanism for HIF-1-mediated vascular endothelial growth factor expression. *Mol Cell Biol* 2001;21:3995–4004.

28. Leppert JT, Lam JS, Yu H, *et al*. Targeting the vascular endothelial growth factor pathway in renal cell carcinoma, a tissue array based analysis. *J Clin Oncol* 2005;23:16S (abstract 4536).

29. Luster AD. Chemokines—chemotactic cytokines that mediate inflammation. *N Engl J Med* 1998;338:436–445.

30. Lyons JF, Wilhelm S, Hibner B, *et al*. Discovery of a novel Raf kinase inhibitor. *Endocr Relat Cancer* 2001;8:219–225.

31. Maranchie JK, Vasselli JR, Riss J *et al*. The contribution of VHL substrate binding and HIF1-alpha to the phenotype of VHL loss in renal cell carcinoma. *Cancer Cell* 2002;1:247–255.

32. Maxwell PH, Wiesener MS, Chang GW *et al*. The tumour suppressor protein VHL targets hypoxia-inducible factors for oxygen-dependent proteolysis. *Nature* 1999;399:271–275.

33. Mendel DB, Laird AD, Xin X *et al*. In vivo antitumor activity of SU11248, a novel tyrosine kinase inhibitor targeting vascular endothelial growth factor and platelet-derived growth factor receptors: determination of a pharmacokinetic/pharmacodynamic relationship. *Clin Cancer Res* 2003;9:327–337.

34. Morice MC, Serruys PW, Sousa JE *et al*. A randomized comparison of a sirolimus-eluting stent with a standard stent for coronary revascularization. *N Engl J Med* 2002;346:1773–1780.

35. Motzer RJ, Rini BI, Michaelson MD *et al*. Phase 2 trials of SU11248 show antitumor activity in second-line therapy for patients with metastatic renal cell carcinoma (RCC). *J Clin Oncol* 2005;23:16S (abstract 4508).

36. Mullins IM, Slingluff CL, Lee JK *et al*. CXC chemokine receptor 3 expression by activated CD8+ T cells is associated with survival in melanoma patients with stage III disease. *Cancer Res* 2004;64:7697–7701.

37. Pantuck AJ, Zeng G, Belldegrun AS *et al*. Pathobiology, prognosis, and targeted therapy for renal cell carcinoma: exploiting the hypoxia-induced pathway. *Clin Cancer Res* 2003;9:4641–4652.

38. Ratain MJ, Eisen T, Stadler WM *et al* . Final findings from a Phase II, placebo-controlled, randomized discontinuation trial (RDT) of sorafenib (BAY 43–9006) in patients with advanced renal cell carcinoma (RCC) *J Clin Oncol* 2005;23:16S (abstract 4544).

39. Ratain MJ, Flaherty KT, Stadler WM *et al*. Preliminary antitumor activity of BAY 43–9006 in metastatic renal cell carcinoma and other advanced refractory solid tumors in a

phase II randomized discontinuation trial (RDT). *J Clin Oncol* 2004;22:14S (abstract 4501).

40. Reckamp KL, Burdick MD, Strieter RM *et al*. The importance of the CXCR3/CXCR3 ligand biological axis in metastatic renal cell carcinoma. *Proc Am Assoc Cancer Res* 2005;46:1092 (abstract 4627).

41. Rini B, Rixe O, Bukowski R *et al*. AG-013736, a multi-target tyrosine kinase receptor inhibitor, demonstrates anti-tumor activity in a phase 2 study of cytokine-refractory, metastatic renal cell cancer (RCC). *J Clin Oncol* 2005;23;16S (abstract 4509).

42. Risau W. Mechanisms of angiogenesis. *Nature* 1997;386: 671–674.

43. Semenza GL. Targeting HIF-1 for cancer therapy. *Nat Rev Cancer* 2003;3:721–732.

44. Spigel DR, Hainsworth JD, Sosman A *et al*. Bevacizumab and erlotinib in the treatment of patients with metastatic renal carcinoma (RCC): update of a phase II multicenter trial. *J Clin Oncol* 2005;23;16S (abstract 4540).

45. Strieter RM. Chemokines: not just leukocyte chemoattractants in the promotion of cancer. *Nat Immunol* 2001;2:285–286.

46. Strieter RM, Belperio JA, Arenberg DA *et al*. CXC chemokine in angiogenesis. In: Universes in Delicate Balance: Chemokines and the Nervous System. R.M. Ransohoff, K. Suzuki, A.E.I. Proudfoot, and W.F. Hickey, Eds. Elsevier Science B.V., Amsterdam, The Netherlands, 2002, p. 129.

47. Strieter RM, Polverini PJ, Kunkel SL *et al*. The functional role of the ELR motif in CXC chemokine-mediated angiogenesis. *J Biol Chem* 1995;270:27348–27357.

48. Yang JC, Haworth L, Sherry RM *et al*. A randomized trial of bevacizumab, an anti-vascular endothelial growth factor antibody, for metastatic renal cancer. *N Engl J Med* 2003;349:427–434.

49. Yu Y, Sato JD. MAP kinases, phosphatidylinositol 3-kinase, and p70 S6 kinase mediate the mitogenic response of human endothelial cells to vascular endothelial growth factor. *J Cell Physiol* 1999;178:235–246.

50. Zhong H, Chiles K, Feldser D *et al*. Modulation of hypoxia-inducible factor 1alpha expression by the epidermal growth factor/phosphatidylinositol 3-kinase/PTEN/AKT/FRAP pathway in human prostate cancer cells: implications for tumor angiogenesis and therapeutics. *Cancer Res* 2000;60: 1541–1545.

51. Zundel W, Schindler C, Haas-Kogan D *et al*. Loss of PTEN facilitates HIF-1-mediated gene expression. *Genes Dev* 2000;14:391–396.

11c
Signal Transduction Inhibitors in Renal Cell Cancer

Andrea Mancuso and Cora N. Sternberg

Introduction

Renal cell carcinoma (RCC) accounts for approximately 3% of adult malignancies and 90–95% of neoplasms arising from the kidney.[1] Surgery is the treatment of choice at initial presentation for patients with a good performance status, even though approximately 30% of patients present with metastatic disease and one-third develop metastasis during follow-up.[2] Immunotherapy with interferon (IFN) and interleukin-2 (IL-2) have produced responses in approximately 15% of patients, with a median time to progression (TTP) of 2–4 months and little benefit in overall survival (approximately 3 months).[3]

A greater understanding of the molecular biology of cancer has led to successful development of various biological and angiosuppressive therapies. Promising results have been reported in second line treatment with vascular endothelial growth factor receptor (VEGFR)- and platelet-derived growth factor receptor (PDGFR)-inhibiting drugs, reporting TTP ranging between 4 and 9 months (SU011248, Bay 43-9006, AG-013736). While confirmatory studies are ongoing, other novel approaches [mammalian target of rapamycin (mTor) inhibitors] have drawn enthusiasm and international attention. This chapter, analyzing basic translational research principles, will summarize the available data on the use of these new therapeutic approaches in RCC.

Biological Basis of New Therapeutic Approaches

Recent developments in understanding the molecular biology of RCC have led to the development of new agents directed against tyrosine kinases (TKs), antigens, and portions of the hypoxic response pathway[4,5] (Table 11c-1). Many studies have demonstrated that overexpression of the epidermal growth factor receptor (EGFR) and its ligands epidermal growth factor (EGF) and tumor growth factor (TGF)-α occurs frequently in RCC and is associated with cancer aggressiveness[6-11] (Fig. 11c-1). EGFR signaling blockade decreases the proliferation of RCC cells *in vitro* and *in vivo* and provides a sound basis for the clinical evaluation of EGFR inhibitors in RCC.[12,13]

Over 75% of RCCs (sporadic histology) are characterized by loss of the von Hippel–Lindau (VHL) tumor suppressor gene, which results in an increased concentration of hypoxia inducible factor-1 (HIF-1). HIF-1 is a central transcriptional factor which regulates the expression of a battery of genes, the products of which are critical components of tumor progression (e.g., VEGFR, PDGFR, KIT, and Flt3 receptors) (Fig. 11c-2). These multiple biological pathway inhibitors provide a large number of striking data in the treatment of refractory RCC.

Tumor progression is also stimulated by growth factors through the phosphatidylinositol-3-kinase (PI3K)–AKT–mTOR signal transduction pathway.[14]

Anti-Epidermal Growth Factor Receptor Therapies

The EGFR is a transmembrane receptor involved in cell proliferation, growth, migration, invasion, and survival. The receptor, belonging to the ErbB family, is structurally composed of three principal domains: an extracellular ligand-binding domain, a transmembrane domain, and an intracellular domain with intrinsic TK activity.[15] Several EGFR inhibitors have been developed in recent years, which can be mainly categorized into two classes: monoclonal antibodies to the extracellular domain of the EGFR (e.g., Cetuximab, ABX-EGF) or small molecules that are inhibitors of the intracellular tyrosine kinase (TKI) domain by interfering with autophosphorylation by adenosine triphosphate (ATP; e.g., ZD1839, OSI-774). Treatment with monoclonal antibodies will be treated extensively in Chapter 11f and the results obtained with this second class of molecules in RCC will be considered.

ZD1839 and OSI-774 are selective ErbB-1 and reversible inhibitors; Drucker et al. in a Phase II trial exploring the efficacy of ZD1839 (Iressa) monotherapy reported negative results in 18 patients; 13 patients (81%) had progression of disease within 4 months of the start of therapy.[16] Considering these negative results, monotherapy trials have been abandoned

TABLE 11c-1. Principal signal transduction inhibitors for metastatic renal carcinoma.[a,b]

Agent	Mechanism of action/ molecular target	Administration	Development stage
Iressa	TKI: EGFR	Oral	Phase II
Tarceva	TKI: EGFR	Oral	Phase I/II
SU11248	Multitarget TKI	Oral	Phase III
Bay 43-9006	TKI: RAF	Oral	Phase II/III
GW572016	TKI: EGFR, ErbB-1-2	Oral	Phase III
PTK787	TKI: VEGFR	Oral	Phase I
Imatinib	TKI: c-kit, PDGFR, Bcr-Abl	Oral	Phase II
CCI-779	TKI: mTOR	Intravenous	Phase III
SU5416	TKI: VEGF	Intravenous	Closed
Bortezomib	26S proteasome inhibitor	Intravenous	Phase II

[a] Monoclonal antibody approaches have not been reported (see Chapter 11f).
[b] TKI, tyrosine kinase inhibitor; EGFR, epidermal growth factor receptor; VEGFR, vascular endothelial growth factor receptor; PDGFR, platelet-derived growth factor receptor; mTOR, mammalian target of rapamycin; VEGF, vascular endothelial growth factor.

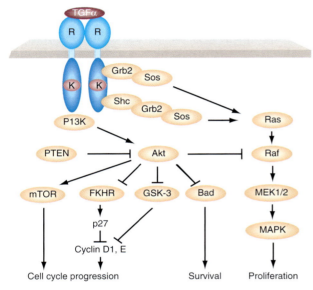

FIGURE 11c-1. Epidermal growth factor receptor signaling. (Courtesy of Mendelsohn J et al. J Clin Oncol 2003: 21: 2787–2799.)

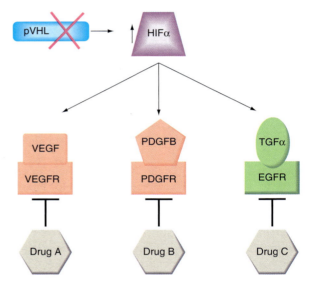

FIGURE 11c-2. Therapeutic targets of the von Hippel–Lindau tumor suppressor protein (pVHL) pathway. (Courtesy of Kim WY et al. J Clin Oncol 2004; 22: 4991–5004.)

and the drug is under investigation in combination trials with a highly potent inhibitor of VEGF receptor-2 TK activity (AZD2171 and SU11248);[17] two phase I trials published by Van Cruijsen et al. and Ronnen et al. on, respectively, 70 and 11 patients published at ASCO 2006 show encouraging preliminary response data. A Phase II trial is planned.[18, 19]

No monotherapy efficacy data on RCC are available with OSI-774 (Tarceva). This has been evaluated in several other solid tumors (including renal cancers) with farnesyl transferase inhibitors on the basis of preclinical data indicating an additive cytotoxic effect.[20] Phase II/III ongoing trials have explored the combination of erlotinib and bevacizumab (see Chapter 11f).

Several preclinical studies are exploring the potential of other TKIs in RCC (PKI-166, GW-2016, EKB-569, and CI-1033). PKI-166 is a dual ErbB-1/ErbB-2 inhibitor that

appears promising considering the possibility of its double mechanism of action, directly on receptor and on tumor suppressor genes.[21]

Multiple Biological Pathway Inhibitors

SU11248

SU11248 (sunitinib, Sutent) is an oral multitargeted receptor tyrosine kinase (RTK) inhibitor with antitumor and antiangiogenic activities through targeting of the PDGFR-ß, VEGFR-2, KIT, and Flt3 receptors.[22, 23] SU11248 has shown antitumor activity by inhibiting RTKs expressed by cancer cells directly involved in cancer proliferation and survival and RTKs expressed on endothelial or stromal cells (pericytes) that support cancer growth.[24] VEGFR-2 is expressed in the endothelium of blood vessels[25] and PDGFR-ß is expressed in the tumor stroma.[26] SU11248's targets are believed to play an important role in the growth and survival of human RCC, especially considering its very vascular nature.

In two independent Phase II single-arm multicenter trials, Motzer et al. reported positive results of SU11248, 50 mg/day in patients with metastatic RCC who had failed cytokine therapy with IL-2 or IFN. Patients with a good or intermediate prognosis received treatment in 6-week cycles, with 4 weeks on and 2 weeks off therapy. In these trials (in total, 169 patients) the partial response rate was around 40% with 25% of patients experiencing stable disease for 3+ months. The median TTP/progression-free survival (PFS) ranged between 8.2 and 8.7 months; median survival (more than 16 months) was particularly noteworthy when compared to prior studies in the second-line setting (Table 11c-2). Adverse events were mostly Grade 1 and 2 and included fatigue, nausea, diarrhea, and stomatitis. Grade 3/4 neutropenia and hyperlipasemia complicated treatment in 15–20% of patients.[27,28]

Based on these data, sunitinib was approved by the Food and Drug Administration (FDA) for advanced RCC in January 2006 and the confirmative randomized Phase III trial of sunitinib versus IFN-α has been presented at the 2006 Annual Meeting of the American Society of Clinical Oncology (ASCO). In this study 750 patients were randomized between two well-balanced arms. Sunitinib demonstrated a significant advantage as compared to IFN-α in disease PFS [11 months vs. 5 months; hazard ratio (HR) = 0.415, $p < 0.000001$] and overall response rate (37% vs. 9%; $p < 0.000001$). Although survival endpoints were still immature, the HR was 0.65 ($p < 0.02$) in favor of sunitinib. Motzer et al. concluded that sunitinib is the new standard of care for metastatic RCC and that inhibition of VEGFR (and PDGFR) must be considered the principal therapeutic targets for RCC.[29]

AG-013736

AG-013736 (axitinib) is an oral multitarget RTK inhibitor with potent effects, especially against VEGF receptors 1 and 2 and the PDGF-β receptor (Fig. 11c-3). Significant activity of AG-013736 was reported by Rini in a Phase I/II study in metastatic cytokine refractory renal cancer.[30] In this study, patients were treated with repeat 4-week cycles of AG-013736 at 5 mg twice daily. Of 52 patients enrolled 24 (46%) achieved a partial response by RECIST Criteria. At a median follow-up of 18 months, 16 (31%) patients progressed and 6 (12%) discontinued therapy due to adverse events. Of 24 responding patients 21 remain on study with response or stable disease. The median time to progression has not been reached, and only three patients with a partial response (PR) have relapsed after more than 232 days of therapy. Grade 3/4 hypertension was the most important related toxicity observed in 15% of patients. There were no cases of neutropenia or thrombocytopenia above Grade 1.

In 13 of the patients an ancillary study was conducted to monitor vascular tumor flow using qualitative and quantitative computed tomography (CT) perfusion for visceral and nonvisceral metastases and to evaluate the effect of antiangiogenic therapy on serum biological parameters (VEGFs, VEGFR-1, and VEGFR-2).[31] Decreasing tumor perfusion was observed in all patients responding to therapy and in patients with stable or progressive disease the intratumoral flow reduction was strongly correlated with clinical improvement. No correlation was observed between responders, nonresponders, and biological parameters.

These data show that AG-013736 has substantial objective and biological activity. Treatment with this drug is well tolerated and toxicity is manageable. Further trials of AG-013736 are ongoing in combination and in refractory RCC.

TABLE 11c-2. SU11248: activity versus other second line agents.[a]

	Number of patients	ORR (%)	SD (%)	TTP/PFS (months)
SU11248 Motzer Trial 1	63	40	28	8.7
SU11248 Motzer Trial 2	106	42	24	8.2
Bay 43-9006 targets	905	2	78	6
AG-013736	52	46	38	12+
CCI-779	106	7	64	6
IL-2[b]	65	5	NR	NA
IFN-α[b]	48	2	NR	NA
Avastin (high dose)[c]	39	10	NR	4.8
Placebo[c]	40	0	NR	2.5
Avastin/erlotinib/imatinib	83	13	63	9.8
Avastin/erlotinib	63	25	61	18
Multiple agents in Phase II trials[d]	137	3	NR	2.9

[a] ORR, objective response rate; TTP, time to progression; PFS, progression-free survival; NR, not reported; NA, not applicable.
[b] Escudier B et al. J Clin Oncol 1999; 17: 2039–2043.
[c] Yang JC et al. N Engl J Med 2003; 349: 427–434.
[d] Motzer RJ et al. J Clin Oncol 2004; 22: 454–463.

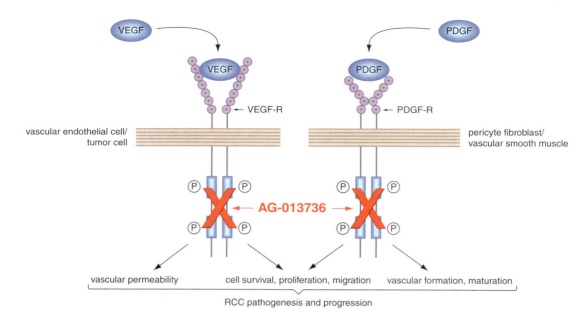

FIGURE 11c-3. Mechanism of action of AG-013736. (Courtesy of Rini B et al. ASCO meeting, 2005, oral presentation.)

BAY 43-9006 (Sorafenib)

BAY 43-9006 (sorafenib) is an oral agent that was designed as a c- and b-raf kinase inhibitor. The Ras/Raf signaling pathway is a mediator of tumor cell proliferation and angiogenesis. Recently, sorafenib has been found to inhibit several RTKs, among them VEGFR-2, PDGFR-β, FLT-3, and c-KIT. In 2005 final results of a randomized discontinuation study with sorafenib 400 mg twice a day in 202 RCC patients revealed that 71% of patients had ≥25% tumor shrinkage or disease stabilization in the first 12 weeks of treatment; 8 (4%) patients had independently confirmed partial responses. The stable patients were then randomized to receive sorafenib or placebo for another 12 weeks; 50% were progression free at 24 weeks compared with 18% of patients randomized to placebo ($p = 0.0077$). PFS was 24 weeks and 6 weeks respectively for patients treated with sorafenib or placebo ($p = 0.0087$).

Dermatological toxicity was the most common adverse event, followed by fatigue and diarrhea. Hand-foot syndrome was the most common Grade 3 toxicity, but with an incidence of <15%. Grade 3 hypertension was observed in <25% of patients and was manageable with oral medications. Sixteen (8%) patients discontinued the treatment due to severe adverse events.[32]

These encouraging results led to a Phase III randomized trial, known as TARGET (Treatment Approaches in RCC Global Evaluation Trial). In 905 patients failing one prior systemic therapy, with good or intermediate prognosis, ECOG performance and status 0–1 were entered. The primary aim of the trial was to assess overall survival in patients with clear cell RCC.[33] In addition to tumor control in 80%, sorafenib significantly prolonged PFS and overall survival (OS) compared with placebo. Of most interest was the improvement in survival (first and second planned interim

analysis, ASCO 2006) in the sorafenib arm of approximately 35% (19.3 months) versus a median of 14.3 months for those on placebo (HR = 0.74, $p = 0.010$). The safety profile was favorable in all subsets of patients stratified according to Motzer's risk groups.[34] Sorafenib demonstrated clinical benefit without adversely impacting overall health-related quality of life and had a positive impact on individual symptoms.[35]

Doppler ultrasonography with perfusion software (vascular recognition imaging) seems to be able to predict the drug efficacy: a decrease in tumor vascularization results related to the CT scan response at 6 weeks and this new cost-effective and simple noninvasive imaging technique is under investigation.[36]

This represents the largest randomized study thus far in advanced RCC. It is positive in its primary endpoint in the first two planned interim analyses. The difference is clinically relevant. Toxicity is manageable. No data are available concerning poor risk patients. Sorafenib can be recommended for cytokine failures meeting the eligibility criteria in this study.

Regarding first line therapy for RCC, a randomized Phase II trial was presented. Escudier et al. randomized 189 untreated patients over 7 months to receive continuous oral sorafenib 400 mg twice a day or IFN 9 million units three times weekly, with an option of dose escalation (600 mg sorafenib twice a day) or crossover from IFN to sorafenib upon disease progression. Data are premature for efficacy analysis considering a median observation time from randomization of 5.3 months and a blinded independent assessment completed in only 52 patients.[37]

Phase II studies with sorafenib in combination with cytokines (IFN-α) as first-line treatment have also been recently published. The overall response rate of 20–40% for the combination of sorafenib and IFN in advanced RCC appears greater than expected with either IFN or sorafenib alone. Toxicity is typical of IFN. Further studies with this combination are needed to confirm these data.[38,39]

PTK787/ZK222584

PTK787/ZK222584 (valatinib), a specific oral inhibitor of the VEGFR TKs is under development as an angiogenesis inhibitor for the treatment of various cancers. In metastatic refractory RCC, a Phase I trial established that it was generally well tolerated at dose levels of 300–1500 mg with partial or minor responses in 19% of patients, while 60% attained stable disease.[40] In this trial, the median TTP was 5.3 months and the median estimated OS was 21.5 months. Changes in tumor blood flow evaluated with dynamic contrast-enhanced magnetic resonance imaging (DCE-MRI) significantly correlated with improved clinical outcomes, but these data need to be confirmed in a larger phase II study.

GW572016 (Lapatinib, Tykerb)

GW572016 (lapatinib) is an oral TK inhibitor (member of the 4-anilinoquinoline class) that is a potent dual inhibitor of the EGFRs, ErbB-1 and ErbB-2.[33] It is orally bioavailable (45–60%), is metabolized by the liver, and has activity in multiple preclinical models and clinical trials with no evidence of cardiac toxicity.[41] A Phase III trial was completed in patients who expressed either the EGFR or Her-2 by centralized immunohistochemistry (IHC) and who had one prior line of immunotherapy. Patients were randomized between lapatinib and hormonal therapy (HT). Results were presented on 416 patients at the 2006 ASCO meeting. TTP was 15.3 weeks for lapatinib versus 15.4 weeks for HT (HR = 0.94; p = 0.60) and median OS was 46.9 weeks for lapatinib versus 43.1 weeks for HT (HR = 0.88; p = 0.29). In the major subgroup of 241 patients with EGFR overexpressed disease (3+ by IHC), the median TTP was 15.1 weeks for lapatinib versus 10.9 weeks for HT (HR = 0.76; p = 0.06) and the median OS was 46.0 weeks for lapatinib versus 37.9 weeks for HT (HR = 0.69; p = 0.02).[42] The EGFR/ErbB-2 dual targeted inhibitor, lapatinib appeared to prolong overall survival compared to hormone therapy in this subset of patients. with 3* expression by IHC. Although lapatinib has also shown preliminary activity in the treatment of brain metastases in some solid tumors, based upon these results in a subset analysis it is unlikely to be brought forward in the treatment of RCC.

Imatinib Mesylate (Gleevec)

The mechanism of action of imatinib mesylate consists of inhibition of the constitutively active kinase activity of Bcr-Abl by binding to the nucleotide-binding site, thereby blocking access to ATP and inhibiting signaling pathways associated with proliferation. Imatinib, moreover, selectively inhibits two other tyrosine kinases, c-kit and PDGF receptor. This latter finding has provided the rationale for treating patients

with RCC. Of note, high expression of the PDGFR and c-kit has also been observed in sarcomatoic specific subtypes.[43]

Despite this background, monotherapy results have been somewhat disappointing in RCC. No major responses were observed in a Phase II study with a median TTP of 3 months. Adverse events were tolerable. Notably, only one tumor (8%) expressed c-kit by immunohistochemistry.[44]

Given the minimal toxicity of this drug, combination trials of imatinib mesylate with bevacizumab and erlotinib or with IFN-α have been developed. Phase I/II preliminary results of the combination of bevacizumab 10 mg/kg every 2 weeks, erlotinib 150 mg, and imatinib are available. Dose escalations were presented initially by Hainsworth et al. (ASCO 2005) and subsequently by Spigel et al. (ECCO 13).[45,46] Diarrhea (29%, Grade 3/4) was the dose-limiting toxicity and other Grade 3/4 toxicities were rash (27%), nausea/vomiting (13%), hypertension (2%), bleeding (2%), proteinuria (2%), and fatigue (6%). Grade 1/2 toxicities included rash (77%), diarrhea (69%), nausea (61%), fatigue (54%), vomiting (31%), and proteinuria (23%). Among 91 patients treated in the Phase II portion of this study, 83 were evaluable for response with a 10-month follow-up: 76% of patients had a PR or minor response/stable disease with PFS of 9.8 months. These results indicate activity with this three-drug regimen. Further follow-up of all of the 91 patients is necessary prior to drawing further conclusions.

Another Phase II combination study of IFN-α and imatinib reported negative results with a response rate of only 7%, a median time to progression of 2 months, and significant toxicities.[47] On these bases further studies of IFN-α and imatinib appear not recommendable in patients with metastatic RCC.

SU5416 (Semaxanib)

SU5416 is a small organic molecule that noncompetitively inhibits the phosphorylation of the VEGF TK receptor Flk-1. Whereas PTK787/ZK222584 inhibits all three isoforms of VEGFR, SU5416 inhibits VEGFR-1 and VEGFR-2. It is delivered intravenously twice weekly.

In Phase I/II studies, single agent SU5416 was well tolerated, but the antitumor response was low, particularly in RCC patients (no PRs, 25% SD).[48] In combination with IFN-α the drug exhibits biological activity as evidenced by significant declines in serial VEGF and plasminogen activator inhibitor-1 plasma levels, but the 1-year relapse free survival of 6% and an adverse toxicity profile (three on-study deaths) have diminished enthusiasm for new additional studies.[49]

mTor Inhibitors

Temsirolimus (CCI-779) is a rapamycin analogue that inhibits mTOR kinase, a regulator of HIF-1α causing G_1 cell cycle arrest.[50] A Phase II dose escalation study of single-agent temsirolimus was performed in 110 patients with refractory RCC, evaluating doses of 25-250 mg. Despite a relative response (RR) of only 7%, the overall tumor growth control was 70% and TTP was 6 months. A minimum of 15 patients remained on study >1 year.[51] There was a suggestion of improved survival in patients with intermediate and poor prognostic risk factors according to Motzer's classification of prognostic groups.[34] A Phase I study of temsirolimus in combination with IFN-α was reported. This was a dose escalation study in advanced RCC patients who had received no more than two prior systemic therapies. A total of 71 patients were enrolled; 96% had undergone prior nephrectomy and 55% had prior immunotherapy. The maximum tolerated dose was 15 mg of temsirolimus weekly in combination with 6 mIU of IFN-α subcutaneously three times weekly. Dose-limiting toxicities were fatigue, stomatitis, and nausea and vomiting. Among all treated patients, there were 8 (11%) PRs and 21 (30%) patients with SD. The median TTP was 9.1 months.[52]

Temsirolimus maintained these promising results in a recent Phase III study in patients with previously untreated poor-prognosis metastatic RCC as single agent versus combined therapy with IFN-α versus IFN-α alone.[53]

Of the 626 patients enrolled, 442 deaths occurred at the time of the report. Patients treated with temsirolimus had a statistically longer survival than those treated with IFN (10.9 vs. 7.3 months, $p = 0.0069$). OS of patients treated with IFN and temsirolimus + IFN was not statistically different (10.9 vs. 8.4, $p = 0.69$). The three most frequently occurring adverse events $\geq$ Grade 3 in patients treated with temsirolimus were asthenia (12–30%), anemia (20–40%), and dyspnea (10%). In conclusion, single-agent temsirolimus significantly increased OS in first-line poor-risk advanced RCC patients compared with IFN, with an acceptable safety profile.[53]

Everolimus (RAD 001) and another mTOR inhibitor AP23573 are potential new targeted drugs for RCC. In two recent Phase I/II studies with these drugs a duration of response (up to 12 months) was observed, but confirmatory studies are needed.[54,55]

Other Novel Signal Transduction Inhibitors

Bortezomib (Velcade, PS-341) is part of a new class of therapeutic agents targeting the 26S proteasome of the ubiquitin-proteasome degradation system. This system is the major extralysosomal pathway responsible for intracellular protein degradation in eukaryotes and plays an important role in the regulation of the cell cycle and in the development and growth of tumor cells.

Many Phase I/II trials of bortezomib in patients with metastatic RCC have been conducted on the basis of observed antitumor activity and the potential role of this agent in antiangiogenesis. In a Phase II trial, Kondagunta et al.

reported an 11% PR rate (95% CI, 3–25%) and SD in 14 (38%; 95% CI, 23–55%) of 37 assessable patients. The four patients with PR had response durations of 8, 8+, 15+, and 20+ months. Grade 2 or 3 sensory neuropathy was present in 10 patients (53%). One patient in the 1.5 mg/m^2 group had Grade 3 sensory neuropathy.[56]

Two other independent Phase II trials of PS 341 confirm the drug's activity (5–10%) in refractory RCC patients. However, considering the modest activity and toxicity profile (fatigue in 50% and neurotoxicity in 28%) other studies with single agent bortezomib are probably not warranted.[57,58] However, it may still be interesting to explore the activity in a subpopulation of patients (non-clear-cell histology and wild type VHL gene, biologically more responding to bortezomib) and in combination therapies with IFN-α or new agents targeting the VEGF pathway.[59]

Discussion

Remarkable progress has been made in a very short time in a disease that was not responsive to most therapies. RECIST criteria may be less useful with newer biological agents that slow the progression of disease without necessarily responding to strict objective parameters. Increases in PFS, changes in tumor blood flow, and measurement of other biological parameters will become increasingly important. In addition, a rational and innovative drug design is needed to evaluate biologics.

There are still many unanswered questions. When can therapy be stopped and is there a rebound phenomenon when these agents are discontinued? Are they effective in high-risk patients and what are the effects on the primary tumor? Future trials will include comparison between the various compounds and combinations with upstream targets such as HIF and mTOR, and with cytokines such as IL-2. There is little information on the long-term effects of these agents and whether or not cytokines are useful afterward. These agents have been studied predominantly in clear cell carcinoma, so we do not have information on their effectiveness in other histologies.

Conclusions

There is an increasing awareness that validation of therapeutic targets is necessary for the discovery of new drugs and for verification of their success. There is a strong rationale for targeting multiple pathways, particularly angiogenesis pathways in RCC. Molecular profiling is heralding the future of prognosis, staging, and treatment. Second line therapy for cytokine refractory RCC is an unmet medical need and agents will shortly be approved (sorafenib, sunitinib) for this indication.

Further exploration of biological targets, angiogenesis inhibition, and EGFR antagonists is providing new possibilities. Efforts to improve results and to find better first line treatment will include an international effort to identify prognostic factors. The next few years should be characterized by new rational treatment strategies based on inhibition of specific biological pathways that will hopefully culminate in a better understanding of the causes of RCC, its prevention, and hopefully its cure.

References

1. Linehan WM, Zbar B. Focus on kidney cancer. Cancer Cell 2004; 6(3): 223–228.
2. Patel NP, Lavengood RW. Renal cell carcinoma: natural history and results of treatment. J Urol 1978; 119: 722–726.
3. Sternberg CN. Metastatic renal cell cancer treatments. Drugs Today 2003; 39(Suppl C): 39–59.
4. Mancuso A, Sternberg CN. What's new in the treatment of metastatic kidney cancer? BJU Int 2005; 95(9): 1171–1180.
5. Cohen HT, McGovern FJ. Renal-cell carcinoma. N Engl J Med 2005; 353(23): 2477–2490.
6. Gomella LG, Anglard P, Sargent ER, Robertson CN, Kasid A, Linehan WM. Epidermal growth factor receptor gene analysis in renal cell carcinoma. J Urol 1990; 143: 191–193.
7. Hofmockel G, Riess S, Bassukas ID, Dammrich J. Epidermal growth factor family and renal cell carcinoma: expression and prognostic impact. Eur Urol 1997; 31: 478–484.
8. Ishikawa J, Maeda S, Umezu K, Sugiyama T, Kamidono S. Amplification and overexpression of the epidermal growth factor receptor gene in human renal-cell carcinoma. Int J Cancer 1990; 45: 1018–1021.
9. Petrides PE, Bock S, Bovens J, Hofmann R, Jakse G. Modulation of pro-epidermal growth factor, pro-transforming growth factor alpha and epidermal growth factor receptor gene expression in human renal carcinomas. Cancer Res 1990; 50: 3934–3939.
10. Everitt JI, Walker CL, Goldsworthy TW, Wolf DC. Altered expression of transforming growth factor-alpha: an early event in renal cell carcinoma development. Mol Carcinog 1997; 19: 213–219.
11. Price JT, Wilson HM, Haites NE. Epidermal growth factor (EGF) increases the in vitro invasion, motility and adhesion interactions of the primary renal carcinoma cell line. Eur J Cancer 1996; 32A: 1977–1982.
12. Asakuma J, Sumitomo M, Asano T, Asano T, Hayakawa M. Modulation of tumor growth and tumor induced angiogenesis after epidermal growth factor receptor inhibition by ZD1839 in renal cell carcinoma. J Urol 2004; 171: 897–902.
13. Prewett M, Rothman M, Waksal H, Feldman M, Bander NH, Hicklin DJ. Mouse-human chimeric anti-epidermal growth factor receptor antibody C225 inhibits the growth of human renal cell carcinoma xenografts in nude mice. Clin Cancer Res 1998; 4: 2957–2966.
14. Pantuck AJ, Zeng G, Belldegrun AS, Figlin RA. Pathobiology, prognosis, and targeted therapy for renal cell carcinoma: exploiting the hypoxia-induced pathway. Clin Cancer Res 2003; 9(13): 4641–4652.
15. Mendelsohn J, Baselga J. The EGF receptor family as targets for cancer therapy. Oncogene 2000; 19: 6550–6565.
16. Drucker B, Bacik J, Ginsberg M et al. Phase II trial of ZD1839 (IRESSA) in patients with advanced renal cell carcinoma. Invest New Drugs 2003; 21: 341–345.
17. Van Cruijsen H, Voest EE, van Herpen CM, Hoekman K, Witteveen PO, Punt CJ, Puchalski TA, Fernandes N, Koehler M, Giaccone G. Phase I clinical evaluation of AZD2171 in combination with gefitinib (Iressa), in patients with advanced tumors. J Clin Oncol 2005; 23(16S): abstract 3030.
18. Van Cruijsen H, Voest EE, Van Herpen CM, Hoekman K, Witteveen PO, Tjin-A-ton ML, Punt CJ, Puchalski T, Milenkova T, Giaccone G. Phase I evaluation of AZD2171, a highly potent, selective VEGFR signaling inhibitor, in combination with gefitinib, in patients with advanced tumors. J Clin Oncol 2006; 24(18S): abstract 3017.
19. Ronnen EA, Kondagunta GV, Lau C, Fischer P, Ginsberg MS, Baum M, Kim ST, Chen I, Baum CM, Motzer RJ. A phase I study of sunitinib malate (SU11248) in combination with gefitinib in patients with metastatic renal cell carcinoma (mRCC). J Clin Oncol 2006; 24(18S): abstract 4537.
20. Ma CX, Croghan G, Reid J, Hanson L, Mandrekar S, Marks R, Adjei A, Furth A. A phase I trial of the combination of erlotinib and tipifarnib in patients with advanced solid tumors. J Clin Oncol 2005; 23(16S): abstract 3000.
21. Fujimoto E, Yano T, Sato H, Hagiwara K, Yamasaki H, Shirai S, Fukumoto K, Hagiwara H, Negishi E, Ueno K. Cytotoxic effect of the Her-2/Her-1 inhibitor PKI-166 on renal cancer cells expressing the connexin 32 gene. J Pharmacol Sci 2005; 97(2): 294–298.
22. Abrams TJ, Murray LJ, Pesenti E et al. Preclinical evaluation of the tyrosine kinase inhibitor SU11248 as a single agent and in combination with "standard of care" therapeutic agents for the treatment of breast cancer. Mol Cancer Ther 2003; 2: 1011–1021.
23. O'Farrell AM, Abrams TJ, Yuen HA et al. SU11248 is a novel FLT3 tyrosine kinase inhibitor with potent activity in vitro and in vivo. Blood 2003; 101: 3597–3605.
24. Nakopoulou L, Stefanaki K, Panayotopoulou E et al. Expression of the vascular endothelial growth factor receptor-2/Flk-1 in breast carcinomas: correlation with proliferation. Hum Pathol 2002; 33: 863–870.
25. de Jong JS, van Diest PJ, van der Valk P, Baak JP. Expression of growth factors, growth inhibiting factors, and their receptors in invasive breast cancer. I: An inventory in search of autocrine and paracrine loops. J Pathol 1998; 184: 44–52.
26. Mendel DB, Laird AD, Xin X et al. In vivo antitumor activity of SU11248, a novel tyrosine kinase inhibitor targeting vascular endothelial growth factor and platelet-derived growth factor receptors. Clin Cancer Res 2003; 9: 327–337.
27. Motzer RJ, Rini BI, Michaelson MD et al. Phase 2 trials of SU11248 show antitumor activity in second-line therapy for patients with metastatic renal cell carcinoma. J Clin Oncol 2005; 23(16S): abstract 4508.
28. Motzer RJ, Rini BI, Michaelson MD et al. Sunitinib malete (SU11248) shows antitumor activity in patients with metastatic renal cell carcinoma: updated results from phase II trials. EJC 2005; 3(2): abstract 797.

29. Motzer RJ, Hutson TE, Tomczak P, Michaelson MD, Bukowski RM, Rixe O, Oudard S, Kim ST, Baum CM, Figlin RA. Phase III randomized trial of sunitinib malate (SU11248) versus interferon-alfa (IFN-α) as first-line systemic therapy for patients with metastatic renal cell carcinoma (mRCC). J Clin Oncol 2006; 24(18S): abstract LBA3.

30. Rini B, Rixe O, Bukowski R, Michaelson MD, Wilding G, Hudes G, Bolte O, Steinfeldt H, Reich SD, Motzer R. AG-013736, a multi-target tyrosine kinase receptor inhibitor, demonstrates anti-tumor activity in a phase 2 study of cytokine-refractory, metastatic renal cell cancer. J Clin Oncol 2005; 23(16S): abstract 4509.

31. Rixe O, Meric J, Bloch J, Gentile A, Mouawad R, Adam V, Buthiau D, Khayat D. Surrogate markers of activity of AG-013736, a multi-target tyrosine kinase receptor inhibitor, in metastatic renal cell cancer. J Clin Oncol 2005; 23(16S): abstract 3003.

32. Ratain MJ, Eisen T, Stadler WM, Flaherty KT, Gore M, Desai A, Patnaik A, Xiong HQ, Schwartz B, O'Dwyer P. Final findings from a phase II, placebo-controlled, randomized discontinuation trial (RDT) of sorafenib (BAY 43–9006) in patients with advanced renal cell carcinoma (RCC). J Clin Oncol 2005; 23(16S): abstract 4544.

33. Eisen T, Escudier B, Szczylik C, Stadler WM, Schwartz B, Shan M, Bukowski RM. Randomized phase III trial of the Raf kinase and VEGFR inhibitor sorafenib (BAY 43–9006) in patients with advanced renal cell carcinoma. J Clin Oncol 2006; 24(18S): abstract 4524.

34. Motzer RJ, Bacik J, Murphy BA, Russo P, Mazumdar M. Interferon-alfa as a comparative treatment for clinical trials of new therapies against advanced renal cell carcinoma. JCO 2002; (20): 289–296.

35. Danda R, Gondek K, Song J, Cella D, Bukowski RM, Escudier B. A comparison of quality of life and symptoms in kidney cancer patients receiving sorafenib versus placebo. J Clin Oncol 2006; 24(18S): abstract 4534.

36. Lamuraglia M, Lassau N, Chami L, Jaziri S, Schwartz B, Leclere J, Escudier B. Doppler ultrasonography with perfusion software and contrast agent injection as a tool for early evaluation of metastatic renal cancers treated with the Raf kinase and VEGFR inhibitor: a prospective study. J Clin Oncol 2005; 23(16S): abstract 3069.

37. Escudier B, Szczylik C, Demkow T, Staehler M, Rolland F, Negrier S, Hutson TE, Scheuring UJ, Schwartz B, Bukowski RM. Randomized phase II trial of the multi-kinase inhibitor sorafenib versus interferon (IFN) in treatment-naïve patients with metastatic renal cell carcinoma (mRCC). J Clin Oncol 2005; 23(16S): abstract 4501.

38. Ryan CW, Goldman BH, Lara PN, Beer TM, Drabkin HA, Crawford E. Sorafenib plus interferon-α2b (IFN) as first-line therapy for advanced renal cell carcinoma (RCC): SWOG 0412. J Clin Oncol 2005; 23(16S): abstract 4525.

39. Gollob J, Richmond T, Jones J, Rathmell WR, Grigson G, Watkins C, Peterson B, Wright J. Phase II trial of sorafenib plus interferon-alpha 2b (IFN-α2b) as first- or second-line therapy in patients (pts) with metastatic renal cell cancer (RCC). J Clin Oncol 2005; 23(16S): abstract 4538.

40. Potti A, George DJ. Tyrosine kinase inhibitors in renal cell carcinoma. Clin Cancer Res 2004; 10: 6371S–6376S.

41. Wood ER, Truesdale AT, McDonald OB et al. Unique structure for epidermal growth factor receptor bound to GW572016 (lapatinib): relationships among protein conformation, inhibitor off-rate, and receptor activity in tumor cells. Cancer Res 2004; 64(18): 6652–6659.

42. Ravaud A, Gardner J, Hawkins R, Von der Maase H, Zantl N, Harper P, Rolland F, Audhuy B, Machiels J, El-Hariry I. Renal Cell Cancer Study Group and GSK CoreT. Efficacy of lapatinib in patients with high tumor EGFR expression: results of a phase III trial in advanced renal cell carcinoma (RCC). J Clin Oncol 2006; 24(18S): abstract 4502.

43. Castillo M, Petit A, Mellado B, Palacin A, Alcover JB, Mallofre C. C-kit expression in sarcomatoid renal cell carcinoma: potential therapy with imatinib. J Urol 2004; 171(6 Pt 1): 2176–2180.

44. Vuky J, Fotoohi M, Isacson C et al. Phase II trial of imatinib mesylate (formerly known as STI-571) in patients with metastatic renal cell carcinoma (RCC). Proc Am Soc Clin Oncol 2003; 22(416): abstract 1672.

45. Hainsworth JD, Sosman JA, Spigel DR, Patton JF, Thompson DS, Sutton V, Hart LL, Yost K, Greco FA. Bevacizumab, erlotinib, and imatinib in the treatment of patients (pts) with advanced renal cell carcinoma (RCC): a Minnie Pearl Cancer Research Network phase I/II trial. J Clin Oncol 2005; 23(16S): abstract 4542.

46. Spigel DR, Hainsworth JD, Sosman JA, Patton JF, Thompson DS, Edwards D, Sutton V, Hart LL, Yost K, Greco FA. Bevacizumab, erlotinib, and imatinib in the treatment of patients (pts) with advanced renal cell carcinoma (RCC): update of a Minnie Pearl Cancer Research Network phase I/II trial. EJC 2005; 3(2): abstract 796.

47. Polite BN, Desai AA, Peterson AC, Manchen B, Stadler WM. A phase II study of imatinib mesylate (IM) and interferon-alpha (IFNA) in metastatic renal cell carcinoma. J Clin Oncol 2005; 23(16S): abstract 4689.

48. Kuenen BC, Tabernero J, Baselga J et al. Efficacy and toxicity of the angiogenesis inhibitor SU5416 as a single agent in patients with advanced renal cell carcinoma, melanoma, and soft tissue sarcoma. Clin Cancer Res 2003; 9(5): 1648–1655.

49. Lara PN, Quinn DI, Margolin K et al. SU5416 plus interferon alpha in advanced renal cell carcinoma: a phase II California Cancer Consortium Study with biological and imaging correlates of angiogenesis inhibition. Clin Cancer Res 2003; 9(13): 4772–4781.

50. Hay N, Sonenberg N. Upstream and Downstream of m-Tor. Genes Devel 2004; 18: 1926–1945.

51. Atkins MB, Hidalgo M, Stadler WM et al. Randomized phase II study of multiple dose levels of CCI-779, a novel mammalian target of rapamycin kinase inhibitor, in patients with advanced refractory renal cell carcinoma. J Clin Oncol 2004; 22: 909–918.

52. Smith JW, Yo K-J, Dutcher J et al. Update of a phase I study of intravenous CCI-779 given in combination with interferon-a to patients with advanced renal cell carcinoma. J Clin Oncol 2004; 22(14S): abstract 4513.

53. Hudes G, Carducci M, Tomczak P, Dutcher J, Figlin R, Kapoor A, Staroslawska E, O'Toole T, Park Y, Moore L. A phase 3, randomized, 3-arm study of temsirolimus (TEMSR) or interferon-alpha (IFN) or the combination of TEMSR + IFN in the treatment of first-line, poor-risk patients with advanced

renal cell carcinoma (adv RCC). J Clin Oncol 2006; 24(18S): abstract LBA4.

54. Tabernero J, Rojo F, Burris H, Casado E, Macarulla T, Jones S, Dimitrijevic S, Hazell K, Shand H, Baselga J. Phase I study with tumor molecular pharmacodynamic (MPD) evaluation of dose and schedule of the oral mTOR-inhibitor everolimus (RAD001) in patients (pts) with advanced solid tumors. J Clin Oncol 2005; 23(16S): abstract 3007.

55. Rivera VM, Kreisberg JI, Mita MM, Goldston M, Knowles HL, Herson J, Rowinksy E, Bedrosian CL, Tolcher A. Pharmaco-dynamic study of skin biopsy specimens in patients (pts) with refractory or advanced malignancies following administration of AP23573, an mTOR inhibitor. J Clin Oncol 2005; 23(16S): abstract 3033.

56. Kondagunta GV, Drucker B, Schwartz L et al. Phase II trial of bortezomib for patients with advanced renal cell carcinoma. J Clin Oncol 2004; 22(18): 3720–3725.

57. Drucker BJ, Schwartz L, Bacik J et al. Phase II trial of PS-341 shows response in patients with advanced renal cell carcinoma. Proc Am Soc Clin Oncol 2003; 22: abstract 1550.

58. Davis NB, Taber DA, Ansari RH et al. A phase II trial of PS-341 in patients with renal cell cancer (RCC). Proc Am Soc Clin Oncol 2003; 22: abstract 1551.

59. An J, Fisher M, Rettig MB. VHL expression in renal cell carcinoma sensitizes to bortezomib (PS-341) through an NF-kappaB-dependent mechanism. Oncogene 2005; 24(9): 1563–1570.

11d
Cytotoxic Chemotherapy for Metastatic Renal Cell Cancer

Walter M. Stadler

Introduction

Cytotoxic chemotherapy is generally considered to be ineffective in metastatic renal cancer. This impression is well supported by a long history of negative Phase II studies using traditional cytotoxic agents and as reviewed in several monographs (Yagoda et al., 1993; Amato 2000; Motzer and Russo 2000; George and Stadler 2003).

Table 11d-1 provides a compilation of many of these studies, most of which were performed prior to the current modern era of "molecularly targeted therapy." In this context it is perhaps best to consider classic cytotoxic therapy as therapy that targets DNA replication and repair pathways. In fact, dysregulated growth, which requires dysregulated DNA replication, and lack of apoptosis following inadequate DNA repair can be considered a sine qua non of the cancer phenotype. In many ways, therefore, cytotoxic compounds are as "targeted" to these dysregulated pathways in cancer cells as are the broad spectrum kinase inhibitors that are targeted to dysregulated angiogenesis and signal transduction pathways and that are reviewed in other chapters. Although these newer agents are showing great promise in renal and other solid tumors, it should not be forgotten that cytotoxic chemotherapy is responsible for much of the success in modern oncology.

This chapter will thus focus on both traditional and more novel cytotoxic compounds targeted at the DNA replication and repair mechanisms and their role in metastatic renal cancer. Although none of these agents is the standard of care for renal cancer at this time, tantalizing data provide hope that subsets of patients with renal cancer will be identified that may benefit from this approach. The discussion will thus focus on the most promising classes of agents, mechanisms of resistance potentially amenable to modification, and issues of trial design and tumor heterogeneity that are critical to identifying the populations most likely to benefit.

Chemotherapy Resistance Mechanisms in Renal Cancer

It is perhaps instructive to first consider why renal cancer is less responsive to the classic cytotoxic drugs than most other solid tumors. Although no single mechanism is likely to explain resistance to all of the diverse agents evaluated to date, the fact that the disease arises from an organ that is responsible for filtering and excreting a variety of endogenous as well as exogenous toxins is at least partly responsible. For example, the proximal renal tubule, from which most renal cancers are hypothesized to arise expresses high levels of the MDR1 (ABCB1) gene whose protein product, P-glycoprotein, is responsible for secretion of a variety of toxic natural products (Ernest et al., 1997). Renal cell cancer, likewise, expresses high levels of MDR1 and thus can be expected to be resistant to multidrug-resistance gene (MDR)-mediated compounds including the natural products paclitaxel, doxorubicin, daunorubicin, and actinomycin B (Fojo et al., 1987).

It is thus perhaps interesting that vinblastine enjoyed a long history as a modestly effective agent for this disease. More modern studies demonstrate, however, that it does not have appreciable antitumor activity. For example, two randomized studies of interferon versus interferon plus vinblastine failed to show any advantage with the addition of vinblastine (Neidhart et al., 1991; Fossa et al., 1992b). Furthermore, only one objective response was observed in 80 patients treated with vinblastine alone and only one additional response was observed when the potent P-glycoprotein inhibitors cyclosporin A or high-dose tamoxifen were added (Samuels et al., 1997). Since hyperbilirubinemia, a pharmacodynamic marker for MDR inhibition, was observed in this study, it is likely that MDR1 overexpression is not solely responsible for the resistant phenotype. In fact, other members of ABC transporters are also overexpressed in this disease as

TABLE 11d-1. Response rates of selected single agent chemotherapy.

Agent	Reference	Number of patients	Overall response (%)
Bortezomib	Davis et al., 2004	37	11
	Kondagunta et al., 2004	21	5
Bleomycin	Johnson et al., 1975	15	0
	Haas et al., 1976	8	37
	Hahn et al., 1977	7	0
Carboplatin	Tait et al., 1988	19	0
	Trump and Elson, 1990	18	0
Cisplatin	Rodriguez and Johnson, 1978	23	0
	Merrin, 1979	10	0
Cyclophosphamide	Kiruluta et al., 1975	10	0
	Hahn et al., 1979	44	4
	Wajsman et al., 1980	12	0
Dactinomycin	Hahn et al., 1981	61	2
2-Deoxycoformycin	Venner et al., 1991	18	0
	Witte et al., 1992	25	0
Docetaxel	Venner et al., 1991	18	0
Doxorubicin	O'Bryan et al., 1977	38	5
liposomal	Law et al., 1994b	14	0
	Skubitz, 2002	11	0
Epirubicin	Fossa et al., 1982	20	0
	Benedetto et al., 1983	19	0
Estramustine	Swanson and Johnson, 1981	16	0
Etoposide	Hahn et al., 1979	43	2
Flavopiridol	Stadler et al., 2000	35	6
	Van Veldhuizen et al., 2005	34	12
Floxuridine/FUDR	Hrushesky et al., 1990	56	20
	Damascelli et al., 1990	42	14
	Merrouche et al., 1991	14	0
	Dexeus et al., 1991	40	10
	Richards et al., 1991	29	0
	Budd et al., 1992	26	8
	Conroy et al., 1993	28	14
5-Fluorouracil	Zaniboni et al., 1989	14	0
	Schulof et al., 1991	27	7
	Ahlgren et al., 1993	35	11
	Kish et al., 1994	61	5
Fludarabine	Balducci et al., 1987	30	0
	Shevrin et al., 1989	15	0
Gemcitabine	Rohde et al., 1996	37	8
	Mertens et al., 1993	37	8
Hydroxyurea	Stolbach et al., 1981	19	5
Ifosfamide	Fossa and Talle, 1980	11	9
	Heim et al., 1981	10	20
	De Forges et al., 1987	16	0
	Bodrogi et al., 1988	9	0
Irinotecan	Fizazi et al., 2003	42	0
Irofulven	Berg et al., 2001	12	0
Ixabepilone	Fojo et al., 2005	57	14
Melphalan	Falkson, 1993	8	0
Methotrexate	Baumgartner et al., 1980	8	25
Mitomycin	Stewart et al., 1987	12	25
Mitotane	Hogan et al., 1981	12	0
Mitoxantrone	De Jager et al., 1984	20	0
	Taylor et al., 1984	49	0
	van Oosterom et al., 1984	29	0
	Gams et al., 1986	48	0
PALA	Natale et al., 1982	15	0
Paclitaxel	Einzig et al., 1991	18	0
Pemetrexed	Thodtmann et al., 2003	32	9
Pyrazoloacridine	Kuebler et al., 2001	18	6
Razoxane	Braybrooke et al., 2000	38	0

TABLE 11d-1. (continued).

Agent	Reference	Number of patients	Overall response (%)
Rebeccamycin	Hussain et al., 2003	24	8
Suramin	La Rocca et al., 1991	10	0
	Motzer et al., 1992	26	4
Temozolamide	Park et al., 2002	12	0
Thiotepa	Hahn et al., 1977	7	14
Topotecan	Law et al., 1994a	14	0
Troxacitabine	Townsley et al., 2003	33	6
UCN-01	Rini et al., 2004	21	0
Vinblastine	Hahn et al., 1977	10	0
	Kuebler et al., 1984	19	16
	Zeffren et al., 1984	10	0
	Tannock and Evans, 1985	14	0
	Crivellari et al., 1987	21	9
	Elson et al., 1988	35	9
	Fossa et al., 1992a	26	4
	Samuels et al., 1997	80	1
	Chico et al., 2001	39	0
Vindesine	Wong et al., 1977	17	0
	Fossa et al., 1983	24	0
Vinorelbine	Canobbio et al., 1991	14	0
	Wilding et al., 1993	24	4

well as in normal renal tubules (Schaub et al., 1999) as are multiple glutathione *S*-transferases (Volm et al., 1993; Oudard et al., 2002; Chuang et al., 2005). All likely contribute to the normal kidney's physiological ability to excrete and inactivate toxins and all likely contribute to the inherent resistance of this disease to many cytotoxic chemotherapy drugs.

Nucleoside Analogs in Renal Cancer

Given the above discussion, it is perhaps not surprising that the classic cytotoxic agents with the most consistent activity in renal cancer across multiple studies have been the nucleoside analogs. Resistance to these agents is traditionally not associated with increased drug efflux or metabolism by typical detoxifying enzymes. A long history of studies with the pyrimidine analog 5-fluorouracil (5-FU) or its congeners has repeatedly suggested that this drug has some antitumor activity (see Table 11d-1, for example). Nevertheless, in the largest multiinstitutional study, the overall objective response rate was only 5% and numerous studies with traditional 5-FU potentiating agents have not convincingly demonstrated any incremental benefit over 5-FU alone (Kish et al., 1994). It is none-the-less interesting that small studies with the pyrimidine analogs gemcitabine and troxacitabine also revealed low level activity (Mertens et al., 1993; De Mulder et al., 1996; Moore et al., 2001). To this end, we undertook a series of studies investigating the combination of gemcitabine and 5-FU (Rini et al., 2000; Desai et al., 2002; George et al., 2002; Ryan et al., 2002). The initial study reported an overall response rate of 17%, which was not improved by

the addition of cisplatin, interleukin (IL)-2 and interferon, or thalidomide. Other studies substituting oral capecitabine for 5-FU confirmed these data (Stadler et al., 2004; Waters et al., 2004). A retrospective review also suggested that overall survival in patients treated with gemcitabine/5-FU-based regimens was better than expected from a prognostic factor controlled historical cohort (Stadler et al., 2003). Nevertheless, the hypothesized benefit was felt to be insufficient to justify larger Phase III confirmatory trials.

Similarly, a combination of gemcitabine and adriamycin has been reported to be very active in poorly differentiated sarcomatoid renal cancers (Nanus et al., 2004). Although this is somewhat at odds with the earlier discussion regarding MDR1 expression and adriamycin resistance, enrollment of a specific renal cancer subset on these trials could explain the observation (see below).

Other Agents with Potential Activity in Renal Cancer

Another agent that has had potential activity in renal cancer is ixabepilone. Ixabepilone is an epothilone and microtubule stabilizing agent with a mechanism of action similar to the taxanes and binding to the same pharmacophore on tubulin (Pellegrini and Budman, 2005). One advantage over taxanes, however, is that preclinical studies suggest that it is not a substrate for P-glycoprotein (Goodin et al., 2004). A Phase II study at the National Cancer Institute (NCI) revealed an overall objective response rate of 14% in 57 patients (Fojo et al., 2005). Associated laboratory studies strongly suggested that tumors with wild-type von Hippel–Lindau (VHL) were the ones most likely to respond and confirmatory trials are underway.

These observations raise the possibility that other tubule interacting agents can be rationally investigated in renal cancer. To this end, kinesin has been considered an attractive anticancer pharmacological target. Kinesin is an ATP-dependent enzyme and tubule-associated protein essential for completion of cell division (Pellegrini et al., 2005). A number of kinesin inhibitors are in preclinical and clinical development and clinical data are eagerly awaited.

Finally, if we broaden our definition of cytotoxic and DNA targeting agents to include specific cell cycle inhibitors, additional compounds deserve mention. Flavopiridol is a nonspecific cyclin-dependent kinase inhibitor with potent antitumor activity in preclinical models. Two separate studies have reported modest clinical activity, with differences between the studies possibly due to differences in the schedule of drug administration (Stadler and Ratain, 2000; Van Veldhuizen et al., 2005). On the other hand, another cyclin-dependent kinase inhibitor that is also a protein kinase C inhibitor, UCN-01, did not lead to any objective responses or to any apparent prolongation of time to progression in a small Phase II trial (Rini et al., 2004).

Tumor Heterogeneity and Chemotherapy Benefit

Despite some of the encouraging data discussed above, the most successful cytotoxic or DNA targeted agents have led to objective responses in only 10–15% of renal cancer patients. Under the assumption that these are the only patients benefiting from the treatment, an assumption that may not be correct (see below), this is clearly not sufficient to qualify as standard therapy or even sufficient to justify definitive Phase III trials. Nevertheless, if the benefiting population can be identified a priori, even some of the current options could become viable treatments. For example, as noted above, the combination of gemcitabine and doxorubicin has been reported to be particularly effective in patients with aggressive "sarcomatoid" renal cancer. Unfortunately, "sarcomatoid" renal cancer is not recognized as a distinct subtype in the most recent pathological categorization and is likely a poorly differentiated version of any one of the well-described pathological variants (Kovacs et al., 1997). More importantly, from a clinical perspective, there is little consensus as to the pathological criteria necessary for defining "sarcomatoid" renal cancers.

Molecular subtyping is thus more likely to be successful. The benefit from ixabepilone, for example, has already been hypothesized to be limited to those patients whose tumors are VHL wild type. Furthermore, expression profiling has identified several putative subgroups above and beyond the well-described pathological variants (Takahashi et al., 2001,

2003). Molecular subtyping of patient tumors in clinical trials may thus very well identify a population more likely to benefit from one or another treatment. In addition to such empiric "brute force" approaches, more hypothesis-directed identification of putative benefiting populations should also be considered. Certainly there is an increasing understanding of the molecular determinants of sensitivity even for the classic cytotoxic agents such as 5-FU. This knowledge raises clear testable hypotheses in regards to patients most likely to benefit from a specific treatment.

Clinical Trial Design and Endpoints

Trials with DNA targeting agents have typically been conducted as uncontrolled single arm studies with a standardized objective response as the endpoint. This is perfectly reasonable under the assumption that these drugs will cause tumor cell kill and tumor shrinkage as their major mechanism leading to patient benefit. Although this is a reasonable assumption, it may not always be correct. Several studies have shown that the "objective partial response rate" is a rather poor surrogate for eventual clinical benefit as assessed by improvement in survival (Ratain and Eckhardt 2004). For example, patients who experience a brief 31% tumor shrinkage sufficient for a Response Evaluation Criteria In Solid Tumors (RECIST)-based response may not necessarily enjoy subsequent improvement in survival. On the other hand, if a drug inhibits growth without causing tumor shrinkage, survival may be enhanced even in the absence of an "objective response." This effect is certainly plausible in renal cancer as interferon leads to a 10% objective response rate and yet has been demonstrated to improve survival in modestly sized Phase III trials (Coppin et al., 2000). This is statistically possible only if more than the 10% of patients experiencing a response are benefiting from the treatment.

The DNA-targeting and cytotoxic agents certainly also inhibit growth in preclinical models, and there are suggestions that low-dose continuous exposure to such agents may have antiangiogenic effects as well (Kerbel and Kamen 2004). Therefore, the concept that a cytotoxic agent could inhibit growth without causing tumor shrinkage is not inconsistent with the current understanding of cancer biology and drug pharmacology.

The major problem with evaluating growth-inhibitory drugs is that a historical control is not always appropriate. Specifically, for the standard objective response endpoint, the null hypothesis, namely, that an inactive drug or a placebo will lead to a 0% response rate, is a well established fact with very narrow confidence intervals (despite the well-described spontaneous regressions in this disease). On the other hand, the appropriate endpoint for a growth inhibitory drug is a measure of time to progression. This endpoint is, however, highly dependent on the methodology for assessing progression, the frequency at which the methodology is applied, and the patient population enrolled. As such, time to progression is rarely if ever appropriately compared to a historical control. Thus, studies that assess agents hypothesized to inhibit growth will typically have to be performed in a controlled manner, even the earlier phases of drug development. Although a full discussion is beyond the scope of this chapter, various approaches including randomized Phase II designs with a "pick the winner" approach and/or enrichment designs such as the randomized discontinuation trial design have been described (Stadler et al., 2000).

Conclusions

In summary, no cytotoxic or DNA-targeted agent can yet be considered to be a standard of care in metastatic renal cancer. Nevertheless, there are true hints of significant activity, especially with the pyrimidine analogs and the novel tubule inhibitor ixabepilone. Although neither is likely to benefit a majority of the kidney cancer population, the available data suggest that a benefiting population can be identified, thus making them more viable treatment alternatives. These data also suggest that continued trials with DNA targeting, DNA repair targeting, and cell cycle-directed agents are useful endeavors, especially when coupled with molecular subtyping of the treated population. Finally, broader consideration of possible drug mechanisms and clinical trial designs including the possibility that even the "cytotoxic" agents may be growth inhibitory should be considered during clinical trial design.

References

Ahlgren, J. D., J. Lokich, et al., (1993). Protracted infusional 5FU (PIF): a well tolerated regimen in metastatic renal cell carcinoma (MRC): A Mid-Atlantic Oncology Program (MOAP) study. *Proc Am Soc Clin Oncol* 12: 244.

Amato, R. J. (2000). Chemotherapy for renal cell carcinoma. *Semin Oncol* 27(2): 177–186.

Balducci, L., B. Blumenstein, et al. (1987). Evaluation of fludarabine phosphate in renal cell carcinoma: a Southwest Oncology Group Study. *Cancer Treat Rep* 71(5): 543–544.

Baumgartner, G., R. Heinz, et al. (1980). Methotrexate-citrovorum factor used alone and in combination chemotherapy for advanced hypernephromas. *Cancer Treat Rep* 64(1): 41–46.

Benedetto, P., T. Ahmed, et al. (1983). Phase II trial of 4′epi-adriamycin for advanced hypernephroma. *Am J Clin Oncol* 6(5): 553–554.

Berg, W. J., L. Schwartz, et al. (2001). Phase II trial of irofulven (6-hydroxymethylacylfulvene) for patients with advanced renal cell carcinoma. *Invest New Drugs* 19(4): 317–320.

Bodrogi, I., M. Baki, et al. (1988). Ifosfamide chemotherapy of metastatic renal cell cancer. *Semin Surg Oncol* 4(2): 95–96.

Braybrooke, J. P., K. J. O'Byrne, et al. (2000). A phase II study of razoxane, an antiangiogenic topoisomerase II inhibitor, in renal cell cancer with assessment of potential surrogate markers of angiogenesis. *Clin Cancer Res* 6(12): 4697–4704.

Budd, G. T., S. Murthy, et al. (1992). Time-modified infusion of floxuridine in metastatic renal cell carcinoma (mRCC). *Proc Am Assoc Cancer Res* 33: 220.

Canobbio, L., F. Boccardo, et al. (1991). Phase II study of navelbine in advanced renal cell carcinoma. *Eur J Cancer* 27(6): 804–805.

Chico, I., M. H. Kang, et al. (2001). Phase I study of infusional paclitaxel in combination with the P-glycoprotein antagonist PSC 833. *J Clin Oncol* 19(3): 832–842.

Chuang, S. T., P. Chu, et al. (2005). Overexpression of glutathione S-transferase alpha in clear cell renal cell carcinoma. *Am J Clin Pathol* 123(3): 421–429.

Conroy, T., L. Geoffrois, et al. (1993). Simplified chronomodulated continuous infusion of floxuridine in patients with metastatic renal cell carcinoma. *Cancer* 72(7): 2190–2197.

Coppin, C., F. Porzsolt, et al. (2000). Immunotherapy for advanced renal cell cancer. *Cochrane Database Syst Rev* (3): CD001425.

Crivellari, D., S. Tumolo, et al. (1987). Phase II study of five-day continuous infusion of vinblastine in patients with metastatic renal-cell carcinoma. *Am J Clin Oncol* 10(3): 231–233.

Damascelli, B., A. Marchiano, et al. (1990). Circadian continuous chemotherapy of renal cell carcinoma with an implantable, programmable infusion pump. *Cancer* 66(2): 237–241.

Davis, N. B., D. A. Taber, et al. (2004). Phase II trial of PS-341 in patients with renal cell cancer: a University of Chicago phase II consortium study. *J Clin Oncol* 22(1): 115–119.

De Forges, A., J. P. Droz, et al. (1987). Phase II trial of ifosfamide/mesna in metastatic adult renal carcinoma. *Cancer Treat Rep* 71(11): 1103.

De Jager, R., P. Cappelaere, et al. (1984). An EORTC phase II study of mitoxantrone in solid tumors and lymphomas. *Eur J Cancer Clin Oncol* 20(11): 1369–1375.

De Mulder, P. H., L. Weissbach, et al. (1996). Gemcitabine: a phase II study in patients with advanced renal cancer. *Cancer Chemother Pharmacol* 37(5): 491–495.

Desai, A. A., N. J. Vogelzang, et al. (2002). A high rate of venous thromboembolism in a multi-institutional phase II trial of weekly intravenous gemcitabine with continuous infusion fluorouracil and daily thalidomide in patients with metastatic renal cell carcinoma. *Cancer* 95(8): 1629–1636.

Dexeus, F. H., C. J. Logothetis, et al. (1991). Circadian infusion of floxuridine in patients with metastatic renal cell carcinoma. *J Urol* 146(3): 709–713.

Einzig, A. I., E. Gorowski, et al. (1991). Phase II trial of taxol in patients with metastatic renal cell carcinoma. *Cancer Invest* 9(2): 133–136.

Elson, P. J., L. K. Kvols, et al. (1988). Phase II trials of 5-day vinblastine infusion (NSC 49842), L-alanosine (NSC 153353), acivicin (NSC 163501), and aminothiadiazole (NSC 4728) in patients with recurrent or metastatic renal cell carcinoma. *Invest New Drugs* 6(2): 97–103.

Ernest, S., S. Rajaraman, et al. (1997). Expression of MDR1 (multidrug resistance) gene and its protein in normal human kidney. *Nephron* 77(3): 284–289.

Falkson, C. I. (1993). New formulation intravenous melphalan in the treatment of patients with metastatic renal cancer. *Invest New Drugs* 11(1): 93.

Fizazi, K., F. Rolland, et al. (2003). A phase II study of irinotecan in patients with advanced renal cell carcinoma. *Cancer* 98(1): 61–65.

Fojo, A. T., D. W. Shen, et al. (1987). Intrinsic drug resistance in human kidney cancer is associated with expression of a human multidrug-resistance gene. *J Clin Oncol* **5**(12): 1922–1927.

Fojo, A. T., M. E. Menefee, et al. (2005). A translational study of ixabepilone (BMS-247550) in renal cell cancer (RCC): assessment of its activity and demonstration of target engagement in tumor cells. *Proc Am Soc Clin Oncol* **24**: (abstract 4541).

Fossa, S. D. and K. Talle. (1980). Treatment of metastatic renal cancer with ifosfamide and mesnum with and without irradiation. *Cancer Treat Rep* **64**(10–11): 1103–1108.

Fossa, S. D., B. Wik, et al. (1982). Phase II study of 4'-epidoxorubicin in metastatic renal cancer. *Cancer Treat Rep* **66**(5): 1219–1221.

Fossa, S. D., L. Denis, et al. (1983). Vindesine in advanced renal cancer. A study of the EORTC Genito-urinary Tract Cancer Cooperative Group. *Eur J Cancer Clin Oncol* **19**(4): 473–475.

Fossa, S. D., J. P. Droz, et al. (1992a). Vinblastine in metastatic renal cell carcinoma: EORTC phase II trial 30882. The EORTC Genitourinary Group. *Eur J Cancer* **28A**(4–5): 878–880.

Fossa, S. D., G. Martinelli, et al. (1992b). Recombinant interferon alfa-2a with or without vinblastine in metastatic renal cell carcinoma: results of a European multi-center phase III study. *Ann Oncol* **3**(4): 301–305.

Gams, R. A., O. Nelson, et al. (1986). Phase II evaluation of mitoxantrone in advanced renal cell carcinoma: a Southeastern Cancer Study Group Trial. *Cancer Treat Rep* **70**(7): 921–922.

George, C. M. and W. M. Stadler. (2003). The role of systemic chemotherapy in the treatment of kidney cancer. *Kidney Cancer*. Norwell, MA: Kluwer Academic Publishers.

George, C. M., N. J. Vogelzang, et al. (2002). A phase II trial of weekly intravenous gemcitabine and cisplatin with continuous infusion fluorouracil in patients with metastatic renal cell carcinoma. *Ann Oncol* **13**(1): 116–120.

Goodin, S., M. P. Kane, et al. (2004). Epothilones: mechanism of action and biologic activity. *J Clin Oncol* **22**(10): 2015–2025.

Haas, C. D., C. A. Coltman, Jr., et al. (1976). Phase II evaluation of bleomycin. A Southwest Oncology Group study. *Cancer* **38**(1): 8–12.

Hahn, D. M., S. C. Schimpff, et al. (1977). Single-agent therapy for renal cell carcinoma: CCNU, vinblastine, thioTEPA, or bleomycin. *Cancer Treat Rep* **61**(8): 1585–1587.

Hahn, R. G., M. Bauer, et al. (1979). Phase II study of single-agent therapy with megestrol acetate, VP-16-213, cyclophosphamide, and dianhydrogalactitol in advanced renal cell cancer. *Cancer Treat Rep* **63**(3): 513–515.

Hahn, R. G., C. B. Begg, et al. (1981). Phase II study of vinblastine-CCNU, triazinate, and dactinomycin in advanced renal cell cancer. *Cancer Treat Rep* **65**(7-8): 711–713.

Heim, M. E., R. Fiene, et al. (1981). Central nervous side effects following ifosfamide monotherapy of advanced renal carcinoma. *J Cancer Res Clin Oncol* **100**(1): 113–116.

Hogan, T. F., D. L. Citrin, et al. (1981). A preliminary report of mitotane therapy of advanced renal and prostate cancer. *Cancer Treat Rep* **65**(5–6): 539–540.

Hrushesky, W. J., R. von Roemeling, et al. (1990). Circadian-shaped infusions of floxuridine for progressive metastatic renal cell carcinoma. *J Clin Oncol* **8**(9): 1504–1513.

Hussain, M., U. Vaishampayan, et al. (2003). A phase II study of rebeccamycin analog (NSC-655649) in metastatic renal cell cancer. *Invest New Drugs* **21**(4): 465–471.

Johnson, D. E., R. A. Chalbaud, et al. (1975). Clinical trial of bleomycin (NSC-125066) in the treatment of metastatic renal carcinoma. *Cancer Chemother Rep* **59**(2 Pt 1): 433–435.

Kerbel, R. S. and B. A. Kamen. (2004). The anti-angiogenic basis of metronomic chemotherapy. *Nat Rev Cancer* **4**(6): 423–436.

Kiruluta, G., A. Morales, et al. (1975). Response of renal adenocarcinoma to cyclophosphamide. *Urology* **6**(5): 557–558.

Kish, J. A., M. Wolf, et al. (1994). Evaluation of low dose continuous infusion 5-fluorouracil in patients with advanced and recurrent renal cell carcinoma. A Southwest Oncology Group Study. *Cancer* **74**(3): 916–919.

Kondagunta, G. V., B. Drucker, et al. (2004). Phase II trial of bortezomib for patients with advanced renal cell carcinoma. *J Clin Oncol* **22**(18): 3720–3725.

Kovacs, G., M. Akhtar, et al., (1997). The Heidelberg classification of renal cell tumours. *J Pathol* **183**(2): 131–133.

Kuebler, J. P., T. F. Hogan, et al., (1984). Phase II study of continuous 5-day vinblastine infusion in renal adenocarcinoma. *Cancer Treat Rep* **68**(6): 925–926.

Kuebler, J. P., G. W. King, et al., (2001). Phase II study of pyrazoloacridine in metastatic renal cell carcinoma. *Invest New Drugs* **19**(4): 327–328.

La Rocca, R. V., C. A. Stein, et al., (1991). A pilot study of suramin in the treatment of metastatic renal cell carcinoma. *Cancer* **67**(6): 1509–1513.

Law, T. M., D. H. Ilson, et al., (1994a). Phase II trial of topotecan in patients with advanced renal cell carcinoma. *Invest New Drugs* **12**(2): 143–145.

Law, T. M., P. Mencel, et al., (1994b). Phase II trial of liposomal encapsulated doxorubicin in patients with advanced renal cell carcinoma. *Invest New Drugs* **12**(4): 323–325.

Merrin, C. E. (1979). Treatment of genitourinary tumours with cis- dichlorodiammineplatinum(II): experience in 250 patients. *Cancer Treat Rep* **63**(9–10): 1579–1584.

Merrouche, Y., S. Negrier, et al., (1991). Phase II study of continuous circadian infusion FUDR in metastatic renal cell cancer (RCC). *Eur J Cancer Clin Oncol* **27**.

Mertens, W. C., E. A. Eisenhauer, et al., (1993). Gemcitabine in advanced renal cell carcinoma. A phase II study of the National Cancer Institute of Canada Clinical Trials Group. *Ann Oncol* **4**(4): 331–332.

Moore, M. J., K. Chi, et al., (2001). A phase II study of troxacitabine in patients with advanced and/or metastatic renal cell carcinoma. NCIC CTG IND.119. *Proc Am Soc of Clin Oncol* **20**:193a (abstract 768).

Motzer, R. J. and P. Russo. (2000). Systemic therapy for renal cell carcinoma. *J Urol* **163**(2): 408–417.

Motzer, R. J., D. M. Nanus, et al., (1992). Phase II trial of suramin in patients with advanced renal cell carcinoma: treatment results, pharmacokinetics, and tumor growth factor expression. *Cancer Res* **52**(20): 5775–5779.

Nanus, D. M., A. Garino, et al., (2004). Active chemotherapy for sarcomatoid and rapidly progressing renal cell carcinoma. *Cancer* **101**(7): 1545–1551.

Natale, R. B., A. Yagoda, et al., (1982). Phase II trial of PALA in hypernephroma and urinary bladder cancer. *Cancer Treat Rep* **66**(12): 2091–2092.

Neidhart, J. A., S. A. Anderson, et al., (1991). Vinblastine fails to improve response of renal cancer to interferon alfa-n1: high response rate in patients with pulmonary metastases. *J Clin Oncol* **9**(5): 832–837.

O'Bryan, R. M., L. H. Baker, et al., (1977). Dose response evaluation of adriamycin in human neoplasia. *Cancer* **39**(5): 1940–1948.

Oudard, S., C. Levalois, et al., (2002). Expression of genes involved in chemoresistance, proliferation and apoptosis in clinical samples of renal cell carcinoma and correlation with clinical outcome. *Anticancer Res* **22**(1A): 121–128.

Park, D. K., C. W. Ryan, et al., (2002). A phase II trial of oral temozolomide in patients with metastatic renal cell cancer. *Cancer Chemother Pharmacol* **50**(2): 160–162.

Pellegrini, F. and D. R. Budman. (2005). Review: tubulin function, action of antitubulin drugs, and new drug development. *Cancer Invest* **23**(3): 264–273.

Ratain, M. J. and S. G. Eckhardt. (2004). Phase II studies of modern drugs directed against new targets: if you are fazed, too, then resist RECIST. *J Clin Oncol* **22**(22): 4442–4445.

Richards, F., M. R. Cooper, et al., (1991). Continuous 5-day (D) intravenous (IV) FUDR infusion for renal cell carcinoma (RCC): a phase I-II trial of the Piedmont Oncology Association. *Proc Am Soc Clin Oncol* **10**: 170.

Rini, B. I., N. J. Vogelzang, et al., (2000). Phase II trial of weekly intravenous gemcitabine with continuous infusion fluorouracil in patients with metastatic renal cell cancer. *J Clin Oncol* **18**(12): 2419–2426.

Rini, B. I., V. Weinberg, et al., (2004). Time to disease progression to evaluate a novel protein kinase C inhibitor, UCN-01, in renal cell carcinoma. *Cancer* **101**(1): 90–95.

Rodriguez, L. H. and D. E. Johnson. (1978). Clinical trial of cisplatinum (NSC 119875) in metastatic renal cell carcinoma. *Urology* **11**(4): 344–346.

Rohde, D., P. H. De Mulder, et al., (1996). Experimental and clinical efficacy of 2′, 2′-difluorodeoxycytidine (gemcitabine) against renal cell carcinoma. *Oncology* **53**(6): 476–481.

Ryan, C. W., N. J. Vogelzang, et al., (2002). A phase II trial of intravenous gemcitabine and 5-fluorouracil with subcutaneous interleukin-2 and interferon-alpha in patients with metastatic renal cell carcinoma. *Cancer* **94**(10): 2602–2609.

Samuels, B. L., D. R. Hollis, et al., (1997). Modulation of vinblastine resistance in metastatic renal cell carcinoma with cyclosporine A or tamoxifen: a cancer and leukemia group B study. *Clin Cancer Res* **3**(11): 1977–1984.

Schaub, T. P., J. Kartenbeck, et al., (1999). Expression of the MRP2 gene-encoded conjugate export pump in human kidney proximal tubules and in renal cell carcinoma. *J Am Soc Nephrol* **10**(6): 1159–1169.

Schulof, R., J. Lokich, et al., (1991). Phase II trial of protracted infusional 5-FU (PIF) for metastatic renal cell carcinoma. *Proc Am Soc Clin Oncol* **10**: 170.

Shevrin, D. H., T. E. Lad, et al., (1989). Phase II trial of fludarabine phosphate in advanced renal cell carcinoma: an Illinois Cancer Council Study. *Invest New Drugs* **7**(2–3): 251–253.

Skubitz, K. M. (2002). Phase II trial of pegylated-liposomal doxorubicin (Doxil) in renal cell cancer. *Invest New Drugs* **20**(1): 101–104.

Stadler, W. M. and M. J. Ratain. (2000). Development of target-based antineoplastic agents. *Invest New Drugs* **18**(1): 7–16.

Stadler, W. M., N. J. Vogelzang, et al., (2000). Flavopiridol, a novel cyclin-dependent kinase inhibitor, in metastatic renal cancer: a University of Chicago Phase II Consortium study. *J Clin Oncol* **18**(2): 371–375.

Stadler, W. M., D. Huo, et al., (2003). Prognostic factors for survival with gemcitabine plus 5-fluorouracil based regimens for metastatic renal cancer. *J Urol* **170**(4 Pt 1): 1141–1145.

Stadler, W. M., S. Halabi, et al., (2004). A phase II study of gemcitabine and capecitabine in patients with metastatic renal cell cancer: A report of Cancer and Leukemia Group B #90008. *Proc Am Soc Clin Oncol* **23**: 384 (abstract 4515).

Stewart, D. J., N. Futter, et al., (1987). Mitomycin-C and metronidazole in the treatment of advanced renal-cell carcinoma. *Am J Clin Oncol* **10**(6): 520–522.

Stolbach, L. L., C. B. Begg, et al., (1981). Treatment of renal carcinoma: a phase III randomized trial of oral medroxyprogesterone (Provera), hydroxyurea, and nafoxidine. *Cancer Treat Rep* **65**(7–8): 689–692.

Swanson, D. A. and D. E. Johnson. (1981). Estramustine phosphate (Emcyt) as treatment for metastatic renal carcinoma. *Urology* **17**(4): 344–346.

Tait, M., J. Abrams, et al., (1988). Phase II carboplatin (CBDCA) for metastatic renal cell cancer with a standard dose (SD) and a calculated dose (CD) according to renal function. *Proc Am Soc Clin Oncol* **7**: 125.

Takahashi, M., D. R. Rhodes, et al., (2001). Gene expression profiling of clear cell renal cell carcinoma: gene identification and prognostic classification. *Proc Natl Acad Sci USA* **98**(17): 9754–9759.

Takahashi, M., X. J. Yang, et al., (2003). Molecular subclassification of kidney tumors and the discovery of new diagnostic markers. *Oncogene* **22**(43): 6810–6818.

Tannock, I. F. and W. K. Evans. (1985). Failure of 5-day vinblastine infusion in the treatment of patients with renal cell carcinoma. *Cancer Treat Rep* **69**(2): 227–228.

Taylor, S. A., D. D. Von Hoff, et al., (1984). Phase II clinical trial of mitoxantrone in patients with advanced renal cell carcinoma: a Southwest Oncology Group study. *Cancer Treat Rep* **68**(6): 919–920.

Thodtmann, R., T. Sauter, et al., (2003). A phase II trial of pemetrexed in patients with metastatic renal cancer. *Invest New Drugs* **21**(3): 353–358.

Townsley, C. A., K. Chi, et al., (2003). Phase II study of troxacitabine (BCH-4556) in patients with advanced and/or metastatic renal cell carcinoma: a trial of the National Cancer Institute of Canada-Clinical Trials Group. *J Clin Oncol* **21**(8): 1524–1529.

Trump, D. L. and P. Elson. (1990). Evaluation of carboplatin (NSC 241240) in patients with recurrent or metastatic renal cell carcinoma. *Invest New Drugs* **8**(2): 201–203.

van Oosterom, A. T., S. D. Fossa, et al., (1984). Mitoxantrone in advanced renal cancer: a phase II study in previously untreated patients from the EORTC Genito-Urinary Tract Cancer Cooperative Group. *Eur J Cancer Clin Oncol* **20**(10): 1239–1241.

Van Veldhuizen, P. J., J. R. Faulkner, et al., (2005). A phase II study of flavopiridol in patients with advanced renal cell carcinoma: results of Southwest Oncology Group Trial 0109. *Cancer Chemother Pharmacol* **56**(1): 39–45.

Venner, P., E. A. Eisenhauer, et al., (1991). Phase II study of 2′-deoxycoformycin in patients with renal cell carcinoma.

A National Cancer Institute of Canada Clinical Trials Group study. *Invest New Drugs* **9**(3): 273–275.

Volm, M., M. Kastel, et al., (1993). Expression of resistance factors (P-glycoprotein, glutathione S-transferase-pi, and topoisomerase II) and their interrelationship to proto-oncogene products in renal cell carcinomas. *Cancer* **71**(12): 3981–3987.

Wajsman, Z., S. Beckley, et al., (1980). High dose cyclophosphamide in metastatic renal cell cancer. *Proc Am Soc Clin Oncol* **21**: 423.

Waters, J. S., C. Moss, et al., (2004). Phase II clinical trial of capecitabine and gemcitabine chemotherapy in patients with metastatic renal carcinoma. *Br J Cancer* **91**(10): 1763–1768.

Wilding, G., J. Kirkwood, et al., (1993). Phase II trial of navelbine in metastatic renal cancer. *Proc Am Soc Clin Oncol* **12**: 253.

Witte, R. S., C. Walsh, et al., (1992). Evaluation of deoxycoformycin in patients with advanced renal cell carcinoma. An ECOG pilot study. *Invest New Drugs* **10**(1): 49–50.

Wong, P. P., A. Yagoda, et al., (1977). Phase II study of vindesine sulfate in the therapy for advanced renal carcinoma. *Cancer Treat Rep* **61**(9): 1727–1729.

Yagoda, A., D. Petrylak, et al., (1993). Cytotoxic chemotherapy for advanced renal cell carcinoma. *Urol Clin North Am* **20**(2): 303–321.

Zaniboni, A., E. Simoncini, et al., (1989). Phase II trial of 5-fluorouracil and high-dose folinic acid in advanced renal cell cancer. *J Chemother* **1**(5): 350–351.

Zeffren, J., A. Yagoda, et al., (1984). Phase I-II trial of a 5-day continuous infusion of vinblastine sulfate. *Anticancer Res* **4**(6): 411–413.

11e
Cell-Based Vaccines for Renal Cell Carcinoma

Dolores J. Schendel and Bernhard Frankenberger

Introduction

Features in the natural history of renal cell carcinoma (RCC) are consistent with the recognition and targeting of RCCs by immune-mediated mechanisms. A number of observations support this assumption. Spontaneous regression of primary or metastatic lesions was observed in a number of documented cases.[48] Spontaneous regression rarely led to long-lasting cures and regression did not necessarily occur for all lesions in patients with multiple metastases. Additional evidence is based on the beneficial effects of cytokine therapies in some patients. Systemic cytokine treatment of RCC patients with recombinant interleukin 2 (IL-2), interferon-α (IFN-α), or both in combination, induced partial or complete remission of tumors in some patients.[53,68] These two cytokines influence the activities of several different cell populations that may contribute to successful antitumor immunity, including monocytes, lymphocytes, and dendritic cells (DCs). Many cytokine-induced remissions were transient and usually not all lesions responded to therapy. The reasons why only some tumor sites in an individual patient were susceptible to immune attack remain unclear. To date, the types of immune response responsible for spontaneous and cytokine-induced regression in RCCs have not been clearly identified.

Some insight into the potential mechanisms of antitumor immunity can be deduced from analyses of tumor tissues. Immunohistochemical studies of RCCs, particularly those of the clear cell type (cRCC), revealed abundant lymphocytic infiltrates in many tumors.[80,81] Cells of both the innate and adaptive immune systems were found in the tumors in situ (Fig. 11e-1). The tumor-infiltrating populations were rich in lymphocytes of the T cell lineage and included both CD4+ and CD8+ lymphocyte subsets. Natural killer (NK) cells were also found to be prevalent in some but not all cRCCs.[73] B lymphocytes were present in only small numbers in RCC infiltrates. Functional studies of tumor-infiltrating lymphocytes (TILs) isolated from RCCs demonstrated that infiltrating lymphocytes belonging to both the NK and T cell families had the capacity to recognize tumor cells in vitro through the secretion of cytokines and activation

of cytotoxic mechanisms.[71] Antitumor responses were also identified using peripheral blood mononuclear cells (PBMCs) of RCC patients that were activated in vitro.[71] Comparisons of the function and specificity of various subpopulations of TILs and activated lymphocytes derived from PBMCs provided substantial insight into the cellular and molecular basis of antitumor responses to RCCs.

The Cellular and Molecular Basis of Anti-Renal Cell Carcinoma Immunity

Natural Killer Cells Recognizing Renal Cell Carcinomas

As components of innate immunity, NK cells play a role in the first line of defense against tumors (Fig. 11e-2). Little is understood about NK cells infiltrating RCCs and their impact on successful antitumor immunity. The ability to study NK cells has improved greatly through the availability of NK receptor-specific monoclonal antibodies. Characterization of renal tissues using an antibody specific for an activating receptor that is constitutively expressed by all NK cells revealed that NK cells were prevalent in some cRCC tissues but there were fewer NK cells in normal kidney parenchyma.[73] NK cell isolates from freshly resected tumors showed differences in expression of inhibitory receptors when compared to circulating NK cells in autologous PBMCs. The differences in composition of NK cells in two different compartments of the same individual indicated that only selected NK cells infiltrated cRCCs. Furthermore, cRCCs could be divided into two categories in which one group of tumors had high percentages of NK cells whereas the other group of RCCs had only sparse numbers of NK cells among the total lymphocytes.[74] NK cells purified from the two types of infiltrates differed in their cytotoxic capacity, whereby those from infiltrates with abundant NK cells displayed cytotoxicity following a short culture ex vivo with IL-2 whereas the others were

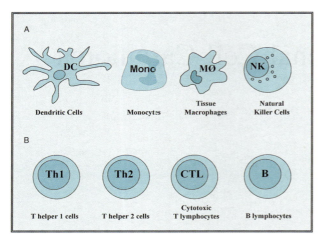

FIGURE 11e-1. Cells of the innate (**A**) and adaptive (**B**) immune system. Innate immunity refers to nonspecific defense mechanisms that come into play immediately or within hours of an antigen's appearance in the body. This first line of defense includes barriers to infection (such as skin), soluble antimicrobial proteins (acute phase proteins, lysozymes, cytokines, and the complement system), phagocytic cells (dendritic cells, monocytes, and macrophages), and natural killer (NK) cells. Adaptive (acquired) immunity refers to antigen-specific immune responses. The development of adaptive immune responses is more complex and takes several days to offer protection. The specific antigen that initiates an adaptive response must first be taken up by antigen-presenting cells (APCs), such as dendritic cells (DCs), and processed and presented for stimulation of T cells. Once a specific antigen has been recognized, the adaptive immune system uses a variety of mechanisms to eliminate the source of antigen. Two types of adaptive immune response can be called into play. When T helper 1 (Th1) cells are activated by APCs, they secrete cytokines that support the development of cytotoxic T lymphocytes (CTLs) that can directly kill antigen-expressing target cells. Th1 cells can also activate antigen-expressing monocytes/macrophages to eliminate intracellular sources of antigen, such as intracellular pathogens that have been taken up by phagocytosis. These responses are designated as cellular immunity. When T helper 2 (Th2) cells are activated by APCs, they secrete cytokines that support B lymphocytes to differentiate into antibody-producing cells that secrete immunoglobulins. This is designated as humoral immunity. Adaptive immunity also includes development of "memory" that allows future responses against the specific antigen to occur quickly and more efficiently. Memory is provided by long-lived antigen-specific T and B lymphocytes. There is an intersection between innate and adaptive immunity since cells of the innate immune system play a critical role in the activation of cells of the adaptive immune system. In particular, the function of DCs to stimulate naive T cells and to provide important cytokines for development of adaptive immune responses bridges innate and adaptive immunity.

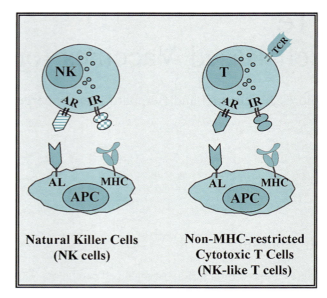

FIGURE 11e-2. Non-MHC-restricted cytotoxic effector cells. NK cells are part of the innate immune defense against neoplastic growth. The cytotoxic activity of NK cells is determined by a balance between signals delivered to activating receptors (ARs) and inhibitory receptors (IRs) that are coexpressed on individual NK cells. One group of ARs, designated as natural cytotoxicity receptors (NCRs), represents the only NK-specific receptors known to date. The activating ligands (ALs) expressed by tumor cells for these receptors remain to be identified. NK cell activation can be impaired or prevented upon simultaneous engagement of IRs with their respective ligands on target cells. IRs recognize MHC class I molecules and their activation can abolish signaling by ARs. MHC class I molecules, encoded by HLA-A, -B, -C, -E, and -G alleles of the MHC, serve as the ligands for different IRs expressed by NK cells. This allows NK cells to distinguish a diverse set of MHC class I allotypes. This is an important mechanism in the defense against tumors, since downregulation of specific MHC class I allotypes by tumor cells may allow them to escape adaptive immunity. In addition to their killing properties, NK cells can secrete several cytokines, including IFN-γ. By secreting IFN-γ, NK cells can influence the function of dendritic cells to secrete cytokines that favor the differentiation of Th1 cells and inhibit the differentiation of Th2 cells, leading to improved cellular immunity against tumors. Lymphocytes of the T cell lineage that are stimulated with high levels of IL-2, in the absence of T cell receptor stimulation, acquire the capacity to kill target cells and to secrete cytokines in a non-MHC-restricted manner. They do not use their T cell receptors to recognize target cells. Like NK cells, these T cells are negatively regulated by MHC class I molecules, leading to their designation as NK-like T cells. NK-like T cells express ARs and IRs that are distinct from those expressed by NK cells.

noncytotoxic. Although only a small number of cases were analyzed, no patients with distant metastases were found in the group of cRCCs from which functional NK cells could be recovered, suggesting that immune control may be more effective in this subset of RCCs. Why different

cRCCs accommodate phenotypic and functionally distinct subsets of NK cells is not understood. Different tumor microenvironments may have attracted specific subpopulations of NK cells or influenced their retention, function, or survival.

Non-Major Histocompatibility Complex-Restricted Tumor-Infiltrating Lymphocytes and Lymphokine-Activated Killer Cells

When TILs were isolated from primary RCCs or metastatic lesions and expanded *ex vivo* for several weeks in culture with IL-2, cytotoxic effector cells with two different patterns of specificity were detected. Some TILs killed a broad spectrum of target cells whereas others were limited in the target cells they recognized.[71] Both types of cytotoxic TILs killed autologous RCC cells, albeit to varying degrees. Broadly reactive TILs often attacked autologous normal cells and they killed allogeneic tumor cells irrespective of histological origin. A prominent characteristic of these TILs was their killing of major histocompatibility complex (MHC) class I-negative target cells, demonstrating that they were not restricted by MHC molecules for target cell recognition. A comprehensive study of TIL-derived lymphocyte clones isolated from different RCC infiltrates revealed that the majority of lymphocytes displayed broad specificity.[7,42]

If PBMCs of RCC patients were cultured *in vitro* with high concentrations of IL-2, a population of cytotoxic effector cells was generated that also displayed a similar broad killing specificity. Due to their activation by IL-2, such effector cells were designated as lymphokine-activated killer (LAK) cells.[66] LAK cells also killed various tumor lines having no matched MHC molecules, establishing their non-MHC-restricted specificity. It is difficult to judge whether LAK cells and TILs showing non-MHC-restricted specificity represent distinct effector cell types. Since RCCs are highly vascularized, culture of TIL isolates in medium containing IL-2 may have led to activation of LAK cells in contaminating PBMCs. LAK cells with broad antitumor activity were also generated from PBMCs of healthy individuals, demonstrating that their activation was independent of prior tumor cell contact.[71] Early studies of adoptive cell therapy demonstrated that LAK cells were able to induce regression of tumors in some RCC patients.[59,67,76,91]

Phenotyping of broadly reactive TILs and LAK cells showed that they were mixtures of lymphocytes, containing both CD3[-]NK cells and CD3[+]T cells.[36,57,61,62] The function of these fractions in LAK cells was analyzed following separation of cells according to phenotype: the strongest cytotoxic potential resided in the CD3[-] NK cell fraction. Broad cytotoxic activity with concurrent killing of MHC class I-negative target cells was also ascribed to CD3[+]CD8[+] cells and CD3[+]CD4[-]CD8[-] LAK cells whereas most CD3[+]CD4[+] cells were not found to be cytotoxic. Our own studies of LAK-derived T cells demonstrated that purified CD4[+] T cells could mediate non-MHC-restricted killing of target cells, including RCCs.[19] In summary, these observations revealed that both CD4[+] and CD8[+] cells with broad killing specificity could be classified as non-MHC-restricted cytotoxic T cells, or simply as NK-like T cells (Fig. 11e-2).

We discovered that RCC cells could be partially protected from killing by NK-like T cells if they expressed adequate levels of particular MHC molecules.[19,70] Treatment of RCC cells with IFN-γ increased MHC class I surface expression overall and induced a concurrent resistance to killing by both NK cells and NK-like T cells. Resistance was associated with increased expression of HLA-C and HLA-E molecules by the tumor cells. Resistance to both effector cell populations could be reversed by the addition of MHC class I-specific antibody, again leading to killing of the RCC cells. Interestingly, although NK-like T cells behaved like NK cells with respect to negative regulation by MHC class I molecules, they did not express any known NK inhibitory receptors that interact with specific MHC class I allotypes, such as specific HLA-C and HLA-E molecules. They also did not express activating receptors characteristic of NK cells. The fact that these T cells were activated through cytokine stimulation and they did not display antigen specificity places their function, like that of NK cells, in the category of innate immunity.

Major Histocompatibility Complex-Restricted T Cell Responses Directed Against Renal Cell Carcinomas

The third type of cytotoxic effector cell that was found in some RCC patients had an MHC-restricted pattern of cytotoxicity, limiting the target cells it recognized[71] (Fig. 11e-3). MHC-restricted cytotoxic T-lymphocytes (CTLs) were detected only rarely among TIL isolates, but the presence of these cells would be masked if non-MHC-restricted cells were present in the uncloned infiltrates since the NK-like T cells would show broad killing specificity. In a few instances, CD3[+]CD8[+] TIL lines or clones were found that killed autologous tumor cells but usually not normal autologous cells. Their killing of RCCs could be blocked by MHC class I-specific antibody. They also did not kill MHC class I-negative cell lines, thereby distinguishing them from the non-MHC-restricted killing of NK-like T cells. Some CTLs also recognized several allogeneic RCC lines that shared MHC class I molecules with the tumor cells against which the CTLs were initially primed. Since MHC-restricted T cells recognize peptide epitopes that are presented by MHC molecules, they can kill only target cells that display the same MHC–peptide ligands. Although TILs that recognized MHC–peptide ligands shared by different RCCs were found occasionally, most MHC-restricted CD8[+] CTLs of RCC patients appeared to recognize epitopes that were only expressed by autologous tumor cells. On occasion, MHC-restricted CD4[+] T cells recognizing RCCs were also found. The activity of these T cells could be blocked by antibody specific for MHC class II molecules.

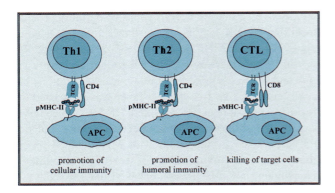

FIGURE 11e-3. Functions of MHC-restricted T cells. Immune recognition by antigen-specific T lymphocytes occurs through surface interactions involving a specific T cell receptor (TCR) on the lymphocyte and an antigen on the target cell. Unlike antibodies, TCRs do not recognize intact antigens. With few exceptions, they recognize only fragments of antigens, in the form of peptides that are presented on the cell surface by molecules of the major histocompatibility complex (MHC). The ability of T cells to recognize antigen only when it is presented by MHC molecules is called "MHC restriction." MHC class I and class II proteins have evolved to deal with different sets of antigens. Exogenous antigens such as bacteria, toxins, cellular debris, and molecules shed from tumor cells are present in extracellular body fluids. Antigen-presenting cells (APCs) take them up by phagocytosis, endocytosis, or receptor-mediated mechanisms. Within the cell they are degraded into peptides and presented by class II molecules (pMHC-II). Endogenous antigens that originate inside the cell, such as viral proteins or mutated and oncogenic proteins in tumor cells, are degraded in the cytosol and presented by class I molecules (pMHC-I). MHC class I molecules also present peptides derived by proteolysis of normal cellular proteins (self-peptides). Thus, the complete internal environment of a cell, consisting of self as well as foreign proteins, is displayed at the cell surface by peptides bound to class I molecules. T cells survey the pMHC ligands presented by APCs. Complexes containing normal self peptides generally are ignored while complexes containing foreign peptides activate T cells via their TCRs. CD4 and CD8 molecules act as accessory adhesion molecules by binding to class II or I molecules, respectively, on APCs. Activated CD4-positive T helper 1 (Th1) cells secrete cytokines, such as IFN-γ, that promote cellular immunity and support activities of macrophages and cytotoxic T lymphocytes (CTLs). Activated T helper 2 (Th2) cells secrete cytokines that favor the promotion of humoral immunity. MHC-restricted CD8-positive CTLs secrete molecules, such as perforin and granzymes, that directly damage the target cells to which they bind. MHC class I molecules are expressed constitutively by nearly all nucleated cells, so that CTLs are able to recognize and destroy almost any cell type, including tumor cells, if they present the appropriate peptide–MHC complexes.

Renal Cell Carcinoma Ligands Recognized by Major Histocompatibility Complex-Restricted T Cells

There is a paucity of information regarding the specific peptides that are presented by MHC molecules on RCCs and recognized by patient-derived antigen-specific CTLs. A few

MHC-restricted CD4[+] T cells were isolated and characterized from RCC patients, but the specific peptides they recognized were not defined.[20,51] Recent studies showed that RCC patients often had circulating CD4[+] T cells in their PBMCs that recognized peptides derived from the cancer germline MAGE-6 protein and the tyrosine kinase receptor, EphA2, in association with particular MHC class II molecules.[64,84]

More success was achieved in the identification of several peptide ligands for MHC-restricted CD8[+] CTLs recognizing RCCs. Using cDNA expression cloning, nine peptide ligands were identified that were recognized by CTLs derived from different RCC patients. The kinds of molecules that were discovered revealed an intriguing array of proteins that served as sources of peptides for CTL recognition of RCCs. Two peptides were derived from alternative open reading frames of normal cellular proteins,[63,65] a third was generated through reverse strand transcription,[87] while a fourth peptide was generated by posttranslational protein splicing.[30] Three additional peptides were derived from mutated proteins.[9,23,94] A further peptide was derived from a protein that is normally expressed only in testis tissue and thereby belongs to the group of cancer germline antigens.[24] Using a modified approach, the CAIX/G250 protein, which is expressed in a majority of cRCCs, was shown to contain a peptide that was presented by HLA-A2 molecules and recognized by patient-derived CTLs.[88] This is the only peptide among the nine that would be expected to be commonly displayed by RCCs from HLA-A2[+] patients and might be more broadly applicable for therapeutic use.

In the development of vaccination strategies for patients with RCC, creating protocols that activate and maintain the effector functions of all these lymphocyte subsets may lead to immune responses with improved clinical benefit for RCC patients. For this reason, the design of vaccine strategies for RCC not only should attempt to induce immune responses *de novo* but also should harness the complex mechanisms of antitumor immunity that already exist in many RCC patients.

Modulation of Immunity to Renal Cell Carcinoma by Vaccination

General Features of Renal Cell Carcinoma Vaccines

The goal in developing vaccines for RCC is to mobilize the inherent capacity of the immune system to recognize and destroy these tumor cells. Although vaccines are classically considered to prevent disease by inducing protective immunity prior to the encounter of an individual with a pathological agent, studies have shown that tumor vaccines can also be beneficial in a therapeutic setting in patients who already have malignant disease.[2,89] Nevertheless, producing effective therapeutic vaccination regimens is a major challenge. On the one hand, vaccines should be able to harness preexisting effector mechanisms in patients who have developed natural immune responses to their tumors, which may have been downregulated in the course of disease. On the other hand, vaccines should also have the capacity to mobilize new immune responses that can efficiently eliminate tumor cells. Since different vaccination strategies can activate different types of immune response, it is important in the preclinical phase to fully characterize the lymphocyte populations activated by any particular vaccine form in order to better understand its impact on antitumor immunity. Because immune responses can vary among tumor types, attaining representative information for RCC subtypes is also

critical. Furthermore, this information is necessary to select the appropriate immune monitoring tools to detect immune responses and to correlate their contributions to changes in clinical status during vaccination trials.

Improved understanding of the molecular and cellular basis of antitumor immunity has led to a continual evolution in the development of vaccine approaches for RCC (Fig. 11e-4). Two types of cell-based vaccine, utilizing either tumor cells or dendritic cells, have been developed for clinical testing. With the more recent identification of appropriate molecular targets, peptide-based vaccines now become feasible for RCC.

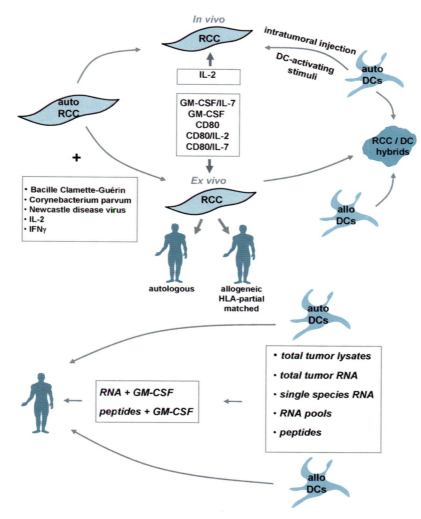

FIGURE 11e-4. Vaccine strategies for RCC. The initial development of vaccines for RCC used autologous tumor cells that were prepared from freshly resected tumor cells that were reapplied with various adjuvants. A second approach used genetic engineering of tumor cells, either in vivo or ex vivo, to allow them to express cytokines or costimulatory molecules to improve their immunogenicity. Tumor cells modified ex vivo were applied to autologous patients or to allogeneic patients selected to be partially matched with the gene-modified RCC vaccines. In another approach, tumor cells were fused to dendritic cells (DCs) to provide them with the superior priming capacity of these professional antigen-presenting cells; here both autologous and allogeneic DCs have been used for hybrid cell formation. Likewise, both autologous and allogeneic DCs have been used directly as vaccines following loading with various sources of tumor-associated antigens. The methods of genomics and proteomics are providing information about specific antigens that can be used to target RCCs for adaptive immune responses. This now allows cell-free vaccination to be studied, based on the use of RNA or peptides with adjuvant. Specific details on studies applying these various vaccine strategies are discussed in detail in the text.

Tumor Cell-Based Vaccines for Renal Cell Carcinoma

Initial vaccine strategies for RCC concentrated on approaches using tumor cells themselves to provide mixtures of tumor-associated antigens (TAAs) as immunizing agents. Under some circumstances, autologous tumors may be able to elicit responses to molecular composites of TAAs characteristic of individual tumors. Thus, even unique mutations that occur in normal cell proteins could serve as epitopes for MHC-restricted CTL recognition, as evidenced by the identification of mutated peptide ligands for several CTLs isolated from RCC patients described above. If allogeneic tumor cells are utilized, development of specific T cell-mediated immunity relies on the presence of target molecules that are shared among various RCCs. More recent data from CTL recognition studies and molecular TAA identification support the validity of this contention for RCCs. Based on these observations, three types of tumor cell-based vaccine have been pursued for RCC: autologous tumor cells with or without adjuvant, autologous gene-modified tumor cells, and allogeneic gene-modified tumor cells.

Autologous Tumor Cell Vaccines and Adjuvant

Failure of naturally occurring immune responses to control RCC growth led to initial considerations to apply surgically resected autologous tumor cells as vaccines, with or without adjuvant, to boost antitumor immunity in patients. Several trials utilized autologous, or occasionally allogeneic, irradiated tumor cells that were combined with different immune adjuvants, including bacillus Calmette–Guérin, *Corynebacterium parvum*, or Newcastle disease virus. These approaches, collectively designated as active specific immunotherapy, were tested in a number of different studies in patients with locally advanced disease or with distant metastases.[14,72] Some studies also included application of systemic cytokines (IL-2 and/or IFN-α) subsequent to vaccination. Many of the vaccinated patients developed delayed type hypersensitivity (DTH) responses to their autologous tumor cells, which served as a measure of T cell reactivity, and early indications suggested clinical benefit for some patients with regression of metastatic lesions. Despite evidence of induction of T cell responses to autologous tumor cells, there was no improvement in disease-free survival or overall survival in the vaccinated groups.

These studies demonstrated safety and feasibility with toxicities mostly of Grade I or II, with some exceptions due to the effects of IL-2. Bioactivity, as measured by vaccine-induced DTH responses upon challenge with autologous tumor cells or by the development of CTL responses directed against tumor cells, was found in some patients in every study where antitumor activity was assessed. Long-term application of these types of vaccine was not possible because of limitations in numbers of tumor cells available

from individual patients. Little insight was gained into the nature of immune responses that were induced through these vaccines because of the limited immune monitoring that was performed prevaccination and postvaccination. Although vaccine toxicities in all these studies were demonstrably low in comparison to the well-known side effects of systemic cytokine therapies, the clinical benefit was also lower in patients with advanced disease. The failure of these approaches to provide improved clinical benefit spurred the development of alternative strategies for the treatment of patients with advanced disease.

More recently, results were reported for a Phase III randomized trial in nonmetastatic patients who were vaccinated with autologous tumor cells that were pretreated with IFN-γ and tocopherol acetate, which served as a radical scavenger to protect cell membranes during the incubation period with cytokine. Thereafter, the tumor cells were repeatedly freeze–thawed to produce cell lysates that were applied to more than 150 patients and compared to an equally large group of untreated patients.[40] In contrast to the various trials in patients with advanced disease, this trial demonstrated improved 5-year and 70-month progress-free survival rates. Unfortunately, the loss of many patients in the trial and the missing determination of overall survival rates are major deficits in the evaluation of the results.[21] Assessments of DTH or other parameters of antitumor reactivity were not reported for this trial. Therefore, further studies are needed to determine how this approach impacts on antitumor immunity and whether it will prolong patient survival.

Gene-Modified Tumor Cell Vaccines

A number of Phase I/II trials explored the use of autologous tumor cells that were directly altered to secrete cytokines or to display costimulatory molecules in order to improve their immunogenicity.[55] Based on animal studies,[16] autologous tumor cells were genetically modified to express granulocyte-macrophage colony-stimulating factor (GM-CSF) for vaccine application in RCC patients with metastatic disease.[78] The capacity of GM-CSF-secreting tumor cells to induce antitumor responses in mice was attributed to their ability to induce inflammatory reactions at the vaccination site, eventually recruiting DCs that utilized injected tumor cells as sources of TAAs for sensitization of T lymphocytes. Biopsies of the vaccine injection sites of RCC patients receiving GM-CSF-secreting autologous tumor cells showed infiltrations of macrophages, DCs, eosinophils, neutrophils, and T cells. The DTH sites induced by challenge with tumor cells revealed prominent CD4+ and CD8+ lymphocytic infiltrates as well as infiltration by eosinophils. Extensive immunological analyses of the T cell responses in PBMCs of these patients documented the development of both MHC-restricted CD4 and CD8 responses with multiple specificities.[51,94] These studies demonstrated that this vaccine strategy was capable of inducing polyvalent adaptive T cell responses.

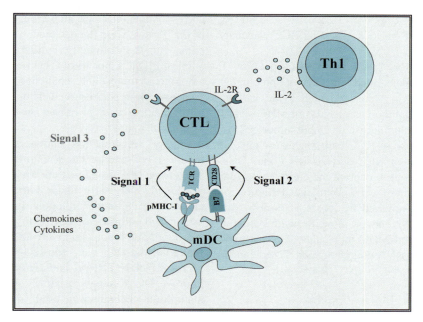

FIGURE 11e-5. T cell activation. Activation of T cells, such as CD8-positive CTLs, which leads to clonal expansion and differentiation into activated effector cells, requires several important signals. The first signal (signal 1) is mediated by the engagement of the T cell receptors (TCRs) of naive T cells with cognate peptide–MHC complexes on antigen-presenting cells (APCs). This interaction determines the antigen specificity of the adaptive immune response. The second signal (signal 2) is not antigen specific and is delivered through the interaction of B7 molecules expressed by APCs with CD28 receptors expressed by T cells. When T cells receive signal 1 and signal 2, they begin to express additional receptors that can bind cytokines, such as IL-2. The cytokine signaling for this step is sometimes referred to as signal 3. Activated CD4-positive T helper 1 cells (Th1 cells) that have been stimulated by MHC class II/peptide complexes and B7 costimulatory molecules on APCs are activated to secrete cytokines, including IL-2, that support the proliferation and function of CD8-positive CTLs. Engagement of the TCR of CD8-positive CTLs with MHC class I/peptide complexes alone (signal 1 in the absence of signal 2) is one mechanism known to induce T cell anergy in cells making their first contact with antigens. The failure of many tumor cells to deliver signal 2 may allow them to escape immune elimination by inducing T cell anergy. Genetic engineering of tumor cells to provide signal 2 and/or signal 3 can help to overcome this deficit.

Nevertheless, only 1 of 18 patients showed an objective clinical response.

Alternatively, genetic modification of tumor cells to express costimulatory molecules may allow tumor cells to directly initiate immune responses.[4,12,86] A clinical trial using autologous RCCs modified to express CD80, in combination with systemic IL-2, was shown to be safe with toxicities comparable to those found with IL-2 alone.[3] DTH responses upon challenge with autologous tumor cells were found in some patients and biopsies of the DTH sites showed infiltrates of CD4+ and CD8+ T cells. Furthermore, increased numbers of T cells producing IFN-γ were found to be circulating in peripheral blood of vaccinated patients. These changes revealed that this vaccine regimen modulated antitumor immunity in patients with advanced disease.

An alternative strategy to preparing autologous vaccines for every patient is to employ gene-modified allogeneic tumor cells to vaccinate selected patients who are partially MHC matched with the vaccine cells in order to allow T cell recognition of common MHC–peptide ligands shared with patient tumor cells. To improve immunogenicity, allogeneic tumor cell lines can also be genetically engineered to express costimulatory molecules, such as CD80 or CD86, alone or

in combination with cytokines.[22] Several ongoing trials are currently evaluating such strategies.

The finding that expression of GM-CSF in RCCs led to DC recruitment that seemed to be critical for antitumor immunity and clinical response spurred the development of vaccine strategies directly employing DCs in RCC patients (Fig. 11e-5).

Dendritic Cell-Based Vaccines for Renal Cell Carcinoma

DCs have attained a position of central interest due to their ability to generate MHC–peptide ligands for both CD4+ and CD8+ T cells. Their expression of an array of costimulatory molecules and secretion of immune stimulatory cytokines provide them with an unsurpassed ability to activate naive T cells.[1,11,28,77] This allows them to support the optimal development of MHC-restricted T cell responses. In addition, DCs can directly activate NK cells and support their proliferation if they secrete IL-2 or IL-12. DC vaccine development has become feasible through a better understanding of how DCs can be prepared in large numbers *ex vivo*. Recent efforts have explored the use of various types of RCC vaccines utilizing DCs.

The potential of DCs to induce RCC-specific T cell responses was demonstrated in several preclinical studies.[10,29,31,35,35,54,82] DCs were provided with various sources of TAAs for presentation as peptides in MHC class I and class II molecules, including use of viable tumor cells to form hybrids with DCs, use of RCC cell lysates for pulsing of DCs, and introduction of RCC-derived RNA into DCs. All of these methods attempt to capture the entire composite of TAAs expressed by tumor cells. With the definition of specific TAAs that are expressed by RCCs, it is now also feasible to load DCs with one or more defined synthetic peptides binding to selected MHC molecules. Alternatively, single species or pools of RNA encoding such TAAs can be introduced into DCs.

Dendritic Cell–Tumor Cell Hybrids

Viable tumor cells were fused with DCs to generate cell hybrids that combined the full mRNA and protein content of RCCs with the superior antigen-presenting capacity of DCs.[6] One widely cited trial in RCC patients using allogeneic DCs fused with autologous tumor cells was retracted and merits no further consideration.[44,45] Two independent studies also evaluated this approach.[8,50] Most of the patients showed DTH responses following vaccination and some clinical responses were observed. The only side effect noted was low-grade fever. Interestingly, improvement in DTH responses specific for several recall antigens occurred, providing evidence for an overall improvement in the immune system. Because there seemed to be some effect on the natural course of disease, this vaccine strategy might be useful in patients with less advanced disease. However, the technical difficulty in generating hybrids of good quality has shifted emphasis to the use of DCs that are directly loaded with various sources of TAA.

Dendritic Cells Loaded with Tumor Cell Lysates

Several trials used immature DCs pulsed with tumor cell lysates as vaccines for RCC patients with advanced disease.[5,27,56,60] In some cases the DCs were also pulsed with the foreign protein, keyhole limpet hemocyanin (KLH), in order to support activation of Th1 responses. In addition, KLH served as a surrogate marker to assess the induction of specific T cell responses from naive lymphocytes since humans would not be naturally exposed to this protein. Some patients also received systemic low-dose IL-2. While KLH reactivity was induced in the patients receiving the

corresponding vaccines, alterations in immunological profiles of the patients were not detected, based on measures of autologous tumor cytotoxicity, cytokine production, or proliferation of PBMCs, nor were DTH responses induced following autologous tumor cell challenge. Also objective clinical responses were not observed. Thus, this vaccine strategy was insufficient to have an impact on either antitumor immunity or clinical status.

Further research has shown that immature DCs can induce T cell anergy rather than lymphocyte activation.[28,77] Therefore, the use of mature DCs as vaccines is strongly warranted. Two early Phase I trials used lysates prepared either from cultured autologous tumors or derived from an established allogeneic RCC line as sources of TAAs for pulsing of autologous immature DCs, along with KLH. In the first trial, the DCs were subsequently matured using tumor necrosis factor (TNF)-α and prostaglandin E_2 was added to improve DC homing capacity.[33] A more complex cytokine maturation cocktail was used in the second trial.[34] The applied DCs had mature phenotypes. Both trials demonstrated feasibility without adverse effects and signs of immunological reactivity were found in most patients subsequent to vaccination. A few patients showed objective clinical responses. Interestingly, two patients showing complete responses received DCs loaded with lysates prepared from autologous metastatic lesions, indicating that the antigenic composition of metastatic cells was perhaps better suited to stimulate clinically effective T cell responses.[34] All patients who were tested showed DTH responses to KLH and antigen-specific T cell responses directed against RCC-associated antigens were often detected, with the strongest responses appearing in patients showing objective clinical responses. After 32 months of follow-up, 8 of 35 patients were still alive, suggesting that this vaccine strategy could impact the disease course in patients with advanced RCC.

Allogeneic mature DCs pulsed with tumor lysates were also evaluated based on the presumption that antigen transfer would occur *in vivo* between the vaccine cells and autologous DCs of the patients.[32] Some patients also received cyclophosphamide to reduce systemic immune suppression. Tumor lysates were prepared either from autologous tumor cells or from a defined RCC line when autologous tumor was not available. The DCs were also pulsed with KLH. Subsequent to vaccination, immune responses to KLH and tumor cells were weak. Two patients who showed stronger T cell responses both received cyclophosphamide, indicating that this pretreatment was having an impact on the capacity of patients to develop better antitumor immunity. The differences between poor adaptive immune responses in patients vaccinated with allogeneic DCs versus the better responses seen utilizing autologous DCs[34] suggest that TAA transfer from vaccine DCs to patient DCs *in vivo* does not correctly mimic the effects achieved with direct autologous DC vaccination.

Dendritic Cells Pulsed with Tumor-Derived RNA

Vaccines based on RNA-pulsed DCs are at early stages of development for RCC. Preclinical studies showed that DCs pulsed with RNA derived from RCC tumor tissue were very effective at inducing tumor-specific T cells *in vitro*.[26,31] These T cells recognized RCCs but not normal kidney parenchyma cells. Furthermore, CTL responses specific for peptides derived from telomerase reverse transcriptase (TERT), which was expressed by the tumor cells, were induced by the DCs. A second preclinical study confirmed these observations and revealed that both whole tumor-derived RNA and amplified tumor messenger RNA could be used instead of mRNA purified from RCC cells to stimulate tumor-specific CTL responses.[29] Instead of preparing RNA from tumor tissue of each individual patient, RNA may also be prepared from a well-characterized RCC cell line providing a generic source of TAAs.[25] A particular advantage of this "generic" strategy is that the composite TAAs expressed by a selected RCC line can be defined in detail using RNA quantification and protein expression and the efficiency of TAA transfer into DCs can be assessed.[39] Furthermore, specific immune monitoring tools can be appropriately designed for clinical studies.

To date, few studies have used RNA-based DC vaccines in RCC patients with advanced disease. A first study used autologous tumor-derived RNA as the source of TAAs, which was naturally taken up by immature DCs.[32] The DCs were not matured *ex vivo* before injection. This study demonstrated the feasibility of this approach and revealed no toxicity. Clinical responses could not be evaluated because most of these advanced disease patients received subsequent alternative treatments. Nevertheless, tumor-related mortality was unexpectedly low in this small group of patients. Monitoring of the immune responses induced by RNA-transduced DCs revealed an effective stimulation of polyclonal T cell responses directed against autologous and some allogeneic tumor cells as well as against defined TAAs common to several RCCs. The demonstration that antigen-specific T cells were induced *in vivo* against several defined molecules shared by multiple RCCs opens the possibility of utilizing these TAAs as specific molecular targets in future DC vaccine approaches.

A more recent study used immature DCs that were loaded with autologous tumor-derived RNA via electroporation and then matured with a cytokine cocktail. These mature DCs were applied to some patients who were also treated 4 days prior to vaccination with an IL-2-diphtheria toxin conjugate in order to reduce T regulatory cells that might inhibit antitumor responses.[15] This study demonstrated that regulatory T cells could be dramatically reduced in the patients by the IL-2-toxin conjugate and that higher numbers of CD8+ T cells were detected in these patients versus patients receiving vaccination alone. Clinical responses were not reported for this study.

Profiling of Renal Cell Carcinoma to Identify Tumor-Associated Antigens

Extensive effort was invested to identify peptides seen by RCC-specific CTLs in the hopes of finding candidate TAAs that could be used for peptide-based vaccines for RCC patients. Unfortunately, the identified CTL epitopes were often unique to autologous tumor cells, making them unsuitable for general vaccine strategies. Therefore, a variety of new approaches have been utilized to identify potential TAAs in RCCs by the use of "reverse immunology." Instead of using immune cells to identify TAAs, tumors are first profiled for their expression of potential target molecules, which are then evaluated for their ability to elicit T cell responses. Reverse immunology utilizes the modern technologies of high-throughput genomics and proteomics to search for shared molecules in RCCs and interesting candidates are now being identified that are being further characterized for their capacity to induce effective T cell responses.

A number of candidate proteins that were found to be overexpressed in other tumor types were assessed for RCC expression at the mRNA level using reverse transcriptase polymerase chain reaction (RT-PCR).[22] Other candidate molecules were studied at the protein level by immunohistochemistry of RCC tissue arrays using corresponding antibodies.[41,47,93] Peptides that were presented at the cell surface by RCCs were eluted from MHC molecules and identified by mass spectrometry.[43,79] Global studies of proteins that were highly expressed in RCCs were made using proteome analysis and cDNA arrays were used to assess mRNA transcripts that were overexpressed by tumor cell lines or freshly resected tumor tissues as compared to normal control samples.[41,46,83,93]

An attractive integrated approach combined cDNA array analysis with peptide elution to identify molecules that were overexpressed in RCCs compared to control tissues, while at the same time identifying the actual peptides that were processed and presented by MHC molecules at the tumor cell surface.[90] In a final step, T cell responses to corresponding synthetic peptides were evaluated. By comparing a series of RCCs using this integrated approach it was possible to identify several TAAs shared by RCC that could be used to develop peptide-based vaccines to treat multiple RCC patients. In addition, this strategy also identified patient-specific peptides that could be employed for individualized vaccines.

The combined information from all these approaches has identified a variety of molecules that showed overexpression in RCCs compared to normal control cells when samples of numerous patients were analyzed. Therefore, they are potential candidates for broad-based immunotherapies. For example, CAIX/G250, survivin, PRAME, adipophilin, insulin-like growth factor-binding protein-3, and epidermal growth factor receptor merit further study for their capacity to induce T cell immunity and tumor regression *in vivo*.[79]

Peptide-Pulsed Dendritic Cells

More recently, peptide-loaded DCs have been considered as vaccine candidates for RCC patients, but no clinical studies have been reported to date. While immature DCs are extremely efficient at internalizing antigens that allow formation of MHC class I and class II peptide–MHC ligands, their failure to express sufficient levels of costimulatory molecules can lead to anergy of T cells. Immature DCs can also induce regulatory T cells that inhibit antitumor immunity.[28,77,95] Therefore, it is important to utilize mature DCs for peptide vaccination. DCs that are loaded with synthetic peptides *in vitro*, in an environment free of inhibitory factors released by tumor cells, may provide a useful vaccination tool. This approach is limited, however, to peptides that have been demonstrated to bind to particular MHC allotypes, thereby restricting the patients who can be treated by such vaccines. Furthermore, the short half-life of peptide–MHC ligands created by external peptide loading is a significant disadvantage. Because immune responses directed against single peptide–MHC ligands may select for outgrowth of tumor variants that no longer express these ligands, it is important to employ multiple peptide–MHC ligands in such vaccine strategies. The incorporation of peptides binding to both MHC class I and class II molecules would be an important advance. Improved knowledge about potential TAAs expressed by RCCs now makes this form of vaccination feasible for evaluation in RCC patients. The first experiments exploring use of peptides derived from adipophilin protein and the c-Met and Her-2/neu oncoproteins have been made *in vitro*.[10,69,75]

Cell-Free Vaccines Using Peptides or RNA with Adjuvant

Cell-free vaccines employing either synthetic peptides or RNA, applied with an immune adjuvant, such as GM-CSF, are also in development. These approaches are based on the mechanism of adjuvant recruitment of antigen-presenting cells, such as DCs, to the vaccination site where they can take up peptides or RNA molecules and then migrate to draining lymph nodes.[1] Here DCs can effectively prime T cell responses after undergoing further maturation. Comparative studies using the same peptides loaded onto DCs or applied in a cell-free form *in vivo* will provide the necessary information to determine which approach is most beneficial for patients. Equally interesting would be comparisons of RNA-pulsed DCs with injected RNA plus adjuvant. Of these two options, peptide vaccines would provide the simplest and least expensive form of vaccine therapy, but RNA would have the advantage of bypassing the limitations of strong patient selection, since multiple peptides binding to different MHC allotypes can be generated from the corresponding proteins encoded by the RNAs.

Future Perspectives

Currently not enough information is available to determine which type of cell-based vaccine will induce immune responses that are clinically most relevant in RCC. To date, the types of immune monitoring that have been performed in most clinical trials have not been detailed enough to determine whether both innate and adaptive immune responses were initiated *de novo* during vaccination and whether preexisting effector mechanisms were reactivated and mobilized for attack of tumor cells. More extensive immune monitoring is needed to identify those vaccine approaches that can best improve the clinical outlook for patients and to reveal the contributions of innate and adaptive immune responses to clinical efficacy. Even if optimal activation of immune responses has been achieved, variations in antigen expression by tumors of different types, among individual tumors of the same type, and even among cells of an individual tumor will play a critical role in determining the success or failure of T cell-mediated tumor elimination. Therefore, inclusion of analyses of tumor cells with respect to MHC and TAA expression is important.[37] In addition, new approaches are needed to overcome the immune suppression that inhibits development of effective immunity in patients with advanced disease.[17] Some studies have approached this problem by treating the patients with cyclophosphamide[32] or an IL-2-diphtheria toxin conjugate[15] to eliminate regulatory T cells. Extensive immune monitoring of the vaccine study employing the IL-2-toxin conjugate revealed that some regulatory T cells could be dramatically reduced prior to vaccination but they reappeared in equal numbers after several months; thus long-term suppression was not achieved. Because the IL-2-toxin conjugate could also kill activated effector cells it could not be applied after vaccination to control newly developing regulatory T cells. Therefore, it will be important to find other markers that can be used to distinguish these two subsets of lymphocytes and allow their differential regulation *in vivo* over time.

The greatest potential for RCC vaccines certainly lies in the adjuvant setting and the treatment of minimal residual disease where the immune system of the patients retains better function and only reduced tumor burdens must be eliminated. A certain risk with all immunotherapies exists in the danger that the immune system may be so actively engaged for tumor defense that the regulatory threshold controlling autoimmune responses will be exceeded, leading to damage of normal tissues. In fact, recent clinical trials of adoptive cell therapy suggest that true clinical benefit may be achieved only when the immune responses in patients are so potent that a substantial degree of autoimmunity is also present.[13,18] Some hope that tumor-specific targeting may allow autoimmunity to be avoided is provided by the observation that T cell receptor transcripts characteristic for tumor-specific CTLs were highly overrepresented in RCCs *in situ* but adjacent regions of normal kidney tissue did not show infiltration by these CTLs.[38] Therefore, the immune system is capable of making an important distinction between malignant and normal tissue in some cases; whether this will hold true for most RCC-associated responses remains to be determined.

It can be foreseen that future treatment regimens for metastatic RCC will use a combination of immunotherapies.[49,52] For example, adoptive cell therapy may be applied to reduce major tumor burdens using mixtures of various types of effector cells. Systemic application of cytokines, such as IL-15, can be used to support adoptive cell therapy.[85] Patients can be pretreated with other agents designed to eliminate cells causing immune suppression.[15,18,58,95] At a later stage, patients can then be regularly vaccinated to maintain effective immunity in order to prevent the development of new metastases. It has already been demonstrated that this type of combination immunotherapy is particularly effective in animal models.[92,95] Furthermore, immunotherapies can be combined with other small molecule inhibitors that impact directly on the growth of tumors as long as they do not interfere with immune cell function. By retarding tumor progression, sufficient time may be won to allow the immune system to generate adequate immune responses following vaccination. These immune responses may, in turn, mediate tumor regression.

Although the vaccines tested to date have not yielded the anticipated benefits for RCC patients, their potential roles in adjuvant settings, their application in patients with reduced tumor burdens following surgery or other therapies, and their inclusion as components of combination therapies emphasize the importance of vaccine development for RCC.

References

1. Adema GJ, de Vries I, Punt CJ, *et al.* Migration of dendritic cell based cancer vaccines: in vivo veritas? *Curr Opin Immunol* 2005;17(2):170–174.
2. Antonia S, Mule JJ, Weber JS. Current developments of immunotherapy in the clinic. *Curr Opin Immunol* 2004;16(2):130–136.
3. Antonia SJ, Seigne J, Diaz J, *et al.* Phase I trial of a B7-1 (CD80) gene modified autologous tumor cell vaccine in combination with systemic interleukin-2 in patients with metastatic renal cell carcinoma. *J Urol* 2002;167(5):1995–2000.
4. Antonia SJ, Seigne JD. B7-1 gene-modified autologous tumor-cell vaccines for renal-cell carcinoma. *World J Urol* 2000;18(2):157–163.
5. Arroyo JC, Gabilondo F, Lorente L, *et al.* Immune response induced in vitro by CD16- and CD16+ monocyte-derived dendritic cells in patients with metastatic renal cell carcinoma treated with dendritic cell vaccines. *J Clin Immunol* 2004;24(1):86–96.
6. Avigan D. Dendritic cell-tumor fusion vaccines for renal cell carcinoma. *Clin Cancer Res* 2004;10:6347–6352.
7. Balch CM, Riley LB, Bae YJ, *et al.* Patterns of human tumor-infiltrating lymphocytes in 120 human cancers. *Arch Surg* 1990;125:200–205.
8. Barbuto JA, Ensina LF, Neves AR, *et al.* Dendritic cell-tumor cell hybrid vaccination for metastatic cancer. *Cancer Immunol Immunother* 2004;53(12):1111–1118.
9. Brandle D, Brasseur F, Weynants P, *et al.* A mutated HLA A2 molecule recognized by autologous cytotoxic T lymphocytes on a human renal cell carcinoma. *J Exp Med* 1996;183(6): 2501–2508.
10. Brossart P, Stuhler G, Flad T, *et al.* Her-2/neu-derived peptides are tumor-associated antigens expressed by human renal cell and colon carcinoma lines and are recognized by in vitro induced specific cytotoxic T lymphocytes. *Cancer Res* 1998;58(4):732–736.
11. Cerundolo V, Hermans IF, Salio M. Dendritic cells: a journey from laboratory to clinic. *Nat Immunol* 2004;5(1):7–10.
12. Chen L, Ashe S, Brady WA, *et al.* Costimulation of antitumor immunity by the B7 counterreceptor for the T lymphocyte molecules CD28 and CTLA-4. *Cell* 1992;71:1093–1102.
13. Childs R, Chernoff A, Contentin N, *et al.* Regression of metastatic renal-cell carcinoma after nonmyeloablative allogeneic peripheral-blood stem-cell transplantation [see comments]. *N Engl J Med* 2000;343(11):750–758.
14. Crusinberry R, Williams RD. Immunotherapy of renal cell cancer. *Semin Surg Oncol* 1991;7(4):221–229.
15. Dannull J, Su Z, Rizzieri D, *et al.* Enhancement of vaccine-mediated antitumor immunity in cancer patients after depletion of regulatory T cells. *J Clin Invest* 2005;115(12):3623–3633.
16. Dranoff G, Jaffee E, Lazenby A, *et al.* Vaccination with irradiated tumor cells engineered to secrete murine granulocyte-macrophage colony-stimulating factor stimulates potent, specific, and long-lasting anti-tumor immunity. *Proc Natl Acad Sci USA* 1993;90(8):3539–3543.
17. Dudley ME, Rosenberg SA. Adoptive-cell-transfer therapy for the treatment of patients with cancer. *Nat Rev Cancer* 2003;3(9):666–675.
18. Dudley ME, Wunderlich JR, Robbins PF, *et al.* Cancer regression and autoimmunity in patients after clonal repopulation with antitumor lymphocytes. *Science* 2002;298(5594): 850–854.
19. Falk CS, Noessner E, Weiss EH, *et al.* Retaliation against tumor cells showing aberrant HLA expression using lymphokine activated killer-derived T cells. *Cancer Res* 2002;62(2):480–487.
20. Finke JH, Rayman P, Alexander J, *et al.* Characterization of the cytolytic activity of CD4+ and CD8+ tumor-infiltrating lymphocytes in human renal cell carcinoma. *Cancer Res* 1990;50: 2363–2370.
21. Fishman M, Antonia S. Specific antitumour vaccine for renal cancer. *Lancet* 2004;363(9409):583–584.
22. Frankenberger B, Pohla H, Noessner E, *et al.* Influence of CD80, interleukin-2, and interleukin-7 expression in human renal cell carcinoma on the expansion, function, and survival of tumor-specific CTLs. *Clin Cancer Res* 2005;11(5):1733–1742.
23. Gaudin C, Kremer F, Angevin E, *et al.* A hsp70-2 mutation recognized by CTL on a human renal cell carcinoma. *J Immunol* 1999;162(3):1730–1738.
24. Gaugler B, Brouwenstijn N, Vantomme V, *et al.* A new gene coding for an antigen recognized by autologous cytolytic T lymphocytes on a human renal carcinoma. *Immunogenetics* 1996;44(5):323–330.

25. Geiger C, Regn S, Weinzierl A, *et al*. A generic RNA-pulsed dendritic cell vaccine strategy for renal cell carcinoma. *J Transl Med* 2005;3:29–43.

26. Gilboa E, Vieweg J. Cancer immunotherapy with mRNA-transfected dendritic cells. *Immunol Rev* 2004;199:251–263.

27. Gitlitz BJ, Belldegrun AS, Zisman A, *et al*. A pilot trial of tumor lysate-loaded dendritic cells for the treatment of metastatic renal cell carcinoma. *J Immunother* 2003;26(5):412–419.

28. Granucci F, Zanoni I, Feau S, *et al*. Dendritic cell regulation of immune responses: a new role for interleukin 2 at the intersection of innate and adaptive immunity. *EMBO J* 2003;22(11):2546–2551.

29. Grunebach F, Muller MR, Nencioni A, *et al*. Delivery of tumor-derived RNA for the induction of cytotoxic T-lymphocytes. *Gene Ther* 2003;10(5):367–374.

30. Hanada K, Yewdell JW, Yang JC. Immune recognition of a human renal cancer antigen through post-translational protein splicing. *Nature* 2004;427(6971):252–256.

31. Heiser A, Maurice MA, Yancey DR, *et al*. Human dendritic cells transfected with renal tumor RNA stimulate polyclonal T-cell responses against antigens expressed by primary and metastatic tumors. *Cancer Res* 2001;61(8):3388–3393.

32. Holtl L, Ramoner R, Zelle-Rieser C, *et al*. Allogeneic dendritic cell vaccination against metastatic renal cell carcinoma with or without cyclophosphamide. *Cancer Immunol Immunother* 2005;54(7):663–670.

33. Holtl L, Rieser C, Papesh C, *et al*. Cellular and humoral immune responses in patients with metastatic renal cell carcinoma after vaccination with antigen pulsed dendritic cells. *J Urol* 1999;161(3):777–782.

34. Holtl L, Zelle-Rieser C, Gander H, *et al*. Immunotherapy of metastatic renal cell carcinoma with tumor lysate-pulsed autologous dendritic cells. *Clin Cancer Res* 2002;8(11):3369–3376.

35. Inaba K, Turley S, Iyoda T, *et al*. The formation of immunogenic major histocompatibility complex class II-peptide ligands in lysosomal compartments of dendritic cells is regulated by inflammatory stimuli. *J Exp Med* 2000;191(6):927–936.

36. Itoh K, Tilden AB, Balch CM. Lysis of human solid tumor cells by lymphokine-activated natural killer cells. *J Immunol* 1986;136:3910–3015.

37. Jager E, Jager D, Knuth A. Clinical cancer vaccine trials. *Curr Opin Immunol* 2002;142:178–182.

38. Jantzer P, Schendel DJ. Human renal cell carcinoma antigen-specific CTLs: antigen-driven selection and long-term persistence in vivo. *Cancer Res* 1998;58(14):3078–3086.

39. Javorovic M, Pohla H, Frankenberger B, *et al*. RNA transfer by electroporation into mature dendritic cells leading to reactivation of effector-memory cytotoxic T lymphocytes: a quantitative analysis. *Mol Ther* 2005;12:734–743.

40. Jocham D, Richter A, Hoffmann L, *et al*. Adjuvant autologous renal tumour cell vaccine and risk of tumour progression in patients with renal-cell carcinoma after radical nephrectomy: phase III, randomised controlled trial. *Lancet* 2004;363(9409):594–599.

41. Kim HL, Seligson D, Liu X, *et al*. Using protein expressions to predict survival in clear cell renal carcinoma. *Clin Cancer Res* 2004;10(16):5464–5471.

42. Kim T-Y, Von Eschenbach AC, Filaccio MD, *et al*. Clonal analysis of lymphocytes from tumor, peripheral blood, and nontumorous kidney in primary renal cell carcinoma. *Cancer Res* 1990;50:5263–5268.

43. Kruger T, Schoor O, Lemmel C, *et al*. Lessons to be learned from primary renal cell carcinomas: novel tumor antigens and HLA ligands for immunotherapy. *Cancer Immunol Immunother* 2005;54(9):826–836.

44. Kugler A, Stuhler G, Walden P, *et al*. Regression of human metastatic renal cell carcinoma after vaccination with tumor cell-dendritic cell hybrids [see comments]. *Nat Med* 2000;6(3):332–333.

45. Kugler A, Stuhler G, Walden P, *et al*. Retraction: Regression of human metastatic renal cell carcinoma after vaccination with tumor cell-dendritic cell hybrids. *Nat Med* 2003;9(9):1221.

46. Lam JS, Belldegrun AS, Figlin RA. Tissue array-based predictions of pathobiology, prognosis, and response to treatment for renal cell carcinoma therapy. *Clin Cancer Res* 2004;10: 6304–6309.

47. Lam JS, Leppert JT, Belldegrun AS, *et al*. Novel approaches in the therapy of metastatic renal cell carcinoma. *World J Urol* 2005;23(3):202–212.

48. Lokich J. Spontaneous regression of metastatic renal cancer. Case report and literature review. *Am J Clin Oncol* 1997;20(4):416–418.

49. Lou Y, Wang G, Lizee G, Kim GJ, *et al*. Dendritic cells strongly boost the antitumor activity of adoptively transferred T cells in vivo. *Cancer Res* 2004;64(18):6783–6790.

50. Marten A, Renoth S, Heinicke T, *et al*. Allogeneic dendritic cells fused with tumor cells: preclinical results and outcome of a clinical phase I/II trial in patients with metastatic renal cell carcinoma. *Hum Gene Ther* 2003;14(5):483–494.

51. Mautner J, Jaffee EM, Pardoll DM. Tumor-specific CD4+ T cells from a patient with renal cell carcinoma recognize diverse shared antigens. *Int J Cancer* 2005;115(5):752–759.

52. Michael A, Pandha HS. Renal-cell carcinoma: tumour markers, T-cell epitopes, and potential for new therapies. *Lancet Oncol* 2003;4(4):215–223.

53. Motzer RJ, Bander NH, Nanus DM. Renal-cell carcinoma. *N Engl J Med* 1996;335(12):865–875.

54. Mulders P, Tso CL, Gitlitz B, *et al*. Presentation of renal tumor antigens by human dendritic cells activates tumor-infiltrating lymphocytes against autologous tumor: implications for live kidney cancer vaccines. *Clin Cancer Res* 1999;5(2):445–454.

55. Nabel GJ. Genetic, cellular and immune approaches to disease therapy: past and future. *Nat Med* 2004;10(2):135–141.

56. Oosterwijk-Wakka JC, Tiemessen DM, Bleumer I, *et al*. Vaccination of patients with metastatic renal cell carcinoma with autologous dendritic cells pulsed with autologous tumor antigens in combination with interleukin-2: a phase 1 study. *J Immunother* 2002;25(6):500–508.

57. Ortaldo JR, Mason A, Overton R. Lymphokine-activated killer cells. Analysis of progenitors and effectors. *J Exp Med* 1986;164:1193–1205.

58. Overwijk WW. Breaking tolerance in cancer immunotherapy: time to ACT. *Curr Opin Immunol* 2005;17(2):187–194.

59. Palmer PA, Vinke J, Evers P, *et al*. Continuous infusion of recombinant interleukin-2 with or without autologous lymphokine activated killer cells for the treatment of advanced renal cell carcinoma. *Eur J Cancer* 1992;28A(6–7): 1038–1044.

60. Pandha HS, John RJ, Hutchinson J, *et al.* Dendritic cell immunotherapy for urological cancers using cryopreserved allogeneic tumour lysate-pulsed cells: a phase I/II study. *BJU Int* 2004;94(3):412–418.

61. Parmiani G. An explanation of the variable clinical response to interleukin 2 and LAK cells. *Immunol Today* 1990;11: 113–115.

62. Phillips JH, Lanier LL. Dissection of the lymphokine-activated killer phenomenon. Relative contribution of peripheral blood natural killer cells and T lymphocytes to cytolysis. *J Exp Med* 1986;164:814–825.

63. Probst-Kepper M, Stroobant V, Kridel R, *et al.* An alternative open reading frame of the human macrophage colony-stimulating factor gene is independently translated and codes for an antigenic peptide of 14 amino acids recognized by tumor-infiltrating CD8 T lymphocytes. *J Exp Med* 2001;193(10):1189–1198.

64. Rayman P, Wesa AK, Richmond AL, *et al.* Effect of renal cell carcinomas on the development of type 1 T-cell responses. *Clin Cancer Res* 2004;10:6360–6366.

65. Ronsin C, Chung-Scott V, Poullion I, *et al.* A non-AUG-defined alternative open reading frame of the intestinal carboxyl esterase mRNA generates an epitope recognized by renal cell carcinoma-reactive tumor-infiltrating lymphocytes in situ. *J Immunol* 1999;163(1):483–490.

66. Rosenberg S. Lymphokine-activated killer cells: a new approach to immunotherapy of cancer. *J Natl Cancer Inst* 1985;75:595–603.

67. Rosenberg SA, Lotze MT, Muul LM, *et al.* A progress report on the treatment of 157 patients with advanced cancer using lymphokine-activated killer cells and interleukin-2 or high-dose interleukin-2 alone. *N Engl J Med* 1987;316:889–897.

68. Rosenberg SA, Yang JC, Topalian SL, *et al.* Treatment of 283 consecutive patients with metastatic melanoma or renal cell cancer using high-dose bolus interleukin 2 [see comments]. *JAMA* 1994;271:907–913.

69. Schag K, Schmidt SM, Muller MR, *et al.* Identification of C-met oncogene as a broadly expressed tumor-associated antigen recognized by cytotoxic T-lymphocytes. *Clin Cancer Res* 2004;10(11):3658–3666.

70. Schendel DJ, Falk CS, Nossner E, *et al.* Gene transfer of human interferon gamma complementary DNA into a renal cell carcinoma line enhances MHC-restricted cytotoxic T lymphocyte recognition but suppresses non-MHC-restricted effector cell activity. *Gene Ther* 2000;7(11):950–959.

71. Schendel DJ, Oberneder R, Falk CS, *et al.* Cellular and molecular analyses of major histocompatibility complex (MHC) restricted and non-MHC-restricted effector cells recognizing renal cell carcinomas: problems and perspectives for immunotherapy. *J Mol Med* 1997;75(6):400–413.

72. Schirrmacher V. Clinical trials of antitumor vaccination with an autologous tumor cell vaccine modified by virus infection: improvement of patient survival based on improved antitumor immune memory. *Cancer Immunol Immunother* 2005;54(6):587–598.

73. Schleypen JS, Von Geldern M, Weiss EH, *et al.* Renal cell carcinoma-infiltrating natural killer cells express differential repertoires of activating and inhibitory receptors and are inhibited by specific HLA class I allotypes. *Int J Cancer* 2003;106(6):905–912.

74. Schleypen JS, Baur N, Kammerer R, *et al.* Cytotoxic markers and frequency predict functional capacity of natural killer cells infiltrating renal cell carcinoma. *Clin Cancer Res* 2006;12(3):719–725.

75. Schmidt SM, Schag K, Muller MR, *et al.* Induction of adipophilin-specific cytotoxic T lymphocytes using a novel HLA-A2-binding peptide that mediates tumor cell lysis. *Cancer Res* 2004;64(3):1164–1170.

76. Schoof DD, Gramolini BA, Davidson DI, *et al.* Adoptive immunotherapy of human cancer using low-dose recombinant interleukin 2 and lymphokine-activated killer cells. *Cancer Res* 1988;48:5007–5010.

77. Schuler G, Schuler-Thurner B, Steinman RM. The use of dendritic cells in cancer immunotherapy. *Curr Opin Immunol* 2003;15(2):138–147.

78. Simons JW, Jaffee EM, Weber CE, *et al.* Bioactivity of autologous irradiated renal cell carcinoma vaccines generated by *ex vivo* granulocyte-macrophage colony- stimulating factor gene transfer. *Cancer Res* 1997;57(8):1537–1546.

79. Stevanovic S. Identification of tumour-associated T-cell epitopes for vaccine development. *Nat Rev Cancer* 2002;2(7): 514–520.

80. Stoerkel SF. Classification of renal cell carcinoma based on morphologic and cytogenetic correlations. In: Bukowski RM, Finke JH, Klein EA, Eds. *Biology of Renal Cell Carcinoma*, 1st ed. New York: Springer-Verlag, 1995: 3–12.

81. Stoerkel S, Keymer R, Steinbach F, *et al.* Reaction patterns of tumor infiltrating lymphocytes in different renal cell carcinomas and oncocytomas. *Prog Clin Biol Res* 1992;378:217–223.

82. Su Z, Dannull J, Heiser A, *et al.* Immunological and clinical responses in metastatic renal cancer patients vaccinated with tumor RNA-transfected dendritic cells. *Cancer Res* 2003;63(9):2127–2133.

83. Sultmann H, von Heydebreck A, Huber W, *et al.* Gene expression in kidney cancer is associated with cytogenetic abnormalities, metastasis formation, and patient survival. *Clin Cancer Res* 2005;11:646–655.

84. Tatsumi T, Kierstead LS, Ranieri E, *et al.* MAGE-6 encodes HLA-DRbeta1*0401-presented epitopes recognized by CD4+ T cells from patients with melanoma or renal cell carcinoma. *Clin Cancer Res* 2003;9(3):947–954.

85. Teague RM, Sather BD, Sacks JA, *et al.* Interleukin-15 rescues tolerant CD8+ T cells for use in adoptive immunotherapy of established tumors. *Nat Med* 2006;12(3):335–341.

86. Townsend SE, Allison JP. Tumor rejection after direct costimulation of CD8+ T cells by B7-transfected melanoma cells. *Science* 1993;259:368–370.

87. Van den Eynde BJ, Gaugler B, Probst-Kepper M, *et al.* A new antigen recognized by cytolytic T lymphocytes on a human kidney tumor results from reverse strand transcription. *J Exp Med* 1999;190(12):1793–1800.

88. Vissers JL, De Vries, I, Schreurs MW, *et al.* The renal cell carcinoma-associated antigen G250 encodes a human leukocyte antigen (HLA)-A2.1-restricted epitope recognized by cytotoxic T lymphocytes. *Cancer Res* 1999;59(21):5554–5559.

89. Waldmann TA. Immunotherapy: past, present and future. *Nat Med* 2003;9(3):269–277.

90. Weinschenk T, Gouttefangeas C, Schirle M, *et al.* Integrated functional genomics approach for the design of patient-

individual antitumor vaccines. *Cancer Res* 2002;62(20): 5818–5827.

91. Weiss GR, Margolin KA, Aronson FR, *et al*. A randomized phase II trial of continuous infusion interleukin-2 or bolus injection interleukin-2 plus lymphokine-activated killer cells for advanced renal cell carcinoma. *J Clin Oncol* 1992;10(2):275–281.

92. Wrzesinski C, Restifo NP. Less is more: lymphodepletion followed by hematopoietic stem cell transplant augments adoptive T-cell-based anti-tumor immunotherapy. *Curr Opin Immunol* 2005;17(2):195–201.

93. Young AN, Amin MB, Moreno CS, *et al*. Expression profiling of renal epithelial neoplasms: a method for tumor classification and discovery of diagnostic molecular markers. *Am J Pathol* 2001;158(5):1639–1651.

94. Zhou X, Jun DY, Thomas AM, *et al*. Diverse CD8+ T-cell responses to renal cell carcinoma antigens in patients treated with an autologous granulocyte-macrophage colony-stimulating factor gene-transduced renal tumor cell vaccine. *Cancer Res* 2005;65(3):1079–1088.

95. Zou W. Regulatory T cells, tumour immunity and immunotherapy. *Nat Rev Immunol* 2006;6:295–307.

11f
Monoclonal Antibody-Based Therapy

Axel Bex, Simon Horenblas, and Gijsbert C. de Gast

Introduction

The idea of applying antigen–antibody binding in the diagnosis and treatment of cancer dates back to Ehrlich's "magic bullet theory" introduced in 1896. Antibodies may bind in a highly selective manner to tumors reducing or even eliminating adverse effects generally observed with cytotoxic chemotherapy. A breakthrough for the application of targeted monoclonal antibodies (mAbs) was the development of hybridoma technology. In 1975 Nobel laureates Georges Köhler and Cesar Milstein reported a procedure of "continuous cultures of fused cells secreting antibodies of predefined specificity" that allowed mAbs to be produced on a large scale.[1] Fusions of mouse myeloma cells with lymphocytes from murine spleens formed so-called hybridoma cells after *in vitro* immunization with the desired antigen. These cultured hybrid cells produce mAbs, typically immunoglobulin G. As they are produced by a single B cell the mAbs are homogeneous with identical antigen-binding sites. Most experience has been gained in the use of murine mAbs. Unfortunately, murine mAbs are extremely immunogenic and their application was invariably followed by stimulation of human antimouse antibodies (HAMA) precluding repeated or long-term use. Eventually, techniques were introduced to "humanize" mAbs and chimeric (murine/human), humanized, and completely human mAbs were produced. Other difficulties became evident. Apart from a variable specificity of mAbs, recognition of mAb-loaded cells by the immune system appeared to be more complex than initially thought. Antigen presentation is heterogenic and mAbs have a limited ability to penetrate tumor tissue. Additionally, a cell may protect itself through a variety of mechanisms against antibody-mediated cellular cytotoxicity or complement activation.

It was therefore not before 1997 that the first mAb targeted against cancer was approved by the Food and Drug Administration (FDA). Since then several mAbs have been approved by the FDA for hematological malignancies and breast cancer and a large number of mAbs are currently being investigated in clinical trials.

Monoclonal Antibodies in Renal Cell Carcinoma

Generally, mAbs investigated for the treatment of metastatic renal cell carcinoma (RCC) interfere with tumor-associated antigens. These antigens are preferentially expressed on malignant cells and to a lesser degree on normal cells. The targeted antigens can be specific epitopes expressed on cells or substances produced by cells, such as growth factors. The most specific tumor-associated antigen in RCC is carboanhydrase IX (CAIX), while growth factors and their receptors such as vascular endothelial growth factor (VEGF), vascular endothelial growth factor receptor (VEGFR), or epidermal growth factor receptor (EGFR) are commonly expressed by a variety of tumors. The antigen-binding site of the mAb targets these antigens upon which several mechanisms may lead to destruction of the tumor cell. Thus mAbs recognize growth factors or receptors, can induce apoptosis, and can bind to tumor cells exposing them as targets to immunological effector cells. An exception is the mAb against cytotoxic T lymphocyte antigen number 4 (CTLA-4). It is not targeting a tumor-associated antigen, but interferes with the immune system resulting in immunostimulation, which is more potent than interferon (IFN)-α or interleukin (IL)-2. This effect may be beneficial in RCC. The most direct mechanism of mAbs is a direct cytotoxic effect through interference with vital cell functions. In antibody-dependent cell-mediated cytotoxicity (ADCC), Fc receptor-bearing macrophages, neutrophils, or natural killer (NK) cells recognize antibody-coated tumor cells. Binding of an mAb to its antigen may also elicit lysis of a tumor cell by activating the complement pathway referred to as complement-dependent cytotoxicity (CDC). Apart from using unconjugated mAbs, the antibodies can be labeled (conjugated) with cytotoxic agents such as chemotherapy or a radionuclide. To reduce nontarget organ toxicity conjucated mAbs should preferentially target antigens almost exclusively expressed by tumor cells. Therefore in clear cell RCC the mAb-G250 recognizing CAIX can be ideally used for radioimmunoimaging and radioimmunotreatment.

TABLE 11f-1. Monoclonal antibodies in the treatment of renal cell cancer.[a]

Product administration	Target	Mechanism of action	Type mAb
Bevacizumab IV	VEGF	Binds circulating VEGF	Humanized IgG$_1$
VEGF-trap IV	VEGF	Binds circulating VEGF	Fully human IgG$_1$
Cetuximab IV	EGFR	Binds EGFR	Chimeric IgG
ABX-EGF IV	EGFR	Binds EGFR	Fully human IgG$_2$
CG250 IV	CAIX	Binds to CAIX	Chimeric IgG
MDX-010 IV	CTLA-4	Binds to CTLA-4	Human IgG$_1$

[a]mAB, monoclonal antibody; IgG, immunoglobulin G; IV, intravenous; VEGF, vascular endothelial growth factor; EGFR, epidermal growth factor receptor; CAIX, carboanhydrase IX; CTLA-4, cytotoxic T lymphocyte antigen number 1.

Five mAbs are currently being investigated in clinical trials for the treatment of RCC, though more are undergoing preclinical evaluation. An overview is given in Table 11f-1.

In the following each mAb is presented with its specific mechanism of action and its current clinical status with a focus on outcome, toxicity, limitations, and future applications.

Bevacizumab

Mechanism of Action

Bevacizumab (Avastin, Genentech, Inc., San Francisco, CA) is a recombinant human monoclonal antibody that binds and neutralizes all biologically active isoforms of VEGF (also known as VEGF-A). Bevacizumab was created by transferring the VEGF-binding complementary-determining regions of a murine antibody to a humanized immunoglobulin G$_1$.[2]

Recent research in the underlying biology of RCC has identified a rationale for a monoclonal antibody against VEGF in RCC. VEGF is a dimeric glycoprotein and belongs to the platelet-derived growth factor (PDGF) superfamily, which includes VEGF-A, -B, -C, - D, and -E. It mediates several functions that are important for both normal and tumor angiogenesis such as increased microvascular permeability and reversal of endothelial cell senescence with division, migration, and protection from apoptosis.[3] The VEGF gene encodes four isoforms of which VEGF165 is the isoform with optimal bioavailability and potency.[4] VEGF interacts with transmembrane tyrosine kinase receptors on the cell surface. Of these receptors VEGFR-2 plays a key role in mediating the proangiogenic effects of VEGF, but VEGFR-1 and -3 are also binding VEGF.[5] Most patients with clear cell RCC have loss of von Hippel–Lindau (VHL) protein primarily due to mutation of the VHL gene, resulting in an impaired breakdown of hypoxia-inducible factor (HIF)-1α.

HIF-1α dimerizes with HIF-1β and leads to transcription of hypoxia-inducible genes, including VEGF, epidermal growth factor (EGF), PDGF, basic fibroblast growth factor (bFGF), and transforming growth factor-α (TGF-α). The binding of TGF-α or EGF to the EGFR seems to trigger mitogenic signal transduction.[6] Evaluation of these inappropriate signal transduction pathways has identified VEGF and its related growth factors as logical therapeutic targets for novel single agents in RCC. These agents can be divided into agents with miscellaneous VEGF effects, monoclonal antibodies, and small molecules.[3,7] Consequently, there are several potential strategies to inhibit VEGF in RCC, of which binding and neutralization of all biologically active isoforms of VEGF by an mAb is one of the approaches. In a recent investigation tissue microarrays of clear cell tumors ($n = 340$) and papillary RCC specimens ($n = 42$) were evaluated regarding expression of VEGF-A, VEGF-C, VEGF-D, VEGFR-1, VEGFR-2, and VEGFR-3.[8] When examining the angiogenesis pathway it was concluded that patients with papillary RCC may be considered for therapies targeting the VEGF-A pathway while patients with clear cell subtypes may be more likely to benefit from receptor kinase inhibitors targeting VEGFR-3.

Clinical Results

After Phase I trials of bevacizumab in patients with advanced tumors demonstrated that no grade 3 or 4 toxicities occurred, it was subsequently investigated in a Phase II trial in patients with metastatic clear cell RCC. Most of the current knowledge and further study designs are based on the results of this randomized Phase II trial, in which 116 patients with progressive metastatic RCC were included.[9] The majority of the patients had prior systemic cytokine therapy with IL-2. Patients were assigned to receive either placebo, low-dose bevacizumab (3 mg/kg), or high-dose bevacizumab (10 mg/kg) given intravenously every 2 weeks until progression occurred. The study was designed to detect a 2-fold increase of the time to progression with either dose of bevacizumab versus placebo. Ultimately, only the high-dose arm showed significant results. Four of 39 patients had a partial response (PR) [10% objective response rate (OR)]. With high-dose bevacizumab a significant prolongation of the time to progression was observed compared to placebo (4.8 versus 2.5 months). However, this Phase II trial was not designed with survival as the endpoint and patients on the placebo arm were crossed over to bevacizumab after disease progression. Hypertension grade 3 with high-dose bevacizumab was observed in 21% of patients, but no life-threatening toxicities or death.

These results demonstrated that bevacizumab may result in a low OR while still potentially delaying progression and prolonging survival. Interestingly, many of the novel agents demonstrating effectivity, including small inhibiting molecules, demonstrated a similar pattern. The OR is low but there may be a significant prolongation of progression-free survival. This has led to study designs that combine bevacizumab with small inhibiting molecules that act in synergy with other pathways involved. A trial involved patients who had previously been treated with cytokines and combined bevacizumab at 10 mg/kg intravenously every 2 weeks with erlotinib 150 mg orally daily, an inhibiting molecule of EGF.[10,11] This combination was chosen to target two pathways critical in the biology of clear cell RCC. Of the 63 patients treated with advanced clear cell RCC, 32% were previously treated with IL-2 or IFN-α. Fifteen of 59 evaluable patients (25%) had objective responses (PR 14) and 36 patients (61%) had SD. The median duration of treatment was 8 months and 26 patients received >12 months of therapy. The median progression free survival was 11 months while the median survival has not been reached. The 1-year progression free survival was 80% for the group of responders and 27% for those with SD. Grade 3 toxicity included diarrhea in 13%, rash in 13%, and nausea/vomiting in 10%. These results are encouraging and will be further updated. In a Phase I trial escalating doses of imatinib were added to the combination of bevacizumab and erlotinib.[12] Imatinib, a PDGF receptor antagonist, targets a third pathway of RCC and was tolerated up to a dose of 400 mg orally daily. The trial continues as a Phase II trial.

To investigate the role of bevacizumab in the first-line treatment for metastatic clear cell RCC in conjunction with initial systemic therapy with cytokines two Phase III trials were initiated and have completed recruitment. Results have not yet been published. IFN-α-2b is regarded as the standard first line therapy and in an intergroup Phase III trial patients with metastatic clear cell RCC without prior systemic therapy were randomly assigned to IFN-α-2b at a dose of 9×10^6 IU three times weekly or to bevacizumab 10 mg/kg intravenously every 2 weeks in combination with the same schedule of IFN-α-2b.[13] The trial is designed to detect an improvement in survival from 13 to 17 months in favor of the combination.

A total of 700 patients will be enrolled and a similar Phase III trial is currently being conducted in Europe with IFN-α-2a.[3]

Vascular Endothelial Growth Factor-Trap

Mechanism of Action

The mechanism of action of VEGF-trap (Regeneron Pharmaceuticals, Tarrytown, NY) is comparable to that of bevacizumab although its affinity to VEGF is reported to be 100-fold higher.[14] It is an entirely human fusion protein engineered by fusing a VEGFR-1 Ig domain and a VEGFR-2 Ig domain to human IgG$_1$.[3]

Clinical Results

Hitherto VEGF trap has been investigated only in a Phase I dose-finding study in patients with refractory solid tumors including nine patients with RCC.[15] Currently further investigation is needed to establish its clinical utility in clear cell RCC.

Cetuximab

Mechanism of Action

Cetuximab (Erbitux, ImClone, NY) is a chimeric (murine/human) monoclonal antibody against EGFR. The rationale for targeting this receptor is based on a high (70–90%) incidence of EGFR expression in patients with RCC.[17] Together with EGFR expression, ligands of EGFR such as TGF-α are upregulated and blockade of this autocrine loop is a strategy in clear cell RCC.

Clinical Results

Cetuximab (C225) has been investigated in a Phase II trial including 55 evaluable patients with advanced RCC.[16] Intravenous loading doses of 400 or 500 mg/m^2 were followed by weekly maintenance doses of 250 mg/m^2. None of the patients developed an objective response. The time to progression was comparable to historical controls treated with IFN-α and, as a consequence, it was concluded that further investigation of cetuximab in RCC is not warranted.

ABX-EGF

Mechanism of Action

Like cetuximab, ABX-EGF (AbgenixInc, Fremont, CA; Amgen Inc., Thousand Oaks, CA) targets EGFR. It is a high-affinity fully human IgG$_2$ mAb that completely blocks binding of EGF and TGF-α to the EGFR and leads to internalization of the receptor in EGFR-expressing RCC.[6,7] As a result, EGFR-dependent cellular functions and autocrine loops are interrupted.

Clinical Results

In a dose-escalating trial the antitumor activity and toxicity of ABX-EGF were evaluated in patients with metastatic RCC.[6] Eighty-eight patients were treated with ABX-EGF doses of 1.0, 1.5, 2.0, or 2.5 mg/kg weekly without a loading dose as an intravenous infusion over 60 min. After a series of eight weekly treatments, response was evaluated and stable or responding patients received as many as five series of eight weekly treatments. All patients either failed cytokine treatment with IL-2 or IFN-α or were unable to receive or were intolerant of cytokine therapy. EGFR immunostaining was performed on 76 tumor biopsy specimens and 69 (91%) were positive. Three patients had an objective response [two partial responses (PR) and one complete response (CR)] and two patients had regression without qualifying for PR. Forty-four patients (50%) had sudden death (SD) after 8 weeks. The median progression-free survival was 100 days. An acneiform rash was the principal adverse effect and occurred in 68–100% of the patients who received at least three doses of ABX-EGF at 1.0–2.5 mg/kg/week. The objective response rate was low in patients previously treated with cytokines with a median time to progression of less than 4 months. It was concluded that the highly consistent toxicological, pharmacokinetic, and parmacodynamic profiles of ABX-EGF were encouraging. It may be that the low objective response rate was due to the select patient group of whom most belonged to the intermediate or high-risk group and were heavily pretreated. No further trials have been published investigating ABX-EGF in metastatic RCC.

cG250

Mechanism of Action

cG250 is an mAb (WG-250; Rencarex) that recognizes G250, also known as carbonic anhydrase IX (CAIX).[17] CAIX is a membrane-associated carbonic anhydrase that is potentially involved in regulating cell proliferation in response to hypoxic conditions. Additionally, it may play a role in oncogenesis and tumor progression. cG250-mAb was constructed by immunization of mice with human RCC homogenates. The original murine G250-mAb was highly immunogenic. CAIX is highly expressed in RCC but is absent in most normal tissues except gastric mucosa epithelial cells. Studies on tumor-bearing kidneys revealed a selective uptake of cG250-mAb in CAIX-expressing cells versus antigen-negative cells. A high uptake of cG250 and a low dose to obtain tumor saturation provided the

basis for several studies on metastatic RCC. Apart from imaging in conjunction with[111] In or[131]I, cG250 can be used for treatment of metastatic RCC either in conjugation with[131]I or[90]Y for radioimmunotherapy or unconjugated as mAb directed against CAIX. In preclinical studies G250 was upregulated by IFN-α and IFN-γ,[18] which may increase its use as target, and the chimeric cG250-mAb induced strong antibody-dependent cellular cytotoxicity (ADCC).[7]

Clinical Results

In a dose-escalating study, 12 patients were treated with cG250 labeled with trace[131] I and unlabeled cG250 in weeks 1 and 5.[7,19] CG250 gamma camera imaging was performed at doses of 5, 10, 25, and 50 mg/m². After the first 6-week cycle one patient had a CR and eight patients had SD. In a similar Phase I dose-escalation study ^{131}I-cG250 was investigated in 12 patients with metastatic RCC. In this study one PR and one SD were obtained.[20] Unconjugated cG250 was recently investigated in a Phase II trial in 36 patients with advanced RCC.[21] During 12 weeks of treatment with 50 mg intravenously per week toxicity was mild. The median survival was 16 months with one CR and five SDs. Trials with unconjugated cG250 in combination with either IL-2 or IFN-α in pretreated patients resulted in moderate objective responses[22] and side effects were mainly cytokine induced. Further studies with chimeric G250-mAb are ongoing.

MDX-010

Mechanism of Action

MDX-010, a human monoclonal IgG$_1$ antibody against CTLA-4, is an immunostimulator more potent than IFN-α or IL-2.[23] CTLA-4 has an immunoregulatory function reducing an already ongoing antigen-specific immune response. It is constitutively expressed on CD4$^+$, IL-2R$^+$ T regulatory cells, which play a role in peripheral tolerance mechanisms. T-lymphocytes express both costimulatory (CD28) and inhibitory (CTLA-4) receptors that are engaged by the B7 family of ligands. Therefore blocking CTLA-4 receptor engagement by a monoclonal antibody may unbalance this antagonistic network in favor of lymphocyte activation.

CTLA-4 knockout mice display a T cell proliferative phenotype due to unlimited T cell proliferation (CD4 and CD8$^+$ T cells). Short-term CTLA-4 blockade can be achieved by aCTLA-4 antibodies, which can result in rejection of low immunogenic tumors and induction of autoimmune disease in animals. Recent human studies in melanoma patients[23] showed that autoimmune disease (AID: ulcerative colitis, dermatitis, uveitis, hepatitis) occurred in 40–50% of patients, which was generally transient and dependent of the dose of aCTLA-4. Autoimmune toxicity generally developed several weeks after aCTLA-4 treatment. Tumor responses, including CRs, occurred only in patients with AID. These studies suggest that a patient-tailored dose of aCTLA-4 on the basis of AID as surrogate marker of response may increase the antitumor response rate.

Clinical Results

In a Phase II trial, 41 patients with advanced RCC were given MDX-010 every 3 weeks.[24] Cohort A ($n = 21$) received 3 mg/kg once, followed by 1 mg/kg. Cohort B ($n = 20$) received all doses at 3 mg/kg. In 12 patients autoimmune toxicities primarily occurred. One patient in cohort A responded (5%) while 5 of 20 patients in cohort B (20%) had a PR. All responses were partial with a duration of 4–18 months. Half of the responding patients had previous treatment with IL-2. It may be that the immunostimulatory response induced by IL-2 is aggrevated by MDX-010 in that it interferes with the immunoregulatory function of CTLA-4 reducing an already ongoing antigen-specific immune response. As in the melanoma study, responding patients were among those showing autoimmune manifestations. MDX-010 antibody can induce partial remissions in RCC associated with clinical autoimmune breakthrough events. Further studies will be needed to investigate toxicity and the combination of MDX-010 antibody with cytokines.

Future Perspectives

The field of mAb therapy of metastatic RCC is expanding fast. Currently five mAbs are being investigated in clinical trials. Apart from cetuximab, they have demonstrated some degree of efficacy as single agents in Phase I and II trials of metastatic RCC. Bevacizumab is currently being investigated in two large Phase III trials sufficiently powered to determine if bevacizumab in combination with IFN-α will be superior as a first-line treatment when compared to IFN-α alone. No results are available yet, but these large multicenter trial designs indicate that after 25 years the treatment of metastatic RCC with cytokines is challenged. If the experience gained for mAbs with other malignancies is repeated for RCC, then it will be likely that mAbs will be used in combination with other mAbs, small inhibiting molecules, cytokines, and chemotherapy to increase efficacy by interfering with a number of vital pathways. Such a promising combination may be bevacizumab and erlotinib. However, currently only data from, at best, Phase II trials have been reported and only a few have been published as full journal articles to date. Most of the current data have been presented as abstracts and median survival has either not yet been reached or not been analyzed. As a consequence, randomized Phase III trials will have to be performed to establish the role of mAbs in the first- and second-line treatment of metastatic RCC.

References

1. Kohler G, Milstein C. Continuous cultures of fused cells secreting antibody of predefined specificity. Nature 256(5517), 495–497, 1975.
2. Yang JC. Bevacizumab for patients with metastatic renal cancer: An update. Clin Cancer Res 10, 6367s–6370s, 2004.
3. Rini BI, Small EJ. Biology and clinical development of vascular endothelial growth factor-targeted therapy in renal cell carcinoma. J Clin Oncol 23(5), 1028–1043, 2005.
4. Rini BI. VEGF-targeted therapy in metastatic renal cell carcinoma. The Oncologist 10, 191–197, 2005.
5. Srinivasan R, Linehan WM. Targeted for destruction: The molecular basis for development of novel therapeutic strategies in renal cell cancer. J Clin Oncol 23(3), 410–412, 2005.
6. Rowinsky EK, Schwartz GH, Gollob JA, Thompson JA, Vogelzang NJ, Figlin R, et al. Safety, pharmakokinetics, and activity of ABX-EGF, a fully human anti-epidermal growth factor receptor monoclonal antibody in patients with metastatic renal cell cancer. J Clin Oncol 22(15), 3003–3015, 2004.
7. Amato RJ. Renal cell carcinoma: review of novel single-agent therapeutics and combination regimens. Ann Oncol 2005; 16: 7–15.
8. Leppert JT, Lam JS, Yu H, Seligson DB, Dong J, Horvath S, et al. Targeting the vascular endothelial growth factor pathway in renal cell carcinoma: A tissue array based analysis. Proc Am Soc Clin Oncol 23, 386s, 2005 (abstract 4536).
9. Yang JC, Haworth L, Sherry RM, Hwu P, Schwartzentruber DJ, Topalian SL, et al. A randomized trial of bevacizumab, an anti-vascular endothelial growth factor antibody, for metastatic renal cancer. N Engl J Med 349(5), 427–434, 2003.
10. Hainsworth JD, Sosman JA, Spigel DR, Schwert RC, Carrell DL, Hubbard F, et al. Phase II trial of bevacizumab and erlotinib in patients with metastatic renal carcinoma (RCC). Proc Am Soc Clin Oncol 23, 381, 2004 (abstract 4502).
11. Spigel DR, Hainsworth JD, Sosman J, Raefsky EL, Meluch AA, Edwards D, et al. Bevacizumab and erlotinib in the treatment of patients with metastatic renal carcinoma (RCC): Update of a phase II multicenter trial. Proc Am Soc Clin Oncol 23, 387s, 2005 (abstract 4540).
12. Hainsworth JD, Sosman J, Spigel DR, Patton JF, Thompson DS, Sutton V, et al. Bevacizumab, erlotinib, and imatinib in the treatment of patients (pts) with advanced renal cell carcinoma (RCC): A Minnie Pearl Cancer Research Network phase I/II trial. Proc Am Soc Clin Oncol 23, 388s, 2005 (abstract 4542).
13. Rini BI, Halabi S, Taylor J, Small EJ, Schilsky RL. Cancer and Leukemia Group B 90206: A randomized phase III trial of interferon-alpha or interferon-alpha plus anti-vascular endothelial growth factor antibody (bevacizumab) in metastatic renal cell carcinoma. Clin Cancer Res 10, 2584–2586, 2004.
14. Holash J, Davis S, Papadopoulos N. VEGF-Trap: A VEGF blocker with potent antitumor effects. Proc Natl Acad Sci USA 99, 11393–11398, 2002.
15. Dupont J, Schwartz L, Koutcher J. Phase I and pharmacokinetic study of VEGF trap administered subcutaneously (sc) to patients with advanced solid malignancies. Proc Am Soc Clin Oncol 23, 197, 2004 (abstract 3009).
16. Motzer RJ, Amato R, Todd M, Hwu WJ, Cohen R, Baselga J, et al. Phase II trial of antiepidermal growth factor receptor antibody C225 in patients with advanced renal cell carcinoma. Invest New Drugs 21(1), 99–101, 2003.

17. Lam JS, Pantuck AJ, Belldegrun A, Figlin R. G250: A carbonic anhydrase IX monoclonal antibody. Curr Oncol Rep 7(2), 109–115, 2005.

18. Brouwers AH, Verel I, van Eerd JEM, Visser GWM, Steffens MG, Oosterwijk E, et al. Interferons can upregulate the expression of the tumor associated antigen G250-MN/CA IX, a potential target for (radio)immunotherapy of renal cell carcinoma. Cancer Biother Radiopharm 18, 539–547, 2003.

19. Wiseman GA, Scott AM, Lee F. Chimeric G250 (cG250) monoclonal antibody phase I dose escalation trial in patients with advanced renal cell carcinoma (RCC). Proc Am Soc Clin Oncol 20, 257s, 2001 (abstract 1027).

20. Steffens MG, Boerman OC, De Mulder PH. Phase I radioimmunotherapy of metastatic renal cell carcinoma with 131-I-labeled chimeric monoclonal antibody G250. Clin Cancer Res 5(10 Suppl), 3268s–3274s, 1999.

21. Bleumer I, Knuth A, Oosterwijk E, Hofmann R, Varga Z, Lamers C. A phase II trial of chimeric monoclonal antibody G250 for advanced renal cell carcinoma patients. Br J Cancer 90, 985–990, 2004.

22. van Spronsen DJ, De Mulder PH. New developments in the treatment of metastatic renal cell carcinoma. Ned Tijdschr Oncol 2(3), 110–116, 2005.

23. Phan GQ, Yang JC, Sherry RM, Hwu P, Topalian SL, Schwartzentruber DJ, et al. Cancer regression and autoimmunity induced by cytotoxic T lymphocyte-associated antigen 4 blockade in patients with metastatic melanoma. Proc Natl Acad Sci USA 100(14), 8372–8377, 2003.

24. Yang JC, Beck KE, Blansfield JA, Tran KQ, Lowy I, Rosenberg SA. Tumor regression in patients with metastatic renal cancer treated with monoclonal antibody to CTLA4 (MDX-010). Proc Am Soc Clin Oncol , 166s, 2005 (abstract 2501).

11g
Hematopoietic Stem Cell Transplantation: Allogeneic Immunotherapy for Cancer

Andreas E. Lundqvist and Richard W. Childs

Introduction

Early studies investigating immunotherapy for renal cell carcinoma (RCC) were initially driven by this tumor's long track record of being refractory to conventional chemotherapy and radiotherapy. Over the past two decades, therapies designed to boost immunity against cancer have played an increasing role in the treatment of this malignancy. RCC is unusual among solid tumors in that it responds to various immunotherapy approaches. Immune boosting therapies including high-dose interleukin-2 (IL-2) and/or interferon-α (IFN-α) and the administration of autologous lymphokine activated killer (LAK) cells with IL-2 can induce regression lasting >10 years in some patients with metastatic disease.[1,2] Unfortunately, high-dose IL-2 treatment has proven to have considerable toxicity and its antitumor effects are restricted to a relatively small subset of patients. The adoptive transfer of tumor-infiltrating lymphocytes (TIL) has been utilized as a method to more specifically target the immune system against RCC.[3,4] Immunotherapy with activated TIL and moderate doses of IL-2 have been used successfully and have been reported to incur less toxicity and lower costs compared to high-dose IL-2 protocols.[5]

Advances in our knowledge of antigens that characterize specific malignancies have led to the use of vaccine strategies using purified tumor-associated antigens (TAA), DNA-encoding protein antigens, and/or protein-derived peptides. In contrast to melanoma, where close to 20 tumor-associated antigens have been described, only a handful of RCC-associated antigens has thus far been characterized. Peptides derived from two of these antigens, G250-MN/CA IX and RAGE-1, have been shown to generate cytotoxic T lymphocytes (CTL) capable of lysing RCC cells *in vitro*.[6,7] Among the more popular strategies used in cancer immunotherapy is vaccination with antigen-loaded dendritic cells (DC). Recently, a Phase I trial demonstrated expansion of RCC-specific T cells following vaccination with DCs transfected with RNA isolated from RCC; this vaccine was shown to induce T cell responses directed against G250 but not against self-antigens expressed on normal renal tissues.[8]

Although data from many preclinical and animal-based cancer immune boosting strategies have provided promising results, the majority of immunotherapy trials have thus far failed to induce clinically meaningful regression of cancer when applied to humans. Defects in the immune system of the tumor-bearing host may in part be responsible for the low response rates seen with treatments attempting to boost autologous immunity to cancer. Strategies to overcome tumor-induced immune suppression or other tumor escape mechanisms are being intensively investigated. Defects in human lymphocyte antigen class I antigen-processing machinery including downregulation or complete loss of TAP and β$_2$-microglobulin represent a common method by which tumors escape T cell immunity.[9] Downregulation of Fas expression and upregulation of Fas ligand expression is another mechanism used by RCC cells to suppress immune recognition.[10] Allogeneic immunotherapy, which replaces the recipient's defective immune system with that of a healthy donor, could potentially overcome some of these barriers.

Allogeneic Stem Cell Transplantation

Over the past few decades allogeneic hematopoietic stem cell transplantation (HCT) has evolved from a treatment of last resort to an accepted treatment option for patients with hematological malignancies who are early in the course of their disease. Myeloablative conditioning was initially believed to be the main contributor eradicating hematological malignancies, with transplantation of donor hematopoietic stem cells given primarily to restore bone marrow function wiped out by dose-intensive conditioning. Although the human histocompatibility antigen system was not understood, it was believed with early transplants that successful bone marrow engraftment required some genetic similarity between the donor and the recipient. In one of the first allogeneic stem cell transplants attempted, a patient with acute lymphoblastic leukemia received an HCT from an identical twin following high-dose total body irradiation. Although full hematological recovery occurred, the leukemia ultimately relapsed, demonstrating that completely matched (i.e., syngeneic) donor marrow cells could restore hematopoietic function after lethal irradiation but failed to maintain a disease remission. Subsequent efforts to improve transplant outcome by preventing disease relapse through intensification of the conditioning regimen have proven largely unsuccessful, mostly as a consequence of increased transplant-associated toxicities. However, an important observation from a number of transplant studies reported in the 1980s showed disease relapse occurred less frequently with allogeneic compared to autologous transplants.[11–13] This and other observations heightened the awareness of the role played by donor immune cells in controlling residual disease after allogeneic HCT. Today, allogeneic HCT is accepted as a powerful type of immunotherapy with the capacity to cure a variety of hematological malignancies, including those that have become completely resistant to cytotoxic chemoradiotherapy.

Graft-versus-Leukemia

Observations that provided some of the earliest indirect evidence of a donor immune-mediated graft-versus-leukemia (GVL) effect after allogeneic HCT include the following:

- Myeloablative conditioning frequently fails to eradicate all leukemic cells in patients who ultimately are cured by the transplant.[14]
- Hematological disease relapse is lower after allogeneic HCT compared to autologous transplantation.[14, 15]
- The risk of disease relapse is higher in recipients of syngeneic transplants (where no antigen disparity exists) compared to nonsyngeneic HLA-matched transplants.[16]
- The risk of leukemic relapse is lower in patients who develop graft-versus-host disease (GVHD).[17, 18]
- The risk of leukemia relapse increases when T cells are removed from the allograft to prevent GVHD.[19, 20]

Direct evidence supporting the existence of the GVL effect was demonstrated in the late 1980s when patients with CML who had relapsed after allogeneic HCT were induced back into remission following a donor lymphocyte infusion (DLI).[21–23]

Although allogeneic HCT can be curative for a variety of hematological malignancies, older and debilitated patients with medical comorbidities have historically been precluded from conventional (myeloablative) transplantation due to substantial and frequently fatal toxicities associated with dose-intensive conditioning. With an increased awareness and confidence in the power of the graft-versus-tumor (GVT) effect, investigators have recently developed allogeneic transplant regimens that utilize reduced-intensity conditioning [so called reduced-intensity stem cell transplantation

(RIST), often also referred to as "minitransplantation" or "nonmyeloablative transplantation"] to test the hypothesis that engrafting donor immune cells, without myeloablative conditioning, will be sufficient to cure some cancers.[24] Reduced intensity conditioning regimens use immunosuppressant agents to allow donor engraftment while reducing chemotherapy- and radiotherapy-associated toxicities. Initial trials of this approach conducted in the late 1990s were used in patients with hematological malignancies that had a track record of sensitivity to the GVL effect.[25, 26] Preliminary data on the safety of this approach have been encouraging, with retrospective studies suggesting RIST to be a safer treatment alternative compared to myeloablative transplantation. Most centers have reported early transplant-related mortality rates of <15% in debilitated and older patient cohorts that are usually precluded from conventional HCT because of an unacceptable mortality risk (i.e., <40%). Importantly, the GVT effects that occur after these transplants have been shown to induce remissions in a significant proportion of patients with hematological malignancies, including acute and chronic leukemias, multiple myeloma, and relapsed lymphomas.[27] An important caveat is that disease status at transplantation has a major impact on outcome following RIST for hematological malignancies. Patients with acute leukemia and intermediate/high-grade lymphomas who are first induced into a remission with chemotherapy can be cured with an allogeneic RIST; in contrast, patients with rapidly progressing chemotherapy refractory acute lymphocytic leukemia (ALL) or acute myeloid leukemia (AML) are much less likely to benefit from such low-intensity transplants.

Following RIST, patients typically have a transient period where both donor and patient myeloid and lymphoid cells are detectable in the blood and bone marrow. This condition is referred to as "mixed chimerism." In contrast to the full donor myeloid and lymphoid chimerism that follows myeloablative HCT, mixed chimerism appears to induce donor tolerance to recipient tissue, leading to a decreased risk of acute GVHD.[28] However, other desirable donor immune effects, such as GVL, are less likely to occur until donor lymphocytes predominate in the blood and mixed chimerism disappears.[29] As a consequence, the majority of RIST HCT regimens incorporate strategies to accelerate conversion from mixed to full donor chimerism by discontinuation of GVHD prophylaxis and the infusion of donor lymphocytes.

Graft-versus-Renal Cell Carcinoma

The evidence that RCC is responsive to the immune system as well as its unfavorable overall prognosis has prompted investigators to explore alternative methods of targeting immune cells against this malignancy.[1, 30, 31] Investigators first pursued RIST HCT in metastatic RCC following reports that hematological malignancies could be cured via the anticancer immune effects that occurred after these types of transplants. Because myeloablative conditioning is associated with considerable risk of morbidity and mortality, and since RCC is refractory to chemotherapy, investigators developed a RIST approach as a safer platform to investigate whether this tumor would be susceptible to the antineoplastic effects of engrafting donor immune cells.

Graft-versus-solid tumor effects resulting in partial and sometimes complete regression of metastatic kidney cancer have been reported by investigators using a variety of different RIST approaches [32-37] (Table 11g-1). All these transplant regimens focus on maximizing GVT effects by inducing rapid donor immune engraftment while minimizing the time patients receive GVHD prophylaxis with cyclosporine or tacrolimus (Fig. 11g-1). At the National Heart, Lung and Blood Institute (NHLBI), 10 of the first 19 patients (54%) experienced tumor regression, including 7 partial responses and 3 complete responses;[33] the first patient treated remains without evidence of disease >8 years after transplantation (Fig. 11g-2). GVT effects were delayed by a median of 4 months after the transplantation, usually occurring following cyclosporine tapering and after T cell chimerism had converted from mixed to predominantly full donor origin. As observed in patients with hematological malignancies, GVT effects occurred most commonly in patients with a history of acute GVHD, although on some occasions complete disease regression was observed in patients who never developed acute or chronic GVHD. This observation provides indirect evidence that donor T cells can be directed against polymorphic minor histocompatibility antigens expressed broadly on malignant and normal host tissues as well as to antigens restricted to the tumor (Fig. 11g-3). Indeed, minor histocompatibility antigen-specific T cell clones that recognize RCC cells in vitro have been isolated from patients with metastatic RCC undergoing a RIST;[38] studies to identify RCC-specific antigens using T cell clones isolated from responding patients are ongoing.[39] The observation that disease regression occurred in patients who had previously failed IL-2 and IFN further suggest

these responses were mediated by engrafting donor immune cells rather than through a nonspecific inflammatory cytokine effect. The mechanisms accounting for disease regression in responding patients as well as the identification of RCC antigens targeted by the donor immune system are intense areas of investigation. Once defined, we will likely see the development of allogeneic HCT regimens that specifically target donor immune cells against the tumor while avoiding potentially harmful GHVD.

Response rates to allogeneic HCT for metastatic RCC have been extremely variable, ranging from 0 to 57%. The familiarity of transplant centers with this approach as well as the use of differing selection criteria to determine patient eligibility have likely contributed to this variability in response. Better markers of disease prognosis and treatment response are needed in order to prognosticate those patients who are mostly likely to benefit from an allogeneic HCT. The accrual of patients with extremely short survivals as well as those who have rapidly growing tumors clearly limits the efficacy of allogeneic HCT for patients with metastatic RCC. Because GVT effects are typically delayed by months after transplantation, patients with rapidly progressing disease frequently fail to benefit from a RIST. In general, patients with metastatic RCC appear to tolerate RIST well. Nevertheless, regimen-related mortality rates of 10–15% persist, largely as the consequence of severe acute GVHD. In addition, only 25% of patients have an HLA-matched sibling, limiting the procedure to a relatively small percentage of patients. Therefore, trials investigating the feasibility of using HLA-matched unrelated donors (who are more readily available than HLA-matched siblings) are currently being pursued and, if successful, could expand the application of allogeneic RIST for RCC.

Although the delay by months until the onset of GVT effects hinders the efficacy of RIST, this procedure nonetheless represents a valuable treatment option in carefully selected patients with metastatic RCC. An analysis

TABLE 11g-1. Clinical trials of allogeneic hematopoietic stem cell transplantation for metastatic RCC.[a]

Reference	N	Conditioning	GVHD Prophylaxis	aGVHD (%)[b]	cGVHD (%)	NRM (%)	Response (%)
Childs et al.[33]	19	Flu + Cy	CSA ± MMF	10 (53)	4 (21)	2 (11)	3 CR, 7 PR (53)
Rini et al./Artz et al.[36,71]	18	Flu + Cy	Tac + MMF	3 (16)	7 (39)	6 (33)	4 PR (22)
Bregni et al.[32]	7	Flu + Thio	CSA + MTX	6 (86)	5 (71)	1 (14)	4 PR (57)
Nakagawa et al.[72]	9	Flu/Cla + Bu + ATG	CSA	4 (44)	4 (44)	0 (0)	1 PR (11)
Ueno et al.[37]	15	Flu + Mel	Tac + MTX	7 (47)	4 (27)	5 (33)	1 CR, 2 PR (20)
Hentschke[c] et al.[34]	10	Flu + TBI ± ATG	CSA + MMF	5 (50)	3 (30)	4 (40)	0 (0)
Massenkeil et al.[73]	7	Flu + Cy + ATG	CSA ± MMF	2 (29)	4 (57)	1 (14)	1 PR (14)
Tykodi et al.[74]	8	Flu + TBI	CSA + MMF	4 (50)	4 (50)	1 (13)	1 PR (13)
Blaise et al.[75]	25	Flu + Bu + ATG	CSA	(42)[b]	(60)[b]	(9)[b]	2 PR (8)
Pedrazzoli[d] et al.[35]	7	Flu + Cy	CSA + MTX	0 (0)	NA	2 (29)	0 (0)

[a]Flu, fludarabine; Cy, cyclophosphamide; Thio, thiotepa; Cla, cladribine; Bu, busulfan; ATG, antithymocyte globulin; Mel, melphalan; TBI, total body irradiation; CSA, cyclosporine; MTX, methotrexate; Tac, tacrolimus; MMF, mycophenolate mofetil; NA, not applicable; CR, complete response; PR, partial response.

[b]Grade II or higher.

[c]Regression of some metastases.

[d]All patients died at or before day 80.

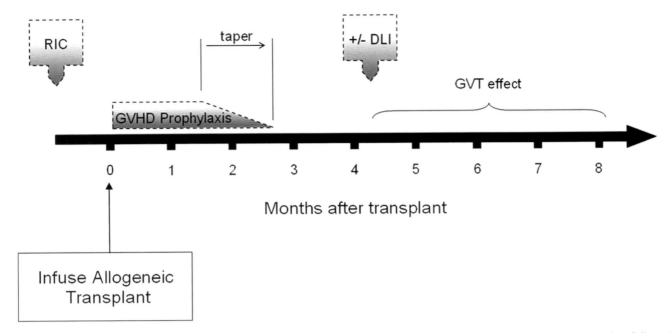

FIGURE 11g-1. Typical reduced-intensity allogeneic transplant strategy for metastatic RCC. Rapid tapering of cyclosporine followed by donor lymphocyte infusions ± IFN-α therapy is used to enhance donor immune-mediated graft-versus-tumor (GVT) effects. RIC, reduced-intensity conditioning; GVHD, graft-versus-host disease; DLI, donor lymphocyte infusion.

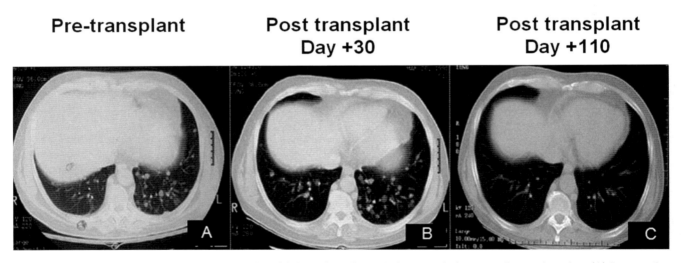

FIGURE 11g-2. Durable GVT effect against metastatic RCC following allogeneic hematopoietic stem cell transplantation. (A) Pretransplant. (B) Multiple pulmonary metastases were noted to initially increase slightly by 30 days posttransplant then (C) disappeared completely by 4 months posttransplant. The patient remains without evidence of metastatic disease >8 years following transplantation.

of published studies shows a modest overall response rate after RIST of about 25% and a complete response (CR) rate of about 8%. In patients with IL-2 and/or IFN refractory disease, allogeneic HCT represents an immune-based treatment modality with the potential to achieve prolonged disease-free survival. Additionally, even in patients who fail to reach partial response (PR) by conventional staging criteria, prolongation of survival with stable or slowly progressive disease may be possible. The incorpo-

ration of drugs that inhibit angiogenesis in the immediate months following transplantation [i.e., vascular endothelial growth factor (VEGF) tyrosine kinase inhibitors or anti-VEGF monoclonal antibodies] could potentially be used to incur disease stability in the time needed for GVT effects to be induced. A RIST trial assessing the impact of anti-VEGF monoclonal antibody therapy following donor engraftment is currently under investigation at the NHLBI.

Donor T-Cells Mediating GVT Effects

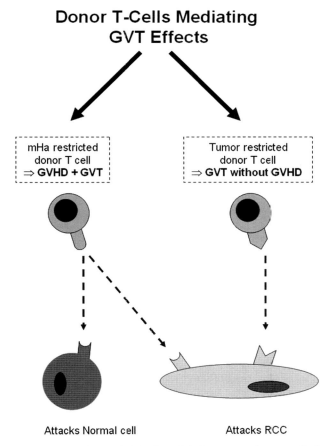

FIGURE 11g-3. Allogeneic T cells and their target antigens mediating graft-versus-tumor (GVT) effects. Donor T cells targeting minor histocompatibility antigens (mHa) expressed on both normal tissues and the tumor mediate GVT effects in association with graft-versus-host disease (GVHD). In contrast, donor T cells recognizing antigens restricted to the tumor mediate GVT effects in the absence of GVHD. RCC, renal cell carcinoma cells.

Graft-versus-Host Disease

GVHD is a frequent donor immune-mediated complication of allogeneic HCT in which allogeneic T cells attack the patient's organs and tissue.[40] GVHD occurring within the first 100 days of transplantation is called acute GVHD; although acute GVHD can be eliminated by corticosteroids and other immunosuppressive therapies, in some cases this process can be unrelenting and fatal. Chronic GVHD by definition occurs more than 100 days after HCT and presents clinically with symptoms similar to those observed with autoimmune diseases such as SICCA syndrome, lupus, and scleroderma-like skin changes. Although significant advances have been made in both the prevention and treatment of this complication, acute and chronic GVHD remain a major obstacle to successful transplant outcome. The most important factor predicting the risk of GVHD is human leukocyte antigen (HLA) disparity between the donor and recipient.[41] Nevertheless, 20–50% of patients transplanted with a completely

HLA matched donor graft may still develop GVHD due to differences in minor histocompatibility antigens. At present, more than 10 minor histocompatibility antigens have been characterized in humans.[42] An example of such an antigen shown to play a clinically significant role in human transplantation is the male-specific HY antigen. During acute GVHD, male patients transplanted with female allografts have an increase in the frequency of T cells targeting male-specific minor histocompatibility antigens.[43] Importantly, such patients also appear to have a lower risk of disease relapse after transplantation.[44] In fact, animal studies as well as studies in humans have provided compelling evidence that minor histocompatibility antigens expressed on tumor cells serve as targets for GVL effects in the allogeneic transplantation setting.[45] The clinical observation of tumor regression occurring concomitant with acute GVHD provides indirect evidence that minor histocompatibility antigens expressed on RCC cells may also be a target for the GVT effect.

It is important to consider that allogeneic HCT is a double-edged sword. The good side is the GVL/GVT effect and the bad side is GVHD. Unfortunately, these two events are often closely linked together. This is best evidenced by studies showing a decreased risk of disease relapse in patients who develop GVHD compared to those who do not.[12,17,18,46] A retrospective analysis of >2000 patients receiving HLA-identical sibling HCT showed both acute and chronic GVHD were associated with a reduction in the risk of disease relapse.[17] Thus, the negative aspect of GVHD is offset to a substantial degree by the enhanced GVL/GVT effects associated with this complication. The close association of GVHD with GVT is evidenced in transplant trials incorporating strategies to prevent acute GVHD, where T cell depletion of the allograft or the use of additional immunosuppressive agents has been shown to increase the risk of leukemia relapse.[19,20,47–49]

Improving Allogeneic Stem Cell Transplantation: Reducing Graft-versus-Host Disease and Enhancing Graft-versus-Tumor Effects

An ongoing research goal is to separate GVT and GVHD effects. The observation that some patients experience GVT effects without GVHD suggests that this goal could someday be achieved. Methods to selectively deplete alloreactive T cells that cause GVHD while preserving T cells with antitumor and antiviral effects are currently being investigated in clinical trials.[50,51] In animal models it has been established that antigen-presenting cells (APC) play a major role in the initiation of GVHD.[51,53] Consequently, significant research is devoted to target molecules involved in host APC/donor T cell interactions. Studies have focused on impairing the migratory function of APC by blocking either chemokine receptor signaling or accessory molecules that are known to be important in the priming of T cells.[54]

Both clinical studies and studies in mouse models suggest that T helper type 1 (Th1) CD4 T cells provide help in inducing GVHD while T helper type 2 (Th2) CD4 T cells may reduce GVHD.[55,56] Thus, a shift from a Th1 to Th2 cytokine profile may be preferable and is currently being evaluated in clinical transplant trials. Recently, mesenchymal stem cells have been found to reduce the incidence and severity of GVHD. This type of stem cell was shown to induce a more antiinflammatory or tolerant phenotype (Th1 to Th2 shift). Specifically, it caused mature dendritic cells to decrease tumor necrosis factor-α (TNF-α) secretion to increase interleukin-10 (IL-10) secretion.[57] Serum levels of IL-10 and TNF-α are known to play a major role in the outcome in allogeneic HCT. For example, IL-10 has a dose-dependent effect on the GVHD lethality mediated by $CD4^+$ or $CD8^+$ T cells, such that high doses accelerate lethality, while low amounts of bioavailable IL-10 are protective.[58] In contrast, a high serum concentration of TNF-α is correlated with increased GVHD.[59] Another area of investigation is the use of regulatory T cells to induce tolerance in recipients of allogeneic stem cell transplant. Substantial evidence indicates that donor $CD4^+CD25^+$ regulatory T cells can suppress GVHD lethality in animal models.[60,61] Edinger et al. demonstrated in a mice model of leukemia and lymphoma that $CD4^+CD25^+$ regulatory T cells suppress the early expansion of alloreactive donor T cells and their capacity to induce GVHD without abrogating their GVT effector function.[62] Thus, $CD4^+CD25^+$ regulatory T cells potentially could be used to separate GVHD from GVT activity incurred by donor T cells. Along the same line, APCs cultured in presence of IL-10 have been shown to induce the differentiation of regulatory T cells. Sato et al. demonstrated that a single injection of these "regulatory APCs" could protect mice from acute GVHD and leukemia relapse.[63] Memory CD4 T cells have been implemented to protect from GVHD as opposed to naive CD4 T cells. Memory $CD4^+$ T cells have also been investigated as a method to protect from GVHD while preserving GVT. Chen and colleagues showed tumor antigen-primed memory $CD4^+$ T cells inhibit tumor growth *in vivo* but do not induce GVHD in a third-party recipient.[64] Based on these data, clinical trials investigating the impact of regulatory or memory T cells on GVHD and GVT effects in humans with malignancies undergoing a RIST will likely be forthcoming.

Infusion of killer IgG-like receptor (KIR) mismatched natural killer (NK) cells is associated with enhanced control of AML relapse and decreased risk of GVHD.[65] Recently, RCC has also been demonstrated to be susceptible to KIR mismatched NK cell lysis.[66] This observation provides the basis for future clinical trials investigating the adoptive infusion of allogeneic KIR-incompatible NK cells in patients with metastatic RCC following HLA mismatched and in some cases HLA-matched allogeneic HCT.

Although the use of allogeneic HCT has provided the evidence that the GVT effect can extend beyond hematological malignancies to the treatment of solid tumors, relatively few complete responses have been observed. Research in allogeneic HCT is increasingly dedicated to enhancing GVT effects. Evidence that GVT effects can be enhanced has been shown in mice vaccinated with modified tumor cells following allogeneic HCT.[67,68] Furthermore, experimental animal studies have demonstrated an increased GVT effect in recipients after allogeneic HCT incorporating dendritic cell vaccination and as well as adoptive transfer of tumor or minor histocompatibility specific T cells.[69,70] It is anticipated that allogeneic HCT trials incorporating the above-mentioned methods to prevent GVHD while targeting the donor immune system against the malignancy will be forthcoming in the near future. These new strategies will hopefully decrease regimen-related toxicities and improve the efficacy of allogeneic RIST for solid tumors.

References

1. Rosenberg SA, Lotze MT, Muul LM, et al. Observations on the systemic administration of autologous lymphokine-activated killer cells and recombinant interleukin-2 to patients with metastatic cancer. N Engl J Med 1985;313(23):1485–1492.
2. Rosenberg SA, Yang JC, Topalian SL, et al. Treatment of 283 consecutive patients with metastatic melanoma or renal cell cancer using high-dose bolus interleukin 2. JAMA 1994;271(12):907–913.
3. Brouwenstijn N, Gaugler B, Kruse KM, et al. Renal-cell carcinoma-specific lysis by cytotoxic T-lymphocyte clones isolated from peripheral blood lymphocytes and tumor-infiltrating lymphocytes. Int J Cancer 1996;68(2):177–182.
4. Bukowski RM, Sharfman W, Murthy S, et al. Clinical results and characterization of tumor-infiltrating lymphocytes with or without recombinant interleukin 2 in human metastatic renal cell carcinoma. Cancer Res 1991;51(16):4199–4205.
5. Goedegebuure PS, Douville LM, Li H, et al. Adoptive immunotherapy with tumor-infiltrating lymphocytes and interleukin-2 in patients with metastatic malignant melanoma and renal cell carcinoma: a pilot study. J Clin Oncol 1995;13(8):1939–1949.
6. Oehlrich N, Devitt G, Linnebacher M, et al. Generation of RAGE-1 and MAGE-9 peptide-specific cytotoxic T-lymphocyte lines for transfer in patients with renal cell carcinoma. Int J Cancer 2005;117(2):256–264.
7. Vissers JL, De Vries IJ, Schreurs MW, et al. The renal cell carcinoma-associated antigen G250 encodes a human leukocyte antigen (HLA)-A2.1-restricted epitope recognized by cytotoxic T lymphocytes. Cancer Res 1999;59(21):5554–5559.
8. Su Z, Dannull J, Heiser A, et al. Immunological and clinical responses in metastatic renal cancer patients vaccinated with tumor RNA-transfected dendritic cells. Cancer Res 2003;63(9):2127–2133.
9. Seliger B, Atkins D, Bock M, et al. Characterization of human lymphocyte antigen class I antigen-processing machinery defects in renal cell carcinoma lesions with special emphasis on transporter-associated with antigen-processing down-regulation. Clin Cancer Res 2003;9(5):1721–1727.

10. Uzzo RG, Rayman P, Kolenko V, et al. Mechanisms of apoptosis in T cells from patients with renal cell carcinoma. Clin Cancer Res 1999;5(5):1219–1229.

11. Bacigalupo A, Van Lint MT, Frassoni F, Marmont A. Graft-versus-leukemia effect following allogeneic bone marrow transplantation. Br J Haematol 1985;61(4):749–751.

12. Weiden PL, Sullivan KM, Flournoy N, Storb R, Thomas ED. Antileukemic effect of chronic graft-versus-host disease: contribution to improved survival after allogeneic marrow transplantation. N Engl J Med 1981;304(25):1529–1533.

13. Woods WG, Neudorf S, Gold S, et al. A comparison of allogeneic bone marrow transplantation, autologous bone marrow transplantation, and aggressive chemotherapy in children with acute myeloid leukemia in remission. Blood 2001;97(1):56–62.

14. Zittoun RA, Mandelli F, Willemze R, et al. Autologous or allogeneic bone marrow transplantation compared with intensive chemotherapy in acute myelogenous leukemia. European Organization for Research and Treatment of Cancer (EORTC) and the Gruppo Italiano Malattie Ematologiche Maligne dell'Adulto (GIMEMA) Leukemia Cooperative Groups. N Engl J Med 1995;332(4):217–223.

15. Gorin NC, Labopin M, Fouillard L, et al. Retrospective evaluation of autologous bone marrow transplantation vs allogeneic bone marrow transplantation from an HLA identical related donor in acute myelocytic leukemia. A study of the European Cooperative Group for Blood and Marrow Transplantation (EBMT). Bone Marrow Transplant 1996;18(1):111–117.

16. Gale RP, Champlin RE. How does bone-marrow transplantation cure leukaemia? Lancet 1984;2(8393):28–30.

17. Horowitz MM, Gale RP, Sondel PM, et al. Graft-versus-leukemia reactions after bone marrow transplantation. Blood 1990;75(3):555–562.

18. Weiden PL, Flournoy N, Thomas ED, et al. Antileukemic effect of graft-versus-host disease in human recipients of allogeneic-marrow grafts. N Engl J Med 1979;300(19):1068–1073.

19. Goldman JM, Gale RP, Horowitz MM, et al. Bone marrow transplantation for chronic myelogenous leukemia in chronic phase. Increased risk for relapse associated with T-cell depletion. Ann Intern Med 1988;108(6):806–814.

20. Marmont AM, Horowitz MM, Gale RP, et al. T-cell depletion of HLA-identical transplants in leukemia. Blood 1991;78(8):2120–2130.

21. Bar BM, Schattenberg A, Mensink EJ, et al. Donor leukocyte infusions for chronic myeloid leukemia relapsed after allogeneic bone marrow transplantation. J Clin Oncol 1993;11(3):513–519.

22. Kolb HJ, Mittermuller J, Clemm C, et al. Donor leukocyte transfusions for treatment of recurrent chronic myelogenous leukemia in marrow transplant patients. Blood 1990;76(12):2462–2465.

23. Porter DL, Roth MS, McGarigle C, Ferrara JL, Antin JH. Induction of graft-versus-host disease as immunotherapy for relapsed chronic myeloid leukemia. N Engl J Med 1994;330(2):100–106.

24. Feinstein L, Sandmaier B, Maloney D, et al. Nonmyeloablative hematopoietic cell transplantation. Replacing high-dose cytotoxic therapy by the graft-versus-tumor effect. Ann NY Acad Sci 2001;938:328–337; discussion 37–39.

25. Giralt S, Estey E, Albitar M, et al. Engraftment of allogeneic hematopoietic progenitor cells with purine analog-containing chemotherapy: harnessing graft-versus-leukemia without myeloablative therapy. Blood 1997;89(12):4531–4536.

26. Slavin S, Nagler A, Naparstek E, et al. Nonmyeloablative stem cell transplantation and cell therapy as an alternative to conventional bone marrow transplantation with lethal cytoreduction for the treatment of malignant and nonmalignant hematologic diseases. Blood 1998;91(3):756–763.

27. Storb RF, Champlin R, Riddell SR, Murata M, Bryant S, Warren EH. Non-myeloablative transplants for malignant disease. Hematology (Am Soc Hematol Educ Program) 2001:375–391.

28. Imamura M, Tsutsumi Y, Miura Y, Toubai T, Tanaka J. Immune reconstitution and tolerance after allogeneic hematopoietic stem cell transplantation. Hematology 2003;8(1):19–26.

29. Childs R, Clave E, Contentin N, et al. Engraftment kinetics after nonmyeloablative allogeneic peripheral blood stem cell transplantation: full donor T-cell chimerism precedes alloimmune responses. Blood 1999;94(9):3234–3241.

30. Kradin RL, Kurnick JT, Lazarus DS, et al. Tumour-infiltrating lymphocytes and interleukin-2 in treatment of advanced cancer. Lancet 1989;1(8638):577–580.

31. Topalian SL, Rosenberg SA. Therapy of cancer using the adoptive transfer of activated killer cells and interleukin-2. Acta Haematol 1987;7(Suppl 1):75–76.

32. Bregni M, Dodero A, Peccatori J, et al. Nonmyeloablative conditioning followed by hematopoietic cell allografting and donor lymphocyte infusions for patients with metastatic renal and breast cancer. Blood 2002;99(11):4234–4236.

33. Childs R, Chernoff A, Contentin N, et al. Regression of metastatic renal-cell carcinoma after nonmyeloablative allogeneic peripheral-blood stem-cell transplantation. N Engl J Med 2000;343(11):750–758.

34. Hentschke P, Barkholt L, Uzunel M, et al. Low-intensity conditioning and hematopoietic stem cell transplantation in patients with renal and colon carcinoma. Bone Marrow Transplant 2003;31(4):253–261.

35. Pedrazzoli P, Da Prada GA, Giorgiani G, et al. Allogeneic blood stem cell transplantation after a reduced-intensity, preparative regimen: a pilot study in patients with refractory malignancies. Cancer 2002;94(9):2409–2415.

36. Rini BI, Zimmerman T, Stadler WM, Gajewski TF, Vogelzang NJ. Allogeneic stem-cell transplantation of renal cell cancer after nonmyeloablative chemotherapy: feasibility, engraftment, and clinical results. J Clin Oncol 2002;20(8):2017–2024.

37. Ueno NT, Cheng YC, Rondon G, et al. Rapid induction of complete donor chimerism by the use of a reduced-intensity conditioning regimen composed of fludarabine and melphalan in allogeneic stem cell transplantation for metastatic solid tumors. Blood 2003;102(10):3829–3836.

38. Warren EH, Tykodi SS, Murata M, et al. T-cell therapy targeting minor histocompatibility Ags for the treatment of leukemia and renal-cell carcinoma. Cytotherapy 2002;4(5):441.

39. Takahashi Y, Mena O, Srinivasan R, et al. Minor histocompatibility antigen (mHa) specific T-cells with cytotoxicity against autologous tumor cells can be isolated from patients with renal cell carcinoma having a GVT effect after nonmyeloablative hematopoietic cell transplantation. ASH abstracts 2003;Poster Session 765-II (2594).

40. Ferrara JL, Deeg HJ. Graft-versus-host disease. N Engl J Med 1991;324(10):667–674.

41. Hansen JA, Yamamoto K, Petersdorf E, Sasazuki T. The role of HLA matching in hematopoietic cell transplantation. Rev Immunogenet 1999;1(3):359–373.

42. Falkenburg JH, van de Corput L, Marijt EW, Willemze R. Minor histocompatibility antigens in human stem cell transplantation. Exp Hematol 2003;31(9):743–751.

43. Mutis T, Gillespie G, Schrama E, Falkenburg JH, Moss P, Goulmy E. Tetrameric HLA class I-minor histocompatibility antigen peptide complexes demonstrate minor histocompatibility antigen-specific cytotoxic T lymphocytes in patients with graft-versus-host disease. Nat Med 1999;5(7):839–842.

44. Gratwohl A, Hermans J, Niederwieser D, van Biezen A, van Houwelingen HC, Apperley J. Female donors influence transplant-related mortality and relapse incidence in male recipients of sibling blood and marrow transplants. Hematol J 2001;2(6):363–370.

45. Perreault C, Jutras J, Roy DC, Filep JG, Brochu S. Identification of an immunodominant mouse minor histocompatibility antigen (MiHA). T cell response to a single dominant MiHA causes graft-versus-host disease. J Clin Invest 1996;98(3):622–628.

46. Sullivan KM, Weiden PL, Storb R, et al. Influence of acute and chronic graft-versus-host disease on relapse and survival after bone marrow transplantation from HLA-identical siblings as treatment of acute and chronic leukemia. Blood 1989;73(6):1720–1728.

47. Keever CA, Small TN, Flomenberg N, et al. Immune reconstitution following bone marrow transplantation: comparison of recipients of T-cell depleted marrow with recipients of conventional marrow grafts. Blood 1989;73(5):1340–1350.

48. Michallet M, Perrin MC, Belhabri A, et al. Impact of cyclosporine and methylprednisolone dose used for prophylaxis and therapy of graft-versus-host disease on survival and relapse after allogeneic bone marrow transplantation. Bone Marrow Transplant 1999;23(2):145–150.

49. Roux E, Helg C, Dumont-Girard F, Chapuis B, Jeannet M, Roosnek E. Analysis of T-cell repopulation after allogeneic bone marrow transplantation: significant differences between recipients of T-cell depleted and unmanipulated grafts. Blood 1996;87(9):3984–3992.

50. Amrolia PJ, Muccioli-Casadei G, Yvon E, et al. Selective depletion of donor alloreactive T cells without loss of antiviral or antileukemic responses. Blood 2003;102(6):2292–2299.

51. Solomon SR, Tran T, Carter CS, et al. Optimized clinical-scale culture conditions for ex vivo selective depletion of host-reactive donor lymphocytes: a strategy for GvHD prophylaxis in allogeneic PBSC transplantation. Cytotherapy 2002;4(5):395–406.

52. Matte CC, Liu J, Cormier J, et al. Donor APCs are required for maximal GVHD but not for GVL. Nat Med 2004;10(9):987–992.

53. Shlomchik WD, Couzens MS, Tang CB, et al. Prevention of graft versus host disease by inactivation of host antigen-presenting cells. Science 1999;285(5426):412–415.

54. Murai M, Yoneyama H, Harada A, et al. Active participation of CCR5(+)CD8(+) T lymphocytes in the pathogenesis of liver injury in graft-versus-host disease. J Clin Invest 1999;104(1):49–57.

55. Blazar BR, Korngold R, Vallera DA. Recent advances in graft-versus-host disease (GVHD) prevention. Immunol Rev 1997;157:79–109.

56. Fowler DH, Kurasawa K, Smith R, Eckhaus MA, Gress RE. Donor CD4-enriched cells of Th2 cytokine phenotype regulate graft-versus-host disease without impairing allogeneic engraftment in sublethally irradiated mice. Blood 1994;84(10):3540–3549.

57. Aggarwal S, Pittenger MF. Human mesenchymal stem cells modulate allogeneic immune cell responses. Blood 2005;105(4):1815–2822.

58. Blazar BR, Taylor PA, Panoskaltsis-Mortari A, et al. Interleukin-10 dose-dependent regulation of CD4+ and CD8+ T cell-mediated graft-versus-host disease. Transplantation 1998;66(9):1220–1229.

59. Holler E, Kolb HJ, Moller A, et al. Increased serum levels of tumor necrosis factor alpha precede major complications of bone marrow transplantation. Blood 1990;75(4):1011–1016.

60. Cohen JL, Trenado A, Vasey D, Klatzmann D, Salomon BL. CD4(+)CD25(+) immunoregulatory T cells: new therapeutics for graft-versus-host disease. J Exp Med 2002;196(3):401–406.

61. Taylor PA, Lees CJ, Blazar BR. The infusion of ex vivo activated and expanded CD4(+)CD25(+) immune regulatory cells inhibits graft-versus-host disease lethality. Blood 2002;99(10):3493–3499.

62. Edinger M, Hoffmann P, Ermann J, et al. CD4+CD25+ regulatory T cells preserve graft-versus-tumor activity while inhibiting graft-versus-host disease after bone marrow transplantation. Nat Med 2003;9(9):1144–1150.

63. Sato K, Yamashita N, Baba M, Matsuyama T. Regulatory dendritic cells protect mice from murine acute graft-versus-host disease and leukemia relapse. Immunity 2003;18(3):367–379.

64. Chen BJ, Cui X, Sempowski GD, Liu C, Chao NJ. Transfer of allogeneic CD62L- memory T cells without graft-versus-host disease. Blood 2004;103(4):1534–1541.

65. Ruggeri L, Capanni M, Casucci M, et al. Role of natural killer cell alloreactivity in HLA-mismatched hematopoietic stem cell transplantation. Blood 1999;94(1):333–339.

66. Igarashi T, Wynberg J, Srinivasan R, et al. Enhanced cytotoxicity of allogeneic NK cells with killer immunoglobulin-like receptor ligand incompatibility against melanoma and renal cell carcinoma cells. Blood 2004;104(1):170–177.

67. Anderson LD Jr, Savary CA, Mullen CA. Immunization of allogeneic bone marrow transplant recipients with tumor cell vaccines enhances graft-versus-tumor activity without exacerbating graft-versus-host disease. Blood 2000;95(7):2426–2433.

68. Teshima T, Mach N, Hill GR, et al. Tumor cell vaccine elicits potent antitumor immunity after allogeneic T-cell-depleted bone marrow transplantation. Cancer Res 2001;61(1):162–171.

69. Ji YH, Weiss L, Zeira M, et al. Allogeneic cell-mediated immunotherapy of leukemia with immune donor lymphocytes to upregulate antitumor effects and downregulate antihost responses. Bone Marrow Transplant 2003;32(5):495–504.

70. Zoller M. Tumor vaccination after allogeneic bone marrow cell reconstitution of the nonmyeloablatively conditioned tumor-bearing murine host. J Immunol 2003;171(12):6941–6953.

71. Artz AS, Van Besien K, Zimmerman T, et al. Long-term follow-up of nonmyeloablative allogeneic stem cell transplantation for renal cell carcinoma: The University of Chicago Experience. Bone Marrow Transplant 2005;35(3):253–260.

72. Nakagawa T, Kami M, Hori A, et al. Allogeneic hematopoietic stem cell transplantation with a reduced-intensity conditioning

regimen for treatment of metastatic renal cell carcinoma: single institution experience with a minimum 1-year follow-up. Exp Hematol 2004;32(7):599–606.

73. Massenkeil G, Roigas J, Nagy M, et al. Nonmyeloablative stem cell transplantation in metastatic renal cell carcinoma: delayed graft-versus-tumor effect is associated with chimerism conversion but transplantation has high toxicity. Bone Marrow Transplant 2004;34(4):309–316.

74. Tykodi SS, Warren EH, Thompson JA, et al. Allogeneic hematopoietic cell transplantation for metastatic renal cell carcinoma after nonmyeloablative conditioning: toxicity, clinical response, and immunological response to minor histocompatibility antigens. Clin Cancer Res 2004;10(23):7799–7811.

75. Blaise D, Bay JO, Faucher C, et al. Reduced-intensity preparative regimen and allogeneic stem cell transplantation for advanced solid tumors. Blood 2004;103(2):435–441.

11h
Bisphosphonate Treatment for Osteolytic Bone Metastases Associated with Renal Cell Carcinoma

Fred Saad and Allan Lipton

Introduction

Renal cell carcinoma (RCC) claims more than 100,000 lives worldwide each year, and the incidence of RCC has increased by approximately 40% over the past 30 years.[1,2] Although fewer patients with RCC develop bone metastases compared with patients with other solid tumors, including breast and prostate cancer, the prognosis for patients with metastatic RCC is very poor (Table 11h-1).[3] The median survival after diagnosis of bone metastases in this patient population is only 6 months.[3]

Bone lesions associated with RCC are predominantly osteolytic; they are the result of increased osteoclast activity accompanied by a concomitant decrease in osteoblastic activity and thus lead to an abnormally high rate of bone resorption resulting in extensive bone loss. Patients with bone metastases from advanced RCC typically experience significant skeletal morbidity including hypercalcemia, severe bone pain that requires palliative radiotherapy, pathological fractures, and spinal cord compression. In an observational study of 31 patients with bone metastases from RCC who did not receive bisphosphonate treatment, approximately 81% required radiotherapy to bone, and 42% experienced a long-bone fracture over 5 years of follow-up.[4] Moreover, patients experienced 2.5–4.0 skeletal-related events (SREs) per year.[4] These events are especially debilitating and have been associated with diminished health-related quality of life (HRQOL).[5] Therefore, there is a need to develop treatments that will effectively prevent skeletal complications in these patients.

The majority of therapies that are currently used to treat patients with RCC do not treat bone metastases. Interferon and interleukin-2 (IL-2), the current standards of care, yield response rates of 11–17% and median survivals of 15–20 months.[6] However, neither of these therapies treats or prevents the skeletal metastases that contribute to the considerable disease morbidity. Zoledronic acid, a nitrogen-containing bisphosphonate (N-BP), was recently shown to significantly reduce the incidence of SREs, reduce the risk of developing skeletal complications, and delay the time to progression of bone lesions in a retrospective subset analysis of 74 patients with RCC in a randomized, double-blind, placebo-controlled clinical trial.[7]

Because bisphosphonates are inhibitors of osteoclast-mediated bone resorption, they are effective in the treatment of a variety of bone diseases. They bind avidly to the bone mineral, accumulate in the bone mineral matrix at sites of active metabolism, and inhibit the bone-resorbing activity of osteoclasts.[8] Furthermore, bisphosphonates have been shown to inhibit osteoclastogenesis in vitro and in vivo,[9,10] and preclinical studies suggest that bisphosphonates possess antitumor activity and may potentially prevent tumor metastasis to bone and delay disease progression in the bone.[11,12]

Physiology of Bone Remodeling

Adult bone normally undergoes continual remodeling through the coordinated interactions of osteoclasts and osteoblasts, which alternately resorb and repair bone, respectively.[13] These activities are mediated by numerous growth factors that are released by the mineralized bone matrix during this process (Fig. 11h-1A).[13] Systemic hormones within the bone microenvironment, including parathyroid hormone, parathyroid hormone-related protein (PTHrP), thyroxine, and cytokines including IL-1, IL-6, and IL-11, participate in osteolysis by inducing the expression of the receptor activator of nuclear factor κB ligand (RANKL) on immature osteoblasts and stromal cells. The binding of RANKL to its receptor, RANK, on the surface of immature osteoclasts initiates signaling pathways that eventually lead to the maturation of osteoclast precursors and promotion of osteoclast survival. Mature osteoclasts secrete proteases and acids that dissolve the bone mineral matrix and release it into the extracellular space. As a result of osteoclast-mediated bone resorption, growth factors including transforming growth factor-β (TGF-β) and insulin-like growth factor II are released from the bone matrix.

TABLE 11h-1. Prevalence of metastatic bone disease.

Primary cancer	5-year world prevalence (millions)	Incidence of bone metastasis (%)	Median survival from diagnosis of bone metastases (months)
Lung	1.39	30–40	6
Breast	3.86	65–75	19–25
Prostate	1.55	65–75	12–53
Myeloma	0.14	70–95	6–54
Renal	0.48	20–25	6
Melanoma	0.53	14–45	6
Thyroid	0.48	60	48

Source: Adapted with permission from Lipton.[3]

Osteoblasts are bone-forming cells (Fig. 11h-1B).[13] The maturation of osteoblasts is less well understood; however, several systemic factors including parathyroid hormone, prostaglandins, and local factors within the bone microenvironment including TGF-β and insulin-like growth factors stimulate the growth and differentiation of osteoblasts.[13] Osteoblasts secrete the collagen-rich extracellular matrix that serves as the site for the deposition of hydroxyapatite crystals that form the bone. When tumors metastasize to the bone, the complex interplay between osteoclasts and osteoblasts becomes disregulated, thus leading to bone loss, irregular bone deposition, and compromised skeletal integrity.

Tumor Metastasis to the Bone and Formation of Lytic Lesions

The skeleton is the most common site of metastasis in many advanced cancers.[14] This is most likely because the bone is a site of high blood flow that is necessary for tumor cell dissemination. The bone is also the site of numerous growth factors that once released, stimulate tumor cell growth and proliferation. The process of metastasis to the bone has been described by a "seed and soil" mechanism; in this way, the tumor cells act as a seed with the potential to grow on a rich soil, the bone. The metastatic process is initiated

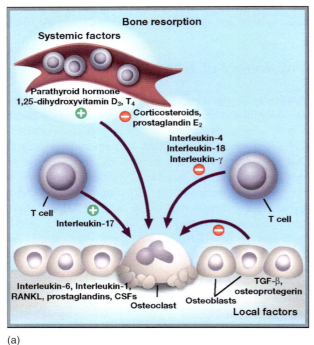

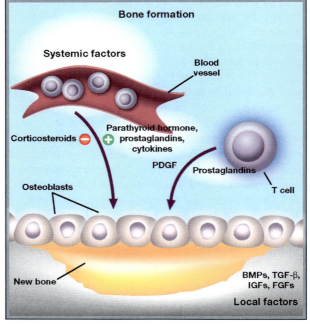

(a)   (b)

FIGURE 11h-1. Both local and systemic factors induce the maturation and activity of the bone-resorbing osteoclasts (**A**) and bone-forming osteoblasts (**B**). T$_4$, thyroxine; RANKL, receptor activator of nuclear factor-κB ligand; CSFs, colony-stimulating factors; TGF, transforming growth factor; PDGF, platelet-derived growth factor; BMPs, bone morphogenetic proteins; IGFs, insulin-like growth factors; FGFs, fibroblast growth factors. (Adapted with permission from Roodman.[13])

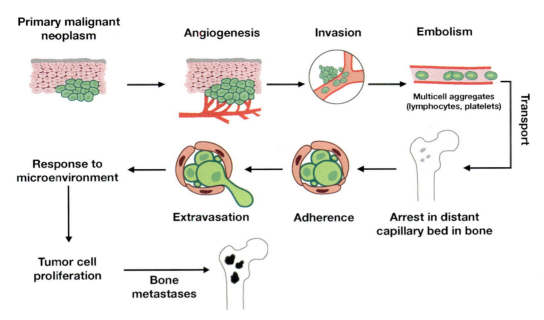

FIGURE 11h-2. Mechanism of tumor cell metastasis from the primary site to the bone. (Adapted with permission from Guise and Mundy.[15])

when primary tumor cells detach from their place of origin by secreting proteolytic enzymes (i.e., matrix metalloproteinases) and/or by loss of adhesion molecule expression (i.e., integrins; Fig. 11h-2).[15] The angiogenic nature of tumors induces the formation of new blood vessels allowing the cells to enter the circulation. Eventually, the tumor cells escape the circulation, invade the marrow stroma, adhere to the endosteal surface of the bone, and proliferate.

Evidence suggests that osteolysis is one of the first steps in establishing bone metastases (Fig. 11h-3).[16] Tumor cells secrete factors including TGF-β, PTHrP, and IL-6 that activate osteoclast activity. The osteoclasts, in turn, degrade the mineralized bone to release additional growth factors including TGF-β and IL-6, which are necessary for tumor cell growth and proliferation. Moreover, evidence from preclinical studies of melanoma and breast cancer cell lines suggests that tumor cells may release proteinases such as matrix metalloproteinases to aid in the degradation of mineralized bone.[16, 17] As a result of this cycle, the normal homeostasis of the bone is disrupted, and excess bone resorption ensues.

Once a metastatic site has been established, lytic lesions ensue primarily through the activity of the osteoclasts rather than the tumor cells. Evidence from studies with breast cancer suggests that PTHrP, which is likely released from most solid tumors, stimulates osteoclast maturation. PTHrP induces the expression of RANKL on marrow stromal cells, thus activating osteoclast maturation through binding of RANKL to its receptor RANK on the osteoclast precursor (Fig. 11h-4).[13] As osteoclasts degrade bone, TGF-β is released; this cytokine increases the production of PTHrP in tumor cells. This "vicious cycle" of bone destruction leads to increases in local calcium levels, which in turn promote tumor growth and PTHrP production. Therefore, once estab-lished, lytic metastases progress rapidly through the release of bone-derived growth factors that stimulate tumor growth and bone destruction.

Consequences of Skeletal-Related Events on Patients and Healthcare Providers

Lytic bone lesions cause significant skeletal morbidity and can have a deleterious impact on HRQOL.[5] Patients with bone lesions from RCC have a particularly high risk of developing SREs. Data from a large multicenter trial in patients ($n = 773$) with bone metastases from lung cancer and other solid tumors, including RCC, showed that the proportion of patients in the placebo arm within the RCC subset who experienced an SRE on study was higher than that reported in any other patient subset,[18–20] thus highlighting the aggressive nature of bone metastases from RCC. After 21 months of follow-up, 79% of RCC patients who had received placebo experienced at least one SRE compared with 46% of the overall trial population who received placebo.[18, 19] These data indicate that the osteolytic lesions associated with RCC are clinically aggressive and that patients with bone involvement have elevated bone metabolism, presumably due at least in part to the systemic release of PTHrP.

The most common SREs in patients with RCC have been shown to be bone pain requiring palliative radiotherapy and long bone fractures (Table 11h-2).[4,7] Zekri et al.[4] investigated skeletal complications from bone metastases in 31 patients with bone metastases from RCC. Over the 5-year observational period, >80% of patients required palliative radiotherapy for bone pain, and 42% of patients experienced long-bone fractures. Moreover, 32 (44%) of the 72 patients in this study

PRIMARY TUMOR

MICROMETASTASES

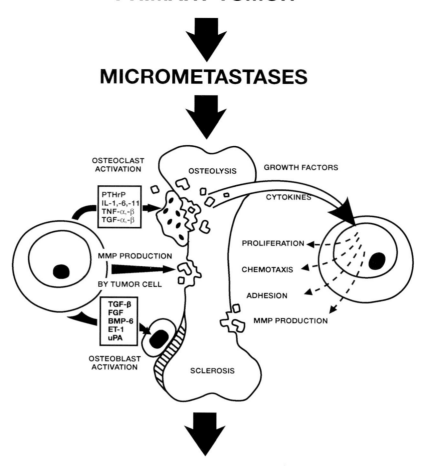

FIGURE 11h-3. Pathophysiology of the formation of bone metastases. PTHrP, parathyroid hormone-related protein; IL, interleukin; TNF, tumor necrosis factor; TGF, transforming growth factor; FGF, fibroblast growth factor; BMP, bone morphogenetic protein; ET, endothelin; uPA, urokinase-type plasminogen activator. (Adapted with permission from Orr et al.[16])

who did not have metastatic bone disease developed hypercalcemia of malignancy during the 5-year observation period.

Lytic bone lesions reduce bone integrity and load-bearing capacities and thus cause pathological fractures that often require surgery. Pathological fractures are especially devastating when they occur in load-bearing bones including the femur or the pelvis and often necessitate prolonged hospital stays. Because the majority of metastatic fractures never heal, they are associated with a particularly poor outcome. Mobility is often restored through surgical procedures, which have an overall postoperative fatality rate of approximately 4%.[21] Vertebral fractures are associated with chronic back pain and loss of height and stature; therefore, these fractures can lead to functional impairment and disability.[22] Deformed vertebrae decrease rib cage support and, thus, result in restricted lung volume and reflux esophagitis.

Bone pain is the most common cancer-associated pain. More than 75% of patients with advanced metastatic disease experience pain, and approximately 45% of patients have

inadequate pain control.[23] Pain is often poorly localized and is characterized as a burning, aching, or stabbing discomfort.[24] Cancer pain is often the result of lesions that arise in the nervous system or tissue injury that results in a release of a variety of chemical mediators that activate nociceptors.[25] Tumor cell-derived factors including TGF-β, IL-1, and IL-6 may also excite or sensitize primary afferent neurons.[23] Therapies for the management of other cancer-related pain include analgesics and radiotherapy. Radiation to bone is used for palliation of severe bone pain that is refractory to analgesics and provides transient relief in approximately 80% of patients.[26] Severe bone pain has a significant impact on HRQOL. Weinfurt et al.[5] found that radiation to bone had the broadest impact on HRQOL; therefore, this endpoint appears to be a reliable surrogate for bone pain. Moreover, patients experienced declines in emotional well being after radiation to bone or pathological fractures.

Skeletal-related events also have a considerable impact on healthcare costs. Cost assessment analyses indicate that within the United States SREs contribute to 10–16% of the

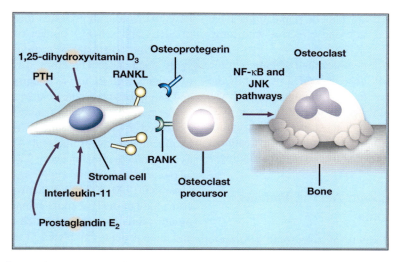

FIGURE 11h-4. Maturation of osteoclast precursors through the activation of the expression of RANKL. RANKL, receptor activator of nuclear factor-κB ligand; PTH, parathyroid hormone; NF-κB, nuclear factor-κB; JNK, jun N-terminal kinase. (Adapted with permission from Roodman.[13])

TABLE 11h-2. Skeletal-related events in patients with renal cell carcinoma ($n = 31$).

SRE[a]	Patients, n (%)	Number of events
Radiotherapy	25 (81)	37
Long bone fracture	13 (42)	15
Hypercalcemia[b]	9 (29)	16
Orthopedic surgery	9 (29)	12
Spinal cord compression	4 (13)	4

Source: Adapted with permission from Zekri et al.[4]

[a]SRE, skeletal-related event.

[b]An additional 32 patients without metastatic bone disease developed hypercalcemia during the 5-year observation period.

total treatment costs for patients with breast cancer, prostate cancer, or multiple myeloma.[27–29] Therefore, reducing the number and incidence of SREs in patients with RCC may reduce healthcare costs.

Current treatment options for patients with RCC include biological therapeutics including IL and interferon. However, these therapies have little effect on preventing bone metastases or skeletal complications. Because approximately 20% of patients with RCC have metastatic disease at diagnosis, there is a need for improved therapies that treat and prevent SREs.[4] The use of bisphosphonates in these patients can delay or prevent skeletal complications, thus providing important and meaningful clinical benefits.[30]

Bisphosphonates in the Treatment of Bone Metastases from Renal Cell Cancer

Bisphosphonates are potent inhibitors of osteoclast-mediated bone resorption and have become an important class of drugs for the treatment of bone metastases. Bisphosphonates may reduce bone resorption through several mechanisms including induction of osteoclast apoptosis, inhibition of osteoclast maturation, and decreased osteoclast activity.[3] During bone resorption, bisphosphonates are released and internalized by osteoclasts, thereby inhibiting their lytic activity and inducing apoptosis. Nitrogen-containing bisphosphonates such as zoledronic acid exert their effects through inhibition of enzymes in the biosynthetic mevalonate pathway, thus inhibiting prenylation of guanosine triphosphate-binding proteins, including Ras, Rho, and Rac.[8,31] These signaling proteins are involved in cell proliferation, survival, membrane trafficking, and cytoskeletal organization and are necessary for osteoclast function. Inhibition of bone resorption by N-BPs may also occur through the inhibition of both osteoclastogenesis and the recruitment of osteoclast progenitors to the bone. Bisphosphonates have also demonstrated antitumor potential[32–34] and have been shown to inhibit tumor cell adhesion and invasion of the bone matrix.[35]

Zoledronic acid is a new-generation N-BP that significantly reduces skeletal morbidity in patients with bone metastases secondary to breast cancer, prostate cancer, lung cancer, and a variety of other solid tumors including RCC.[19,20,30,36]

Extensive clinical trials in these patient populations have shown that zoledronic acid is safe and effective with long-term use.[37]

More recently, Yuasa et al.[38] demonstrated that minodronic acid, a third generation N-BP, dose dependently inhibits the growth of RCC cells in vitro. In vivo, minodronic acid was shown to enhance the antitumor effect of interferon on RCC cell growth ($p < 0.05$). Although these preclinical studies suggest that minodronic acid may be effective in the treatment of RCC, clinical studies are needed to verify these findings.

Clinical Trials of Zoledronic Acid in Patients with Renal Cell Carcinoma

The long-term efficacy and safety of zoledronic acid were recently investigated in a randomized, double-blind, placebo-controlled, Phase III trial in patients ($n = 773$) with bone metastases from solid tumors other than breast cancer or prostate cancer, including RCC.[19] Over the 21-month study period, zoledronic acid reduced the number of patients experiencing one or more SREs while on study, significantly delayed the median time to the first SRE, significantly reduced the annual incidence of SREs, and significantly reduced the risk of developing an SRE by multiple event analysis. A separate evaluation of the subset of patients with

RCC in this trial showed that there was a very high incidence of SREs and a heavy burden of disease from bone metastases in these patients compared with patients in the overall study population. Therefore, a retrospective subset analysis of patients with RCC was undertaken to evaluate the efficacy and safety of zoledronic acid in these patients.[7]

The retrospective subset analysis reported by Lipton et al.[7] examined 74 patients with RCC who were randomized to treatment with zoledronic acid (4 mg or 8/4 mg), administered as a 15-minute infusion every 3 weeks, or placebo; all patients also received daily oral supplements of calcium (500 mg) and vitamin D (400–500 IU). Patients who completed the 9-month core phase of the trial could extend their treatment for up to 21 months; nine patients continued for an additional 12 months and three patients completed 21 months of therapy.[18] Efficacy conclusions were not drawn from the 8/4-mg treatment group.

Baseline disease characteristics and patient demographic factors for the RCC subset were well balanced between the 4-mg zoledronic acid ($n = 27$) and placebo arms ($n = 19$; Table 11h-3).[7] The primary efficacy endpoint was the percentage of patients who experienced at least one SRE on study; SREs were defined as pathological fracture, radiotherapy to bone, surgery to bone, and spinal cord compression. Secondary efficacy endpoints included mean annual SRE incidence (i.e., skeletal morbidity rate), time

TABLE 11h-3. Patient demographics and baseline disease characteristics.

Characteristic	Zoledronic acid ($n = 27$)	Placebo ($n = 19$)
Median age, years	64	65
Sex, n (%)		
Male	18 (67)	17 (89)
Female	9 (33)	2 (11)
Primary therapy, n (%)		
Immunotherapy[b]	17 (63)	9 (47)
Hormonal therapy	1 (4)	1 (5)
Median time from initial diagnosis to study entry, months[c]	25.5	21.2
ECOG performance status, n (%)		
≤ 1	21 (78)	18 (95)
≥ 2	5 (19)	1 (5)
Number of lesions at study entry (%)		
Unknown	1 (4)	1 (5)
1–3	21 (78)	12 (63)
4–6	4 (15)	4 (21)
7–9	1 (4)	2 (11)
Previous SRE, n (%)		
Yes	22 (81)	18 (95)
No	5 (19)	1 (5)
Baseline serum creatinine, n (%)		
Normal (<1.4 mg/dl)	17 (63)	9 (47)
Abnormal (≥ 1.4 mg/dl)	10 (37)	10 (53)

Source: Adapted with permission from Lipton et al.[7]
[a]ECOG, Eastern Cooperative Oncology Group; SRE, skeletal-related event.
[b]Denotes interferon- and/or interleukin-based immunotherapy, with or without additional chemotherapeutic agents.
[c]Twenty-eight days in a month.

TABLE 11h-4. Best bone response by treatment group.

Response	Patients, n (%)	
	Zoledronic acid (n = 27)	Placebo (n = 19)
Partial response	2 (7)	0
No change	11 (41)	4 (21)
Progression	6 (22)	10 (53)
Not evaluable	8 (30)	5 (26)

Source: Adapted with permission from Lipton et al.[18]

to first SRE, multiple event analysis, time to progression of bone lesions, hypercalcemia of malignancy, and overall survival.

Skeletal Complications

Zoledronic acid was significantly more effective than placebo in preventing SREs in the RCC subset. Over 21 months, zoledronic acid significantly reduced the proportion of patients with any SRE by almost 50% (41% versus 79% for placebo; $p = 0.011$).[18] Moreover, zoledronic acid consistently reduced the proportion of patients with each type of SRE (unpublished data, 2002). The most common SREs experienced by patients were pathological fracture and radiation to bone. Zoledronic acid also significantly prolonged the time to first SRE.[18] The median time to first SRE for patients in the placebo group was 72 days from study entry; the time to first SRE was delayed by 352 days in the patients treated with zoledronic acid (median 424 days, $p = 0.007$).[18] The median time to first pathological fracture was also significantly delayed for patients receiving zoledronic acid (median not reached versus 168 days for placebo), and the mean annual incidence of SREs was significantly reduced by approximately 18% (2.58 versus 3.13 events per year for placebo, $p = 0.009$). These results demonstrate the aggressive nature of lytic lesions associated with RCC and the clinical benefit provided by zoledronic acid.

Based on Andersen-Gill multiple event analysis, zoledronic acid significantly reduced the risk of developing SREs for patients with RCC. Compared with patients in the placebo group, patients treated with zoledronic acid had a 58% overall reduction in the risk of SREs throughout the 21-month trial (risk ratio = 0.418; 95% confidence interval = 0.215, 0.812; $p = 0.010$). This risk reduction was greater in the RCC subset compared with a 31% risk reduction in the overall patient population.[18] These results highlight not only the efficacy of zoledronic acid treatments but also the acute impact of RCC on the skeleton.

Bone Lesion Response and Progression

Not only did zoledronic acid prevent SREs, but it also had clinically observable effects on bone lesions in patients with RCC (Table 11h-4).[18] After 21 months of treatment, two

(7%) patients in the RCC subset had partial responses in their bone lesions compared with no patients in the placebo arm. Overall, 41% of patients receiving zoledronic acid had stable disease compared with 21% of patients receiving placebo. This increased incidence of bone lesion response during bisphosphonate therapy is consistent with prior reports in patients with osteolytic lesions from breast cancer where pamidronate was shown to significantly increase bone lesion response rates (34% bone lesion response versus 19% for placebo; $p = 0.002$).[39] Moreover, zoledronic acid significantly extended the time to progression of bone lesions (median 586 days versus 89 days for placebo, $p = 0.014$).[18] This is the first demonstration of a significant delay of bone lesion progression by a bisphosphonate in a randomized, placebo-controlled trial and suggests that zoledronic acid may have antitumor effects in patients with metastatic RCC. A trend toward improved survival was also observed (median survival 347 days versus 218 days for placebo, $p = 0.104$), suggesting that progression of visceral metastases and overall disease progression may also have been delayed in patients treated with zoledronic acid compared with those receiving placebo.

Zoledronic Acid Safety

Despite the potential for cancer-related renal impairment in patients with RCC, zoledronic acid was well tolerated in the RCC subset. The adverse-event profile for patients treated with zoledronic acid was similar to that for patients receiving placebo. Adverse events occurring more frequently in patients treated with zoledronic acid included nausea, fatigue, pyrexia, arthralgia, anorexia, and rigors. These events are consistent with the effects of the acute-phase reaction that is known to occur in some patients following initial bisphosphonate infusion. Acute phase reactions occur in approximately 10–15% of patients receiving bisphosphonates, are typically more common after the first few infusions of bisphosphonates, and rarely occur following subsequent infusions (unpublished data, 2005).

Because many patients with RCC have had a nephrectomy for treatment of their primary cancers, it is necessary to preserve function in the remaining kidney.[40] For this reason, renal function was closely monitored over the course of the trial. Notably, the incidence of renal-related adverse events was similar between patients receiving zoledronic acid and those receiving placebo (22% versus 20% for placebo).[18] The most commonly reported renal adverse events for patients receiving zoledronic acid were hematuria (11%), hyperuricemia (6%), and renal failure (6%).[18] Therefore, at the 4 mg dose, zoledronic acid appears safe for use in most patients with RCC.

Osteonecrosis of the jaw (ONJ) is a complication associated with standard chemotherapy and long-term steroid use. However, several cases of ONJ have been reported in patients who were receiving bisphosphonates.[41–46] Before starting bisphosphonate therapy, patients with concomitant risk factors for ONJ, which include cancer diagnosis, chemotherapy, radiotherapy, or corticosteroid use and comorbid conditions, should have a dental examination. Patients are also advised to avoid invasive dental procedures during bisphosphonate therapy because recovery may be prolonged. Even though the true incidence of osteonecrosis is not known, the condition appears to be rare, and a direct causal relationship between bisphosphonates and ONJ has not been established. No patients with RCC in this subset analysis developed ONJ.

Conclusions

Bone metastases are present in approximately 35% of patients with metastatic RCC and represent a source of significant skeletal morbidity.[4] Lytic bone lesions from RCC are clinically aggressive, and the median survival from time of diagnosis of bone metastases is only 6 months.[3] Most patients with metastatic RCC require radiotherapy to palliate bone pain and more than half experience pathological fractures. Overall, these patients have a high incidence of SREs and an increased risk of developing SREs compared with patients with other primary tumors. Interferon and IL-2, the current standard of care for the treatment of patients with RCC, do not adequately treat bone metastases. Therefore, new treatment options are necessary to reduce the skeletal morbidity associated with metastatic RCC.

Bisphosphonates are the current standard treatment for the clinical management of bone metastases from a variety of solid tumors. In particular, zoledronic acid has demonstrated efficacy in preventing SREs in patients with bone metastases from RCC.[7] Zoledronic acid significantly reduced the incidence of SREs, delayed the time to first SRE and first pathological fracture, and reduced the risk of developing SREs compared with placebo. Zoledronic acid was also shown to significantly delay bone lesion progression in patients with RCC. To date, zoledronic acid is the only bisphosphonate that has been shown to be effective in reducing skeletal complications in patients with RCC.

Patients with RCC appear to be particularly sensitive to the effects of zoledronic acid compared with other tumor types; this may be attributed to the potential antiangiogenic effects of this bisphosphonate. RCC is a highly vascularized tumor, and reducing tumor angiogenesis may inhibit tumor cell growth and proliferation. Preclinical studies have demonstrated that zoledronic acid inhibits testosterone-stimulated vascular regrowth in rat ventral prostate and inhibits tumor angiogenesis in the long bones of mice bearing 5T2 multiple myeloma cells.[47,48] In August 2004, the European Medicines Agency granted orphan drug status to BAY 43-9006 (Bayer Pharmaceuticals Corporation, West Haven, CT, and Onyx Pharmaceuticals, Inc., Richmond, CA) for the treatment of RCC.[49] BAY 43-9006 is a novel Raf kinase and vascular endothelial growth factor receptor inhibitor that specifically inhibits tumor angiogenesis. Another vascular endothelial growth factor receptor inhibitor, PTK787/ZK 222584, has demonstrated antiangiogenic activity in a murine RCC model.[50] Therefore, therapies that target tumor cell angiogenesis may be particularly effective at inhibiting renal cell tumor progression.

Clinical trials are ongoing to investigate the potential role of bisphosphonates in the prevention of bone metastases. Identifying patients at high risk of metastases and early intervention with bisphosphonates may eventually lead to a reduction in metastases and improved survival in these patients. This would be welcome for patients with RCC who have such a poor prognosis and minimal treatment options.

References

1. Parkin DM, Bray F, Ferlay J, Pisani P. Global cancer statistics, 2002. *CA Cancer J Clin* 2005;55:74–108.
2. Ries LAG, Eisner MP, Kosary CL, *et al. SEER Cancer Statistics Review, 1975–2000.* National Cancer Institute, Bethesda, MD. Available at http://seer.cancer.gov/csr/1975_2000. Accessed July 6, 2004.
3. Lipton A. Pathophysiology of bone metastases: How this knowledge may lead to therapeutic intervention. *J Support Oncol* 2004;2:205–213.
4. Zekri J, Ahmed N, Coleman RE, Hancock BW. The skeletal metastatic complications of renal cell carcinoma. *Int J Oncol* 2001;19:379–382.
5. Weinfurt KP, Li Y, Castel LD, *et al.* The significance of skeletal-related events for the health-related quality of life of patients with metastatic prostate cancer. *Ann Oncol* 2005;16:579–584.
6. McDermott DF, Regan MM, Clark JI, *et al.* Randomized phase III trial of high-dose interleukin-2 versus subcutaneous interleukin-2 and interferon in patients with metastatic renal cell carcinoma. *J Clin Oncol* 2005;23:133–141.
7. Lipton A, Zheng M, Seaman J. Zoledronic acid delays the onset of skeletal-related events and progression of skeletal disease in patients with advanced renal cell carcinoma. *Cancer* 2003;98:962–969.
8. Rogers MJ, Gordon S, Benford HL, *et al.* Cellular and molecular mechanisms of action of bisphosphonates. *Cancer* 2000;88(Suppl):2961–2978.
9. Van Beek ER, Lowik CW, Papapoulos SE. Bisphosphonates suppress bone resorption by a direct effect on early osteoclast precursors without affecting the osteoclastogenic capacity of osteogenic cells: the role of protein geranylgeranylation in

the action of nitrogen-containing bisphosphonates on osteoclast precursors. *Bone* 2002;30:64–70.

10. Clohisy DR, O'Keefe PF, Ramnaraine ML. Pamidronate decreases tumor-induced osteoclastogenesis in osteopetrotic mice. *J Orthop Res* 2001;19:554–558.

11. Corey E, Brown LG, Quinn JE, *et al*. Zoledronic acid exhibits inhibitory effects on osteoblastic and osteolytic metastases of prostate cancer. *Clin Cancer Res* 2003;9:295–306. Erratum: *Clin Cancer Res* 2003;9:1574–1575.

12. Green J, Gschaidmeier H, Yoneda T, Mundy G. Zoledronic acid potently inhibits tumour-induced osteolysis in two models of breast cancer metastasis to bone [abstract]. *Ann Oncol* 2000;11(Suppl 4):14 (abstract 50P).

13. Roodman GD. Mechanisms of bone metastasis. *N Engl J Med* 2004;350:1655–1664.

14. Coleman RE. Skeletal complications of malignancy. *Cancer* 1997;80(Suppl):1588–1594.

15. Guise TA, Mundy GR. Cancer and bone. *Endocr Rev* 1998;19:18–54.

16. Orr FW, Lee J, Duivenvoorden WC, Singh G. Pathophysiologic interactions in skeletal metastasis. *Cancer* 2000;88(Suppl):2912–2918.

17. Sanchez-Sweatman OH, Lee J, Orr FW, Singh G. Direct osteolysis induced by metastatic murine melanoma cells: role of matrix metalloproteinases. *Eur J Cancer* 1997;33:918–925.

18. Lipton A, Seaman J, Zheng M. Efficacy and safety of zoledronic acid in patients with bone metastases from renal cell carcinoma. Presented at What Is New in Bisphosphonates? Seventh Workshop on Bisphosphonates—From the Laboratory to the Patient; March 24–26, 2004; Davos, Switzerland. Poster 28.

19. Rosen LS, Gordon D, Tchekmedyian NS, *et al*. Long-term efficacy and safety of zoledronic acid in the treatment of skeletal metastases in patients with nonsmall cell lung carcinoma and other solid tumors: a randomized, phase III, double-blind, placebo-controlled trial. *Cancer* 2004;100:2613–2621.

20. Saad F, Gleason DM, Murray R, *et al*. Long-term efficacy of zoledronic acid for the prevention of skeletal complications in patients with metastatic hormone-refractory prostate cancer. *J Natl Cancer Inst* 2004;96:879–882.

21. Fourneau I, Broos P. Pathologic fractures due to metastatic disease. A retrospective study of 160 surgically treated fractures. *Acta Chir Belg* 1998;98:255–260.

22. Van der Klift M, De Laet CE, McCloskey EV, Hofman A, Pols HA. The incidence of vertebral fractures in men and women: the Rotterdam Study. *J Bone Miner Res* 2002; 17: 1051–1056.

23. Sabino MAC, Mantyh PW. Pathophysiology of bone cancer pain. *J Support Oncol* 2005;3:15–24.

24. Coleman RE. Metastatic bone disease: clinical features, pathophysiology and treatment strategies. *Cancer Treat Rev* 2001;27:165–176.

25. Woolf CJ, Salter MW. Neuronal plasticity: increasing the gain in pain. *Science* 2000;288:1765–1769.

26. Hoegler D. Radiotherapy for palliation of symptoms in incurable cancer. *Curr Probl Cancer* 1997;21:129–183.

27. McKiernan JM , Delea TE, Liss M, *et al*. Impact of skeletal complications on total medical care costs in prostate cancer patients with bone metastases [abstract]. *Proc Am Soc Clin Oncol* 2004;23:531 (abstract 6057).

28. Delea T, McKiernan J, Liss M, *et al*. Effects of skeletal complications on total medical care costs in women with bone metastases of breast cancer [abstract]. *Bone* 2004;34:S86 (abstract 68).

29. Delea T, McKiernan J, Liss M, *et al*. Cost of skeletal complications in patients with multiple myeloma [abstract]. Presented at the IXth Annual International Workshop on Multiple Myeloma, May 23–27, 2003, Salamanca, Spain.

30. Michaelson MD, Rosenthal DI, Smith MR. Long-term bisphosphonate treatment of bone metastases from renal cell carcinoma. *J Clin Oncol* 2004;22:4233–4234.

31. Luckman SP, Hughes DE, Coxon FP, Graham R, Russell G, Rogers MJ. Nitrogen-containing bisphosphonates inhibit the mevalonate pathway and prevent post-translational prenylation of GTP-binding proteins, including Ras. *J Bone Miner Res* 1998;13:581–589.

32. Aparicio A, Gardner A, Tu Y, Savage A, Berenson J, Lichtenstein A. In vitro cytoreductive effects on multiple myeloma cells induced by bisphosphonates. *Leukemia* 1998;12:220–229.

33. Senaratne SG, Pirianov G, Mansi JL, Arnett TR, Colston KW. Bisphosphonates induce apoptosis in human breast cancer cell lines. *Br J Cancer* 2000;82:1459–1468.

34. Lee MV, Fong EM, Singer FR, Guenette RS. Bisphosphonate treatment inhibits the growth of prostate cancer cells. *Cancer Res* 2001;61:2602–2608.

35. Boissier S, Ferreras M, Peyruchaud O, *et al*. Bisphosphonates inhibit breast and prostate carcinoma cell invasion, an early event in the formation of bone metastases. *Cancer Res* 2000;60:2949–2954.

36. Rosen LS, Gordon D, Kaminski M, *et al*. Long-term efficacy and safety of zoledronic acid compared with pamidronate disodium in the treatment of skeletal complications in patients with advanced multiple myeloma or breast carcinoma: a randomized, double-blind, multicenter, comparative trial. *Cancer* 2003;98:1735–1744.

37. Ali SM, Esteva FJ, Hortobagyi G, *et al*. Safety and efficacy of bisphosphonates beyond 24 months in cancer patients. *J Clin Oncol* 2001;19:3434–3437.

38. Yuasa T, Nogawa M, Kimura S, *et al*. A third-generation bisphosphonate, minodronic acid (YM529), augments the interferon alpha/beta-mediated inhibition of renal cell cancer cell growth both in vitro and in vivo. *Clin Cancer Res* 2005;11:853–859.

39. Hortobagyi GN, Theriault RL, Lipton A, *et al*. Long-term prevention of skeletal complications of metastatic breast cancer with pamidronate. *J Clin Oncol* 1998;16:2038–2044.

40. Lipton A, Colombo-Berra A, Bukowski RM, Rosen L, Zheng M, Urbanowitz G. Skeletal complications in patients with bone metastases from renal cell carcinoma and therapeutic benefits of zoledronic acid. *Clin Cancer Res* 2004;10(Suppl): 6397S–6403S.

41. Marx RE. Pamidronate (Aredia) and zoledronate (Zometa) induced avascular necrosis of the jaws: a growing epidemic. *J Oral Maxillofac Surg* 2003;61:1115–1117.

42. Wang J, Goodger NM, Pogrel MA. Osteonecrosis of the jaws associated with cancer chemotherapy. *J Oral Maxillofac Surg* 2003;61:1104–1107.

43. Pogrel MA. Bisphosphonates and bone necrosis. *J Oral Maxillofac Surg* 2004;62:391–392.

44. Migliorati CA. Bisphosphonates and oral cavity avascular bone necrosis. *J Clin Oncol* 2003;21:4253–4254.

45. Carter GD, Goss AN. Bisphosphonates and avascular necrosis of the jaws. *Aust Dent J* 2003;48:268.

46. Ruggiero SL, Mehrotra B, Rosenberg TJ, Engroff SL. Osteonecrosis of the jaws associated with the use of bisphosphonates: a review of 63 cases. *J Oral Maxillofac Surg* 2004;62:527–534.

47. Fournier P, Boissier S, Filleur S, *et al*. Bisphosphonates inhibit angiogenesis in vitro and testosterone-stimulated vascular regrowth in the ventral prostate in castrated rats. *Cancer Res* 2002;62:6538–6544.

48. Croucher PI, De Raeve H, Perry MJ, *et al*. Zoledronic acid treatment of 5T2MM-bearing mice inhibits the development of myeloma bone disease: evidence for decreased osteolysis, tumor burden and angiogenesis, and increased survival. *J Bone Miner Res* 2003;18:482–492.

49. 04 August 2004—-EMEA grants orphan drug designation of BAY 43–9006 for the treatment of renal cell carcinoma. Press release: Bayer Pharmaceuticals Corporation, West Haven, CT, and Onyx Pharmaceuticals, Inc., Richmond, CA.

50. Drevs J, Müller-Driver R, Wittig C, *et al*. PTK787/ZK 222584, a specific vascular endothelial growth factor-receptor tyrosine kinase inhibitor, affects the anatomy of the tumor vascular bed and the functional vascular properties as detected by dynamic enhanced magnetic resonance imaging. *Cancer Res* 2002;62:4015–4022.

11i
Therapeutic Counseling for the Medical Management of Renal Cell Carcinoma

Brant A. Inman and Bradley C. Leibovich

Introduction

This chapter will attempt to review the various nonsurgical therapies for renal cell carcinoma (RCC) from the perspective of the particular patient and the treating physician. We will consider two main settings of medical therapy: (1) adjuvant therapy for the high-risk postnephrectomy patient and (2) salvage therapy for the patient with metastatic RCC. The overriding goal will be to provide a practical framework for the responsible management of patients with aggressive RCCs.

To better understand our approach to patient management and to accurately interpret the results of the clinical trials that we will be citing, we feel that three brief detours are required. The first detour deals with treatment outcomes: What is it we are trying to achieve? The second deals with prognostication: How do we predict who is going to do poorly? The last deals with genetic testing: Who should we test for hereditary RCC? The answers to these three questions will form the foundation of our discussion of therapeutic counseling.

Endpoints in Oncology

Understanding therapeutic endpoints is critical to the management of patients with advanced cancer. Endpoints are used pervasively in oncology—from clinical trials to patient decision making—and their interpretation can be a source of confusion and discordance for both patients and physicians alike. For the purpose of this review, a therapeutic endpoint is defined as a target result that is sought by either the patient or physician during the management of the patient's cancer. Some of the more important endpoints used in assessing the treatment of advanced RCC patients are discussed below.

Response Rate

A reduction in tumor size has been used as a surrogate marker for treatment efficacy for a very long time. The rationale is simple: if a malignant tumor is getting larger it is likely unresponsive to the active treatment regimen and if it is shrinking it is likely responding to treatment. Mathematical modeling of tumor response to treatment began in the late 1950s and continued into the 1960s in an attempt to more accurately describe the response of a tumor to treatment.[1,2] Shortly thereafter physicians started asking the critical question: What is an objective tumor response? After many years of individual effort and differing opinion, in 1979 the World Health Organization (WHO) formally introduced a tumor response classification system as an outgrowth of numerous similar systems that were being developed in a variety of solid tumors.[3,4] The original WHO system had four response categories: (1) *complete response*—indicating the disappearance of all known disease, (2) *partial response*—indicating a decrease in tumor burden of 50% or more, (3) *progressive disease*—indicating an increase in tumor burden of 25% or more, and (4) *no change (also known as stable disease)*—indicating a tumor burden that has not decreased by $\geq 50\%$ or increased by $\geq 25\%$. These criteria were meant to be applied to both measurable and nonmeasurable disease and were considered rough estimates given the recognized possibility of measurement error.[5] Response rates are usually an endpoint in Phase II clinical trials.

Numerous problems have been noted by trialists attempting to apply the original WHO criteria to modern clinical trials. The minimum number of tumor lesions that need to be recorded is unclear. Whether or not growth in a solitary tumor should constitute progressive disease when other tumor sites are stable is unknown. The relevance of three-dimensional tumor volume measurements is unclear (the original WHO categories relied on unidimensional or bidimensional measurement).[6] And perhaps the most relevant point for our discussion on RCC is that new molecular therapeutics may provide a survival benefit without resulting in tumor shrinkage.[7] An attempt to reconcile these and other problems has led to a report from a new multinational consensus group—the Response Evaluation Criteria in Solid Tumors (RECIST) group—on the appropriate evaluation of tumor response to treatment.[8] In this report, *target lesions* have been defined as all measurable tumor sites, up to a maximum of 5 tumors per organ or a maximum of 10 total lesions. If more than 10 lesions are present, the lesions that have the longest unidimensional diameter should be included as the target lesions. A partial response has been redefined as a ≥30% reduction in the sum of the longest dimension of all the target lesions and progression has been redefined as a ≥20% increase in this same measurement. To reduce the possibility of overoptimism in response rate reporting, the RECIST group has maintained the WHO suggestion that all complete and partial responses must be confirmed by a repeated assessment of target lesion sizes after a period of at least 4 weeks. Other important details regarding the assessment of tumor response are outlined in this report but are beyond the scope of this chapter.

Whether or not tumor shrinkage is correlated with cancer-specific survival is a matter of great controversy. This issue is of some practical importance because the treatment response rates observed in uncontrolled Phase II clinical trials will often dictate whether or not the new treatment regimen is explored in a larger controlled Phase III clinical trial. Recent evidence from the lung cancer literature suggests that Phase II response rates do not necessarily correlate with Phase III median survival estimates.[9] Numerous authors have cautioned about these types of comparisons, however, because analysis of survival by tumor response can produce extremely biased and misleading results.[10–12] Two major errors have been noted in these comparisons. First, the usual statistical methods used for detecting a difference in survival between two groups are incorrect when applied to responders and nonresponders. This is because guarantee time bias causes falsely favorable survival curves for the responder group and falsely unfavorable survival curves for the nonresponders, particularly if many patients die early in the follow-up protocol. Better techniques would include the Mantel–Byar and landmark methods.[13,14] Second, longer survival in the responders is misinterpreted as evidence that tumor response equates to prolonged survival or, even worse, that the treatment is effective. The response of a set of patients to a given treatment regimen may simply be a marker for patients with good prognosis tumors. In other words, it is a self-fulfilling prophesy that patients who respond to a treatment will survive longer than those who do not.[14] A dramatic example of this problem was developed by Nathan Mantel who showed that responders outlive nonresponders even for a treatment that worsens survival.[12] The best way to know with certainty whether a treatment regimen prolongs survival is the randomized controlled trial.

Duration of Response

In the original WHO guidelines, the duration of a complete response was defined as the period of time from the first recording of the complete response to the first recording of progressive disease and the duration of a partial response (also known as overall response duration) was defined as the period of time from the first treatment date to the first recording of disease progression.[4] The RECIST group maintained the definition for complete response duration but redefined the overall response duration as the time period from the first demonstration of a partial response to the first demonstration of progressive disease.[8] They also defined the duration of stable disease as the period of time from the first treatment date to the first recording of progressive disease (i.e., the original WHO overall response definition). The duration of stable disease is similar to the progression-free survival time that is discussed below. It is important to note that all these time periods will depend on the time interval between assessments of disease response. Studies that assess outcomes frequently may find somewhat shorter durations of response than studies that assess outcomes infrequently.

Progression-Free Survival

Progression-free survival was not defined in the original WHO publication but has recently become a measurement of major importance in clinical trials. Noncytoreductive anticancer agents—which includes various antiangiogenic and immunotherapeutic agents used in the treatment of RCC—may result in improved survival without shrinking the target tumor lesions.[15] Response rates would therefore be inappropriate surrogate endpoints for these agents and the duration of time from treatment initiation until disease progression or disease-related death (i.e., progression-free survival time) would be a better measure of treatment efficacy. The use of progression-free survival as an endpoint in uncontrolled trials should be done cautiously as there is no comparison group for judging treatment efficacy. It is recommended that the progression-free survival time of a comparable group of untreated patients be estimated prior to starting an uncontrolled clinical trial of a new treatment regimen in order to reduce the chance of overoptimism.[8] This being said, a new multinomial stopping rule that uses progression-free survival for uncontrolled Phase II trials appears to be more efficient than the traditional Fleming or Gehan stopping rules.[16] Potential benefits to the patient resulting from this new multinomial stopping rule include minimizing exposure to potentially toxic drugs and a decreased likelihood of falsely rejecting an active drug.

Recurrence-Free Survival

This endpoint is applicable to those patients who are rendered disease free by some primary intervention and then followed or treated with an adjuvant treatment regimen. Recurrence-free survival (RFS, also known as disease-free survival) is defined as the period of time that a patient is alive and free of disease following a primary treatment regimen.[17] Patients who die of causes other than the cancer in question are usually, but not always, censored. In competing risks survival analysis, for instance, competing outcomes are not censored. It has been shown in colorectal cancer that RFS is perhaps the endpoint most sensitive to a treatment effect while still accounting for any imbalance in adverse event-related deaths.[18] The Food and Drug Administration (FDA) has recently approved the use of several chemotherapy drugs based on the 3-year RFS data from Phase III randomized trials.

Median Survival

Median survival is a more stringent measure of treatment efficacy than response rates and relatively few chemotherapy clinical trials are able to demonstrate statistically significant differences across treatment arms in this parameter.[19] This is because median survival estimates have an important relationship to the treatment response rate. The treatment response rate is an important determinant of survival for most (but not all) chemotherapeutic agents and if it falls to levels less than 50%, the median survival measured in the treatment arm will principally reflect the survival outcomes of the nonresponding patients.[19] It is therefore unusual that the median survival rates will be different across treatment arms if the treatment response rate is less than 50%, even if the response rates between the groups are statistically significantly different. It is possible to have a difference in median survival but no difference in 5-year survival if the treatment regimen only delays an inevitable cancer death.

Survival at 5 and 10 Years

This is the gold standard criterion for cancer treatment assessment and all the endpoints previously discussed should be considered surrogate endpoints of this measure. Two forms of this endpoint exist: (1) *cancer-specific survival* (also known as disease-specific survival) where only patients who die from the cancer at study are considered failures and (2) *overall survival* where all patients who die are considered failures. When the cancer treatment is safe and the chances of dying from competing causes is high, as in prostate cancer, cancer-specific survival is the best endpoint to measure. Contrarily, when the disease process is highly lethal or when treatment-related mortality is significant, overall survival is an equally important endpoint. A cancer treatment regimen is potentially efficacious if there is a cancer-specific survival advantage for the treated patient population. However, if the treatment is very toxic and many treatment-related deaths occur, the 5-year cancer-specific survival advantage will occur in the absence of a 5-year overall survival advantage. In this case efficacy will have been lost.

The importance of measuring survival endpoints should be emphasized. Although surrogate endpoints may allow a reduction in sample size or a reduction in trial duration—both of which improve clinical trial efficiency and are primarily financial benefits—there are many examples where misleading results have been obtained because of undo reliance on surrogate endpoints in clinical trials.[20] Fleming and DeMets first wrote "a correlate does not a surrogate make."[20] Yet, despite the publication of formal criteria for validating surrogate endpoints, few have undergone the rigorous evaluation proposed.[21] For this reason, survival endpoints should be obtained by cancer investigators whenever possible.

Quality of Life

Quality of life is becoming an increasingly important endpoint for cancer clinical trials.[22, 23] It has been realized that a chemotherapy regimen that improves symptoms and reduces suffering may provide clinical benefit to patients even if they do not survive any longer.[24, 25] New methodologies are being developed to better assess the impact of cancer treatment on the quality of life of both curable and incurable patients. One such methodology is the *quality-adjusted time without symptoms of disease and toxicity of treatment* (Q-TWIST). The Q-TWIST methodology has made survival analyses possible while considering the impact of treatment (or lack thereof) on the quality of life.[26, 27]

One interesting observation that has recently been made is that quality of life may be a surrogate marker for the efficacy of immunotherapy. In a German study of 22 patients receiving either interleukin (IL)-2 or interferon (IFN)-α_{2A} for progressive metastatic RCC, a rapid decrease in quality of life (as measured by the EORTC QLQ-C30 questionnaire) was associated with improved therapeutic efficacy of the treatment regimen.[28] We are unaware of any independent confirmation of this observation.

Despite the undeniable importance of quality of life as a cancer treatment outcome, one important point warrants emphasis: most patients with cancer, especially if they are young, report that they would accept an intensive treatment regimen associated with considerable side-effects and elevated risk even if there was a very small (i.e., <5%) chance of cure.[29, 30]

Predicting Oncological Outcomes

Prognosis is evidently of paramount importance to the cancer patient. An accurate prediction of a cancer patient's future outcome can be tremendously useful. Decisions regarding adjuvant therapy, disease monitoring, and possible enrollment in clinical trials all hinge on prognosis. Patients who are predicted to do well after standard therapy would likely not receive an adjuvant treatment and would be screened less often for recurrence. On the other hand, patients predicted to do poorly would likely receive adjuvant therapy (if an effective adjuvant therapy existed for the cancer in question) and would be followed much more closely for recurrent cancer. This approach is called risk-directed therapy.

Clinical Survival Prediction

Historically, the physician's main preoccupation was to arrive at a diagnosis and institute a treatment, if one existed. The modern physician has added a new skill to his repertoire: the prediction of patient outcome. In the case of cancer patients, these predictions are not always very good. For example, when physicians attempt to predict the survival of terminally ill cancer patients (median survival of 4 weeks), they are correct within 1 week in only 25% of cases.[31] In the majority of studies that have assessed this issue, the major problem appears to be overestimation of the anticipated survival time.[32,33] Despite its inaccuracy, a physician's "best guess" has been shown in multiple studies to be superior to any other single general predictor of survival (such as performance status, cachexia, symptoms, and laboratory tests).[34,35]

Survival Prediction in Advanced Cancer Patients

The physician's clinical survival prediction can be markedly improved by considering some of the other information that is routinely available in the patient's chart. Items that are commonly associated with a worsened cancer-specific survival are poor performance status, anorexia or weight loss, dyspnea or dysphagia, edema, delirium, high leukocyte or low lymphocyte counts, elevated platelet counts, low serum albumin, and elevated serum lactate dehydrogenase (LDH) levels. Several groups have developed simplified prognostic tools for advanced cancer patients and two of these, the *palliative prognostic score* and the *palliative prognostic index*, have generated the most interest.[36–38] Both use a combination of laboratory tests and clinical assessment to arrive at their score, but only the *palliative prognostic score* incorporates the survival prediction of the clinician into its algorithm. The positive and negative predictive values for the *palliative prognostic index* prediction of 6-week survival were shown by one group to be 0.89 and 0.60, respectively, although this is clearly dependent on the population of palliative patients at study.[35] The authors of this study noted that after they had used the index for a brief while, the positive and negative predictive values for their own predictions of 6-week survival were superior to the index at 0.90 and 0.67, respectively![35] The take-home message is that mathematical tools are not always more accurate than the clinical judgment of an informed and experienced physician.

Survival Prediction in Renal Cell Carcinoma

There were many early attempts to define prognostic factors for RCC. One of the earliest comprehensive prognostic tools was presented by Störkel et al. in 1989.[39] Since that time,

numerous prognostic tools have been developed for specifically predicting the outcomes of patients with RCC.[?,40–43,45–50] We have outlined the principal features of selected prognostic tools in Table 11i-1. Upon examining this table it should be immediately clear that there is no RCC prediction tool that is perfect for every situation. Each prediction tool is distinct by virtue of the patient population that it is targeting and the outcome it is meant to predict. Other important factors that cause differences in the various prognostic tools are (1) the characteristics of the referral patient population of the institution that developed the tool, (2) the number of patients studied, (3) the variables that were evaluated in the statistical modeling phase (i.e., not all centers collect and analyze the same clinicopathological variables), and (4) the statistical methodology used to derive the tool.

External validation studies have been carried out for only a few of the RCC prognostic tools. For metastatic cases, the Motzer score has been shown to be of prognostic value in an independent patient population, though several other predictors of survival independent of the Motzer score were identified.[52] The Störkel score and the UCLA Integrated Staging System (UISS) have also been validated in independent patient cohorts.[53,54] However, it should be noted that a European multiinstitutional comparative study of nonmetastatic prognostic tools showed the Kattan nomogram to be superior to the UISS, the residual renal function (RRF) score, and the Johns Hopkins score.[55] The SSIGN score was not examined in this study because tumor necrosis was not assessed in many patients in the study. Given that tumor necrosis has been demonstrated to be of prognostic importance in several different patient populations,[46,56,57] one wonders if the results would have been different if necrosis had been routinely assessed and the SSIGN score included. It is clear that a large multiinstitutional collaboration is needed to independently assess the performance of the various prognostic tools and variables in order to identify a prognostic tool for each important clinical setting that will be the international staging standard. These efforts are already underway.

Genetic Testing for Hereditary Renal Cell Carcinoma

RCC can be sporadic or inherited. The management of inherited RCC is usually quite different than the sporadic forms because multifocality, bilaterality, and recurrence are more common and because a targeted approach to therapy can be used.[58,59] Patients presenting with a strong family history of kidney cancer, with tumors at a young age, with multiple synchronous or metachronous tumors, or with other phenotypic characteristics of an inherited RCC syndrome should undergo genetic screening.[60] Table 11i-2 shows the key clinical features of the genetic syndromes that are currently recognized to be associated with renal tumors. Testing for von Hippel–Lindau (vHL) mutations, *MET* mutations, and chromosomal translocations is available. Familial linkage analysis for chromosome 1q is also possible if many family members are affected. The input of an expert medical geneticist is essential for these syndromes.

Adjuvant Therapy for High-Risk Postnephrectomy Renal Cell Carcinoma

To address the issue of postnephrectomy adjuvant therapy we need to know who is at risk of progression, what we will do to reduce the chance of recurrence, and how we will monitor these patients for recurrence.

Who Is at High Risk for Postnephrectomy Recurrence and Death?

The majority of patients with RCC who are treated with nephrectomy will be cured. This contemporary reality is a result of the fact that most patients—roughly 70% in the Mayo Clinic series—present with localized renal masses (≤pT2) that are usually easily removed.[61] The remaining 30% of patients are not so lucky. These patients present with more aggressive tumors that demonstrate extrarenal tumor extension, adrenal gland invasion, tumor thrombi, or regional lymph node involvement.[61–63] Not all of these patients develop metastases and die, however. Identifying those who will is the first step to risk-stratified treatment of RCC.

This is where the prognostic tools discussed in the previous section become important. These tools can help to distinguish patients who are truly at increased risk of metastases and death from those who are not.[42–46] Table 11i–1 shows that the most important postoperative prognostic factors for tumor progression or death are increasing pathological tumor stage, increasing tumor size, regional lymph node involvement, clear cell subtype, and increasing nuclear grade. If the tumor was of clear cell histology, both the Mayo[44] and the Memorial Sloan-Kettering Cancer Center (MSKCC)[46] predictive tools for RCC RFS would be appropriate because we are interested in the risk of both metastases and survival. If the tumor was of papillary or chromophobe histology, the UISS[42] and MSKCC[45] prognostic tools for RCC survival could be used. The downside of these two instruments is that they are not designed to specifically predict survival for these two histological RCC types or the development of metastases. The only indications for using the preoperative prognostic tools proposed by Cindolo et al.[40] or Yaycioglu et al.[41] would be the rare cases of RCC that are treated by radiofrequency ablation, cryotherapy, or laparoscopically with tissue morcellation. We do not recommend routine laparoscopic renal tumor morcellation because of the possibility of tumor spillage,[64,65] the loss of valuable pathological information,[66] and the fact that it does little to reduce postoperative symptoms.[67]

None of the tools in Table 11i–1 are designed specifically to predict the occurrence of a local recurrence and, to our knowledge, no such prognostic tool exists. The risk of a local recurrence increases with increasing size and stage of the primary renal tumor, the presence of bilaterality and multifocality, the presence of regional lymph node or systemic metastases, the method used to treat the primary tumor, and the presence of genetic syndrome-associated RCC. Following radical nephrectomy, isolated renal fossa recurrences occur in roughly 1% of initially nonmetastatic patients. A much higher proportion of patients undergoing cytoreductive nephrectomy for metastatic RCC will develop fossa recurrences (up to 50%).[68,69] The general consensus seems to be that complete surgical resection of the fossa recurrence is the best treatment for the patient when technically possible.[68,70] The 1-year RFS rate for surgically resected renal fossa recurrences is only 50–65%, which is explained by the high incidence of concomitant systemic metastases.[68,70] Whether immunotherapy or radiotherapy is of benefit in this situation is controversial, but most series have not shown a major benefit.[68,70–73] The local recurrence rate for partial nephrectomy is approximately 3%, with the exception of patients with vHL disease who will recur in over 80% of cases.[74] The majority of patients with post-partial nephrectomy local recurrences can be cured with repeat nephrectomy (either partial or radical).

Does an Effective Postnephrectomy Adjuvant Therapy for Renal Cell Carcinoma Exist?

The previous chapters in this book have examined in detail the mechanisms and evidence supporting the various medical therapies for RCC. Here we present the key data concerning the efficacy of these agents as adjuvant therapy.

Radiation

A few small retrospective studies have suggested that radiation therapy may be an effective adjuvant treatment for patients with locally advanced RCC.[73,75–77] This is not the general consensus, however.[78] A Finnish randomized controlled trial of 33 Gy of radiation prior to nephrectomy did not show any advantage for the radiation arm.[79] Similarly, a Danish randomized controlled trial showed that 50 Gy of adjuvant radiation therapy is not effective in preventing cancer recurrence in high-risk RCC patients.[80] This trial also showed a 44% major complication rate in the radiotherapy-treated patients and nearly 20% of these complications contributed directly to patient death. Other groups have also reported toxicity, carcinogenicity, and a lack of efficacy for renal radiation.[81,82] Modern radiotherapy, with its higher doses and possible lower toxicity, may theoretically give better results than these, but this remains to be proven. There is one recent study that has suggested some efficacy of radiotherapy as a primary treatment for patients who were not surgical candidates but its patient numbers are small and its efficacy modest.[83]

TABLE 11i-1. Contemporary survival prediction tools for renal cell carcinoma.[a]

Source of prognostic tool	Preoperative		Postoperative								Metastatic		
	Europe[40]	Johns Hopkins	Mainz[42]	UCLA[42]	Mayo[43]	Mayo[44]	MSKCC[45]	MSKCC[46]	Mayo[47]	MSKCC[48]	MSKCC[49]	UCLA[50]	Germany[51]
Commonly used name	RRF score	–	Störkel score	UISS	SSIGN score	–	Kattan nomogram	–	–	Motzer score	–	SANI score	–
Type of tool	Score	Score	Score	Categories	Score	Score	Nomogram	Nomogram	Score	Score	Score	Score	Score
Number of patients studied	660	296	431	477	1801	1671	612	701	727	670	251	173	425
Target population	All RCC + nephrec. + unilateral + N0 + M0	All RCC + nephrec. + unilateral + N0 + M0 + IVC (–)	All RCC + nephrec.	All RCC + nephrec.	ccRCC + nephrec. + unilateral	ccRCC + nephrec. + unilateral + M0 + M0	All RCC + nephrec. + unilateral + N0 + M0	ccRCC + nephrec. + unilateral + N0	All RCC + nephrec.	All RCC	All RCC + failed immunoTx	All RCC + nephrec. + IL-2	All RCC + first line immunoTx
Outcome predicted	RFS	RFS	OS	OS	CSS	RFS	RFS	RFS	CSS	OS	OS	CSS	OS
Predictive accuracy (internal validation)	–	–	0.80	–	0.84	0.82	0.74	–	0.67	–	–	–	–
Predictive accuracy (external validation)	0.62[55]	0.59[55]	–	0.68[55]	–	–	0.71[55]	0.82[46]	–	–	–	–	–
Primary tumor variables													
TNM or Robson stage			X	X	X	X	X	X					
Lymph nodes					X	X					X	X	
Fuhrman or Thoenes grade			X	X	X	X		X	X				
Necrosis					X	X		X	X				
Size	X	X			X	X	X	X					
Histological subtype		X	X				X						
Sarcomatoid features												X	
Tumor thrombus									X				
Vascular invasion								X					
Growth form	X		X										

Variable	1	2	3	4	5	6	7	8	9	10
Metastasis variables										
Presence of metastases							X	X		
Bone metastases		X			X					
Liver metastases	X	X			X					
Multiple metastases	X	X			X					
Nephrectomy metastases time	X				X					
Complete metastasis resection					X					
Patient variables										
Age									X	
Performance status			X	X				X		
Symptoms					X	X				X
Lactate dehydrogenase	X			X						X
Calcium			X	X						
Hemoglobin			X	X						
Neutrophil count	X									
C-reactive protein	X									
TSH		X		X						
Nephrectomy status										

[a]RFS, recurrence-free survival; CSS, cancer-specific survival; OS, overall survival; RCC, renal cell carcinoma; ccRCC, clear cell renal cell carcinoma; nephrec., nephrectomy; IL-2, interleukin 2; immunoTx, first line immunotherapy; TSH, thyroid-stimulating hormone.

TABLE 11i-2. Hereditary renal cell carcinoma syndromes.[a]

Syndrome	Genetic problem	Renal tumors	Other clinical features
vHL disease[184,185]	vHL gene dysfunction (3p25) Type 1 vHL Loss of function mutations Pheochromocytoma rare	ccRCC (multiple, bilateral)	Tumors Cerebellar/spinal hemangioblastoma Epididymal/broad ligament cystadenoma Endolymphatic sac tumor Pancreatic endocrine tumors Pheochromocytoma Retinal hemangioma Cysts Epididymis Kidney Pancreas
	Type 2 vHL Missense mutations Pheochromocytoma common		
Familial clear cell RCC syndrome with chromosome 3 translocation[60,186,187]	Chromosome 3 translocations t(3;8)(p14:q24) t(3;6)(p13:q25.1) t(3;6)(q12:q15) t(3;4)(p13:p16) t(2;3)(q35:q21) t(2;3)(q33:q21) t(2;3)(q33:q21) t(1;3)(q32:q13.3)	ccRCC (multiple, bilateral)	Bladder cancer Gastric cancer Pancreatic cancer Thyroid cancer (FHIT translocations)

Familial clear cell RCC syndrome[188,189]	?	ccRCC (solitary)	
Hereditary papillary RCC[190-192]	c-MET protooncogene mutation (7q31-34); Trisomy 7 is common	pRCC Type 1 (hundreds)	Biliary tract cancer; Bladder cancer; Breast cancer; Lung cancer; Malignant melanoma; Pancreatic cancer; Stomach cancer
Hereditary leiomyomatosis and RCC[193,194]	Fumarate hydrogenase mutations (1q42.3-43)	pRCC Type 2 (solitary, aggressive); cdRCC; Oncocytoma	Bladder cancer; Breast cancer; Leiomyomas (cutaneous, uterine)
Familial papillary thyroid-papillary renal carcinoma[195]	1q21	pRCC Type 1; Oncocytoma	Papillary carcinoma of the thyroid
Birt-Hogg-Dubé syndrome[196-198]	17p12-q11.2	Oncocytic RCC; Oncocytoma; Chromophobe RCC	Skin tumors; Acrochordoma; Fibro folliculoma; Trichodiscoma; Other lesions; Colon cancer; Lung disease (bronchiectasis, cysts, pneumothorax); Renal cysts
Familial oncocytoma[199,200]	?	Oncocytoma	Renal cysts
Familial renal hamartomas associated with hyperparathyroidism-jaw tumor[201,202]	1q21-q23	pRCC Type 1; Adult Wilms' tumor; Renal hamartoma	Hyperparathyroidism (adenoma or carcinoma); Ossifying fibroma of the jaw; Renal cysts

[a]VHL, von Hippel-Lindau; RCC, renal cell carcinoma; ccRCC, clear cell renal cell carcinoma; pRCC, papillary renal cell carcinoma; cdRCC, collecting duct renal cell carcinoma.

Medroxyprogesterone Acetate

Medroxyprogesterone acetate has been used in the treatment of RCC for decades.[84] The treatment was an outgrowth of initial experiments in hamsters that suggested that hormonotherapy could induce regression of renal cortical tumors.[85] Retrospective studies have shown mixed results as to the potential benefit of adjuvant medroxyprogesterone acetate for nonmetastatic cases of RCC.[86,87] To our knowledge, the only randomized trial to test this agent in the adjuvant setting is an Italian study conducted in the early 1980s.[88] This trial enrolled 120 postnephrectomy patients with nonmetastatic disease and randomized them to 500 mg of medroxyprogesterone acetate per day or observation. After 5 years of follow-up, medroxyprogesterone acetate did not produce a survival advantage for any patient subgroup. The presence of steroid receptors on the renal tumors appeared to be associated with an decreased relapse rate in the treated group (29% vs. 42%), but this was not statistically significant. The majority of the patients treated with medroxyprogesterone acetate in this trial experienced side effects including loss of libido (42% of men), a >10 kg weight gain (22%), hypertension (10%), hirsuitism (5% of women), and amenorrhea (5% of women).

Bacillus Calmette-Guérin and Tumor Cells

Bacillus Calmette-Guérin (BCG) can be mixed with tumor cells to create an active tumor-specific immunotherapy.[89] An Italian randomized controlled trial evaluated this type of immunotherapy as an adjuvant treatment to radical nephrectomy in patients with nonmetastatic RCC.[90] No serious toxicity or improvement in survival was observed in patients treated with this vaccine. Other groups have confirmed that tumor vaccines can be safely administered in the adjuvant setting but that they do not improve survival.[91]

Interleukin-2

IL-2 has been tested as adjuvant monotherapy in one randomized controlled trial. This trial, published by the Cytokine Working Group, randomized 69 high-risk RCC patients who had undergone complete resection of their disease to high-dose IL-2 or observation.[92] After following the patients for a median of 22 months, the trial was closed early due to lack of treatment efficacy.

Interferon-α

Three randomized clinical trials have evaluated the utility of IFN-α adjuvant to nephrectomy in high-risk patients but only two have been published. Messing at al. randomized 283 nonmetastatic postnephrectomy patients to 12 cycles of lymphoblastoid interferon (IFN-$α_{NL}$) or observation.[93] This form of IFN-α was chosen based on study results that were available in the early 1980s when the trial was initially planned.[94] With a median follow-up of 10 years, there was no demonstrable difference in survival between the two groups. Grade 4 toxicity was observed in 10% of patients on IFN-$α_{NL}$. In a similar trial, Pizzocaro et al. randomized 247 postnephrectomy patients to intramuscular IFN-$α_{2A}$ or observation and followed this group for a median of 5 years.[95] There was no difference in overall survival or RFS between the treatment and observation arms. Roughly 25% of IFN-$α_{2A}$-treated patients required a dose reduction or drug cessation due to toxicity.

Combination Immunochemotherapy

A recently published German trial randomized 203 patients with high-risk nonmetastatic RCC to observation or treatment with a combination of subcutaneous IL-2, subcutaneous IFN-α, and intravenous 5-fluorouracil (5-FU).[96] Surprisingly, the 5-year overall survival rate was worse for the treated patients than for the observed patients (58% vs. 76%, p = 0.03). The RFS rates were not significantly different. No formal evaluation of toxicity was reported.

Autologous Tumor Vaccine

The only treatment regimen that has shown efficacy as an adjuvant therapy for high-risk postnephrectomy RCC is the autologous tumor vaccine. Preliminary studies for autologous tumor vaccines showed promise and led to a multiinstitutional Phase III clinical trial.[54,97] This German trial randomized 379 patients to an autologous tumor vaccine or observation.[54] The 70-month progression-free survival rate was higher in the vaccine group than in the control group (72% vs. 59%, p = 0.02). When analyzed by subgroups, the group of patients with pT2 tumors did not appear to benefit from the vaccine while those patients with pT3 tumors did. A multivariate analysis showed that the most important predictors of progression-free survival were increasing Störkel score [hazard ratio (HR) = 2.5], absence of vaccine treatment (HR = 1.6), increasing tumor size (HR = 1.2), increasing age (HR = 1.04), and female gender (HR = 0.6). Perhaps just as important as the survival advantage is the fact that the side effects observed in the vaccine and control groups were almost identical, indicating that the autologous tumor vaccine is very safe. This treatment is not widely available at this time.

On the Horizon

There are many new molecular treatments that are undergoing evaluation in clinical trials. Oncophage (HSPPC-96) is a vaccine produced from heat-shock protein complex 96 of surgically resected RCCs. Initial trials have been completed and a large Phase III trial is underway.[98] The Phase III trial was very popular with patients and it rapidly accrued 1491 patients of which 644 were randomized to the vaccine or observation. Rencarex (WX-cG250) is a monoclonal antibody that targets carbonic anhydrase IX (CAIX). It is being tested clinically in two types of studies: (1) it is being tagged with radioactive molecules (^{131}I, ^{111}In, ^{90}Y, ^{17}Lu, or ^{186}Re) and used as targeted radiotherapy,[99,100] and (2) it is being used "cold" as a potential method of recruiting the immune system for tumor destruction.[101] Early results for this drug are mixed and a large Phase III trial is underway.[102]

Putting It all Together: What to Tell the Patient at High Risk of Recurrence

Consider a patient who will require surgery for a nonmetastatic renal mass. The first order of business is to establish (1) the renal function (present and future) of the patient, (2) whether the patient is likely to have an inherited form of RCC or not, and (3) whether the tumor is multifocal or bilateral. Patients at risk of renal failure or with syndromes are best managed with partial nephrectomy if possible. In fact, partial nephrectomy is probably a good policy for any renal mass less than 7 cm that can be technically removed without ablation of the entire kidney.[103]

It should now be clear that autologous tumor vaccines currently have the best evidence of efficacy in the adjuvant setting. Unfortunately, these vaccines are not currently widely available. The patient and clinician are therefore left with four general options for adjuvant therapy: (1) observation with intervention once disease recurs, (2) enrolling in a clinical trial that is assessing a new form of adjuvant therapy for RCC, (3) trying a therapy that has been shown to be effective in metastatic RCC but that has not yet been assessed in the adjuvant setting, and (4) using a form of adjuvant therapy that has previously been shown to be ineffective in a randomized controlled trial.

To decide what is best for the patient, the physician must use the information gathered in the perioperative period to predict how likely the patient is to have recurrent renal cancer. If the patient has clear cell RCC, the physician can use the Mayo or MSKCC prognostic tools from Table 11i–1 to estimate the RFS of the patient. Papillary and chromophobe RCC should be assessed with different prognostic tools. If the estimated RFS at 5 years is greater than 75%, the patient will not likely benefit from any form of adjuvant therapy and close observation with intervention at recurrence is probably the best policy. Management of the patient with an intermediate risk of recurrence (50–75% RFS at 5 years) is uncertain and a case-by-case approach is recommended. However, if the estimated RFS is less than 50% at 5 years, the patient shown be considered "high risk" and is likely to benefit from an *effective* adjuvant therapy. If the autologous tumor vaccine was available, this would be the cohort to use it in. A good second option is enrolling the patient in a randomized controlled trial. The patient will access new adjuvant treatment regimens that have often shown some efficacy in metastatic disease. If the patient refuses the clinical trial but still desires some form of adjuvant therapy, the next best option would probably be the use of the new agent bevacizumab (Avastin). Bevacizumab and the combination of bevacizumab and erlotinib (Tarceva) have both shown efficacy in a Phase II clinical trial in metastatic RCC.[104,105] A Phase III trial of bevacizumab–IFN-α versus IFN-α alone is currently underway.

Salvage Therapy for Metastatic Renal Cell Carcinoma

Metastatic RCC is one the most treatment-resistant malignancies.[7] It is beyond the scope of this chapter to review all the treatments that have been tried and that have failed in treating metastatic RCC. Rather, we will comment very briefly on agents that we feel are of historical importance and on the few agents that have shown promise in treating RCC.

Traditional Therapeutic Agents for Treating Metastatic Renal Cell Carcinoma

Hormonal Therapy

Hormonal therapy has been used extensively in metastatic RCC since the late 1960s.[84] Agents that have been tried include tamoxifen,[106] medroxyprogesterone acetate,[107–109] and androgens.[110,111] None of these agents has been proven effective.

Chemotherapy

Numerous chemotherapeutic agents have been tried and failed in RCC.[112,113] The apparent cause is the presence of multidrug resistance genes.[114,115] Multidrug resistance has been correlated with poor prognosis and several attempts to reverse it have been published.[116,117] Newer chemotherapy agents may improve this dismal track record somewhat. Various chemotherapy combinations using gemcitabine have shown better antitumoral activity with the gemcitabine–5-FU combination being the most promising.[118,120]

Interferon-α

IFN-α is one of the two pillars of contemporary immunotherapy for RCC (the other being IL-2) and has been shown to provide benefit in many Phase III randomized controlled trials.[121] Response rates of roughly 15% are typically observed in metastatic RCC, but only 5% of patients have a complete response.[122] The median duration of a response is only 10 months.[123] IFN-α has been unsuccessfully combined in Phase III trials with vinblastine,[124,125] IL-2,[126,127] IL-2 and 5-FU,[106] IL-2 and tamoxifen,[128] and IFN-γ.[129] A beneficial effect has been proven when IFN-α is combined with cytoreductive radical nephrectomy.[130,131] Some groups have suggested that the results for IFN-α immunotherapy may be improved by combining it with 13-*cis*-retinoic acid, but this has not been the experience of all groups.[125,132–134] The results of the Phase III trial combining bevacizumab and IFN-α are eagerly awaited. Lastly, one important advantage for IFN-α is that its efficacy is independent of the route of administration.

Interferon-γ

The only randomized trial in RCC to compare a new agent to placebo was conducted by the Canadian Urologic Oncology Group.[135] This trial compared IFN-γ to placebo and demonstrated a 7% response rate in placebo-treated patients. This is something other clinical trialists should keep in mind when planning Phase III trials for metastatic RCC.[136]

Interleukin-2

IL-2 was first reported as an immunotherapeutic agent for RCC in 1985.[137] The optimal dose and method of administration have been debated and Phase III trials have shown two advantages for high-dose IL-2: a modest increase in the durability of response and a slightly higher response rate.[127,138,139] However, overall survival is not better for high-dose IL-2 and there is a significant amount of toxicity associated with this regimen.[140,141] The following agents have been assessed in Phase III trials and proven to be of little benefit when combined with IL-2: lymphokine-activated killer cells,[142,143] tumor-infiltrating lymphocytes,[144] IFN-α,[126,127] IFN-α and 5-FU,[106,125] and IFN-α and tamoxifen.[128] A recent four-arm randomized controlled trial conducted by the French Immunotherapy group has shown that immunotherapy with IL-2, IFN-α, or both does not improve the survival of patients with an intermediate prognosis.[145]

New Therapeutic Agents for Treating Metastatic Renal Cell Carcinoma

Thalidomide

Thalidomide has been tried as an antiangiogenic agent in metastatic RCC.[146,147] The results of Phase II studies of thalidomide monotherapy are modest.[148] Combinations of thalidomide and various other agents (such as IL-2) are being assessed in Phase II and III clinical trials.[149]

Bevacizumab

Bevacizumab is a monoclonal antibody that targets vascular endothelial growth factor (VEGF) and therefore acts as an antiangiogenic agent. A Phase II trial from the National Cancer Institute (NCI) randomized 116 patients to bevacizumab or placebo and showed a significant improvement in progression-free survival for the treated arm.[104] Phase III trials for this agent are underway.[150] The

toxicity profile of this drug is good and it is FDA approved for colorectal cancer.

Erlotinib

Erlotinib is an epidermal growth factor receptor (EGFR) tyrosine kinase inhibitor. It has been tested in a Phase II trial in combination with bevacizumab.[105,151] Of the 63 patients that received the bevacizumab/erlotinib combination, 25% had an objective response and 61% had stable disease (RECIST criteria). The median survival for the cohort was 11 months. A Phase II neoadjuvant study for metastatic RCC prior to cytoreductive nephrectomy is planned.

Sutinib

Sutinib is a tyrosine kinase inhibitor of VEGF-receptor 2 (VEGFR-2) and platelet-derived growth factor receptor B (PDGFR-B). Two Phase II trials with a combined patient count of 169 have been conducted in patients who had failed prior cytokine therapy.[152,153] The partial response rate was 40% and the median progression-free survival time was 8 months. These results are impressive considering the cohort at study. The toxicities of the drug appear to be minimal and a Phase III trial is ongoing.[154]

Sorafenib

Sorafenib has a dual mechanism of action: it inhibits Raf kinase and it is a tyrosine kinase inhibitor of VEGFR-2, VEGFR-3, and PDGFR-B.[155,156] A Phase III trial of sorafenib versus best supportive care has been completed.[157] A total of 769 patients were randomized and the 3-month progression-free rate was significantly higher in treated patients (79% vs. 50%). The side-effect profile is acceptable and long-term follow-up is eagerly awaited.[158–160] Sorafenib has recently been approved by the FDA for kidney cancer.

Temsirolimus

Temsirolimus is a specific inhibitor of the mammalian target of rapamycin (mTOR). A Phase II trial of temsirolimus was conducted in 111 patients with metastatic RCC.[161] This trial demonstrated a response rate of 7% and a median time to progression of 6 months. The toxicities of the drug were acceptable and a Phase III trial has accrued but has not yet been reported.

Zoledronic Acid

Zoledronic acid is a powerful bisphosphonate that can be effective in treating bone metastases.[162] This drug has been shown to be effective in treating RCC that has metastasized to bone.[163,164] There is even some evidence that zoledronic acid may have some antitumoral effects in RCC.[165]

Putting It all Together: What to Tell the Patient at High Risk of Progression

The management of the patient with metastases from RCC is difficult. The traditional agents used to treat this disease have not been proven to provide much long-term benefit. Newer agents that specifically target angiogenesis, growth factors, and intracellular signaling have shown very promising results in Phase II trials. Multiple Phase III trials are in progress for these newer drugs but none has been formally completed and published. The options for patients with metastatic RCC are therefore 4-fold: (1) surgical removal of all resectable disease, including the diseased kidney (discussed elsewhere in this book), (2) traditional immunotherapy, (3) participation in a clinical trial, and (4) best supportive care. We are advocates of shared informed decision making in all aspects of cancer management.[166]

The SANI score from Table 11i–1 can help predict which patients will have a good outcome with high-dose IL-2 treatment. Otherwise, the tool for metastatic RCC from the Mayo Clinic or the MSKCC Motzer score are probably the most appropriate ways of assessing patient risk. Although all of these patients are at high risk of dying from RCC, some patients carry a particularly poor prognosis. Informing patients of their prognosis is a very important task that should be done gently and with understanding because the diagnosis of an incurable cancer is likely to be one of the most significant events in a patient's life.[167] It is not always appropriate to divulge the entire story in one visit and occasionally active silence with an invitation for renewed discussion at another visit may be the best course of action.[168]

Patients who are young or otherwise healthy are usually the best candidates for aggressive treatment. For this group, a clinical trial employing one the novel agents is probably the best course of action. For the patient who is unwilling to be randomized, immunotherapy with IL-2 or IFN-α is a second option that may be worth pursuing. The patient must recognize that these agents are unlikely to lead to cure and may be associated with significant toxicity. Older and sicker patients may be good candidates for randomized controlled trials because the newer agents have toxicity profiles that are less concerning. Standard immunotherapy doses need to be reduced in the elderly, but age alone does not appear to affect prognosis.[169]

In 5–10% of cases, the histological variant of RCC that has metastasized will not be clear cell RCC. It is important to recognize these other subtypes because they generally do not respond well to conventional immunotherapy. The distribution of the variant histological subtypes of RCC and their survival are different in the metastatic setting than in the localized setting (Table 11i-3).[170,171] Despite the fact that metastases develop more commonly in collecting duct RCC than in papillary RCC and that localized papillary RCC is usually associated with a good prognosis, the reverse relationship is noted in metastatic RCC.[170,172,172–174] Collecting duct carcinoma appears to be resistant to conventional immunotherapy and chemotherapy, but some favorable responses have been noted with the combinations of taxotere-carboplatin and gemcitabine-cisplatin.[175] No therapy has been reported to be advantageous for patients with metastatic papillary or chromophobe RCC. Sarcomatoid RCC is an aggressive form of RCC that is found in association with other histological subtypes and that metastasizes rapidly.[176] IL-2 may be of benefit in this population,[177] but the combination of gemcitabine and doxorubicin has also shown promise.[178]

Lastly, an important role for the physician to play in the management of a patient with an incurable malignancy is to help the patient prepare for death.[179,180] Physicians and patients have differing views about what is important in the palliative setting and physicians should be aware of this.[30,181] A patient may want to try alternative remedies that may be costly and unlikely to provide benefit. The responsible doctor should honestly advise the patient but be supportive if the advice is not followed.[182] Physicians should strive to

TABLE 11i-3. Renal cell carcinoma histological subtypes.[a]

| RCC histological subtype | Incident cases[203] | | Metastatic cases[170,177] | | Systemic treatment |
	Proportion	5-year CSS	Proportion	Median survival(months)	
Clear cell	81%	72%	92%	12	IL-2, IFN-α,bevacizumab, erlotinibsutinib, sorafenibtem-sirolimus
Papillary	14%	91%	2.25%	5.	?
Chromophobe	5%	88%	1.5%	29	?
Collecting duct	0.2%	20%[b]	3.25%	11	Gemcitabine + cisplatin,taxotere + carboplatin
Sarcomatoid features	5%	30%[b]	?	10	Gemcitabine + doxorubicin,IL-2

[a]RCC, renal cell carcinoma;CSS, cancer-specific survival; IL-2, interleukin-2; IFN-α, interferon-α.
[b]Two-year cancer-specific survival.

maintain patient autonomy as long as is possible.[183] Whether or nor family members should be part of the process should be decided on an individual basis, but is rarely a wrong decision. A team approach is the best approach for managing the palliative patient because all the resources of the health care system can be maximally utilized to improve the quality of the patient's remaining time.

Conclusions

The management of high-risk nonmetastatic RCC and metastatic RCC is changing. Unfortunately, for the time being, the multiple new promising agents tested in Phase II trials have not been adequately tested in Phase III trials to unequivocally prove their efficacy. Furthermore, some agents that have been shown to be efficacious are not commercially available. This leaves the patient with the option of a clinical trial or the alternative of traditional immunotherapy. The horizon is bright, but the current situation has, for the moment, remained largely unchanged.

References

1. Brindley CO, Markoff E, Scheneiderman MA. Direct observation of lesion size and number as a method of following the growth of human tumors. *Cancer* 1959;**12**(1):139–146.
2. Priore RL. Using a mathematical model in the evaluation of human tumor response to chemotherapy. *J Natl Cancer Inst* 1966;**37**(5):635–647.
3. World Health Organization. WHO handbook for reporting results of cancer treatment. WHO offset publication No. 48. Geneva: World Health Organization, 1979.
4. Miller AB, Hoogstraten B, Staquet M, Winkler A. Reporting results of cancer treatment. *Cancer* 1981;**47**(1):207–214.
5. Moertel CG, Hanley JA. The effect of measuring error on the results of therapeutic trials in advanced cancer. *Cancer* 1976;**38**(1):388–394.
6. James K, Eisenhauer E, Christian M, et al. Measuring response in solid tumors: unidimensional versus bidimensional measurement. *J Natl Cancer Inst* 1999;**91**(6):523–528.
7. Stadler WM. Targeted agents for the treatment of advanced renal cell carcinoma. *Cancer* 2005;**104**(11):2323–2333.
8. Therasse P, Arbuck SG, Eisenhauer EA, et al. New guidelines to evaluate the response to treatment in solid tumors. European Organization for Research and Treatment of Cancer, National Cancer Institute of the United States, National Cancer Institute of Canada. *J Natl Cancer Inst* 2000;**92**(3):205–216.
9. Chen TT, Chute JP, Feigal E, Johnson BE, Simon R. A model to select chemotherapy regimens for phase III trials for extensive-stage small-cell lung cancer. *J Natl Cancer Inst* 2000;**92**(19):1601–1607.
10. Oye RK, Shapiro MF. Reporting results from chemotherapy trials. Does response make a difference in patient survival? *JAMA* 1984;**252**(19):2722–2725.
11. Anderson JR, Cain KC, Gelber RD. Analysis of survival by tumor response. *J Clin Oncol* 1983;**1**(11):710–719.
12. Mantel N. An uncontrolled clinical trial–treatment response or spontaneous improvement? *Control Clin Trials* 1982;**3**(4):369–370.
13. Mantel N, Byar DP. Evaluation of response-time data involving transient states: an illustration using heart-transplant data. *J Am Stat Assoc* 1974;**69**(345):81–86.
14. Buyse M, Piedbois P. On the relationship between response to treatment and survival time. *Stat Med* 1996;**15**(24): 2797–2812.
15. Pazdur R. Response rates, survival, and chemotherapy trials. *J Natl Cancer Inst* 2000;**92**(19):1552–1553.
16. Zee B, Melnychuk D, Dancey J, Eisenhauer E. Multinomial phase II cancer trials incorporating response and early progression. *J Biopharm Stat* 1999;**9**(2):351–363.
17. Chua YJ, Sargent D, Cunningham D. Definition of disease-free survival: this is my truth-show me yours. *Ann Oncol* 2005;**16**(11):1719–1721.
18. Sargent DJ, Wieand HS, Haller DG, et al. Disease-free survival versus overall survival as a primary end point for adjuvant colon cancer studies: individual patient data from 20,898 patients on 18 randomized trials. *J Clin Oncol* 2005;**23**(34):8664–8670.
19. Lokich J. Tumor response and survival end points in clinical trials: a clinician's perspective. *Am J Clin Oncol* 2004;**27**(5):494–496.
20. Fleming TR, DeMets DL. Surrogate end points in clinical trials: are we being misled? *Ann Intern Med* 1996;**125**(7):605–613.
21. Prentice RL. Surrogate endpoints in clinical trials: definition and operational criteria. *Stat Med* 1989;**8**(4):431–440.
22. Feldstein ML. Quality-of-life-adjusted survival for comparing cancer treatments. A commentary on TWiST and Q-TWiST. *Cancer* 1991;**67**(3 Suppl):851–854.
23. Tassinari D, Panzini I, Sartori S, Ravaioli A. Surrogate outcomes in quality-of-life research: where will we end up? *J Clin Oncol* 2003;**21**(9):1894–1895; author reply 1895.
24. Verweij J. The benefit of clinical benefit: a European perspective. *Ann Oncol* 1996;**7**(4):333–334.
25. Bowcock SJ, Shee CD, Rassam SM, Harper PG. Chemotherapy for cancer patients who present late. *BMJ* 2004;**328**(7453):1430–1432.
26. Cole BF, Gelber RD, Goldhirsch A. Cox regression models for quality adjusted survival analysis. *Stat Med* 1993;**12**(10): 975–987.
27. Messori A, Trippoli S. Can the Q-TWiST method provide information on patients' preferences without collecting preference data from the patients? Quality-Adjusted Time Without Symptoms or Toxicity. *J Clin Oncol* 1998;**16**(11):3716–3717; author reply 3718.
28. Atzpodien J, Kuchler T, Wandert T, Reitz M. Rapid deterioration in quality of life during interleukin-2- and alpha-interferon-based home therapy of renal cell carcinoma is associated with a good outcome. *Br J Cancer* 2003;**89**(1): 50–54.
29. Fagerlin A, Zikmund-Fisher BJ, Ubel PA. Cure me even if it kills me: preferences for invasive cancer treatment. *Med Decis Making* 2005;**25**(6):614–619.
30. Slevin ML, Stubbs L, Plant HJ, et al. Attitudes to chemotherapy: comparing views of patients with cancer with those of doctors, nurses, and general public. *BMJ* 1990;**300**(6737):1458–1460.
31. Glare P, Virik K, Jones M, et al. A systematic review of physicians' survival predictions in terminally ill cancer patients. *BMJ* 2003;**327**(7408):195.

32. Vigano A, Dorgan M, Bruera E, Suarez-Almazor ME. The relative accuracy of the clinical estimation of the duration of life for patients with end of life cancer. *Cancer* 1999;**86**(1):170–176.

33. Parkes CM. Accuracy of predictions of survival in later stages of cancer. *BMJ* 1972;**2**(5804):29–31.

34. Maltoni M, Nanni O, Derni S, et al. Clinical prediction of survival is more accurate than the Karnofsky performance status in estimating life span of terminally ill cancer patients. *Eur J Cancer* 1994;**30A**(6):764–766.

35. Morita T, Tsunoda J, Inoue S, Chihara S. Improved accuracy of physicians' survival prediction for terminally ill cancer patients using the palliative prognostic index. *Palliat Med* 2001;**15**(5):419–424.

36. Morita T, Tsunoda J, Inoue S, Chihara S. The palliative prognostic index: a scoring system for survival prediction of terminally ill cancer patients. *Support Care Cancer* 1999;**7**(3):128–133.

37. Pirovano M, Maltoni M, Nanni O, et al. A new palliative prognostic score: a first step for the staging of terminally ill cancer patients. Italian Multicenter and Study Group on Palliative Care. *J Pain Symptom Manage* 1999;**17**(4):231–239.

38. Maltoni M, Caraceni A, Brunelli C, et al. Prognostic factors in advanced cancer patients: evidence-based clinical recommendations—-a study by the Steering Committee of the European Association for Palliative Care. *J Clin Oncol* 2005;**23**(25):6240–6248.

39. Storkel S, Thoenes W, Jacobi GH, Lippold R. Prognostic parameters in renal cell carcinoma—-a new approach. *Eur Urol* 1989;**16**(6):416–422.

40. Cindolo L, de la Taille A, Messina G, et al. A preoperative clinical prognostic model for non-metastatic renal cell carcinoma. *BJU Int* 2003;**92**(9):901–905.

41. Yaycioglu O, Roberts WW, Chan T, Epstein JI, Marshall FF, Kavoussi LR. Prognostic assessment of nonmetastatic renal cell carcinoma: a clinically based model. *Urology* 2001;**58**(2):141–145.

42. Zisman A, Pantuck AJ, Dorey F, et al. Improved prognostication of renal cell carcinoma using an integrated staging system. *J Clin Oncol* 2001;**19**(6):1649–1657.

43. Frank I, Blute ML, Cheville JC, Lohse CM, Weaver AL, Zincke H. An outcome prediction model for patients with clear cell renal cell carcinoma treated with radical nephrectomy based on tumor stage, size, grade and necrosis: the SSIGN score. *J Urol* 2002;**168**(6):2395–2400.

44. Leibovich BC, Blute ML, Cheville JC, et al. Prediction of progression after radical nephrectomy for patients with clear cell renal cell carcinoma: a stratification tool for prospective clinical trials. *Cancer* 2003;**97**(7):1663–1671.

45. Kattan MW, Reuter V, Motzer RJ, Katz J, Russo P. A postoperative prognostic nomogram for renal cell carcinoma. *J Urol* 2001;**166**(1):63–67.

46. Sorbellini M, Kattan MW, Snyder ME, et al. A postoperative prognostic nomogram predicting recurrence for patients with conventional clear cell renal cell carcinoma. *J Urol* 2005;**173**(1):48–51.

47. Leibovich BC, Cheville JC, Lohse CM, et al. A scoring algorithm to predict survival for patients with metastatic clear cell renal cell carcinoma: a stratification tool for prospective

clinical trials. *J Urol* 2005;**174**(5):1759–1763; discussion 1763.

48. Motzer RJ, Mazumdar M, Bacik J, Berg W, Amsterdam A, Ferrara J. Survival and prognostic stratification of 670 patients with advanced renal cell carcinoma. *J Clin Oncol* 1999;**17**(8):2530–2540.

49. Motzer RJ, Bacik J, Schwartz LH, et al. Prognostic factors for survival in previously treated patients with metastatic renal cell carcinoma. *J Clin Oncol* 2004;**22**(3):454–463.

50. Leibovich BC, Han KR, Bui MH, et al. Scoring algorithm to predict survival after nephrectomy and immunotherapy in patients with metastatic renal cell carcinoma: a stratification tool for prospective clinical trials. *Cancer* 2003;**98**(12):2566–2575.

51. Atzpodien J, Royston P, Wandert T, Reitz M. Metastatic renal carcinoma comprehensive prognostic system. *Br J Cancer* 2003;**88**(3):348–353.

52. Mekhail TM, Abou-Jawde RM, Boumerhi G, et al. Validation and extension of the Memorial Sloan-Kettering prognostic factors model for survival in patients with previously untreated metastatic renal cell carcinoma. *J Clin Oncol* 2005;**23**(4):832–841.

53. Patard JJ, Kim HL, Lam JS, et al. Use of the University of California Los Angeles integrated staging system to predict survival in renal cell carcinoma: an international multicenter study. *J Clin Oncol* 2004;**22**(16):3316–3322.

54. Jocham D, Richter A, Hoffmann L, et al. Adjuvant autologous renal tumour cell vaccine and risk of tumour progression in patients with renal-cell carcinoma after radical nephrectomy: phase III, randomised controlled trial. *Lancet* 2004;**363**(9409):594–599.

55. Cindolo L, Patard JJ, Chiodini P, et al. Comparison of predictive accuracy of four prognostic models for nonmetastatic renal cell carcinoma after nephrectomy: a multicenter European study. *Cancer* 2005;**104**(7):1362–1371.

56. Lam JS, Shvarts O, Said JW, et al. Clinicopathologic and molecular correlations of necrosis in the primary tumor of patients with renal cell carcinoma. *Cancer* 2005;**103**(12):2517–2525.

57. Sengupta S, Lohse CM, Leibovich BC, et al. Histologic coagulative tumor necrosis as a prognostic indicator of renal cell carcinoma aggressiveness. *Cancer* 2005;**104**(3):511–520.

58. Bottaro DP, Linehan WM. Multifocal renal cancer: genetic basis and its medical relevance. *Clin Cancer Res* 2005;**11**(20):7206–7208.

59. Linehan WM, Vasselli J, Srinivasan R, et al. Genetic basis of cancer of the kidney: disease-specific approaches to therapy. *Clin Cancer Res* 2004;**10**(18 Pt 2):6282S–6289S.

60. Takahashi M, Kahnoski R, Gross D, Nicol D, Teh BT. Familial adult renal neoplasia. *J Med Genet* 2002;**39**(1):1–5.

61. Frank I, Blute ML, Leibovich BC, Cheville JC, Lohse CM, Zincke H. Independent validation of the 2002 American Joint Committee on cancer primary tumor classification for renal cell carcinoma using a large, single institution cohort. *J Urol* 2005;**173**(6):1889–1892.

62. Blute ML, Leibovich BC, Lohse CM, Cheville JC, Zincke H. The Mayo Clinic experience with surgical management, complications and outcome for patients with renal cell carcinoma and venous tumour thrombus. *BJU Int* 2004;**94**(1):33–41.

63. Thompson RH, Cheville JC, Lohse CM, et al. Reclassification of patients with pT3 and pT4 renal cell carcinoma improves prognostic accuracy. *Cancer* 2005;**104**(1):53–60.

64. Meng MV, Miller TR, Cha I, Stoller ML. Cytology of morcellated renal specimens: significance in diagnosis and dissemination. *J Urol* 2003;**169**(1):45–48.

65. Fentie DD, Barrett PH, Taranger LA. Metastatic renal cell cancer after laparoscopic radical nephrectomy: long-term follow-up. *J Endourol* 2000;**14**(5):407–411.

66. Rabban JT, Meng MV, Yeh B, Koppie T, Ferrell L, Stoller ML. Kidney morcellation in laparoscopic nephrectomy for tumor: recommendations for specimen sampling and pathologic tumor staging. *Am J Surg Pathol* 2001;**25**(9):1158–1166.

67. Varkarakis I, Rha K, Hernandez F, Kavoussi LR, Jarrett TW. Laparoscopic specimen extraction: morcellation. *BJU Int* 2005;**95(Suppl 2)**:27–31.

68. Itano NB, Blute ML, Spotts B, Zincke H. Outcome of isolated renal cell carcinoma fossa recurrence after nephrectomy. *J Urol* 2000;**164**(2):322–325.

69. Schrodter S, Hakenberg OW, Manseck A, Leike S, Wirth MP. Outcome of surgical treatment of isolated local recurrence after radical nephrectomy for renal cell carcinoma. *J Urol* 2002;**167**(4):1630–1633.

70. Tanguay S, Pisters LL, Lawrence DD, Dinney CP. Therapy of locally recurrent renal cell carcinoma after nephrectomy. *J Urol* 1996;**155**(1):26–29.

71. Sandhu SS, Symes A, A'Hern R, et al. Surgical excision of isolated renal-bed recurrence after radical nephrectomy for renal cell carcinoma. *BJU Int* 2005;**95**(4):522–525.

72. Master VA, Gottschalk AR, Kane C, Carroll PR. Management of isolated renal fossa recurrence following radical nephrectomy. *J Urol* 2005;**174**(2):473–477; discussion 477.

73. Frydenberg M, Gunderson L, Hahn G, Fieck J, Zincke H. Preoperative external beam radiotherapy followed by cytoreductive surgery and intraoperative radiotherapy for locally advanced primary or recurrent renal malignancies. *J Urol* 1994;**152**(1):15–21.

74. Steinbach F, Novick AC, Zincke H, et al. Treatment of renal cell carcinoma in von Hippel-Lindau disease: a multicenter study. *J Urol* 1995;**153**(6):1812–1816.

75. Malkin RB. Regression of renal carcinoma following radiation therapy. *J Urol* 1975;**114**(5):782–783.

76. Stein M, Kuten A, Halpern J, Coachman NM, Cohen Y, Robinson E. The value of postoperative irradiation in renal cell cancer. *Radiother Oncol* 1992;**24**(1):41–44.

77. Kao GD, Malkowicz SB, Whittington R, D'Amico AV, Wein AJ. Locally advanced renal cell carcinoma: low complication rate and efficacy of postnephrectomy radiation therapy planned with CT. *Radiology* 1994;**193**(3):725–730.

78. Forman JD. The role of radiation therapy in the management of carcinoma of the kidney. *Semin Urol* 1989;**7**(3):195–198.

79. Juusela H, Malmio K, Alfthan O, Oravisto KJ. Preoperative irradiation in the treatment of renal adenocarcinoma. *Scand J Urol Nephrol* 1977;**11**(3):277–281.

80. Kjaer M, Iversen P, Hvidt V, et al. A randomized trial of postoperative radiotherapy versus observation in stage II and III renal adenocarcinoma. A study by the Copenhagen Renal Cancer Study Group. *Scand J Urol Nephrol* 1987;**21**(4):285–289.

81. Vogelzang NJ, Yang X, Goldman S, Vijayakumar S, Steinberg G. Radiation induced renal cell cancer: a report of 4 cases and review of the literature. *J Urol* 1998;**160**(6 Pt 1):1987–1990.

82. Finney R. The value of radiotherapy in the treatment of hypernephroma—a clinical trial. *Br J Urol* 1973;**45**(3):258–269.

83. Beitler JJ, Makara D, Silverman P, Lederman G. Definitive, high-dose-per-fraction, conformal, stereotactic external radiation for renal cell carcinoma. *Am J Clin Oncol* 2004;**27**(6):646–648.

84. Bloom HJ. Cancer of the urogenital tract: kidney. The basis for hormonal therapy. *JAMA* 1968;**204**(7):605–606.

85. Bloom HJ, Dukes CE, Mitchley BC. Hormone-dependent tumors of the kidney: II. Effect of endocrine ablation procedures on the transplanted estrogen-induced renal tumor of the Syrian hamster. *Br J Cancer* 1963;**17**:646–656.

86. Satomi Y, Takai S, Kondo I, Fukushima S, Furuhata A. Postoperative prophylactic use of progesterone in renal cell carcinoma. *J Urol* 1982;**128**(5):919–922.

87. Bono AV, Benvenuti C, Gianneo E, Comeri GC, Roggia A. Progestogens in renal cell carcinoma. A retrospective study. *Eur Urol* 1979;**5**(2):94–96.

88. Pizzocaro G, Piva L, Di Fronzo G, et al. Adjuvant medroxyprogesterone acetate to radical nephrectomy in renal cancer: 5-year results of a prospective randomized study. *J Urol* 1987;**138**(6):1379–1381.

89. Hoover HC Jr, Peters LC, Brandhorst JS, Hanna MG Jr. Therapy of spontaneous metastases with an autologous tumor vaccine in a guinea pig model. *J Surg Res* 1981;**30**(4):409–415.

90. Galligioni E, Quaia M, Merlo A, et al. Adjuvant immunotherapy treatment of renal carcinoma patients with autologous tumor cells and bacillus Calmette-Guerin: five-year results of a prospective randomized study. *Cancer* 1996;**77**(12):2560–2566.

91. Dillman RO, Barth NM, VanderMolen LA, et al. Treatment of kidney cancer with autologous tumor cell vaccines of short-term cell lines derived from renal cell carcinoma. *Cancer Biother Radiopharm* 2001;**16**(1):47–54.

92. Clark JI, Atkins MB, Urba WJ, et al. Adjuvant high-dose bolus interleukin-2 for patients with high-risk renal cell carcinoma: a cytokine working group randomized trial. *J Clin Oncol* 2003;**21**(16):3133–3140.

93. Messing EM, Manola J, Wilding G, et al. Phase III study of interferon alfa-NL as adjuvant treatment for resectable renal cell carcinoma: an Eastern Cooperative Oncology Group/Intergroup trial. *J Clin Oncol* 2003;**21**(7):1214–1222.

94. Trump DL, Elson PJ, Borden EC, et al. High-dose lymphoblastoid interferon in advanced renal cell carcinoma: an Eastern Cooperative Oncology Group Study. *Cancer Treat Rep* 1987;**71**(2):165–169.

95. Pizzocaro G, Piva L, Colavita M, et al. Interferon adjuvant to radical nephrectomy in Robson stages II and III renal cell carcinoma: a multicentric randomized study. *J Clin Oncol* 2001;**19**(2):425–431.

96. Atzpodien J, Schmitt E, Gertenbach U, et al. Adjuvant treatment with interleukin-2- and interferon-alpha2a-based chemoimmunotherapy in renal cell carcinoma post tumour nephrectomy: results of a prospectively randomised trial of the

German Cooperative Renal Carcinoma Chemoimmunotherapy Group (DGCIN). *Br J Cancer* 2005;**92**(5):843–846.

97. Repmann R, Goldschmidt AJ, Richter A. Adjuvant therapy of renal cell carcinoma patients with an autologous tumor cell lysate vaccine: a 5-year follow-up analysis. *Anticancer Res* 2003;**23**(2A):969–974.

98. Wood CG, Escudier B, Gorelov S, et al. A multicenter randomized study of adjuvant heat-shock protein peptide-complex 96 (HSPPC-96) vaccine in patients with high-risk of recurrence after nephrectomy for renal cell carcinoma (RCC)– a preliminary report. *J Clin Oncol 2004 ASCO Annu Meet Proc (Post-Meet Ed)*. 2004;**22**(14S):2618.

99. Steffens MG, Boerman OC, de Mulder PH, et al. Phase I radioimmunotherapy of metastatic renal cell carcinoma with 131I-labeled chimeric monoclonal antibody G250. *Clin Cancer Res* 1999;**5**(10 Suppl):3268s–3274s.

100. Brouwers AH, Buijs WC, Oosterwijk E, et al. Targeting of metastatic renal cell carcinoma with the chimeric monoclonal antibody G250 labeled with (131)I or (111)In: an intrapatient comparison. *Clin Cancer Res* 2003;**9**(10 Pt 2):3953S–3960S.

101. Bleumer I, Knuth A, Oosterwijk E, et al. A phase II trial of chimeric monoclonal antibody G250 for advanced renal cell carcinoma patients. *Br J Cancer* 2004;**90**(5):985–990.

102. Brouwers AH, Mulders PF, de Mulder PH, et al. Lack of efficacy of two consecutive treatments of radioimmunotherapy with 131I-cG250 in patients with metastasized clear cell renal cell carcinoma. *J Clin Oncol* 2005;**23**(27):6540–6548.

103. Leibovich BC, Blute ML, Cheville JC, Lohse CM, Weaver AL, Zincke H. Nephron sparing surgery for appropriately selected renal cell carcinoma between 4 and 7 cm results in outcome similar to radical nephrectomy. *J Urol* 2004;**171**(3): 1066–1070.

104. Yang JC, Haworth L, Sherry RM, et al. A randomized trial of bevacizumab, an anti-vascular endothelial growth factor antibody, for metastatic renal cancer. *N Engl J Med* 2003;**349**(5):427–434.

105. Hainsworth JD, Sosman JA, Spigel DR, Edwards DL, Baughman C, Greco A. Treatment of metastatic renal cell carcinoma with a combination of bevacizumab and erlotinib. *J Clin Oncol* 2005;**23**(31):7889–7896.

106. Atzpodien J, Kirchner H, Illiger HJ, et al. IL-2 in combination with IFN-alpha and 5-FU versus tamoxifen in metastatic renal cell carcinoma: long-term results of a controlled randomized clinical trial. *Br J Cancer* 2001;**85**(8):1130–1136.

107. Samuels ML, Sullivan P, Howe CD. Medroxyprogesterone acetate in the treatment of renal cell carcinoma (hypernephroma). *Cancer* 1968;**22**(3):525–532.

108. Bloom HJ. Medroxyprogesterone acetate (Provera) in the treatment of metastatic renal cancer. *Br J Cancer* 1971;**25**(2):250–265.

109. Porzsolt F, Messerer D, Hautmann R, et al. Treatment of advanced renal cell cancer with recombinant interferon alpha as a single agent and in combination with medroxyprogesterone acetate. A randomized multicenter trial. *J Cancer Res Clin Oncol* 1988;**114**(1):95–100.

110. Morales A, Kiruluta G, Lott S. Hormones in the treatment of metastatic renal cancer. *J Urol* 1975;**114**(5):692–693.

111. Papac RJ, Keohane MF. Hormonal therapy for metastatic renal cell carcinoma combined androgen and Provera followed by high dose tamoxifen. *Eur J Cancer* 1993;**29A**(7):997–999.

112. Yagoda A, Abi-Rached B, Petrylak D. Chemotherapy for advanced renal-cell carcinoma: 1983–1993. *Semin Oncol* 1995;**22**(1):42–60.

113. Motzer RJ, Russo P. Systemic therapy for renal cell carcinoma. *J Urol* 2000;**163**(2):408–417.

114. Kanamaru H, Kakehi Y, Yoshida O, Nakanishi S, Pastan I, Gottesman MM. MDR1 RNA levels in human renal cell carcinomas: correlation with grade and prediction of reversal of doxorubicin resistance by quinidine in tumor explants. *J Natl Cancer Inst* 1989;**81**(11):844–849.

115. Rochlitz CF, Lobeck H, Peter S, et al. Multiple drug resistance gene expression in human renal cell cancer is associated with the histologic subtype. *Cancer* 1992;**69**(12):2993–2998.

116. Hofmockel G, Bassukas ID, Wittmann A, Dammrich J. Is the expression of multidrug resistance gene product a prognostic indicator for the clinical outcome of patients with renal cancer? *Br J Urol* 1997;**80**(1):11–17.

117. Yu DS, Sun GH, Ma CP, Chang SY. Cocktail modulator mixtures for overcoming multidrug resistance in renal cell carcinoma. *Urology* 1999;**54**(2):377–381.

118. Rini BI, Vogelzang NJ, Dumas MC, Wade JL, 3rd, Taber DA, Stadler WM. Phase II trial of weekly intravenous gemcitabine with continuous infusion fluorouracil in patients with metastatic renal cell cancer. *J Clin Oncol* 2000;**18**(12):2419–2426.

119. Porta C, Zimatore M, Imarisio I, et al. Gemcitabine and oxaliplatin in the treatment of patients with immunotherapy-resistant advanced renal cell carcinoma: final results of a single-institution phase II study. *Cancer* 2004;**100**(10): 2132–2138.

120. Waters JS, Moss C, Pyle L, et al. Phase II clinical trial of capecitabine and gemcitabine chemotherapy in patients with metastatic renal cell carcinoma. *Br J Cancer* 2004;**91**(10): 1763–1768.

121. Interferon-alpha and survival in metastatic renal carcinoma: early results of a randomised controlled trial. Medical Research Council Renal Cancer Collaborators. *Lancet* 1999;**353**(9146):14–17.

122. Wirth MP. Immunotherapy for metastatic renal cell carcinoma. *Urol Clin North Am* 1993;**20**(2):283–295.

123. van Sponsen DJ, Mulders PF, De Mulder PH. Novel treatments for metastatic renal cell carcinoma. *Crit Rev Oncol Hematol* 2005;**55**(3):177–191.

124. Fossa SD, Martinelli G, Otto U, et al. Recombinant interferon alfa-2a with or without vinblastine in metastatic renal cell carcinoma: results of a European multi-center phase III study. *Ann Oncol* 1992;**3**(4):301–305.

125. Atzpodien J, Kirchner H, Jonas U, et al. Interleukin-2- and interferon alfa-2a-based immunochemotherapy in advanced renal cell carcinoma: a prospectively randomized trial of the German Cooperative Renal Carcinoma Chemoimmunotherapy Group (DGCIN). *J Clin Oncol* 2004;**22**(7):1188–1194.

126. Negrier S, Escudier B, Lasset C, et al. Recombinant human interleukin-2, recombinant human interferon alfa-2a, or both in metastatic renal-cell carcinoma. Groupe Francais d'Immunotherapie. *N Engl J Med* 1998;**338**(18):1272–1278.

127. McDermott DF, Regan MM, Clark JI, et al. Randomized phase III trial of high-dose interleukin-2 versus subcutaneous interleukin-2 and interferon in patients with metastatic renal cell carcinoma. *J Clin Oncol* 2005;**23**(1):133–141.

128. Henriksson R, Nilsson S, Colleen S, et al. Survival in renal cell carcinoma—-a randomized evaluation of tamoxifen vs interleukin 2, alpha-interferon (leucocyte) and tamoxifen. *Br J Cancer* 1998;**77**(8):1311–1317.

129. De Mulder PH, Oosterhof G, Bouffioux C, van Oosterom AT, Vermeylen K, Sylvester R. EORTC (30885) randomised phase III study with recombinant interferon alpha and recombinant interferon alpha and gamma in patients with advanced renal cell carcinoma. The EORTC Genitourinary Group. *Br J Cancer* 1995;**71**(2):371–375.

130. Mickisch GH, Garin A, van Poppel H, de Prijck L, Sylvester R. Radical nephrectomy plus interferon-alfa-based immunotherapy compared with interferon alfa alone in metastatic renal-cell carcinoma: a randomised trial. *Lancet* 2001;**358**(9286):966–970.

131. Flanigan RC, Salmon SE, Blumenstein BA, et al. Nephrectomy followed by interferon alfa-2b compared with interferon alfa-2b alone for metastatic renal-cell cancer. *N Engl J Med* 2001;**345**(23):1655–1659.

132. Fossa SD, Mickisch GH, De Mulder PH, et al. Interferon-alpha-2a with or without 13-cis retinoic acid in patients with progressive, measurable metastatic renal cell carcinoma. *Cancer* 2004;**101**(3):533–540.

133. Aass N, De Mulder PH, Mickisch GH, et al. Randomized phase II/III trial of interferon alfa-2a with and without 13-cis-retinoic acid in patients with progressive metastatic renal cell carcinoma: the European Organisation for Research and Treatment of Cancer Genito-Urinary Tract Cancer Group (EORTC 30951). *J Clin Oncol* 2005;**23**(18):4172–4178.

134. Motzer RJ, Murphy BA, Bacik J, et al. Phase III trial of interferon alfa-2a with or without 13-cis-retinoic acid for patients with advanced renal cell carcinoma. *J Clin Oncol* 2000;**18**(16):2972–2980.

135. Gleave ME, Elhilali M, Fradet Y, et al. Interferon gamma-1b compared with placebo in metastatic renal-cell carcinoma. Canadian Urologic Oncology Group. *N Engl J Med* 1998;**338**(18):1265–1271.

136. Elhilali MM, Gleave M, Fradet Y, et al. Placebo-associated remissions in a multicentre, randomized, double-blind trial of interferon gamma-1b for the treatment of metastatic renal cell carcinoma. The Canadian Urologic Oncology Group. *BJU Int* 2000;**86**(6):613–618.

137. Rosenberg SA, Lotze MT, Muul LM, et al. Observations on the systemic administration of autologous lymphokine-activated killer cells and recombinant interleukin-2 to patients with metastatic cancer. *N Engl J Med* 1985;**313**(23):1485–1492.

138. Yang JC, Sherry RM, Steinberg SM, et al. Randomized study of high-dose and low-dose interleukin-2 in patients with metastatic renal cancer. *J Clin Oncol* 2003;**21**(16):3127–3132.

139. Yang JC, Topalian SL, Parkinson D, et al. Randomized comparison of high-dose and low-dose intravenous interleukin-2 for the therapy of metastatic renal cell carcinoma: an interim report. *J Clin Oncol* 1994;**12**(8):1572–1576.

140. Heywood GR, Rosenberg SA, Weber JS. Hypersensitivity reactions to chemotherapy agents in patients receiving chemoimmunotherapy with high-dose interleukin 2. *J Natl Cancer Inst* 1995;**87**(12):915–922.

141. Margolin KA, Rayner AA, Hawkins MJ, et al. Interleukin-2 and lymphokine-activated killer cell therapy of solid tumors: analysis of toxicity and management guidelines. *J Clin Oncol* 1989;**7**(4):486–498.

142. Rosenberg SA, Lotze MT, Yang JC, et al. Prospective randomized trial of high-dose interleukin-2 alone or in conjunction with lymphokine-activated killer cells for the treatment of patients with advanced cancer. *J Natl Cancer Inst* 1993;**85**(8):622–632.

143. Law TM, Motzer RJ, Mazumdar M, et al. Phase III randomized trial of interleukin-2 with or without lymphokine-activated killer cells in the treatment of patients with advanced renal cell carcinoma. *Cancer* 1995;**76**(5):824–832.

144. Figlin RA, Thompson JA, Bukowski RM, et al. Multicenter, randomized, phase III trial of CD8(+) tumor-infiltrating lymphocytes in combination with recombinant interleukin-2 in metastatic renal cell carcinoma. *J Clin Oncol* 1999;**17**(8):2521–2529.

145. Negrier S, Perol D, Ravaud A, et al. Do cytokines improve survival in patients with metastatic renal cell carcinoma (MRCC) of intermediate prognosis? Results of the prospective randomized PERCY Quattro trial. *J Clin Oncol (Meet Abstr)* 2005;**23**(16 Suppl):LBA4511.

146. Daliani DD, Papandreou CN, Thall PF, et al. A pilot study of thalidomide in patients with progressive metastatic renal cell carcinoma. *Cancer* 2002;**95**(4):758–765.

147. Eisen T, Boshoff C, Mak I, et al. Continuous low dose thalidomide: a phase II study in advanced melanoma, renal cell, ovarian and breast cancer. *Br J Cancer* 2000;**82**(4):812–817.

148. Motzer RJ, Berg W, Ginsberg M, et al. Phase II trial of thalidomide for patients with advanced renal cell carcinoma. *J Clin Oncol* 2002;**20**(1):302–306.

149. Hernberg M, Virkkunen P, Bono P, Ahtinen H, Maenpaa H, Joensuu H. Interferon alfa-2b three times daily and thalidomide in the treatment of metastatic renal cell carcinoma. *J Clin Oncol* 2003;**21**(20):3770–3776.

150. Rini BI, Halabi S, Taylor J, Small EJ, Schilsky RL. Cancer and Leukemia Group B 90206: A randomized phase III trial of interferon-alpha or interferon-alpha plus anti-vascular endothelial growth factor antibody (bevacizumab) in metastatic renal cell carcinoma. *Clin Cancer Res* 2004;**10**(8):2584–2586.

151. Spigel DR, Hainsworth JD, Sosman JA, et al. Bevacizumab and erlotinib in the treatment of patients with metastatic renal carcinoma (RCC): update of a phase II multicenter trial. *J Clin Oncol (Meet Abstr)* 2005;**23**(16 Suppl):4540.

152. Motzer RJ, Michaelson MD, Redman BG, et al. Activity of SU11248, a multitargeted inhibitor of vascular endothelial growth factor receptor and platelet-derived growth factor receptor, in patients with metastatic renal cell carcinoma. *J Clin Oncol* 2006;**24**(1):16–24.

153. Motzer RJ, Rini BI, Michaelson MD, et al. Phase 2 trials of SU11248 show antitumor activity in second-line therapy for patients with metastatic renal cell carcinoma (RCC). *J Clin Oncol (Meet Abstr)* 2005;**23**(16 Suppl):4508.

154. Faivre S, Delbaldo C, Vera K, et al. Safety, pharmacokinetic, and antitumor activity of SU11248, a novel oral multitarget tyrosine kinase inhibitor, in patients with cancer. *J Clin Oncol* 2006;**24**(1):25–35.

155. Ahmad T, Eisen T. Kinase inhibition with BAY 43-9006 in renal cell carcinoma. *Clin Cancer Res* 2004;**10**(18 Pt 2):6388S–6392S.

156. Wilhelm SM, Carter C, Tang L, et al. BAY 43–9006 exhibits broad spectrum oral antitumor activity and targets the RAF/MEK/ERK pathway and receptor tyrosine kinases involved in tumor progression and angiogenesis. *Cancer Res* 2004;**64**(19):7099–7109.

157. Escudier B, Szczylik C, Eisen T, et al. Randomized phase III trial of the Raf kinase and VEGFR inhibitor sorafenib (BAY 43–9006) in patients with advanced renal cell carcinoma (RCC). *J Clin Oncol (Meet Abstr)* 2005;**23**(16 Suppl):LBA4510.

158. Strumberg D, Richly H, Hilger RA, et al. Phase I clinical and pharmacokinetic study of the novel Raf kinase and vascular endothelial growth factor receptor inhibitor BAY 43–9006 in patients with advanced refractory solid tumors. *J Clin Oncol* 2005;**23**(5):965–972.

159. Awada A, Hendlisz A, Gil T, et al. Phase I safety and pharmacokinetics of BAY 43–9006 administered for 21 days on/7 days off in patients with advanced, refractory solid tumours. *Br J Cancer* 2005;**92**(10):1855–1861.

160. Moore M, Hirte HW, Siu L, et al. Phase I study to determine the safety and pharmacokinetics of the novel Raf kinase and VEGFR inhibitor BAY 43–9006, administered for 28 days on/7 days off in patients with advanced, refractory solid tumors. *Ann Oncol* 2005;**16**(10):1688–1694.

161. Atkins MB, Hidalgo M, Stadler WM, et al. Randomized phase II study of multiple dose levels of CCI-779, a novel mammalian target of rapamycin kinase inhibitor, in patients with advanced refractory renal cell carcinoma. *J Clin Oncol* 2004;**22**(5):909–918.

162. Rosen LS, Gordon D, Tchekmedyian S, et al. Zoledronic acid versus placebo in the treatment of skeletal metastases in patients with lung cancer and other solid tumors: a phase III, double-blind, randomized trial–the Zoledronic Acid Lung Cancer and Other Solid Tumors Study Group. *J Clin Oncol* 2003;**21**(16):3150–3157.

163. Lipton A, Colombo-Berra A, Bukowski RM, Rosen L, Zheng M, Urbanowitz G. Skeletal complications in patients with bone metastases from renal cell carcinoma and therapeutic benefits of zoledronic acid. *Clin Cancer Res* 2004;**10**(18 Pt 2):6397S–6403S.

164. Lipton A, Zheng M, Seaman J. Zoledronic acid delays the onset of skeletal-related events and progression of skeletal disease in patients with advanced renal cell carcinoma. *Cancer* 2003;**98**(5):962–969.

165. Saad F, Lipton A. Zoledronic acid is effective in preventing and delaying skeletal events in patients with bone metastases secondary to genitourinary cancers. *BJU Int* 2005;**96**(7):964–969.

166. McNutt RA. Shared medical decision making: problems, process, progress. *JAMA* 2004;**292**(20):2516–2518.

167. Loprinzi CL, Johnson ME, Steer G. Doc, how much time do I have? *J Clin Oncol* 2003;**21**(9 Suppl):5–7.

168. Himelstein BP, Jackson NL, Pegram L. The power of silence. *J Clin Oncol* 2003;**21**(9 Suppl):41.

169. Atzpodien J, Wandert T, Reitz M. Age does not impair the efficacy of immunochemotherapy in patients with metastatic renal carcinoma. *Crit Rev Oncol Hematol* 2005;**55**(3):193–199.

170. Motzer RJ, Bacik J, Mariani T, Russo P, Mazumdar M, Reuter V. Treatment outcome and survival associated with metastatic renal cell carcinoma of non-clear-cell histology. *J Clin Oncol* 2002;**20**(9):2376–2381.

171. Mai KT, Landry DC, Robertson SJ, et al. A comparative study of metastatic renal cell carcinoma with correlation to subtype and primary tumor. *Pathol Res Pract* 2001;**197**(10):671–675.

172. Delahunt B, Eble JN. Papillary renal cell carcinoma: a clinicopathologic and immunohistochemical study of 105 tumors. *Mod Pathol* 1997;**10**(6):537–544.

173. Cheville JC, Lohse CM, Zincke H, Weaver AL, Blute ML. Comparisons of outcome and prognostic features among histologic subtypes of renal cell carcinoma. *Am J Surg Pathol* 2003;**27**(5):612–624.

174. Matz LR, Latham BI, Fabian VA, Vivian JB. Collecting duct carcinoma of the kidney: a report of three cases and review of the literature. *Pathology* 1997;**29**(4):354–359.

175. Gollob JA, Upton MP, DeWolf WC, Atkins MB. Long-term remission in a patient with metastatic collecting duct carcinoma treated with taxol/carboplatin and surgery. *Urology* 2001;**58**(6):1058.

176. Cheville JC, Lohse CM, Zincke H, et al. Sarcomatoid renal cell carcinoma: an examination of underlying histologic subtype and an analysis of associations with patient outcome. *Am J Surg Pathol* 2004;**28**(4):435–441.

177. Cangiano T, Liao J, Naitoh J, Dorey F, Figlin R, Belldegrun A. Sarcomatoid renal cell carcinoma: biologic behavior, prognosis, and response to combined surgical resection and immunotherapy. *J Clin Oncol* 1999;**17**(2):523–528.

178. Nanus DM, Garino A, Milowsky MI, Larkin M, Dutcher JP. Active chemotherapy for sarcomatoid and rapidly progressing renal cell carcinoma. *Cancer* 2004;**101**(7):1545–1551.

179. Abratt RP. A "Good Death" revisited in the context of doctor-patient relationships. *J Clin Oncol* 2003;**21**(9 Suppl):97.

180. Gazelle G. A good death: not just an abstract concept. *J Clin Oncol* 2003;**21**(9 Suppl):95–96.

181. Higginson I, Wade A, McCarthy M. Palliative care: views of patients and their families. *BMJ* 1990;**301**(6746):277–281.

182. Gertz MA, Bauer BA. Caring (really) for patients who use alternative therapies for cancer. *J Clin Oncol* 2003;**21**(9 Suppl):125–128.

183. Davis MP, Davis DD, Smith ML, Cooper K. Just whose autonomy is it? *J Clin Oncol* 2003;**21**(9 Suppl):67–69.

184. Maher ER, Webster AR, Richards FM, et al. Phenotypic expression in von Hippel-Lindau disease: correlations with germline VHL gene mutations. *J Med Genet* 1996;**33**(4):328–332.

185. Friedrich CA. Genotype-phenotype correlation in von Hippel-Lindau syndrome. *Hum Mol Genet* 2001;**10**(7):763–767.

186. Cohen AJ, Li FP, Berg S, et al. Hereditary renal-cell carcinoma associated with a chromosomal translocation. *N Engl J Med* 1979;**301**(11):592–595.

187. van Kessel AG, Wijnhoven H, Bodmer D, et al. Renal cell cancer: chromosome 3 translocations as risk factors. *J Natl Cancer Inst* 1999;**91**(13):1159–1160.

188. Woodward ER, Clifford SC, Astuti D, Affara NA, Maher ER. Familial clear cell renal cell carcinoma (FCRC): clinical features and mutation analysis of the VHL, MET, and CUL2 candidate genes. *J Med Genet* 2000;**37**(5):348–353.

189. Teh BT, Giraud S, Sari NF, et al. Familial non-VHL non-papillary clear-cell renal cancer. *Lancet* 1997;**349**(9055):848–849.

190. Zbar B, Glenn G, Lubensky I, et al. Hereditary papillary renal cell carcinoma: clinical studies in 10 families. *J Urol* 1995;**153**(3 Pt 2):907–912.

191. Schmidt L, Duh FM, Chen F, et al. Germline and somatic mutations in the tyrosine kinase domain of the MET proto-oncogene in papillary renal carcinomas. *Nat Genet* 1997;**16**(1):68–73.

192. Zhuang Z, Park WS, Pack S, et al. Trisomy 7-harbouring non-random duplication of the mutant MET allele in hereditary papillary renal carcinomas. *Nat Genet* 1998;**20**(1):66–69.

193. Wei MH, Toure O, Glenn G, et al. Novel mutations in FH and expansion of the spectrum of phenotypes expressed in families with hereditary leiomyomatosis and renal cell cancer. *J Med Genet* 2006;**43**:18–27.

194. Tomlinson IP, Alam NA, Rowan AJ, et al. Germline mutations in FH predispose to dominantly inherited uterine fibroids, skin leiomyomata and papillary renal cell cancer. *Nat Genet* 2002;**30**(4):406–410.

195. Malchoff CD, Sarfarazi M, Tendler B, et al. Papillary thyroid carcinoma associated with papillary renal neoplasia: genetic linkage analysis of a distinct heritable tumor syndrome. *J Clin Endocrinol Metab* 2000;**85**(5):1758–1764.

196. Khoo SK, Bradley M, Wong FK, Hedblad MA, Nordenskjold M, Teh BT. Birt-Hogg-Dube syndrome: mapping of a novel hereditary neoplasia gene to chromosome 17p12-q11.2. *Oncogene* 2001;**20**(37):5239–5242.

197. Vocke CD, Yang Y, Pavlovich CP, et al. High frequency of somatic frameshift BHD gene mutations in Birt-Hogg-Dube-associated renal tumors. *J Natl Cancer Inst* 2005;**97**(12):931–935.

198. Khoo SK, Kahnoski K, Sugimura J, et al. Inactivation of BHD in sporadic renal tumors. *Cancer Res* 2003;**63**(15):4583–4587.

199. Junker K, Weirich G, Moravek P, et al. Familial and sporadic renal oncocytomas—a comparative molecular-genetic analysis. *Eur Urol* 2001;**40**(3):330–336.

200. Weirich G, Glenn G, Junker K, et al. Familial renal oncocytoma: clinicopathological study of 5 families. *J Urol* 1998;**160**(2):335–340.

201. Szabo J, Heath B, Hill VM, et al. Hereditary hyper-parathyroidism-jaw tumor syndrome: the endocrine tumor gene HRPT2 maps to chromosome 1q21-q31. *Am J Hum Genet* 1995;**56**(4):944–950.

202. Tan MH, Teh BT. Renal neoplasia in the hyperparathyroidism-jaw tumor syndrome. *Curr Mol Med* 2004;**4**(8):895–897.

203. Lohse CM, Cheville JC. A review of prognostic pathologic features and algorithms for patients treated surgically for renal cell carcinoma. *Clin Lab Med* 2005;**25**(2):433–464.

11j
Trends in Medical Management of Renal Cell Cancer

Bernard Escudier

Introduction

Considerable progress has been made in the treatment of renal cell carcinoma (RCC) in the past few years, as demonstrated in the previous chapters. Early diagnosis has been greatly improved, due to new imaging techniques, such as spiraled computed tomography (CT) scans, magnetic resonance imaging (MRI), and positron emission tomography (PET) scanning. Histopathological classifications were reviewed in 2004, and new pathological entities have been described with the help of molecular biology. Treatment of localized tumors is evolving to less aggressive methods, and treatment of metastatic disease is moving from the cytokine era to the targeted agents period. Prognostic factors for both localized and metastatic diseases have been reported, making it possible to better predict patient outcome. New molecular factors have been described and will have to be incorporated in future staging systems, as already proposed by the UCLA group.[1] In this chapter, some future perspectives are outlined.

Classification of Renal Cell Carcinoma

A new classification for RCC was described in 2004. This classification still relies on a histopathological description, with clear cell carcinoma remaining the most common kidney cancer. The major role of vascular endothelial growth factor (VEGF) mutation in this disease has been extensively studied and has led to new targeted therapies that appear to be very promising. Considerable effort has been expended in identifying proteins whose expression is regulated by VEGF: hypoxia-inducible factor (HIF), VEGF receptors, and epidermal growth factor (EGF) receptors have been found to be relevant targets for new treatments. This pathway is still under investigation and should lead to novel agents

in the future. However, histopathology is not sufficient to predict outcome based on classical criteria such as size, grade, tumor necrosis, or vascular invasion. The recognition of the prognostic value of new biomarkers such as carbonic anhydrase CAIX (or G250) or pTEN might help in the near future to better classify these tumors.

Papillary tumors (type I and II), the second cause of renal cancer, are also better understood, and descriptions of several gene mutations in this disease, such as cMet or fumarate hydratase, should allow new therapeutic approaches to be developed in this now well-recognized entity. Despite recent efforts, some tumors remain unclassified, meaning that new tools still have to be developed to improve the pathological classification.

Treatment of Localized Tumors

Although radical nephrectomy remains the gold standard for the treatment of large kidney tumors, even metastatic ones,[2,3] minimal invasive approaches have been extensively developed in the past 10 years. Partial nephrectomy (or nephron-sparing surgery) was initially developed in solitary kidneys. After more than 10 years of follow-up, this technique appears to be safe, with similar carcinological results at 10 years. Thus, partial nephrectomy has now become the standard treatment for tumors less than 4 cm in size, with excellent long-term results. During the same period of time, laparoscopic surgery has become popular. It is now widely used for radical nephrectomy, and its utilization for partial nephrectomy, although still reserved for experimental groups, has increased. It is anticipated that this laparoscopic approach will become the standard treatment for most tumors in the future. New "miniinvasive" techniques, such as radiofrequency or cryoablation, are under evaluation, but preliminary data are encouraging. More follow-up will be necessary before these techniques can be routinely used.

Prognostic Factors

Prognostic factors for RCC have been extensively described in the past decade, and many models for predicting the outcome of RCC have been reported. Most of these models use histopathogy and clinical or biological variables and allow better stratification of both localized and metastatic diseases. The UCLA staging system is the only one to propose a model suitable for both situations. Incorporation of new biomarkers is ongoing, and preliminary data from UCLA suggest that some of these markers, such as CAIX, circulating endothelial cells, may be relevant.[4] However, these sophisticated techniques will probably not be used for many years due to the lack of an easy method to measure them in routine practice. Whether these factors will eventually become useful remains questionable, although tremendous efforts are currently ongoing in large institutions.

Prognostic factors for metastatic renal cell carcinoma (MRCC) are currently being studied by an international kidney staging group, sponsored by the Kidney Cancer Association. This new staging system should be available soon and will help in obtaining a worldwide consensus concerning this disease. However, these prognostic factors will apply to patients treated in the cytokine era. Whether the same factors will be applicable with the new targeted agents is still unclear, and will have to be investigated.

Treatment of Metastatic Disease

Cytokine-Based Therapy

Interleukin 2 (IL-2) and interferon (IFN) were the standard treatment for MRCC in 2005. However, recent studies might change the way patients will be offered these treatments.

- Bolus intravenous IL-2 is the gold standard in the United States. This treatment, despite its toxicity, provides some long-lasting complete remissions. However, no study has ever been able to demonstrate that this treatment provides any benefit in terms of survival over subcutaneous IL-2 as well as over IFN.[4] Based on these considerations, IL-2 should be reserved for patients with good physical status, and probably for those in the good prognostic groups. Recent studies from the Cytokine Working Group show that high expression of CAIX is a good predictor of response to IL-2.[4] The same group also described some pathological features that could help to better determine which patients are the most likely to respond to treatment.[5] A specific study aiming to validate these predictors for response will soon begin in the United States, and might help to determine if high dose IL-2 will remain a standard treatment for MRCC in selected patients.
- A recent study reported at the American Society of Clinical Oncology (ASCO) 2005 by Negrier et al.[6] studied the role of IL-2 and IFN in the intermediate prognostic group, as defined by the French group.[7,8] In this study, called the Percy Quattro study, patients were randomized between medroxyprogesterone acetate, IL-2, IFN, and a combination of both cytokines. This study has failed to demonstrate any survival benefit of IL-2 or IFN in the patients who do not receive these cytokines over those who do receive them. Thus, continuing to give those patients cytokines has become questionable, and should be considered only on a case-by-case basis.
- Finally, the triple regimen of IL-2, IFN, and 5-fluorouracil (5-FU) (the so-called Atzpodien regimen) is still under investigation. This regimen, very popular in the 1990s, has not been validated outside Germany, despite some positive randomized trials. A large study is currently ongoing throughout the United Kingdom and the European Agency for the Treatment of Cancer (EORTC) comparing this triple regimen to IFN. If this study turns out to be positive, the role of this treatment will have to be reconsidered. If not, this combination may no longer be used.

Targeted Agents

A better understanding of the physiology of clear cell carcinoma has led in the past years to a new generation of drugs, aiming at targeting the VEGF/HIF pathway. Through the interaction with the VEGF pathway, these drugs block angiogenesis and could induce either tumor shrinkage and/or tumor necrosis, leading to a delay in tumor growth. The decrease in tumor vascularization has been observed by different radiological approaches including Doppler ultrasound[9] and dynamic CT scans.[10] Results from studies with these new agents have recently been reported and offer new strategic options for patients with MRCC.

- Sorafenib (BAY 43-9006) is a multitarget tyrosine kinase inhibitor that interacts with many receptors on the VEGF pathway, mainly VEGF R2 and platelet-derived growth factor (PDGF). This oral drug has shown promising activity and a good safety profile in MRCC in Phase I/II trials. Recently, Escudier et al. reported[11] the results of a large randomized study, called the Treatment Approaches in Renal Cancer Global Evaluation Trial (TARGET), in patients who had failed a first-line treatment. In this 903 patient study, patients were randomized between sorafenib (400 mg bid) and placebo. Tumor shrinkage has been observed in a large majority of patients and progression-free survival (PFS) has been significantly improved from 3 to 6 months ($p < 0.0001$). Survival data show that patients treated with sorafenib have a 39% increase in overall survival (OS) compared to placebo.[12] This difference is not yet statistically significant since it did not reach the O'Brien–Fleming boundary for significance. A final analysis will be performed after 540 deaths. The efficacy of sorafenib as a first-line treatment in MRCC is currently under investigation through a randomized Phase II trial comparing sorafenib 400 mg bid to IFN, 9 million × 3/week. Data from this study are expected to be available soon.

- SU11248 (sunitinib) is another multitargeted tyrosine kinase inhibitor that has activity in MRCC. Motzer et al.[13,14] reported the results from two consecutive Phases II trialsin more than 160 patients with MRCC who failed first-line cytokine-based therapy. In these studies, high response rates with sunitinib, at 50 mg daily for 4 weeks followed by a 2-week rest period, have been consistently observed around 40%, with an overall survival around 16 months. The activity of this promising drug has been confirmed through a large Phase III trial comparing sunitinib with IFN in untreated patients. In this 750 patient study,[15] PFS was 5 months in the IFN arm compared to 11 months in the sunitinib arm (p <0.000001). In this study, a high response rate was confirmed with 37% of the patients obtaining a partial response by Response Evaluation Criteria in Solid Tumors (RECIST) criteria versus 9% for IFN. As for the Treatment Approaches in Renal Cancer Global Evaluation Trial (TARGET) study, preliminary data on OS show a difference in the curves of survival that is not yet statistically significant. Although sunitinib has been developed with an intermittent dosing, there is a strong rationale to block angiogenesis in a continuous manner. Recently, data with a continuous dosing of 37.5 mg have been presented.[16] The response rate was 14.6%.
- AG013736 is the third drug reported by Rini et al.[17] with impressive activity in 52 patients (a 46% response rate). As with the previous drug, this targeted agent is an oral drug with a good safety profile. The activity of this drug needs to be confirmed in larger randomized studies.
- Bevacizumab (Avastin) is an antibody against VEGF. This drug significantly improves PFS,[18] at a dose of 10 mg/kg every 2 weeks compared to placebo in patients failing high-dose IL-2. In combination with erlotinib and gefitinib, promising response rates have been reported.[19] However, a recent randomized study has failed to show the benefit of the addition of erlotinib over bevacizumab alone in untreated patients.[20] It should be noted that in this randomized Phase II study, PFS with bevacizumab is 8.5 months, which might reflect the good activity of the drug in a first line setting. The results of two large randomized studies in untreated MRCC comparing a combination of IFN and bevacizumab to IFN alone or IFN with a placebo should help to better determine the role of this antibody in the treatment of RCC.
- Temsirolimus (CCI 779) is a mammalian target of rapamycin (mTOR) inhibitor, acting directly on HIF production, a driver for the VEGF pathway. The activity of this drug was reported by Atkins et al. in 2004.[21] Recently, the results of a large Phase III trial in MRCC

patients with poor risk features were reported.[22] In this 626 patient study, IFN, 9–18 million × 3/week, has been compared to temsirolimus alone at 25 mg intravenously weekly and temsirolimus 15 mg intravenously weekly combined with IFN, 6 million × 3/week. OS was significantly better with temsirolimus alone than with IFN, with a 49% improvement from 7.3 to 10.9 months (p = 0.0069); the combined arm did not demonstrate better OS than IFN alone. It must be emphasized that this study was restricted to a group of patients with poor risk characteristics, and thus the activity of this drug will have to be confirmed in the good and intermediate prognostic groups.

Another pathway has been explored in MRCC, the EGF pathway. Despite several negative trials with EGF inhibition as monotherapy, a combination of both VEGF and EGF inhibition has been tested, based on a good scientific rationale. After initial encouraging results in Phase II,[19] two recent randomized studies have been reported that may terminate the further development of this pathway in RCC. The first one[20] failed to show any benefit of adding erlotinib to bevacizumab in a randomized Phase II trial. Still more disappointing are the data presented by Ravaud et al.[23] with lapatinib. A large Phase III trial comparing lapatinib and hormone therapy in cytokine-refractory patients did not show any benefit in time to progression or in OS. However, in patients with high EGF expression, a significant benefit in OS was observed, leaving the question of the potential benefit of inhibition of EGF in selected patients open.

Conclusions

In conclusion, treatment of MRCC is currently moving from the cytokine era to the targeted agent era. Both sorafenib (Nexavar) and sunitinib (Sutent) have recently been approved by the Food and Drug Administration (FDA) and the European Agency for the Evaluation of Medicinal Products (EMEA), and are becoming the standard of care. Temsirolimus (Torisel) should also be approved in the future based on this large randomized study showing survival benefits.

However, many questions remain. The role of cytokines in a selected group of patients still remains, particularly in reaching complete durable remissions that are not obtained with targeted agents. A combination of these agents, either together or with cytokines, has a strong rationale. Many ongoing studies are investigating such combinations. Finally, the benefit of sequential treatment with several targeted agents is still unclear. A single prospective study has been reported so far[24] showing that sunitinib has good activity in patients refractory to bevacizumab.

In addition, new agents will arise that will target one of the receptors or one of the proteins involved in the VEGF/HIF pathway, providing the expectation of future advances.

References

1. Lam JS, Leppert JT, Figlin RA, Belldegrun AS. Role of molecular markers in the diagnosis and therapy of renal cell carcinoma. Urology 2005;66(5 Suppl):1–9.

2. Flanigan RC, Salmon SE, Blumenstein BA et al. Nephrectomy followed by interferon alfa-2b compared with interferon alfa-2b alone for metastatic renal-cell cancer. N Engl J Med 2001;345(23):1655–1659.

3. Mickisch GH, Garin A, van Poppel H et al. Radical nephrectomy plus interferon-alfa-based immunotherapy compared with interferon alfa alone in metastatic renal-cell carcinoma: a randomised trial. Lancet 2001;358(9286): 966–970.

4. McDermott DF, Regan MM, Clark JI et al. Randomized phase III trial of high-dose interleukin-2 versus subcutaneous interleukin-2 and interferon in patients with metastatic renal cell carcinoma. J Clin Oncol 2005;23(1):133–141.

5. Upton MP, Parker RA, Youmans A, McDermott DF, Atkins MB. Histologic predictors of renal cell carcinoma response to interleukin-2-based therapy. J Immunother 2005;28(5): 488–495.

6. Negrier S, Perol D, Ravaud A et al. Do cytokines improve survival in patients with metastatic renal cell carcinoma (MRCC) of intermediate prognosis? Results of the prospective radomized PERCY Quattro trial. J Clin Oncol 2005;23:380s (abstract 4511).

7. Negrier S, Escudier B, Lasset C et al. Interleukin-2, interferon or both in 425 patients with metastatic renal cell cancer: results of a multicenter randomized trial. N Engl J Med 1998;338:1272–1278.

8. Negrier S, Escudier B, Gomez F et al. Prognostic factors of survival and rapid progression in 782 patients with metastatic renal carcinomas treated by cytokines: a report from the groupe français d'immunothérapie. Ann Oncol 2002;13:1460–1468.

9. Lamuraglia M, Lassau N, Chami L et al . Doppler ultrasonography with perfusion software and contrast agent injection as a tool for early evaluation of metastatic renal cancers treated with the Raf kinase and VEGFR inhibitor: a prospective study. J Clin Oncol 2005;23:380s (abstract 3069).

10. Rixe O, Meric J, Bloch J et al. Surrogate markers of activity of AG-013736, a multi-target tyrosine kinase receptor inhibitor, in metastatic renal cell cancer (RCC). J Clin Oncol 2005;23:380s (abstract 3003).

11. Escudier B, Szczylik C, Eisen T et al. Randomized phase III trial of the Raf kinase and VEGFR inhibitor sorafenib (BAY 43–9006) in patients with advanced renal cell carcinoma (RCC). J Clin Oncol 2005;23:380s (abstract 4510).

12. Escudier B, Szczylik C, Eisen T et al. Randomized phase III trial of the multikinase inhibitor sorafenib (BAY43–9006) in patients with advanced renal cell carcinoma (RCC). Eur J Cancer 2005;3:226 (abstract 794).

13. Motzer RJ, Michaelson MD, Redman BG et al. Activity of SU11248, a multitargeted inhibitor of vascular endothelial growth factor receptor and platelet-derived growth factor receptor, in patients with metastatic renal cell carcinoma. J Clin Oncol 2006;24 (1):16–24.

14. Motzer RJ, Rini BI, Bukowski RM et al. Sunitinib in patients with metastatic renal cell carcinoma. JAMA 2006;295(21):2516–2524.

15. Motzer RJ, Hutson TE, Tomczak P et al. Phase III randomized trial of sunitinib malate (SU11248) versus interferon-alfa (IFN-α) as first-line systemic therapy for patients with metastatic renal cell carcinoma (mRCC). J Clin Oncol 2006;24:18S (abstract LBA3).

16. Escudier B, Roigas J, Gillessen S et al. Continuous daily administration of sunitinib malate (SU11248). A phase II study in patients (pts) with cytokine-refractory metastatic renal cell carcinoma (mRCC). ESMO 2006, Istanbul, Turkey (abstract 4360).

17. Rini B, Rixe O, Bukowski R et al. AG-013736, a multi-target tyrosine kinase receptor inhibitor, demonstrates anti-tumor activity in a phase 2 study of cytokine-refractory, metastatic renal cell cancer (RCC). J Clin Oncol 2005;23:380s (abstract 4509).

18. Yang JC, Haworth L, Sherry RM, Hwu P, Schwartzentruber DJ, Topalian SL, Steinberg SM, Chen HX, Rosenberg SA. A randomized trial of bevacizumab, an anti-vascular endothelial growth factor antibody, for metastatic renal cancer. N Engl J Med 2003;349(5):427–434.

19. Hainsworth JD, Sosman JA, Spigel DR et al. Treatment of metastatic renal cell carcinoma with a combination of bevacizumab and erlotinib. J Clin Oncol 2005;23(31):7889–7896.

20. Bukowski R, Kabbinavar F, Figlin R et al. Results of a randomised phase II trial of bevacizumab +/- erlotinib in mRCC. J Clin Oncol 2006;24:18S (abstract 4523).

21. Atkins MB, Hidalgo M, Stadler WM et al. Randomized phase II study of multiple dose levels of CCI-779, a novel mammalian target of rapamycin kinase inhibitor, in patients with advanced refractory renal cell carcinoma. J Clin Oncol 2004;22(5):909–918.

22. Hudes G, Carducci M, Tomczak P et al. A phase 3, randomized, 3-arm study of temsirolimus (TEMSR) or interferon-alpha (IFN) or the combination of TEMSR + IFN in the treatment of first-line, poor-risk patients with advanced renal cell carcinoma (adv RCC). J Clin Oncol 2006;24:18S (abstract LBA4).

23. Ravaud A, Gardner J, Hawkins R et al. Efficacy of Tykerb (lapatinib) in patients with high tumor EGFR expression: results of a phase III trial in advanced renal cell cancer (RCC). J Clin Oncol 2006;24:18S (abstract 4502).

24. Rini BI, George DI, Michaelson MD et al. Efficacy and safety of sunitinib malate in bevacizumab-refractory metastatic renal cell carcinoma. J Clin Oncol 2006;24:18S (abstract 4522).

12
Models of Human Renal Cell Carcinoma

Meaghan L. Douglas and David L. Nicol

Introduction

The dynamic and complex processes involved in tumor growth and progression are difficult to study merely by analysis of clinical specimens. Detailed investigations of the effects of tumor cytokine pathways, particularly in relation to cell cycle and function and tumor/host interactions, including metastasis, angiogenesis, and immunological responses, require model systems that can be controlled and manipulated. These systems are also often necessary to determine the effects and safety of therapeutic strategies before translation into clinical practice.

Principles of Tumor Models

The complexity of tumor biology combined with the variety of models available for cancer study makes it necessary for researchers to have a clear understanding of both the question they wish to ask and how the answer might best be found.[1,2] Within the limits of feasibility—-ethics, required skill, time, and expense—-a model must accurately and repeatedly reflect the tumor of interest, reproducing as many clinical features of the disease as possible or specifically replicating a singular process observed in clinical specimens to be important in the development, growth, progression, or treatment response of the tumor.[3,4] Although it is not possible to completely model any human tumor under experimental conditions,[3] a number of systems, used appropriately and in combination, may be powerful tools in the study of human renal cell carcinoma (RCC).

In simple terms, models are either *in vitro* (cell or tissue culture, using tissue explants, primary or established/immortalized cell lines) or *in vivo* (animal models, with spontaneous, induced, or surgically implanted tumors). There are several principles involved in selecting the most appropriate model for the proposed study (see Table 12-1), including relevance, reproducibility, and feasibility.

Relevance: The Model Must Reflect the Tumor and/or Process under Investigation

There are several aspects to the issue of relevance. As stated earlier, the ideal model would reproduce all the known clinical features of the tumor or tumor feature (e.g., a signaling cascade or metabolic pathway). For *in vitro* models, cell lines need to be characterized and shown to be highly similar, if not identical, to the tumor cells they represent, rather than expressing a different, possibly irrelevant profile of genes. The relevance of many established, widely used cell lines is now questioned: how were these cells derived decades ago and have they changed over time? A leading example is the HeLa cell line, now thought to bear little resemblance to the cancer from which it was initially derived (cervical carcinoma) and shown to have diverged into several unique strains internationally. Global gene expression analysis using microarray or similar techniques provides researchers with the means to verify the relevance of cell lines they intend to use. Direct comparisons between immortalized and primary cell lines can be made with tumor specimens, demonstrating the extent to which cultured cells still represent the tumors from which they were isolated.

For *in vivo* studies, the ideal model replicates all stages of tumor development and progression, arising spontaneously in an animal bearing physiological and genetic similarities to human patients.[4] Genetic events should involve homologous genes and response to treatment in the animal model should accurately predict efficacy and side effects in humans. However, such models are rare and human RCC is no exception.

Another relevant aspect addresses the type of model used for a study. A clear understanding of the limitations of each model system is required when deciding how to test a hypothesis.[1] The choice is not limited to *in vitro* versus *in vivo*: for example, studies of cell migration or invasive ability may both be performed *in vitro* but require different approaches. It may be necessary, even preferable, to use more than one model in an investigation. For this reason, researchers may consider establishing a range of

TABLE 12-1. Principles involved in selecting an appropriate model.

	In vitro		In vivo	
	Primary cells/tissue	Immortalized cell lines	Spontaneous or induced	Surgically implanted, xenografts
Relevance	**Moderate** Cells/tissue derived directly from human tumor	**Low** Cells may have changed over time with repeated passages	**Moderate/high** Tumors homologous to humans but no human cells/tissue involved	**High** Human cells/tissue used but in a nonhuman host
Reproducibility	**Moderate** Differences between patients lead to variability	**High** Cell lines used correctly should exhibit consistent characteristics over repeated experiments	**High** Established model should exhibit consistent characteristics over repeated experiments	**Moderate** Dependent on multiple factors, including operator, cells/tissue used, animals, environment, etc.
Ethics	**Moderate** Requires informed consent of tissue donors	**Low** For commercially available cell lines	**High** Involves animal experimentation, breeding colonies, tumor growth	**High** Involves animal experimentation, surgical procedures, tumor growth
Time	**Moderate** Limited patient availability, time to establish, only limited number of passages	**Low** Frozen stocks on hand, experiments completed over days to weeks, instantly repeatable	**High** Months to years for tumors to develop, need to breed new animals	**Moderate** Using frozen cell lines and purchased animals, tumors grow over weeks rather than months
Cost	**Moderate** Specialized staff for culture and collection of clinical specimens	**Low** Cell lines may be banked for future use, basic equipment and reagents	**High** Breeding colonies and months/years of housing, specialized staff	**Moderate** Using frozen cell lines, shorter housing times, specialized staff
Skill	**Moderate** Experience needed for primary tissues/cells and interactions with tissue donors	**Low** Basic tissue culture techniques	**Moderate** Basic animal husbandry and vivisection	**High** Difficult surgery on animals including anesthesia, resection, etc.

complementary systems, where the weaknesses associated with one technique may be answered using one or more other approaches.

In choosing between *in vitro* and *in vivo* model systems, there is an understanding that *in vivo* models may have greater clinical relevance to the tumor of interest than *in vitro* models. Animal models exhibit many aspects of tumor biology that cannot be replicated in the tissue culture environment at this time. However, with increasing clinical relevance comes increasing complexity: *in vivo* systems are more difficult to establish, operate, and interpret, affecting their reliability and feasibility, as outlined below.

Reproducibility: The Model Must Provide Predictable and Reliable Outcomes

As with any experimental procedure, confidence in the data is based on reproducibility, both within an experiment and across several repetitions of an experiment. However, biological systems, including tumor models, are known for their variability. Reliable data are based partly on the relevance of the model—an *in vivo* system is more likely to reveal real data regarding drug efficacy than an *in vitro* system—but reproducibility may be affected by the quality of experimental animals and their environment. There are many anecdotal accounts of researchers establishing a model

and then, over time, finding inconsistent results possibly related to very subtle changes in breeding stock, housing, diet, personnel, and so on. Similarly, a model established in one laboratory may prove impossible or unreliable in another.

The simplicity of *in vitro* systems offers more control and therefore more reliable data, but possibly less confidence in how those data may be applied to the clinical situation. Regardless of the type of model chosen, reproducibility can be improved by keeping techniques as simple and methodical as possible and ensuring consistency in the source, type, and use of all reagents, consumables, cell lines, and animals. Modifications in any component or procedure must be introduced carefully and with forethought, while changes, even subtle ones, must be documented and their possible impact on the data considered.

Feasibility: The Model Must Be Chosen with Respect to Time, Cost, and Ethical Issues

As discussed earlier, complex models may provide greater relevance but present researchers with other challenges, including ethical considerations, long experimental timeframes, and increased costs. The decision to use an *in vivo* model is not an easy one.

The welfare of experimental animals is paramount in any *in vivo* model design and ethical concerns may rule out certain types of models due to unacceptable levels of pain and distress.[1,5] For example, the use of death as an endpoint is no longer acceptable, making survival curve analyses inappropriate in studying possible treatment regimes. Some researchers or research institutions may find it difficult to justify their involvement in animal experimentation or the use of certain types of animal, such as primates or companion animals (e.g., dogs and cats). Rodents are more accepted as experimental animals, but their relevance to humans and human diseases may, at times, be limited.

In an increasingly competitive research environment, the costs involved in using *in vivo* models may also be prohibitive.[1] Researchers must be highly skilled and diligent in order to successfully complete an *in vivo* study, sometimes spending hours at daily tasks such as monitoring and drug administration. This may require experienced specialist or additional personnel, a cost burden for any laboratory. Animal models may require weeks, months, or years to reach statistically relevant endpoints, requiring expensive maintenance over that time. In particular, spontaneous tumor models require breeding colonies and many months or years for tumors to progress from normal tissue to precancerous lesions to invasive phenotypes. These limitations almost ensure such models are established only in rats or mice, small, social animals able to be housed in relatively large numbers in limited space, with easily met environmental and behavioral requirements and rapid breeding cycles with large litter numbers. *In vivo* models where tumors are induced or surgically implanted are less costly and provide faster results, but again, may require highly trained personnel to establish and maintain. Additionally, the efficacy and/or toxicity of a drug designed for use in humans may not be demonstrated adequately in some *in vivo* models due to differences in metabolism, pharmacokinetic properties, gene expression, and so on.

Therefore, *in vitro* models offer significant advantages in terms of feasibility, enabling high-throughput study at lower cost and over shorter time periods, with fewer ethical concerns. Deriving novel lines from tissue explants is a challenging exercise involving advanced tissue culture techniques and interactions with patients, who must give their informed consent as part of the tissue donation process, and their healthcare providers, who will be concerned to ensure the process of sample collection does not have any negative impact on the health of their patient. Established cell lines, particularly those available commercially or from colleagues, usually require minimal skill, equipment, and approvals (ethical or in regard to genetic modification).

Models of Renal Cell Carcinoma

As mentioned earlier, there are two broad categories into which models may be grouped—*in vitro* and *in vivo*—within which variations in technique and approach offer different means of studying the cancer of interest. Selecting the model most likely to yield useful, verifiable data is an important but difficult process. It is crucial to understand the limitations of each model system and how they affect the subsequent interpretation of findings.[1]

In Vitro Models of Renal Cell Carcinoma

The use of tissue culture-based models in the study of RCC offers, as outlined above, advantages in terms of feasibility and reliability of data. *In vitro* models are suited to answering specific questions under highly controlled conditions. Various aspects of tumor cell biology can be tested *in vitro*, including cell growth and death, migration, adhesion, response to treatment substances, and expression of responsive genes. However, the tissue culture environment lacks clinical relevance: cells in culture do not necessarily "behave" as they would *in vivo*. The influence of culture media, conditions, and culture vessel plastics can be difficult to predict and define.

Established or Immortalized Cell Lines

Researchers may choose between studying primary cells/tissues or established cell lines, each with their own advantages and disadvantages (see Table 12-1). Traditionally, much of the *in vitro* research into cancers like RCC has relied on established or immortalized cell lines available either commercially or by agreement with the laboratory that first isolated them. There is a limited number of well-described, immortalized RCC cell lines from both human and animal sources, available through commercial suppliers, such as the American Type Culture Collection (ATCC) or European Collection of Cell Cultures (ECACC) or from research institutes such as the Memorial Sloan-Kettering Cancer Center of New York (see Table 12-2). The most common cell lines—Caki-1 and Renca, for example—have been used extensively over many years to study RCC.[6–11] In recent times, the provenance of cell lines established decades before has become the topic of debate: how relevant are these cell lines to the tumors they are meant to represent? Many were isolated from metastatic lesions, in some cases, distant sites unusual for RCC. The SN12K-1 cell line,[12] for instance, is known to have been derived from a skin metastasis, whereas RCC is more commonly found in the lungs, viscera, and brain. Other concerns include incomplete documentation on how the cells were derived and handled; if they represent a single homogeneous population of cells; if the cells are truly tumor cells or overgrown populations of fibroblasts or a contaminating cell line like HeLa;[13] whether they have been exposed to potentially harmful infectious agents, such bovine spongiform encephalitis (BSE), human immunodeficiency virus (HIV), or hepatitis; and the extent to which they have been characterized and shown to represent the tumors from which they were derived.

TABLE 12-2. Established RCC or RCC-like cell lines described in the literature.

Cell line	Species	RCC type	Collection	Notes
Caki-1	Human	Clear cell	ATCC: HTB-46	Isolated from metastatic site (skin), 49-year-old male Caucasian patient
Caki-2	Human	Clear cell	ATCC: HTB-47 ECACC: 93120819	Isolated from primary renal tumor, 69-year-old male Caucasian patient
ACHN	Human	Fibroblast?	ECACC: 88100508	Derived from pleural effusion of 22-year-old male patient with metastatic renal adenocarcinoma
RAG	Mouse	Adenocarcinoma	ATCC: CCL-142 ECACC: 89040605	Derived from renal-2a BALB/cd renal adenocarcinoma
Renca	Mouse	Murine renal adenocarcinoma	No longer available from ATCC or ECACC	Derived from spontaneous renal tumor in BALB/c mouse[8]
SK-RC-series	Human	Various	Memorial Sloan-Kettering Cancer Center, New York	Several lines established from primary and metastatic tumors[59]
SMKT-R- series	Human	Clear cell?	Private	See Miyao et al.[15]
RBM1	Human	Metastatic RCC	Private	Isolated from metastatic site (bone), 59-year-old male patient[17] Histological subtype probably PRCC, due to presence of trisomy of chromosome 7 and constitutive expression of c-Met protooncogene
NCI group	Human	Various	Private	See Anglard et al.[60]

[a]RCC, renal cell carcinoma; ATCC, American Type Culture Collection; ECACC, European Collection of Cell Cultures; PRCC, papillary renal cell carcinoma.

For immortalized cell lines, either spontaneous mutation or induction of cell immortality may change key characteristics of the cells. Gene expression profiles may change, leading to findings that prove irrelevant in patients. This concern has led to the suggestion that whole genome assessments of cell lines should be carried out using microarray technology. The extent to which a cell line remains representative of the tumor from which it was originally derived may be evaluated by comparing the gene expression profiles of each cell line against those observed in whole tumors.

Primary Cell Lines and Tissue Explants

An alternative to using established cell lines is to use primary isolates instead. The disadvantages are many. Primary cell cultures can be difficult to establish and usually last only a few passages. This introduces a reliance on the availability of resected, tumor-affected kidneys or metastatic lesions as well as the understanding, generosity, and cooperation of patients, surgeons, pathologists, and clinicians. Comparing data from several primary cell lines can be difficult as each tumor is likely to yield highly variable cell populations, an important consideration in RCC as these tumors are typically heterogeneous. Despite these problems, primary cell lines are more directly relevant and capable of demonstrating important principles in tumor cell biology and response to proposed treatment strategies.[14,15] That is, they are highly similar to the original tumor.

The establishment of primary cell lines may provide the opportunity for the generation of new immortalized lines of RCC where the concerns listed earlier in regard to provenance and relevance may be controlled and tested. Given the spectrum of histological subtypes of RCC,[16] such as clear cell and papillary forms, as well as metastatic sites,[17] the isolation and immortalization of new RCC cell lines should be considered a priority. This would allow researchers to study and compare the differing underlying genetic mechanisms and cytokine expression patterns associated with each RCC subtype or metastatic lesion, improving treatment options and outcomes.

Applications

There is a broad scope for study of in vitro assays using established/immortal and/or primary cell lines. Cell proliferation and death (cytotoxicity, apoptosis, etc.) may be studied using techniques ranging from traditional visual counting of viable cells to colorimetric detection of metabolic or apoptotic by-products to radioisotopic labeling of DNA synthesis during cell replication.[6] Cellular properties that may contribute to tumor growth or metastasis, such as migration, adhesion, and invasion, are frequently tested and studied in vitro using a variety of both simple and sophisticated techniques. Tumor cells may be cocultured with stromal cells to observe chemotactic responses and invasion of interceding membranes or substrates such as Matrigel® may also be observed. In vitro systems are suited for high-throughput and automated analyses and large volume production of tumor antigens for vaccine research. Genetic manipulation—overexpression, silencing, and mutation—is readily possible in cell lines and phenotypical outcomes may be studied. Lastly, cell lines used for in vitro studies may also be used in vivo and vice versa. Xenograft animal models provide an in vivo platform to study cell lines following in vitro work. This may be needed to verify data obtained from tissue culture experiments that remain consistent in the in vivo environment.[6,7,9,17] Further, tumor cells in an animal model—either xenograft or spontaneous—may be isolated and established as cell lines for study *in vitro*, providing opportunities to dissect out individual characteristics for detailed investigation.[15,17,18]

Monolayer Culture

Regardless of the type of cell used, it must be understood that the tissue culture flask differs enormously from the physiological environment in which cells grow. Tumor cells grown in monolayers often do not express proteins observed in tumor sections, particularly proteins involved in cellular interactions, like cell adhesion molecules (e.g., E-cadherin and integrins). This is not a desirable state in which to study tumor cells: they may respond to agents quite differently under these conditions or be more sensitive to apoptotic triggers, distorting our understanding of their strengths and weaknesses.

Spheroid Culture

A new method has been developed to address these problems: multicellular spheroids allow adherent cells to grow in a three-dimensional fashion, albeit still under artificial culture conditions. As the spheroids are able to be fixed and embedded in the same way as tissue samples, immunohistochemical analysis has shown cells grown in this manner express proteins in locations and proportions similar to that shown *in vivo*.[19] Cells grown in monolayers shown to be acutely sensitive to common therapeutic approaches—chemotherapy, radiotherapy, and immunotherapy—display a more resistant, and therefore more relevant, phenotype when grown in spheroids.[19] Although the spheroid technique is more technically challenging and involves labor-intensive analysis, it may allow RCC cells to retain more relevant patterns of gene expression than traditional monolayer culture.[9,20–22] Another drawback is that treatment agents may not penetrate the spheroid adequately or evenly, so this technique may not have widespread application for RCC research but is certainly an interesting new development.

In Vivo Models of Renal Cell Carcinoma

Despite the difficulties involved, animal models remain an essential tool in efforts to better understand and treat cancer.[23,24] The most useful type of animal model for any human disease arises spontaneously and demonstrates the same or very similar clinical and histopathological features and outcomes.[4] Unfortunately, renal neoplasms are rare in most domesticated species. While they are observed more often in pigs, dogs,[25,26] and cats than rabbits and rodents,[27,28] research involving either large livestock animals or animals commonly kept as companions in society have considerable ethical and feasibility issues.

An alternative to the spontaneous animal model of RCC are those models that result from genetic or chemical manipulation, leading to the development of renal cancers. Strains of rat or mouse known to develop spontaneous renal tumors may be used in studies of carcinogens, where loss of heterozygosity (LOH) of a single wild-type allele as a result of chemically induced gene inactivation leads to the appearance of tumors in the kidney. However, studies may also utilize wild-type mice to examine the carcinogenicity of certain compounds and these studies have identified potent renal carcinogens that may be used to induce spontaneous tumors in mice with no known predilection for RCC.

A similar type of model involves the use of genetic manipulation to generate transgenic animals susceptible to renal tumor development. Genes may be overexpressed, silenced, or mutated either transiently or transgenically to study their involvement in normal development and susceptibility to RCC.

The advantages of induced models include a level of control and specificity not available in spontaneous animal models, and, in common with spontaneous models, immune responses may be preserved. However, data from such models are limited by lack of relevance to the clinical situation, the artificial means by which tumor development is triggered and the difficulty involved in developing transgenic animals.

The last and now most widely used form of animal model for studying cancer is the xenograft model, where human tumor cells are implanted in immunocompromised/immunodeficient mice for study *in vivo*.[23,24] Implantation may be either orthotopic—-that is, human tumor cells or tissue may be implanted in the physiologically relevant organ—-or heterotopic, such as subcutaneous implantation. While orthotopic xenografts are considered to have greater clinical relevance than subcutaneous/heterotopic xenografts,[23,24] they are not always possible or feasible: the relevant organ may differ substantially in the animal host compared to human physiology (e.g., human prostate compared to mouse prostate) or the orthotopic site may be technically challenging or ethically unacceptable. Despite their limitations, subcutaneous xenografts continue to provide valuable data in preclinical trials of anticancer drugs.

Xenografts may be achieved using single-cell suspensions of cultured tumor cell lines or by directly implanting pieces of tumor harvested from human patients or other host animals. While the latter method tends to retain many of the architectural, morphological, and genetic/molecular features of the tumor from which it was derived, the likelihood of successful engraftment—-so-called "tumor take"—-is lower compared to cell suspension injections, where poorly differentiated or undifferentiated xenograft tumors are more typical.[24] The advantages and disadvantages of immortalized/established cell lines compared with primary isolates are inherited by these contrasting methods of tumor implantation: xenografts resulting from injections of cultured cells are more likely to be unrepresentative of the tumors from which they were derived due to genetic changes over repeated passages *in vitro* and following the change in environment from *in vitro* to *in vivo*.[24]

Another elegant feature of the xenograft exploits the subtle differences between human and host animal genetic sequences. DNA/RNA and protein studies can be designed to distinguish the expression of human genes/proteins and those of the host, establishing the extent to which stromal components influence or react to tumor growth and vice versa.[12, 29] The advantages and disadvantages of each type of *in vivo* model dictate their usefulness in studies of RCC, including how each model will perform and the quality of the data they yield.

Spontaneous Animal Tumors

Despite the infrequency with which renal cancer arises in rodents, certain inbred strains of rats and mice have proved useful for RCC research (see Table 12-3).

Inactivation of the von Hippel–Lindau (vHL) gene is observed in the majority of clear cell RCC and appears to be the underlying mechanism in the commonest form of hereditary RCC.[30] vHL disease is also associated with the development of tumors in the eye, central nervous system, pancreas, and kidney.[30] vHL inactivation has been observed in over 60% of sporadic RCCs, but there is currently no animal model that reproduces susceptibility to renal neoplasms as a result of mutations in animal homologues of the vHL gene. Mice with one inactive allele for Vhl (the murine homolog of vHL) show no increase in the incidence of renal cancers compared with wild-type mice, even when exposed to known renal carcinogens,[31–33] and homozygous

Vhl mutation is embryonically lethal in rodents.[30, 31, 34] Other human diseases associated with a higher incidence of renal neoplasms include tuberous sclerosis complex (TSC), associated with mutations in the TSC1 and TSC2 genes that encode hamartin and tuberin, respectively;[35, 36] Birt–Hogg–Dubé (BHD) syndrome, related to inactivation of the BHD gene and loss of its protein product, folliculin;[35, 36] hereditary papillary renal cell carcinoma (HPRCC), associated with mutations in the gene for the hepatocyte growth factor (HGF) receptor protein, c-met; and hereditary leiomyomatosis and renal cell carcinoma (HLRCC) syndrome, resulting from mutations in the fumarate hydratase (FH) gene.[35, 36]

Eker Rat

The first animal model of inherited RCC to be described and studied was by Eker in 1954.[37] The original mutation arose spontaneously in an inbred strain of Wistar rats that demonstrated a high incidence of bilateral, multiple renal adenomas inherited in an autosomal-dominant fashion.[33, 36–39] The tumors arise from proximal tubular epithelial cells of the rat kidney, progressing from preneoplastic abnormalities to adenomas and carcinomas. While the Eker rat renal tumors are not histopathologically clear cell RCCs, but are described as chromophilic lesions,[33, 40] they demonstrate extensive neovascularization.

The Eker mutation was later found to result from the inactivation of a single tumor suppressor gene named Tsc2, the rat/mouse homolog of the human tuberous sclerosis complex

TABLE 12-3. Genetic forms of renal cell carcinoma (RCC) and known animal models.

Gene	Protein	Human disease	Animal models
VHL	pVHL	von Hippel–Lindau (vHL) disease Renal lesions: RCC (clear cell), renal cysts Other: hemangioblastomas of central nervous system (CNS) and eyes, pheochromocytomas, pancreatic cysts	None vHL[+/−] mice phenotypically normal Embryonic stem cell teratoma analysis[34]
TSC-1 TSC-2	Hamartin Tuberin	Tuberous sclerosis complex (TSC) Autosomal-dominant disease Renal lesions: RCC (clear cell, papillary, chromophobe and oncocytic), renal angiomyolipomas, polycystic kidney disease (PKD), renal oncocytomas, hamartomas Other: hamartomas of the brain, skin, and heart, mental retardation, seizures, autism	Eker rat:[35, 36] Tsc2[+/Ek] Renal lesions: RCC, renal cysts Other: uterine leiomyoma, lesions in brain and spleen Mice: Tsc1[+/−] and Tsc2[+/−] Renal lesions: RCC Other: liver lesions
BHD	Folliculin	Birt–Hogg–Dubé (BHD) syndrome Autosomal-dominant disease Renal lesions: RCC (chromophobe, oncocytic, clear cell and papillary) Other: benign skin tumors, lung cysts, spontaneous pneumothorax	Nihon rat:[18] Bhd[+/NR] Renal lesions: RCC RCND dog:[36] BHD[+/mut] Renal lesions: RCC Other: skin nodules, uterine leiomyoma
FH	Fumarate hydratase	Hereditary leiomyomatosis and renal cell cancer (HLRCC) Renal lesions: RCC (papillary) Other: skin and uterine leiomyoma	None at this time
PRCC/TFE3 fusion	PRCCTFE3 fusion protein	Subset of papillary RCC (PRCC) with Xp11.2 abnormalities	Frog[61] Specific for interactions between PRCC and Mad2B proteins
Other/unknown	–	Forms of RCC associated with other or as yet unknown underlying genetic changes	Renca murine model, RCC xenografts, etc.[4]

2 (TSC2) gene.[33,38,40] Homozygosity for the Eker mutation is embryonically lethal and heterozygotes develop normally, but inherit a predisposition for the development of neoplasms in the kidney, uterus, and spleen.[40] Renal neoplasms are the most common manifestation with complete penetrance within the first year of life.[40] Although disruption of TSC2, and its related gene TSC1, is known to cause TSC in humans, and this disease is associated with several renal lesions that include RCCs, the low incidence of RCC and the mixed RCC types observed in TSC patients suggest TSC mutations are not as important in the development of human RCC as other genetic defects, such as vHL inactivation.[35]

Knudson used the Eker rat to confirm his "two-hit" hypothesis for the actions of tumor suppressor genes. Heterozygotes (Tsc2$^{+/Ek}$) exposed to renal carcinogens demonstrate LOH in the wild-type allele, leading to loss of tuberin synthesis and renal neoplastic development.

The Eker rat has proven to be a useful model for testing carcinogens,[38,40] but perhaps lacks relevance as a model for human RCC. While the initiating mutation in the Eker rat does not represent that most often observed in human RCC, the model may still be useful for preclinical studies of new treatment modalities. The most common forms of RCC—clear cell and papillary—arise from proximal tubule cells of the kidney: Eker mutation-associated renal tumors in rats and mice also arise from proximal tubule cells.[33,40] Furthermore, studies suggest the downstream effects of TSC loss of function are similar to those observed in VHL mutants—dysregulation of hypoxia inducible factor-α (HIF-α) and increased expression of vascular endothelial growth factor (VEGF)[33,35]—while other similarities have been described, including a higher incidence in males compared to females, overexpression of transforming growth factor-β (TGF-β), and frequent mutations of the p53 gene.[40]

Nihon Rat

Similarly, the Nihon rat is an animal model for BHD syndrome, with inactivating mutations in the rat homolog of the BHD gene.[18] Again, the predisposition for renal tumors is inherited in an autosomal dominant fashion with complete penetrance for RCC by 6 months. Homozygosity is embryonically lethal and heterozygotes demonstrate LOH of the wild-type Bhd allele in renal lesions. Unlike the Eker rat, Nihon rat renal tumors are predominantly clear cell or papillary RCCs,[18] but again, mutation of BHD in human RCC is uncommon.[35] Lastly, an animal model for spontaneous BHD mutation-associated RCC has been described in the German Shepherd breed of dog;[36] for reasons discussed earlier, the feasibility of using such a model is low.

While these spontaneous familial animal models of RCC have many disadvantages, including lack of direct clinical relevance to human tumors and manipulability, these animals do exhibit the full spectrum of tumor development and growth, from precancerous to cancerous lesions. Furthermore, these animals have intact immune systems, enabling studies

of the role immunity plays in inhibition or regression of tumor growth.[4] This is an important point: at this time, the only successful therapeutic regimes approved for the treatment of advanced RCC are based on immunotherapy, using either interferon-α (IFN-α) or interleukin-2 (IL-2).[41–44]

Immunotherapy relies on activation of antitumoral responses normally lacking in RCC due in part to aberrant expression of human leukocyte antigen (HLA) class I and II molecules.[45] IFN-α has been shown to directly inhibit RCC proliferation in vitro and to stimulate host mononuclear cells, but it is also thought to inhibit RCC growth by upregulating the expression of required HLA molecules. IL-2 promotes activation of both T cells and natural killer (NK) cells. Athymic nude mice are congenitally unable to produce T cells; SCID mice cannot produce functional B and T cells due to mutations affecting T cell receptor and immunoglobulin assembly, but retain NK cells, antigen-presenting cells, and normal myeloid cells. Therefore, the efficacy of agents such as IFN-α and IL-2 is limited in immunocompromised/immunodeficient mice and studies of similar immunogenic strategies require animals with intact immune systems.

Induced Models

As mentioned earlier, Eker and Nihon rats may be used in studies of carcinogens, where LOH of the single wild-type allele as a result of chemically induced gene inactivation leads to the appearance of tumors in the kidney.[33,38,40,46] Wild-type mice may also be used to examine the carcinogenicity of certain compounds: studies have identified potent renal carcinogens able to induce spontaneous tumors in mice with no known predilection for RCC.

RCC may also be induced in animals by genetically introducing defects that give rise to tumors in a manner similar to that observed in spontaneous models. The Eker mutation has been reproduced by inactivating the murine homologs for the TSC1 and TSC2 genes (Tsc1 and Tsc2) in wild-type mice, which subsequently develop RCC and hemangiomas of the liver. Furthermore, such transgenic models may target mutations to specific cell populations/tissues/organs or genetic changes may also be placed under the control of inducible promoters to selectively activate or silence genes for study. This may be a more accurate model for sporadic RCC and permits in vivo studies of the effects of embryonically lethal mutations, such as the homozygous vHL knockout, in adult animals.

Xenograft Models—Subcutaneous Implants

The rate at which a tumor grows and how this rate responds to potential treatment strategies are probably two of the most basic questions asked when studying cancer. The subcutaneous xenograft model provides a relatively noninvasive means of measuring tumor growth or regression. By implanting tumor cells or tissue into the subcutaneous space of the mouse flank, repeated measurements of implant size can be made using callipers.[6,7,9,10,24] These models are relatively simple *in vivo* systems and require very little surgical skill to establish. As with all xenograft models, host animals must be immunodeficient/immunocompromised to prevent rejection of the human tumor material. Athymic nude mice are often used as the hairless skin improves visibility of the implanted tumor, but subcutaneous xenografts are also commonly implanted in SCID mice.

While the animal provides an *in vivo* environment in which the growing tumor forms recognizable architectural features, including neovascularization, and allows systemic dosing of drugs, the subcutaneous space does not replicate the environment in which solid tumors such as RCC routinely develop.[1] Many subcutaneous models fail to produce metastases;[1,24] the biological milieu may not match that of the kidney or distant sites such as the lung or viscera. Some studies revealed tumors grown subcutaneously were sensitive to agents that were subsequently found to have no clinical effect: the lack of effect was then confirmed using orthotopic xenograft tumors, demonstrating that subcutaneous tumors may be significantly different from both primary and secondary tumors in the host.[1,24] However, subcutaneous xenografts remain important in preclinical evaluations of novel anticancer treatments aimed at either reducing tumor size (cytotoxic) or slowing tumor growth (cytostatic). For therapeutic strategies targeting processes such as metastasis or angiogenesis, orthotopic xenograft models, or models involving specialized tumor inoculation techniques, are more appropriate.

Orthotopic Xenograft Models

There is evidence to suggest the microenvironment in which a tumor grows influences the genes expressed by tumor cells, the most compelling being microarray studies showing differential gene expression profiles in primary and secondary neoplasms.[23,24,47–49] Implanting tumor cells or tissue into the relevant organ therefore provides a greater degree of clinical relevance.[1,9,23,24] For RCC models, the kidney is not only relevant but relatively easy to work with compared to tumors affecting other organs.[8,9] The kidney is accessible, large, and easily recognized. The blood supply to and from the organ can be temporarily suspended by means of clamps or permanently to allow for nephrectomy. The renal capsule is tough enough to be punctured and made to trap either cells in suspension or minced pieces of tumor tissue without splitting or rupturing. The kidney itself has the capacity to have large pieces of tissue or large volumes of cells implanted directly into the cortex without causing the organ to fail. Lastly, the presence of a contralateral kidney offers researchers an internal control organ as well as redundancy to support normal renal function regardless of damage to or dysfunction of the implanted kidney. While the surgical techniques involved require more skill than is needed in *in vitro* models or subcutaneous

implants, with training, elegant and sophisticated orthotopic models can be established.

Unlike spontaneous models, orthotopic xenografts replicate the later stages of advanced, invasive disease. Local invasion and metastasis are common features,[8,24] although it is sometimes necessary to resect the primary tumor to allow secondary tumors time to develop.[1] As stated above, the kidney is relatively easy to isolate and remove surgically: primary xenografts approaching ethical endpoints (e.g., 1 cm^3 or 10% of the total body weight) may be surgically removed from the animal without compromising normal kidney function, thus extending the time period in which occult metastases may develop into patent lesions.

There are considerable disadvantages to these models.[1,23] It is difficult to monitor or visualize the rate of tumor growth or regression and data tend to be collected only at the time of cull. In addition to the technical challenges, the presence of tumors in the kidney/abdominal compartment and systemic dissemination to vital organs such as the lungs is ethically sensitive. Animals must be carefully monitored for signs of distress or suffering and culled for humane reasons when these welfare issues cannot be avoided.[24] Natural biological variability can confound the data and larger numbers of mice may be required to generate clear, unambiguous results. Orthotopic models are not immune from the phenomenon observed in many subcutaneous tumor models, where researchers in preclinical trials were misled as to the efficacy of a drug or treatment regimen.[1,24]

Some of these disadvantages of orthotopic xenografts may soon be a thing of the past with the introduction of new technologies. By inducing tumor cells to express a fluorescent protein, such as luciferase or green fluorescent protein (GFP), primary tumor growth and dissemination may now be monitored using noninvasive means.[1,23] Positron emission tomography (PET) imaging, magnetic resonance imaging (MRI), and other noninvasive methods of estimating solid tumor growth are also improving how orthotopic models may be utilized.[1,23] The use of such methods is not widespread due to cost and restricted access to such equipment,[1] particularly for immunocompromised animals usually housed in specific pathogen-free (SPF) environments,[23] but efforts to monitor realtime tumor progression *in vivo* continue.

Models for Specific Processes not Related to Primary Tumor Growth or Response to Treatment

Subcutaneous xenograft models rarely metastasize, while orthotopic models frequently exhibit metastatic behavior.[24] While the pattern of metastatic spread is often clinically relevant, involving sites and progressions similar to those observed in humans, it is not always possible to study metastasis in an orthotopic xenograft model. Frequently, the rate at which the primary xenograft grows is too rapid and the host animal must be euthanized before metastasis has occurred or before the secondary tumors are microscopically visible postmortem. As mentioned earlier, nephrectomy of the implanted kidney may provide time for relevant metastatic development, but the process of tumor cell dissemination, implantation, and growth in remote sites can be modeled *in vivo* without the involvement of a primary tumor. Such models are usually referred to as experimental metastasis models, compared to the spontaneous metastasis observed following xenograft implantation.

The usual method of introducing single cell suspensions of cultured tumor cells directly into the circulation of the host animal has been intravenous injection using an easily accessible major vein, such as the tail vein in rodents. Extensive pulmonary metastases have been observed following tail vein injection of various cancer cell lines, including RCC.[1,50,51] As lung metastases are the most common secondary tumors observed in RCC patients, tail vein injection models have been widely used and continue to be used in studying the metastatic potential of cells and the efficacy of antimetastatic treatment strategies. However, there is evidence to suggest these models do not accurately reflect the metastatic properties of all cancer cells. Intravenous injection via the tail vein inevitably leads to tumor cells passing through and becoming trapped in the pulmonary capillary bed before encountering other organs/tissues in the body.[52,53] While introduction of tumor cells via retroorbital injection is a faster, easier method compared to tail vein injection, the resulting dissemination pattern is probably no different from that seen in tail vein-injected animals.[54]

The rapid growth of multiple tumors in the lungs is thought to force euthanasia of the host animal before lesions in other sites become patent.[1] The alternative is to introduce tumor cells to the circulation via systemic intraarterial injection or directly into the left ventricle.[34,52,53,55] These methods are more technically demanding, requiring skill and experience to ensure tumor cells are implanted correctly while avoiding potentially fatal complications in the host animal, such as cardiac tamponade, hemorrhage, and embolism.

Specific sites of metastasis may require the directed implantation of tumor cells in the site of interest. Metastases are known to occur in bone in many tumors, including RCC, but lesions may not develop in animal models in a timely fashion either spontaneously from orthotopic xenografts or experimentally via induced hematogenous dissemination. Direct intratibial injection of tumor cells has been used to establish models for the study of bony metastases in several types of tumor, including RCC.[17] Again, this method is technically challenging: correct, efficient inoculation of the tibia requires skill and experience and noninvasive follow-up during tumor growth requires access to radiological facilities. Furthermore, tumor growth in bone requires greater attention to animal welfare issues: close monitoring of animals is required throughout the experiment.

Clear cell RCC is a notoriously angiogenic solid tumor. The processes underlying neovascularization in RCC may be studied using an orthotopic xenograft model, but for quantitative experiments of antiangiogenic potential, it may be preferable to use a heterotopic *in vivo* model. The improved dorsal air sac assay described by Funahashi et al.[56] has been used in quantifiable *in vivo* evaluations of antiangiogenic therapies for several types of cancer, including RCC.[57] The method involves subcutaneous implantation of a filter chamber in which tumor cells are cultured *in vitro*. Introduction of radiolabeled red blood cells enables comparisons to be made between animals receiving pretreated or untreated tumor cells for the extent to which neovascularization occurs in the area of skin over the implant.

A last example of a model designed to examine specific features of tumors is that described by Rathmell et al. in the study of vHL-mediated tumorigenesis.[34] Conventional animal model studies were not possible due to the embryonic lethality of the homozygous vHL mutation. Rathmell et al. used $Vhl^{-/-}$ murine embryonic stem cells in both *in vitro* and *in vivo* studies to examine the effects of missense mutation of the vHL protein.[34] Teratoma analysis permits examination of three-dimensional cell growth by implanting embryonic stem cells subcutaneously in immunodeficient mice, a blend of *in vitro* and *in vivo* models described earlier.

Conclusions

With roles in both fundamental research into tumor biology and development of new or improved therapeutic strategies, *in vitro* and *in vivo* models of cancer, including RCC, continue to contribute enormously to cancer research worldwide. Exciting new technologies are expanding the scope and potential of cancer models. Combined with a greater understanding of the strengths and limitations of various model techniques, the ability to use models effectively in cancer research is constantly improving.

The most noticeable changes in cancer models include a greater emphasis on the use of *in vitro* models and significant advances in the ethical use of *in vivo* models. Animal welfare concerns remain paramount in the design and use of animal models. Wherever possible, the principles of replacement, reduction, and refinement must be applied. There are now extensive means of investigating many aspects of tumor biology and antineoplastic responses using *in vitro* methods. However, while this has reduced the need for animal models, preclinical trials of both efficacy and safety are not wholly achievable *in vitro*.[1,2,23,24] The *in vivo* model remains a critical step in the drug development process.

The importance of data gained from tumor models, particularly *in vivo* models, requires researchers to thoroughly evaluate and understand the techniques they intend to use. Models and every component used in the model must be as completely characterized as is possible before major studies begin. Variables inherent in each model and each technique should be considered, as described in Table 12-4: the types of model used; relevance, reliability, and feasibility; whether to use primary or immortalized cell lines; whether the cells

TABLE 12-4. Variables to be considered in tumor models.[2,23,24]

Variable	Considerations
Model type	*In vitro, in vivo,* specialized technique, relevance, reproducibility, feasibility
Cell lines	Primary/transient, established/immortalized, human vs. nonhuman
Primary isolates, biopsies	Primary tumor or metastatic site, common or rare type
Immortalized cell lines	Genetic changes due to immortalization and repeated passage
Implantation site	Subcutaneous, heterotopic, orthotopic, other
Endpoints	Humane, relevant, informative, achievable
Statistical relevance	Numbers of animals or replicates, appropriate controls
Presence of feature/target	Gene/protein/feature of interest expressed and functional
Treatment agent	Formulation of agent, delivery, bioavailability, appropriate for humans
Treatment timing	Treatment onset is appropriate for relevant stage of human disease
Postexperimental samples	Method of collection, storage, downstream analysis

or tumor tissue represent the tumor under investigation; and experimental design with respect to endpoints, replicates, clinical relevance, and how samples will be collected, stored, and used effectively and without compromising data. Some of the considerations may be subtle and difficult to predict—-e.g., the bioavailability, efficacy, and toxicity of a drug formulated for use in humans administered *in vitro* or to rodents or whether use of an anesthetic for experimental animal euthanasia will compromise downstream sample analysis—-but without careful planning and forethought, data emerging from tumor model studies are likely to be flawed, misleading, or dismissed.[2,24] These requirements are important core principles of any form of scientific investigation and should not dissuade researchers from using cancer models.

Several published studies on RCC utilize a combination of models to improve our understanding of these challenging and diverse tumors: the papers of Kausch et al. on Ki-67 inhibition,[8,9] the publications of Keyes et al. regarding angiogenic factors in RCC,[10,58] and the study of Rathmell et al.,[34] as mentioned earlier. There is a continuing need for new, more elegant, reliable, and relevant models of RCC to be developed and for existing models to be used in more sophisticated ways, overcoming current limitations and exploiting new technology. Certainly, if an effective means of treating advanced RCC in patients is to be identified in the near future, it will result from the collaborative and clever use of RCC model systems in laboratories dedicated to the cause.

References

1. Bibby MC. Orthotopic models of cancer for preclinical drug evaluation: advantages and disadvantages. Eur J Cancer 2004;40:852–857.

2. Suggitt M, Bibby MC. 50 years of preclinical anticancer drug screening: empirical to target-driven approaches. Clin Cancer Res 2005;11:971–981.

3. Hawk ET, Umar A, Lubet RA, Kopelovich L, Viner JL. Can animal models help us select specific compounds for cancer prevention trials? Recent Results Cancer Res 2005;166:71–87.

4. Hillman GG, Droz JP, Haas GP. Experimental animal models for the study of therapeutic approaches in renal cell carcinoma. In Vivo 1994;8:77–80.

5. Hawkins P. Recognizing and assessing pain, suffering and distress in laboratory animals: a survey of current practice in the UK with recommendations. Lab Anim 2002;36:378–395.

6. Knoll K, Wrasidlo W, Scherberich JE, Gaedicke G, Fischer P. Targeted therapy of experimental renal cell carcinoma with a novel conjugate of monoclonal antibody 138H11 and calicheamicin thetaI1. Cancer Res 2000;60:6089–6094.

7. Chagnon F, Tanguay S, Ozdal OL, Guan M, Ozen ZZ, Ripeau JS, Chevrette M, Elhilali MM, Thompson-Snipes LA. Potentiation of a dendritic cell vaccine for murine renal cell carcinoma by CpG oligonucleotides. Clin Cancer Res 2005;11:1302–1311.

8. Kausch I, Jiang H, Brocks C, Bruderek K, Kruger S, Sczakiel G, Jocham D, Bohle A. Ki-67-directed antisense therapy in an orthotopic renal cell carcinoma model. Eur Urol 2004;46:118–124; discussion 24–25.

9. Kausch I, Jiang H, Ewerdwalbesloh N, Doehn C, Kruger S, Sczakiel G, Jocham D. Inhibition of Ki-67 in a renal cell carcinoma severe combined immunodeficiency disease mouse model is associated with induction of apoptosis and tumour growth inhibition. BJU Int 2005;95:416–420.

10. Keyes K, Cox K, Treadway P, Mann L, Shih C, Faul MM, Teicher BA. An in vitro tumor model: analysis of angiogenic factor expression after chemotherapy. Cancer Res 2002;62:5597–5602.

11. Weiss JM, Shivakumar R, Feller S, Li LH, Hanson A, Fogler WE, Fratantoni JC, Liu LN. Rapid, in vivo, evaluation of antiangiogenic and antineoplastic gene products by nonviral transfection of tumor cells. Cancer Gene Ther 2004;11:346–353.

12. Douglas ML, Reid JL, Hii SI, Jonsson JR, Nicol DL. Renal cell carcinoma may adapt to and overcome anti-angiogenic intervention with thalidomide. BJU Int 2002;89:591–595.

13. O'Brien SJ. Cell culture forensics. Proc Natl Acad Sci USA 2001;98:7656–7658.

14. Kim IY, Lee DH, Lee DK, Kim BC, Kim HT, Leach FS, Linehan WM, Morton RA, Kim SJ. Decreased expression of bone morphogenetic protein (BMP) receptor type II correlates with insensitivity to BMP-6 in human renal cell carcinoma cells. Clin Cancer Res 2003;9:6046–6051.

15. Miyao N, Tsukamoto T, Kumamoto Y. Establishment of three human renal cell carcinoma cell lines (SMKT-R-1, SMKT-R-2, and SMKT-R-3) and their characters. Urol Res 1989;17:317–324.

16. Takahashi M, Yang XJ, Sugimura J, Backdahl J, Tretiakova M, Qian CN, Gray SG, Knapp R, Anema J, Kahnoski R, Nicol D, Vogelzang NJ, et al. Molecular subclassification of kidney tumors and the discovery of new diagnostic markers. Oncogene 2003;22:6810–6818.

17. Weber KL, Pathak S, Multani AS, Price JE. Characterization of a renal cell carcinoma cell line derived from a human bone

metastasis and establishment of an experimental nude mouse model. J Urol 2002;168:774–779.

18. Okimoto K, Kouchi M, Matsumoto I, Sakurai J, Kobayashi T, Hino O. Natural history of the Nihon rat model of BHD. Curr Mol Med 2004;4:887–893.

19. Sier CF, Gelderman KA, Prins FA, Gorter A. Beta-glucan enhanced killing of renal cell carcinoma micrometastases by monoclonal antibody G250 directed complement activation. Int J Cancer 2004;109:900–908.

20. Mayer B, Klement G, Kaneko M, Man S, Jothy S, Rak J, Kerbel RS. Multicellular gastric cancer spheroids recapitulate growth pattern and differentiation phenotype of human gastric carcinomas. Gastroenterology 2001;121:839–852.

21. Song H, Jain SK, Enmon RM, O'Connor KC. Restructuring dynamics of DU 145 and LNCaP prostate cancer spheroids. In Vitro Cell Dev Biol Anim 2004;40:262–267.

22. Walenta S, Doetsch J, Mueller-Klieser W, Kunz-Schughart LA. Metabolic imaging in multicellular spheroids of oncogene-transfected fibroblasts. J Histochem Cytochem 2000;48:509–522.

23. Shaw TJ, Senterman MK, Dawson K, Crane CA, Vander-hyden BC. Characterization of intraperitoneal, orthotopic, and metastatic xenograft models of human ovarian cancer. Mol Ther 2004;10:1032–1042.

24. Kelland LR. Of mice and men: values and liabilities of the athymic nude mouse model in anticancer drug development. Eur J Cancer 2004;40:827–836.

25. Khan KN, Stanfield KM, Trajkovic D, Knapp DW. Expression of cyclooxygenase-2 in canine renal cell carcinoma. Vet Pathol 2001;38:116–119.

26. Lucke VM, Kelly DF. Renal carcinoma in the dog. Vet Pathol 1976;13:264–276.

27. Rabstein LS, Peters RL. Tumors of the kidneys, synovia, exocrine pancreas and nasal cavity in BALB-cf-Cd mice. J Natl Cancer Inst 1973;51:999–1006.

28. Hard GC. Pathology of tumours in laboratory animals. Tumours of the rat. Tumours of the kidney, renal pelvis and ureter. IARC Sci Publ 1990;(99):301–344.

29. Douglas ML, Richardson MM, Nicol DL. Endothelin axis expression is markedly different in the two main subtypes of renal cell carcinoma. Cancer 2004;100:2118–2124.

30. Haase VH. The VHL tumor suppressor in development and disease: Functional studies in mice by conditional gene targeting. Semin Cell Dev Biol 2005;16(4–5):564–574.

31. Gnarra JR, Ward JM, Porter FD, Wagner JR, Devor DE, Grinberg A, Emmert-Buck MR, Westphal H, Klausner RD, Linehan WM. Defective placental vasculogenesis causes embryonic lethality in VHL-deficient mice. Proc Natl Acad Sci USA 1997;94:9102–9107.

32. Kleymenova E, Everitt JI, Pluta L, Portis M, Gnarra JR, Walker CL. Susceptibility to vascular neoplasms but no increased susceptibility to renal carcinogenesis in Vhl knockout mice. Carcinogenesis 2004;25:309–315.

33. Liu MY, Poellinger L, Walker CL. Up-regulation of hypoxia-inducible factor 2alpha in renal cell carcinoma associated with loss of Tsc-2 tumor suppressor gene. Cancer Res 2003;63:2675–2680.

34. Rathmell WK, Hickey MM, Bezman NA, Chmielecki CA, Carraway NC, Simon MC. In vitro and in vivo models analyzing von Hippel-Lindau disease-specific mutations. Cancer Res 2004;64:8595–8603.

35. Henske EP. The genetic basis of kidney cancer: why is tuberous sclerosis complex often overlooked? Curr Mol Med 2004;4:825–831.

36. Cook JD, Walker CL. The Eker rat: establishing a genetic paradigm linking renal cell carcinoma and uterine leiomyoma. Curr Mol Med 2004;4:813–824.

37. Eker R. Familial renal adenomas in Wistar rats; a preliminary report. Acta Pathol Microbiol Scand 1954;34:554–562.

38. Kleymenova E, Walker CL. Determination of loss of heterozygosity in frozen and paraffin embedded tumors by denaturing high-performance liquid chromatography (DHPLC). J Biochem Biophys Methods 2001;47:83–90.

39. Eker R, Mossige J, Johannessen JV, Aars H. Hereditary renal adenomas and adenocarcinomas in rats. Diagn Histopathol 1981;4:99–110.

40. McDorman KS, Wolf DC. Use of the spontaneous Tsc2 knockout (Eker) rat model of hereditary renal cell carcinoma for the study of renal carcinogens. Toxicol Pathol 2002;30:675–680.

41. Mancuso A, Sternberg CN. What's new in the treatment of metastatic kidney cancer? BJU Int 2005;95:1171–1180.

42. Staehler M, Rohrmann K, Bachmann A, Zaak D, Stief CG, Siebels M. Therapeutic approaches in metastatic renal cell carcinoma. BJU Int 2005;95:1153–1161.

43. Maher SG, Condron CE, Bouchier-Hayes DJ, Toomey DM. Taurine attenuates CD3/interleukin-2-induced T cell apoptosis in an in vitro model of activation-induced cell death (AICD). Clin Exp Immunol 2005;139:279–286.

44. Avigan D. Dendritic cell-tumor fusion vaccines for renal cell carcinoma. Clin Cancer Res 2004;10:6347S–6352S.

45. Bukur J, Malenica B, Huber C, Seliger B. Altered expression of nonclassical HLA class Ib antigens in human renal cell carcinoma and its association with impaired immune response. Hum Immunol 2003;64:1081–1092.

46. Patel SK, Ma N, Monks TJ, Lau SS. Changes in gene expression during chemical-induced nephrocarcinogenicity in the Eker rat. Mol Carcinog 2003;38:141–154.

47. Hao X, Sun B, Hu L, Lahdesmaki H, Dunmire V, Feng Y, Zhang SW, Wang H, Wu C, Fuller GN, Symmans WF, Shmulevich I, et al. Differential gene and protein expression in primary breast malignancies and their lymph node metastases as revealed by combined cDNA microarray and tissue microarray analysis. Cancer 2004;100:1110–1122.

48. Reinholz MM, Iturria SJ, Ingle JN, Roche PC. Differential gene expression of TGF-beta family members and osteopontin in breast tumor tissue: analysis by real-time quantitative PCR. Breast Cancer Res Treat 2002;74:255–269.

49. Yanagawa R, Furukawa Y, Tsunoda T, Kitahara O, Kameyama M, Murata K, Ishikawa O, Nakamura Y. Genome-wide screening of genes showing altered expression in liver metastases of human colorectal cancers by cDNA microarray. Neoplasia 2001;3:395–401.

50. Yamazaki S, Morita T, Endo H, Hamamoto T, Baba M, Joichi Y, Kaneko S, Okada Y, Okuyama T, Nishino H, Tokue A. Isoliquiritigenin suppresses pulmonary metastasis of mouse renal cell carcinoma. Cancer Lett 2002;183:23–30.

51. Yoshimura I, Mizuguchi Y, Miyajima A, Asano T, Tadakuma T, Hayakawa M. Suppression of lung metastasis of renal cell

carcinoma by the intramuscular gene transfer of a soluble form of vascular endothelial growth factor receptor I. J Urol 2004;171:2467–2470.

52. Basse P, Hokland P, Heron I, Hokland M. Fate of tumor cells injected into left ventricle of heart in BALB/c mice: role of natural killer cells. J Natl Cancer Inst 1988;80:657–665.

53. Arguello F, Baggs RB, Eskenazi AE, Duerst RE, Frantz CN. Vascular anatomy and organ-specific tumor growth as critical factors in the development of metastases and their distribution among organs. Int J Cancer 1991;48:583–590.

54. Price JE, Barth RF, Johnson CW, Staubus AE. Injection of cells and monoclonal antibodies into mice: comparison of tail vein and retroorbital routes. Proc Soc Exp Biol Med 1984;177: 347–353.

55. Arguello F, Baggs RB, Frantz CN. A murine model of experimental metastasis to bone and bone marrow. Cancer Res 1988;48:6876–6881.

56. Funahashi Y, Wakabayashi T, Semba T, Sonoda J, Kitoh K, Yoshimatsu K. Establishment of a quantitative mouse dorsal air sac model and its application to evaluate a new angiogenesis inhibitor. Oncol Res 1999;11:319–329.

57. Sasamura H, Takahashi A, Yuan J, Kitamura H, Masumori N, Miyao N, Itoh N, Tsukamoto T. Antiproliferative and antiangiogenic activities of genistein in human renal cell carcinoma. Urology 2004;64:389–393.

58. Keyes KA, Mann L, Sherman M, Galbreath E, Schirtzinger L, Ballard D, Chen YF, Iversen P, Teicher BA. LY317615 decreases plasma VEGF levels in human tumor xenograft-bearing mice. Cancer Chemother Pharmacol 2004;53: 133–140.

59. Ebert T, Bander NH, Finstad CL, Ramsawak RD, Old LJ. Establishment and characterization of human renal cancer and normal kidney cell lines. Cancer Res 1990;50:5531–5536.

60. Anglard P, Trahan E, Liu S, Latif F, Merino MJ, Lerman MI, Zbar B, Linehan WM. Molecular and cellular characterization of human renal cell carcinoma cell lines. Cancer Res 1992;52:348–356.

61. van den Hurk WH, Martens GJ, Geurts van Kessel A, van Groningen JJ. Isolation and characterization of the Xenopus laevis orthologs of the human papillary renal cell carcinoma-associated genes PRCC and MAD2L2 (MAD2B). Cytogenet Genome Res 2004;106:68–73.

13
Follow-Up Strategies for Renal Cell Carcinoma After Nephrectomy

Andreas Skolarikos and Gerasimos J. Alivizatos

Introduction

In the era of easily available computed tomography (CT) and ultrasound (US) imaging, the majority of patients undergoing nephrectomy for sporadic renal cell carcinoma (RCC) have incidentally detected, low-stage lesions and are cured by surgery alone (McLaughlin and Lipworth, 2000; Pantuck et al., 2001). However, approximately one-third of patients present with metastatic disease and up to 50% of those treated for localized disease develop metastases (Pantuck et al., 2001). As a consequence, an estimated 11,900 and 1450 patients die from metastatic disease annually in the United States and Canada, respectively (Jemal et al., 2003; National Cancer Institute of Canada, 2002).

No consensus exists on surveillance guidelines after radical or partial nephrectomy for local or advanced RCC. Current protocols are largely empirical and patients are followed postoperatively according to the discretion of the responsible physician with laboratory and radiological evaluations at regular intervals. Large prospective randomized studies testing the most suitable follow-up scheme for these patients are lacking and therefore the following questions still need to be answered:

1. What is the rationale for following up patients treated for RCC?
2. Should surveillance protocols be based only on tumor staging?
3. What evidence is derived from stage-based surveillance protocols after radical nephrectomy?
4. What is the optimal period that follow-up should last?
5. What are the appropriate follow-up schemes?
6. Should patients after nephron-sparing surgery or thermoablative techniques be followed differently compared to patients after radical nephrectomy?
7. How should patients with hereditary RCC be followed?

We review the literature with the intent to answer the above questions and provide a logical scheme for RCC patient follow-up.

What Is the Rationale for Following-up Patients Treated for Renal Cell Carcinoma?

Metastatic disease following surgery for RCC occurs in approximately 40% of patients, who will eventually die of cancer (McLaughlin and Lipworth, 2000). Among patients who develop metastases, 29–54% have pulmonary involvement, 16–27% have bone involvement, 2–10% have brain metastases, and 0.77–1.8% have isolated renal bed recurrences (Sandock et al., 1995; Hafez et al., 1997; Levy et al., 1998; Ljunberg et al., 1999; Stephenson et al., 2004; Gofrit et al., 2001; Fuhrman et al., 1982; Lerner et al., 1996; Itano et al., 2000; Schrodter et al., 2002). The risk of metastasis and local recurrence following radical nephrectomy appears to be related to high tumor stage and grade (Sandock et al., 1995; Hafez et al., 1997; Levy et al., 1998; Ljunberg et al., 1999; Stephenson et al., 2004; Gofrit et al., 2001; Fuhrman et al., 1982; Lerner et al., 1996; Schrodter et al., 2002; Esrig et al., 1992; Tanguay et al., 1996). However, they do occur in patients with less advanced and aggressive tumors as well (0–7% for pT1 tumors, 5.3–26.5% for pT2 tumors, 9% for grade 1 tumors, and 61% for grade 2 tumors) (Sandock et al., 1995; Hafez et al., 1997; Levy et al., 1998; Ljunberg et al., 1999; Stephenson et al., 2004; Gofrit et al., 2001; Fuhrman et al., 1982; Lerner et al., 1996). As a consequence, all patients undergoing surgery for RCC require follow-up.

Untreated local recurrence carries a poor prognosis, with 1-year survival not exceeding 14% (Frydenberg et al., 1994). Surgical resection of isolated fossa recurrences with or without adjuvant radiation or immunotherapy can lead to a 5-year cause-specific survival rate of 36–75% (Itano et al., 2000; Schrodter et al., 2002; Esrig et al., 1992; Tanguay et al., 1996; Sandhu et al., 2005; Kavolius et al., 1998). These rates are superior to the 18% and 13% 5-year cancer-specific survival of patients with solitary local recurrence who are treated with medical therapy or observation, respectively (Itano et al., 2000).

Five-year survival of patients with untreated metastatic disease has been reported to be 2.7–9% (Maldazys et al., 1986; Negrier et al., 2002). However, response rates of 5–20% have been reported with systemic immunotherapy, and encouraging results have been published for metastatic patients who fail cytokine therapy and receive either chemotherapy (Shamash et al., 2003) or antivascular endothelial growth factor antibody (Yang et al., 2003).

Five-year survival following surgery of lung metastasis (either solitary or multiple) when it represents the only site of recurrence ranges from 24% to 60% (Piltz et al., 2002). Surgical resection of isolated brain metastasis resulted in a mean survival of 13.8 months compared to 7 months when surgery is not performed (Decker et al., 1984). The average survival of patients with head and neck metastasis after surgery, radiation, or combined treatment has been reported to be 32.3 months, 19.7 months, and 20.7 months, respectively (Kent and Majumdar, 1985). Solitary metastasis of RCC to the liver is reported to occur in 5.4% of all cases with metastasis (Saitoh et al., 1982). It is unclear whether surgical resection improves survival in these patients, although a 5-year cancer-specific survival of 27% has been reported (Fujisaki et al., 1997). In the rare case in which a patient has a solitary bony metastasis surgical excision of the metastatic site leads to a 5-year survival of 13–30% (Baloch et al., 2000).

Patients who present with symptoms prior to nephrectomy have a worse prognosis compared to patients who are asymptomatic at presentation (Kim et al., 2004; Fergany et al., 2000). However, whether treatment of an asymptomatic recurrence detected on regular follow-up carries a survival advantage over treatment of recurrence detected by symptoms has not been thoroughly studied in the literature (Jansen et al., 2003). Among patients who are operated on for local recurrences, those who present with clinical symptoms have a higher rate of incomplete recurrence resection, positive surgical margins, and poorer survival (Levy et al., 1998).

The above data indicate that follow-up after nephrectomy is recommended in all patients to detect local recurrence and distant metastases as early as possible and to permit additional treatment when indicated and if possible. A discrete proportion of patients with locally recurrent or metastatic disease after nephrectomy for localized RCC will benefit from additional treatment and will eventually be cured.

Since it appears that early intervention may influence survival in low-volume metastatic RCC, it is logical to expect prospective studies in order to define whether waiting for symptoms to appear from the metastatic sites is justified or not (Levy et al., 1998).

Should Surveillance Protocols Be Based Only on Tumor Staging?

Primary tumor characteristics such as pathological stage, tumor size, histological subtype, and nuclear grade are the most important RCC prognostic factors that should be taken into consideration when constructing a surveillance protocol after nephrectomy.

The prognosis is greatly influenced by pathological tumor stage (Sandock et al., 1995; Hafez et al., 1997; Levy et al., 1998; Ljunberg et al., 1999; Stephenson et al., 2004; Gofrit et al., 2001; Tsui et al., 2000). More than 75% of patients who are operated on have organ confined disease (pT1–2), of whom 91% remain relapse free at 5 years (Table 13-1). In contrast, approximately 38% of patients with locally advanced disease (pT3a-b) relapse within 3 years postoperatively (Stephenson et al., 2004). The timing of disease relapse is also associated with pathological stage. Patients with pT3a–b disease tend to have relapse early after nephrectomy, that is, 49% and 83% of recurrences develop within 12 and 24 months postsurgery, respectively. In contrast, 40% of patients with pT1–2 develop recurrence 3 years after surgery. Patients

TABLE 13-1. Five-year cancer-specific/disease-free survival after radical/partial nephrectomy.

	5-year cancer-specific (disease-free) survival					
	pT1a	pT1b	pT2	pT3a	pT3b	*p*-value
Levy et al., 1998[a]	90%[b]		75%	60%		0.001
Ljunberg et al., 1999	95%[b]		87%	52%	37%	<0.001
Hafez et al., 1997[c]		71.4%[b]		30%	55%	0.04
Fergany et al., 2000[c] [d]	97.6%	95%	100%	85%	59%	0.007[b]
Fergany et al., 2000[c] [e]	94.5%	67%	100%	74%	23.5%	
Gofrit et al., 2001[a]	100%	97%	87%	73%[b]		NA[f]
Stephenson et al., 2004[a]	93%[b]		81%	66%	57%	<0.001

[a] Disease free.
[b] Combined results for different stages are presented.
[c] Results of partial nephrectomy series.
[d] Five-year cancer-specific survival.
[e] Ten-year cancer-specific survival.
[f] NA, not available.

with pT3a–b tumors are also at higher risk for relapse at abdominal sites (local and/or systemic relapse) compared to those with pT1–2 disease (Stephenson et al., 2004).

Although tumor grade seems to have a prognostic significance (Fuhrman et al., 1982; Tsui et al., 2000), the inability of the several grading systems to accurately predict survival or metastasis for similarly staged tumors emphasizes the fact that tumor cell differentiation is a less useful tool for prognosis (Fuhrman et al., 1982; Lerner et al., 1996; Jansen et al., 2003; Goldstein et al., 1997).

Several histological subtypes of RCC, such as collecting duct carcinoma, medullary carcinoma, or elements of sarcomatoid differentiation within the tumor, are associated with metastatic potential and decreased survival. However, the prognostic implications of the different histological differentiation of RCCs have not been identified adequately and therefore have not been used in constructing surveillance protocols (Jansen et al., 2003; Amin et al., 2002; Motzer et al., 2002).

A few authors have constructed surveillance protocols based on a combination of prognostic factors. Tumor stage, Fuhrman grade, and performance status were combined in a protocol proposed by investigators at UCLA (Zisman et al., 2002). An the Memorial Sloan–Kettering Cancer Center, Kattan et al. (2001) created a postoperative prognostic nomogram for RCC combining patient symptoms, tumor histology, size, and pathological stage. Investigators from the Mayo Clinic reviewed more than 1800 patients and created a predictive scoring system based on tumor stage, size, grade, and necrosis (SSIGN score) (Frank et al., 2002). These combinations accurately predicted the 5-year probability of treatment failure among patients with newly diagnosed RCC. Their power over the stage-specific strategy for RCC surveillance should be validated in large series and if approved they can be used for follow-up planning.

What Is the Evidence Derived from Stage-Based Surveillance Protocols after Radical Nephrectomy?

Several retrospective studies of stage-based surveillance following radical nephrectomy for localized RCC (pT1–3, N0, Nx, M0) have been published during the past decade. In all of these studies the interval to first metastasis, the site of metastasis, and the method of diagnosis were correlated with the primary tumor stage (Sandock et al., 1995; Levy et al., 1998; Ljunberg et al., 1999; Stephenson et al., 2004; Gofrit et al., 2001) (Table 13-2).

Among 629 patients with pT1 disease treated in these series, 3.2–7% developed metastases at a median time of 35–48 months (Sandock et al., 1995; Levy et al., 1998; Ljunberg et al., 1999; Stephenson et al., 2004; Gofrit et al., 2001). Of those patients who experienced recurrence 0–68.7%

developed pulmonary metastases, out of which 16.6–64% were diagnosed from their symptoms only and 81–100% by the combination of symptoms and chest X-ray. Abdominal metastases occurred in less than 1.6%, of which 0.3% were symptomatic. Bone and brain metastases were diagnosed due to symptoms.

Three hundred and one patients had pT2 disease and 14–27% of these developed metastases at a median time of 25–32 months (Sandock et al., 1995; Levy et al., 1998; Ljunberg et al., 1999; Stephenson et al., 2004; Gofrit et al., 2001). Approximately 50% of these patients developed pulmonary metastases, 11–71.4% of which were diagnosed due to symptoms. All pulmonary metastases were detected by the combination of clinical assessment and chest X-ray. Abdominal metastases occurred in 0–38.5% of the patients, 60–100% of whom had findings in the physical examination, symptoms, or abnormal serum studies, such as liver function tests. Lymph node involvement was detected in 5.8–23% of the patients. All lymph node-positive patients were asymptomatic, were diagnosed via CT scans, and had concomitant metastases at other sites (Sandock et al., 1995; Levy et al., 1998). Bone metastases developed in 17.6–45% of pT2 patients, 67–100% of whom had symptoms at presentation. All these patients were diagnosed with a combination of history, serum alkaline phosphatase, and plain skeletal X-rays. Brain metastases were rare (0–15.4%), developed at a late stage of the disease, and were all symptomatic at presentation.

Among the 351 patients with pT3 disease, 26–54% developed metastases at a median time of 11–22 months (Sandock et al., 1995; Levy et al., 1998; Ljunberg et al., 1999; Stephenson et al., 2004; Gofrit et al., 2001). More specifically, from 162 patients with pT3a disease and 108 patients with pT3b disease, 31–55% and 0–54% developed metastases at a median time of 8.2–32 months and 8–46 months, respectively. In up to 75% of 39 patients with pT3ab tumor, metastatic disease developed at a median time of 11.5–39.7 months. In general, among all the pT3 patients who experienced recurrence, 41.8–63.2% developed pulmonary metastases, of whom 4.1–75% were diagnosed due to symptoms. All pulmonary metastases were detected by a combination of clinical assessment and chest X-ray. Abdominal metastases occurred in 13.9–42.1% of patients, 73.3–100% of whom had findings in the physical examination, symptoms, or abnormal serum studies. Lymph node involvement was detected in 11.6–26.3% of patients. All lymph node-positive patients were asymptomatic, were diagnosed via CT scans, and had concomitant metastases at other sites (Sandock et al., 1995; Levy et al., 1998). Bone metastases developed in 16.27–26.5% of patients, 57–100% of whom had symptoms at presentation. All patients were diagnosed with the combination of history, serum alkaline phosphatase, and plain films. Brain metastases were rare (4.4–11.1%), developed at a late stage of the disease, and were all symptomatic at presentation.

TABLE 13-2. Data derived from stage-based surveillance after radical nephrectomy.

		Sandock et al., 1995[a]	Levy et al., 1998	Ljunberg et al., 1999	Gofrit et al., 2001	Stephenson et al., 2004
Number of patients	pT1	19	113	70	124	303
	pT2	82	64	43	26	84
	pT3	36	109	48	50	108
Recurrence (%)	pT1	0	7	7	3.2	5
	pT2	14.6	27	14	23	16.6
	pT3	52.8	39	54	26	34.25
Median (range) time to recurrence (months)	pT1	–	38 (18–67)	43 (27–60)	48 (22–64)	35 (2–93)
	pT2	29.5 (3.5–97)	32 (3–115)	29.5 (3–144)	28.2 (6–64)	25 (3–95)
	pT3	22 (3–138)	17 (2–88)	17 (2–62)	19.8 (4–55)	11 (1–102)
Pulmonary metastases (total/symptomatic) (%)	pT1	0 (–)	50 (0)	54.5[b] (16.6)	NA[c]	68.7 (64)
	pT2	53.8 (71.4)	52.9 (11)	54.5 (16.6)	NA	NA
	pT3	63.2 (75)	41.8 (11)	53.3 (4.1)	NA	NA
Median (range) time to diagnosis of pulmonary metastases (months)	pT1	–	53 (30–67)	8.5 (3–60)[b]	NA	NA
	pT2	39.6 (6.9–96.6)	31 (4–67)	8.5 (3–60)[b]	NA	NA
	pT3	26.4 (3–138)	14 (5–59)	17 (2–62)	NA	NA
Abdominal metastases (total/symptomatic)[d] (%)	pT1	0 (–)	0 (–)	0 (–)	NA	1.6 (0.3)
	pT2	38.5 (92.3)	29.4 (60)	0 (–)	NA	1.8 (100)
	pT3	42.1 (92.3)	34.8 (73.3)	20 (100)	NA	13.9 (73.3)
Median (range) time to diagnosis of abdominal metastases (months)	pT1	–	–	–	NA	NA
	pT2	12 (3.5–29)	68 (53–83)		NA	NA
	pT3	7.6 (3–18.2)	23.5 (5–67)	13 (3–20)	NA	NA
Bone metastases (total/symptomatic) (%)	pT1	0 (–)	25 (100)	45 (100)[b]	NA	NA
	pT2	38.5 (100)	17.6 (67)	45 (100)[b]	NA	NA
	pT3	26.5 (100)	16.27 (57)	22.2 (100)	NA	NA
Median (range) time to diagnosis of bone metastases (months)	pT1	–	38.5 (35–42)	40 (8–144)[b]	NA	NA
	pT2	37 (3.8–97)	24 (3–115)	40 (8–144)[b]	NA	NA
	pT3	19.8 (3.8–40.5)	7 (3–65)	14.5 (6–36)	NA	NA
Brain metastases (total/symptomatic) (%)	pT1	0 (–)	12.5 (100)	0 (–)	NA	NA
	pT2	15.4 (100)	5.8 (100)	0 (–)	NA	NA
	pT3	11.1 (100)	9.3 (100)	4.4 (100)	NA	NA
Median (range) time to diagnosis of brain metastases (months)	pT1	–	18	–	NA	NA
	pT2	NA	11	–	NA	NA
	pT3	4	17 (9–22)	9.5 (9–10)	NA	NA

[a]T category was based on 1992 TNM classification.
[b]Results for pT1 and pT2 stages were combined in the study of Ljunberg et al. (1999).
[c]NA, no available information.
[d]In parentheses and under the term symptomatic are presented cases that were diagnosed due to positive physical examination, symptom history, or abnormal serum studies.

What Is the Optimal Period that Follow-up Should Last?

Among all studies that presented data on RCC surveillance during the past decade, the latest postnephrectomy pulmonary lesion was detected at 67 months for pT1 tumors, at 60–96.6 months for pT2 tumors, and at 59–137.9 months for pT3 tumors (Sandock et al., 1995; Levy et al., 1998; Ljunberg et al., 1999; Stephenson et al., 2004; Gofrit et al., 2001). The latest abdominal lesion was detected at 97 months for pT1 tumors, at 29.1–92 months for pT2 tumors, and 18.2–79 months for pT3 tumors, respectively. The latest bone lesion was detected at 42–144 months, 96.7–144 months, and 36–65 months in pT1, pT2, and pT3 tumors, respectively (Sandock et al., 1995; Levy et al., 1998; Ljunberg et al., 1999; Stephenson et al., 2004; Gofrit et al., 2001).

In the study of Sandock et al. (1995), 85% of recurrences occurred within the first 3 years, while the remaining 15% occurred between 3.4 and 11.4 years. Ljunberg et al. (1999) showed that 43% of metastases were observed within 1 year, 70% within 2 years, 80% within 3 years, and 93% within 5 years of follow-up. Only 7% of metastases occurred after 5 years and most of them were symptomatic. Stephenson et al. (2004) detected 25% and 21% of pT1 and pT2 recurrences 5 years after surgery. Of pT3a and pT3b recurrences, 4.3% and 7.1% were detected 3 years after surgery in the same study. In addition, while patients with pT3 RCC have a higher risk of metastasis than those with pT1–T2 disease, all three groups are at risk for the same duration (Levy et al., 1998).

These findings suggest that follow-up should be emphasized during the first 3–5 years after nephrectomy. However, the data also indicate that the follow-up of patients after radical nephrectomy should be longer than 5 years, preferably lifelong (Gofrit et al., 2001; Mickish et al., 2001).

Which Appropriate Follow-up Schemes Are Proposed in the Literature?

Guidelines for the surveillance of patients undergoing nephrectomy have been published by several authors in the past decade (Sandock et al., 1995; Hafez et al., 1997; Levy et al., 1998; Ljunberg et al., 1999; Stephenson et al., 2004; Gofrit et al., 2001; Mickish et al., 2001; Uzzo and Novick, 2003) (Table 13-3).

Physical examination and history recording, laboratory studies (full blood count, renal biochemical profile, liver function tests, and alkaline phosphatase), chest X-ray, and abdominal CT scans constitute the urologist's armamentarium.

First assessment is recommended at 4–6 weeks and includes a physical examination to exclude surgical complications, serum creatinine to assess the remaining kidney function, and hemoglobin to assess the recovery of preoperative blood loss. If alkaline phosphatase is abnormal preoperatively, repeat measurements are recommended because recurrent or persistent alkaline phosphatase elevation after surgery suggests distant metastasis or residual tumor (Mickish et al., 2001).

Less than half of the published series propose that patients with pT1–T2 tumors should be evaluated with clinical assessment and chest X-ray every 6 months during the first 3 years and yearly thereafter (Sandock et al., 1995; Ljunberg et al., 1999; Mickish et al., 2001). The remaining studies have recommended a yearly follow-up for these patients (Hafez et al., 1997; Levy et al., 1998; Stephenson et al., 2004; Uzzo and Novick, 2003). All studies agreed that for pT3 tumors, clinical assessment and chest X-ray should be performed every 6 months for the first 3 years and yearly thereafter.

Three out of eight studies have recommended routine abdominal CT in patients with pT2 disease (Hafez et al., 1997; Levy et al., 1998, Uzzo and Novick, 2003) and seven out of eight recommended routine abdominal imaging for pT3a–b disease (Hafez et al., 1997; Levy et al., 1998; Ljunberg et al., 1999; Stephenson et al., 2004; Gofrit et al., 2001; Mickish et al., 2001; Uzzo and Novick, 2003). Interestingly, the reported rate of abdominal relapse in each of these studies was similar in patients with pT1–2 lesions (0–5%) and in patients with pT3a–b lesions (9.2–22%), and therefore the fact that different recommendations for the use of CT scans during follow-up have been proposed is surprising.

Sandock et al. (1995) showed that only 0.73% of patients benefited from routine follow-up CT and, therefore, they recommend CT at suspicion of recurrence based on symptoms or abnormal serum tests. In another study, Levy et al. (1998) showed that 9% of patients with metastases were diagnosed only on the basis of surveillance CT in the absence of symptoms, abnormal serum chemistry, or disease recurrence at another site. Surveillance CT detected no metastases prior to a 29-month period postoperatively, regardless of pathological stage. Therefore, these authors advocated surveillance CT of the abdomen and pelvis at 24 and 60 months. Contrary to the above conclusion, Ljunberg et al. (1999) reported in their series that one of the nine intra-abdominal/retroperitoneal metastases was detected by scheduled CT and they recommended routine CT scans for high-risk patients (e.g., pT3 tumors) at 6 and 12 months. The rest of the studies recommended abdominal CT for pT3a–b tumors every 6 months (Hafez et al., 1997; Mickish et al., 2001), or yearly (Ljunberg et al., 1999; Uzzo and Novick, 2003) up to the second (Hafez et al., 1997; Uzzo and Novick, 2003) or third year (Ljunberg et al., 1999; Mickish et al., 2001) postoperatively and then annually (Mickish et al., 2001) or biannually (Hafez et al., 1997; Stephenson et al., 2004; Uzzo and Novick, 2003).

TABLE 13-3. Surveillance guidelines after nephrectomy proposed during the decade 1995–2005.

	Clinical assessment (history, physical examination, laboratory studies)	Chest X-ray	Abdominal computed tomography
pT1			
Sandock et al., 1995[a]	Every 6 months until 3 years; then yearly	Every 6 months until 3 years; then yearly	Not recommended
Hafez et al., 1997[b]	Yearly	Yearly	Every 2 years for tumors greater than 2.5 cm
Levy et al., 1998	Yearly	Yearly	Not recommended
Ljunberget al., 1999	Every 6 months until 3 years; then yearly	Every 6 months until 3 years; then yearly	Not recommended
Gofrit et al., 2001[b]	Not recommended for pT1a tumors; periodic for pT1b	Not recommended for pT1a tumors; periodic for pT1b	Not recommended for pT1a tumors; periodic for pT1b
Mickish et al., 2001[c]	Every 6 months for 3 years; then every year from 3 to 5 years	Every 6 months for 3 years; then every year from 3 to 5 years	Not recommended
Stephenson et al.,2004[b]	Yearly	Yearly	Not recommended
Uzzo and Novick,2003	Every year or 2 years	Not recommended	Not recommended
pT2			
Sandock et al., 1995	Every 6 months until 3 years; then yearly	Every 6 months until 3 years; then yearly	Not recommended
Hafez et al., 1997[b]	Yearly	Yearly	Every 2 years for tumors greater than 2.5 cm
Levy et al., 1998	Yearly	Yearly	At 24 and 60 months
Ljunberg et al., 1999	Every 6 months until 3 years; then yearly	Every 6 months until 3 years; then yearly	Not recommended
Gofrit et al., 2001[b]	Meticulous periodic follow-up	Meticulous periodic follow-up	Meticulous periodic follow-up
Mickish et al., 2001[c]	Every 6 months for 3 years; then every year from 3 to 5 years	Every 6 months for 3 years; then every year from 3 to 5 years	Not recommended
Stephenson et al., 2004[b]	Yearly	Yearly	Not recommended
Uzzo and Novick, 2003	Every year	Every year	At year 2; then every 2 years
pT3			
Sandock et al., 1995	Every 6 months until 3 years; then yearly	Every 6 months until 3 years; then yearly	Not recommended
Hafez et al., 1996[b]	Yearly	Yearly	Every 6 months until 2 years; then every 2 years
Levy et al., 1998	Every 6 months until 3 years; then yearly	Every 6 months until 3 years; then yearly	At 24 and 60 months
Ljunberg et al., 1999	Every 6 months until 3 years; then yearly	Every 6 months until 3 years; then yearly	At 6 and 12 months
Gofrit et al., 2001[b]	Meticulous periodic follow-up	Meticulous periodic follow-up	Meticulous periodic follow-up
Mickish et al., 2001[c]	Every 6 months for 3 years; then every year from 3 to 10 years	Every 6 months for 3 years; then every year from 3 to 10 years	Every 6 months for 3 years; then every year from 3 to 10 years
Stephenson et al., 2004[b]	Every 6 months until 3 years; then yearly	Every 6 months until 3 years; then yearly	At 6, 12, 24, and 36 months; then every 2 years
Uzzo and Novick, 2003	Every 6 months	Every 6 months	At year 1; then every 2 years

[a]T category was based on the 1992 TNM classification.
[b]Partial nephrectomy was performed in 100% (Hafez et al., 1997), 22.5% (Gofrit et al., 2001), and 21% (Stephenson et al., 2004) of the patients.
[c]European Association of Urology (EAU) proposed guidelines based on literature data.

Should Patients after Nephron-Sparing Surgery or Thermoablative Techniques Be Followed Differently Compared to Patients after Radical Nephrectomy?

Stage-specific survival rates following nephron-sparing surgery are similar to those following radical nephrectomy (Belldegrun et al., 1999). In a review of 14 articles that included 1088 patients who underwent nephron-sparing surgery, disease-free survival was 90–100% after a mean follow-up of 31–78 months, and only 2.1% of these patients had local recurrence (Gofrit et al., 2001).

Hafez et al. (1997) created surveillance guidelines based on nephron-sparing surgery in 327 patients with pT1–3, N0, M0 disease (1992 TNM classification). The incidence of local tumor recurrence for all patients was 4%. None of the pT1 patients developed local recurrence. Local recurrence at a mean interval of 62, 36, and 30 months postoperatively occurred in 2%, 8% and 11% for pT2, pT3a, and pT3b tumors, respectively. All pT2 recurrences occurred more than 4 years after surgery, whereas 70% of pT3 recurrences were detected between 6 and 24 months from surgery. Among all patients, 38.4% were asymptomatic and diagnosed by surveillance CT of the abdomen.

In the same group of patients distant metastases occurred in 4%, 5%, 12%, and 15% in pT1, pT2, pT3a, and pT3b tumors, respectively. Metastases were detected from associated symptoms in 65.8% and by follow-up chest X-ray or abdominal CT in 34.2% of patients. Pulmonary metastases were detected in 44% of patients at a mean of 25 months postoperatively (Hafez et al., 1997). Of these patients 72.7% were symptomatic at the time when the metastasis was diagnosed. All patients with solitary or multiple bone metastases presented with bone pain (Hafez 1997).

Recently the same group of investigators (Fergany et al., 2000) presented their 10-year follow-up of 117 nephron-sparing renal operations, having updated the TNM classification to the one proposed by Guinan et al. in 1997. The local tumor recurrence rate for all patients was 10%, with no recurrence found in pT1a, pT1b, and pT2 tumors. The incidence of local tumor recurrence was 10% and 12% at a mean interval of 105 and 79.5 months for T3a and T3b disease, respectively. Distant metastases occurred in 2%, 29%, 0%, 33%, and 53% at a median follow-up of 20, 51, 41, and 25 months in patients with pT1a, pT1b, pT2, pT3a, and pT3b disease, respectively. Combined local recurrence and distant metastases occurred in 2%, 5%, 20%, 10%, and 12% of patients, respectively. In the above study, recurrence in general was noted in a follow-up period longer than 5 and 10 years after surgery in 41% and 8.8% of patients respectively. This finding illustrates the unpredictable nature of RCC and the need for long-term follow-up (Fergany et al., 2000).

Novick and Derweesh (2005) in a recent review concluded that irrespective of tumor stage, all patients who undergo nephron-sparing surgery should have an annual evaluation, including medical history and physical examination, measurement of serum calcium and alkaline phosphatase, and tests for liver and renal function. The need for radiographic surveillance varied according to the initial stage. Patients with pT1 RCC did not require radiography, as they had a very low risk of recurrent malignancy. An annual chest X-ray was recommended for patients with pT2 or pT3 tumors because the lung was the most common site of metastasis in these groups. Abdominal or retroperitoneal tumor recurrence was uncommon in patients with pT2 RCC, particularly early after nephron-sparing surgery, and these patients required only occasional follow-up abdominal CT (every 2 years) (Novick and Derweesh, 2005). Patients with pT3 RCC had a higher risk of local tumor recurrence, particularly during the first 2 years after surgery, and they benefited from more frequent follow-up abdominal CT schedules that should not differ from those after radical nephrectomy (Novick and Derweesh, 2005).

Various needle ablative procedures have recently being advocated as nephron-sparing minimally invasive treatment for carefully selected patients. These include cryoablation, radiofrequency ablation, high-intensity focused ultrasound, interstitial laser, microwave thermotherapy, and photon irradiation. At present the clinical data are limited and the follow-up is short. The assessment of the effectiveness of therapy by diligent follow-up imaging and/or biopsy of the tumor lesions is still controversial. No specific guidelines on how we should follow the progress of these patients presently exist (Ankem and Nakada, 2005).

How Should Patients with Hereditary Renal Cell Carcinoma Be Followed?

There is a paucity of guidelines in the literature regarding follow-up of patients with hereditary RCC (Duffey et al., 2004). In contrast to sporadic RCCs, hereditary RCCs such as those presented with von Hippel–Lindau disease (vHL), tuberous sclerosis (TS) complex, or hereditary papillary renal cell carcinoma (HPRCC) are often discovered at a younger age in a multicentric and bilateral fashion, and affected individuals face a high and lifelong risk of recurrence (Hwang et al., 2003). Neumann et al. (1998) showed that although renal tumors in vHL disease have an earlier onset, they also have a slower growth rate and higher 10-year survival rate compared to sporadic renal tumors.

Most hereditary RCCs seem to have a minimal metastatic potential when the tumor measures less than 3 cm in diameter. Nephrectomy in these cases is not performed until the largest tumor reaches 3 cm. As a consequence, surveillance of these patients is mainly based on tumor size rather than on tumor histology, location, or multifocality (Duffey et al., 2004; Walther et al., 1999). Patients who exhibit an aggressive phenotype should undergo imaging relatively frequently(every 3–6 months), whereas patients with a mild phenotypemay safely undergo imaging at 2- to 3-year intervals. Physical examination, renal ultrasound, chest X-ray or CT, abdominal imaging with CT or magnetic resonance imaging when patients cannot undergo contrast-enhanced CT, and routine laboratory testing are all used in the follow-up protocols.

Conclusions

RCCs often behave aggressively and are associated with a poor prognosis. One-third of patients have metastatic disease at presentation and approximately 50% of those treated for localized disease will eventually develop metastases. Among these patients, a subset will benefit from salvage surgery or immunotherapy, a fact that emphasizes the need for surveillance following primary surgical treatment.

Most surveillance protocols are based upon the primary tumor stage. Surveillance protocols based on the combination of various prognostic factors require further validation over stage-based protocols.

Patients should be followed similarly after radical or partial nephrectomy while further studies are required for those patients undergoing thermoablation and for those with hereditary types of RCC.

Physical examination, blood profiles, and chest radiography are important follow-up investigations. However, the exact timing at which these investigations should be performed is still debated. The usefulness and the frequency of CT scans in surveillance protocols are also an open debate.

Prospective randomized trials are needed to provide a rational approach to identify treatable recurrences while minimizing unnecessary examinations and patient anxiety.

References

Amin MB, Tamboli P, Javidan J, et al. Prognostic impact of histological subtyping of adult renal epithelial neoplasms: an experience of 405 cases. Am J Surg Pathol 2002; 26: 281–291.

Ankem MK, Nakada SY. Needle-ablative nephron-sparing surgery. BJU Int 2005; 95(Suppl 2): 46–51.

Baloch KG, Grimer RJ, Carter SR, et al. Radical surgery for the solitary bony metastasis from renal-cell carcinoma. J Bone Joint Surg Br 2000; 82: 62–67.

Belldegrun A, Tsui KH, deKernion JB, et al. Efficacy of nephron-sparing surgery for renal cell carcinoma: analysis based on the new 1997 tumor-node-metastasis staging system. J Clin Oncol 1999; 17: 2868–2875.

Choyke PL, Glenn GM, Walther MM, et al. Hereditary renal cancers. Radiology 2003; 226: 33–46.

Decker DA, Decker VL, Herskovic A, et al. Brain metastases in patients with renal cell carcinoma: prognosis and treatment. J Clin Oncol 1984; 2: 169–173.

Duffey BG, Choyke PL, Glenn G, et al. The relationship between renal tumor size and metastases in patients with von Hippel-Lindau disease. J Urol 2004;172: 63–65.

Esrig D, Ahlering TE, Lieskovsky G, et al. Experience with fossa recurrence of renal cell carcinoma. J Urol 1992; 147: 1491–1494.

Fergany AF, Hafez KS, Novick A. Long-term results of nephron sparing surgery for localized renal cell carcinoma: 10-year follow-up. J Urol 2000; 163: 442–445.

Frank I, Blute ML, Cheville JC, et al. An outcome prediction model for patients with clear cell carcinoma treated with radical nephrectomy based on tumor stage, size, grade, and necrosis: the SSIGN score. J Urol 2002; 168: 2395–2400.

Frydenberg M, Gunderson L, Hahn G, et al. Preoperative external beam radiotherapy followed by cytoreductive surgery and intra-operative radiotherapy for locally advanced primary or recurrent renal malignancies. J Urol 1994; 152: 15–21.

Fuhrman SA, Lasky LC, Limas C. Prognostic significance of morphologic parameters in renal cell carcinoma. Am J Surg Pathol 1982; 6: 655–663.

Fujisaki S, Takayama T, Shimada K, et al. Hepatectomy for metastatic renal cell carcinoma. Hepatogastroenterology 1997; 44: 817–819.

Gofrit ON, Shapiro A, Kovalski N, et al. Renal cell carcinoma: evaluation of the 1997 TNM system and recommendations for follow-up after surgery. Eur Urol 2001; 39: 669–675.

Goldstein NS. The current state of renal cell carcinoma grading. Union Internationale Contre le Cancer (UICC) and the American Joint Committee on Cancer (AJCC). Cancer 1997; 80: 977–980.

Guinan P, Sobin LH, Algaba F, et al. TNM staging of renal cell carcinoma. Workgroup No. 3. Union International Contre le Cancer (UICC) and the American Joint Committee on Cancer (AJCC). Cancer 1997; 80: 992–993.

Hafez KS, Novick AC, Campbell SC. Patterns of tumor recurrence and guidelines for followup after nephron sparing surgery for sporadic renal cell carcinoma J Urol 1997; 157: 2067–2070.

Hwang JJ, Uchio EM, Linehan WM, et al. Hereditary kidney cancer. Urol Clin N Am 2003; 30: 831–842.

Itano NB, Blute ML, Spotts B, et al.: Outcome of isolated renal cell carcinoma fossa recurrence after nephrectomy J Urol 2000; 164: 322–325.

Jansen NK, Kim HL, Figlin RA, et al. Surveillance after radical or partial nephrectomy for localized renal cell carcinoma and management of recurrent disease. Urol Clin N Am 2003; 30: 843–852.

Jemal A, Murray T, Samuels A, et al. Cancer statistics 2003. CA Cancer J Clin 2003; 53: 5–26.

Kattan MW, Reuter V, Motzer RJ, et al. A postoperative prognostic nomogram for renal cell carcinoma. J Urol 2001; 166: 63–67.

Kavolius JP, Mastorakos DP, Pavlovich C, et al. Resection of metastatic renal cell carcinoma. J Clin Oncol 1998; 16: 2261–2266.

Kent SE, Majumdar B. Metastatic tumours in the maxillary sinus. A report of two cases and a review of the literature. J Laryngol Otol 1985; 99: 459–462.

Kim HL, Han KR, Zisman A, et al. Cachexia-like symptoms predict a worse prognosis in localized T1 renal cell carcinoma. J Urol 2004; 171: 1810–1813.

Lerner SE, Hawkins CA, Blute ML, et al. Disease outcome in patients with low stage renal cell carcinoma treated with nephron sparing or radical surgery. J Urol 1996; 155: 1868–1873.

Levy DA, Slaton JW. Swanson DA, et al. Stage specific guidelines for surveillance after radical nephrectomy for local renal cell carcinoma. J Urol 1998; 159: 1163–1167.

Ljunberg B, Alamdari FI, Rasmuson T, et al. Follow-up guidelines for nonmetastatic renal cell carcinoma based on the occurrence of metastases after radical nephrectomy. BJU Int 1999; 84: 405–411.

Maldazys JD, de Kernion JB. Prognostic factors in metastatic renal carcinoma. J Urol 1986; 136: 376–379.

McLaughlin JK, Lipworth L. Epidemiologic aspects of renal cell cancer. Semin Oncol 2000; 27(2): 115–123.

Mickish G, Carballido J, Hellsten S, et al. Guidelines on renal cell cancer. Eur Urol 2001; 40: 252–255.

Motzer RJ, Bacik J, Mariani T, et al. Treatment outcome and survival associated with metastatic renal cell carcinoma of non-clear-cell histology. J Clin Oncol 2002; 20: 2376–2381.

National Cancer Institute of Canada. Canadian Cancer Statistics 2002, Toronto, 2002.

Negrier S, Escudier B, Gomez F, et al. Prognostic factors of survival and rapid progression in 782 patients with metastatic renal carcinomas treated by cytokines: a report from the Groupe Francais d' Immunotherapie. Ann Oncol 2002; 13: 1460–1468.

Neumann HP, Bender BU, Berger DP, et al. Prevalence, morphology and biology of renal cell carcinoma in von Hippel-Lindau disease compared to sporadic renal cell carcinoma. J Urol 1998; 160: 1248–1254.

Novick AC, Derweesh I. Open partial nephrectomy for renal tumours: current status. BJU Int 2005; 95(Suppl 2): 35–40.

Pantuck AJ, Zisman A, Belldegrum AS. The changing natural history of renal cell carcinoma. J Urol 2001; 166: 1611–1623.

Piltz S, Meimarakis G, Wichmann MW, et al. Long-term results after pulmonary resection of renal cell carcinoma metastases. Ann Thorac Surg 2002; 73: 1082–1087.

Saitoh H, Nakayama M, Nakamura K, et al. Distant metastasis of renal adenocarcinoma in nephrectomized cases. J Urol 1982; 127: 1092–1095.

Sandhu SS, Symes A, A'Hern R, et al. Surgical excision of isolated renal-bed recurrence after radical nephrectomy for renal cell carcinoma. BJU Int 2005; 95: 522–525.

Sandock DS, Seftel AD, Resnick MI. A new protocol for the followup of renal cell carcinoma based on pathological stage. J Urol 1995; 154: 28–31.

Schrodter S, Hakenberg OW, Manseck A, et al. Outcome of surgical treatment of isolated local recurrence after radical nephrectomy for renal cell carcinoma J Urol 2002; 167: 1630–1633.

Shamash J, Steele JP, Wilson P, et al. IPM chemotherapy in cytokine refractory renal cell cancer. Br J Cancer 2003; 19; 88(10): 1516–1521.

Stephenson AJ, Chetner MP, Rourke K, et al. Guidelines for the surveillance of localized renal cell carcinoma based on the patterns of relapse after nephrectomy. J Urol 2004; 172: 58–62.

Tanguay S, Pisters LL, Lawrence DD, et al. Therapy of locally recurrent renal cell carcinoma after nephrectomy J Urol 1996; 155: 26–29.

Tsui KH, Shvarts O, Smith RB, et al. Prognostic indicators for renal cell carcinoma: a multivariate analysis of 643 patients using the revised 1997 TNM staging criteria. J Urol 2000; 163: 1090–1095.

Uzzo RG, Novick AC. Surveillance strategies following surgery for renal cell carcinoma. In: Belldegrun A, Ritchie AWS, Figlin RA, Eds. Renal and Adrenal Tumors: Biology and Management. New York: Oxford University Press, 2003, pp. 324–330.

Walther MM, Choyke PL, Glenn G, et al. Renal cancer in families with hereditary renal cancer: prospective analysis of a tumor size threshold for renal parenchymal sparing surgery. J Urol 1999; 161(5): 1475–1479.

Yang JC, Haworth L, Sherry RM, et al. A randomized trial of bevacizumab, an anti-vascular endothelial growth factor antibody, for metastatic renal cancer. N Engl J Med 2003; 349: 427–434.

Zisman A, Pantuck AJ, Wieder J, et al. Risk group assessment and clinical outcome algorithm to predict the natural history of patients with surgically resected renal cell carcinoma. J Clin Oncol 2002; 20: 4559–4566.

14
Palliative Treatment in Renal Cell Cancer

Dick Richel

Introduction

Nonlocalized renal cell carcinoma (RCC) usually progresses rapidly with a 5-year survival rate of less than 10%.[1] Because options for systemic treatment for inoperable and metastatic RCC are limited, palliative treatment of symptoms and improvement of quality of life (QOL) are the main goals in this stage of disease. Several effective palliative options are available for treating paraneoplastic syndromes, bleeding, pain, and symptoms related to cytokine therapy.

Paraneoplastic Syndromes in Renal Cell Carcinoma

Approximately 20% of patients with RCC have paraneoplastic syndromes at presentation and 10–40% of patients develop paraneoplastic syndromes during the course of the disease.[2]

Paraneoplastic syndromes represent a constellation of symptoms that results from the release of tumor-associated proteins or the induction of immunological reactions, rather than a consequence of local tumor growth/invasion.

Paraneoplastic symptoms related to tumor cachexia are weight loss, anorexia, fatigue, and hypoalbuminemia. A relationship has been demonstrated between the existence of cachexia-related symptoms and survival.

Other paraneoplastic symptoms include fever, night sweats, hypercalcemia, erythrocytosis, hepatic dysfunction (Stauffer's syndrome), and hypertension.

Hypercalcemia may be induced by a parathyroid-like hormone (PTH) produced by tumor cells (PTH-like peptide) or by osteolysis in case of bone metastasis; erythrocytosis is thought to be the result of the production of erythropoietin by cancer cells, whereas hypertension is probably the result of the aberrant production of renin. In the case of resectable disease, paraneoplastic symptoms disappear after nephrectomy; if symptoms continue, metastatic disease is present.

Symptoms and Treatment

Pain

Pain in cancer patients can be caused by the direct effects of the tumor (e.g., invasion of bone by the tumor, nerve compression) or by complications of treatment. Pain can be divided into three categories based on etiology: somatic, visceral, and neuropathic. This characterization is useful since the approach to treatment for each is different. However, it is important to realize that cancer pain may have multiple etiologies.

Although there are no quantitative biochemical or neurophysiological measures of pain, tools have been devised to assess pain intensity. The visual analog scale, rating pain from 0 to 10, is a useful method for tracking pain intensity in the individual patient and can be recorded repeatedly during pain treatment[3] (Fig. 14-1).

Types of Pain

Somatic Pain

Somatic pain is triggered by potential or real injury to tissues and is the typical pain that we have all experienced acutely or chronically. The area of pain is tender and the pain is localized to the site of injury. Somatic pain is constant and sometimes throbbing or aching. Bone metastasis is the most common cause of somatic pain in patients with cancer.[4]

Visceral Pain

In contrast to somatic pain, visceral pain is poorly localized and is often referred to a distant cutaneous site that may be tender. It may be less constant than somatic pain, occurring in dull, colicky waves. Unlike somatic pain, it is often associated with nausea and diaphoresis.

Neuropathic Pain

Neuropathic pain, caused by damage to nerves, is often described as prolonged, severe, burning, lancinating, or

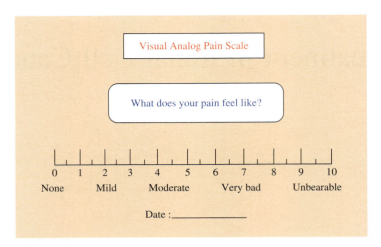

FIGURE 14-1. Visual analog pain scale.

squeezing, and is often associated with focal neurological deficits. It is usually constant but may be interrupted by paroxysms of dramatically increased pain. There may be no area of tenderness, or areas of exquisite sensitivity to normally innocuous stimuli (allodynia). Symptoms and signs of autonomic instability (e.g., tachycardia, sweating) may accompany neuropathic pain. Neuropathic pain is also characterized by its relative resistance to opioids, making it the most challenging type of pain to treat.[5]

Pain Treatment

Local pain has to be treated with local treatments, if possible, such as surgery or radiation.

If pain is caused by the primary tumor a palliative nephrectomy is the treatment of choice. In case of inoperability, local radiation or arterial embolization is an alternative.

Medications are the cornerstone of systemic cancer pain treatment, and their use is aimed at providing the greatest pain relief possible with the fewest number of side effects and the greatest ease of administration. What medications should be used for each person and for each type of cancer pain that should be treated with medications constitutes the art of effective pain relief.

Mild Pain

For mild cancer pain, acetaminophen or nonsteroidal antiinflammatory drugs (NSAIDs), such as aspirin, ibruprofen, and diclofenac, are often used.

Moderate and Severe Pain

For moderate to severe cancer pain, when pain relief is not achieved with acetaminophen or NSAID medications, opioids are the treatment of choice.[6] Opioids are widely used because of their reliability, safety, multiple routes of administration, and ease of titration. Opioids can be used for all types of pain

(i.e., somatic, visceral, neuropathic); although neuropathic pain may be more difficult to treat, a favorable response to opioid-based analgesia is often possible.[7] Almost always, opioid treatment for cancer pain begins with a low dose, and the dosage is increased until pain relief is satisfactory to the person in pain. Weak opioids (codeine, tramadol) are often prescribed in combination with nonopioid analgesics (acetaminophen or NSAIDs). The coanalgesic activity often delays dose escalation or a change to stronger opioids. The first stronger opioid preparations chosen typically have a short half-life and are used on an as needed basis, since initial pain is often episodic and predictable. If pain becomes constant, a sustained-release preparation (available orally for morphine and oxycodone) and transdermally for fentanyl) can be added on a regular dosing schedule.

The side effects of opioid medications include constipation, nausea and vomiting, sleepiness, and respiratory depression. For most people, the nausea effects fade away after taking the medication for a short period of time. Constipation necessitates the use of laxatives from the beginning of treatment.

Breakthrough Cancer Pain

Many people with chronic cancer-related pain experience intermittent flares of pain that can occur even though a person is taking analgesic medications on a fixed schedule for pain control. These severe flares of pain are called breakthrough pain because the pain "breaks through" the regular pain medication. About one-half to two-thirds of patients with chronic cancer-related pain also experience episodes of breakthrough cancer pain.[8]

The characteristics of breakthrough cancer pain vary from person to person, including the duration of the breakthrough episode and possible causes. Generally, breakthrough pain happens fast, and may last anywhere from seconds to minutes to hours. The average duration of breakthrough pain in one study was 30 minutes. This kind of pain can happen unexpectedly for no obvious reason, or it may be triggered by a specific activity, like coughing, moving, or going to the bathroom. Most people who have breakthrough cancer pain experience several episodes a day.

The ideal medication for breakthrough cancer pain should be easily administered, work rapidly, and be excreted from the body within a relatively short period of time, like short acting opioids.[9]

Neuropathic Pain

NSAIDs and opioids are often not sufficient to relieve neuropathic pain. Antidepressants and antiepileptics, such as amitriptyline, carbamazepine, and gabapentine, are the basis for neuropathic pain management.[10]

Bone Pain

Tumor involvement of bone is the most common cause of cancer pain. Common sites of bony metastasis are the vertebral column, skull, humerus, ribs, pelvis, and femur. Local radiotherapy is the treatment of choice. NSAIDs eventually combined with opioids are often effective.

Adjuvant Treatment

Adjuvant drugs in managing cancer pain have not been developed for the treatment of cancer pain but may enhance the activity of analgesics.[11] These include drugs against nausea, anxiety, depression, and seizures and may contribute to neuropathic and bone pain control.

Other adjuvants in cancer pain treatment are corticosteroids and bisphosphonates.

Corticosteroids are the most widely used general purpose adjuvant analgesics. They may ameliorate pain and produce beneficial effects on appetite, nausea, and mood. They provide analgesia from pain syndromes associated with raised intracranial pressure, acute spinal cord compression, superior vena cava syndrome, metastatic bone pain, neuropathic pain due to infiltration or compression by the tumor, and hepatic capsular distention.[12] Patients with advanced cancer who experience pain and other symptoms that may respond to steroids are usually given relatively small doses (dexamethasone, 1–2 mg twice daily). In patients with epidural spinal cord compression, high doses of dexamethasone can be used to manage an acute episode of severe pain.

Bisphosphonate drugs, pamidronate (Aredia), zoledronate (Zometa), clodronate, etidronate, and ibandronate bind to bone hydroxyapatite inhibiting osteoclast activity and are highly effective in the management of metastatic disease to the bone. Recent large, randomized, double-blind studies have demonstrated their efficacy for relieving bone pain as well as for reducing skeletal complications.[13] Most of the current experience related to pain management exists for skeletal metastasis from breast and prostate cancer.

Other Procedures for Pain Relief

Radiotherapy

Radiation, which is also used to treat cancer, can be very helpful in alleviating cancer pain in some circumstances. It can be used to reduce the size of some tumors, which, in turn, takes pressure off the organs and nerves that the tumor touches. It can also be used to treat the pain of cancer that has spread to the bones, brain, blood vessels, nerves, and spine.

Nerve Blocks

Nerve blocks involve the injection of anesthetic medication into specific areas of the body where pain is experienced, notably the nerves. Medications sometimes used for nerve blocks include lidocaine or bupivacaine, used alone or in combination with corticosteroids. Permanent blocks are not usually permanent, but may provide 3–6 months of pain relief. There are other types of nerve blocks that can be used to relieve pain as well.

Radiofrequency Ablation

While the patient is sedated, a radiologist uses a special needle to deliver radiofrequency current into a tumor, which then destroys cancer cells. This procedure has few side effects and can provide pain relief for some kinds of pain for several months. It can also be repeated when necessary.

TENS

TENS stands for transcutaneous electrical nerve stimulation, and it is a low-voltage current that is transmitted to the body via electrodes placed on the skin. A portable battery is the power source. A tingling sensation is felt (and this is adjustable in intensity, for comfort) and for some people pain is reduced where the TENS is applied.

Fatigue

Fatigue is one of the most frequently reported complaints in cancer patients and is directly related to QOL.[14] Cancer patients often complain of a reduced capacity to carry out the normal activities of daily living, slow physical recovery from tasks, and diminished concentration. Fatigue is a subjective condition defined as a patient feeling a lack of energy. In contrast to tiredness in healthy individuals, cancer-related fatigue is perceived as being of greater magnitude, disproportionate to the activity or exertion, and not relieved by rest. About 70% of cancer patients report fatigue during radiotherapy, chemotherapy, and cytokine therapy.

Factors contributing to fatigue are probably multifactorial and may include anemia, weight loss, fever, pain, medication, and infection. In cancer patients, many of these factors are influenced by a frequently disrupted balance between endogenous cytokine levels and their natural antagonists. Indeed, cancer cells and the immune system appear to overexpress a range of cytokines in patients with cancer. Some of these cytokines act as autocrine or paracrine growth factors for the neoplastic tissue while simultaneously causing secondary symptoms related to fatigue

For instance, cancer-associated anemia may be due to a blunted erythropoietin response and/or to cytokines [interleukin (IL)-1, IL-6, tumor necrosis factor (TNF)-α] that suppress erythropoiesis.

Cancer-related fatigue is associated with treatment-related physiological and psychological mechanisms. Physiological mechanisms include reduced aerobic capacity and physical performance as well as muscle wasting, and is aggrevated by inactivity resulting from bed rest and downscale activities. In fact, a vicious circle may occur and account for the persistence of fatigue in the long term.

Psychological factors related to the onset and the persistence of fatigue include anxiety, depression, reduced self-efficacy, sleep disorders, distress, and difficulty in coping.

Although exercise training is reported to be beneficial because it is aimed at improving functional capacity and muscle strength,[5] treatment is often limited to treatment of fatigue-related symptoms, such as anemia, mental depression, and metabolic disorders

Hypercalcemia

Hypercalcemia in patients with cancer is due to increased bone resorption and release of calcium from bone.[16] There are two major mechanisms by which this can occur: osteolytic metastases with local release of cytokines (including osteoclast activating factors) and tumor secretion of parathyroid hormone-related protein (PTHrP). In RCC both mechanisms contribute to the rather high incidence of hypercalcemia.

Hypercalcemia is, in almost all patients, due to an elevation in the physiologically important ionized (or free) calcium concentration. However, 40–45% of the calcium in serum is bound to protein, principally albumin; as a result, increased protein binding can cause an elevation in the serum total calcium concentration without any rise in the serum ionized calcium concentration.

Symptoms of hypercalcemia are dehydration, renal function dysfunction, nausea and vomiting, constipation, abdominal pain, fatigue, and somnolence. The extent of symptoms is a function both of the degree of hypercalcemia and the rate of onset of the elevation in the serum calcium concentration. A serum calcium concentration of 12–14 mg/dl (3–3.5 mmol/liter) may be well tolerated chronically while in acute rise to these concentrations may cause marked changes in sensorium

The treatment of hypercalcemia typically begins with saline administration to produce volume expansion and increase urinary calcium excretion. However, saline therapy rarely normalizes the serum calcium concentrations in patients with more than mild hypercalcemia.

In addition, intravenous administration of bisphosphonates belongs to the standard treatment of cancer-related hypercalcemia.[17]

Bisphosphonates

The bisphosphonates are nonhydrolyzable analogs of inorganic pyrophosphate that adsorb to the surface of bone hydroxyapatite and inhibit calcium release by interfering with the metabolic activity of osteoclasts; they are also cytotoxic to osteoclasts. Pamidronate, zoledronate, ibandronate, and etidronate are the currently available agents that are approved for the treatment of malignancy-associated hypercalcemia.

All of the bisphosphonates are relatively nontoxic compounds and they are more potent than calcitonin and saline in patients with moderately severe hypercalcemia. As such, they have become the preferred agents for the management of malignancy-related hypercalcemia. Their maximum effect occurs in 2–4 days,

Intravenous zoledronate acid is the bisphosphonate of choice for malignancy-associated hypercalcemia because it is more potent than pamidronate and can be administered over a shorter time period (15 minutes as compared to 2 hours).

Symptoms Related to Systemic Treatments in Renal Cell Cancer

Interferon-α

Interferon-α (IFN-α) and IL-2 are frequently used cytokine treatments for metastatic RCC.

The first 2–8 hours after treatment is when acute adverse effects of IFNs occur, but these adverse effects rarely limit treatment. Flu-like symptoms,[18] hypotension or hypertension, tachycardia, and nausea and vomiting are common side effects. With chronic administration, fatigue and anorexia can become severe, and significant weight loss (>10% body weight) can occur.[19] Anxiety, agitation, seizures, and coma have been reported with high-dose schedules and are reversible. These neurological side effects and behavioral/cognitive changes may limit treatment. Mild granulocytopenia (about 50% reduction in counts) develops gradually after the first week of treatment and is rapidly reversible upon drug discontinuation. Autoimmune and immune hemolytic anemia, myelosuppression, and thrombocytopenia may also be rarely seen. Flu-like side effects may be managed with acetaminophen or NSAIDs. Other supportive care may be provided based on the symptoms. In most patients, symptoms will decrease with subsequent doses of IFN.

Interleukin-2

Cardiovascular and hemodynamic adverse effects that resemble septic shock are associated with high-dose IL-2 therapy.[18] High-dose intravenous therapy can lead to hypotension, vascular leak syndrome, and respiratory insufficiency. Support of peripheral vascular resistance with vasopressors, endotracheal intubation, and fluid resuscitation may be necessary during therapy.[20] Acute central nervous system side effects such as psychosis, disorientation, and behavioral changes may be seen with high-dose IL-2 therapy. Other neurological side effects, such as seizures and coma, have been reported in patients with brain metastases. IL-2 treatment should be stopped as soon as neurological toxicity is observed.

Lower-dose intravenous and subcutaneous IL-2 regimens can be administered in an ambulatory care setting with observation after administration for several hours. The severity of adverse effects of lower-dose therapy is dose dependent. Common symptoms include fever, chills, nausea, vomiting, anorexia, malaise, fatigue, myalgia, arthralgia, and pruritus. Prophylaxis treatment includes acetaminophen and histamine type I and II (H_1 and H_2) receptor antagonists.

References

1. Motzer RJ, Bander NH, Nanus DM. Renal cell carcinoma. N Engl J Med 1996; 335:865–875.
2. Kim HL, Belldegrun AS, Freitas DG, Bui MHT, Han KR, Dorey FJ, Figlin RA. Paraneoplastic signs and symptoms of renal cell carcinoma: implications for prognosis. J Urol 2003; 170:1742–1746.
3. Revill SI, Robinson JO, Rosen M, Gogg MI. The reliability of a linear analogue for evaluation of pain. Anaesthesia 1976; 31:1191–1198.
4. Foley KM. The treatment of cancer pain. N Engl J Med 1985; 313:84.
5. Cline MA, Ochoa J, Torebjork HE. Chronic hyperalgesia and skin warming caused by sensitized C nociceptors. Brain 1989; 112:621.
6. McNicol E, Strassels S, Goudas L, et al. Nonsteroidal anti-inflammatory drugs, alone or combined with opioids, for cancer pain: a systematic review. J Clin Oncol 2004; 22:1975.
7. Portenoy RK, Foley KM, Inturrisi CE. The nature of opioid responsiveness and its implications for neuropathic pain: new hypotheses derived from studies of opioid infusions. Pain 1990; 43:273.
8. Portenoy RK, Hagen NA. Breakthrough pain: definition, prevalence and characteristics. Pain 1990; 41(3):273–281.
9. Simmonds MA. Management of breakthrough pain due to cancer. Oncology 1999; 13(8):1103–1108; discussion 1110, 1113–1114.
10. Hegarty A, Portnoy RK. Pharmacotherapy of neuropathic pain. Sem Neurol 1994; 14:213–224.
11. Portenoy RK. Adjuvant analgesics. In: Cherny NI, Foley JM, Eds. Hematology/Oncology Clinics of North America: Pain And Palliative Care, Vol 10. Philadelphia: Saunders, 1996, p. 103.
12. Wooldridge JE, Anderson CM, Perry MC. Corticosteroids in advanced cancer. Oncology 2001; 15:225–234.
13. Body JJ, Bartl R, Burckhardt P, Delmas PD, Diel IJ, Fleisch H, Kanis JA, Kyle RA, Mundy GR, Paterson AH, Rubens RD. Current use of bisphosphonates in oncology. J Clin Oncol 1998; 16(12):3890–3899.
14. Stasi R, Abiani L, Beccaglia P, Terzoli E, Amadori S. Cancer-related fatigue. Cancer 2003; 98:1786–1801.
15. Weert v E, Hoekstra-Weebers J, Otter R, Postema K, Sanderman R, Schans van der C. Cancer-related fatigue: predictors and effect of rehabilitation. The Oncologist 2006; 11:184–196.
16. Ralston SH, Gallacher SJ, Patel U, Campbell J, Boyle IT. Cancer-associated hypercalcemia: morbidity and mortality. Clinical experience in 126 treated patients. Ann Intern Med 1990; 112(7):499–504.
17. Berenson JR. Treatment of hypercalcemia of malignancy with bisphosphonates. Semin Oncol 2002; 29:12.
18. Vial T, Descotes J. Immune-mediated side-effects of cytokines in humans. Toxicology. 1995; 105(1):31–57.
19. Jones TH, Wadler S, Hupart KH. Endocrine-mediated mechanisms of fatigue during treatment with interferon-alpha. Semin Oncol 1998; 25(1 Suppl 1):54–63.
20. Schwartzentruber DJ. Guidelines for the safe administration of high-dose interleukin-2. J Immunother 2001; 24(4):287–293.

15
Future Directions

Jean J.M.C.H. de la Rosette, Cora N. Sternberg, and Hein P.A. van Poppel

Renal cell carcinoma (RCC) represents 2% of the world total of adult malignancies. In the past few decades we have witnessed a steady increase in the incidence of RCC, especially involving tumors that are 2–4 cm in size. The widespread use of abdominal imaging is probably the major contributor to the increasing number of incidentally found tumors: 10% in 1970 versus 61% in 1998. Obviously we now diagnose tumors earlier; therefore, the true incidence may not have increased. This conclusion is supported by autopsy studies in which no significant change in the number of RCCs was found. Moreover, this earlier diagnosis has not resulted in a significant difference in stage presentation.

When looking at the epidemiological data more closely, however, there is a very positive trend toward an improvement in survival. Whereas the 5-year relative survival rate was only 34% in 1954, this almost doubled to 62% by 1996. The major contributor to this is most probably the improvement in surgical treatment of local (advanced) RCC. Expectations for the future contribution of new angiogenesis inhibitors and small molecules to the treatment of RCC are very high.

Radical nephrectomy remains the treatment of choice for RCC that is not well suited to nephron-sparing surgery. Larger tumors, locally advanced tumors, and tumors with extension to the inferior vena cava are best dealt with through open surgery, whereas for smaller less extended tumors laparoscopic radical nephrectomy has become the standard of care. The advantages for the patient are significant and the oncological result is most probably comparable. Both the transperitoneal and extraperitoneal approach can be used, and a laparoscopic team should be able to master both approaches. The availability of laparoscopic radical nephrectomy, however, should not encourage urological surgeons to execute radical laparoscopic nephrectomies in patients who are suitable candidates for nephron-sparing partial nephrectomy. Preservation of renal parenchyma with less risk of progressive renal failure remains the second reason for nephron-sparing surgery, with the first being eradication of disease.

In larger tumors, lymph node dissection and resection of the adrenal gland are probably beneficial to those patients who have microscopic invasion that was not recognized on preoperative imaging. Therefore the debate as to whether lymph node dissection and adrenalectomy belong to classical radical nephrectomy remains unresolved.

Bench surgery to perform nephron-sparing surgery in very difficult cases can be a last possibility, although *in situ* removal of the majority of tumors after clamping and eventually cooling of the kidney is feasible. Open partial nephrectomy is well established, but laparoscopic experts are now able to equal the results of open surgery through the laparoscope. The techniques of resection and hemostasis are still improving, but today, laparoscopic partial nephrectomy should be performed only in centers of expertise and is not the technique of choice for the average urological surgeon.

Since the initiation of nephron-sparing surgery, it has always been advocated that there should be a safety margin of healthy tissue covering the tumor. Numerous data have become available demonstrating that very marginal resections and even enucleations do not predispose patients to local recurrences. The use of frozen sections and microscopic analysis of the surgical margins have proven to be rather unreliable. It is the surgeon's intraoperative responsibility to ensure complete resection of the tumor.

When RCC extends to the inferior vena cava and the patient is without lymph node or distance metastasis, surgical removal remains mandatory. For a tumor thrombus higher than the hepatic veins it is preferable to perform the surgery in collaboration with liver transplant or cardiovascular surgeons to allow a safe complete resection that will still cure a significant number of patients.

In additiom, advanced disease, with direct extension to the adrenal gland, the liver, the spleen, or the colon, requires surgical extirpation, although many patients will a posteriori prove to be metastatic. Surgery is, however, the only chance for cure. The same holds for local recurrence after partial nephrectomy and locoregional recurrence.

Future developments for the surgical treatment of RCC are directed toward minimally invasive treatment modalities. Minimally invasive therapy can, of course, be used when patients have a recurrence in the remnant kidney after partial nephrectomy. While cryosurgery might seem oncologically superior to radiofrequency ablation, there are, at present, still insufficient data and expertise available. As more data become available, it is certain that minimally invasive therapies will be applied more frequently, especially in selected patients with significant comorbidities. Cryosurgery is applied primarily through the laparoscope, and therefore remains more invasive than radiofrequency ablation, which is done percutaneously. At present, minimally invasive techniques are being studied with a focus on extracorporeal tumor ablation using energy sources such as high-intensity focused ultrasound (HIFU) and radiosurgery.

In addition to advances in surgical management, we have recently witnessed significant developments in the field of medical oncology in the treatment of advanced RCC. Targeted therapies provide hope and have demonstrated robust activity in metastatic RCC in several settings. There is an increasing awareness that validation of therapeutic targets is necessary for the discovery of new drugs and for verification of their success. There is a strong rationale for targeting multiple pathways, particularly angiogenesis pathways, in RCC. No direct comparisons of the various agents have been made, and thus all have emerged as promising and viable options for patients with metastatic RCC. It is unclear whether these agents are cross-resistant and whether combination therapy can improve outcome. There are still many questions to be answered. What is the effect of the novel targets on the primary tumor? Is nephrectomy still required? Can we stop angiogenesis inhibitors after documentation of progressive disease or is there a rebound phenomenon? What is the role of these agents in the adjuvant setting, and what is the role of these agents in non-clear cell RCC? Clinical trials of theseagents in the adjuvant setting and in combination are ongoing to optimize the timing, sequence, and combination of therapies in RCC. Molecular profiling is heralding the future of prognosis, staging, and treatment. Further exploration of multiple biological targets such as angiogenesis and mTOR inhibition is providing new possibilities. In the next few years new rational treatment strategies based on inhibition of specific biological pathways will emerge. An important step has already been accomplished based upon the results of well-designed randomized Phase III landmark trials.

Treatment strategies for RCC are guided by etiology and prognosis. The full etiology of RCC, however, is unknown and causative factors have not yet been identified. We are aware that, for example, obesity, smoking, and hypertension are risk factors. At present, however, the evidence for most risk factors is inconsistent or equivocal. In addition, prognosticators of survival in the early and advanced stages of RCC are eagerly awaited. Whereas 25% of patients have metastasis at diagnosis, 30% will develop metastasis after surgery for localized RCC and 40% will die of progression. Current prognostic factors include anatomical, histological, and clinical parameters. We strongly believe that in the future these factors should be integrated with more sophisticated molecular markers of prognosis to establish more accurate methods to predict the likelihood of local recurrence, metastases, and response to treatment. The incorporation of molecular factors will probably yield improved prognostic accuracy beyond what presently exists.

The triad of diagnosis–prognosticator–treatment will eventually guide us toward turning renal cell cancer into a curable or controllable disease.

Index

Printed in the United States of America